Textbook of
Pulmonary Diseases
Sixth Edition
Volume I

Textbook of Pulmonary Diseases

Sixth Edition

Volume I

Edited by

Gerald L. Baum, B.S., M.D.
Medical Director
Israel Lung Association
Professor (Emeritus)
Department of Medicine
Sackler School of Medicine
Tel Aviv University
Tel Aviv, Israel

James D. Crapo, M.D.
Chairman
Department of Medicine
Executive Vice President of Academic Affairs
National Jewish Medical and Research Center
Denver, Colorado

Bartolome R. Celli, M.D.
Professor
Department of Medicine
Pulmonary and Critical Care Division
Tufts University School of Medicine
Chief
Pulmonary and Critical Care Division
St. Elizabeth's Medical Center of Boston
Boston, Massachusetts

Joel B. Karlinsky, M.D.
Associate Professor
Department of Medicine
Division of Pulmonary and Critical Care
Boston University School of Medicine
Assistant Chief
Medical Service
Boston VA Medical Center
Boston, Massachusetts

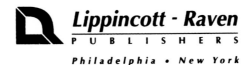

Lippincott - Raven
P U B L I S H E R S
Philadelphia • New York

Acquisitions Editor: Joyce-Rachel John
Developmental Editor: Michelle LaPlante
Manufacturing Manager: Dennis Teston
Production Manager: Lawrence Bernstein
Production Editor: Janice Lochansky
Cover Designer: Karen Quigley
Indexer: Robert Elwood
Compositor: Tapsco Inc.
Printer: Courier Westford

Printed in the United States of America

9 8 7 6 5 4 3 2 1

Library of Congress Cataloging-in-Publication Data

Textbook of pulmonary diseases/edited by Gerald L. Baum. . . [et al.].—6th ed.
    p. cm.
  Includes bibliographical references and index.
  ISBN 0-316-08434-4
  1. Lungs—Diseases. 2. Pleura—Diseases. I. Baum. Gerald L. [DNLM: 1. Lung Diseases.
  WF 600 T355 1997]
  RC756.T48 1997
  616.2′4—DC21
  DNLM/DLC
  for Library of Congress

Care has been taken to confirm the accuracy of the information presented and to describe generally accepted practices. However, the authors, editors, and publisher are not responsible for errors or omissions or for any consequences from application of the information in this book and make no warranty, express or implied, with respect to the contents of the publication.

The authors, editors, and publisher have exerted every effort to ensure that drug selection and dosage set forth in this text are in accordance with current recommendations and practice at the time of publication. However, in view of ongoing research, changes in government regulations, and the constant flow of information relating to drug therapy and drug reactions, the reader is urged to check the package insert for each drug for any change in indications and dosage and for added warnings and precautions. This is particularly important when the recommended agent is a new or infrequently employed drug.

Some drugs and medical devices presented in this publication have Food and Drug Administration (FDA) clearance for limited use in restricted research settings. It is the responsibility of the health care provider to ascertain the FDA status of each drug or device planned for use in their clinical practice.

Contents

I. The Normal Lung

Section II. Diagnostic Methods

Section III. Differential Diagnosis

Section IV. Pulmonary Pharmacology

Section V. Inflammatory and Interstitial Diseases

Section VI. Infectious Diseases

Section VII. Environmental Lung Disease

Subject index follows page 788

Volume 2
Section VIII. Obstructive Lung Disease

Contributing Authors

Muzaffar Ahmad, M.D.   *Professor of Medicine, Department of Medicine, Cleveland Clinic Foundation, 9500 Euclid Avenue Cleveland, Ohio 44195-5014*

Gerald L. Baum, B.S., M.D.   *Professor Emeritus, Department of Medicine, Tel-Aviv University, Sackler School of Medicine, Tel-Aviv University, Ramat Aviv, Medical Director, Israel Lung Association, Tel-Aviv ISRAEL*

Maher A. Baz, M.D.   *Assistant Professor of Medicine, Department of Medicine, Division of Pulmonary and Critical Care Medicine, University of Florida, 1600 SW Archer Road, Gainesville, Florida 32610*

William S. Beckett, M.D., M.P.H.   *Occupational Medicine Division, Department of Environmental Medicine, University of Rochester School of Medicine, 601 Elmwood Avenue, Rochester, New York 14642*

Issahar Ben-Dov, M.D.   *Senior Lecturer, The Pulmonary Institute, Chaim Sheba Medical Center, Tel-Aviv University, Sackler School of Medicine, Tel Hashomer 52621 ISRAEL*

Robert Bilenker, M.D.   *Head, Comprehensive Care and Developmental Pediatrics, Case Western Reserve University School of Medicine; Pediatric Pulmonologist, MetroHealth Medical Center, 2500 MetroHealth Drive, Cleveland, Ohio 44109*

David J. Birnkrant, M.D.   *Assistant Professor, Department of Pediatrics, Case Western Reserve University School of Medicine and Pediatric Pulmonologist, MetroHealth Medical Center, 2500 MetroHealth Drive, Cleveland, Ohio 44109-1998*

Richard J. Blinkhorn, Jr., M.D.   *Assistant Professor of Medicine, Department of Internal Medicine, Case Western Reserve University School of Medicine; and MetroHealth Medical Center, 2500 MetroHealth Drive, Cleveland, Ohio 44109*

Hugh A. Cassiere, M.D.   *Assistant Clinical Instructor in Medicine, Departments of Thoracic Cardiovascular Surgery and Pulmonary and Critical Care Medicine, Winthrop-University Hospital, 259 First Street, Mineola, New York 11501*

Bartolome R. Celli, M.D.   *Professor of Medicine, Department of Medicine, Division of Pulmonary and Critical Care, Tufts University School of Medicine; and Chief, Division of Pulmonary and Critical Care, St. Elizabeth's Medical Center, 736 Cambridge Street, Boston, Massachusetts 02135-2997*

Shan C. Chu, M.D., F.A.C.P.   *Senior Staff Fellow, Pulmonary-Critical Care Medicine Branch, National Heart, Lung, and Blood Institute, National Institutes of Health, 10 Center Drive, MSC 1590, Bethesda, Maryland 20892-1590*

James D. Crapo, M.D.   *Chairman, Department of Medicine, Executive Vice President of Academic Affairs, National Jewish Medical and Research Center, 1400 Jackson Street, Denver, Colorado 80206*

Robert O. Crapo, M.D.   *Professor of Medicine, Department of Medicine, Pulmonary Division, University of Utah School of Medicine; and Medical Director, Pulmonary Lab, LDS Hospital, 8th Avenue and C Street, Salt Lake City, Utah 84143*

Jeffrey L. Curtis, M.D.   *Associate Professor of Internal Medicine, Department of Internal Medicine, The University of Michigan Medical Center, 3916 Taubman center, Ann Arbor, Michigan 48109-0360*

Michael V. Cutaia, M.D.   *Pulmonary Section, University of Pennsylvania, University and Woodland Avenues, Philadelphia, Pennsylvania 19104*

Stephen L. Demeter, M.D. M.P.H.   *Professor of Medicine; and Head of Pulmonary Division, Northeastern Ohio Universities College of Medicine, 4209 State Route 44, Rootstown, Ohio 44272*

Thomas A. Dillard, M.D.   *Associate Professor of Medicine, Department of Medicine and Uniformed Services University of the Health Sciences, Madigan Army Medical Center, MCHJ-MPU (COL.. Dillard), Tacoma, Washington 98431*

Jeffrey M. Drazen, M.D.   *Parker B. Francis Professor of Medicine, Department of Pulmonary and Critical Care, Brigham and Women's Hospital, 75 Francis Street, Boston, Massachusetts 02115*

Raed A. Dweik, M.D.   *Staff Physician, Department of Pulmonary and Critical Care Medicine, Cleveland Clinic Foundation, 9500 Euclid Avenue, Cleveland, Ohio 44195*

N. Tony Eissa, M.D.   *Senior Staff Fellow, Pulmonary-Critical Care Medicine Branch, National Heart, Lung, and Blood Institute, National Institutes of Health, 10 Center Drive, MSC 1590, Bethesda, Maryland 20892-1590*

Jack A. Elias, M.D.   *Professor of Medicine, and, Chief, Section of Pulmonary and Critical Care Medicine, Department of Internal Medicine, Yale University School of Medicine, 333 Cedar Street-105 1CI, New Haven, Connecticut 06520-8057*

Patrick J. Fahey, M.D.   *Professor of Medicine and Anesthesiology, Department of Medicine and Anesthesiology, Loyola University of Chicago, Stritch School of Medicine, 2160 South 1st Avenue, Maywood, Illinois 60153*

M. Elon Gale, M.D.   *Associate Professor of Radiology, Department of Radiology, Boston Veterans Administration Medical Center, 150 South Huntington Avenue, Boston, Massachusetts 02130*

Daniel R. Gale, M.D.   *Department of Radiology, Veterans Affairs Medical Center, 150 South Huntington Avenue, Boston, Massahcusetts 02130*

David R. Graham, M.D., F.R.C.P.   *Department of Respiratory Medicine, Whiston Hospital, Prescot, Merseyside L35 5DR, Liverpool ENGLAND*

Alejandro E. Grassino, M.D.   *Professor of Medicine, Department of Medicine, Notre Dame Hospital, 1560 Sherbrook Street East, I-2158, Montreal, Quebec H2L-4M7, CANADA*

Kurt W. Grathwohl, M.D.   *Senior Fellow, Department of Pulmonary and Critical Care Medicine, Madigan Army Medical Center, MCHJ-MPU (Grathwohl), Tacoma, Washington 98431-5000*

Nicholas J. Gross, M.D., Ph.D.   *Professor of Medicine, Department of Medicine, Loyola University of Chicago, Stritch School of Medicine, Maywood, Illinois 60153*

François Haas, Ph.D.   *Associate Professor of Rehabilitation Medicine, Department of Medicine, Division of Pulmonary and Critical Care Medicine, New York University Medical Center, 400 East 34th Street, New York, New York 10016*

Sheila Sperber Haas, Ph.D.   *Medical, Science Writer, 3 Bedford Street, New York, New York 10014*

James E. Hansen, M.D.   *Professor Emeritus of Medicine, Department of Respiratory and Critical Care Physiology and Medicine, University of California at Los Angeles, Harbor-UCLA Medical Center, Torrance, California 90509*

Nicholas S. Hill, M.D.   *Professor of Medicine, Department of Medicine, Division of Pulmonary, Sleep, and Critical Care Medicine, Rhode Island Hospital, Brown University, 593 Eddy Street, Providence, Rhode Island 02903*

Helen M. Hollingsworth, M.D.   *Associate Professor of Medicine, Division of Pulmonary and Critical Care Medicine, Boston University School of Medicine, R304 Pulmonary Center, 80 East Concord Street, Boston, Massahusetts 02115*

Frederic J. Hoppin, Jr., M.D. *Professor, Department of Medicine and Physiology, Brown University Medical School, Memorial Hospital of Rhode Island, 11 Brewster Street, Pawtucket, Rhode Island 02860*

Yuh Chin Tony Huang, M.D.   *Assistant Professor of Medicine, Department of Medicine, Division of Pulmonary and Critical Care Medicine, Duke University Medical Center, Durham, North Carolina 27710*

Russell D. Hull, M.D., M.B.B.S., M.Sc., F.R.C.P.(c.), F.A.C.P., F.C.C.P.   *Professor of Medicine, Department of Internal Medicine, University of Calgary, Health Sciences Centre, 3330 Hospital Drive NW, Calgary, Alberta T2N 4N1 CANADA*

Gary W. Hunninghake, M.D.   *Professor, Department of Medicine; and Director, Department of Pulmonary, Critical Care, and Occupational Medicine, University of Iowa College of Medicine, 200 Hawkins Drive, Iowa City, Iowa 52242*

Joel B. Karlinsky, M.D.   *Associate Professor of Medicine, Division of Pulmonary and Critical Care Medicine, Pulmonary Center, Boston University School of Medicine; and, Assistant Chief, Medical Service, Boston VA Medical Center, 150 South Huntington Avenue, Boston, Massachusetts 02130*

Jason Kelley, M.D.   *Professor of Medicine, Department of Pulmonary and Critical Care Medicine, University of Vermont College of Medicine, Given C-305, Burlington, Vermont 05405*

Steven G. Kelsen, M.D.   *Professor of Medicine and Physiology, Department of Medicine and Physiology, Division of Pulmonary and Critical Care Medicine, Temple University School of Medicine, Temple University Hospital, 3401 North Broad, Philadelphia, Pennsylvania 19140*

Joel N. Kline, M.D.   *Department of Internal Medicine, Division of Pulmonary, Critical Care, and Occupational Medicine, University of Iowa College of Medicine, 200 Hawkins Drive, Iowa City, Iowa 52246*

R. John Looney, M.D.   *Clinical Immunology Unit, Department of Medicine, University of Rochester Medical Center, 601 Elmwood Avenue, Rochester, New York 14642*

William W. Lunn, M.D.   *Pulmonary Specialist, Pulmonary Specialists of Tyler, 619 South Fleishel, Tyler, Texas 75701*

Joseph P. Lynch, III, M.D.   *Professor of Internal Medicine, Department of Internal Medicine, Division of Pulmonary and Critical Care Medicine, University of Michigan Medical Center, 3916 Taubman Center, Ann Arbor, Michigan 41809-0360*

Neil R. MacIntyre, M.D.   *Professor of Medicine, Respiratory Care Services, Duke University Medical Center, 400 Erwin Road, Durham, North Carolina 27710*

Barry J. Make, M.D.   *Professor of Medicine, Department of Medicine, University of Colorado School of Medicine; and Director, Pulmonary Rehabilitation, National Jewish Medical and Research Center, 1400 Jackson Street, Denver, Colorado 80206-2762*

Bonita T. Mangura, M.D.   *Associate Professor of Clinical Medicine, Department of Medicine, New Jersey Medical School, University of Medicine and Dentistry of New Jersey, 65 Bergen Street, Newark, New Jersey 07107-3001*

John Marini   *Professor, Department of Medicine, University of Minnesota; and, Director, Division of Pulmonary and Critical Care Medicine, St. Paul Ramsey Medical Center, 640 Jackson Street, St. Paul, Minnesota 55101-2595*

F. Dennis McCool, M.D.   *Associate Professor of Medicine, Department of Medicine, Brown University Medical School, Memorial Hospital of Rhode Island, 111 Brewster Street, Pawtucket, Rhode Island 02860*

Reynard J. McDonald, M.D.   *Professor of Clinical Medicine, Department of Clinical Medicine, University of Medicine and Dentistry of New Jersey, University Hospital, 65 Bergen Street, Newark, New Jersey 07107-3001*

Robert R. Mercer, Ph.D.   *Biomedical Engineer, Pathology and Physiology Branch, National Institute of Occupational Safety and Health, 1095 Willowdale Drive, Morgantown, West Virginia 26505*

Scot H. Merrick, M.D.   *Associate Clinical Professor, Department of Surgery, Division of Cardiothoracic Surgery, University of California School of Medicine, 505 Parnassus Avenue, San Francisco, California 94143*

Clifford S. Mitchell, M.D., M.Ph.   *Assistant Professor, Division of Occupational and Environmental Health, Johns Hopkins University, 615 N. Wolfe Street, Room 7041, Baltimore, Maryland 21205*

W.K.C. Morgan, M.D., F.R.C.P.(C)   *Professor of Medicine, Department of Medicine, University Campus-London Health Sciences Centre, 339 Windermere Road, London, Ontario N6A 5A5 CANADA*

Joel Moss, M.D., Ph.D.   *Chief, Pulmonary–Critical Care Medicine Branch, National Heart, Lung, and Blood Institute, National Institutes of Health, 10 Center Drive, MSC 1590, Bethesda, Maryland 20892-1590*

Michael S. Niederman, M.D., F.A.C.P., F.C.C.P., F.C.C.M.   *Director, Medical Intensive Care Unit; Professor, Department of Medicine, SUNY at Stony Brook; and Director, Critical Care Subsection, Division of Pulmonary and Critical Care Medicine, Winthrop-University Hospital, 222 Station Plaza North, Suite 400, Mineola, New York 11501*

Catherine B. Niewoehner, M.D.   *University of Minnesota School of Medicine, Minneapolis VA Medical Center, One Veterans Drive, Minneapolis, Minnesota 55417*

Dennis E. Niewoehner, M.D.   *Professor, Department of Medicine, University of Minnesota; and, Chief, Pulmonary Section, VA Medical Center, One Veterans Drive, Minneapolis, Minnesota 55417*

Robert A. Nonn, M.D.   *Fellow of Pulmonary and Critical Care Medicine, Department of Medicine, Division of Pulmonary and Critical Care Medicine, Loyola Stritch School of Medicine, 2160 S. First Street, Maywood, Illinois, 60153*

Thomas O'Riordan, M.D., M.R.C.P.   *Assistant Professor of Clinical Medicine, Division of Pulmonary and Critical Care Medicine, University of Miami School of Medicine, Miami, Florida 33101*

Claude A. Piantadosi, M.D   *Professor of Medicine, Division of Pulmonary and Critical Care Medicine, Duke University Medical Center, Box 3315, Durham, North Carolina 27710*

Graham F. Pineo, M.D.   *Professor of Medicine and Oncology, Department of Medicine and Oncology, University of Calgary, South Tower, Foothills Hospital, 1403 29th Street NW, Calgary, Alberta T2N 2T9, CANADA*

Udaya B.S. Prakash, M.D.   *Edward W. and Betty Knight Scripps Professor of Medicine, Mayo Medical School and Mayo Graduate School of Medicine; Consultant in Pulmonary, Critical Care, and Internal Medicine; Director of Bronchoscopy, Mayo Clinic and Mayo Medical Center, 200 First Street S.W., Rochester, Minnesota 55905*

Ganesh Raghu, M.D.   *Associate Professor of Medicine, Division of Pulmonary and Critical Care Medicine, University of Washington, Box 356522, Seattle, Washington, 98195*

D. Eugene Rannels, Ph.D.   *Distinguished Professor and Vice Chairman, Department of Cellular and Molecular Physiology, The Pennsylvania State University College of Medicine, 500 University Drive, Hershey, Pennsylvania 17033-0850*

Lee B. Reichman, M.D., M.P.H.   *Professor of Pathology and Preventive Medicine, Department of Preventive Medicine, New Jersey Medical School, National Tuberculosis Center and Community Health, Martland Building, 65 Bergen Street, Newark, New Jersey 07107-3001*

Stephen I. Rennard, M.D.   *Professor of Medicine, Department of Pulmonary and Critical Care Medicine, University of Nebraska Medical Center, 600 South 42nd Street, Omaha, Nebraska 68198-5300*

Judith C. Rhodes, Ph.D.   *Associate Professor of Pathology and Laboratory Medicine, Department of Pathology and Laboratory Medicine, University of Cincinnati College of Medicine, P.O. Box 670529, Cincinnati, Ohio 45267-0529*

Jean Rinaldo, M.D.   *Professor, Vanderbilt University, T-1219 Medical Center North, Nashville, Tennessee 31232*

Mark J. Rosen, M.D.   *Professor of Medicine, Department of Medicine, Albert Einstein College of Medicine, Bronx, New York; and, Chief, Division of Pulmonary and Critical Care Medicine, Beth Israel Medical Center, First Avenue and 16th Street New York, New York 10003*

Sharon I.S. Rounds, M.D.   *Professor of Medicine, Department of Pulmonary and Critical Care Section, Department of Medicine, Providence VA Medical Center, 830 Chalkstone Avenue, Providence, Rhode Island 02908*

Kenneth G. Saag, M.D., M.Sc.   *Assistant Professor of Medicine, Department of Internal Medicine, Division of Rheumatology, University of Iowa College of Medicine, SE 615 GH, Iowa City, Iowa 52242*

Steven A. Sahn, M.D.   *Professor and Director of Medicine, Division of Pulmonary and Critical Care Medicine and Allergy and Clinical Immunology, Medical University of South Carolina, 171 Ashley Avenue, Charleston, South Carolina 29425*

Jonathan M. Samet, M.D., M.S.   *Professor and Chairman, Department of Epidemiology, Johns Hopkins University School of Hygiene and Public Health, 615 North Wolfe Street, Suite 6039 Baltimore, Maryland 21205*

Irwin A. Schafer, M.D.   *Professor, Case Western Reserve University; and, Department of Pediatrics and Genetics, MetroHealth Medical Center, 2500 MetroHealth Drive, Cleveland, Ohio 44109-1998*

Steven M. Scharf, M.D.   *Assistant Professor of Medicine, Department of Medicine, Division of Pulmonary and Critical Care, Long Island Jewish Medical Center, New Hyde Park, New York 11040*

Roslyn F. Schneider, M.D.   *Assistant Professor of Medicine, Department of Medicine, Albert Einstein College of Medicine, 1300 Morris Park Avenue, Bronx, New York 10461*

Robert B. Schoene, M.D.   *Professor of Medicine, Department of Medicine, University of Washington, Harborview Hospital, 325 9th Avenue, Seattle, Washington 98104*

Mark R. Schuyler, M.D.   *Department of Medicine, University of New Mexico School of Medicine, Albuquerque, New Mexico 87131*

Lewis J. Smith, M.D.   *Professor of Medicine, Division of Pulmonary and Critical Care Medicine, Department of Medicine, Northwestern University School of Medicine, 303 East Superior Street, Chicago, Illinois 60611*

David J. Sugarbaker, M.D.   *Associate Professor of Surgery, Department of Thoracic Surgery, Brigham and Women's Hospital, 75 Francis Street, Boston, Massachusetts 02115*

Scott J. Swanson, M.D.   *Professor of Surgery, Department of Thoracic Surgery, Harvard Medical School; and Brigham and Women's Hospital, 75 Francis Street, Boston, Massachusetts 02115*

John W. Swisher, M.D., Ph.D.   *Assistant Professor of Medicine, Department of Medicine, The Pennsylvania State University College of Medicine, 500 University Drive, Hershey, Pennsylvania 17033*

Lynn T. Tanoue, M.D.   *Assistant Professor of Medicine, Pulmonary and Critical Care Section, Department of Internal Medicine, Yale University School of Medicine, 333 Cedar Street, New Haven, Connecticut 06520*

Victor F. Tapson, M.D.   *Medical Director, Duke Lung Transplant Program, Division of Pulmonary and Critical Medicine, Duke University Medical Center, Box 31175 Durham, North Carolina 27710*

Austin B. Thompson, M.D.   *Associate Professor of Medicine, Department of Internal Medicine, University of Nebraska Medical Center, 600 South 42nd Street, Omaha, Nebraska 68198-5300*

Martin J. Tobin, M.D.   *Pulmonary and Critical Care Division, Loyola University of Chicago, Stritch School of Medicine, P.O. Box 1356, Hines, Illinois 60141*

Mark J. Utell, M.D.   *Professor of Medicine and Environmental Medicine, Department of Environmental Medicine; and Associate Chairman for Clinical Affairs, Department of Environmental Medicine, Division of Pulmonary and Critical Care, University of Rochester Medical Center, Strong Memorial Hospital, 601 Elmwood Avenue, Rochester, New York 14642-8692*

Adam Wanner, M.D.   *Professor of Medicine and Chief, Division of Pulmonary and Critical Care Medicine, University of Miami School of Medicine, P.O. Box 016960, Miami, Florida 33101*

Todd H. Wasserman, M.D.   *Radiation Oncology Center, Mallinckrodt Institute of Radiology, Washington University School of Medicine, St. Louis, Montana 63110*

Robert E. Wood, M.D., Ph.D.   *Professor of Pediatrics, Department of Pediatrics, University of North Carolina, CB 7220, Chapel Hill, North Carolina 27599*

Laurel A. Wright, M.D.   *Assistant Professor of Medicine, Department of Pulmonary and Critical Care Medicine, St. Paul Ramsey Medical Center; University of Minnesota, 640 Jackson Street, St. Paul, Minnesota 55101-2595*

Preface to the First Edition

Why another textbook? A few years ago when this work began, I approached the prospective contributors and found that they felt, as I did, that the available compilations and texts were weak in one or another of the major areas in the field of chest diseases. It seemed that by using specialists whose major interests were in these areas and allowing them to be responsible for covering all that they felt belonged in their area, a more complete and current textbook would result. Thus, the authors were assembled with an overall plan to cover the field completely and in a coordinated way with current material being woven into concepts by each author.

The difficulties of such a project are apparent. As part of internal medicine, the study of pulmonary diseases involves a wide variety of disciplines. Anatomy, physiology, immunology, bacteriology, mycology, biochemistry, epidemiology, and pathology, among the basic sciences, must be blended with physical diagnosis, therapeutics, radiology, clinical pathology, physiatry, and psychiatry to present a complete picture of this field of medicine. In addition, emphasis must be placed on the more important problems in public health as they bear on each area. Putting this material into an orderly and readable form is crucial to the value of the book, and providing a complete but selective bibliography is essential to making this a true textbook and not just a review.

In many areas, such as allergic disease and interstitial diseases, extensive background discussions precede the actual clinical presentations. This was done in order to provide sound physiologic basis for the clinical expressions of pathology that direct the activities of the clinician. In addition, embryology of the lung is discussed within the areas of congenital, developmental, and hereditary diseases and in continuity with this material rather than in a remote part of the book where its application would not be directly apparent. For the same reason, details of bronchial and parenchymal anatomy are followed by well-illustrated chapters on emphysema and pulmonary insufficiency.

At the clinical level, the approach to the various infectious diseases is consistent, and it makes use of principles proven reliable in the field of clinical bacteriology as the basis of the approach to viral, rickettsial, and fungal diseases. The mycobacterioses are described in a fresh way which clearly integrates new knowledge of chemotherapy and rehabilitation with established pathogenetic and clinical principles. It is in this historically prime subject in the field of pulmonary diseases that this book offers something that has not been available before. The established treatises dealing with tuberculosis have merely modified and appended the old format to include the subjects of drug therapy, drug resistance, resectional therapy, and rehabilitation based on physical activity early rather than late in the course of treatment. No continuity of approach was projected in such an exposition. By contrast, in this textbook, Drs. Jenkins and Wolinsky have synthesized a discussion that deals with broad principles in light of current information on one hand and provide orderly presentation of details on the other.

Diagnosis is the first subject dealt with in this book, and this is appropriate. Drs. Smith and Kory have developed a unique set of tables at the end of their chapters which should be extremely useful to the student and to the practitioner alike. It is no coincidence that Drs. Amberson, Middleton, and Schwarz have each repeatedly stressed the primacy of accurate diagnosis to many generations of students.

The authors and I have attempted to make this book detailed and current enough to appeal to the sophisticated specialist and clinical researcher and orderly, clearly organized, and well indexed to be of use to the beginning student. Because this book deals with pulmonary diseases primarily, specific discussions of mediastinal diseases other than tumors or gastrointestinal diseases with thoracic manifestations have not been included. Finally, I have written nothing myself, but have devoted my efforts to organization of material and exhortation of the authors.

This textbook is only a beginning, since new work will make much of what is written here obsolete; possibly obsolescence will have set in before publication. Nevertheless, the soundness of the physiologic approach allows for the addition of current knowledge to that discussed here without loss of continuity.

I sincerely hope that this book will, through the authority of the authors' material, stimulate the most important ingredient of any textbook in any field: the curiosity of the student.

G.L.B.
Cincinnati

Preface

The need to publish a new edition of this book has been dictated by an increased understanding of the basic science and clinical aspects of pulmonary diseases.

Many chapters from the previous edition have been continued albeit some of them with new authors. A chapter on Molecular Biology of Pulmonary Disease has been added, reflecting the current emphasis on the genetic basis for an increasing number of abnormalities. Two chapters on Differential Diagnosis have been added to emphasize the clinical aspects and the roentgenologic aspects of common pulmonary syndromes. The chapters dealing with aerosols, theophylline, and surfactant reflect an increasing emphasis on Pulmonary Pharmacology.

The broader world view of tuberculosis is presented in the chapters dealing with mycobacterial disease, which have been written in this edition by the group from the New Jersey Medical School National Tuberculosis Center.

The selection of new authors reflects the trend towards the combination of youth and excellence that characterize the best in recent medical literature. Thus, it is our opinion that this edition of the Textbook is written by the very best clinician/scientists in the world of pulmonary medicine.

Two other circumstances deserve mention. Dr. Wolinsky retired as an editor after the last edition, and Drs. Celli, Crapo, and Karlinsky have joined Dr. Baum in producing what we all hope is a textbook worthy of our readers. And Lippincott-Raven has taken on the responsibility of publishing the book. Thus continuity of the technical excellence of the book is assured.

We all sincerely believe that this edition of the *Textbook of Pulmonary Diseases* maintains the high standard achieved in previous editions and will be of value to students, both undergraduate and those highly experienced in the field of pulmonary medicine.

GLB
JDC
BRC
JBK

Acknowledgments

Of the many people involved in the production of this edition of the *Textbook of Pulmonary Diseases* who deserve our heartfelt thanks, none is in the league of Laurie Anello. This highly professional medical editor has worked with Dr. Wolinsky and Dr. Baum for two editions of the book and gave the sendoff to Drs. Celli, Crapo, Karlinsky, and Baum for this one.

We wish to express our gratitude to the editing staff at Little, Brown, especially Jo-Ann Strangis, who continued in their active and efficient efforts prior to the change in publishers. And since the changeover formally took place, the energetic approach taken by Joyce-Rachel John and Michelle LaPlante of Lippincott-Raven Publishers has been very impressive, and undoubtedly, responsible for this edition appearing on schedule and in the fine shape that it is in. Their help has been consistent, and the results impressive.

A word about Dr. Wolinsky must be said. As the previous editor of the Textbook, Dr. Wolinsky continued to help in the preliminary planning of this edition despite his formal retirement from editorship. His no-nonsense approach and his good sense is expressed in the best of this current edition.

And finally, all four editors wish to express their sincerest gratitude to our authors, new and veteran.

I   THE NORMAL LUNG

Textbook of Pulmonary Diseases, 6th ed.
edited by G.L. Baum, J.D. Crapo, B.R. Celli, and J.B. Karlinsky,
Lippincott–Raven Publishers, Philadelphia, © 1998.

Introduction

The Sociopolitical Response to the Discovery of *Mycobacterium Tuberculosis*

François Haas · Sheila Sperber Haas

"'Children and others, who work in the large cotton factories, are particularly disposed to be affected by contagion of fever, and when such infection is received it is rapidly propagated, not only amongst those who are crowded together in the same departments, but in the families and neighborhoods to which they belong.' However, the warning went unheeded. The passion for financial gains made acquisitive men blind to the fact that they were part of the same social body as the unfortunates who operated their machines. Tuberculosis was, in effect, the social disease of the nineteenth century, perhaps the first penalty that capitalistic society had to pay for the ruthless exploitation of labor."

Rene and Jean Dubos, *The White Plague*

"To combat consumption successfully requires the combined action of a wise government, well-trained physicians, and an intelligent people."

A. S. Knopf, *Tuberculosis as a Disease of the Masses, and How to Combat It*

In the previous edition of this book, we discussed the historical development of tuberculosis, from Fracastoro's critical formulation of the germ theory during the Renaissance to Robert Koch's landmark discovery of *Mycobacterium tuberculosis* in 1882. Discovery of the bacterium, confirming the contagious nature of this epidemic disease, had broad implications that demanded a response from both the medical/scientific community and society as a whole. Because space is limited here, and the developments in medical treatment are already reasonably well-

known, this chapter focuses on the closely interwoven social and political reactions to tuberculosis.

We are doing this in a general textbook on pulmonary diseases because tuberculosis—which infects one third of the world's population—is still the leading infectious killer of adults. It is responsible for 26% of avoidable deaths in developing industrial countries, which face health problems similar to those that confronted countries undergoing industrialization during the 19th century. And it is resurgent now in these same industrialized countries, as past problems—homelessness, overcrowding, inadequate health infrastructure, and disenfranchisement—re-emerge and the pool of patients with drug-resistant tuberculosis, particularly among disenfranchised groups, increases. To these problems must be added the epidemic of HIV infection; tuberculosis is becoming the leading cause of death among affected individuals. Worldwide, tuberculosis will kill 30 million people in this decade, according to the World Health Organization.

Our hope is that this chapter will be "useful to those who want to understand clearly the events which happened in the past and which—human nature being what it is—will, at some time or other and in much the same ways, be repeated in the future."[1]

PERCEPTION OF THE DISEASE

". . . Cleanse the slums, limit the pubs, stop the smoke, clear the air,

F. Haas: Department of Rehabilitation Medicine, New York University Medical Center, New York, New York 10016.

S.S. Haas: New York University Medical Center, New York, New York 10016.

[1]Thucydides (circa 460–400 BC), *The History of the Peloponnesian War.*

And the water, of all the foul things that they bear,
Give food to the needy and good clothing to wear,
Shut up the wild lads who turn night into day,
And succor the women who lead them astray,
When your race is again strong, healthy and fair,
Rely on my word, you'll not find us there,
When struma, syphilis, cancer and gout,
By cleaner living have been driven out,
When lechery's over, carousing and riot,
We'll gladly return to our guinea-pig diet . . ."
James Hurd Keeling (1831–1909), *The Song of the Squirt*

While the industrializing northern Europeans were still relegating tuberculosis contagion to the closet, the Italians and Spanish were returning to strong anticontagion public health legislation—modeled on Lucca's 1699 laws—to protect their citizenry. In Florence, the 1754 edict included the admonition "to take care that the patient does not empty his sputum except into vessels of glass or glazed earthenware, and that these utensils be frequently cleansed and boiled. . ." Naples built a tuberculosis hospital and passed the stringent laws of July 19, 1782, stipulating both precautions during illness and measures to be taken after death.[2] Although these laws were eventually revoked because of the financial burdens they placed on both families and the community, the common people in these regions continued to fear contagion throughout the 19th century.

In contrast, northern Europe and North America had adopted the notion that tuberculosis reflected an inherited constitutional vulnerability and was a disease capable of bestowing genius—the *spes phthisica*—on its victims. The ubiquitous nature of the disease and the long, lingering death it entrained may well have fueled the romantic movement in the arts, making languid consumptive pallor—exemplified by Marie Duplessis, the mistress of Alexandre Dumas *fils* and the model for Marguerite of *The Lady of the Camellias*—highly attractive. Lord Byron, for example, was overheard saying while looking into a mirror, "I look pale. I should like to die of consumption." When asked why, he answered, "Because

the ladies would all say, 'Look at that poor Byron, how interesting he looks dying'" (Dubos and Dubos, 1987).

Although the longstanding notion of inheritability persisted throughout the 19th century, a changing perspective on the source of vulnerability began to surface—particularly in North America and England—in the latter part of the century. Vulnerability was now attached to class and morality. Tuberculosis was becoming a social disease, a ". . . diathesis . . . built up with equal certainty by impure air, drunkenness, and want among the poor, and by dissipation and enervating luxuries among the rich . . ." (Dubos and Dubos, 1987). Since one could now, in that current view, avoid tuberculosis by leading a "good life," it followed that contracting and dying of the disease documented one's inner weakness and intrinsic moral unfitness. Discovery of the tuberculosis bacterium clearly accelerated this trend in both Europe and the United States. A typical example was Dr. S. Adolphus Knopf, an American whose prize-winning tract—*Tuberculosis as a Disease of the Masses, and How to Combat It,* published in 1907—identified those most susceptible to the disease as either the personally depraved, whose alcoholism had temporarily or permanently enfeebled them, or the innocent victims of poverty.

Fertile Conditions for the Spread of Tuberculosis

As the population in Europe moved from rural to urban centers and immigrants inundated the eastern cities of the United States, greedy landlords on both sides of the Atlantic Ocean built dark, cramped living quarters—lacking adequate water, sewage, and ventilation—in the open yards behind apartment buildings. These "back tenements" and "dark rooms" created virulent seedbeds of tuberculosis (Figs. 1 and 2). Ernest Poole, a member of the antituberculosis committee of New York City's Charity Organization Society, described this typical scene in the "lung block" (Fig. 3) in the most crowded part of the city:

> "In a rear tenement a young Roumanian Jew lay dying of consumption. . . . In this room, 10 feet square, six people lay on the floor. . . . The other room was only a closet six feet by seven, with a grated window high up opening on an air shaft 18 inches wide. And in that closet four more people were sleeping" (Huber, 1906).

Another typical house, called the "ink pot," had front and rear tenements five floors high, with a small court between them. One hundred forty-five people, including 23 babies, lived in this building.

> "Up on the third floor, looking down into the court, is a room with two little closets behind it. In one of these a blind Scotchman slept and took the plague in 1894. . . . He died in the hospital. Only a few months later the plague fastened . . . (on) his little daughter. . . . At last she, too, died. Then one year later, in October, a Jew rented this same room. He was taken, and died in the summer. The room was rented . . . in the autumn by a

---

[2] The law of July 19, 1782, from the Kingdom of Naples:
 I. The physician shall report a consumptive patient, under penalty of 300 ducats for the first offense and 10 years' banishment for repetition of it.
 II. The authorities . . . shall inventory . . . the clothing in the patient's room to be identified after his death. . . if any opposition . . . be made, (if the person doing so . . . belongs to the lower class, (he) shall have 3 years in the galleys or in prison, and if of the nobility, 3 years in the castle and a penalty of 300 ducats.
 III. Household goods not susceptible of contamination shall immediately be cleansed and that which are susceptible shall at once be burned and destroyed.
 IV. The authorities . . . shall tear out and replaster the house from cellar to garret, carry away and burn the wooden doors and windows and put in new ones.
 V. Newly built houses shall not be inhabited for 1 year after . . . completion or 6 months after plastering has been done and everything (else) . . . has been finished.
 VI. The poor sick shall at once be removed to a hospital.
 VII. Hospital superintendents must keep clothing and linens for the use of consumptives in separate places.

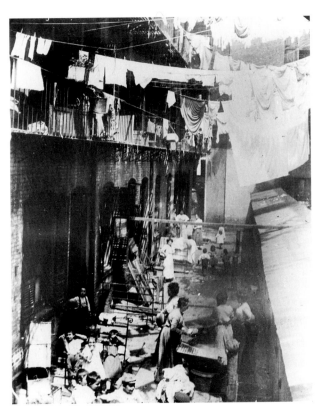

FIG. 1. Tenement house yard. Photograph by Jacob Riis (reproduced with permission of the Museum of the City of New York).

German and his wife. She had the plague already, and died. Then an Irish family came in. The father was a hard, steady worker, and loved his children. . . . But six months later he took the plague. He died in 1901. . . . In the rear house is another plague room. . . . Here, in 1896, lived an old Irish hat maker with his wife, small daughter, his two sons. . . . He took the plague, worked a year or more there on his hats, then died. The cough came on his wife soon after. She suffered long, weary months, only to see at the end her young daughter begin the same suffering. The mother died. The home was shattered. The girl was taken by her aunt, and soon followed her mother. The two sons died of the same disease, spreading it out into other tenements. . . . When the next housekeeper came to this same room with his wife, both were strong and well. The man took the plague in 1899. He still fought for life when all knew he was hopeless . . .; he . . . could . . . only lie alone in one of these closed bed rooms. (There are no fewer than 20 such rooms in this rear house—windowless, six feet by eight.) That winter of 1900 brought the memorable blizzard. While it was raging, a settlement visitor came to his room and found the water pipe burst, the room flooded. The plucky little wife had carried her husband upstairs on her back. A few days later his struggle was ended. The wife is still there'' (Huber, 1906).

Responding to the Threat

Although laws with codes setting minimum ventilation and window areas for individual rooms had been on the books since 1890, greed, indifference, political corruption, inventiveness of landlords, plus the sheer numbers

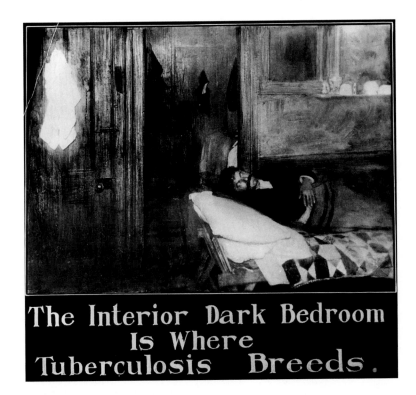

FIG. 2. There were 361,000 such "dark rooms" in New York City. Photograph by Jacob Riis (reproduced with permission of the Museum of the City of New York).

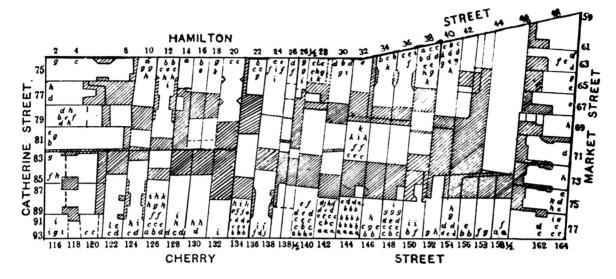

FIG. 3. Ground-plan of the "lung block." The shaded sections are courts and air shafts. Each letter represents a new case of tuberculosis reported to the Health Department between 1894 and 1903 (e.g., *a* represents 1 case in 1894 and *b* represents 1 case in 1895). Because the records do not indicate whether a given case resided in the front or rear tenement, all have been assembled in the front building except at 144 Cherry Street, as there was not enough room. (Huber JB. *Consumption: Its Relation to Man and His Civilization; Its Prevention and Cure.* Philadelphia: JB Lippincott; 1906:147.)

of immigrants, overwhelmed any attempt at enforcement or further reform. During that decade, however, a death rate of 776/100,000 and the knowledge that the "white plague" was reaching out beyond these impoverished neighborhoods added to the urgency for action.

One response to this threat was zealous reform. Progressive reformers such as Jacob A. Riis,[3] the author and photographer of *How the Other Half Lives,* brought the plight of the tenement-dwelling poor in New York City to public notice. One of the most effective of the tenement house reformers in New York, he advocated broad welfare programs to eliminate both poverty and illness and urged programs for remodeling tenement houses, abolishing sweatshops, reducing work hours, outlawing child labor, purifying water, and building parks and playgrounds.

The alternate response was fueled by the conviction that those living in such abominable circumstances found themselves there because they were morally unfit. The designation of "unfit" was applied to those who made the power structure anxious. In the United States, one saw an escalating xenophobia among Americans who feared being outnumbered by aliens who did not share their language, heritage, or democratic institutions. Europeans

feared the revolutionary zeal of the anarchists and socialists among the poor. Throughout the industrial world, the germ of tuberculosis spread by immigrants and the poor became intertwined with the "germs" of radical political reform.

Governments attempted to meet both the social activists' reform agenda and the conservatives' demand for restraining the behavior of the poor, as the same means could be applied to satisfy both. The operative tenets were that the disease was preventable if patients could be removed from society, and that it was curable if patients could be persuaded (or helped) to live properly (or humanely). The first required a political reaction—the development of public health departments and policy, so that patients with tuberculosis could be identified and controlled. The second involved the development of treatment facilities, and accompanying efforts to return these patients to society.

THE POLITICAL RESPONSE

The Local Department of Health

Politically, the results of the debate over the establishment of strong departments of health—which included compulsory identification of the tubercular patient—varied from place to place. But rather than present a superficial survey of these variations, we have opted to focus on New York City, where the establishment of a strong

---

[3]Ironically, although Jacob A. Riis is known as a social reformer who was instrumental in improving living conditions for poor tenement dwellers in New York City, his outrage over these living conditions was reserved for victims of German or Bohemian descent. Virulently anti-Semitic, he castigated Jews for their industriousness even though fully aware that this was exactly what would lift them out of their poverty. He also admonished the Italians, Irish, and Chinese for various perceived sins.

Department of Health and compulsory notification reflected the first clear victory for the group of physicians, politicians, and lay people who were convinced that only through strong administrative control could tuberculosis be contained.

In the United States, state health departments were first established in the mid-19th century. They employed sanitarians—engineers sent out to locate the causal elements in the transmission of disease (then believed to stem from foul-smelling or miasmic conditions). They were to establish uncontaminated water supply systems and uncontaminating sewage systems, and develop efficient and safe disposal for garbage and dead animals.

In the 1890s these sanitarians began to be replaced by public health physicians, whose mandate was broadened to the control of all transmittable diseases. For them, notification of contagious diseases was a necessary step in effective social policy to protect public health. Foremost among the proponents of this kind of social control was Hermann M. Biggs of New York (Fig. 4).

Born in Trumansburg, a small village in the Finger Lakes region of New York State, Biggs took pride in the fact that he was descended from six American-born generations on his father's side and eight on his mother's. Convinced that one's station in life is partly a gift of

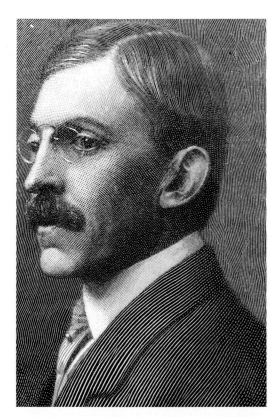

FIG. 4. Hermann M. Biggs, 1859–1923, established the New York City Board of Health Laboratory, set administrative controls for tuberculosis, and introduced diphtheria antitoxin and programs in child health.

inheritance, he grew up with a strong autocratic sense modulated by his father's passion for order. Early in his career, Biggs fastened onto the notion that cleanliness is next to godliness, turning his views on hygiene into a political credo in his baccalaureate thesis at Cornell in 1882 (coincidentally, the year of Koch's discovery of the tuberculosis bacillus): ''Upon recognition and careful observance of hygienic laws depend the healthy physical condition, and so prosperity, not only of individuals and communities, but also of whole states and nations'' (Winslow, 1929).

Biggs received his medical degree from the Bellevue Medical College in 1883, in the first medical class in the United States to take a formal pathology course, which was held in the country's first pathology laboratory.[4] William H. Welch, who founded the laboratory, remembered Biggs as the most active and interested student in the class, often staying late and working on special problems assigned him by Welch.

Biggs' choice of Bellevue was fortunate for other reasons as well. First, the faculty (including Edward Janeway and Francis Delafield as well as Welch), which had already begun to be involved in bacteriologic studies, espoused the highly unpopular hypothesis that all of tuberculosis was one disease, and readily accepted Koch's etiologic discovery of the tuberculosis bacterium. They countered the prevailing view of this microbe, as stated, for example, in the *Report of the Committee on Practical Medicine and Epidemics of the Illinois State Medical Society for 1882–83:* ''. . . mere accompaniments of certain deteriorative changes in organic matter, and possessing no causative relations whatever.'' Second, Bellevue's origin in 1816 as a prison, evolving into a hospital that embodied the notion of providing aid—sometimes forcibly—to the indigent population, provided an orientation that Biggs, probably because of his upbringing, supported unflinchingly. He clearly stated his position several years after entering medical practice, in an address to a meeting of the British Medical Association in Montreal:

> ''The government of the United States is democratic, but the sanitary measures adopted are sometimes autocratic, and the functions performed by sanitary authorities paternal in character. We are prepared, when necessary, to introduce and enforce, and the people are ready to accept, measures which might seem radical and arbitrary, if they were not plainly designed for the public good, and evidently beneficent in their effect'' (Winslow, 1929).

---

[4]The College of Physicians and Surgeons had offered W. H. Welch a faculty position, but refused to build a laboratory in which he could implement the histology and microbiology techniques he had learned in Germany. Bellevue Hospital gave him this laboratory, and he joined the faculty there as Professor of Pathological Anatomy and General Pathology. The College of Physicians and Surgeons, soon realizing its mistake, built a pathology laboratory under T. Mitchell Prudent.

Biggs' first application of bacteriology to a Health Department problem occurred in 1887, when he and T. Mitchell Prudent (then professor of pathology at the College of Physicians and Surgeons, and Biggs' close friend) correctly identified the cholera spirillum in an Italian immigrant who had presented with a clinically doubtful case of cholera and died on board the steamship Britannia. The passengers had been quarantined on the ship, and Asiatic cholera later developed in a considerable number of them.

This incident helped convince Commissioner of Health Joseph D. Bryant of the need to establish a Division of Bacteriology and Disinfection within the Board of Health. In 1888, as a consequence of meetings on the cholera issue between the New York City Health Department and the New York Academy of Medicine, Biggs and Prudent, along with colleagues Drs. Janeway and Loomis, were appointed as consulting pathologists to the New York City Board of Health. In May 1889, Commissioner Bryant asked them to issue a position paper on tuberculosis for the Board.

This document asserted the validity of Koch's findings and declared that tuberculosis was preventable, was not directly inherited, and required direct transmission from sick to healthy individuals. As such, the position paper suggested the following measures: a system of rigid inspection of cattle to prevent public consumption of tainted meat and milk; public education regarding the dangers of pulmonary discharges from tubercular people; and disinfection of rooms and hospital wards occupied, or previously occupied, by tubercular patients. Their report was received coolly by the medical community, with the large majority indicating that no official action was called for.

The Push for Public Health Measures

Because Biggs, Prudden, Commissioner Bryant, and Board President Dr. C. C. Wilson were sufficiently politically astute to realize that any further legislative initiative would be fruitless without public support, they undertook a direct campaign of public education, handing out flyers—issued in several languages—prepared by the pathologists and signed by the Board of Health President and Secretary. (Cultivating a favorable political constituency by means of educational materials would become a hallmark of the campaign waged by Biggs and colleagues to control tuberculosis via a strong Board of Health and compulsory notification.) These flyers detailed the following preventive measures:

"DO NOT—permit consumptive patients to spit on the floor; sleep in a room with a consumptive patient; fail to wash thoroughly the eating utensils of a consumptive patient as soon after eating as possible; mingle a patient's unwashed clothing with the clothing of others; fail to catch the bowel discharges of a consumptive patient with diarrhea in a vessel containing corrosive sublimates; fail

to consult the family physician regarding the social relations (i.e., 'sexual relationships') of people suspected of having consumption; permit mothers suspected of having consumption to nurse; keep, but destroy, household pets suspected of having consumption; fail to cleanse thoroughly the floors, walls, and ceilings of the living and sleeping rooms of consumptive patients at least once in two weeks" (Winslow 1929).

On November 28, 1893, $4\frac{1}{2}$ years after the initial report, the Board again took up the cause of tuberculosis control by asking Dr. Biggs (now Chief Inspector of the Division of Pathology, Bacteriology, and Disinfection) for an updated recommendation. His report—curiously dated the same day as this request—presented seven measures:

"(1) Educate the public via circulars and publications; (2) require notification by public institutions (e.g., asylums, social welfare facilities, hospitals) within 7 days of all persons suffering from pulmonary tuberculosis; (3) appoint special inspectors to ensure effective disinfection of contaminated premises; (4) separate tuberculosis patients from other patients; (5) establish a hospital exclusively for tuberculosis patients; (6) require the Board of Health Department to carry out a diagnostic bacteriologic sputum examination in every case of pulmonary disease of doubtful character; (7) insist that all physicians practicing in this city notify the Board of all pulmonary tuberculosis coming under their professional care (Winslow, 1929)."

This time around, the Board adopted Biggs' plan as "timely and well advised," except for the notification clause addressed to individual physicians. They correctly sensed that the medical profession would not passively accept it. Biggs strategically retreated—temporarily—to "recommending" full notification and counterbalanced by recommending even more stringent treatment of infected dwellings. He required that ". . . the Medical Sanitary Inspectors visit all premises (vacated) . . . by consumptive patients either by death or removal, and shall forward written recommendations as to the cleansing and renovation of the premises. . . . The Board (would) not allow the premises to be occupied by (new renters) . . . until the (recommendations have) been complied with" (Winslow, 1929).

The Board found Biggs' slightly softened position acceptable. On February 15, 1894, the *Sun* newspaper wrote that "the Board of Health formally declared war upon consumption when it adopted Professor Hermann Biggs' plan of campaign." However, the article, noting the parallel to the Naples law of 1792 (see footnote 2)—which had punished nonreporting physicians with 10 years of banishment and punished those who resisted the intervention of authority with 3 years in the galleys—stated that ". . . the Board *will not yet compel* (the authors' emphasis) physicians to report their consumptive patients. That will come later on" (Winslow, 1929).

Grumbling by the New York medical establishment—whose members saw the handwriting on the wall—was not yet followed by organized resistance. However, repercussions were felt elsewhere. Philadelphia's College of Physicians—over the objections of Dr. L. F. Flick, the compassionate pioneer of Pennsylvania's antituberculosis movement, and Dr. William Osler—met on January 12, 1894, and presented an antinotification edict to their municipal Board of Health, ostensibly because ''the attempt to register consumptives and to treat them as the subjects of contagious disease would be . . . stamping (these unfortunates) as the outcasts of society . . . (and) not lead to any measures of real value not otherwise obtainable. . . .'' (Winslow, 1929).

Notification: Friends and Enemies

Overt hostility between the New York Board of Health and the medical establishment broke out in earnest the following year, but the Board held firm and eventually—on January 19, 1897—Biggs saw his vision become reality in an amendment to the sanitary code:

> ''Section 225. That pulmonary tuberculosis is hereby declared to be an infectious and communicable disease, dangerous to the public health. It shall be the duty of every physician in this city to report to the Sanitary Bureau in writing the name, age, sex, occupation, and address of every person having such disease who has been attended or who has come under the observation of such physician for the first time within 1 week of such time. . . .'' (Winslow, 1929).

The medical profession's response to what they saw as a loss of authority and possible income was immediate. Dr. George Shrady's editorial in the influential *Medical Record* minced no words:

> ''The real obnoxiousness of this amendment to the sanitary code is its offensively dictatorial and defiantly compulsory character. . . . The profession as a whole has watched with jealous eye the encroachments of the Board upon many of the previously well-recognized privileges of the medical attendant. . . .'' (Winslow, 1929).

And in a follow-up editorial he accused the Board of wanting ''. . . to assume official control of the cases after they have been reported, thus not only . . . directly interfering with the physician in the diagnosis and treatment of the patient, but . . . possibly depriving him of one of the means of a legitimate livelihood'' (Winslow, 1929). (Ironically, Shrady—as a consulting physician to the Board—had written an editorial in the 1983 *Medical Record* endorsing the original compulsory notification regulation for cases diagnosed in public institutions. Why he eventually changed sides is unclear, although he did voice the views of a considerable faction of physicians.)

This feared loss of income because of anticipated interference by the Board of Health was paramount in the resistance of the medical profession, both to the notification program and to the establishment of tuberculosis hospitals. Physicians felt that the eradication or limitation of this disease would dramatically shrink the income-producing population of tuberculosis patients, and that improved public health facilities would attract many of the remaining patients. They blamed elimination of the income assessment previously used to qualify patients for these facilities—now leaving it up to individual honesty—for ''distributing the best care below market cost.''[5] The welfare cheat, who can afford to pay but pretends poverty (a recurrent image in the United States), was evoked: ''Dispensary patients leave their carriages and servants around the nearby corner of a street'' (Fox, 1974).

The issue came to a head in March 1897. The Medical Society of the County of New York unanimously protested the view of tuberculosis as infectious and communicable, and stated ''that in the judgment of this society the recent edict of the Board of Health in relation to compulsory reporting of cases of tuberculosis is unnecessary, inexpedient and unwise'' (Winslow, 1929).

The West Side German Dispensary resolved that the view of tuberculosis as a communicable disease ''is not entirely correct, (and that) . . . to grant the Health Board officials further powers . . . in regard to the removal of those subjects of tuberculosis . . . would be an interference that would be alike humiliating to the physician and intolerable to the patient and his family'' (Winslow, 1929). The *Medical Record* asserted, ''It would now appear that the time has come for the Health Board to rescind the obnoxious regulation, in order that it may, as formerly, work in harmony with the wishes of the profession.'' Arthur M. Jacobus in his presidential address to the County Society accused the Health Department of ''usurping the duties, rights, and privileges of the medical profession'' (Fox, 1974).

Despite this bellicose posturing, Prudden described the opposition as the ''little scattering of a gang of purps'' [sic] who longed for the ''good old times when a patient with tuberculosis could be lulled into a sense of security. . . .'' (Fox, 1974). Biggs attributed this medical opposition to ''timidity, selfishness and ignorance.''

However, the local medical societies did not speak for all physicians in New York City. The Medical Association (the local branch of the American Medical Association, or AMA) was already competing for physician support in two other extremely sensitive areas: the right to consult with homeopaths, and the right to advertise and sell proprietary remedies. Both rights were favored by the local societies, but stringently opposed by the AMA's code of ethics. The split of the medical community on the

---

[5]Feared loss of income by physicians was a recurrent concern. A 1904 report from the tuberculosis clinic at Gouverneur Hospital, in an attempt to counter this apprehension, noted: ''We are sure that the medical profession is not being impoverished because people are treated free. Occasionally we have a well-dressed child, but the appearance of some other member of the family outweighs the first impression of competence.''

notification issue fell along these predrawn organizational alliances.

The pro-notification group included members of the New York Academy of Medicine, the state's most prestigious group of physicians. The Academy contingent worked behind the scenes for a compromise. The Academy's Committee of Eight, with Biggs' friends Prudden and Janeway as spokesmen, suggested that the Board of Health "might wisely delay the enforcement of compulsory notification but should adopt more stringent measures for the care of all sputum." The full Academy accepted this motion that the Board delay, but not rescind, enforcement of compulsory notification of tuberculosis patients. With Shrady leading the outraged physicians and Biggs leading the notification forces, an agreement was forged to leave the new but gently enforced regulation on the books in return for an official consulting board, chosen by the Academy, to advise the Board of Health. (This new board came into being in 1898.)

The medical societies, however, would not accept the Academy compromise. Both the New York County and Kings County Medical Societies tried to push bills through the state legislature calling to rescind that provision of the New York City charter empowering the municipal Board of Health to deal with tuberculosis as an infectious disease. They had gone to Albany believing that the Republican-dominated legislature would be eager to discredit the Board of Health as a means of diminishing the power of Tammany Hall.[6] But because the notification controversy had divided Republican physicians just as it had other physician subgroups, the legislators saw no clear gain in restricting New York City's Board of Health on this issue. Although a legislative committee was appointed for show, in actual fact the issue was quickly dropped. Thus, a strong, well-organized minority with access to sufficient patronage and publicity—like Biggs and his colleagues—was able to achieve its goals over the objections of a poorly organized majority.

The primacy of New York City's Board of Health in this realm can be attributed to public health innovators who—by need, inclination, or both—were intensely political and selectively partisan and had cultivated ties to the various power bases. Joseph Bryant had connections with the Democratic organization. Dr. Alvah H. Doty, Health Officer of the Port of New York, was close to the Republican organization. Prudden had ties to the anti-Tammany reformers, and Biggs himself had a warm relationship with C. F. Murphy, then Tammany district leader and subsequently county leader.

Once notification was finally the rule, Biggs, Prudden, and their allies were careful to develop a favorable constituency among their fellow physicians. This was done in part by increasing the Board's importance in the city's medical economy, which was particularly influential because of the economic depression afflicting the country during the century's final decade. The Board paid out approximately $250,000 yearly in part-time and full-time salaries. In 1897, for example, in a politically popular move, the Board hired 192 physicians as school inspectors, with each one receiving $30 per month to spend 40 minutes a day in neighborhood schools. (The move was practical as well as politically prudent. On the first day alone they examined 4225 children and found among them 14 cases of diphtheria, 3 of measles, and 55 of parasitic disease.)

The reformers also avoided antagonizing the general population. They separated the antidisease and antipoverty issues. Prudden, in an article in *Harper's Magazine* in March 1894 entitled "Tuberculosis and Its Prevention," said that the tuberculosis bacilli lived in the "thick pile carpets" belonging to the rich and to those others who also accepted the "tyranny of things." And they remained neutral in the controversy about society's responsibility to the poor, and in debates about heredity versus environment, self-help versus charity, fit versus unfit, and the movement against health abuses in the workplace.

They also gained the loyalty of that 80% of the New York City population who were either foreign-born or first-generation Americans by printing educational circulars in a variety of languages (initially German, Italian, and Yiddish, and eventually Bohemian, Finnish, Polish, Slovakian, Ruthenian, Swedish, Armenian, Spanish, and Chinese), and making sure that Board of Health personnel who visited the homes of tubercular patients either spoke their native language or were accompanied by an interpreter who did.

Furthermore, so as not to exacerbate the alienation of opposing physicians, the Board of Health's eventual enforcement was, as promised, cautious, selective, and politically wise. During the first decade of compulsory notification, only six "recalcitrant" physicians were fined.

In retrospect, the Board of Health's compulsory notification directive was successful. Reported cases of tuberculosis increased from 8559 in 1898 to 32,065 in 1910, and sputum examinations increased from 2920 to 40,000 during this same period.

The forum in which the antituberculosis public health crusaders had fought for compulsory notification was the political arena. As such, it required the resolution of political conflicts and use of the bargaining process to transform positions into legislated public policy and workable administrative arrangements. Although similar battles were fought in most industrialized communi-

---

[6]Tammany Hall, led at that time by Richard Cocker, was the political oligarchy—associated with corruption and governmental mismanagement—that ruled New York City at the turn of the 20th century. The Board of Health evolved mainly during Tammany's control of City Hall.

ties, the successful achievement of compulsory notification in New York was unique. (For example, although Sir Robert Philip first pressed for compulsory notification in Britain as early as 1890, it took 20 years to be enacted into law.)

The medical profession in New York City could take pride in the international recognition they received for their success in identifying tubercular patients. In 1901 Robert Koch told Biggs, "I wish to cite the example of the American people, who of their own free will accepted the limitation of their liberties in the interest of public health," and recommended the New York model to the "study and imitation of all municipal sanitary authorities" (Fox, 1974). This model, in fact, dominated medical and public debate so thoroughly that it helped bring about an international medical and public consensus about the communicability of tuberculosis and the importance of notification.

THE CRUSADE

National Organizations

The world's first international medical congress, which met in Paris in 1867, included presentations on tuberculosis, among them Jean-Antoine Villemin's classic work on its specificity and communicability. Afterward, international congresses devoted specifically to tuberculosis were held at regular intervals until the end of the century.

This latter period also saw the emergence of national organizations—made up of medical, lay, and government personnel—to battle the disease. The first of these national organizations, called "A Society for the Establishment of Sanatoria for the Consumptive Poor," was established in Austria in 1890. Organizations in Denmark ("National League for the Campaign Against Tuberculosis") and France ("French League Against Tuberculosis") were established in 1891, and then Germany, Belgium, England, Portugal, Italy, and Canada rapidly followed suit.

A large, variegated country like the United States initially produced local antituberculosis organizations, with Philadelphia in the lead. On April 22, 1892, Dr. Lawrence F. Flick gathered 25 people, mostly lay persons, in his office, carefully excluding everyone who was inimical to the contagious theory of tuberculosis, to form the first American organization dedicated to combatting tuberculosis. With Flick as president, it became incorporated in 1895 as the Pennsylvania Society for the Prevention of Tuberculosis and set itself the following objectives: (1) to spread the gospel of contagiousness (still far from universally accepted) through public education; (2) to provide the poor with hospital treatment; (3) to visit poor patients and supply the necessary materials for protecting those they lived with; (4) to cooperate with the Board of Health's preventive measures; and (5) to lobby for appropriate public health laws. After the establishment of this unique antituberculosis group, another one finally followed in Ohio in 1901; then in quick succession associations were incorporated in six more states, including New York, and 11 local societies were formed.

The initial impetus to form a national association came not from the medical establishment, but from the Medico-Legal Society of the City of New York, a group of lawyers, scientists, and physicians who had organized a national meeting in 1900 to discuss state laws relating to the disease and its treatment. This meeting had heralded a shift in emphasis from treating individual patients to controlling the disease in society, a point of view that had been accepted a decade earlier in Canada and several European countries.

Between 1900 and 1903, Clark Bell (nonmedical president of the Medico-Legal Society) led an abortive attempt to parlay this meeting into a permanent, all-inclusive national organization. However, it failed because of territorial squabbles between physicians and lay persons. These often bitter conflicts arose between the AMA-supported organizations—representing practicing physicians' predominant emphasis (motivated by self-interest) on what they felt should be a purely medical approach to the disease—and organizations supported by public health officials and social workers dedicated to educational and legislative weapons for controlling the disease.

One of these conflicts erupted over an AMA-supported International Congress on Tuberculosis planned to be held Paris in 1904. On December 5, 1903, the *Journal of the American Medical Association* published a letter calling attention to the impropriety of proposed American congresses by "certain groups of little-known people who independently had been soliciting support, lay and political, for conflicting congresses." The AMA called for the formation of the following:

> ". . .a committee with power to act to consider the conditions existing with regard to the proposed Tuberculosis Congress and other National Antituberculosis Associations in the United States; also to consider the formation of a National Committee to represent this country at the International Congress at Paris, and that the members of this conference will abide by the action of the Committee; also that the Committee had power to add to its membership . . ." (Knopf, 1922).

The formative meeting took place, fittingly, in Philadelphia on March 28, 1904. Present on the medical side were the profession's foremost luminaries in the fight against tuberculosis: Edward Livingston Trudeau, S. A. Knopf, Henry Bowditch's son Vincent (founder of the first sanatorium in Massachusetts), Lawrence Flick, Sir William Osler, William Welch, and Hermann Biggs. Although physicians were heavily in the majority, all parties present resolved to coalesce into a national organization. Thus, the committee that was initially formed to head off anti-

AMA competition became a stepping stone to the formation of an inclusive national organization. On June 6th, in Atlantic City, New Jersey, the United States Society for the Study and Prevention of Tuberculosis[7]—with Trudeau as its first president in recognition of his past achievements—was born; it comprised a broad alliance of health care workers, politicians, clergy, employers, and philanthropists.

The International Movement

At this same time, the international movement was materializing. The first step had been taken at the 1899 International Congress, held in Berlin, with the granting of official recognition to lay government and voluntary organizations as part of the expanding drive against tuberculosis. The Congress of 1902, again in Berlin, formalized acceptance of these organizations by creating the Central Bureau for the Prevention of Tuberculosis (soon renamed the International Antituberculosis Association). Headquartered in Berlin and composed of representatives appointed by national organizations and governments, the Association's work was interrupted by World War I, then resumed with 24 member nations. Renamed the International Union Against Tuberculosis (IUAT) and based in Paris, the IUAT—currently with 114 member countries—continues to organize international meetings and publishes the *Bulletin of the International Union Against Tuberculosis*. Its expanded mission eventually called for the following:

> "All countries wishing to eradicate tuberculosis to decide among themselves on the methods, to agree on the most effective weapons, and to forge and implement them jointly against the common enemy. . . . Antituberculosis measures must some day be standardized . . ., but first it is necessary for the research workers to make a thorough investigation of the problem in order to provide governments with the necessary information. It is in this spirit and for these ends that we wish to create an International Union Against Tuberculosis" (Rouillon, 1982).

It was also at this meeting that the double red cross, as suggested by Dr. Gilbert Sersiron of the French national association, became the unofficial—and in 1928 the official—international symbol[8] of the voluntary movement to control tuberculosis. The cross, associated with the Christian Crusades, was the ideal symbol for what was viewed as an international "crusade" against this killer disease. Eradication was the common goal, although individual eradication campaigns reflected their national gestalt.

The Crusade in America

Because Americans typically viewed tuberculosis as a disease of the poor, the unfit, and the ethnically inferior, the campaign here took on an evangelical aura fed by the melding of three judgmental philosophies that stemmed, respectively, from the following: (1) the ascetic Protestant-capitalist tradition based on the Calvinistic doctrine of predestination[9]; (2) the converse view that individuals are responsible for their actions; and (3) a newly emerging corollary of Darwinian evolution whose precept was survival of the morally and physically fittest for the good of the human race—the biologic equivalent of the Calvinistic doctrine of predestination. Despite the obvious differences between these three social views, they all identified a subclass—the *same* subclass—as needing help.

Central to ascetic Protestantism (and those sects, such as Puritanism and Methodism, that derive from Calvinism) is the two-point doctrine of predestination: (1) God chooses before birth those to be saved and those destined for eternal damnation. (2) God's choice can only be guessed at by looking for signs of His grace. Although ascetic Protestants professed to disdain the pursuit of wealth as an end in itself, when it was attained as the fruit of one's labor, it was surely a sign of God's blessing. So the rich were confident that their wealth documented their place among the chosen, and they found the damned equally recognizable simply because of their poverty. Tuberculosis was easily woven into this fabric; the chosen did not fall ill, while those afflicted with tuberculosis were clearly among the damned.

A group opposing this deterministic view held that individuals could control where and how they lived. People who chose to live in filth, or were too unambitious or lazy to find work outside the crowded tenement districts, bore full responsibility if they contracted tuberculosis.

The third version—of the "defective" patient, the "Darwinian" point of view in relation to tuberculosis—was expressed in an article in the *Atlantic Monthly* by the noted Boston physician Henry Bowditch:

> "We must confess the sad and unwelcome truth that (some children) are doomed to an early death . . . by the diseased condition of the parents, sometimes . . . alas! due to their own or their ancestors' previous excesses. . . . 'For the sins of the fathers are visited upon the

---

[7]This organization was renamed the National Tuberculosis Association in 1904 and is with us still as the American Lung Association.

[8]This double cross symbolized Christian Jerusalem in the second century AD. Eventually appearing in Byzantium as a "Greek cross," it entered the Hungarian coat of arms in 1074 when the Byzantine Emperor gave it to Hungary's King Geasa I. Then, in 1099, Godefroy de Bouillon, Prince of Lorraine, added it to his banner to commemorate his Crusaders' capture of Jerusalem. Almost a millennium later, this cross was adopted as an emblem by the Free French in World War II. Since it has become associated with the antituberculosis movement, some countries have replaced it with a culturally more meaningful symbol (double red crescent or red lion and sun).

[9]Even a cursory discussion is beyond the scope of this chapter. The interested reader is referred to Erich Fromm, *Escape From Freedom* (New York: Avon Books; 1965) and Max Weber, *The Protestant Ethic and the Spirit of Capitalism* (New York: Charles Scribner's Sons; 1958).

children unto the third and fourth generation.' Such children die early; **and this is exactly right. The race would constantly deteriorate were it otherwise** (*authors' emphasis*). . . . Only to strength and perfect health belongs the highest life, which alone has as its birthright the will and the power to contribute to the continuance of the human race'' (Bowditch, 1869).

As all three viewpoints regarded the tubercular patient as inferior—whether damned by God, by his ancestors, or by his own actions—the National Association for the Study and Prevention of Tuberculosis found it easy to integrate them. The organization embarked on a campaign of propaganda, education, and aid dedicated not only to controlling tuberculosis, but also to developing a power base to control what was becoming a major industry. (By 1950, for example, the antituberculosis program in the United States approached $500 million.)

The *Confidential Bulletin,* the organization's internal newsletter, urged a concerted effort to recruit employers into the antituberculosis crusade because of their influence over their workers. Employers, selfishly motivated, were easily persuaded to join. On the one hand, the need to keep a healthy work force led these ''captains of industry'' to confront the ''captain of all these men of death.'' Some large corporations built ''cure'' facilities for their workers. The Standard Oil Company of New Jersey, for example, built such a pavilion at the Loomis Sanatorium in the Catskill Mountains of New York. (Ironically, during and after the industrial revolution it had been the blind drive for wealth—and thus evidence of God's grace—with its exclusive focus on profits and consequent disregard for humane working conditions, that had created an environment so favoring the spread of the disease.) And on the other hand, at a time when labor was becoming more restive and militant, this health crusade taught that passive obedience to employers was in the worker's best interest. Because the National Association viewed the city-dwelling poor as morally inadequate and thus in need of society's vigilance, they offered hygiene and morals in one basket. Lectures on tuberculosis, housing, and working conditions went hand in hand with such lectures as ''The Amusement Problem: Snares of Amusements, Saloons, Dance Halls and Burlesque Theaters.'' And the urban masses themselves were given the following admonitions:

Don't spit on the floor of your shop.
When you spit, spit in the gutters or spittoon.
Don't cough without holding a handkerchief or your hand over your mouth.
Don't drink whiskey, beer, or other intoxicating drinks.
Whatever thou take in hand, remember the end and thou shall never do amiss.
Whatever is worth doing is worth doing well.

Because health and personal conduct were now intertwined, coming down with tuberculosis became plainly unpatriotic: ''Community health is essential to national preparedness. Now is the time to show that wasteful sickness can be prevented.''

Consistent with the prevailing capitalistic mentality, public participation in the fight against tuberculosis took the concrete form of donations to finance the different programs. The very first appeal for public funds was a small-scale effort mounted in Denmark, based on Einar Holboell's idea of selling special stamps or seals to raise money. In 1907, one of these seals reached the notice of photographer and social reformer Jacob A. Riis, whose ensuing article in an American magazine sparked the idea here. Emily P. Bissell of Wilmington, Delaware, who had read the article, commissioned the artist Howard Pyle to design a seal that she sold to raise $3000, financing construction of an eight-bed tuberculosis cabin. She then persuaded the American Red Cross to apply the idea nationwide, and they raised $135,000 in 1907 and $200,000 in 1908. For the next decade, the seal campaign was a joint Red Cross and National Tuberculosis Association effort. Then in 1919 the Red Cross gave full proprietorship and responsibility to the National Tuberculosis Association, which used the seal to raise $4 million that year. By 1950, the Christmas Seal program, as it came to be known, raised $20 million a year.

MEDICAL CARE

Compulsory notification and the social welfare movement were necessary, but not sufficient, weapons in the fight against tuberculosis. Once identified, tubercular patients needed treatment—whether they wanted it or not. The form that treatment took was tied to economic level, and patients were segregated by race. The wealthy were often treated at home by a private physician, to whom they paid a standard fee. Private funds were also required for sanatorium treatment, which promised a cure in return for subservient obedience. The majority of poor patients relied on public dispensaries combined with some sort of home care. The municipal hospitals cared for patients who were either terminally ill, noncompliant, or indigent.

The Sanatorium Movement

The history of the sanatorium movement has been well documented, if somewhat idealized, and the reader is referred to the ample literature on this subject for a detailed review. The summary here provides the outlines.

Sanatoria had sprung up in central Europe during the last half of the 19th century, then spread to coastal and riverside areas of Great Britain; after 1882 they crossed the Atlantic to America. Philosophically, sanatoria fell into two groups. One adhered to the motto of the Hotel/Sanatorium at Davos, Switzerland—*mox sani* (''the merry are soon well'')—illustrated in Thomas Mann's

The Magic Mountain. The other upheld the motto of Brehmer's Sanatorium at Gobersdorf—*die Patienten kommen nicht um zich zu amusiren sondern um geheilt zu werden* ("patients do not come here to amuse themselves but to be cured")—agonizingly portrayed in A. E. Ellis's *The Rack.*

The latter approach, incorporating the same Puritan ethic that permeated the National Association, better suited the American psyche. Patients entering sanatoria here implicitly agreed to a bargain: medical advice, treatment, and nursing care in exchange for complete submission to a rigorously demanding institutional authority. Although the sanatorium life was often romanticized in European literature, in reality it meant sacrificing dignity for the uncertain prospect of a cure. Patients typically entered an Orwellian society in which they became a number, divested of all sense of individuality via a combination of ideologic and psychologic assaults.

The experience was unchanged decades later when Marshall McClintock, who became a long-term resident of the Adirondack Cottage Sanatorium, described his arrival. On entering he was handed a rule book inscribed with his number (8027), which he was required to read and sign. He noted, "I felt worse than ever. Like a prisoner. And the book was full of rules, lots of rules" (McClintock, 1931).

Some patients viewed sanatoria as oases because they provided a refuge from sweat shops and squalid tenements. But the rigidly regimented life (not by accident reminiscent of monastic routine) often quickly became untenable, especially when it came to segregation of the sexes. Sex was believed to be both a major factor in the development of tuberculosis (". . . girls with the tuberculosis diathesis do not have the same moral stamina that girls in robust health have. . . . This explains . . . why so many prostitutes are tubercular" [Peters, 1909]), and a result of tuberculosis "toxemia," which was regarded as ". . . effective in the direction of causing sexual irritability" (Fishberg, 1919). The harshness of sanatorium rules caused between 10% and 30% of these patients to leave within their first month.

Society replicated its inequalities and prejudices in the health care system in general, and in the sanatoria in particular. Blacks, for example, whose death rate from tuberculosis was twice that of whites, were completely barred from sanatorium treatment. When Lawrence F. Flick defended the initial nonsegregation policy at White Haven Sanatorium in Pennsylvania, the white patients there threatened to leave:

> "As there is nothing in your advertising literature sent to patients . . . that they would be expected to associate with Negroes; we think it is an injustice to live in daily contact with them . . . (and) we do not think it desirable for the White and Black Races to mix" (Bates, 1992).

Flick, to his credit, pitted his principles against the economic survival of the institution he had helped found.

But the sanatorium board voted against him and issued a new rule: "No Negroes will be admitted to the sanatorium." In response, Flick resigned as medical director.

Patients who were poor and/or addicted to alcohol were also looked down on. These elitist attitudes are illustrated by the Otisville Sanatorium in New York, which had been built at Hermann Biggs' urging and embodied his autocratic notions. It was the first municipal sanatorium in the United States and, unlike most sanatoria, had a "work cure" to prevent "the cultivation of habits of idleness." Biggs objected to the rest cure enforced at various other sanatoria on the grounds that their successful cases often consisted of "converting a sick tuberculosis individual into a fairly healthy loafer" (Winslow, 1929). (There was also a practical aspect, because inmates who were earning their keep to some degree reduced operating costs.)

Alcoholics were the most "worthless" patients of all. The rather terse notice sent to patients newly accepted at the Otisville Sanatorium included the following: "If under the influence of liquor, or smelling of the same, you will be rejected." The antituberculosis movement was obsessed with alcohol, which in the United States was viewed as the prime nonbacterial factor contributing to the disease. (One can speculate as to the role of the antituberculosis movement in the development of Prohibition.)

Whether or not sanatorium treatment was effective in curing tuberculosis—it was never scientifically evaluated—in reality, the great majority of patients never had the opportunity to experience it. (By 1954, for example, when the incidence of tuberculosis was well on the wane, the 130,000 existing sanatorium beds could accommodate only half of the patients with active disease. Some of those unable to find space, or unwilling to submit to the demeaning regimen, went to the Colorado mountains or the southwestern desert, where large and desolate tent colonies—known as "bugsvilles" or "lunger's camps"—had been set up beyond town limits. The colony at Tucson, Arizona, for example, located 1 mile beyond the last bus stop and with no running water and only primitive sewage conditions, was a place of "lost souls and lingering death." Those remaining in the city most often sought help via dispensaries and home care, and as a last resort entered a local municipal hospital.

The Dispensary

Antituberculosis dispensaries first appeared in Europe several years after the discovery, if not universal acceptance, of the communicability of the disease. The initial one was established in Edinburgh, Scotland, by Sir Robert Philip. In 1900, Ernest Malvoz established the second dispensary in Liège, Belgium, with Albert Calmette doing the same in Lille, France, in 1901. The first American dispensary, the Henry Phipps Institute in Philadelphia, opened in 1903, and was followed soon after by Gouverneur and Bellevue Hospitals in New York City. The 1904 Bellevue Report described the dispensary as providing the following: (1) careful and thorough medical attention; (2) systematic investigation and supervision of the patient's home conditions; (3) education of both patient and family; and (4) evaluation of the social and economic conditions affecting the medical aspects of each case (Miller, 1904). Figure 5 shows the Bellevue Dispensary's first 5 months of activity.

Although all dispensaries shared these same basic aims, each institution had its individual perspective. At Bellevue, for example, "careful and thorough medical atten-

REPORT OF THE TUBERCULOSIS DIVISION OF THE BELLEVUE HOSPITAL OUT-PATIENT DEPARTMENT.

From January 1 to May 31, 1904.

Number of new patients treated	210
Number of visits to clinic by all patients	850
Number of visits by nurses in the homes	593
Number of cases untraced	39
Number of patients sent to hospitals	89
Number of patients under observation May 1	91
Number of patients given material assistance	139

Summary of Material Assistance.

SOURCE.	NUMBER OF PATIENTS	ASSISTANCE.	
		Quarts Milk.	Dozen Eggs.
Bellevue Hospital	35	920	685
N. Y. Diet Kitchens	19	1,836	....
Strauss Depots	8	570	...
Charity Organization Society	37	General Relief	
Ass'n for Improving Condition of the Poor	16	"	
United Hebrew Charities	4	"	
Miscellaneous Organizations	20	"	

Total milk given, 3,326 quarts—cost	$166 00
Total eggs given, 685 dozen—cost	144 00
Total cost of milk and eggs	$310 00

It will be noted from the above report that of the 210 patients treated, 39, or 19 per cent., were untraced in their homes. These are almost all lodging-house cases, whom it is very difficult to manage from the dispensary. They should all be sent to hospitals, if not willingly, then compulsorily, by authority of the Health Department.

FIG. 5. Expenses incurred by the Bellevue Hospital outpatient tuberculosis clinic during its first 5 months. (Miller JA. The tuberculosis clinic of the Bellevue Hospital outpatient department. In: Lambert A, Draper WK, Curtis BF, Woolsey G. *Medical and Surgical Report of Bellevue and Allied Hospitals in the City of New York,* 1904;1:204–205.)

tion" involved collecting sputum for analysis by the Department of Health, making a probable diagnosis, and instructing the patient—both orally, and with written instructions for home use—as to nature of the disease and the needed precautions. Patient and family education was an ongoing responsibility of the physicians and nurses, and was supported with printed circulars. The 1904 Bellevue Report observed that each patient "is now a center of information in regard to the general principles of healthful living" (Miller, 1904). In contrast, the 1904 Gouverneur Report noted, "We have distributed very little literature. It has seemed to us that what patients know they will talk about, and that those with whom we work are usually more confused than helped by printed information" (Bradford and Seymour, 1904).

Both dispensaries prescribed a daily diet that started with a minimum of 2 quarts of milk and 4 raw eggs and increased to 3 quarts of milk and 10 eggs. (Very few patients were thought to benefit from more.) Patients were given a cuspidor and pocket sputum pouches free of charge. However, medication played a very minor role at Bellevue, whereas Gouverneur regularly used therapeutic agents such as strychnine, cod-liver oil, and ichthyol, and heroin was touted to control cough.

Patients at Bellevue were seen weekly, and their weight, temperature, pulse, and general condition were recorded. If needed, patients could be admitted to Bellevue's tent cottage (Fig. 6). The dispensary could also refer patients to an appropriate sanatorium and/or charitable organization. Investigation and supervision of the patient's home situation was done by home visits. In France, Calmette trained former tuberculosis patients for these visits, whereas the Phipps Institute and the New York City hospitals used visiting nurses. The year that the Phipps Institute dispensary opened, Dr. Lawrence L. Flick, soul of Philadelphia's antituberculosis movement, wrote, "Tactful, kind supervision by a well-trained woman soon brings the most ignorant consumptive under control" (Bates, 1992).

As stated in the Bellevue Report, the aim of the visit was "to arrange the whole domestic economy to the best interest of the patient, and to provide against dangers of infection to his household and associates" (Miller, 1904). This included instructions for room ventilation, disinfection, expectoration, and general hygiene. Plans for taking the "rest cure" outdoors were made and, where possible, outdoor sleeping accommodations were constructed (Figs. 7 and 8). If a home was found to be completely unsuitable, the visiting nurse could insist that the patient be moved to a more healthful location.

As well-meaning as these health efforts were, patients did not always welcome them, as the following letter to Dr. Flick at the Phipps Institute indicates:

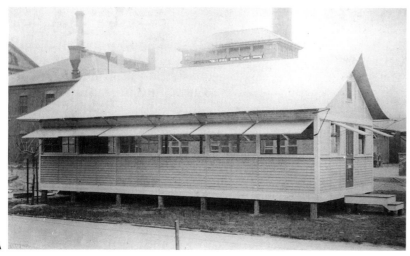

A

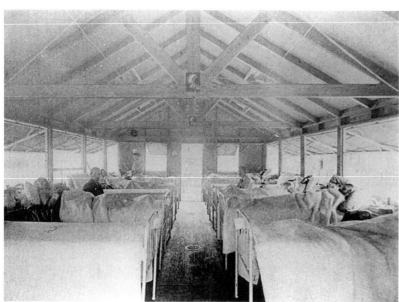

B

FIG. 6. Top: The tent cottage at Bellevue Hospital. **Bottom:** A tent interior, with gas light and steam heat. (Lambert A, Draper WK, Curtis BF, Woolsey G. *Medical and Surgical Report of Bellevue and Allied Hospitals in the City of New York,* 1904;1:204–205.)

"And doc, I now right to you to tell you, that you sent 2 nearses here to see Katie MiCarty and I would like to know, if you can tell who sent you a letter about my doarter. . . . I would like to tell your's nearses to pleas not bother a bout my business, for there is only one cure for my child and that is in heven" (Bates, 1992).

Just as it is today, patient compliance was of great concern to these public health pioneers. The 1904 Gouverneur Hospital Report notes the following:

"The intelligence of these patients varies greatly. . . . Some at once sense the situation and work with us. . . . Among our most intelligent are the schoolchildren, who take kindly to the idea that they are in training as important as any athlete. On the other hand, there are those who come when they feel the need, and stay away at the slightest improvement."

In the Phipps Institute's second annual report, Dr. Flick's earlier optimism that patients could easily be swayed to lead a "proper" life style with "tactful and kind supervision" had been replaced: "Considerable pressure is brought to bear on patients to induce them to practice preventive measures when they seem reluctant to do so. . . . When, ultimately, they are found to be intractable, they are discharged from the institute" (Bates, 1992).

The Municipal Hospital

For these disobedient patients, only the municipal institutions remained. As early as 1896, the AMA was urged to promote a network of state hospitals where "indigent consumptives who were careless in their hygienic habits could forcibly be confined." The Rhode Island Commission, charged in 1911 with building such an institution there, listed "confinable" offenses as follows: being found a public nuisance; noncompliance; homelessness; friendlessness; dependency; dissolute behavior; dissi-

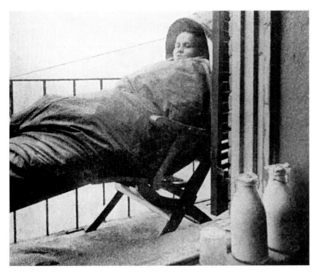

FIG. 7. Fighting tuberculosis on the fire escape. (Lambert A, Draper WK, Curtis BF, Woolsey G. *Medical and Surgical Report of Bellevue and Allied Hospitals in the City of New York,* 1904;1:204–205.)

pated and vicious behavior; residence in a lodging house or public institution with refusal to enter one's assigned hospital; living at home in unfavorable sanitary conditions, thus posing a danger to the family; and insisting on being discharged from a hospital against medical advice.

The New York Department of Health designated Riverside Hospital on North Island as the facility for involuntary confinement of all tubercular patients whose dissipated and vicious habits presented a danger to the community. But it failed both as a prison and as a hospital, as was typical of municipal efforts in the early 20th century. Riverside was often short of sputum cups, at the time a staple in the fight against contagion. It failed to give instruction in, or enforce, hygienic measures. Discipline was lax, bed rest was not enforced, and patients spent their days playing cards and wandering about.

In 1913, a report on 25 municipal facilities in five major cities (issued by the Committee on Hospitals for Advanced Cases of Tuberculosis of the National Association for the Study and Prevention of Tuberculosis) observed that, as in almshouses, patients would admit themselves as the weather grew cold and leave as soon as temperatures improved.[10] These institutions made no attempt to provide even rudimentary treatment or enforce the rules designed to prevent contagion. They were also cited for permitting patients to leave to visit friends and relatives. These municipal facilities, the Association concluded, served as "a place of last resort to the narrow group of cases in the extreme stages of physical and economic helplessness" (Rothman, 1993).

HOW EFFECTIVE WAS THE PUBLIC HEALTH INITIATIVE?

The death rate from tuberculosis between 1880 and 1920 decreased throughout the industrial world. In New York State, for example, it declined from almost 400/100,000 to just over 100/100,000, and in Wales and England from 200/100,000 to 100/100,000. The respective public health movements and national associations regarded this decline with pride and attributed it to their public health measures—that is, the education and isolation of an increasing proportion of patients.

This self-congratulatory attitude has been challenged on the grounds that these measures simply happened to coincide with a decline in tuberculosis deaths that reflected the larger cycles of the disease, a decline that was in reality not even accelerated by the public initiative. And a closer examination of death rates between 1800 (the start of reasonably accurate data) and 1950 (when effective antibacterial agents were first used) indicates that a constant decline in tuberculosis mortality had begun well before the interventions described above, and continued to fall at the same constant rate even after the health initiatives were put in place. Thomas McKeown and R. G. Record, among others, attribute this constant decline in tubercular deaths to a general improvement in social conditions during the period (improved housing, sanitation, and nutrition). Their position is based on two negative-inference arguments.

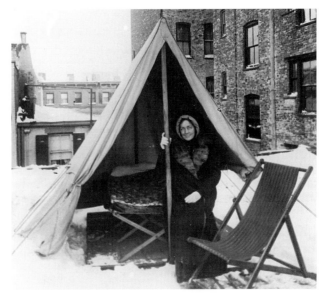

FIG. 8. Fighting tuberculosis on the roof. Photograph by Jacob Riis (reproduced with permission of the Museum of the City of New York).

---

[10]I (F.H.) remember a spring day in my childhood (in the early 1950s) when I accompanied my father to his job as Director of the Pulmonary Rehabilitation Program at Bellevue Hospital. A panhandler approaching our car suddenly recognized my father and apologized. That winter I saw him again, this time in Bellevue. My father explained that every year, he would check into the hospital when the weather turned cold, stay for the winter, then leave in the spring.

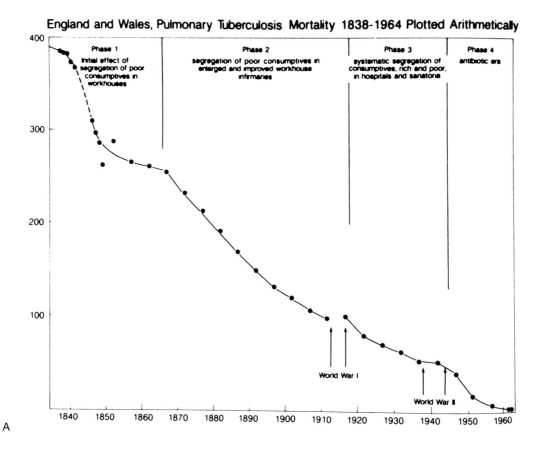

A

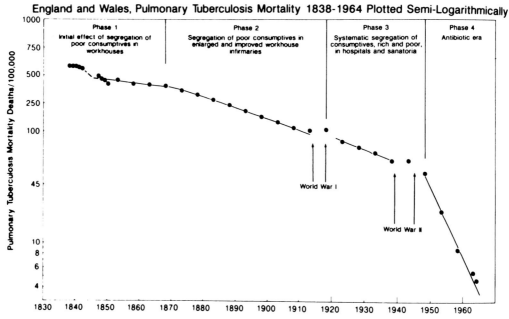

B

FIG. 9. Top: Arithmetic graph of tuberculosis mortality in England and Wales. **Bottom:** Semilogarithmic graph of the same data. (Wilson LG. The historical decline of tuberculosis in Europe and America: its causes and significance. *J Hist Med Allied Sci* 1990;45:390.)

The first is that the slope of the mortality line did not grow steeper with each new public health initiative (Fig. 9, *top*), indicating that these initiatives apparently had no significant effect. The second argument is that the slope of the death rate remained nearly constant despite the increasing proportion of patients receiving treatment. Throughout most of this period, in any given decade the incidence of tuberculosis continuously decreased, while the number of patients isolated and treated remained fairly constant. (In New York, for example, it held steady at about 15,000 per decade.) Because this meant an increasingly greater proportion of patients were being treated, the death rate should have decreased more and more rapidly if the treatments were successful. But again the slope of the line appears constant, suggesting that these medical and social interventions were not having a significant impact.

In contrast, the public health and medical interventionists argue that their policies *did* accelerate the decrease in tuberculosis deaths. Leonard Wilson provides mathematical support for this view using the same data from England and Wales (Fig. 9, *bottom*). He argues that the decreasing mortality was not constant, but rather declined exponentially. And when the mortality data are plotted semilogarithmically, four distinct segments of increasing slope emerge. The discontinuity in the lines corresponds to the World Wars. The accelerated decrease in death rate, indicated by the steeper slope of each segment, coincides with better isolation of tubercular patients from the healthy population. A similar plot can be obtained from New York City data (Fig. 10), in which the steepest drop (1918–1922) immediately followed the opening of three large tuberculosis hospitals. Subsequently, the decline in deaths returned to approximately its previous steady exponential rate. (Those hypothesizing that the continued drop in tuberculosis deaths was a consequence of continuously improving social conditions could also view the two World Wars—during which the death rate soared in response to dramatically deteriorating social conditions—as perverse retrospective experiments favoring their hypothesis.)

In our opinion, these conflicting observations actually illustrate two coincidental and superimposed mechanisms, one reflecting human interventions and the other reflecting the innate rhythms of the disease. On the one hand, a slow steady decline representing the effects of social improvements was interspersed with periods of accelerated decline consistent with the introduction of new antituberculosis initiatives. Disease epidemics, however, have their own natural and characteristic ebb and flow. For tuberculosis, these dynamics are dictated by the three types of postinfectious responses (Fig. 11). In most people who are infected, the disease does not develop further. Those remaining in the infectious pool separate into the relatively small group of "fast" (primary progressive) tuberculosis, and the larger group of "slow" (reactivation) tuberculosis. The early phase of an epidemic obviously represents the fast cases, and thus the death rate is high. As the epidemic progresses, the "slow" component becomes dominant and dictates a time unit of many decades, with the typical tuberculosis epidemic operating on a protracted time scale of 100 years or more. During this long-term phase, the death rate flattens substantially.

Current thought suggests that the rising phase of the ongoing epidemic in Europe and North America started

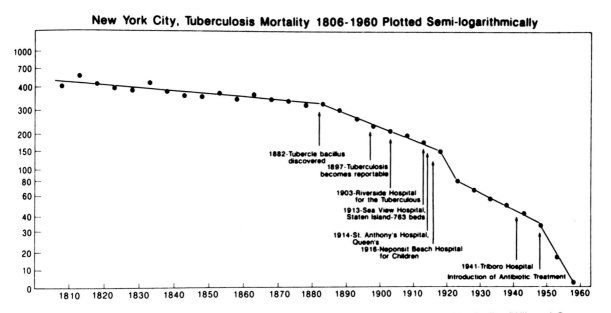

FIG. 10. Mortality in New York City between 1806 and 1960 plotted semilogarithmically. (Wilson LG. The historical decline of tuberculosis in Europe and America: its causes and significance. *J Hist Med Allied Sci* 1990;45:393.)

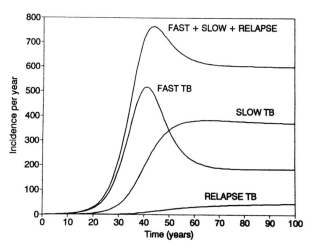

FIG. 11. A numerical simulation of a tuberculosis epidemic initiated by one infectious case at time zero in a disease-free, susceptible population of 200,000. The simulation illustrates the relative contributions of the three categories of tuberculosis (fast, slow, and relapse) to the incidence rate of this disease. A decline occurs in the absence of change in any parameter, and is simply the consequence of the intrinsic dynamics of transmission. (Blower SM, McLean AR, Porco TC, Small PM, et al. The intrinsic transmission dynamics of tuberculosis epidemics. *Nat Med* 1995; 1:820.)

when population densities exceeded transmission threshold levels. This coincided with the development of industrialization and the consequent vast migration from rural to industrial areas in both Europe and North America, and the inundation of North America by massive numbers of immigrants looking for a better life. After peaking in the early 19th century, deaths would have been expected to decrease as a consequence of the unique dynamics of a tuberculosis epidemic. Because the medical innovations and improved social conditions outlined here (with respect to hygiene and nutrition) happened to coincide with this declining phase, they were constrained to operate within—and thus appear muted by—the slow response time dictated by the intrinsic dynamics of the epidemic.

CONCLUSION

The discovery of *Mycobacterium tuberculosis* was essential for the development of an antituberculosis technology. The accumulation of new knowledge that followed precipitated an atmosphere of optimism, with the expectation that the means for detection and elimination of this single agent would ultimately achieve elimination of a feared and widespread disease. The irony is that altruism and charity played only a minor role in society's eventual attempts at controlling the tuberculosis epidemic. It was the often greedy fear of economic loss, combined with the anxiety of self-protection, that drove the campaign against this disease.

The leading edge of the current tuberculosis epidemic

coincided with the initial phase of the Industrial Revolution, and its crest coincided with the subsequent apotheosis of unrestrained capitalism. The initial stimulus for the development of a societal antituberculosis initiative, therefore, came from the need to protect the investment and profits of the owning class. In the early phase, when large numbers of laborers migrated from farms to industrialized centers and the jobs there required little special training, workers were cheap and easily replaceable. In this kind of labor market, the health of individual workers was of little concern to employers. Eventually, however, the reserve of potential workers from rural areas shrank while the demand for skilled labor increased, so that employers had to spend significantly more to retain their workers. It became financially meaningful not to lose employees. (This cycle of an epidemic of tuberculosis coinciding with rapid industrialization, dense migration from rural to urban slum districts, and the exploitation of laborers, which characterized the Industrial Revolution in Western Europe and North America, is recurring now in Latin America, Asia, and Africa.)

The second catalyst in the antituberculosis movement came from the gradual realization by physicians that the untreated and unsupervised poor were a real threat, not only to their fellow poor living alongside them in squalor, but to the middle and upper classes as well:

> "Then the poor servants of the well-to-do, if there be consumption in their own homes, are likely to bring infection into the families of their masters; as are also poor consumptive workmen who are employed upon repairs in the homes of the rich. There is in fact, no limit to the extent to which the disease may be disseminated from its primal base—the home of poor sufferers" (Huber, 1906).

The foot soldiers of the antituberculosis crusade—the compassionate nurses and physicians who dealt directly with patients—often participated for altruistic reasons, but the development of effective public health programs often had little to do with compassion and altruism and were, in fact, determined by hard economic concerns and fears. The antituberculosis program was enabled by scientific progress, brought to fruition through the deft amalgamation of public fears and self-interest, and facilitated by the skillful political manipulations of ambitious men to overcome what Castiglioni, in his 1933 *History of Tuberculosis,* called ". . . the short-sighted interests of a few who, in all times and every land, tried to sacrifice the public good to the selfish motive of the minority."

The crusade achieved its success by playing on society's fears and bigotry. Because the poor were a ready target, the antituberculosis campaign purposefully emphasized and perpetuated the stereotype of the poor tenement dweller as an immoral drunkard who was sexually promiscuous and lazy, and reinforced the general notion that the tubercular patient was the cause, rather than the victim, of disease. This stereotype was a critical element in galvanizing and financing the public health campaign to eliminate tuberculosis. The dynamics of this campaign aptly illustrated Hermann Biggs' conviction: ''Public health is purchasable and within natural limitations, any community can determine its own death rate'' (Winslow, 1929).

BIBLIOGRAPHY

Bates B. *Bargaining for Life: A Social History of Tuberculosis, 1876– 1938.* Philadelphia: University of Pennsylvania Press; 1994. *Concentrates on the social aspects of the tuberculosis story, especially in Pennsylvania.*

Blower SM, McLean AR, Porco TC, Small PM, et al. The intrinsic transmission dynamics of tuberculosis epidemics. *Nat Med* 1995; 1:816–821. *Presents a good model of a hypothetical tuberculosis epidemic.*

Bowditch H. Consumption in America. *Atlantic Monthly* 1869. *Expounds on the important role of fresh, clean air in the prevention of consumption.*

Bradford SS, Seymour NG. Report of the tuberculosis clinic at Gouverneur Hospital. In: Lambert A, Draper WK, Curtis BF, Woolsey G. *Medical and Surgical Report of Bellevue and Allied Hospitals in the City of New York,* 1904;1. *Together with the Miller article, this offers a unique view of the city hospitals' dealings with tuberculosis on an outpatient basis.*

Caldwell M. *The Last Crusade: The War on Consumption, 1862–1954.* New York: McMillan; 1988. *The history of tuberculosis in the United States from a social perspective.*

Castiglioni A. *History of Tuberculosis.* New York: Medical Life Press; 1933. *A well-written history of the disease prior to the advent of antibiotics.*

Committee on Hospitals for Advanced Cases of Tuberculosis. *Transactions of the Ninth Annual Meeting of the National Association for the Study and Prevention of Tuberculosis,* 1913. *An evaluative survey indicting municipal tuberculosis facilities.*

Davis AL. History of the sanatorium movement. In: Rom W, Garay S, eds. *Tuberculosis.* Boston: Little, Brown; 1996:35–54. *A concise history of the sanatorium movement.*

Dubos R, Dubos J. *The White Plague: Tuberculosis, Man and Society.* New Brunswick, NJ: Rutgers University Press; 1987. *The classic book on the history of tuberculosis.*

Fishberg M. *Pulmonary Tuberculosis.* Philadelphia: Lea and Febiger; 1919. *Incorporates the conviction that tuberculosis could act as an aphrodisiac.*

Fox DM. Social policy and city politics: tuberculosis reporting in New York, 1889–1900. *Bull Hist Med* 1974;49:169–195. *A detailed analysis of the factors leading to New York's preeminence in tuberculosis reporting at the turn of the 20th century.*

Haas F, Haas SS. The history of tuberculosis from the Renaissance to 1900. In: Baum G, Wolinsky J, eds. *Textbook of Pulmonary Diseases.* 5th ed. Boston: Little, Brown; 1993:xix–xiii. *The history of tuberculosis prior to the discovery of* Mycobacterium tuberculosis.

Huber JB. *Consumption: Its Relation to Man and His Civilization; Its Prevention and Cure.* Philadelphia: JB Lippincott; 1906. *State-of-the-art medical textbook of the period.*

Knopf SA. *A History of the National Tuberculosis Association: The Anti-tuberculosis Movement in the United States.* New York: National Tuberculosis Association; 1922. *Written by one of the luminaries in the fight against tuberculosis in the United States.*

McClintock M. *We Take to Bed.* New York: Jonathan Cape and Harrison Smith; 1931. *A first-person report of the sanatorium experience.*

McKeown T. *The Role of Medicine: Dream, Mirage, or Nemesis?* London: The Rock Carling Fellowship; 1976. *The premise is that socioeconomic changes are more important than medical breakthroughs to society's health.*

Miller JA. The tuberculosis clinic of the Bellevue Hospital outpatient department. In: Lambert A, Draper WK, Curtis BF, Woolsey G. *Medical and Surgical Report of Bellevue and Allied Hospitals in the City of New York,* 1904;1:204–205. *Together with the article by Bradford and Seymour, this offers a unique view of the city hospitals' dealings with tuberculosis on an outpatient basis.*

Peters WH. The sexual factor in tuberculosis. *N Y Med J* 1909;89:116– 120. *Associates tuberculosis with moral weakness.*

Rhode Island State Commission on Tuberculosis. *Report on Hospitals for Advanced Cases.* Providence, 1911:34–36. *How politicans viewed tubercular patients at the turn of the century.*

Riis JA. *How the Other Half Lives: Studies Among the Tenements of New York.* New York: Dover; 1971 (reprint edition). *The plight of the tenement poor in the 1890s.*

Rothman SM. Seek and hide: public health departments and persons with tuberculosis, 1890–1940. *J Law Med Ethics* 1993;21:289–295. *The antitubercular health campaign seen from the liberal lawyer's point of view.*

Rouillon A. The international union against tuberculosis: a general view. *Bull Int Union Against Tuberculosis* 1982;57:196–197. *A short history of the IUAT.*

Wilson LG. The historical decline of tuberculosis in Europe and America: its causes and significance. *J Hist Med Allied Sci* 1990;45: 366–396. *A balanced history of the causes of decline in tuberculosis mortality in the 19th and early 20th centuries.*

Winslow CEA. *The Life of Hermann M. Biggs, M.D.: Physician and Statesman of the Public Health.* Philadelphia: Lea and Febiger; 1929. *A very thorough and overly flattering portrait of the mastermind of the New York City Health Department's war on tuberculosis.*

Textbook of Pulmonary Diseases, 6th ed.
edited by G.L. Baum, J.D. Crapo, B.R. Celli, and J.B. Karlinsky,
Lippincott–Raven Publishers, Philadelphia, 1998.

CHAPTER

1

Normal Anatomy and Defense Mechanisms of the Lung

Robert R. Mercer · James D. Crapo

INTRODUCTION

Inhalation of approximately 10,000 L of air is necessary to meet the daily gas exchange requirements of the adult human lung. The normal lung has an extraordinary respiratory reserve. Arterial oxygenation commonly improves with exercise, and even under heavy work conditions, pulmonary gas exchange in a normal adult is rarely a cause of limitation to aerobic performance. To accomplish the efficient extraction of oxygen and exchange of carbon dioxide, the lung has an internal surface area approximately equal to that of a tennis court. The upper and lower respiratory tracts act to condition the inhaled air, and the lung has developed unique defense pathways to allow it to maintain its fine, delicate gas exchange surface while being continuously exposed to potentially injurious reactive or infectious agents in inhaled air. This chapter reviews the normal anatomy of the human lung and focuses on the unique structural characteristics that allow the lung to maintain normal function while being continuously exposed to inhaled reactive gases and particles.

THE NORMAL RESPIRATORY TRACT

Two normal adult lungs at maximal capacity contain 5 to 6 L of air and weigh an average of 850 g in men and 750 g in women. Blood makes up a substantial fraction of the lung weight, and *in vivo* the lungs have been estimated to contain as much as 360 mL of blood. Lung weight is approximately 1% of total body weight in a normal adult.

R. R. Mercer: Pathology and Physiology Branch, National Institute of Occupational Safety and Health, Morgantown, West Virginia 26505.
J. D. Crapo: Department of Medicine, National Jewish Medical and Research Center, Denver, Colorado 80206.

Ninety percent of the volume of the lungs is made up of gas exchange regions or lung parenchyma, whereas lung weight is approximately equally divided between the parenchyma and structures other than parenchyma (airways and large vessels).

The right lung is commonly slightly larger than the left, comprising about 53% of the volume of both lungs on average. Each lung is completely covered by a visceral pleura. The visceral pleura subdivides each lung, although incompletely, into lobes. The right lung has three lobes, and the left is divided into two lobes. Incomplete fissures between the lobes commonly allow for some collateral ventilation between lobes. The bronchopulmonary segments are defined by the primary segmental bronchi that branch off the lobar bronchi. Lobar segments are not commonly subdivided by pleura. There are 10 segments in the right lung (Fig. 1) and eight in the left. Common terminology identifies 10 segments in each lung, with the first and second (apical posterior) segments of the left upper lobe being a combined segment and the anterior basal and medial basal segments being combined in the left lower lobe. The left lingula is anatomically part of the left upper lobe and is not commonly separated by a pleura-containing fissure. The fissure separating the right middle lobe from the right upper lobe is termed the *horizontal fissure* and can occasionally be recognized as a horizontal line on an anterior-posterior chest radiograph. The oblique or major fissures separating the upper and lower lobes of both the left and right lungs can be identified on lateral chest radiographs. The left major fissure commonly lies slightly apically and anteriorly to the right major fissure (Fig. 2). However, this apparent position can be easily altered by small variations in the orientation of a left lateral chest radiograph.

A common variant in the lobation of the lung is the presence of a horizontal fissure partially demarcating the

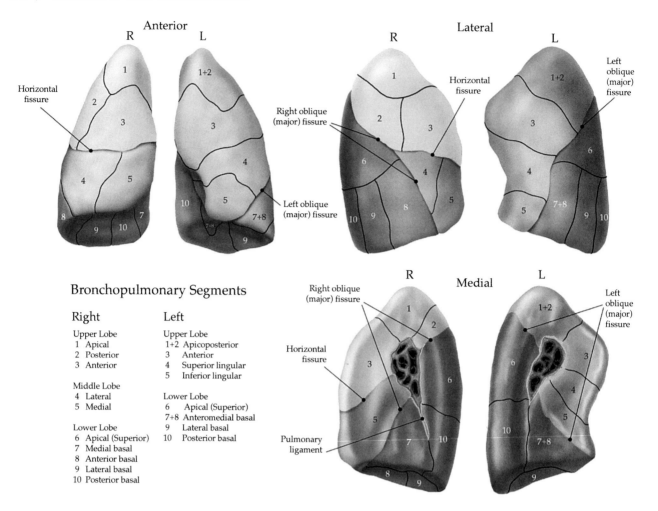

FIG. 1. Location of bronchopulmonary segments from anterior, lateral, and medial views. *See color plate 1.*

superior segment of either the right or left lower lobes. Another variant occurs when during development the azygos vein moves into the apical portion of the right pleural cavity. This displaces parietal pleura into the lung, producing a fissure in the apex of the upper lobe of the right lung. This partially separated lung lobe, known as an *azygos lobe,* occurs in slightly less than 1% of the population. The lingula of the left lung may also be demarcated by an anomalous fissure.

Contours along the lung surfaces for the heart, mediastinal structures, and major vessels are illustrated in Fig. 1. A fold of tissue containing connecting tissue and vessels that extends inferiorly from the hilum on both sides is termed the *pulmonary ligament.*

Pleura

The normal visceral pleura is a thin translucent sheet of mesothelial tissue. It is contiguous with the parietal pleura at the hilum, the parietal pleura being the surface covering of the chest wall. Pleural spaces are filled with a minimal amount of fluid ranging from 1 to 20 mL. The movement of fluid into and out of the pleural space depends on the combined effects of hydrostatic, colloid osmotic, and tissue pressures in the parietal and visceral pleura. The parietal pleura contains lymphatics that drain into the internal mammary artery, periaortic arteries, and diaphragmatic lymph nodes. Pleural fluid is thought to arise primarily from the capillaries lining the parietal pleura. This fluid circulates back across the parietal pleura, where it is cleared by lymphatics. Tracer studies have suggested that the parietal pleura accounts for most fluid movement into and out of the pleural spaces under normal conditions. Visceral pleural capillaries and visceral pleural lymphatics do not normally play a major role in fluid fluxes through the pleural space.

In total, the driving force withdrawing fluid from pleural spaces is greater than the net force moving fluid out of the pleural capillaries and into the pleural spaces. This results in the pleural space remaining relatively dry. Fluid does not normally accumulate in the pleural space unless hydrostatic pressure is elevated in the pulmonary capillary

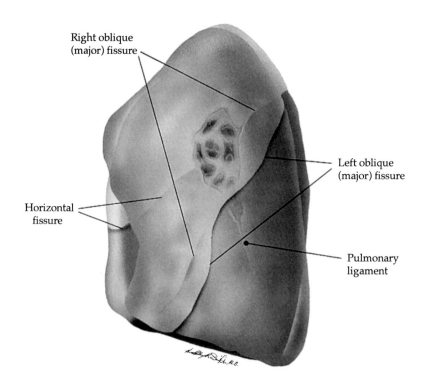

Right oblique (major) fissure

Horizontal fissure

Left oblique (major) fissure

Pulmonary ligament

FIG. 2. Left lateral view of the lungs. Partially translucent image of the left lung allows the right lung to be seen. The location of the major fissures and the horizontal fissure of the right lung are illustrated in the positions in which they would appear on a left lateral chest radiograph. Note that the major fissure on the right side lies slightly anterior and apical to the major fissure on the left side. *See color plate 2.*

bed or an inflammatory condition of the pleura causes protein leakage into perivascular and pleural spaces, decreasing the oncotic pressure gradient and thereby the major force favoring extraction of fluid from the pleural spaces.

Anatomically, the pleura is made up of mesothelium. Mesothelial cells are characterized by their long microvilli, up to 2 μm in length. These cells contain desmosomal intracellular attachments (macular adherens) and also intermediate filaments in their cytoplasm (cytokeratin). Mesothelial cells have a well-developed endoplasmic reticulum, which suggests that they are metabolically active. Beneath the mesothelial cells is a thin, loose connective tissue structure containing both capillaries and lymphatics. There is also a deeper layer of elastic fibers between the relatively thin visceral pleura and the immediately subjacent alveolar septal tissues. The parietal pleura has a similar architecture, except that the underlying connective tissue layer is substantially thicker and overlies intercostal muscle, fat, and vascular structures.

Lung Lymphatics

Tissue fluids in the lung move centrally toward the hilum. In alveolar tissue, alveolar septal junctions create spaces through which fluid is thought to move until it reaches the walls of an airway or vascular structure in which lymphatic structures are present. These intrapulmonary lymphatics, termed *deep lymphatics,* drain the bronchovascular bundles toward the lung hilum. The superficial pleural lymphatics carry fluid along the pleural surfaces to the point at the hilum

where the visceral pleura reflects into the parietal pleura. These superficial lymphatics also follow interlobular septa and thereby interconnect with the deep pulmonary lymphatic system. The deep pulmonary lymphatic system can be clearly identified anatomically beginning at about the level of respiratory bronchioles.

Lymph nodes are abundant in the pulmonary hilum and along the trachea and extrapulmonary bronchi. Lymphatic fluid drains through anastomosing channels that connect these lymph nodes and moves upward along the trachea. The lymphatics on the right side re-enter the systemic circulation through the subclavian vein near its junction with the jugular vein. Pulmonary lymphatics on the left side return to the systemic circulation through the thoracic duct or by directly emptying into the left subclavian vein.

Four major groups of lymph nodes exist in the lung. These include intrapulmonary nodes adjacent to lobar, segmental, and smaller bronchi and small nodes (1 to 3 mm) located in subpleural regions, often at junctions with interlobular septa. Extrapulmonary nodes are situated in the subcarinal region near the bifurcation of the main bronchi. They are also found along the walls of the trachea and main bronchi. The intrapulmonary nodes, which are part of either the pleura or small intrapulmonary airways, are termed *N1 nodes.* Extrapulmonary nodes along the main bronchi may also be termed *N1.* Subcarinal and ipsilateral tracheal nodes are termed *N2,* whereas contralateral hilar, tracheal, or bronchial nodes are termed *N3.*

The lung also can contain aggregates of lymphoid tissue along all levels of large and small airways. This tissue is called *bronchus-associated lymphoid tissue (BALT).*

BALT contains lymphoid follicles with germinal centers but does not have the fibrous capsule and capsular sinus characteristic of lymph nodes. The question has been raised as to whether BALT occurs normally in humans or rather develops only after stimulation. Its specific role in immune regulation is not yet well defined.

Upper Respiratory Tract

The upper respiratory tract plays a critical role in conditioning air entering the lungs. Most of the air moving through the nasal cavity has turbulent flow characteristics. In addition, air moving downward into the trachea encounters a right-angle turn at the posterior nasopharynx (Fig. 3). Because of these characteristics of nasopharyngeal anatomy and air flow dynamics, most airborne particulate matter and highly reactive gases impact or are absorbed along the mucosal surfaces and so are removed in the upper airways. Aggregates of lymphoid tissue in the posterior pharynx (pharyngeal tonsils) also play a role in clearing the large amounts of airborne material deposited in the nose and other regions of the upper respiratory tract. Most airborne materials deposited in the upper airway tract are moved posteriorly along the nasal mucous coat to the posterior pharynx, where the secretions are eventually swallowed. The upper respiratory tract also plays a role in warming and humidifying the air. This process is continued in the large airways. For gases of low reactivity and particles of 1 μm in size, upper respiratory tract clearance is less efficient. A significant fraction of these airborne pollutants is deposited in the small airways and alveolar regions.

Trachea and Bronchi

The trachea and main bronchi contain U-shaped rings of hyaline cartilage. The dorsal wall of the trachea is made up of a smooth muscle coat (the trachealis muscle). The main bronchi are fully encircled with cartilage for only four to six generations. Thereafter, the cartilaginous rings of intrapulmonary bronchi contain islands of cartilage that are not contiguous. The number and size of these cartilaginous islands diminish as the airways become smaller and more peripheral. This organizational pattern of cartilage has the advantage of assisting in an effective cough mechanism. The cough is initiated when intrapulmonary pressure is raised against a closed glottis, causing the smaller bronchi to narrow in size. The abrupt opening of the glottis with the onset of cough leads to high pressure and rapid flow through narrow airways, which can facilitate removal of obstructing secretions. Under normal breathing conditions, the intrapulmonary bronchi do not collapse because they are tethered to surrounding alveolar tissue with elastic and cartilaginous interconnections. The

incomplete cartilage rings provide support for the intrapulmonary airways while still permitting them to narrow.

Intrapulmonary bronchi contain a subepithelial elastic layer. Outside this, smooth muscle bundles form a narrow spiral around the airways, with the smooth muscle extending to the level of the respiratory bronchiole. The tight spiral organization of the smooth muscle causes airway narrowing when the smooth muscle contracts. A loose connective tissue layer surrounds the muscular coat, and bronchial glands and cartilage plates lie in this space.

The bronchial epithelium is a stratified epithelium that includes a number of cell types. Predominant among these are secretory cells, which in the large airways are primarily mucus-secreting cells. Ciliated epithelial cells and nonciliated basal cells make up the other two major airway epithelial cell types. The bronchial epithelium also contains neurosecretory cells, termed *Kultschitsky cells* or *K cells*. They are similar to the Kultschitsky cells found in the gastrointestinal tract. These cells, which occur singly or in clusters of four to 10 cells termed *neuroepithelial bodies,* are thought to have a neuroendocrine secretory function. These endocrine cells are found in both bronchi and bronchioles. Kultschitsky cells are most distinctively recognized by their large numbers of fine, dense core granules aggregated in the basal part of the cells. The granules are secreted basally into the peribronchial connective tissue and surrounding smooth muscle. Various products identified with the neuroendocrine cells influence smooth muscle contraction, secretion of mucus, and ciliary beat.

Cilia are the principal means for clearing inhaled toxicants deposited in the mucous lining layers of the nasal passages and airways. Dysfunction in cilia is known to predispose individuals to respiratory infections and bronchiectasis. Ciliated cells are densely distributed in the airways, and the cilia greatly increase their apical surface area. The plasma membrane surface of the cilia accounts for approximately 80% of the plasma membrane surface in airways. Thus, the cilia themselves are a primary filter and/or target for inhaled toxicants that react with cell membranes. In the serous fluid layer in which they beat, the cilia make up 40%–50% of the volume. Each ciliated cell contains approximately 200 cilia; these beat in a biphasic stroke consisting of a fast forward flick and a slower recovery motion. Coordinated strokes by adjacent ciliated cells produce a proximally directed wave of motion in the mucous lining layer. The beating cilia produce mucociliary transport rates that vary from approximately 20 mm/min in the large bronchi to a distinctly slower rate of approximately 1 mm/min in the bronchioles. This gradient in transport rates has been assumed to be the result of a corresponding gradient in ciliary density, with fewer cilia in the small airways and greater numbers in the larger airways, to prevent piling up of mucus on the relatively small surface area of the larger airways. However, direct measurements of the density of ciliated cells

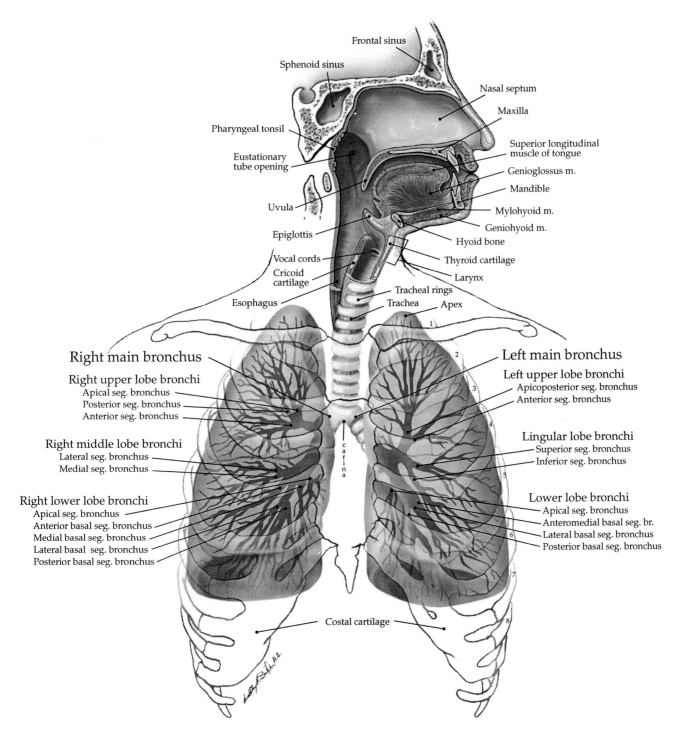

FIG. 3. Anatomy of the upper and lower respiratory tracts.

and their cilia do not support this hypothesis. The mechanism or mechanisms responsible for the higher transport rate of mucus in larger airways remain to be determined.

Ciliated cells not only mechanically move mucus but also have a secretory function. These epithelial cells contain ion pumps that move sodium away from the bronchial lumen and chloride toward it. This allows water to follow the resulting osmotic gradient and thereby control the thickness and viscosity of the serous fluid layer. Proteins controlling this ion flux are encoded by the cystic fibrosis transmembrane conductance regulator (CFTR) gene. This gene is a highly regulated chloride channel in the apical membrane of ciliated epithelial cells. Mutations in this gene cause cystic fibrosis.

Mucous cells (goblet cells) and mucous glands both produce mucus, but the volume coming from glands is substantially greater than that derived from mucous cells under normal conditions. The mucous glands are compound tubular glands lining the submucosa of the bronchi between cartilage plates. The glands are connected by a secretory tubule to the airway lumen. Plasma cells are often found around these secretory tubules. The plasma cells contain both IgA and IgG, although the primary immunoglobulin in mucus is 11S secretory IgA. Two IgA molecules, both of which are produced by plasma cells, are joined by the J protein. These molecules are then complexed with a secretory piece by epithelial cells lining the secretory tubules, and the complex is transported into the tubular lumen and into the mucous layer.

Examples of airway epithelium and mucous layer architecture from human bronchi are shown in the electron micrographs of Fig. 4. Characteristic profiles of ciliated and goblet cells are illustrated in Fig. 4A. In Fig. 4B, a goblet cell is in the process of secreting into the mucous lining layer. The mucous lining layer in this micrograph has a well-defined electron-dense surface film at the top of the sol layer. Examples of other secretory and basal cells in human airways are shown in Fig. 5. Secretory cells other than goblet cells are typically found in highly clustered groups, as illustrated in Fig. 5A, showing a group of secretory cells containing electron-dense granules. A basal cell with numerous desmosomes (d) and keratin filaments (f) appears in Fig. 5B. An intermediate cell (I) with the same features as a basal cell (i.e., desmo-

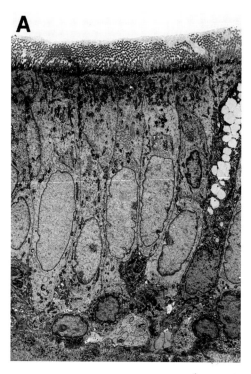

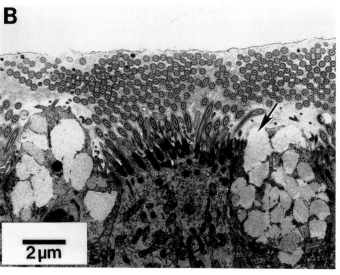

FIG. 4. Electron micrographs of the airway epithelium and mucous lining layers from human bronchi. **A:** Ciliated cells showing mitochondria concentrated in the apical portion of the cell and cilia extending into the mucous lining layer. One goblet cell is shown with its secretory granules distributed across the upper half of the cell. **B:** Two goblet cells in the process of releasing electron-lucent secretory granules from their apical surface into the mucous lining (arrow). This micrograph also illustrates a region in which the gel (or electron-dense) layer above the cilia is absent. (Reproduced with permission from Mercer RR, Russell ML, Roggli VL, Crapo JD. Am J Respir Cell Mol Biol 1994;10:613–624.)

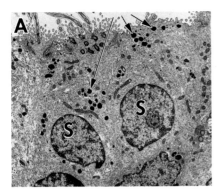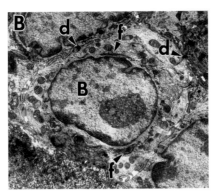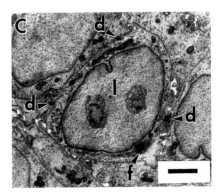

FIG. 5. Electron micrographs of secretory, basal, and intermediate cells from human bronchi. **A:** Secretory cells (*S*) containing electron-dense granules (*arrows*). **B:** Several desmosomes (*d*) and keratin filaments (*f*) of a basal cell (*B*). **C:** An intermediate cell (*I*) with the same features as a basal cell (i.e., desmosomes, keratin filaments, and a high nucleus-to-cytoplasm ratio) but no basement membrane contact. Whereas a prominent nucleolus is typically found in basal cell nuclei, two nucleoli, as illustrated in the intermediate cell in C, were noted only in intermediate cells. *Bar* at the bottom right represents 2 μm. (Reproduced with permission from Mercer RR, Russell ML, Roggli VL, Crapo JD. *Am J Respir Cell Mol Biol* 1994;10:613–624.)

somes, keratin filaments, and a high nucleus-to-cytoplasm ratio) but no basement membrane contact is shown in Fig. 5C. The layered arrangement of cells in human bronchi is principally attributable to the basal cell layer, which accounts for approximately 90% of the cell surfaces making contact with the basement membrane. In the pseudostratified epithelium of human bronchi, the average basement membrane contact of a ciliated, goblet, or other secretory cell is significantly smaller than that of basal cells. The large concentration of keratin filaments and hemidesmosomes found in basal cells suggests that these cells play a primary role in the attachment of columnar cells to the basal lamina.

Mucous Lining Layers

It has long been known that the lung clears or removes inhaled particulate matter by means of a mucociliary escalator mechanism. The mucous lining of the lung airways is composed of at least two physically and morphologically distinct layers: an underlying serous layer, in which the cilia beat (sol layer), is blanketed by a viscous layer (gel layer). Whether a continuous gel layer exists throughout the airways is a matter of debate. In general, studies focusing on the nasal epithelium and upper airways have found a continuous blanket, whereas studies focusing on more distal airways and bronchioles have not. More recent studies have demonstrated that the mucous lining layer of the airways contains a surface-active film at the air-fluid interface in addition to the two layers originally described.

The bronchial epithelium plays a critical role in both producing and moving mucus out of the lung. The rate of movement of mucus is slowest in the small airways and fastest in the large bronchi and trachea. The normal adult produces substantial quantities of lung secretions daily, virtually all of which are transported by ciliary clearance to the posterior pharynx, where they are unconsciously swallowed. The outer layer of the mucous coat is a highly viscous gel containing glycoproteins with molecular weights of several million daltons. In addition to mucous glycoproteins, the airways secretions contain immunoglobulins (primarily IgA), proteinase inhibitors, and antibacterial proteins (lysozyme and lactoferrin). Sixty to eighty percent of the cells in the airway epithelium are ciliated cells; the remaining cells are either basal or secretory cells.

Methods for preserving the mucous lining layer have included direct visual observation on dissected airway specimens, fixation by immersion, vascular perfusion fixation, quick freezing, and osmium tetroxide vapor fixation. Of these different methods of preservation, vascular perfusion fixation is the most generally applicable, as mechanical disruption from immersion or airway instillation of fixative is eliminated. Because the extensive capillary bed of the lungs is used to place the fixative in the immediate vicinity of the fluid lining layers, this method has been shown to improve significantly the preservation of mucous lining layers in the airways and the surface-active film of the alveolar region. Figure 6 demonstrates the changes in the mucous lining layer along the respiratory tract of a lung fixed by a combination of osmium vapor and vascular perfusion fixation. The gel layer is present in the airways from the trachea to the bronchi. In the distal and terminal bronchioles, the gel layer is attenuated and not always present. Tubular myelin and other surfactant debris are commonly found in both the gel layer of the upper airways (trachea to bronchi) and near the surface of the sol layer of the more distal airways, where the gel layer may be absent.

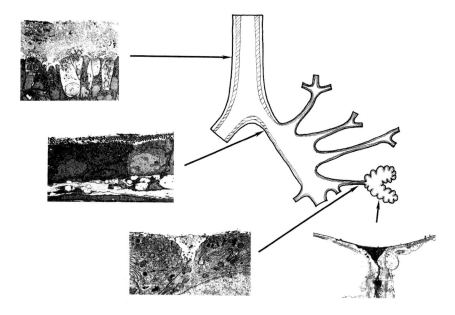

FIG. 6. Changes in the mucous lining layer along one airway path from trachea to alveolar surface. The thickness decreases from 10 to 20 μm in the trachea to 0.1 μm on the alveolar surface.

Bronchioles

Bronchioles are defined by the absence of cartilaginous structures in the bronchial wall. Smooth muscle continues along bronchiolar walls and reaches the terminal bronchioles. The bronchial smooth muscle spirals around the airways and does not form a continuous coat in the bronchial wall. Thus, there is no true muscular mucosa in bronchi. The connective tissue surrounding bronchial walls is termed the *lamina propria*. The lamina propria includes vascular structures, lymphatics, loose fibrous tissue, and modest numbers of inflammatory cells. Adipose tissue may also be found in the walls of bronchi, particularly in older individuals.

The airway epithelium of bronchioles is simple columnar and is made up of two primary types of cells, ciliated cells and nonciliated secretory cells. The latter cell type commonly is termed a *Clara cell*. Unlike the arrangement in the bronchial epithelium, ciliated cells and Clara cells in the bronchioles have extensive contact with both the luminal and basement membrane surfaces. Mucus-secreting cells are not found in bronchioles under normal conditions. Chronic exposure to tobacco smoke can cause proliferation of mucous cells, which are then found in bronchioles and likely account for the higher density of viscous small-airway secretions in smokers. The production of mucus in small airways in response to chronic irritation is an adaptive response that would have the effect of absorbing or reacting with inhaled pollutants, thereby providing better protection of the underlying bronchiolar epithelium. The function of Clara cells is still being defined. These cells are thought to be involved in production of the thin serous fluid that normally lines small airways, in the detoxification of chemicals depositing in small airways, and in regulating the immune or inflammatory responses in airways. Their products include surfactant apoproteins A, B, and D, antileukoproteinase, and a unique 10-kD protein that has been found to bind to environmental pollutants. Clara cells are also thought to be a stem cell involved in the regeneration or repair of epithelial injury in bronchioles.

The number of cells per unit area of epithelial basement membrane for human airways is shown in Fig. 7. The cells populating the airway epithelium change significantly as the airways narrow and a transition occurs from a pseudostratified epithelium (with an extensive population of basal and goblet cells) to a simple columnar epithelium in bronchioles. The pseudostratified arrangement of cells in the epithelium of human bronchi creates a total epithelial cell density almost twice that of the more distal bronchioles. In addition, the cell composition changes, from larger numbers of goblet and basal cells in bronchi to larger numbers of Clara cells in bronchioles.

Bronchial Branching

A terminal bronchiole represents, on average, 16 generations or branchings from the trachea. Most of the path lengths are shorter and can consist of as few as six to eight generations. The longest path length is the axial path to the posterior caudal tip of the right lower lobe, with 20 to 25 generations. Human lung airways are characterized by an asymmetric, dichotomous branching pattern in which the two (or three) daughter branches at most junctions are not of the same diameter and do not form a consistent, symmetric branching angle with the parent airway (Fig. 8). Pulmonary arteries follow the airways, whereas pulmonary veins lie in the boundaries between gas exchange units. This position allows the veins to accept blood from multiple adjacent gas exchange units (Fig. 9). An important result of the vascular supply following the airways is that each segmental bron-

HUMAN AIRWAY CELL DENSITY

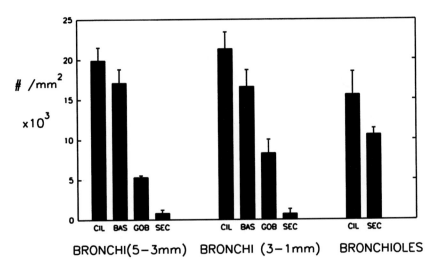

FIG. 7. The number of cells per unit area of epithelial basement membrane for human airways. Human airway cell populations change dramatically from the pseudostratified epithelium of bronchi, which have a large proportion of basal (*bas*) and goblet (*gob*) cells, to the simple columnar epithelium of bronchioles, composed primarily of ciliated (*cil*) and secretory (*sec*) cells.

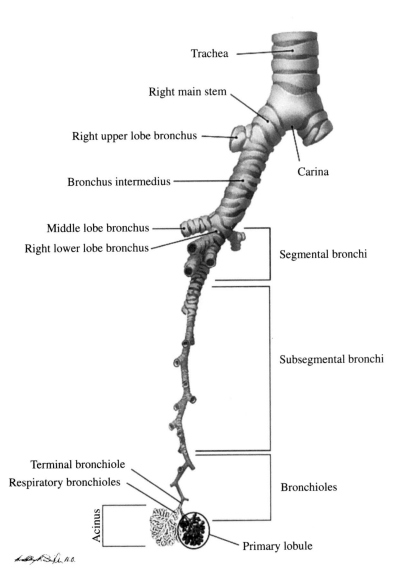

FIG. 8. Airway anatomy of the human tracheobronchial tree. This figure illustrates typical branching along one of the longer paths to a right lower lobe segment. In the normal human lung, there are approximately five to 15 branch points from a segmental bronchus to a terminal bronchiole. In a completely binary, symmetric branching system, 14 to 15 branch points from the trachea would be required to create the 40,000 terminal bronchioles in a human lung. Because many paths are shorter, there are also path lengths with greater than 15 branch points from the trachea. Segmental bronchi are characterized by the presence of cartilaginous plates in their walls, whereas bronchioles contain smooth muscle in their walls but no cartilage. *See color plate 3.*

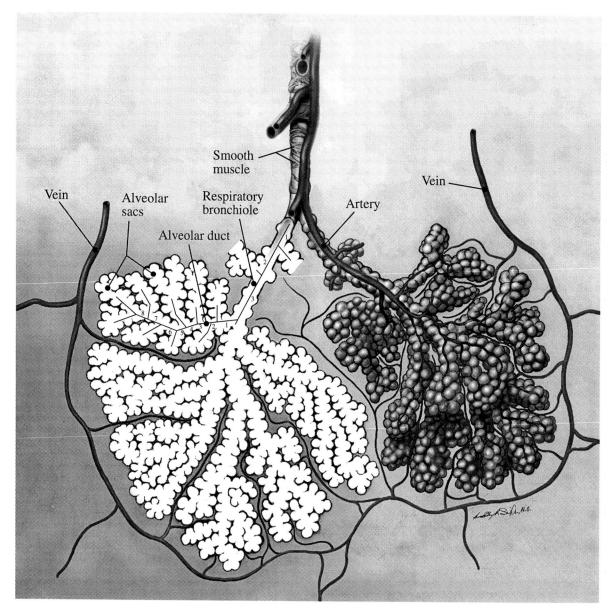

FIG. 9. Vascular supply and branching anatomy of the human acinus. Respiratory bronchioles typically show up to three branch points, whereas alveolar ducts have up to nine branches. Pulmonary arterioles travel with the respiratory bronchioles and alveolar ducts into the center of the acinus. The capillary network radiates outward from the arterioles to form anastomoses with the venous system, for which the major channels lie on the surface of the acinus.

chus with its pulmonary segment has its own vascular supply. Thus, a pulmonary segment can be resected as an anatomically discrete subdivision. Resection of one or more pulmonary segments does not compromise the blood flow to adjacent lung segments.

Acini

All the gas exchange structures distal to a single terminal bronchiole represent an acinus. Thus, an acinus is a parenchymal lung unit in which all structures participate in gas exchange. The human lung fairly consistently has three generations of respiratory bronchioles that are followed by a number of divisions of alveolar ducts. Rats have from three to 13 divisions of alveolar ducts, and the human lung has a similar alveolar ductal architecture, with approximately nine generations of alveolar ducts.

A typical normal human lung contains approximately 30,000 to 40,000 terminal bronchioles and, by definition, the same number of acini. Each acinus is approximately 6 mm in diameter and has a volume of approximately 0.50 mm^3. Acini vary substantially in size and typically contain 10,000 to 12,000 alveoli (Table 1).

TABLE 1. *Structural characteristics of the normal human lung*

Volumes (gas)	
Upper respiratory tract	20 cm³
Airways	
Bronchi	88 cm³
Bronchioles	23 cm³
Alveolar region	5018 cm³
Numbers	
Terminal bronchioles	30–40,000
Acini	30–40,000
Alveoli	500×10^6
Cells (alveolar region)	20×10^9
Epithelial cells	
Upper respiratory tract	560×10^6
Bronchi	7200×10^6
Bronchioles	3300×10^6
Alveolar region	$52,000 \times 10^6$
Surface areas	
Upper respiratory tract	104 cm²
Bronchi	1300 cm²
Bronchioles	1100 cm²
Alveolar epithelium	1,022,000 cm²
Alveolar capillaries	720,000 cm²
One alveolus	121,000 μm²

In older literature, divisions of the lung into primary and secondary lobules is described. The primary lobule refers to all respiratory tissue distal to a final respiratory bronchiole, and thus contains only alveolar ducts and alveolar sacs. Some animal species, such as the rat, have only rudimentary respiratory bronchioles, and in this situation a primary lobule is a useful concept to define aspects of ventilation and gas distribution in specific lung units. In the human, the primary lobule is not a very useful concept, because the acinus divides into multiple respiratory bronchioles and a high degree of collateral ventilation occurs between these subunits. Secondary lobules are lung units delineated by connective tissue septa; they are about 1 cm³ in size. They form structures that are clearly visible on the pleural or cut surface of the lung. The secondary lobule is supplied by a bronchiole with a diameter of about 1 mm that divides into five to 12 terminal bronchioles, and thus into a similar number of acini.

Alveoli

The gas exchange region of the lung is made up of approximately 500,000,000 alveoli having a total surface area of approximately 100 m². These alveoli are highly vascularized, with the alveolar septal capillary bed having a vascular surface area of approximately 70 m². The normal alveolar septa are approximately 10 μm thick. The alveolar air-capillary barrier is made up of variable thin and thick segments. The thin segment is composed of an alveolar epithelium, a fused epithelial and endothelial basement membrane, and a capillary endothelium. Because both type I epithelial cells and capillary endothelial cells are highly attenuated, the combined thickness of this air-blood barrier can be as little as 0.5 μm. The alveolar walls contain connective tissue, primarily collagen, which weaves through the capillary mesh. This and other cellular and acellular components of the interstitium create the thicker portions of the alveolar septal walls. Three-dimensional reconstructions of alveolar septal walls from rats have demonstrated that the alveolar entrance rings are particularly rich in both collagen and elastin. Alveolar mouths form the boundary of alveolar ducts (Fig. 10), and their entrance rings are linked together into a connective tissue structure that spirals down alveolar ducts, providing a connection between the openings or mouths of individual alveoli. Elastic tissue is most prominent along the alveolar duct openings. Collagen strands or fibers interlace across the alveolar walls and connect adjacent alveoli along a single alveolar duct as well as connect alveoli between two adjacent alveolar ducts.

Based on morphologic evidence of collagen and elastin distributions and the effects of surfactant depletion on the structure of alveoli and alveolar ducts, Wilson and Bachofen developed a model of lung micromechanics comparing the contributions of alveoli and alveolar ducts to lung elasticity. This model suggests that elastic components abundant in the walls of alveolar ducts are primarily responsible for the function of alveolar ducts, whereas surface tension effects are primarily responsible for the tension in alveoli. Three-dimensional reconstructions of alveoli and alveolar ducts as transpulmonary pressure is raised from 0 to 30 cm H_2O demonstrate that at low lung volumes alveoli make up 80% of the parenchymal lung volume and dominate the gas volume changes. As pulmonary pressure increases, the contributions to changes in volume by both alveoli and alveolar ducts converge (Fig. 11). This suggests that at high lung volumes connective tissue elements, both between and within the alveolar ducts, come under tension and act to equalize further changes in volume between alveoli and alveolar ducts. This both limits overextension of alveoli and enhances lung stability by distributing stress among all contributing units of an alveolar duct interconnected by elastic and collagenous structures.

The alveolar epithelium is covered primarily by type I and type II epithelial cells. The characteristics of the alveolar septal wall in normal human lung is shown in Fig. 12. Type I epithelial cells are thin squamous epithelial cells having an average surface area of approximately 7000 μm² (Table 2). Their highly attenuated cytoplasm has an average thickness of only 0.36 μm. The alveolar epithelium contains approximately equal numbers of type I and type II cells. The type II cell is cuboidal in shape and is commonly found at junctions of alveolar septa and along the alveolar surfaces surrounding intrapulmonary vascular and airway structures. Alveolar type II epithelial cells have conspicuous mitochondria and an extensive Golgi apparatus, indicating a high synthetic role for these

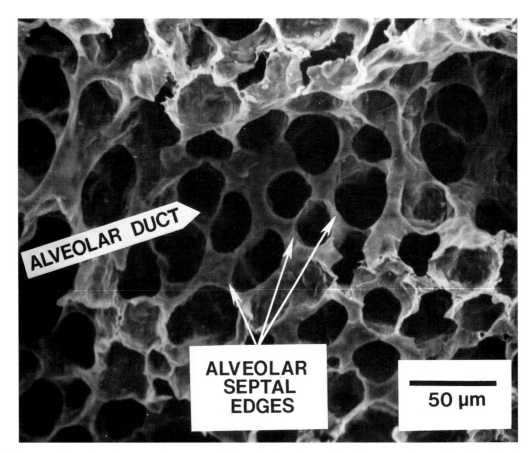

FIG. 10. Scanning electron micrograph of the alveolar duct region from a rat lung. The alveolar duct walls are made up of alveolar mouth openings surrounded by flattened alveolar septal edges forming the entrance rings around the alveolar openings. The primary collagen and elastin network lining the alveolar ducts is under tension in this fully expanded lung.

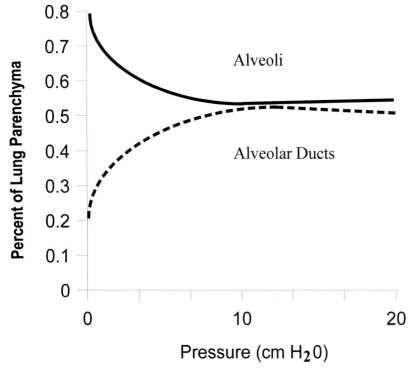

FIG. 11. Volume ratios of alveoli and alveolar ducts as a function of the transpulmonary extending pressure. These pressure-volume relationships were determined using morphometric point-counting procedures to estimate the relative contributions of alveoli and alveolar ducts during lung expansion. At low lung volumes, alveoli make up the majority (80%) of the lung parenchyma. As lung volume increases, alveolar ducts initially show the greatest change in volume, and they increase from 20% to almost 50% of the volume of the lung parenchyma. At about 10 cm of water pressure, the two curves converge, showing that changes in volume of these two compartments are proportionally similar from intermediate to high lung volumes or pressures. The convergence of these two curves at higher pressures suggests that the connective tissue elements within and between the alveolar ducts are under tension and help stabilize the lung by equally distributing further increases in lung volume.

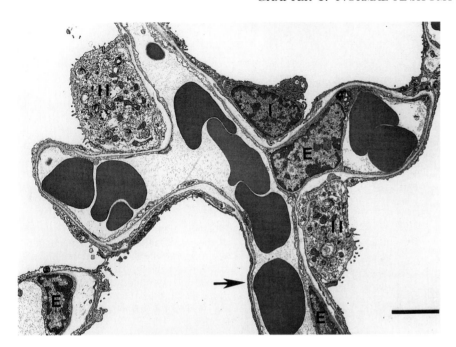

FIG. 12. Transmission electron micrograph showing the alveolar septum from a normal human lung. An efficient exchange of O_2 and CO_2 between inspired air and red blood cells is promoted by the large gas exchange surface with minimal distances (*arrow*) across the epithelial, interstitial, and endothelial components of the alveolar septa. *I*, type I alveolar epithelial cell; *II*, type II alveolar epithelial cell; *c*, capillary endothelial cell. Bar = 1 μm. (Reproduced with permission from Crapo et al. *Am Rev Respir Dis* 1982; 125:740–745.)

cells. They are characterized chiefly by the presence of large numbers of small microvilli on the apical surface (Fig. 13) and of unique secretory granules, known as *lamellar bodies.* Each type II cell contains 100 to 200 lamellar bodies. These are composed of tightly packed whirls of surfactant, which give these bodies their lamellar appearance on cross-section. The continued secretion of lamellar contents replenishes surfactant at the alveolar air-liquid interface. Alveolar type II cells are connected to adjacent type I cells with a relatively impermeable tight junction. These junctions contain three to five junctional strands on electron microscopy of freeze-fracture replicas. Type II cells have four known primary functions: (1) They secrete surfactant. (2) They act as an ion pump, moving fluid from the alveolar spaces into the subjacent interstitial spaces. Type II cells move sodium from the alveolar lumen to the interstitium via an apical sodium channel regulated by cyclic AMP. Water passively follows the sodium movement. (3) They repair alveolar injury. These cells are the progenitor cells for alveolar epithelium and can regenerate alveolar type I epithelium.

(4) They control alveolar inflammation. Type II alveolar epithelial cells secrete antiinflammatory cytokines. They also secrete antioxidants, including the extracellular superoxide dismutase enzyme. Type II cells have been shown to secrete nitric oxide by the activation of nitric oxide synthase. The secretion of both antioxidant enzymes and nitric oxide by type II cells is induced by the proinflammatory cytokines interferon-γ and tumor necrosis factor-α, suggesting a role for these cells in the control of inflammatory functions.

The shape of alveoli *in vivo* approximates a smooth partial circle. Smoothing of the folds on the alveolar surface is accomplished by folding of alveolar septal membranes into the capillaries and by filling of tissue depressions with alveolar lining fluid containing surfactant at its surface. Changes in alveolar size are thought to occur primarily by folding and unfolding of the alveolar pleats, and this process minimizes stress tension on alveolar septal cells.

Stability of alveoli with their small radius of curvature requires a highly surface-active material at the air-liquid interface. La Place's Law describes the relationship of the alveolar pressure (P) required to keep an alveolus open with alveolar surface tension (τ) and radius of curvature (r):

$$P = 2 \tau/r$$

According to this principle, as the radius falls during exhalation, the surface tension must also fall, or the required pressure to maintain open alveoli would rise. As alveolar pressure falls during exhalation, this scenario would result in alveolar collapse with each breath. Surfactant prevents alveolar collapse. As the radius of alveoli decreases, the surfactant phospholipids are packed more

TABLE 2. *Characteristics of alveolar septal cells in normal human lung*

	No. in both lungs	Average cell surface area	Average cell volume
Alveolar epithelial cells			
Type I	19×10^9	6900 μm²	2400 μm³
Type II	32×10^9	250 μm²	800 μm³
Capillary endothelial cells	73×10^9	1000 μm²	600 μm³

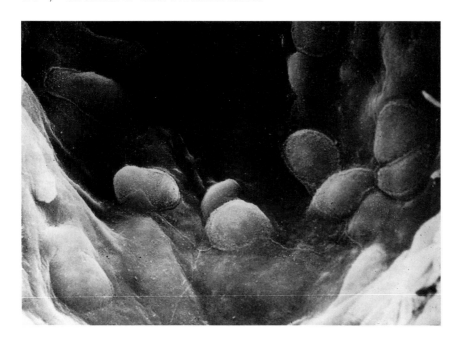

FIG. 13. Scanning electron micrograph of the alveolar septal surface showing several type II alveolar epithelial cells surrounded by type I epithelium. Type II cells are identified by their distinctive microvilli. In this micrograph, the overlying surfactant layer was removed by fixatives.

tightly and surface tension is reduced. Thus, alveolar surface tension and the radius of alveoli *in vivo* fall synchronously, and alveolar stability is maintained.

Surfactant is a complex mixture of lipids and proteins synthesized by alveolar type II epithelial cells. The primary lipids include saturated phosphatidylcholine and phosphatidylglycerol. Surfactant also contains a number of proteins, three of them identified as surfactant proteins A, B, and C. Each of these facilitates the spreading and recycling of surfactant. A fourth surfactant protein, SP-D, is produced and secreted by type II cells but is not known to be a part of surfactant. It is thought to play a role in antibacterial defense.

The proportion of the alveolar septum of the human lung that is interstitium is substantially greater than in many other species, as shown in Fig. 14. The alveolar interstitium increases as a function of age in both rodents and humans. The high amount of interstitium in the human lung likely reflects the substantially longer life span of the human and exposure to environmental air pollutants. The lungs of children have substantially less interstitial connective tissue and interstitial matrix elements than do adult human lungs (Fig. 14.) The alveolar macrophages on the alveolar surfaces in a normal nonsmoking human make up only about 3% of total alveolar cells. The number of alveolar macrophages is substantially elevated in smokers and can be 10% of the alveolar septal cells. The normal human alveolus has a diameter of about 225 μm and a surface area of 120,000 μm^2; it is made up of 148 endothelial cells, 106 interstitial cells, and 107 epithelial cells (types I and II) and contains 12 alveolar macrophages. The comparative cellular anatomy of an average alveolus from the mouse to the human is shown in Fig. 15. The relative cell composition of the alveolar septa is similar across species. The larger alveoli of larger species are generally contain more cells of the same average size rather than larger cells. The differences in cellular size and shape between cells of different function are dramatic, as shown in Table 2, with the alveolar type I epithelial cell being four times larger than a capillary endothelial cell and having a sixfold greater surface area. Thus, cellular function, not species or organ size, determines characteristics of each class of cell.

Pulmonary Circulation

The main pulmonary artery and the next several generations of pulmonary arteries with diameters greater than 0.5 cm are called *elastic arteries.* The walls of these vessels contain multiple concentric elastic lamina as well as smooth muscle and collagen layers. These vessels enter the lung at the hilum and lie adjacent to and branch with each of the bronchi. Arteries with diameters ranging from 0.1 to 0.5 cm are termed *muscular pulmonary arteries.* These vessels contain circular smooth muscle located between an internal and external elastic lamina. Muscular pulmonary arteries begin at the level of smaller bronchi, have the same approximate diameter as the bronchi, and travel and branch with the bronchi. These arteries continue to follow bronchioles and respiratory bronchioles and enter into the center of the acinus, branching with alveolar ducts. Their size decreases as they move peripherally, and by the time they reach the acinus they are substantially smaller than the alveolar ducts.

Pulmonary veins travel in the peripheral walls of acini and along the connective tissue planes of sublobular and lobular septa. Thus, blood enters the acinus alongside the airways and then moves outward across the acinus to the periphery, where pulmonary veins collect blood from

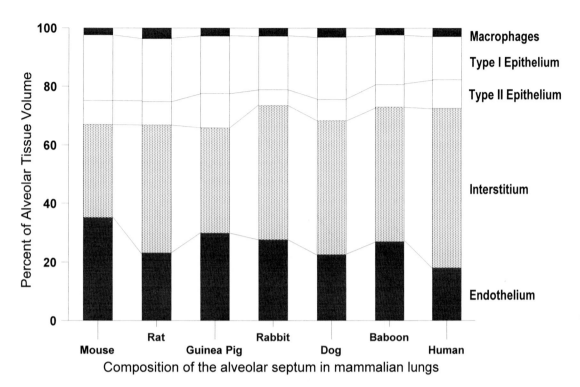

Composition of the alveolar septum in mammalian lungs

FIG. 14. Composition of the tissues of the alveolar region in mammalian lungs. The ratios of endothelium, interstitium, epithelium, and alveolar macrophages are shown. Note that the human lung has proportionally more interstitium than do the other species illustrated. This is likely related to the extensive environmental pollutants to which human lungs are exposed, leading to microscopic fibrotic interstitial reactions.

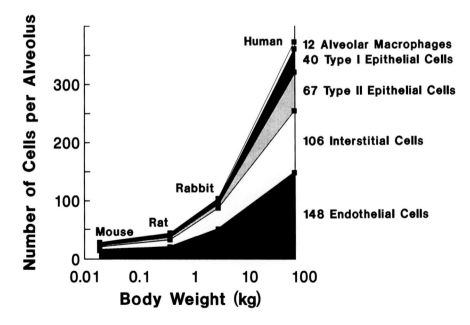

FIG. 15. The cellular makeup of alveoli in mouse, rat, rabbit, and human. Numbers along the right vertical axis correspond to the data for human lungs. The typical human alveolus is made up of almost 400 cells.

multiple adjacent acini. Each vein drains a much larger zone than is supplied by a single small muscular pulmonary artery.

A separate circulation and nutrient supply to the bronchi and the walls of their adjacent pulmonary arteries arises from the systemic circulation via bronchial arteries. These arteries come directly from the aorta or from the internal mammary, subclavian, or intercostal arteries. This systemic arterial supply to the bronchi travels as small vessels in the walls of the bronchi and extends to the level of the bronchioles. Bronchial veins exist only in the most central bronchi and empty into the azygos and hemiazygos veins. The remainder of the bronchial arterial circulation drains into pulmonary veins and moves by that circuit to the left atrium.

The relative surface areas and volumes of different components of the pulmonary vascular bed are given in Table 3. The volume of blood in the lung is normally approximately equally distributed between the arterial system, capillary network, and venous system. Ninety-six percent of the pulmonary vascular surface area is in the capillary bed. The capillary network has the capacity for substantial expansion if all capillary beds are recruited and functional, as under conditions of exercise. When the capillary network is fully recruited, the proportion of the pulmonary blood volume in the capillary bed can increase from 30% to 50%–60%.

The pulmonary vascular system is a low-pressure circulation, and the pulmonary arteries are substantially more distensible than are systemic arteries. Pulmonary veins are also highly distensible at relatively low transmural pressures. Distensibility of the pulmonary vascular bed makes it possible for the blood volume to change readily in response to vasomotor stimuli or hydrostatic/orthostatic conditions. The pulmonary vascular bed acts as a capacitance reservoir for the left side of the heart. Sufficient blood is contained in the elastic reservoir to support two to three heartbeats. Pulmonary blood volume can increase 30% during a change of position from standing to lying. Up to half of the pulmonary blood volume can be forced out of the lungs by Valsalva's maneuver (increasing intrathoracic pressure against a closed glottis).

The vertical height of a normal human lung is about 25 cm, with the hilum situated about one-third the distance from the top of the lungs (Fig. 2). Pulmonary capillary pressure varies from the top to the bottom of the lung. With an average pulmonary arterial pressure of 20 cm H_2O, the pulmonary arterial pressure from the top to the bottom of the lung varies from 12 cm H_2O to 36 cm H_2O. Pulmonary venous pressure varies from approximately 0 at the top of the lung to 24 cm H_2O at the bottom, with a mean pressure of 6 to 8 cm H_2O at the hilum. Thus, with a highly distensible pulmonary vascular bed, pulmonary blood volume is preferentially distributed toward the dependent portions of the lung. The effects of gravity and distensibility are balanced by vasomotor tone regulating blood flow across the pulmonary vascular bed. Because muscular arteries extend into the acinus, local vasomotor control can influence distribution of blood flow to each lung unit and thereby determine the ventilation-perfusion ratio of each of these units.

Blood flow in the pulmonary capillaries is pulsatile except under conditions of severe pulmonary hypertension. Blood flow in the capillary network has been estimated to have a velocity averaging about 1000 μm/sec.

The pulmonary capillary bed is made up of an extensive network of interconnected small tubules. There has been substantial debate regarding whether pulmonary capillary blood flow is best modeled as tubular flow or sheet flow. Anatomically, as illustrated in Fig. 16, the capillary bed is a combination of the two. The capillary network crosses multiple alveoli as blood flows from the central arteriole in an acinus to the venules at the acinar margins. This creates a fairly long path length over which gas exchange can occur. The average transit time of a red cell through the pulmonary capillary bed has been estimated to be 0.1 to 0.5 sec. Under normal resting conditions, red blood cells are fully saturated with oxygen during the first third of their transit through the pulmonary capillary bed. The lung has a sufficient gas exchange reserve that even heavy exercise does not produce arterial desaturation, and in fact increased blood flow throughout the entire capillary bed generally results in an increased arterial partial pressure of oxygen (PaO_2) under conditions of exercise. Red cells are likely to leave the capillary bed not fully saturated with oxygen only when the inspired oxygen tension is low or when disease prevents adequate ventilation of individual gas exchange units. One of the important ventilation-perfusion regulatory pathways in the lung is hypoxic pulmonary vasoconstriction. Relative hypoxemia in small gas exchange units leads to constriction of the corresponding muscular pulmonary arteries, which maintains balanced ventilation-perfusion ratios. The pulmonary venous system also contains smooth muscle and has been shown to be equally sensitive to vasoactive mediators, thus regulating venous pooling in the lung.

The pulmonary capillary bed acts as an efficient filter of the systemic vascular system. Approximately three quarters of the blood volume of the body is contained in the systemic venous system. This blood passes through the pulmonary capillary bed on each circulation, and any microemboli forming in the systemic venous system will

TABLE 3. *Human pulmonary vascular system*

Vessel	Surface area	Volume
Arteries > 500 μm	0.4 m^2	68 cm^3
Arterioles 13–500 μm	1.0 m^2	18 cm^3
Capillaries	70 m^2	60–200 cm^3
Venules 13–500 μm	1.2 m^2	13 cm^3
Veins > 500 μm	0.1 m^2	58 cm^3

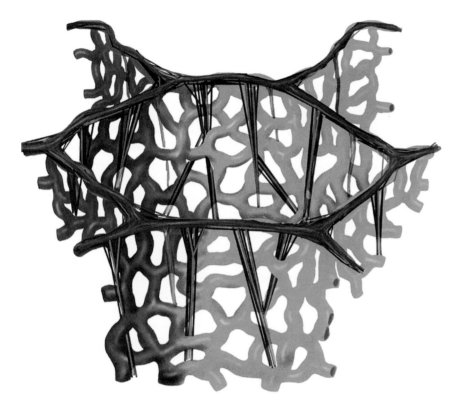

FIG. 16. Schematic illustration of the pulmonary capillary bed showing the high density of short, highly interconnected capillary segments in the alveolar walls. The distribution of collagen and elastin fibers in the lung parenchyma is also shown. The drawing illustrates the high concentrations of connective tissue fibers along the alveolar duct septal edges that form the alveolar duct walls. Elastin fibers tend to be located over the major collagen bundles lining the alveolar entrance rings. Thus, the alveolar entrance rings are rich in both elastin and collagen. The alveolar walls contain thin collagen strands that interconnect adjacent alveoli by weaving between capillary segments.

therefore be filtered by the lung. These microemboli produce no dysfunctional or pathologic effects in the lung and are rapidly cleared by lytic pathways or the pulmonary reticuloendothelial system. The physiologic effects of resection of one lung clearly demonstrate that up to half the pulmonary vascular system can be obstructed or removed without serious change in the hemodynamics of the remaining pulmonary vascular bed. This design of the pulmonary vascular system allows it to be an efficient filter of the body's blood supply.

Capillary endothelial cells form a continuous lining of alveolar capillaries. These cells are connected by tight junctions that, however, are more permeable to macromolecules than are the junctions between airway epithelial cells. Endothelial cell junctions contain one to three junctional strands, in which discontinuities exist. In comparison, airway epithelial cell junctions have three to five junctional strands. In addition, because alveolar type I epithelial cells are substantially larger (Table 2) and cover a much greater surface area per cell than do capillary endothelial cells, the total junctional area over which fluid and macromolecular transport can occur is substantially lower at the alveolar epithelium than it is along the pulmonary capillary endothelium. The impermeability of the alveolar epithelium to fluid and electrolyte movement explains why pulmonary vascular congestion (failure of the left side of the heart) leads to pulmonary interstitial edema substantially sooner than intra-alveolar pulmonary edema occurs.

The pulmonary capillary epithelium has a number of metabolic functions. Because it is the only capillary bed that receives the entire blood flow of the body during each circulation, the pulmonary capillary bed is in a critical position to regulate reactive bloodborne materials. Pulmonary endothelium plays a role in either activating or degrading a number of vasoactive mediators. Some substances are metabolized by enzymes on the capillary endothelial cell surface, whereas others require uptake into the endothelial cells. For example, angiotensin-converting enzyme (ACE) converts angiotensin I to angiotensin II on the surface of pulmonary capillaries, producing a vasoconstrictive molecule of substantially greater physiologic potency. The same enzyme, ACE, inactivates bradykinin. Bradykinin is a highly potent, locally released vasodilator, and its inactivation in the lung prevents it from causing systemic hypotension. Other mediators, such as serotonin and norepinephrine, are metabolized by endothelial cells but require uptake into the cellular cytoplasm. Pulmonary capillary endothelium also synthesizes prostacyclin and tissue plasminogen activator. These cells are a rich source of thrombomodulin, a cell surface protein with anticoagulant properties. The endothelium secretes nitric oxide, a local vasorelaxant, and secretes endothelins, which are potent vasoconstrictor peptides. Vascular endothelium metabolizes adenonucleotides and both prostaglandins E_2 and $F_{2\alpha}$. Vascular endothelium also plays a role in regulating phagocytic cell function via the expression of cell surface adhesion

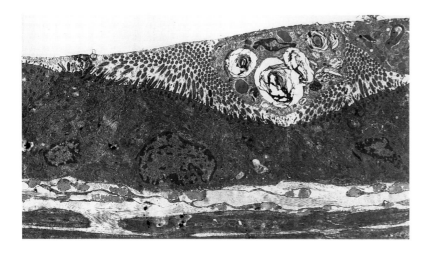

FIG. 17. Electron micrograph of an airway macrophage beneath the electron-dense lining layer of a rat bronchiole.

molecules. The adhesion molecules interact with receptors on phagocytic cells and regulate the movement of phagocytic cells through the vascular bed as well as their migration into subjacent tissues.

Alveolar Macrophages

Alveolar macrophages are the principal means by which the lungs process the normal burden of inhaled particles. Alveolar macrophages are also secretory and regulatory cells and prevent injurious actions of other lung cells. For instance, it has recently been demonstrated that macrophage engulfment of neutrophils significantly contributes to the resolution of pulmonary inflammation. Once phagocytosis of the ingested particle has been accomplished by alveolar macrophages, the cell and/or toxicant is eliminated by internal digestion or mucociliary transport of the macrophage to the oropharynx. In an additional mechanism, particle-laden macrophages have been shown to traverse the interstitial spaces to reach the mediastinal lymph nodes. Figure 17 demonstrates an airway macrophage beneath the electron-dense lining layer of a rat bronchiole. Airway macrophages are approximately five times more numerous per unit of airway surface area than they are per unit of alveolar surface (Table 4). However, because of the large surface area of the alveolar gas exchange region, alveolar macrophages account for approximately 99% of total air space macrophages.

Alveolar macrophages are unique mononuclear phagocytes. These cells contain numerous lysosomes in their cytoplasm, consume oxygen and secrete neutral proteases

at a high rate, and are more active than other tissue macrophages. Although these cells are individually active, they are poor antigen-presenting cells and poor accessory cells. The primary antigen-presenting cell in the lung is a dendritic cell. The primary role of alveolar macrophages is thought to be in defense of alveoli against dust and pathogens. They appear to be able to carry out this role without activating excessive inflammatory processes in the alveolar septa. The vast majority of antigens reaching the small airways and alveolar septa are processed without activation of lymphocyte-based immune recognition and neutrophils. The lung contains very few lymphocytes in alveolar septa.

Alveolar macrophages arise in bone marrow. There is also an interstitial macrophage pool in the lung, and alveolar macrophages proliferate on the alveolar surfaces. Regeneration of the alveolar macrophage population has been shown to occur in all three of these sites.

Mast Cells

Mast cells are a normal, albeit small, component of lung cells. They are identified by the presence of numerous membrane-bound intracytoplasmic granules with variable intragranular inclusions. These granules are 0.6 to 0.8 μm in diameter. The cells also have long filiform microvilli on the surface. Mast cells have high-affinity IgE membrane-bound receptors that are specific for inhaled allergens. On activation, these cells release allergic mediators, such as histamine, prostaglandin D_2 (PGD_2) and leukotriene C_4 (LTC_4). Mast cells also produce neutral proteases (tryptase and chymase), lysosomal enzymes, myeloperoxidase, eosinophil chemotactic factor of anaphylaxis, high-molecular-weight neutrophil chemotactic factor, and heparin. Although the specific role of mast cells is unclear, they clearly play a role in airways secretory and bronchoconstrictor responses of hypersensitivity reactions such as anaphylaxis, hay fever, and asthma. Increased numbers

TABLE 4. *Macrophage distribution and number*

Region	Density on surface (No./cm^2)	Total No. (millions per both lungs)
Airways	25,000 ± 6400	62 ± 8
Alveoli	5861 ± 1860	5990 ± 1900

of mast cells are found in pulmonary edema and pulmonary fibrosis.

Neutrophils

Neutrophils are terminally differentiated cells that are distributed in the bone marrow, blood, and tissue compartments. In the normal lung, neutrophils are almost exclusively found within the circulation, and almost half of the total body circulating neutrophils may be marginated along the walls of pulmonary capillaries and venules. Neutrophils are found in significant numbers in the pulmonary tissue spaces only in cases of pulmonary inflammation, such as in the adult respiratory distress syndrome (ARDS). Migration into tissue spaces occurs in response to chemotactic agents produced by invading microorganisms, toxin-derived products, and complement-activated chemoattractants, such as C5. Following phagocytosis, invading organisms are killed within neutrophils by an oxidant-mediated mechanism, by microbicidal proteins contained in neutrophil granules, or both. In the oxidant-mediated process, a membrane-bound NADPH oxidase generates O_2^-, which can enzymatically or spontaneously dismute to generate H_2O_2. These species react to form hydroxyl radical, another potent oxidant. These agents individually or in combination kill bacteria. Neutrophil granules contain a host of bactericidal agents, including myeloperoxidase, cathepsin G, acid hydrolases, elastase, and lysozyme.

Eosinophils

Eosinophils are not normally present in lung tissue spaces. However, the presence of significant numbers of these cells and their synthesis products has been shown to occur in allergically induced lung inflammation, and they are believed to play a major role in the development of reactive airways disease.

Eosinophils develop in the bone marrow and are transported via the circulation to the tissue spaces of the gastrointestinal and respiratory tracts. The host defense function is less well defined for eosinophils than for neutrophils. Eosinophils may be capable of some bactericidal activity. However, the principal function of these cells is likely their antiparasitic activity. Eosinophils synthesize and secrete potent inflammatory mediators, such as platelet-activating factor and LTC_4.

Innervation of the Lung

Motor neurons in the pulmonary nervous system influence airway tone, pulmonary blood flow, and secretion of mucus. Sensory neurons modulate the cough reflex, the Hering-Breuer reflex, and responses to irritant dusts and gases, and they may respond to interstitial fluid pressure. In addition, a variety of neural peptides released by afferent nerves may modulate airway tone, vascular tone, and airway secretions.

The primary motor and sensory innervation of the lung comes from the vagus nerve (cranial nerve X). In addition, sympathetic fibers arising from the second to the fourth thoracic sympathetic ganglia innervate the lung. Fibers from both the vagus nerve and the thoracic sympathetic plexus comingle as they enter the hilum of the lung and then divide into plexuses that follow bronchi, arteries, and veins. Along the airways, the nerve plexuses lie both internally and externally to the cartilage, with the larger external plexus containing ganglia along the first three bronchial divisions. Nerve fibers continue in airway walls to the level of respiratory bronchioles.

The arterial nerve plexus travels in the media and distally reaches the full extent of muscular arterioles. The venous nerve plexus reaches all the way to the visceral pleura and even supplies subpleural alveolar walls.

In addition, small unmyelinated nerve fibers have been identified in alveolar walls. They are rare, and their source has not been clearly identified. These fibers are thought to represent J (juxtacapillary) receptors, which in animals have been shown to respond to interstitial fluid pressure and certain chemicals. They cause a transitory reflex apnea and shallow rapid respiration.

The primary motor innervation for the lung is parasympathetic (cholinergic). Stimulation of the vagus nerve leads to bronchoconstriction and enhanced secretion of mucus. These actions are blocked by atropine. Parasympathetic nerves arising from the vagus nerve synapse in the ganglia of the first generations of intrapulmonary bronchi. The primary neural inhibitor of bronchial muscular tone is vasoactive intestinal peptide (VIP). This neuropeptide is stored and released by parasympathetic neurons and may coexist with acetylcholine. Thus, the same group of neurons may release acetylcholine, which contracts airway smooth muscle, and VIP, which counteracts the action of acetylcholine to act as a bronchodilator. There are multiple examples of neurotransmitters with opposing actions being released from common nerve elements in the lung; for example, neuropeptide Y, a bronchial and vascular constrictor, coexists in pulmonary adrenergic nerves with norepinephrine. The complex interactions of the parasympathetic, sympathetic, and nonadrenergic, noncholinergic (NANC) nervous systems in the lung and the coexistence of opposing neurotransmitters has made the study of neural control of lung function difficult. It is clear, however, that motor innervation of the airways is predominantly parasympathetic and that there is no significant direct adrenergic innervation of bronchial smooth muscle.

The NANC nerve supply to the lung is thought to regulate primarily mucous secretion and bronchial blood flow. NANC nerves can be either inhibitory or excitatory, and their function is not yet well characterized. The inhibitory functions include relaxation of bronchial smooth muscle, perhaps by the release of nitric oxide or VIP. VIP is a potent relaxant of human bronchi *in vitro* but appears to have little effect on smaller airways. Excitatory responses of the NANC system include bronchoconstriction, possibly mediated by the release of tachykinins, such as substance P. By means of neural stains and electron microscopy, unmyelinated nerve fibers have been shown to pass through the airway epithelial basement membrane and be distributed between columnar bronchial epithelial cells. These fibers contain neuropeptides thought to be released as a reflex response to activation of local irritant receptors. The major neuropeptides identified in the lung are shown in Table 5. In addition, Kultschitsky neuroendocrine cells may play a role in afferent nerve function. These cells have been found to release neuroactive peptides, including serotonin, calcitonin, and bombesin.

Neural control of the pulmonary vascular system has been a substantial area of investigation. Despite this, the role of the nervous system in regulating blood flow in the human lung is not well understood. Nerves arising from both the sympathetic and parasympathetic systems innervate the pulmonary vascular system. In most animals, adrenergic supply of the pulmonary arterial system predominates over cholinergic innervation. Electric stimulation of the nerves of the lung has been shown to cause both vasoconstriction and vasodilation. Pulmonary arterioles are thought to be the primary site for pulmonary vascular resistance. The pulmonary venous system is well innervated and may also play a role in regulating resistance and capacitance of the pulmonary vascular system. Sympathetic stimulation in animals has been shown to cause pulmonary venous constriction.

The sensory system in the lung travels upward through both the vagus nerve and the thoracic sympathetic plexus. Receptors in the main bronchi mediate the cough reflex. Small airways contain irritant receptors that respond to irritant gases, irritant dust, and mechanical stimuli to produce bronchoconstriction, hyperventilation, and chest discomfort. The Hering-Breuer reflex involves mechanoreceptors located in airway walls. These receptors increase their rate of firing under stretch and thus inhibit the central inspiratory center as a progressive reflex response to lung expansion. The nerves mediating this reflex are thought to be located in the smooth muscle of the bronchial walls.

RESPIRATORY TRACT DEFENSE MECHANISMS

For the exchange of gases, conditioning of inspired air, and defense against inhaled toxicants to be accomplished simultaneously, highly synergistic interactions between respiratory tract clearance and secretion and biochemical and cellular defense mechanisms are required. In the normal lung, defense functions are mediated by epithelial cells of the airways and alveolar regions, resident alveolar macrophages, and numerous proteins in the extracellular spaces and mucous lining layers. Resident lung macrophages carry out the normal tasks of lung defense by selective phagocytosis of foreign particles; secretion of proteases, oxygen free radicals, and cytokines; and antigen presentation. In the presence of toxicants or other pathologic conditions, infiltration of bloodborne phagocytes, such as neutrophils, and toxicant-specific immunologic mechanisms, such as antibody production by B lymphocytes and cellular cytotoxic actions by T lymphocytes, augment the normal defense functions. Inflammatory cells recruited into the lungs tend to produce indiscriminate injury to resident lung cells and tissues by nonselective release of proteases, oxygen free radicals, and other cytotoxic agents. The lung appears to be designed to clear normal levels of inhaled pollutants without activating these inflammatory patterns, but it can activate them when more severely stressed.

Deposition of Inhaled Gaseous Toxicants

Because the physical mechanisms of transport and chemical uptake vary significantly between different airborne toxicants, no single approach can be used to estimate the pulmonary uptake of all inhaled agents. For instance, formaldehyde and ozone are both highly reactive gaseous toxicants with an inspiratory uptake of greater than 90%. However, the solubility of formaldehyde in aqueous biologic solutions is approximately 12 times greater than that of ozone. Because of their different solubilities, the critical target sites of injury for formaldehyde and ozone are at opposite ends of the respiratory tract. The major sites of uptake and toxic reactions of formaldehyde are in the nose and other parts of the upper respiratory tract. The uptake of formaldehyde in the upper respiratory tract is so rapid that virtually none of it reaches the lower respiratory tract. In contrast, because of the lower solubility of ozone, more of it reaches the lower respiratory tract. Significant uptake of ozone does occur in the nasal passages and upper respiratory tract; however,

TABLE 5. *Neuropeptides in the human lung*

Neuropeptide	Functions
Vasoactive intestinal peptide	Enhanced secretion
	Bronchorelaxation
Peptide histidine methionine	Bronchorelaxation
	Vasorelaxation
Neurokinin A	Vasorelaxation
Substance P	Enhanced secretion
Calcitonin gene-related peptide	Enhanced secretion
Neuropeptide K	Bronchoconstriction
Neuropeptide Y	Bronchoconstriction
	Vasoconstriction
	Decreased secretion

this uptake is associated with reaction of ozone with components of the thick mucous layer lining this region. The site of greatest injury from inhalation of ozone, and similar oxidant gases, is the alveolar epithelium at the transition between airways and the gas exchange region. In this region, the surface lining fluids are thin, so that the probability of ozone reacting directly with the underlying alveolar epithelial cells is greater. The critical respiratory targets and the toxic responses to all airborne pollutants depend on their inhaled concentrations, the resulting concentration gradient in different regions of the respiratory tract, and the effects of scrubbing and/or detoxification of the reactive gas by the mucous lining layer overlying the epithelial layer in each region.

Deposition of Inhaled Particles

The alveolar septal region is continually bombarded by a variety of organic and inorganic materials ranging from transition metals to animal and human proteins. Although the upper respiratory tract and upper airways filter most inhaled particulate matter, it is well documented that particles of 1 μm in size are not effectively filtered by the upper respiratory tract and that a significant fraction of these particles deposit on the intrapulmonary airways or reach the alveolar region. Normal ambient air can contain on the order of 10,000 respirable particles, defined as less than 10 μm in size with a mass median aerodynamic diameter (MMAD) of 0.3 μm, per cubic centimeter. Up to 30% of these particles deposit on medium and small airways, and about 10% deposit in the alveolar region. Thus, if a minute ventilation of 10 L is assumed, 30 million particles deposit per minute on smaller airways and 10 million particles deposit per minute on alveoli and alveolar ducts. Although the human lung contains 500 million alveoli, the particles tend to deposit proximally, and the load can be estimated to be up to one particle per minute per alveolus in the proximal alveolar ducts. The lung handles this steady, normal load of particulate matter without inducing inflammatory amplification.

These same pollutants would cause a strong inflammatory reaction if injected into another organ, yet they appear to cause virtually no reaction in alveolar septa in normal lungs. This is remarkable when one considers that the alveolar-capillary gas exchange membrane in most regions is thinner than 1 μm. If the organic and inorganic materials reaching the airways and alveolar surface were to stimulate the type of inflammatory reactions that occur in many other tissues, white cells would be rapidly recruited into these spaces and a progressive inflammation would result, leading to acute bronchitis, acute alveolitis, and/or interstitial fibrosis. The absence of an injurious response to normal lung particle burdens appears to be the result, in part, of the unique role of resident lung defense cells, such as alveolar macrophages. Each alveolus contains an average of 12 macrophages, which are thought to process all particles reaching this region under normal conditions. Alveolar macrophages have been shown to have a blunted capacity for antigen presentation and mitogen production compared with other monocytic phagocytes, and thus they are able to process inhaled particles without stimulating excessive immunologic responses or lung inflammation. The lipids and/or proteins of the alveolar surface lining layer have been shown to have anti-inflammatory actions. High particle loads given experimentally have been shown to overload these and other anti-inflammatory defense mechanisms and induce alveolar inflammation. The dose-response relationship for the onset of particle-induced inflammation is not known, nor are the mechanisms controlling this process.

Pulmonary disorders in which particle deposition and/or clearance plays a major role include hypersensitivity pneumonitis, silicosis, asbestosis and other mineral fiber disorders, and a number of metal- and organic antigen-specific disorders. In most of these cases, the biologic association between toxicant dose and health effects has been clearly demonstrated.

Epidemiologic studies demonstrate a significant association between particulate exposure and increases in hospital admissions, morbidity, and mortality. Children, whose small airways are potentially more susceptible to particle-induced inflammation and limitations of air flow, are thought to be at high risk. Airborne particulate levels as low as 150 μg/m^3 are statistically associated with increases in elementary school absenteeism. The association between particle concentration and increased mortality appears to be maximal when the experimental results are averaged over a 3- to 5-day period. Such studies have been the primary means of identifying human health risks associated with particle inhalation. These studies taken as a whole suggest that ambient levels of particles on the order of 100 μg/m^3 are associated with adverse health effects. Each increase of 10 μg/m^3 in the PM$_{10}$ (particulate matter with an aerodynamic diameter of 10 μm) is associated with an approximate 1% increase in mortality. The increased mortality appears to occur largely among the sick and elderly. The underlying biologic mechanisms responsible for these epidemiologic associations have not been determined. Interactions between particles and other pollutants, such as sulfur dioxide and nitrogen dioxide, and the effects of climate have been suggested as critical factors. High levels of trace metals in the particulate matter from urban and industrial sources have been suggested as possible causative agents. Table 6 illustrates the significant differences that exist in trace element composition between air sampled at a remote natural site and in various North American cities. In cities with a large number of anthropogenic sources, the potentially toxic trace elements of nickel, copper, and zinc are present at substantial levels. Particle samples from natural sites that are not

TABLE 6. *Comparison of ambient dust concentrations*

Trace element	Grand Canyon, Arizona	Houston, Texas	Washington, D.C.	Ottawa, Canada
Nickel, ng/m^3	0.1	5.0	1.0	4.4
Copper, ng/m^3	0.3	16.0	3.4	73.0
Zinc, ng/m^3	0.6	102.0	13.9	114.0
Selenium, ng/m^3	0.2	0.2	2.5	0.3
Arsenic, ng/m^3	0.2	0.1	0.6	0.5
Total mass PM$_{10}$	9400.0	29,000.0	34,900.0	44,500.0

PM$_{10}$, particulate matter <10 μm in aerodynamic diameter (ng/m^3).

contaminated by anthropogenic sources do not contain significant levels of these elements.

Deposition of inhaled particles occurs according to physical mechanisms of inertial impaction, gravitational sedimentation, diffusion, and interception. A variety of factors, such as aerosol particle size, density, shape, hygroscopic/hydrophobic character, and electrostatic charge, may also play important roles in determining how these mechanisms control the location and efficiency of deposition in the lungs. Because particles are present in a range of sizes and shapes, an aerosol is typically described by a size distribution or a mass/count weighted mean. In toxicologic evaluations, the Mass Median Aerodynamic Diameter (MMAD) is typically used to describe an aerosol in terms of the aerodynamic behavior of its particles, site(s) of particle deposition, and deposited mass. Particles in the size range of 1 to 10 μm deposit with relatively high efficiency in the upper respiratory tract and large airways, where inertial deposition is driven by high flow rates. Particles in the size range of 0.01 to 0.1 μm deposit by diffusion and are primarily taken up in the alveolar regions, where the large surface area enhances deposition by diffusion and sedimentation. The small airways do not have a single dominant mechanism of deposition.

Both empiric and mathematical approaches have been used to assess the dosimetry of inhaled particles. Direct measurements of deposition demonstrate that the human upper respiratory tract efficiently removes particles with an Mass Median Aerodynamic Diameter (MMAD) of approximately 5 μm. For particles in the 1- to 5-μm range, the total respiratory tract (upper respiratory tract plus conducting airways plus gas exchange region) deposition efficiency is on the order of 20%. Mathematically based estimates of the alveolar deposition efficiency of inhaled 1- and 5-μm aerosol particles are 5.2% and 17%, respectively.

Because of the nature of the mechanisms of deposition, deposited particles are not uniformly distributed on respiratory tract surfaces. Aerosols have been shown to deposit preferentially on the ridges of airway bifurcations, both in theoretical models and in direct observation of aerosol behavior using airways casts. Experimental observations of ciliary activity and mucous flow suggest that the concentration of particles on the ridges of airway bifurcations could, in part, result from trapping of particles on these ridges as they are cleared from more distal airways. Particles on airway ridges or branch points are cleared with a half-life of approximately 1 hour.

Particles deposited in the airways are rapidly cleared by the mucociliary escalator and by airway macrophages. Within 24 hours, most particles with a diameter of 1 μm are cleared from the airways. Particles initially deposited in the alveolar region are primarily cleared by macrophage phagocytosis. Clearance from the alveolar region is considerably slower than clearance from the airways, and removal of insoluble particles may require weeks to months.

Immunologic Responses

Immunologic responses can be classified as nonspecific or innate immune responses (actions of macrophages, monocytes, lymphocytes, and granulocytes) or agent-specific immune responses (immunologic memory of T and B cells). The innate defense mechanisms include a combination of phagocytosis and cytotoxic effects by effector cells and activation of the complement cascade. In the adaptive response, a large population of antigen-specific lymphocytes is produced that results in a potentially greater and prolonged immune system response. The adaptive response occurs when an antigen derived from the toxicant exposure is processed and presented by a dendritic cell, macrophage, or monocyte to a lymphocyte. The lymphocyte then undergoes clonal expansion to produce large numbers of cells that are specific for the particular toxic agent. Cytotoxic T-cell production occurs by this process when major histocompatibility (MHC) is expressed by the antigen-presenting cells in association with toxicant-derived antigen. Activated T cells produce numerous cytokines, such as tumor necrosis factor, that significantly enhances the immune response and the inflammatory responses of resident lung cells. Antibodies specific to the antigen are produced by B cells, which are stimulated by the interleukins to produce memory cells and plasma cells.

The effects of inhaled particles on human health are likely to involve inflammation, hypersensitization, and immunologic memory of T and B cells. These mechanisms are capable of amplifying injury initiated by repeated, low-dose exposures to antigens and therefore have the potential to produce significant effects at ambient levels of exposure. The pulmonary immune system differs from the systemic immune system in its ability to produce localized cell-mediated immune responses on repeated exposure to inhaled antigenic materials. Such localized response may play a significant role in hypersensitivity pneumonitis. Particles that contain metals have been shown to produce these responses. For instance, nickel and other transition metals are highly toxic and known to produce delayed hypersensitivity. Recent studies indicate that T-cell recognition of metal-complexed haptens plays a role in T-lymphocyte immune responses.

The airway epithelium and the alveolar epithelium are the primary lung surfaces on which inhaled toxicants may be initially distributed and/or react. The airway epithelium is a likely critical target site for an inhaled toxicant, as it is the first cellular barrier to inhaled toxicants and the most densely populated of the target surfaces. These aspects are offset to a large extent by the protection afforded by the thick mucous layer overlying airway epithelial cells and the efficient ciliary propulsion system. The alveolar epithelium of the gas exchange region has a large surface with a relatively low density of cells covered by a thin surface film. The thin surface film of the alveolar epithelial layer constitutes a critical site of possible action for pollutants not filtered by proximal airways. The outermost region of the respiratory path is the pleura, and this site is typically involved in toxic processes only after secondary transport following initial uptake of the reactive substance in more proximal air spaces. At each level, the presence or absence of adverse effects of inhaled particles and reactive gases is primarily determined by the unique immune response system in the lung.

BIBLIOGRAPHY

Ansfield M, Benson B. Identification of the immunosuppressive components of canine pulmonary surface active material. *J Immunol* 1980; 125:1093–1098. *This study was one of the first to demonstrate the immunosuppressive nature of surfactant.*

Barry BE, Crapo JD. Patterns of accumulation of platelets and neutrophils in rat lungs during exposure to 100% and 85% oxygen. *Am Rev Respir Dis* 1985;132:548–555. *This study demonstrates that platelet and neutrophil accumulation play a significant role in the differentiation of response between lethal and adaptive oxygen exposure.*

Boyden EA. *Segmental Anatomy of the Lungs: A Study of the Patterns of the Segmental Bronchi and Related Pulmonary Vessels.* New York: McGraw-Hill; 1955. *The classic description of the many variations in segmental anatomy in the human lung.*

Butcher EC. Leukocyte-endothelial cell recognition: three (or more) steps to specificity and diversity. *Cell* 1991;67:1033–1036. *Review describing the sequential steps of leukocyte recruitment.*

Cox G, Crossley J, Xing Z. Macrophage engulfment of apoptotic neutrophils contributes to the resolution of acute pulmonary inflammation in vivo. *Am J Respir Cell Mol Biol* 1995;12:232–237. *Study demonstrating that macrophages play a key role in limiting lung toxicity from neutrophil recruitment.*

Crapo JD, Barry BE, Gehr P, Bachofen M, Weibel ER. Cell number and cell characteristics of the normal human lung. *Am Rev Respir Dis* 1982;126:332–337. *This study reports the number and types of cells in each component of the alveolar septum and defines the structural characteristics of each cell type.*

Ettensohn D, Roberts N. Human alveolar macrophage support of lymphocyte responses to mitogens and antigens. *Am Rev Respir Dis* 1983;

18:516–522. *Description of the role that pulmonary macrophages play in mitogen and antigen processing.*

Harmsen AG, Muggenburg BA, Snipes MB, Bice DE. The role of macrophages in particle translocation from lungs to lymph nodes. *Science* 1985;230:1277–1280. *Study using novel techniques to demonstrate the lymph node-mediated clearance of particles by macrophages.*

Hasleton PS. *Spencers Pathology of the Lung.* 5th ed. New York: McGraw-Hill; 1996. *A comprehensive pulmonary pathology textbook with excellent chapters on lung anatomy.*

Horsfield K, Cumming G. Morphology of the bronchial tree in man. *J Appl Physiol* 1968;24:373–383. *The classic study in which latex airway casts were measured to determine the sizes and branching characteristics of the entire bronchial tree.*

Mercer RR, Crapo JD. Three-dimensional reconstruction of the rat acinus. *J Appl Physiol* 1987;63:785–794. *The three-dimensional relationships of airway, vascular, and alveolar structures are defined, including the branching pattern of alveolar ducts.*

Mercer RR, Crapo JD. Spatial distribution of collagen and elastin fibers in the lungs. *J Appl Physiol* 1990;69:756–765. *This study defines the unique locations and spatial relationships of collagen and elastin in the lungs and their functions in lung structure and physiology.*

Mercer RR, Russell ML, Roggli VL, Crapo JD. Cell number and distribution in human and rat airways. *Am J Respir Cell Mol Biol* 1994; 10:613–624. *Airway epithelial cells are quantified in terms of both distribution along the airways and individual cell structures.*

Meyrick B, Sturgess J, Reid L. A reconstruction of the duct system and secretory tubules of the human bronchial submucosal glands. *Thorax* 1969;24:729–736. *A thorough anatomic description of the mucous secretory system in the human airways.*

Morrow PE. Dust overloading of the lungs: update and appraisal. *Toxicol Appl Pharmacol* 1992;113:1–13. *Appraisal of the significance of lung burden in evaluation and/or production of toxicity.*

Pump KK. Morphology of the acinus of the human lung. *Dis Chest* 1969;56:126–134. *A classic study of the structure and function of the human acinus.*

Richardson JB. Nerve supply to the lungs. *Am Rev Respir Dis* 1979;119: 785–802. *Excellent description of the efferent and afferent pulmonary nervous systems.*

Schlesinger RB. Comparative deposition of inhaled aerosols in experimental animals and humans: a review. *J Toxicol Environ Health* 1985; 15:197–214. *In-depth comparision of deposition patterns based on collection of data from a number of sources.*

Schürch S, Gehr P, Im Hof V, Geiser J, Green F. Surfactant displaces particles toward the epithelium in airways and alveoli. *Respir Physiol* 1990;80:17–32. *One of the first studies to demonstrate that the mucous lining layer of the airways has surfactant-like surface tension-lowering properties.*

Sibille Y, Reynolds HY. Macrophages and polymorphonuclear neutrophils in lung defenses and injury. *Am Rev Respir Dis* 1990;141:471–501. *Review of the unique functions of lung phagocytic cells.*

Stone KC, Mercer RR, Gehr P, Stockstill B, Crapo JD. Allometric relationships of cell numbers and size in the mammalian lung. *Am J Respir Cell Mol Biol* 1992;6:235–243. *Characteristics of cell size and structure across species show remarkable similarity from small to large lungs.*

Thurlbeck WM, Churg AM, eds. *Pathology of the Lung.* 2nd ed. New York: Thieme Medical Publishers; 1995. *An excellent, comprehensive text including detailed chapters on lung anatomy and development.*

Weibel ER. *Morphometry of the Human Lung.* New York: Academic; 1963. *The classic monograph on lung structure, from airway structure and branching to the alveolus.*

Weibel ER, Knight B. A morphometric study on the thickness of the pulmonary air-blood barrier. *J Cell Biol* 1967;21:367. *A classic study, fully characterizing the air-blood tissue barrier in the lung and the structural elements that facilitate gas exchange.*

Wilson TA, Bachofen H. A model for mechanical structure of the alveolar duct. *J Appl Physiol* 1992;52:1064–1070. *An excellent model based on biochemical and structural analysis defining the interrelated compliance of alveoli and alveolar ducts and their gas distribution during normal ventilation.*

Yeh HC, Phalen RF, Raabe OG. Factors influencing the deposition of inhaled particles. *Environ Health Perspect* 1976;15:147–156. *Introductory review of the critical factors determining particle deposition in the lungs.*

Textbook of Pulmonary Diseases, 6th ed.
edited by G.L. Baum, J.D. Crapo, B.R. Celli, and J.B. Karlinsky,
Lippincott–Raven Publishers, Philadelphia, © 1998.

CHAPTER

2

Control of Ventilation

Steven G. Kelsen

INTRODUCTION

The respiratory system, along with cardiovascular structures, operates as part of an intricate organization controlled by the central nervous system (CNS) to ensure optimal cell performance, providing sufficient oxygen to meet metabolic requirements and removing enough carbon dioxide so that cell function is not impaired by excessive changes in hydrogen ion concentration. The major function of the respiratory system is to maintain the arterial tension of oxygen (PaO_2) and carbon dioxide ($PaCO_2$) within acceptable limits in the face of changing metabolic needs and environmental conditions. To achieve this, the system is equipped with multiple sensors that monitor changes in blood chemistry (chemoreceptors) and changes in the mechanical properties of the lung and chest wall (mechanoreceptors). The chemoreceptors and mechanoreceptors allow ventilation to be continuously readjusted in accordance with metabolic needs, despite changes in body posture that alter the mechanical advantage or movement of the respiratory muscles. In addition, these receptors coordinate the contraction and relaxation of the respiratory muscles, so that adequate gas exchange is carried out with minimum expenditure of energy.

In addition, the respiratory chemoreceptors and mechanoreceptors participate in a protective network that adjusts the pattern of breathing and the mechanical conditions of the airways to minimize the deleterious effects on the lung of inhaled, noxious material.

Ventilation, unlike blood pressure and cardiac output, can be controlled consciously (voluntarily) as well as automatically (involuntarily). Indeed, the pathways for voluntary and automatic control of the respiratory muscles are anatomically separate. Voluntary as well as automatic control is essential for using the respiratory muscles in speech. In humans, afferent information continuously fed back to the CNS by mechanoreceptors in the airways, lungs, and chest wall allows the force of contraction of the respiratory muscles to be coordinated smoothly in volitional acts.

Besides inputs from respiratory system sensors, ventilation is influenced by projections from the vasomotor neurons to respiratory neurons and by signals received from thermoreceptors and vascular receptors. The multiplicity of inputs to the respiratory neurons ensures that ventilation is maintained when disease affects one or more afferent pathways or when the perception of some sensory cue is blunted by a depressed state of consciousness (e.g., sleep or anesthesia). However, conflicting demands and signals from different receptors may be responsible for dyspnea, a common symptom in respiratory disease.

CENTRAL RESPIRATORY NEURONS

The precise organization of the central respiratory neurons is still a matter of contention. Although there may be respiratory pacemaker cells in which spontaneous changes in transmembrane potential occur, in the intact system, the respiratory rhythm depends on interconnections between different respiratory neurons.

Because breathing is preserved in anesthetized animals even after removal of the brain rostral to the pons, it is believed that the neurons on which respiratory rhythm

---

S. G. Kelsen: Division of Pulmonary Medicine, Temple University Hospital, Philadelphia, Pennsylvania 19140.

critically depends are located in the bulbopontine region. Many investigators believe that the essential features of the respiratory rhythm remain even after separation of the pons from the medulla, and that the central pattern generator must be anatomically located within the confines of the medulla. There is evidence, however, that pontine neurons, particularly the complex composed of the nucleus parabrachialis medialis (NPBM) and the Kölliker-Fuse nucleus (KFN), as well as nuclei in the tegmentum (magnocellular and gigantocellular nuclei), significantly modify breathing.

In addition to these pontine and medullary respiratory neuronal aggregates, neurons with activity that is modulated by respiration can be found all through the brain stem intermixed with nonrespiratory neurons. It also has been shown that when breathing is stimulated, respiratory modulation of the activity of these neurons decreases according to level of anesthesia and sleep state.

A number of neurons whose firing patterns demonstrate a respiratory modulation but whose phase relationships with phrenic motor activity and with one another differ have been identified in the brain stem. Some of these neurons project to the spinal cord (bulbospinal) and are therefore true premotor cells. The remainder have axons that project to other parts of the brain (propriobulbar). Only the function of the bulbospinal neurons has been determined with any degree of certainty. It is generally believed, however, that the propriobulbar cells actively inhibit or excite other neurons involved in the respiratory cycle. The precise function of these propriobulbar neurons remains under investigation, although it is generally agreed that they are organized into networks whose complicated interactions determine the level of excitation of the bulbospinal neurons and produce respiratory phase switching.

MEDULLARY RESPIRATORY NEURONS

The respiratory neurons in the medulla seem to be aggregated into two groups (Fig. 1). One collection, the ventral respiratory group (VRG), forms a longitudinal column of neurons in the ventrolateral part of the medulla. It extends rostrally from the upper border of the spinal cord almost to the bulbopontine boundary. The other group, the dorsal respiratory group (DRG), is more circumscribed anatomically. It is located in a more medial and dorsal part of the medulla in the region of the ventrolateral nucleus of the tractus solitarius (NTS) and extends from the obex about 2.5 mm rostrally.

The nuclei of the solitary tract appear to function as relay stations for important respiratory and cardiovascular information. Afferents from pulmonary stretch receptors and carotid chemoreceptors and baroreceptors appear to synapse for the first time in the brain at this location.

Dorsal Respiratory Group

The DRG contains almost entirely inspiratory neurons. One kind of inspiratory neuron, the I_a neuron, like the phrenic motor neurons, demonstrates an augmenting pattern of firing that peaks at end-inspiration. Axons from these cells decussate in the medulla at or immediately rostral to the obex and connect with phrenic and inspiratory intercostal motor neurons in the spinal cord. Collaterals are sent to the ipsilateral inspiratory neurons in the VRG, but a few also are distributed to the expiratory neurons in the VRG.

The firing of I_b neurons, as of I_a neurons, occurs primarily in inspiration but, in contrast to the discharge of I_a neurons, is augmented by inputs from pulmonary stretch receptors. In animals, the discharge peak of I_b is not as sharp and the decline in activity during expiration is slower than for I_a. In the absence of excitatory input from vagal stretch receptors, however, the discharge patterns of I_a and I_b neurons are similar.

Like I_a neurons, some of the I_b neurons project to the spinal cord. Those I_b neurons that do not project to the cord appear to undergo extensive axonal arborization in

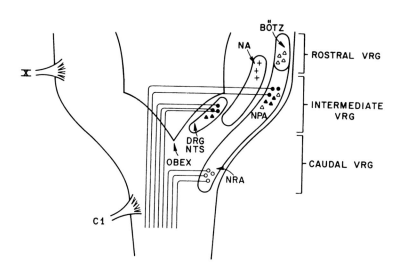

FIG. 1. Schematic depicting the organization of medullary respiratory neurons in the dorsal and ventral respiratory groups (DRG and VRG, respectively). Structures on one side only are shown. Axons from inspiratory bulbospinal neurons in the nucleus tractus solitarius (NTS) and the nucleus para-ambigualis (NPA) decussate rostral to the obex and extens caudally in the contralateral cord. Axons from expiratory bulbospinal neurons in the nucleus retroambigualis (NRA) decussate caudal to the obex. Bötz = Bötzinger complex in the nucleus retrofacialis; NA = nucleus ambigualis.

the NTS. I_b neurons seem to be responsible for the shortening of inspiratory time induced by lung inflation. Their responsiveness to stretch-receptor input is less during expiration than during inspiration.

The DRG also contains late-onset inspiratory neurons that reach their peak firing rate in the transition from inspiration to expiration. Their activity, like that of I_b neurons, is facilitated by stretch-receptor activity. These neurons may participate in the short phase of graded inhibition of inspiratory activity seen with volume changes occurring toward the terminal portion of inspiration.

Recently, a small number of early-expiratory neurons have been observed in the DRG (and possibly also in the VRG) intermingled with inspiratory cells. They begin their firing shortly before the end of inspiration and reach peak discharge rates quickly, and then their activity slowly diminishes during expiration, disappearing before inspiration begins. Increases in lung volume slow the rate of decline in activity of these cells, whereas prevention of lung inflation does the opposite. The activity of these neurons is related to postinspiration inspiratory activity (PIIA), which occurs in the diaphragm and intercostal and laryngeal muscles and retards expiratory flow and the rate of lung deflation.

Ventral Respiratory Group

The VRG in the medulla comprises several anatomically and probably functionally distinct populations (Fig. 1). One classification divides the neurons of the VRG into three aggregates: the nucleus retroambigualis (NRA), the nucleus para-ambigualis (NPA), and the nucleus retrofacialis (NRF).

The nucleus ambigualis (NA) is composed primarily of subnuclei of motor neurons innervating the laryngeal, pharyngeal, and facial muscles. This nucleus also contains the vagal motor neurons innervating the bronchial smooth muscles and the smooth muscles of the thoracic and abdominal viscera. These neurons are almost completely inactive during deep anesthesia, suggesting that they are not essential to respiratory rhythmogenesis.

The NPA is located in the region medial to the NA and 1 mm caudal to 3.5 mm rostral to the obex. The NPA is composed primarily of premotor inspiratory neurons, but some expiratory cells are present.

Most of the inspiratory neurons of the NPA (like I_a cells in the DRG) fire in a ramplike fashion, with peak activity occurring at the conclusion of the inspiratory phase. The NPA also contains a few inspiratory propriobulbar, so-called early-burst neurons. These cells begin to discharge slightly before the onset of the phrenic discharge, peak rapidly, and then demonstrate a decline and disappearance of activity in the latter half of inspiration. They send no projections to spinal motor neurons, but they have a rich pattern of arborization with expiratory neurons in the contralateral NRA, whose activity they appear to inhibit.

The activity of other neurons in the VRG (located in the NRA and NRF) is mainly directed to expiration. The expiratory neurons in the NRA demonstrate a slowly augmenting pattern of activity, with peak discharge late in expiration. Input from pulmonary stretch receptors prolongs the time of firing of these neurons. Hypercapnia causes these neurons to discharge earlier in inspiration and increases the steepness with which their rate of discharge rises. Lesioning experiments indicate that neurons in the NRA are the sole source of expiratory premotor neurons but are not of fundamental importance in generating the respiratory rhythm.

Respiratory neurons in the NRF (also called the *Bötzinger complex*) and in an area immediately rostral to it, called the *pre-Bötzinger complex,* have been described. Bötzinger neurons discharge mainly in expiration with a slowly augmenting firing pattern that peaks at end-expiration. They send projections to the DRG on the opposite side and seem to inhibit the inspiratory neurons located there. On the other hand, pre-Bötzinger neurons fire during inspiration, demonstrate pacemaker-like activity, and appear to be exclusively propriobulbar in type. In the neonatal rat, lesions in this pre-Bötzinger complex eliminate respiratory rhythmogenesis. Some pharyngeal motor neurons also can be found in the NRF.

Interrelationship Between Dorsal and Ventral Respiratory Groups

The precise interactions between the DRG and VRG remain unclear. Earlier studies indicated that inspiratory neurons of the DRG projected to the VRG, but a reciprocal connection was not apparent. These studies suggested that the central pattern generator was composed only of inspiratory cells and was located in the DRG. In this view, the DRG was the prime mover in the genesis of the respiratory rhythm, dominating the cells in the VRG and governing their activity. More recent studies indicate that cells from the VRG (Bötzinger complex) may inhibit inspiratory neurons in the DRG. Ablation experiments eliminating either the entire DRG or the Bötzinger complex in the VRG do not eliminate rhythmogenesis, indicating that substantial redundancy is present in the system.

The functional significance of the interconnections between groups of inspiratory cells in the DRG and VRG is also unclear. These interconnections may serve to synchronize the timing of neuronal firing in anatomically separate locations. For example, midline incisions through the medulla are associated with asynchronous firing of the two phrenic nerves.

TIMING OF RESPIRATORY MOTOR ACTIVITY

During inspiration, firing rates increase monotonically in both inspiratory propriobulbar and bulbospinal neurons. Early in expiration, inspiratory propriobulbar neurons are silenced, but the activity of inspiratory bulbospinal neurons stops only momentarily, reappearing after a brief period of silence and then gradually declining as expiration proceeds. This PIIA corresponds in time to the period of firing of early-expiratory neurons in the DRG and VRG. Expiratory bulbospinal neurons are silent during this early phase of expiration, whereas inspiratory propriobulbar neurons are actively inhibited. Furthermore, because the time course of inhibition of the respiratory propriobulbar neurons is similar to the time course of activity of the early-expiratory units, it has been suggested that the respiratory rhythm is caused by inhibition of an inspiratory ramp generator by these early-expiratory neurons.

Based on these observations, it has been proposed that expiration be divided into two phases, E_I and E_{II}. The E_I phase corresponds to the period of PIIA, whereas the E_{II} phase corresponds to the period in which PIIA is absent and expiratory neuronal activity may be present. In some situations, PIIA may extend throughout expiration, suggesting that the respiratory rhythm does not depend on the occurrence of activity in expiratory neurons.

PIIA appears to be associated with "braking" of expiratory air flow by contraction of the inspiratory muscles. Increases in PIIA and prolongations in E_I occur, for example, when the larynx is bypassed so as to decrease upper airway resistance. PIIA (E_I) is markedly reduced or eliminated by vagotomy, suggesting that mechanoreceptors that sense lung volume and/or tracheal air flow are important inputs. Hypercapnia decreases the duration of E_I, whereas hypoxia appears to do the reverse. Increases in PIIA may contribute to the increase in functional residual capacity (FRC) observed during hypoxia.

Respiratory timing can be significantly affected by the rostral pontine pneumotaxic center, which comprises the NPBM and KFN. This structure contains a number of neurons that have different patterns of firing: inspiratory, expiratory, or phase-spanning. When the vagi are intact, discharge patterns in the NPBM are mainly tonic, but they become more clearly phasic after vagotomy. Both the VRG and the DRG send projections to the pneumotaxic center, so that the respiratory activity seen in this center appears to be of medullary origin. Depending on the region involved, stimulation of the pneumotaxic center can either terminate or prolong inspiration. Stimulation of the dorsolateral region terminates inspiration. The earlier in inspiration the stimulation is applied, the stronger is the stimulus needed. If the pneumotaxic center is lesioned and the vagi are cut, an apneustic breathing pattern develops in anesthetized animals that is characterized by prolonged inspiratory time. If time is allowed for recovery, however, and the animal regains consciousness, breathing loses its apneustic quality. If the animal is then given anesthesia or allowed to go to sleep, the apneustic pattern returns. These observations suggest the lack of importance of the pneumotaxic center in generating the respiratory pattern, and indicate that an interaction between states of alertness and the activity of higher brain centers and the brain stem bulbopontine respiratory neurons can significantly affect respiratory rhythm.

It is not clear whether some or any of the different respiratory neurons described in fact make up the central pattern generator. Three different ways in which the central respiratory pattern may be produced in the brain have been proposed. In one, the pattern generator is composed only of inspiratory neurons; an inspiratory ramp continues until it is terminated by the activity of off-switch neurons. The off-switch neurons are triggered after some predetermined time or after the inspiratory ramp reaches some threshold level of activity. Both trigger and ramp neurons could be stimulated by hypoxia and hypercapnia. In this scheme, inspiration is a self-terminating process carried out by cells whose activity is confined to inspiration.

In a second hypothesis, the central pattern generator may include both inspiratory and expiratory cells affected by chemical drives causing tonic increases in the activity of each. The increasing ramplike discharge seen in inspiratory intercostal and phrenic nerves may result from a gradual decline in inhibition rather than a gradual increase in excitation. This hypothesis is based on the observation that during apnea induced by hypocapnia, decreases in PO_2 elicit inspiratory tonic activity. Progressive decreases in PO_2 during apnea elicit progressive increases in tonic inspiratory activity until at a critical level of hypoxia the respiratory rhythm reappears. On the other hand, hypocapnia under hyperoxic conditions produces continuous firing of expiratory neurons, which increases as PCO_2 rises until rhythmic breathing resumes. This suggests hypoxia exerts an excitatory effect predominantly on inspiratory activity, and that hypercapnia affects expiratory motor activity.

The third idea is that respiratory rhythmogenesis arises in the antagonistic activity of inspiratory and early-expiratory neurons and does not depend on the activity of conventional expiratory neurons that peaks late in the expiratory phase.

PATTERN OF MOTOR OUTFLOW TO THE INSPIRATORY MUSCLES

The firing of the bulbospinal inspiratory neurons projecting to the diaphragm and intercostal muscles increases progressively throughout inspiration and is terminated abruptly (off-switching). The ramplike increase in activity of these bulbospinal neurons (the central inspiratory activ-

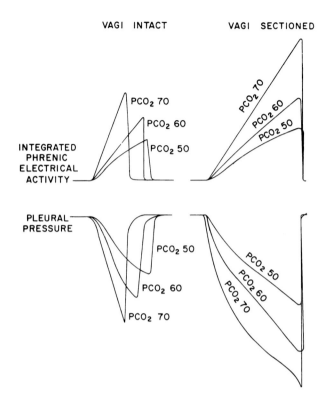

FIG. 2. Effect of hypercapnia on the duration of the phrenic nerve electrical activity integrated as a moving time average and its rate of increase and the pleural pressure waveform. Note the similarity in shape of the integrated phrenic neurogram and the pleural pressure tracing. Following bilateral vagotomy, the duration of inspiration remains relatively constant despite the progressive increase in PCO_2.

ity) causes a progressive increase in excitation of the inspiratory muscles and hence their force of contraction (Fig. 2). The electrical and mechanical analogues of central inspiratory activity are, respectively, the integrated activity of the phrenic neurogram and diaphragmatic electromyogram (EMG) and the pleural pressure waveform. The progressively augmenting shape of central inspiratory activity allows the inspiratory musculature to overcome the progressive increase in elastic recoil of the lung during inspiration despite progressive shortening and a decrease in the intrinsic ability of the inspiratory muscles to generate force (i.e., the length-tension relationship).

Control of the rate of rise in central inspiratory activity and hence the rate of lung inflation differs from control of inspiratory off-switching. Both chemical (e.g., hypoxia and hypercapnia) and nonchemical (e.g., thermal and mechanoreceptor afferents) inputs affect the steepness of the ramp of central inspiratory activity. On the other hand, the timing of inspiratory off-switching depends largely on inputs from pulmonary stretch receptors and from higher CNS structures, such as the NPBM and the KFN.

In anesthetized animals, phasic increases in lung volume resulting from the ramp of central inspiratory activity progressively increase pulmonary stretch-receptor activ-

ity. Integration of inputs from pulmonary stretch receptors and projections reflecting the intensity of the central inspiratory activity by as yet incompletely described pools of neurons terminates inspiration. Vagotomy eliminates stretch-receptor input, prolonging inspiration and increasing tidal volume, but the rate of rise in central inspiratory activity and hence the rate of inspiratory air flow are virtually unchanged. On the other hand, hypoxia and hypercapnia increase the steepness of the ramp of inspiratory activity and hence increase the rate of inspiratory air flow and tidal volume, but they have little effect on the duration of inspiration and frequency of breathing.

When the vagus is intact, so that respiratory neurons receive input from the stretch receptors as well as inputs reflecting central inspiratory activity, the duration of inspiration is reduced, because the inspiratory off-switch is activated earlier. Because central inspiratory activity increases with time, more stretch-receptor input (i.e., a greater change in lung volume) is needed early in inspiration to terminate a breath. This accounts for the curvilinear relationship between tidal volume (V_t) and inspiratory time (t_{insp}) that has been noted in studies of anesthetized animals (Fig. 3).

Consistent with these observations is the idea that ventilatory responses to hypercapnia and hypoxia depend on the sensitivity of both stretch receptors and chemoreceptors. Chemoreceptor sensitivity, because it influences the rate of increase in central inspiratory activity, is more

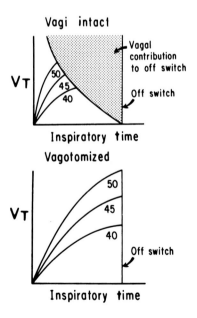

FIG. 3. Effect of lung volume information in determining off-switch and, hence, t_{insp}. Vagal input allows the off-switch threshold to be reached earlier in inspiration. The numbers refer to the PCO_2 with the vagi intact. Inspiratory time declines and tidal volume rises with increasing hypercapnia. Without lung volume information (vagotomy), t_{insp} is fixed.

closely related to the average level of air flow during inspiration than to minute ventilation. That is, the change in the ratio of tidal volume to inspiratory time, rather than the change in ventilation itself, most closely reflects chemical drive. On the other hand, the change in inspiratory time as a fraction of total breath duration indicates the activity of stretch receptors.

Although ventilation is conventionally thought to be equal to tidal volume times frequency (f), the concept of central respiratory neuronal organization suggests that ventilation should more realistically be considered to be the product of the following:

$$\frac{V_T}{t_{insp}} \times \frac{t_{insp}}{t_{insp} + t_{exp}}$$

where t_{insp} is inspiratory time and t_{exp} is expiratory time.

Some studies in humans have tried to separate neural and chemical responses to hypoxia and hypercapnia by analyzing ventilatory responses with this approach. In some cases, depressed ventilatory responses to CO_2 seem to be caused by altered mechanoreceptor function rather than by depressed chemosensitivity.

It is important to remember that this concept originated from experiments carried out in anesthetized animals and accordingly does not include the effects on breathing of inputs eliminated by anesthesia. These additional inputs, occurring during both wakefulness and sleep, may greatly distort the basic relationships between the medullary respiratory neurons observed in animals during anesthesia. Thus, in awake humans, increases in breathing frequency produced by hypercapnia and hypoxia are associated mainly with a shortening of expiratory time, whereas inspiratory time remains relatively constant. Rapid-eye-movement (REM) sleep is associated with an irregular breathing pattern and seems to eliminate ventilatory increases to hypercapnia, but not to hypoxia. In non-REM sleep, breathing is more regular, but responses to changes in CO_2 remain lower than during wakefulness.

Even in anesthetized animals, influences from thermal and circulatory receptors can affect breathing. For example, temperature increases accelerate the frequency of breathing without changing tidal volume.

CENTRAL CHEMORECEPTORS

When CO_2-enriched gas is inspired, ventilation increases. The increase in ventilation tends to minimize the rise in $PaCO_2$. Because the amount of CO_2 delivered to the chemoreceptors depends on the CO_2 carried to them by the arterial blood, the $PaCO_2$ determines the PCO_2 in the immediate environment of the chemoreceptors.

The effect of increases in ventilation on $PaCO_2$ can be determined by the following equation:

$$PaCO_2 = \frac{\dot{V}CO_2 \times K}{\dot{V}A} + PiCO_2$$

where $\dot{V}CO_2$ is the metabolic production of CO_2 each minute, $\dot{V}A$ is the alveolar ventilation, $PiCO_2$ is the partial pressure of inspired CO_2, and K is a proportionality constant.

It can be seen that the greater the increase in ventilation caused by a change in $PiCO_2$, the lower is the $PaCO_2$. In conscious humans, central chemoreceptors located within the medulla account for 70%–80% of the increase in ventilation. The peripheral chemoreceptors account for the remainder of the increase in ventilation when CO_2-enriched gas is inspired and for all the increase in ventilation produced by hypoxia.

The exact location of the central chemoreceptors is still disputed, although most experimental data indicate that they (1) are distinct from the inspiratory motor neurons themselves, (2) are not located in the dorsal and ventral groups described earlier, and (3) respond to changes in hydrogen ion concentration of brain interstitial fluid but also may respond directly to changes in PCO_2 (perhaps through a change in intracellular pH).

Studies in which drugs and temperature probes have been applied to the ventrolateral surface of the medulla have demonstrated abrupt and striking ventilatory effects, suggesting that many of the neurons comprising the central chemoreceptors or their associated axons may be located near the surface. Chemoreceptor activity can be influenced from three different superficial areas (Fig. 4). Recent studies suggest that respiratory cells near the ventral surface are intermingled with cells that also have significant vasomotor effects. Many agents that increase ventilation when applied superficially to the ventral medullary surface (e.g., nicotine, acetylcholine, kainic acid) also raise blood pressure. On the other hand, agents that decrease respiration when similarly applied (e.g., τ-amino butyric acid, taurine, enkephalins) also decrease blood pressure. Nonetheless, discrete areas have been described from which either respiratory or vasomotor effects predominate (e.g., the nucleus paragigantocellularis, a collection of cells close to the ventral medulla).

The crucial experiments in which activity from the central chemoreceptors would be directly recorded have never been performed. Hence, it has been possible to

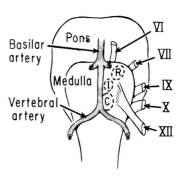

FIG. 4. Ventrolateral medulla and its rostral (R), intermediate (I), and caudal (C) chemosensitive areas.

evaluate central chemoreceptor activity only indirectly. This is usually accomplished by measuring the increase in ventilation or phrenic nerve activity produced when the PICO₂ is changed. Changes in ventilation theoretically should be related to changes in hydrogen ion concentration in the brain, but this concentration cannot be measured easily, either in humans or in animals. Instead, changes in ventilation are conventionally related to the measured levels of PaCO₂. This kind of indirect estimation of central chemoreceptor activity is valid only under restricted circumstances and only if certain assumptions are made. It is assumed, for example, that in a steady state, after CO₂ has been inspired for 10 to 20 minutes, changes in PaCO₂ reflect changes in the hydrogen ion concentration of the brain. By the Henderson-Hasselbalch equation, hydrogen ion concentration in the brain, as in other tissues, varies according to the ratio PCO_2/HCO_3^-, where PCO_2 is the partial pressure of CO₂ at the chemoreceptor in the interstitial fluid and HCO_3^- is the bicarbonate concentration of the medullary interstitial fluid. Hence, increases in bicarbonate concentration decrease hydrogen ion concentration, whereas decreases in bicarbonate concentration have the opposite effect.

The relationship between arterial PCO₂ and PCO₂ in the brain interstitial fluid depends on cerebral venous PCO₂ and therefore on cerebral blood flow. The greater the cerebral blood flow, the smaller the difference between PCO₂ in arterial blood and in interstitial fluid. As cerebral blood flow increases with PCO₂, the change in ventilation produced by a change in PaCO₂ depends on the CO₂ responsiveness of cerebral blood vessels as well as on the sensitivity of the central chemoreceptors. This may be a significant factor in patients with cerebrovascular disease.

Changes in blood bicarbonate levels are not immediately mirrored in the brain interstitial fluid. In addition, evidence suggests that hydrogen ion concentration in interstitial fluid is actively regulated by cellular pumps at the blood-brain barrier or by the metabolism of brain cells. This means that in metabolic acidosis or alkalosis, neither PaCO₂ nor hydrogen ion concentration in blood may reliably indicate the status of hydrogen or bicarbonate ion concentrations in interstitial fluid.

The stimulatory effect of acid injected into the blood on the peripheral chemoreceptors lowers PCO₂. Because the transfer of PCO₂ between blood and brain interstitial fluid is faster than the transfer of hydrogen or bicarbonate ions, the brain interstitial fluid may actually become alkaline when the blood PCO₂ is acutely made acidic. Direct administration of acid into the cerebrospinal fluid to bypass the blood-brain barrier increases the hydrogen ion concentration in brain interstitial fluid and drives the PaCO₂ down by stimulating central chemoreceptors.

With chronic acid-base disturbances, hydrogen ion changes in cerebrospinal fluid are usually qualitatively the same as those in the blood but are quantitatively less.

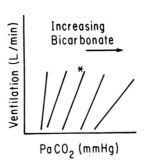

FIG. 5. Effect of changes in blood bicarbonate on the relationship between ventilation and PCO₂. The asterisk indicates the response line at the usual level of HCO_3^-.

The effect of chronic metabolic acidosis and alkalosis on ventilatory responses to CO₂ is shown in Fig. 5. It can be seen that in metabolic acidosis the level of ventilation is greater at any given level of PCO₂, whereas in metabolic alkalosis ventilation decreases. These changes in ventilation reflect the altered level of bicarbonate in the brain interstitial fluid. If the same ventilation results are plotted as a function of hydrogen ion concentration in brain interstitial fluid, the response lines are identical.

In humans and animals, increases in PCO₂ over a wide range cause a virtually linear increase in ventilation. At levels of PaCO₂ >80 to 100 mmHg, the response to hypercapnia diminishes and may plateau. Decreases in PaCO₂ below the usual level depress ventilation. In anesthetized and sleeping animals and humans, artificial hyperventilation with progressively reduced PCO₂ eventually produces apnea. In a normal, awake human, however, active voluntary hyperventilation rarely causes apnea. In most cases, when voluntary hyperventilation is suspended, the increase in ventilation persists for perhaps 30 to 50 seconds. The persistence of ventilation in awake subjects at low levels of PCO₂ has been attributed to a ''wakefulness drive'' caused by the continued impingement of other stimuli (e.g., noise, mechanoreceptor input, and light input) on the respiratory neurons. However, continuation of phrenic nerve activity at low levels of PCO₂ has been described even in anesthetized animals made to hyperventilate actively by electrical stimulation of the carotid body nerves. This effect, which has been attributed to persisting reverberations in medullary respiratory neuron circuits, probably contributes to the wakefulness drive and helps stabilize breathing.

PERIPHERAL CHEMORECEPTORS

Sensors in both the carotid body (innervated by the ninth cranial nerve) and the aortic body (innervated by the tenth cranial nerve) respond to hypoxia by increasing ventilation. If the carotid and aortic bodies are removed, hypoxia depresses breathing. In most species, the increase in ventilation with hypoxia is more a consequence of carotid than of aortic body activity. The carotid body also responds, to a limited extent, to changes in PCO_2 and hydrogen ion concentration, and it appears to be particularly important in the immediate increase in ventilation seen in metabolic acidosis. However, the increase in peripheral chemoreceptor activity caused by CO_2 appears to be inconsequential under hyperoxic conditions.

With decreases in PaO_2, afferent fibers from the carotid body increase their discharge hyperbolically. Reduction in PO_2 rather than in O_2 content in the arterial blood is mainly responsible for the increasing activity. The biochemical and physiologic mechanism that allows the carotid body to respond to even relatively mild hypoxia has not been completely elucidated, but some details are known. Although blood flow in the carotid body is unusually high, so is the metabolic rate. Vascular shunts through the carotid body as well as its high metabolic rate may produce areas of hypoxia within the carotid body, even when the arterial blood is fully saturated with O_2. Measurements of carotid body PO_2 have shown some extremely low tensions, but the range of tensions is wide. Cytochrome enzymes within the carotid body may have an especially low affinity for O_2, thus accounting for the sensitivity of the carotid body to changes in PO_2. Although the primary function of the peripheral arterial chemoreceptors is to transduce changes in arterial PO_2, PCO_2, and/or hydrogen ion levels into nerve signals, there is no general agreement as to how this is accomplished, nor is it known whether all stimuli act through a common mechanism.

Ultrastructural studies of the carotid and aortic bodies demonstrate the presence of two distinct types of cells. Afferent nerve terminals from the carotid sinus nerve appose type I glomus cells, which contain abundant, dense, clear-cored synaptic vesicles, mitochondria, and conspicuous rough endoplasmic reticulum. The cytology of type II (sustentacular) cells resembles that of Schwann cells. They envelop the afferent terminal-glomus cell complex.

Whereas it was originally proposed that the afferent terminals are chemosensitive and that the type I cells function as modulatory interneurons, subsequent studies have suggested that the integrity of the glomus cells (type I and perhaps type II cells) is essential for the process of chemoreception. After the glomus cells are destroyed, nerve endings alone seem unable to respond to physiologic stimuli.

Glomus cells (type I cells) contain a variety of agents, including acetylcholine, norepinephrine, dopamine, and 5-hydroxytryptamine. Recent immunocytochemical studies also have shown the presence of at least three polypeptides in the carotid body of cats and rats (i.e., substance P, vasoactive intestinal polypeptide [VIP], and enkephalins), suggesting that neuropeptides may play important roles in the transmission of nerve signals. Substance P, a member of the tachykinin group of polypeptides, has been proposed as a general transmitter/modulator for primary afferent fibers sensing nociceptive stimuli. In addition, substance P enhances the discharge of carotid body preparations in vivo and in vitro. These excitatory effects of substance P are dose-dependent, seem to be slow in onset, and last several seconds after intracarotid administration. Hypoxic excitation of the carotid body is markedly attenuated by substance P antagonists. The mechanism(s) for sensing O_2 in the carotid body remains unclear. However, hypoxia depolarizes type I cells and increases cytosolic calcium, perhaps through effects on O_2-sensitive, voltage-gated potassium channels and cytochrome protein(s) with a low affinity for O_2. Depolarization of glomus cells in turn causes neurotransmitter release and activation of sinus nerve afferent terminals.

Efferent discharge to the carotid body from the CNS depresses afferent activity provoked by hypoxia. This efferent inhibition may prevent saturation of the carotid body response, allowing the carotid body to respond to a wider range of PO_2 than it could otherwise. In part, efferent control depends on sympathetic nervous regulation of carotid body blood flow. However, other inhibitory efferent fibers that have no effect on the carotid body vasculature are also present.

With hypoxia, ventilation, like carotid body activity, increases hyperbolically (Fig. 6). Also, changes in PCO_2 seem to enhance the ventilatory response to hypoxia, and vice versa (i.e., CO_2 and hypoxia interact multiplicatively). Single carotid body fibers respond to both CO_2 and hypoxia, so that some of the interaction of hypoxia and hypercapnia occurs at the cellular level in the sensor

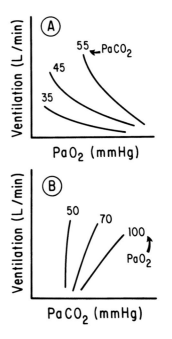

FIG. 6. Effect of changing $PaCO_2$ on (A) the ventilatory response to hypoxia and (B) the ventilatory response to hypercapnia.

itself. However, other evidence suggests that convergence of input from central and peripheral chemoreceptors at the level of the CNS helps enhance the interaction of hypoxia and hypercapnia as ventilatory stimulants. Experimental studies on the effect of carotid nerve stimulation in different phases of breathing show that carotid body discharge is more effective in stimulating breathing during inspiration than during expiration. Carotid body discharge varies spontaneously during the breathing cycle as a result of variations in PaO_2. The relationship between oscillations in carotid body activity and phase of breathing depends on the circulation time between the lungs and the carotid body. Thus, changes in cardiac output theoretically might affect both the level and pattern of breathing. When central chemoreceptor activity and the response to CO_2 have been eliminated by destruction of the ventrolateral medullary surfaces, input from the carotid body alone is sufficient to maintain rhythmic breathing. Both central and peripheral chemoreceptors respond proportionally as the level of PCO_2 is altered. Some studies suggest that increases in the rate of change of CO_2 but not in the rate of change of PO_2 also stimulate the carotid body.

RESPIRATORY SENSORY RECEPTORS

The receptors of the lungs and airways are innervated through the vagi and superior laryngeal and trigeminal nerves, and respond, as in other hollow visceral structures, to irritation of the lining layers and changes in distending forces. The mechanoreceptors associated with the respiratory muscles are innervated by spinal nerves and, like those in other skeletal muscles, monitor changes in joint movement and in the length and tension of the muscle itself.

Pulmonary Receptors

There are basically three types of pulmonary receptors: stretch receptors in the smooth muscles of the airway, irritant receptors in the airway epithelium, and J (juxta-capillary) receptors situated in the lung interstitium.

Stretch Receptors

Stretch receptors are innervated by large myelinated fibers. As the lung is inflated, these receptors inhibit inspiration, promote expiration, and initiate the Hering-Breuer reflex. In animals, lung inflation cuts short inspiration and produces expiratory apnea; the duration of apnea is proportional to the degree of inflation.

Direct measurements of stretch-receptor activity indicate that stretch receptors in humans are excited by even small changes in lung volume during quiet breathing. In humans, however, unlike what occurs in animals, vagal

blockade to abolish stretch-receptor input does not affect breathing frequency or tidal volume at rest. Vagal blockade in both humans and animals does, however, prevent the increase in breathing frequency that occurs when ventilation is stimulated by hypercapnia or hypoxia and tidal volume is larger.

In animals, stretch-receptor activity helps to preserve tidal volume whenever the usual movements of the lung are hindered by changes in airways resistance or respiratory system compliance. Anything that retards lung inflation diminishes inspiratory inhibitory stretch-receptor activity. Therefore, inspiration is prolonged and tidal volume tends to approach its usual level when the airway is obstructed or respiratory compliance is reduced, despite mechanical interference. When expiration is hindered and lung deflation slowed, increased stretch-receptor activity heightens the force of contraction of the expiratory muscles and also prolongs expiratory time. Both these stretch-receptor actions tend to prevent mechanical impediments to expiration from increasing end-expiratory volume and, as a consequence, decreasing the resting length of the inspiratory muscle. Stretch-receptor activity, by promoting full expiration, helps preserve inspiratory muscle function.

Although stretch receptors are not important in humans in shaping resting breathing patterns, they may help maintain tidal volume when breathing is stimulated or lung or chest-wall mechanical performance is impaired. The increase in breathing frequency caused by stretch-receptor activity in animals and during stimulated breathing in humans decreases the work of breathing of the respiratory muscles, conserving the energy that has to be expended to produce gas exchange. Although it is well-known that peripheral inputs from lung mechanoreceptors strongly affect the timing of respiratory motor activity, at the present time it is difficult to separate clearly the ventilatory effects of the pulmonary stretch-receptor afferents from those of other vagal sensory components (e.g., irritant and C-fiber afferents). However, changes in vagal afferent activity elicited by phasic lung volume changes seem to control predominantly the duration of inspiration, whereas tonic inputs predominantly affect the duration of expiration.

Irritant Receptors

Irritant receptors, like the stretch receptors, are innervated by myelinated fibers, whereas unmyelinated fibers supply the J receptors. Unlike the stretch receptors, both irritant and J receptors are rapid-adapting (within seconds). Neither irritant nor J receptors have a pattern of firing that is related to the phases of inspiration and expiration. Consequently, it is believed that neither receptor has an important influence in determining the pattern of breathing at rest.

Mechanical stimulation of the airways or the inhalation of potentially noxious agents (e.g., particulate matter, nitrogen dioxide, sulfur dioxide, ammonia, and antigens) seems to excite irritant receptors and produce airway constriction. Stimulation of irritant receptors augments the activity of the inspiratory neurons and, by interaction with the stretch receptors, promotes rapid, shallow breathing. This pattern of breathing, in combination with airway constriction, may limit penetration of dangerous agents into the lung and prevent them from reacting with the gas-exchanging surfaces.

The inspiratory augmenting effect of irritant-receptor excitation and the increase in breathing frequency it produces may help maintain ventilation in asthmatic patients, even when the work of breathing is massively increased.

Irritant receptors can be excited by traction on the airways and are stimulated if atelectasis reduces lung compliance. These receptors seem to cause augmented breathing and the large sighs that occur sporadically during normal breathing, and help to open collapsed areas of the lung. As a consequence, irritant receptors help maintain adequate gas exchange.

J Receptors

J receptors are stimulated by pulmonary interstitial edema, but they also can be activated by various chemical agents, such as histamine, halothane, and phenyldiguanide. Activation of the J receptors causes laryngeal closure and apnea, followed by rapid, shallow breathing. When pulmonary edema develops as a result of exercise, J receptors seem to depress the activity of the exercising limbs by a somatic reflex involving cingulate gyrus. J receptors, together with irritant receptors, may be responsible for the tachypnea seen in patients with pulmonary embolus, pulmonary edema, and pneumonia.

Laryngeal Receptors

Mechanoreceptors and chemoreceptors in the upper airway reflexively affect the level and pattern of breathing, motor outflow to the upper airway and chest-wall muscles, and airway tone. The best-studied of the upper airway receptors are the laryngeal receptors. In fact, all areas of the laryngeal mucosa and deeper structures contain sensory nerve endings. Several types of laryngeal receptors have been described: (1) pressure receptors, (2) "drive" receptors, and (3) cold receptors.

Pressure receptors, the most numerous of the laryngeal receptors, are activated by increases in negative (intraluminal less than extraluminal pressure) or positive transmural pressure. Pressure receptors fire in response to both dynamic and static pressure changes, and are slow-adapting. Approximately, two thirds of the pressure receptors respond to negative pressure; the remaining third respond to positive pressure. Approximately one half of laryngeal pressure receptors demonstrate a respiratory modulation in the absence of air flow in the isolated, bypassed upper airway, suggesting that they respond to laryngeal muscle shortening in response to descending motor drive. These so-called drive receptors fire primarily during inspiration. Their firing pattern is diminished by paralysis of the intrinsic muscles of the larynx.

Reflexes elicited by laryngeal pressure receptors tend to stabilize the upper airway, retard its tendency to collapse in response to subatmospheric pressure, and reestablish its patency following occlusion. Laryngeal pressure receptors reflexively activate upper airway muscles while inhibiting inspiratory muscles of the chest wall. Negative transmural airway pressure reflexes increase the activity of inspiratory upper airway muscles (e.g., genioglossus, sternohyoid, cricothyroid, levator alae nasi, posterior arytenoids), advance the onset of the upper airway-muscle EMG relative to that of the diaphragm, increase the duration of inspiration and expiration, and decrease the average rate of rise of diaphragmatic and inspiratory intercostal EMG activity. (Normally, activation of upper airway muscles occurs 50 to 100 ms before the outset of diaphragmatic activation.) Reflex responses to negative pressure in the upper airway mediated by pressure receptors may explain the greater tidal volume, expiratory time, and ventilation during nasal than in tracheostomy breathing in conscious animals and humans.

In contrast to pressure receptors, laryngeal cold receptors are silent near body temperature but are activated by decreases in laryngeal temperature to 34°C or below. When active, cold receptors demonstrate a phasic, inspiratory firing pattern and, in contrast to pressure receptors, appear to adapt rapidly. Cold receptors appear to be located superficially in the mucosa on the edge of the vocal cords near the arytenoid process. Increases in lower airway resistance elicited by laryngeal cooling may be mediated by these receptors.

Finally, mechanical or chemical irritation of the larynx (e.g., probe contact or application of acid) elicits cough, laryngeal closure, bronchoconstriction, an increase in tracheal production of mucus, and a decrease in heart rate and blood pressure. These reflex responses to laryngeal irritation suggest that laryngeal chemoreceptors and mechanoreceptors function to protect the lower airway from aspiration or inhalation of toxic fumes.

Of interest, reflex responses to laryngeal stimulation appear to be state-dependent and are qualitatively different during wakefulness and sleep. For example, in the dog, application of distilled water to the larynx during wakefulness consistently elicits cough and bronchoconstriction. In contrast, the same maneuver performed during REM sleep does not stimulate cough, but rather elicits apnea and bradycardia.

Chest-Wall Receptors

Three types of receptors in the chest wall—joint, tendon, and spindle receptors—signal changes in the force exerted by the respiratory muscles and movement of the chest wall. Specialized Ruffini receptors, as well as pacinian and Golgi organs, are present in joints. Joint-receptor activity, which can be consciously perceived, varies with the degree and rate of change of rib movement.

Inputs arising from muscular receptors, both proprioceptive (particularly muscle spindle) and nociceptor afferent (types III and IV) endings, influence the level and timing of respiratory activity. Proprioceptor afferents (chiefly from the intercostal and abdominal muscles) project to the phrenic motor neurons, where their effect is on firing rate only, and to medullary respiratory neurons in the DRG and NRA, where their predominant effect is on respiratory timing.

Tendon organs in the intercostal muscles and diaphragm monitor the force of muscle contraction and produce an inspiratory inhibitory effect. It was once thought that tendon organ activity was provoked only by unusual levels of muscle force, but it is now believed that tendon organs are stimulated by even small changes in force. Tendon organ input may be important in regulating both intercostal muscle and diaphragmatic contraction during breathing at rest.

Muscle spindles, which are abundant in the intercostal muscles but scarce in the diaphragm, are involved in several kinds of intercostal respiratory reflexes and also help coordinate breathing during changes in posture and speech.

Figure 7 shows schematically the operation of the spindle and its neural connections. Spindles are located on intrafusal muscle fibers aligned in parallel with extrafusal fibers, which move the ribs. Motor innervation of the extrafusal fibers originates in alpha motor neurons, whereas the intrafusal fibers receive motor innervation from gamma (fusimotor) motor neurons. Passive stretch of an intercostal spindle by lateral flexion of the trunk, for example, increases spindle afferent activity and acti-

vates a monosynaptic segmental reflex that causes contraction of the parent extrafusal fiber and restores the upright position. The spindles also can be stretched by an efferent fusimotor discharge, which causes contraction and shortening of the intrafusal fiber itself. Some fusimotor fibers fire phasically, so that their rate of discharge rises during inspiration and falls during expiration; other fusimotor fibers are tonically active. The cerebellum determines the balance between tonically and phasically active fusimotor fibers. Without phasic fusimotor activity, spindle discharge would decrease when the extrafusal fibers contract during inspiration. Simultaneous activation of fusimotor and alpha motor neurons causes the spindles to be under continuous stretch during inspiration and enhances the contribution made by the intercostal muscles to respiration. If inspiratory movements are impeded, afferent activity from a spindle innervated by a phasically active fusimotor fiber is enhanced, thus increasing inspiratory muscle force and helping to preserve tidal volume. Activity from lower intercostal muscle spindles, through an intersegmental spinal reflex, also enhances diaphragmatic contraction, allowing the diaphragm to contribute to the compensatory increase in muscle force that occurs when respiratory movements are hindered. In contrast, stretch of the intercostal spindles in the midthoracic region of the chest decreases the duration of inspiration and diminishes the force of inspiratory muscle contraction. This reflex may cut short ineffective inspirations. Ineffective inspirations sometimes are seen in the newborn when the negative intrathoracic pressure produced by powerful diaphragmatic contraction causes paradoxical inward movement of the flexible infant rib cage.

Of considerable importance, spindle afferents reach the highest level of the central nervous system, the sensorimotor cortex. Projection of spindle afferent activity to the cerebral cortex allows respiratory muscle length and tension to be sensed consciously and modulated with great precision, thereby allowing complex volitional acts to be performed (e.g., speaking, playing a wind instrument). Spindle afferent activity also likely contributes to the sense of breathlessness. It has been suggested that dyspnea occurs when spindle afferent activity is "high" relative to the intensity of central motor activity to the inspiratory muscles. This concept, which has been termed *length-tension inappropriateness,* explains the dyspnea that arises in the setting of lung diseases that increase inspiratory muscle load and impede muscle shortening. Of interest, the sense of breathlessness can be affected in patients with chronic obstructive pulmonary disease (COPD) by application of vibratory stimuli to the intercostal muscles, which changes spindle afferent activity. Dyspnea is ameliorated by vibratory stimuli applied in phase with muscle contraction and worsened when the vibratory stimulus is applied out of phase with muscle contraction.

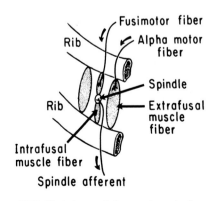

FIG. 7. Intercostal muscle spindle.

Integration of Afferent Input

Although it is clear that afferent input to the medullary respiratory neurons from mechanoreceptors in the lungs, respiratory muscles, and cardiovascular and thermal regulatory systems (and even the exercising limbs) have significant effects on breathing, the precise manner in which these inputs are integrated is poorly understood. However, the changes in respiratory motor activity elicited by changes in these inputs are not stereotyped. The reflex responses to these inputs may affect the motor output to some respiratory muscles more than others. Pulmonary stretch-receptor input inhibits chest-wall muscle activity (i.e., diaphragm and external intercostal muscles) but increases the activity of the upper airway-dilating muscles (i.e., posterior cricoarytenoid) and the chest-wall expiratory muscles. Even more interesting, some receptors seem to have opposing effects on muscles that normally act as agonists. For example, stimulation of esophageal mechanoreceptors by balloon distension of the distal esophagus reflexively inhibits diaphragmatic activity, both costal and vertebral, but enhances external intercostal activity.

CONTROLLED SYSTEM EFFECTS ON REGULATION OF BREATHING

The translation of the output of the inspiratory neurons to ventilation involves, as shown in Fig. 8, the successive transformation of nerve impulses to muscle electrical activity, muscle shortening, force, and then ventilation. Usually, moderate changes in the mechanical properties of

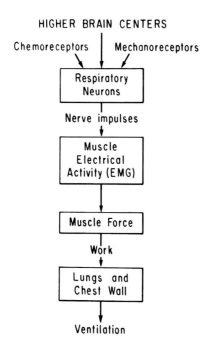

FIG. 8. Steps by which respiratory neural activity is translated into ventilation.

the muscles or chest bellows have little or no effect on the resting blood gas tensions. Compensating effects by the chemoreceptor and mechanoreceptor reflexes, conscious adjustments, and the intrinsic force-velocity relationships of the muscles themselves allow the force of contraction to increase whenever the rate of contraction is slowed. In the presence of sufficiently severe chest disease, however, gas exchange is inadequate despite all efforts to compensate.

Even when the compensatory responses prove ultimately to be adequate, changes in mechanical conditions (or metabolic rate) cause a transient period in which gas exchange is disturbed and gas tensions are abnormal. The degree to which blood gas tensions deviate from normal in such situations depends on the volume and arrangement of the body stores of O_2 and CO_2.

CO_2 is contained in the body in large amounts as gas in the lungs, but mainly in the form of bicarbonate and carbonate solutions in blood and tissues. O_2, on the other hand, is stored in much smaller amounts in alveolar gas, in solution, and in combination with hemoglobin and myoglobin. Disturbances in gas exchange cause small changes in PCO_2 because of the large size of the CO_2 stores, but large changes in PO_2.

Rates of change of PO_2 and PCO_2 depend not only on the volume of gas stores, but also on organization—that is, the way O_2 and CO_2 contained in different body tissue compartments are linked by the circulation, rates of perfusion, and metabolic rates in the various body compartments—and the ability of the tissues in each compartment to bind CO_2 and O_2.

The rate at which peripheral and central chemoreceptors respond to changes in inspired CO_2 and O_2 depends on the arrangement of the body gas stores. The small size of the arterial compartment and the high rate of carotid body blood flow allow peripheral chemoreceptors to respond quickly to changes in both O_2 and CO_2. The larger CO_2 stores of the brain cause the central chemoreceptors to respond more slowly to changes in inspired CO_2. This difference in response time of central and peripheral chemoreceptors has been used to distinguish the contribution of each receptor to the CO_2 response.

TESTS OF CHEMORECEPTOR SENSITIVITY

When lung function is normal, the sensitivity of the peripheral and central chemoreceptors to CO_2 can be evaluated by measuring the ventilatory response to inspired CO_2. In the conventional steady-state test, the inspired CO_2 is increased in steps, and ventilation at each step is related to the change in $PaCO_2$. Sensitivity to CO_2 is determined from the slope of the line relating ventilation to CO_2. Although the central chemoreceptors are readily accessible to CO_2, the size of cerebral CO_2 stores increases the time required for ventilation to reach a steady state when PCO_2 changes. Usually, the inspired CO_2 concentrations at each step must be maintained constant for 10 to 20 minutes to ensure equilibration. Relative rates of equilibration of PCO_2 in arterial and brain venous blood (Fig. 9) indicate that $PaCO_2$ reaches its steady-state level long before the venous PCO_2. It is apparent from Fig. 9 that if ventilation, which closely tracks cerebral venous PCO_2, is measured too soon, chemosensitivity will be underestimated.

When CO_2 is rebreathed from a bag containing CO_2 at the mixed venous level together with O_2, arterial and venous blood equilibrate more rapidly. After a brief transition period, PCO_2 at all sites in arterial, cerebral, and mixed venous blood and alveolar air rises at the same rate. Consequently, the rate of change of PCO_2 in alveolar air can be used as an index of the rate of change in PCO_2 in the central chemoreceptors. The exact length of the transition period depends on the size of the rebreathing bag. When the volume of the rebreathing bag is about the same as the vital capacity, chemosensitivity can be estimated by continuous recording of ventilation and PCO_2 after 45 to 60 seconds of rebreathing. Measurements for wide variations in PCO_2 can be obtained in a few minutes. Estimates obtained by this rebreathing method agree with those obtained by the more prolonged steady-state technique. However, the rebreathing tests measure CO_2 sensitivity at much higher levels of PCO_2 than are usually encountered. Moreover, differences have been noted between rebreathing and steady-state ventilatory response to CO_2 when metabolic acidosis or alkalosis is present. With the steady-state technique, moderate alkalosis and acidosis produce larger changes in the position of the ventilatory response line but relatively small changes in its slopes, whereas the reverse is true in the rebreathing tests. The explanation for this difference is obscure, but it may be related to the different levels of PCO_2 at which steady-state and rebreathing tests are performed.

The average ventilatory response to CO_2 is about 2.5 L/min/mmHg in normal adult men. It is somewhat less in women than in men and tends to decline with advanced age. It varies greatly between individuals but is much more constant in repeated measurements from a single subject. Some of this variability is caused by differences in personality, genetic makeup, and body size, and it is reduced when the CO_2 response is corrected for differences in vital capacity.

Cortical activity is known to affect the response to CO_2. Ventilatory responses to CO_2 measured with the subject's eyes open are greater than ventilatory responses to CO_2 measured with the subject's eyes shut.

TESTS OF PERIPHERAL CHEMORECEPTORS

The peripheral chemoreceptors also respond to CO_2 and contribute about 20%–30% of the total ventilatory increase observed when CO_2 is inhaled. Because peripheral chemoreceptors react rapidly to changes in CO_2, peripheral chemoreceptor responses have been evaluated by measuring the immediate increase in ventilation caused by a few breaths of inspired CO_2 or by measuring the immediate decrease in ventilation observed when CO_2 is abruptly removed.

The response to hypoxia, like the response to hypercapnia, can be measured by either rebreathing or steady-state techniques. Because of the prominent effects of CO_2 on breathing, it is important to keep the CO_2 constant while the response to hypoxia is measured. Because O_2 stores are small, the peripheral chemoreceptor response to O_2 also can be evaluated by measuring the effect on ventilation of a few breaths of N_2 or 100% O_2.

No matter how it is measured, the ventilatory response to hypoxia is curvilinear, making quantitation difficult. The response can be made linear, however, by relating ventilation to the reciprocal of PO_2 or to the arterial O_2 saturation.

There are insufficient data to establish the range of normal values of the ventilatory response to hypoxia; however, available information indicates that it is closely related to the metabolic rate and is at least as variable as the CO_2 response.

Prolonged periods of hypoxia, particularly early in life, are associated with depression of the chemoreceptor response to hypoxia. The ventilatory response to hypoxia is reduced in native residents of regions at high altitudes and in children with congenital cyanotic heart disease. The carotid body appears to be larger in native residents of high altitudes. The change in size may be caused by increased carotid body vascularity, which raises PO_2 and decreases responsiveness.

In the newborn, hypoxia causes only a transient increase in ventilation, which then subsides to nearly prehypoxic levels. It has been recently appreciated that in adult humans, hypoxia lasting for as short a time as 5 minutes produces a gradual reduction in ventilation from its initial peak level.

The initial increase in ventilation is of course mediated by the carotid body. The subsequent decrease seems to

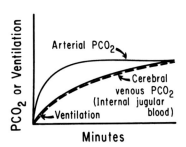

FIG. 9. Changes of ventilation, $PaCO_2$, and cerebral venous $PaCO_2$ when inspired CO_2 is changed.

represent a depressant effect of hypoxia on central respiratory neurons by hypoxia-induced increases in cerebral blood flow and probably the release of inhibitory neuromodulators, such as adenosine.

Lung disease or respiratory muscle weakness can depress ventilatory responses to chemical stimuli. The depressant effect seems to be greater for the response to CO_2 than for the response to hypoxia. As a result of studies in which airway resistance was increased by requiring subjects to breathe through external resistance, either during inspiration or expiration, it was suggested that the inspiratory work of breathing at a given level of PCO_2 is fixed, so that when the ratio of inspiratory muscle work to ventilation is increased by disease, ventilation decreases. The hypercapnia observed in severe obstructive lung disease was explained by the increase in flow-resistive work associated with chronic airway obstruction.

More recent studies have indicated that small increases in airway resistance have little effect on resting ventilation or CO_2 response in normal subjects and may even heighten ventilation. The mechanisms responsible for the preservation of ventilation under these circumstances could include intrinsic properties of the respiratory muscles, increased inspiratory augmenting output from lung and chest-wall mechanoreceptors, readjustment in the sequence of contractions of the respiratory muscles so that mechanical advantage of the muscles and their coordination is improved, and increased inspiratory drive originating from the motor cortex. This last mechanism may depend on the conscious perception of changes in airway resistance. It is interesting that the ability to detect changes in airway resistance varies, decreasing with increasing airway resistance, and that it decreases further when airway obstruction is chronic than when it is acute.

Because mechanical changes may limit the ventilatory response to chemical stimuli, other methods of assessing the output of respiratory motor neurons have been devised. Two methods have been employed: measurement of occlusion pressure and EMG of the diaphragm. Neither is perfect, but both are useful under certain circumstances.

In the measurement of occlusion pressure, the force of contraction of the inspiratory muscles under quasi-isometric conditions is determined as follows: The airway is momentarily blocked at the beginning of inspiration, and the negative pressure developed during inspiration is measured. In conscious subjects, the reproducibility of the response is greater when the airways are occluded for just a fraction of a second. The occlusion pressure increases with hypercapnia and hypoxia and can be related to change in PCO_2 and PO_2 to estimate chemosensitivity.

Airway occlusion at FRC produces a no-flow state at the relaxed position of the respiratory system. The absence of air flow and prevention of significant volume change during inspiration prevent increases in airway resistance or decreases in compliance from affecting this index of respiratory output. In patients with mechanical abnormalities of the ventilatory pump caused by diseases of the lung or chest wall, occlusion pressure therefore more accurately reflects the neuromuscular drive to breathe than does ventilation.

Because the tensions developed by the inspiratory muscles theoretically depend on their initial length, the occlusion pressure in patients with lungs hyperinflated by disease may not reflect respiratory drive accurately. Increased FRC in animals reduces occlusion pressure responses. However, studies in conscious humans in whom FRC has been changed by altering body position show little effect on occlusion pressure, even when changes in FRC are fairly large (1000 mL). A conscious person apparently maintains constant muscle tension successfully, despite changes in initial muscle length, by altering neural output.

Measurement of the electrical activity of the diaphragm is probably the most direct way of evaluating respiratory neuronal output. This can be accomplished by passing a catheter containing electrodes down the esophagus and positioning the electrodes so that they straddle both surfaces of the diaphragm.

Various ways have been devised to quantitate diaphragmatic electrical activity measured this way. In the method most used currently, diaphragmatic activity is integrated over small intervals of time (100 to 200 ms), and the average activity per time limit is recorded (the so-called moving average). Electrical activity measured in this way depends on the exact positions of the electrodes in relation to the diaphragm during breathing, so that it is difficult to compare one individual with another. It is possible, however, to use this method to determine the effect of different therapeutic interventions in the same person.

CLINICAL IMPLICATIONS

The most important cause of respiratory failure is derangement of lung mechanics. However, respiratory failure does not develop in all patients, even those with severe impairment of pulmonary function. It has long been suspected that those patients who have the poorest chemosensitivity are the ones in whom CO_2 retention is most likely to develop when the performance of the chest bellows is reduced. The evidence for this is indirect. For example, normal offspring of hypercapnic subjects with COPD demonstrate significantly lower ventilatory and occlusion pressure responses to hypoxia and hypercapnia (~60% lower) than do normal offspring of eucapnic subjects with COPD.

The CO_2 sensitivity of children who have retained CO_2 because of upper airway obstruction resulting from hypertrophy of the adenoids and tonsils is depressed, even after the tonsils and adenoids have been removed. Asthmatic patients who have retained CO_2 during an asthmatic attack also show persistently low ventilatory responses to CO_2,

TABLE 1. *Conditions sometimes associated with depressed responses to hypercapnia and hypoxia*

Genetic factors
Obesity-hypoventilation syndrome
Bulbar poliomyelitis
Metabolic alkalosis
Parkinson's disease
Narcotic addictions (temporary)
Myxedema
Bilateral spinothalamic lesions
Severe hepatic failure

TABLE 3. *Conditions associated with increased responses to carbon dioxide and/or hypoxia*

Hyperthyroidism
Salicylism
Fever
Hemodialysis for uremia
Luft's syndrome
Pregnancy
Mild hepatic failure

even after recovery from the asthmatic episode. Moreover, subjects who have had asphyxial, near-fatal episodes of asthma display lower ventilatory and occlusion pressure responses to hypoxia than do either age-matched normal subjects or asthmatic subjects with no history of near-fatal episodes.

There is also a small group of subjects who retain CO_2 even though lung function is normal. In some of these patients, the cause of the depressed CO_2 sensitivity is not known, but in others it seems to be associated with specific diseases, certain metabolic abnormalities, such as alkalosis, or the long-term administration of respiratory depressant drugs, such as methadone. These conditions are summarized in Table 1. In a few conditions listed in Table 2, only the ventilatory response to hypoxia is depressed. Individuals with these conditions are able to maintain blood gas tensions within usual limits because of their normal CO_2 drive. However, when CO_2 sensitivity is reduced by the administration of drugs (e.g., premedication before surgery), significant hypoxemia can develop. Depressed ventilatory responses to hypoxia may also increase the tendency for CO_2 retention to develop in COPD and may be a risk factor for acute mountain sickness.

Certain conditions seem to predispose to heightened responses to CO_2 or hypoxia, even when the lungs are normal. These conditions are listed in Table 3.

Abnormalities in mechanoreceptor function also can influence gas exchange. Patients with chronic airway obstruction who breathe with small tidal volumes tend to retain CO_2, whereas those who breathe with larger tidal volumes do not. The small tidal volumes are caused by abbreviated inspiratory time and perhaps by heightened pulmonary or chest-wall receptor activity. Heightened mechanoreceptor activity may also be responsible for dys-

pnea in some patients with interstitial lung disease, as vagal blockade at times alleviates this sensation.

EFFECTS OF SLEEP ON VENTILATION

State-related changes in CNS activity associated with the transition from wakefulness to sleep exert complex effects on ventilatory control that profoundly affect the level and pattern of breathing. In general, withdrawal of cortical and higher CNS influences that provide excitatory inputs to the medullary respiratory neurons during wakefulness cause the chemical regulation of ventilation to assume greater importance.

The transition from wakefulness to slow-wave sleep (i.e., stages 1, 2, 3, and 4 non-REM) is associated with increases in $PaCO_2$ and decreases in PO_2, an increase in the threshold of the ventilatory response to CO_2, and elimination of the ''dog leg'' in the ventilatory response to CO_2 attributable to the wakefulness drive. In normal subjects, elimination of wakefulness drives and decreases in chemosensitivity typically increase $PaCO_2$ and decrease PO_2 by 4 to 8 mmHg. Small reductions in PCO_2 in the order of 4 to 6 mmHg regularly induce apnea in normal subjects, in contrast to what occurs during wakefulness, when breathing persists despite marked hypocapnia. Steady-state changes in PCO_2 during slow-wave sleep appear to be inversely related to the magnitude of the ventilatory response to CO_2 during wakefulness.

Breathing during stages 1 and 2 of slow-wave (i.e., light) sleep is frequently periodic and often characterized by apnea (i.e., cessation of air flow for >10 seconds) with or without occlusion of the airway (see below). Periodic breathing resembles the Cheyne-Stokes respiration occurring during wakefulness. On the other hand, stages 3 and 4 of non-REM sleep are generally characterized by a slow, deep, regular pattern of breathing. Interestingly, this phase of sleep is associated with a greater depression of ventilatory responses to CO_2 and O_2 than are stages 1 and 2.

Breathing during REM sleep is rapid and irregular, with marked variation in the duration of inspiration and expiration, tidal volume, and average inspiratory air flow rate. Periods of hyperpnea appear to coincide with REM sleep. Electrical activity (EMG) of the rib cage and upper airway respiratory muscles is profoundly depressed in

TABLE 2. *Conditions associated mainly with a decreased response to hypoxia*

Narcotic addictions (long-term)
Carotid endarterectomy
Cyanotic congenital heart disease
Familial dysautonomia
Semistarvation
Arnold-Chiari syndrome

REM sleep, in keeping with the marked muscular atonia observed in the limb muscles. Diaphragmatic EMG activity is relatively spared, but abrupt, irregular periods of inhibition during inspiration may occur. A disproportionate reduction in intercostal relative to diaphragmatic activity in REM sleep leads to paradoxical inward movement of the rib cage on inspiration. Profound inhibition of upper airway muscle electrical activity considerably increases upper airway resistance. Ventilatory responses to CO_2 and O_2 are at their lowest during this stage of sleep. In subjects with underlying lung disease, the greatest disturbances in PaO_2 and $PaCO_2$ occur during this stage of sleep, presumably because of the rapid, shallow pattern of breathing, increased ratio of volume of dead space to tidal volume, and uncoordinated pattern of rib cage and abdominal movement.

Periodic Breathing During Sleep

Recent studies have suggested several possible mechanisms for the periodic breathing and airway occlusion that occur during the transition from wakefulness to light sleep, each of which causes instability in the ventilatory control system. First, removal of the wakefulness drive depresses ventilation, with concomitant large and rapid increases in PCO_2 and reductions in PO_2 that stimulate peripheral and central chemoreceptors. Second, alterations in blood gas tensions and mild reductions in metabolic activity that decrease CO_2 production and O_2 consumption increase plant gain—that is, the change in blood gas tensions induced by a given change in ventilation. Increased plant gains in stage 1 and stage 2 sleep may offset the mild reductions in ventilatory responses to CO_2 and O_2 that occur during these stages and increase controller gain. Third, progressive increases in respiratory effort during occlusive apnea lead to arousal, the primary mechanism whereby occlusive apnea is terminated. Collapse of the upper airway and arousal destabilize breathing by producing large and rapid changes in PCO_2 and PO_2. Fourth, arousal may be followed by a rapid return to sleep, removal of the wakefulness drive, and rapid deterioration in blood gases. Cycles of airway occlusion and arousal superimposed on sleep-related changes in controller gain may be mutually reinforcing and lead to sustained, progressively amplifying oscillations in breathing and blood gas tensions. Breathing in stages 3 and 4 of sleep is likely to be more stable than in stages 1 and 2, because overall controller gain may be diminished and because changes in ventilation caused by external stimuli are less likely than in stages 1 and 2. Depression of CO_2 and O_2 chemosensitivity in stages 3 and 4 may more than offset increases in plant gain.

Changes in respiration with periods of apnea, profound arterial desaturation, and disturbed sleep appear to be especially common in patients with congestive heart fail-

ure. Periodic breathing in these subjects may be explained by a prolongation in circulation time with information delays and increases in plant gain as a result of decreases in pulmonary stores of O_2 related to pulmonary edema.

Airway Occlusion During Sleep

The pathogenesis of airway occlusion during sleep has now been elucidated. Patency of the upper airway during sleep depends on a balance between the subatmospheric "sucking" pressures in the posterior nasopharyngeal space generated by the inspiratory muscles of the chest wall and the opposing dilating forces generated by the upper inspiratory airway muscles, which tend to enlarge and "stiffen" the upper airway. In essence, collapse of the upper airway during inspiration occurs when there is an imbalance of forces in favor of the subpharyngeal pressures. Collapse of the upper airway therefore depends on three factors: (1) activity of the dilator muscles, (2) intraluminal airway pressure, and (3) mechanical properties of the passive upper airway.

The activity of the respiratory skeletal muscles of the upper airways, which originate on the mandible, tongue, larynx, and hyoid bone and dilate the upper airway (i.e., genioglossus, geniohyoid, sternohyoid, posterior arytenoids, cricothyroid), demonstrate a respiratory modulation—that is, the EMG and tension of these muscles increase during inspiration, thereby augmenting the caliber of the upper airway and its tendency to remain patent. Hypercapnic and hypoxic chemical stimuli to breathing increase upper airway muscle electrical activity (e.g., genioglossus, posterior arytenoids) in a manner qualitatively similar to that seen in the pump muscles of the chest wall. All stages of sleep are associated with depression of EMG activity of upper airway muscles at any given level of PO_2 or PCO_2 out of proportion to changes in chest-wall muscle EMG. REM sleep is associated with the greatest inhibition of upper airway muscle electrical activity, in keeping with the generalized muscular atonia that occurs during this stage of sleep. Airway collapse during sleep is favored, therefore, by depression of the electrical activity of dilating upper airway muscles. Re-establishment of airway patency in the setting of obstructive apnea requires arousal and increases in upper airway EMG activity. Of interest, administration of alcohol in amounts that have no effect on ventilation or pattern of breathing depress genioglossus EMG activity during eucapnia or hypercapnia. This finding may explain the greater tendency for obstructive sleep apnea to develop after alcohol ingestion or sedative use.

In addition, end-expiratory lung volume (FRC) oscillates during periodic breathing and demonstrates progressive reduction during the several breaths preceding occlusion. Reductions in lung volume *per se* reduce the cross-sectional area of the posterior nasopharynx and increase the mechanical advantage of the inspiratory muscles of the chest wall (i.e., the inspiratory pressure generated for a given EMG activity is increased).

Classic control system theory indicates that increased controller gain predisposes to control system instability and oscillation. However, it seems likely that the precise mechanisms by which periodic breathing with apnea develop during sleep vary from individual to individual and may depend on the magnitude of the wakefulness drive, the propensity to awaken and undergo rapid, state-related changes in ventilation, and the proclivity of the upper airway to collapse.

BIBLIOGRAPHY

Altose MD, et al. Effects of hypercapnia on mouth pressure during airway occlusion in conscious man. *J Appl Physiol* 1976;40:338. *Study demonstrating that the airway occlusion pressure increases linearly in conscious subjects during progressive hypercapnia and is augmented by an acute increase in resistance to air flow.*

Altose MD, et al. Effects of hypercapnia and inspiratory flow-resistive loading on respiratory activity in chronic airways obstruction. *J Clin Invest* 1977;59:500. *Study comparing airway occlusion responses to progressive hypercapnia and inspiratory resistance in normal subjects and patients with chronic obstructive lung disease. Subjects with chronic hypercapnia have a blunted occlusion pressure response to hypercapnia and to acute application of respiratory resistive load.*

Arkinstall WW, et al. Genetic differences in the ventilatory response to inhaled CO_2. *J Appl Physiol* 1974;36:9. *A careful comparison of variability in the ventilatory response to progressive hypercapnia carried out by examining rebreathing in identical and fraternal twins. Identical twins demonstrate less variability than fraternal twins, indicating a genetic basis to the response.*

Aubier M, et al. Central drive in acute respiratory failure of patients with chronic obstructive pulmonary disease. *Am Rev Respir Dis* 1980;122:191. *Important study demonstrating that airway occlusion pressure is heightened in patients with COPD who are in respiratory failure and decreases progressively as subjects improve clinically. This finding indicates that patients with COPD who are in acute respiratory failure have a heightened neuromuscular drive to breathe because of abnormalities in lung function and blood gas tensions.*

Bianchi AL, Denavit-Saubie M, Champagnat J. Central control of breathing in mammals: neuronal circuitry, membrane properties, and neurotransmitters. *Physiol Rev* 1995;75:1. *Extremely comprehensive review characterizing respiratory neuronal firing pattern, anatomic organization, and synaptic connection. It contains a wealth of information about central control of breathing and neuronal circuitry.*

Chapman KR, Gothe BB, Cherniack NS. Possible mechanisms of periodic breathing during sleep. *J Appl Physiol* 1988;64:1000. *In this interesting study, Cheyne-Stokes-like periodic breathing was produced in awake human subjects by manipulation of inspired O_2, demonstrating that instability in blood gas tensions predisposes to period breathing.*

Cherniak NS. Potential role of optimization in alveolar hypoventilation and respiratory instability. In: von Euler C, Lagercrantz H, eds. *Neurobiology of the Control of Breathing.* New York: Lippincott-Raven; 1987;45–50. *Interesting discussion of potential optimization of respiratory drive and timing to minimize sense of breathlessness, inspiratory effort, or work of breathing.*

Cherniack NS, Altose MD. Respiratory response to ventilatory loading. In: Hornbein TF, ed. *Regulation of Breathing;* part II. New York: Marcel-Dekker; 1981:905–987 (*Lung Biology in Health and Disease;* vol 17). *Important review article demonstrating the breathing responses to resistive and elastic loads.*

Cherniack NS, Longobardo GS. CO_2 and O_2 gas stores of the body. *Physiol Rev* 1970;50:196. *The definitive word on O_2 and CO_2 gas stores in the body and their importance in the control of breathing.*

Clark FJ, von Euler C. On the regulation of depth and rate of breathing.

J Physiol 1972;222. *Classic article demonstrating the role of vagal stretch receptors in breathing in anesthetized animals.*

Corda M, von Euler C, Lennerstrand G. Reflex and cerebellar influences on alpha and on "rhythmic" and "tonic" gamma activity in the intercostal muscle. *J Physiol* 1966;184:898. *Classic article demonstrating coactivation of muscle spindles and intercostal muscles and indicating that central respiratory motor drive projects to muscle spindle gamma efferents.*

Cormack RS, Cunningham DJC, Gee JBL. The effect of carbon dioxide on the respiratory response to want of oxygen in man. *Q J Exp Physiol* 1957;42:303. *Classic article demonstrating the interaction between hypercapnic and hypoxic drives in humans. Beautiful data.*

Euler C von. The functional organization of the respiratory phase-switching mechanisms. *Fed Proc* 1977;36:2375. *Early but still relevant article describing the role of vagal stretch receptors on inspiratory "off-switch" mechanisms.*

Euler C von, et al. Effects of lesions in the parabrachial nucleus on the mechanisms for central and reflex termination of inspiration in the cat. *Acta Physiol* 1976;96:324. *Study demonstrating the importance of the parabrachial nucleus (i.e., the pneumotaxic center) on inspiratory "off-switch" mechanisms.*

Feldman JL, Smith JC. Neural control of respiratory pattern in mammals: an overview. In: Dempsey J, Pack AI, eds. *Regulation of Breathing.* 2nd ed. New York: ; 1995:39–69 (*Lung Biology in Health and Disease;* vol 79). *Excellent recent review of the central control of breathing. A must for those interested in the topic.*

Feldman JL, Speck DF. Interactions among inspiratory neurons in dorsal and ventral respiratory groups in cat medulla. *J Neurophysiol* 1983;49:472. *Important neurophysiologic study demonstrating connections and functional interactions between neurons of the dorsal and ventral respiratory groups.*

Fleetham JA, Arnup ME, Anthonisen NR. Familial aspects of ventilatory control in patients with chronic obstructive pulmonary disease. *Am Rev Respir Dis* 1984;129:3. *Important study demonstrating that ventilatory and occlusion pressure responses to hypoxia are smaller in offspring of hypercapnic subjects with COPD than in offspring of eucapnic subjects. The study also shows that impaired chemosensitivity to hypoxia plays a role in the development of respiratory failure in patients with COPD.*

Gleeson K, Zwillich W, White DP. The influence of increasing ventilatory effort on arousal from sleep. *Am Rev Respir Dis* 1990;142:295. *Important study demonstrating that arousal in non-REM sleep is related to the magnitude of the inspiratory effort, and explaining why subjects wake up in the setting of airway occlusion.*

Goldring RM, et al. Respiratory adjustment to chronic metabolic alkalosis in man. *J Clin Invest* 1967;47:188. *Classic article demonstrating the effects of chronic metabolic alkalosis on the ventilatory response to hypercapnia.*

Guz A, et al. The role of vagal inflation reflexes in man and other animals. In: Poster R, ed. *Breathing: Hering-Breuer Centenary Symposium.* London: Churchill; 1970:315–336. *Excellent, still relevant discussion of the role of vagal stretch receptor reflexes in humans.*

Hanly PJ, et al. The effect of oxygen on respiration and sleep in patients with congestive heart failure. *Ann Intern Med* 1989;111:777. *Interesting study indicating that periodic breathing is extremely common in patients with congestive heart failure and is corrected with supplemental O_2.*

Hirshman CA, McCullough RE, Weil JV. Normal values for hypoxic and hypercapnic ventilatory drives in man. *J Appl Physiol* 1975;38:1095. *Important study showing wide variability in hypoxic and hypercapnic ventilatory responses in normal subjects.*

Hudgel DW, Weil JV. Asthma associated with decreased hypoxic ventilatory drive: a family study. *Ann Intern Med* 1974;80:623. *Examination of family members of an index case with asthma and respiratory failure. Family members, like index case, showed depressed ventilatory drive in response to hypoxia.*

Irsigler GB. Carbon dioxide response lines in young adults: the limits of the normal response. *Am Rev Respir Dis* 1976;114:529. *Classic study showing distribution of the ventilatory response to hypercapnia in 126 healthy African medical students.*

Kawakami Y, et al. Familial factors affecting arterial blood gas values and respiratory chemosensitivity in chronic obstructive pulmonary disease. *Am Rev Respir Dis* 1982;125:420. *Examination of arterial blood gas tension during a prolonged period in patients with COPD, showing that changes in blood gas tension in patients correlate with occlusion pressure responses to hypoxia in the adult sons.*

Kelsen SG, Altose MD, Cherniack NS. The interaction of lung volume and chemical drive on respiratory muscle EMG and respiratory timing. *J Appl Physiol* 1977;42:287. *Study demonstrating that in anesthetized animals, the distribution of respiratory motor outflow to inspiratory and expiratory muscles is determined by the interaction of chemical drive and vagal afferent activity.*

Khoo MCK, Gottschalk A, Pack AI. Sleep-induced periodic breathing and apnea: a theoretical study. *J Appl Physiol* 1991;70:2014. *Interesting theoretical study that explains the pathogenesis of periodic breathing and apnea during sleep. A must read for those interested in the sleep apnea syndrome.*

Kikuchi Y, Okabe S, Tamura G, et al. Chemosensitivity and perception of dyspnea in patients with a history of near-fatal asthma. *N Engl J Med* 1994:330:1229. *Important article suggesting that blunted respiratory responses to chemoreceptor and mechanoreceptor afferents predispose to respiratory failure and death in asthma.*

Kronenberg RS, Drage CW. Attenuation of the ventilatory and heart rate responses to hypoxia and hypercapnia in aging in normal man. *J Clin Invest* 1973;52:1812. *Study demonstrating that ventilatory responses to hypoxia and hypercapnia diminish with aging in normal humans.*

Lopez-Barneo J, et al. Chemotransduction in the carotid body: K^+ current modulated by PO_2 in type I chemoreceptor cells. *Science* 1988; 241:581. *Study of the electrophysiology of isolated type I carotid body cells that provides potential mechanism to explain depolarization of glomus cells during hypoxia.*

Milic-Emili J, Whitelaw WA, Grassino AE. Measurements and testing of respiratory drive. In: Hornbein TF, ed. *Regulation of Breathing;* part II. New York: Marcel-Dekker;1981:675–743 (*Lung Biology in Health and Disease;* vol 17). *Good review of this topic. Easy to understand.*

Mitchell RA, et al. Stability of cerebrospinal fluid pH in chronic acid-base disturbances in blood. *J Appl Physiol* 1965;20:443. *Classic article showing the relative lack of change of cerebrospinal fluid acid-base status despite changes in the arterial blood.*

Monti-Block L, Eyzaguirre C. Effects of methionine-enkephalin and substance P on chemosensory discharge of the cat carotid body. *Brain Res* 1985;338:297. *Study indicating that neuropeptides act as neurotransmitters in the carotid body to excite sensory nerve activity.*

Mountain R, Zwillich C, Weil J. Hypoventilation in obstructive lung disease: the role of familial factors. *N Engl J Med* 1978;298:521. *Classic article demonstrating that ventilatory responses to hypoxia and hypercapnia are lower in normal offspring of hypercapnic subjects with COPD than in offspring of eucapnic subjects and indicating that familial factors play a role in chemosensitivity and the pathogenesis of respiratory failure in COPD.*

Onal E, Lopata M. Periodic breathing and the pathogenesis of occlusive sleep apneas. *Am Rev Respir Dis* 1982;126:676. *Interesting study showing Cheyne-Stokes-like oscillations in the electrical activity of the tongue and diaphragm in subjects with obstructive sleep apnea.*

Pack AI. Changes in respiratory motor activity during rapid eye movement sleep. In: Dempsey JA, Pack AI, eds. *Regulation of Breathing.* 2nd ed. New York: 1995:983–1010 (*Lung Biology in Health and Disease;* vol 79). *Review article dealing with changes in respiratory muscle electrical activity during sleep and their functional importance.*

Paintal AS. The nature and effects of sensory inputs into the respiratory centers. *Fed Proc* 1977;36:2428. *Nice review of the several vagal sensory endings in the respiratory tract and their stimuli and reflex effects.*

Patrick JM, Howard A. The influence of age, sex, body size, and lung size on the control and pattern of breathing during CO_2 inhalation in Caucasians. *Respir Physiol* 1972;16:337. *Description of variables that influence the ventilatory response to CO_2 and the pattern of breathing.*

Rebuck AS, Slutsky AS. Measurement of ventilatory response to hypercapnia and hypoxia. In: Hornbein TF, ed. *Regulation of Breathing;* part II. New York: Marcel-Dekker;1981:745–904 (*Lung Biology in Health and Disease;* vol 17). *Easily understood review article. A good place to begin before attempting to make these measurements yourself.*

Shannon R. Reflexes from respiratory muscle and costovertebral joints. In: Cherniack NS, Widdicombe JG, eds. *Control of Breathing;* part I. Washington, DC: American Physiological Society; 1986:431–447 (*Handbook of Physiology;* section 3, *The Respiratory System;* vol II).

Sibuya M, et al. Effect of chest vibration on dyspnea in patients with chronic respiratory disease. *Am J Respir Crit Care* 1994;149:1235. *Interesting article demonstrating that application of in-phase vibratory stimuli to the intercostal muscle diminishes dyspnea in patients with COPD, and showing the importance of afferent information arising from the muscles of the chest wall in respiratory sensation.*

Skatrud JD, Dempsey JA. Interaction of sleep state and chemical stimuli in sustaining rhythmic ventilation. *J Appl Physiol* 1983;55:813. *Study demonstrating that mild reductions of PCO_2 consistently induce apnea in normal subjects during sleep.*

Textbook of Pulmonary Diseases, 6th ed.
edited by G.L. Baum, J.D. Crapo, B.R. Celli, and J.B. Karlinsky,
Lippincott–Raven Publishers, Philadelphia, 1998.

CHAPTER

3

Respiratory Functions of the Lung

Claude A. Piantadosi · Yuh-Chin Tony Huang

INTRODUCTION

When the human body is at rest, the lungs receive 5 L of pulmonary blood flow and nearly 5 L of fresh gas/min. The blood in the circulation exchanges metabolic gases within the lung's approximately 300 million alveoli, each of which is about 300 μm in diameter. The alveoli provide a huge surface area of approximately 75 m^2 for gas exchange, with a thickness of <0.5 μm. The alveoli are intertwined with a complex pulmonary capillary network having a surface area of approximately 50 m^2. In the pulmonary capillaries, the erythrocytes traverse the microcirculation in about three quarters of a second. Within the first third of this brief transit time, oxygen and carbon dioxide exchange is such that as the blood exits from the pulmonary capillaries, the concentrations of oxygen and carbon dioxide in the erythrocyte are in equilibrium with those of the alveoli. This system is relatively simple but highly efficient and capable of accommodating as much as a sixfold increase in the rate of blood flow and a twenty-fold increase in the rate of oxygen consumption by the body. The first portion of this chapter describes how the lungs match ventilation with blood flow to insure efficient gas exchange under normal and diseased conditions.

VENTILATION

The adult human lung is described most simply as a system containing conducting airways and the air spaces, or alveoli. The conducting airways consist of bronchi

(cartilaginous airways) and bronchioles (noncartilaginous airways), but they contain no alveoli and therefore do not participate in gas exchange. They constitute the "anatomic dead space." Generally speaking, beginning with the trachea, the conducting airways comprise the first 19 generations of bronchi, ending in terminal bronchioles (Fig. 1). Each terminal bronchiole subtends a terminal respiratory unit, or acinus. The acinus consists of respiratory bronchioles that have alveoli arising from their walls, and alveolar ducts that are lined with alveoli. These structures constitute the "respiratory zone" of the lung, and comprise generations 20 through 27 in Fig. 1. The respiratory zone makes up most of the lung, and for the adult, its volume is approximately 3000 mL.

The Weibel lung model of Fig. 1 conveniently includes some obvious simplifications. For example, some respiratory bronchioles conduct gas in series to more distal respiratory bronchioles and their alveolar ducts and alveoli. In some regions of the human lung, there are fewer than 27 bifurcations from the trachea to the alveoli, whereas other regions contain more than 27 bifurcations. This type of airway branching is known as an *irregular dichotomous pattern*. The presence of shorter pathways may be one of the mechanisms by which gas exchange is sufficient to support life even when tidal volume is less than the dead space, as occurs during high-frequency ventilation.

Despite its limitations, the simple lung model works quite well for simulating the gas exchange behavior of the lung under resting conditions. The utility of the approach is shown in Fig. 2, where the Weibel model is used to examine the nature of gas flow in the lung. The model indicates little change in the total cross-sectional area of the airways until the terminal bronchioles are reached, where the cross-sectional area increases dramatically. The physical effect of this rapid increase in cross-sectional area is to decrease the forward velocity of the

C. A. Piantadosi and Y. C. T. Huang: Division of Pulmonary and Critical Care Medicine, Duke University Medical Center, Durham, North Carolina 27710.

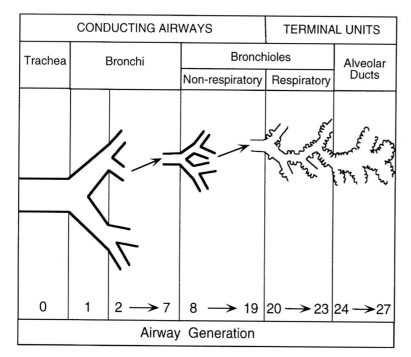

FIG. 1. Weibel's lung model. Note that generation number begins with the trachea. For details, see text. (Adapted and reprinted with permission from Weibel ER. *Morphometry of the Human Lung.* Berlin: Springer-Verlag; 1963:111.)

gas flow dramatically, such that the primary mechanism of gas transport changes from convective to "diffusive" in the regions of terminal bronchioles. Indeed, molecular diffusion of the gas phase is essentially the only mechanism of gas entry into the alveoli.

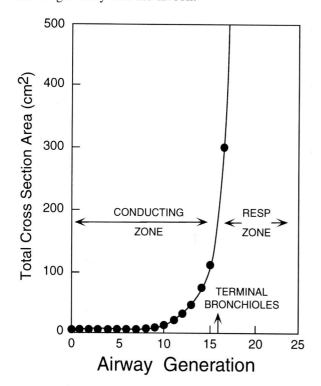

FIG. 2. Diagram of total cross-sectional area of the airways in the respiratory (*resp*) zone. The rapid increase in cross-sectional area in the respiratory zone is predicted from Weibel's model (Fig. 1). (Reprinted with permission from West JB. *Respiratory Physiology—The Essentials.* 4th ed. Baltimore: Williams & Wilkins; 1990.)

Alveolar Ventilation and Dead Space

The alveolar ventilation ($\dot{V}A$) is the amount of fresh inspired air reaching the alveoli per minute. It can be calculated by subtracting the ventilation not involved in gas exchange (dead space ventilation, $\dot{V}D$) from total ventilation (or minute ventilation, $\dot{V}E$).

$$\dot{V}A = f(V_T - V_D) = \dot{V}E - \dot{V}D$$

where f is the respiratory rate; V_T is tidal volume; and V_D is the dead space. Because an appreciable part of each tidal volume does not reach the regions of the lungs in which gas exchange occurs, this fraction of the tidal volume is exhaled largely unchanged and comprises the dead space of the breath. Therefore, it is useful to think of dead space as a fraction of the tidal volume (V_D/V_T) when evaluating the efficiency of carbon dioxide elimination.

Another way to measure the alveolar ventilation in normal subjects is by way of the alveolar ventilation equation:

$$\dot{V}A = \dot{V}CO_2/P_ACO_2 \times K$$

where $\dot{V}CO_2$ is the volume of CO_2 exhaled per minute, P_ACO_2 is the partial pressure of CO_2 in the alveoli, and K is a proportionality constant (0.863). Because in normal lungs the PCO_2 of alveolar gas and that of arterial blood ($PaCO_2$) are virtually identical, the $PaCO_2$ can be used in the equation to substitute for the P_ACO_2. The same equation also can be used in patients with underlying lung disease, but the solution would yield the "effective" alveolar ventilation. This value is not the same as the alveolar ventilation defined by the anatomic dead space. The "effective" alveolar ventilation would be the volume of fresh inspired gas involved in gas exchange with the capillary blood. Regardless of how it is measured, it is the alveolar ventilation, and not the total ventilation, that determines the effectiveness of CO_2 elimination. This principle can be illustrated by the example of a patient with severe lung disease requiring mechanical ventilation. Such a patient may require as much as 20 L/min of total ventilation to maintain an acceptable PCO_2, because the majority of the gas is used to ventilate air spaces in the lung that are not perfused with pulmonary arterial blood.

Components of the Dead Space

The *anatomic dead space* is the internal volume of the conducting airways from the nose and mouth to the terminal bronchioles. In adults, the anatomic dead space in milliliters is approximately equal to the ideal body weight in pounds. The value increases slightly as lung volume increases or with agents that relax smooth muscle and dilate the airways. Anatomic dead space is also greater during hyperventilation and during exercise, because radial traction is exerted on the bronchi by the surrounding parenchyma of the lung. This traction increases the caliber of the conducting airways.

The volume of the anatomic dead space can be determined easily by Fowler's method (Fig. 3). For this measurement, the patient takes a single inspiration of 100% oxygen, and the nitrogen concentration at the mouth is measured during a slow exhalation. Initially, pure oxygen from the dead space is measured (phase I); nitrogen con-

centration begins to rise as the dead space gas is washed out by the alveolar gas (phase II). Then, an almost uniform gas concentration is recorded, which represents alveolar gas (phase III). The nitrogen concentration of the final part of the expiration (phase IV) rises because the small airways progressively close at the bases of the lungs. The anatomic dead space is calculated by transforming phase II into an ideal square front (vertical dashed line) and determining the expired volume on the abscissa. The anatomic dead space is not measured routinely in the clinical pulmonary function laboratory because it has little diagnostic value.

Whereas anatomic dead space is determined solely by the structure of the lung, physiologic dead space represents the part of the lungs not involved in carbon dioxide elimination. It is equivalent to the "wasted" ventilation, a term preferred by some authors because physiologic dead space is neither "physiologic" nor "dead." Physiologic dead space can be calculated from the Bohr equation:

$$V_D/V_T = (P_ACO_2 - P_ECO_2)/P_ACO_2$$

where A and E refer to alveolar and mixed expired gas, respectively. In subjects with normal lungs, the PCO_2 of alveolar gas (P_ACO_2) and that of arterial blood (P_aCO_2) are virtually identical, so that the P_aCO_2 is often substituted for the P_ACO_2.

The volume of the physiologic dead space is about the same as the anatomic dead space for the normal lung. In the presence of ventilation-perfusion mismatch, however, physiologic dead space increases, mainly from ventilation

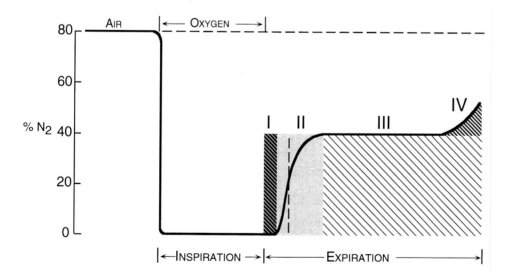

FIG. 3. A single-breath N_2 washout analysis to calculate anatomic dead space. The subject is requested to take a deep breath of O_2 and breathe out slowly and evenly. At the beginning of expiration, pure O_2 (0% N_2) is expired (phase I). This is followed with a rapidly rising N_2 concentration, which represents the washout of the remainder of the dead space gas by alveolar gas, and then by pure alveolar gas (phase III). The N_2 concentration in the last part of the expiration (phase IV) rises because of the progressive closure of the small airways at the bases of the lungs. The anatomic dead space is calculated by transforming phase II into a rectangle and determining the expired volume on the abscissa. (Reproduced with permission from Forster RE, et al., eds. *The Normal Lung: Physiological Basis of Pulmonary Function Tests.* 3rd ed. Chicago: Year Book; 1986.)

of lung units with abnormally high ventilation-perfusion ratios. The inspired air that enters these lung units is less effective in eliminating carbon dioxide from the venous blood and produces marked inefficiency of exchange between the blood and gas phases.

Distribution of Ventilation

Regional Distribution of Ventilation

In normal human lung, the alveolar ventilation is not distributed uniformly throughout the air spaces. Using a radioactive tracer gas (e.g., ^{133}Xe) to assess gas distribution, the ventilation per unit volume of the lung in normal upright individuals is found to be the greatest near the base and becomes progressively lower toward the apex. When the subject lies supine, this difference decreases, but the ventilation of the dependent (posterior) lung exceeds that of the nondependent (anterior) lung. In the lateral decubitus position, the dependent lung also is ventilated more effectively.

The topographic distribution of ventilation in the upright lung may be explained by the pleural pressure gradient (Fig. 4). Experimental studies in the upright position show that there is a gradient of intrapleural pressure of 0.6 to 0.7 cm H_2O per centimeter of vertical distance such that the intrapleural pressure is more negative in the upper compared with the lowermost regions of the lungs. The lower transpulmonary pressure (intra-alveolar pressure minus intrapleural pressure) at the base of the upright lung produces two effects: First, the volume of the alveoli at the base is lower, as indicated by the pressure-volume

curve at the bottom of Fig. 4. Second, the change in volume for a small change in transpulmonary pressure is greater, because the alveoli are operating on a steeper part of the pressure-volume curve (i.e., the compliance is greater). Thus, the ventilation measured as change in volume per resting volume is greater at the base than at the apex.

The dependent portion of the lung receives more ventilation when a breath is initiated from the functional residual capacity (FRC). If a normal subject makes a small inspiration from residual volume (RV), however, most of the ventilation goes to the apex of the upright lung. This is because the intrapleural pressures in the lowermost lung regions become positive and exceed intra-alveolar pressure, causing the small airways to close. A small decline in transpulmonary pressure that does not exceed the critical opening pressure of the small airways does not allow gas to enter the extreme base of the lung, and only the apex is ventilated (Fig. 4).

The volume at which the basal airways close on exhalation (probably in the region of the respiratory bronchioles) is called the *closing volume*. This closure occurs only at lung volumes below FRC in young normal subjects, but the lung volume at which closing begins increases with advancing age and obesity. This is one of the reasons why the dependent portions of the lungs of older and heavier individuals are more susceptible to atelectasis under conditions that decrease the FRC, such as general anesthesia.

The factors that contribute to vertical gradient of intrapleural pressure are complex. In small animals with compliant thoracic cages, the effects of gravity on the

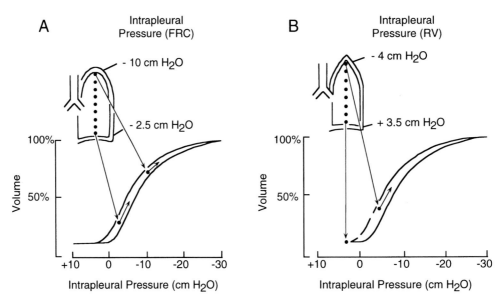

FIG. 4. The topographic distribution of ventilation of the upright lung. **A:** An inspiration from FRC. **B:** An inspiration from RV. (Reproduced with permission from West JB. *Respiratory Physiology—The Essentials.* 4th ed. Baltimore: Williams & Wilkins; 1990.)

shape of the chest wall appears to be the major determinant of the pressure gradient. In contrast, in large animals with less compliant rib cages, the weight of the lung appears to be the major factor causing the regional gradient of intrapleural pressure and, hence, regional variations in transpulmonary pressure. It also should be noted that in large animals, factors other than lung weight also contribute to the regional distribution of ventilation. For example, the vertical gradient of intrapleural pressure evident in dogs studied in the supine position disappears when they are turned to the prone position. Voluntary breathing with different groups of respiratory muscles also affects the distribution of intrapleural pressure and regional ventilation. Thus, a complete explanation for the nonuniformity of ventilation and the regional differences in intrapleural pressure should take into account the effects not only of lung weight but also of the physical stresses on the lung tissue and thorax.

Unlike the topographic distribution of ventilation, the distribution of ventilation in small regions of the lung cannot be measured easily, because it is beyond the resolution of existing external detectors, such as gamma cameras. Several physiologic factors cause uneven ventilation at the lobular or even the acinar level of the lung.

Time Constants

The time constant of a unit of the lung is determined by the product of its resistance and compliance. Lung units with different time constants inhale and exhale at different rates. A lung unit with a long time constant (i.e., greater resistance and compliance) does not completely fill by the end of inspiration and empties slowly during expiration. In contrast, a lung unit with a short time constant (i.e., smaller resistance and compliance) fills and empties rapidly. The higher the respiratory rate, the greater the discrepancy in filling and emptying between these two kinds of units, and thus the greater the inhomogeneity of ventilation.

When a lung unit with a long time constant is located adjacent to a lung unit with a short time constant, the unit with the long time constant may withdraw gas from the adjacent lung unit with a short time constant rather than fresh inspired gas. This "to and fro" behavior is known as *pendelluft,* and it can occur in abnormal lungs. In addition, a lung unit with a short time constant may receive a higher proportion of dead space gas, which reduces its alveolar ventilation. This effect is prominent in chronic obstructive lung disease, in which compliant lung units with extremely long time constants behave essentially as dead space.

Structural Asymmetry

The inherent asymmetry of the anatomy of the lung produces lung units of different sizes. As expected, smaller lung units receive greater penetration of gas by diffusion than larger units. As a consequence, incomplete mixing of gases may occur in the larger unit, a behavior functionally similar to that caused by stratified inhomogeneity (see below). This mechanism becomes most prominent in bullous lung diseases.

Stratified Inhomogeneity

Another reason for uneven ventilation of small lung units is a gradient of gas concentration along the small airways. This condition is called *stratified inhomogeneity.* Inspired gas reaches approximately the region of the terminal or respiratory bronchioles by convective flow, but gas flow over the rest of the distance to the alveoli is accomplished principally by molecular diffusion within the airways. When airway calibers are altered (e.g., in centrilobular emphysema), the process of gas diffusion may be incomplete for each breath. Thus, alveoli more distal to the conducting airways are less well ventilated than proximal alveoli.

The overall inhomogeneity of ventilation of the lung can be estimated in the laboratory using single-breath or multiple-breath washout techniques. For example, a single breath of air can be inspired containing a small concentration of a chemically inert, relatively insoluble gas (e.g., helium or methane) and then slowly and evenly exhaled into a spirometer or flow meter while concentration of the tracer gas is recorded continuously. Nonuniformity of ventilation can be assessed by measuring the slope of the alveolar plateau (phase III) in Fig. 3. A multiple-breath technique also can be used based on the rate of washout of nitrogen gas when pure oxygen is breathed (nitrogen washout). Inhomogeneity can be judged by the number of breaths required to obtain 90% of the equilibrium value compared with the number calculated assuming the tidal gas is distributed uniformly.

Factors Counteracting Ventilation Inhomogeneity

Several mechanisms tend to preserve the uniform distribution of ventilation in the lung. One of these mechanisms is the *pendelluft* phenomenon described above. Another mechanism is gas exchange through collateral air channels between adjacent lung units. *Collateral ventilation* can occur between alveoli (pores of Kohn), neighboring terminal units, contiguous lobules (canals of Lambert), and foramina of Martin. The factors affecting flow through these channels, including lung volume and the PCO_2 in alveolar gas, have been studied in several species of experimental animals. Studies in humans, however, are limited. It appears that in normal subjects breathing near FRC there is little gas flow going through collateral channels. Collateral flow becomes more important in determining the mechanical behavior and distribution of ventilation of lungs with airway obstruction.

Another factor that tends to improve uniformity of ventilation is the *interdependence* of peripheral lung units. This concept originates from the observation that contiguous lung units are attached integrally to each other by the connective tissue framework of the lung parenchyma. The behavior of one unit must therefore influence the behavior of its neighbors. This framework serves to offset the tendency for regional differences in compliance to make lung units larger or smaller than they should be for optimal performance. Finally, the pulsatile action of the heart promotes mixing of gas by imparting physical motion to the surrounding lung tissue. The effects of such *cardiogenic mixing* on distribution of ventilation, however, are probably quite small compared with the other factors mentioned above.

PERFUSION

The pulmonary circulation consists of a pump (the right ventricle), a distribution system (arteries and arterioles), a gas exchange surface (the capillary bed), and a collecting system (venules and veins). In a normal-sized adult, the pulmonary circulation contains about 500 mL of blood, of which approximately 150 mL is in the capillary bed. The capillary bed opposes the alveolar epithelium and provides an extensive interface for the uptake of oxygen and elimination of carbon dioxide. It is a readily expandable bed that can tolerate blood flow of several times the resting cardiac output with only a small rise in the pressure (Table 1).

TABLE 1. *Pulmonary and systemic hemodynamic variables during rest and moderate exercise in a normal adult man*

Condition	Rest (sitting)	Exercise
Oxygen consumption	300	2000 mL/min
Blood flow		
Cardiac output	6.3	16.2 L/min
Heart rate	70	135 beats/min
Stroke volume	90	120 mL/beat
Intravascular pressure		
Pulmonary arterial pressure	20/10	30/11 mmHg
Mean	14	20 mmHg
Left atrial pressure, mean	5	10 mmHg
Brachial arterial pressure	120/70	155/78 mmHg
Mean	88	112 mmHg
Right atrial pressure, mean	3	1 mmHg
Resistances		
Pulmonary vascular resistance	1.43	0.62 units[a]
Systemic vascular resistance	13.5	6.9 units[a]

[a] Units = mmHg/L/min.

Hemodynamic Properties of the Pulmonary Circulation

The pressure within the pulmonary circulation is quite low (about one fifth of that of the systemic circulation), although the blood flow to the lungs is comprised of the entire cardiac output. This feature of the pulmonary circulation is responsible for much of its special behavior. A comparison of pulmonary and systemic hemodynamic variables at rest in the normal adult is given in Table 1. The following three concepts about pressure in the pulmonary vessels are important to understanding the behavior of the pulmonary circulation.

Intravascular Pressure

The actual blood pressure inside the lumen of any vessel referenced to atmospheric pressure is the intravascular pressure. Some intravascular pressures, such as pulmonary arterial pressure and pulmonary venous pressure, can be measured directly by placing catheters into the bloodstream at specific points. Pulmonary capillary pressure, on the other hand, is difficult to measure directly. In fact, there is still uncertainty about the exact values of capillary pressure in the pulmonary circulation. Obviously, as blood flows from the pulmonary arterioles through the capillaries to the pulmonary venules, the capillary pressure must be less than arteriolar and greater than venular pressure. In clinical practice, capillary pressure can be estimated by wedging a catheter into a lobar branch of pulmonary artery. The "wedge" pressure measured under conditions of "no flow" reflects pressure downstream within the vascular network at the site of the next freely communicating channels, that is, pulmonary capillaries or small pulmonary venules.

Transmural Pressure

Transmural pressure is the difference between the pressure inside a vessel and the pressure in the tissue around it (perivascular pressure). Transmural pressure is related to the diameter of the vascular lumen. For example, the pressure around the pulmonary arteries and veins is approximately equal to the intrapleural pressure. The pressure around the capillaries is approximately the intra-alveolar pressure. It is this difference in transmural pressure that leads to the different behavior of alveolar and extra-alveolar vessels under conditions such as lung inflation (discussed later). At the capillary level, the transmural pressure is also an important determinant of the rate of transudation of fluid across the capillary bed.

Pulmonary Driving Pressure

Driving pressure is the difference in intravascular pressure between one point in a vessel and another point downstream. It is the pressure involved in overcoming the frictional resistance that impedes blood flow between two points. The driving pressure for the pulmonary circulation is the difference between the intravascular pressure in the main pulmonary artery and that immediately after the pulmonary circulation in the left atrium.

It is important to recognize the differences among these three pressures. For example, if mean pulmonary arterial pressure is 15 mmHg and mean left atrial pressure is 5 mmHg, the driving pressure across the lung would be 10 mmHg (15 − 5). In the presence of mitral stenosis, the mean left atrial pressure may rise to 20 mmHg and the mean pulmonary pressure to 30 mmHg. In this case, the driving pressure for the pulmonary circulation remains at 10 mmHg, but the behavior of the circulation has changed dramatically. The work of the right ventricle has doubled and the transmural pressure at each point along the pulmonary circulation is increased (assuming no change in extravascular pressures), so that pulmonary edema is more likely to develop. There are also situations in which increased pulmonary arterial pressure is associated with normal pulmonary capillary pressure (e.g., primary pulmonary hypertension). In such cases, there is unusually high resistance in the arteries or arterioles. There may be evidence of severe right ventricular strain and failure without an additional tendency for fluid transudation across the pulmonary capillary bed.

Because the pulmonary circulation is a low-pressure system, the pulmonary arteries, both large and small, contain much less smooth muscle than comparable vessels in the systemic circulation. Two exceptions to this generalization occur in the normal lung. One exists in the fetus, where the pulmonary artery connects with the aorta via the patent ductus arteriosus, and therefore the pulmonary artery is exposed to systemic pressures. Another exception occurs in long-term residents of high altitudes, who have elevated pulmonary arterial pressures through the mechanism of chronic hypoxic pulmonary vasoconstriction. As a consequence, these individuals have increased amounts of smooth muscle in the walls of their pulmonary arteries. The extension of vascular smooth muscle into distal pulmonary arteries is found in arterioles as small as 20 μm in diameter.

Different segments of the pulmonary vessels are subject to different perivascular pressures, which strongly influences their internal calibers. This effect occurs because intravascular pressures in the pulmonary circulation are low and vascular diameter depends heavily on transmural pressure. Extrapulmonary vessels are exposed to subcostal pleural pressure modified by local mechanical effects. These extrapulmonary vessels include the large pulmonary arteries and pulmonary veins. Intrapulmonary vessels, on the other hand, can be exposed to perivascular pressures ranging from those at the pleura to those at the alveolus, depending on their anatomic location.

Intrapulmonary Vessels

Differences in the behavior of intrapulmonary vessels were first observed by Macklin, who showed that the volume of the larger vessels increased with lung inflation and decreased with deflation. These observations were extended by Howell and associates, who used the surface tension differential produced by kerosene to separate larger from smaller vessels. These investigators observed that positive-pressure inflation of the lungs compressed small vessels, which were not filled by kerosene, while larger kerosene-containing vessels were expanded.

Intrapulmonary vessels can be divided into alveolar, corner, and extra-alveolar vessels, depending on the perivascular pressures to which they are exposed. The *alveolar vessels* are largely capillaries contained within the interstitium that separates adjacent alveoli. The pressure to which they are exposed is very close to alveolar pressure. When the lung expands, the alveolar walls unfold and the connective tissue elements around them are rearranged. This process compresses the alveolar vessels.

Corner vessels are located at sites where three alveoli meet and therefore are insulated from the surrounding alveolar pressure. These corner vessels are usually about 30 μm in diameter. Morphologic evidence suggests that corner vessels are contained within pleats in the alveolar septa. At low lung volume, the cell structures and connective tissue elements are displaced inward away from the surface of the alveoli. Thus, the enfolded capillaries behave like extra-alveolar vessels, because they are not exposed to alveolar pressure. When the septa unfold, however, the same capillaries behave like alveolar vessels, because the pressure around them is now much closer to the pressure in the adjacent alveoli. Functionally, such corner vessels are probably the vessels that remain open in the zone 1 lung (see below).

The *extra-alveolar vessels,* by definition, are vessels not affected by changes in alveolar pressure but that do enlarge during lung inflation. These vessels can be arteries, arterioles, veins, venules, or precapillaries. The key anatomic feature of the extra-alveolar vessels is their location within a perivascular interstitial space surrounded by a connective tissue sheath. Measurements of pressure with micropipettes inserted into the perivascular interstitial spaces have revealed pressures that are slightly more negative than pleural pressure. The perivascular interstitial pressures become even more negative as the lungs inflate, resulting in dilation of extra-alveolar vessels.

Pressure-Flow Relationships in the Lung

In the upright position, the relationship between pressure and flow in the normal pulmonary circulation is not linear. This is a consequence of the distensibility of the vessels and recruitment of additional vessels when flow is increased. This principle is readily demonstrated in the isolated lung preparation. If pulmonary blood flow is plotted against pulmonary arterial pressure while pulmonary venous pressure and transpulmonary pressure (alveolar pressure minus intrapleural pressure) are held constant (thus fixing lung volume), the slope of the line describing the pulmonary vascular resistance decreases until it reaches a constant value.

Two mechanisms are responsible for the fall in pulmonary vascular resistance in the above system. These are vascular recruitment, that is, the opening of previously closed blood vessels, and distention, or an increase in the caliber of the open vessels. Figure 5 shows experimental data from lungs (of dogs) quick frozen in situ that indicate the importance of recruitment as the pulmonary arterial pressure is raised from low values. The number of open capillaries per millimeter of length of alveolar wall increased from about 25 to >50 as the pulmonary arterial pressure was raised from 0 to nearly 15 cm H_2O. Figure 5 also shows the importance of distention of pulmonary capillaries. The mean width of the capillaries increased from about 3.5 to nearly 7 μm as the capillary pressure was increased to approximately 50 cm H_2O. Beyond that, very little change in diameter occurs with increases in pressure.

The mechanisms of recruiting pulmonary capillaries are not fully understood. As the pulmonary arterial pressure is increased, it has been suggested that the critical opening pressures of various arterioles are overcome successively. In a dense network of numerous interconnected capillary segments, it can be shown that individual capillary segments require a very small critical pressure before flow begins. Because the network contains a distribution of these critical pressures, recruitment can occur over a large range of arterial pressures. For example, in a network with as many elements as the human pulmonary capillary bed, a critical pressure on the order of only 0.02 cm H_2O for individual segments would be required to recruit vessels over a range of arterial pressures from 0 to 30 cm H_2O. Such a very small critical pressure could result from the basic flow properties of blood, especially when red blood cells fill the capillary lumen.

Just where and how critical opening occurs in pulmonary microvessels is debatable. The variation in red blood cell concentration within areas supplied by single arterioles is probably sufficient to account for the variation between areas supplied by different arterioles. This suggests that recruitment may occur at the capillary rather than the arteriolar level. This would be consistent with the notion that blood flow to the gas-exchanging regions of the lung is regulated at the alveolar level. Thus, under special conditions (e.g., regional gas trapping and edema), closure of alveolar vessels by pericapillary forces may divert blood flow from one pulmonary capillary to another.

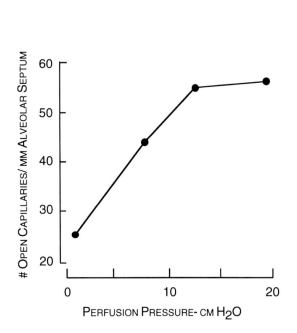

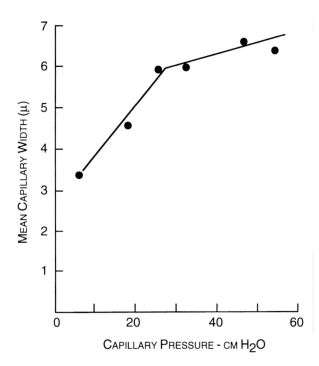

FIG. 5. Left panel: Importance of recruitment of pulmonary capillaries as the pulmonary arterial pressure is raised. (Reproduced with permission from Warrell DA, Evans JW, Clarke RO, Kingaby GP, West JB. Pattern of filling in the pulmonary capillary bed. *J Appl Physiol* 1972;32:346–356.)
Right panel: Importance of distention of pulmonary capillaries as their pressure is increased. (Reproduced with permission from Glazier JB, Hughes JMB, Maloney JE, West JB. Measurements of capillary dimensions and blood volume in rapidly frozen lungs. *J Appl Physiol* 1969;26:65–76.)

The mechanism by which pulmonary capillaries distend is related simply to the ability of the alveolar wall to bulge when the transmural pressure is raised in the capillaries. It has sometimes been argued that the mechanism of distention of pulmonary capillaries cannot be analogous to the behavior of some systemic capillaries. For example, in frog mesentery, the intracapillary pressure can be raised to 100 mmHg without measurable distention. This apparent capillary rigidity, however, can be explained by the support offered by the surrounding interstitial tissue rather than by the stiffness of the capillary walls themselves. This kind of support for the capillaries by the interstitial tissue is lacking in the alveolar region of the lung. One analogy sometimes used to describe the pulmonary capillary network is that of Swiss cheese: the open holes are supported by the cheese around them. Indeed, photomicrographs of pulmonary capillaries in rapidly frozen lungs at high intracapillary pressures show remarkable distention. This finding supports the notion that pulmonary capillaries are passively distensible with increased transmural pressure.

When the capillary pressure is raised to very high levels, the capillary walls are damaged. This damage allows protein or red blood cells to leak out, causing high-permeability pulmonary edema or even frank hemorrhage. In rabbits, this occurs at a capillary transmural pressure of about 40 mmHg, and the ultrastructural changes in the lungs include disruption of the capillary endothelial layer, the alveolar epithelial layer, or both. Because the calculated stress across the interstitium is very high under these conditions, the phenomenon is known as *stress failure*.

There are five conditions in which stress failure of capillaries may be involved. These are as follows: (1) Increased pressure causes high-permeability edema—for example, neurogenic pulmonary edema or high-altitude pulmonary edema (HAPE)—in which the pulmonary edema is of the high-permeability type despite an increased capillary pressure. In neurogenic pulmonary edema, the increased capillary pressure is related to excessive sympathetic activity. In HAPE, intense hypoxic vasoconstriction raises pressure in small pulmonary arterioles. The vasoconstriction, however, is heterogeneous, and some capillaries are not protected by arterial constriction and are exposed to high pressure. The stress failure hypothesis in HAPE is supported by the patchy distribution of pulmonary edema and the observation that exercise at high altitude is a provocative factor. (2) Increased pressure causes hemorrhage—for example, exercise-induced pulmonary hemorrhage in race horses and possibly top-notch human athletes. Pulmonary systolic pressures as high as 120 mmHg can develop in race horses while galloping. The fact that increased capillary pressure causes bleeding rather than high-permeability edema may be related to the very abrupt rise in pressure. (3) Increased pressure causes edema and hemorrhage—for example, in mitral stenosis and pulmonary veno-occlusive disease. (4)

Overinflation or hyperinflation of the lung increases the longitudinal tension in the alveolar wall, some of which is transmitted to the capillary wall. This could explain the increased capillary permeability at high lung volumes. The increased permeability is caused by high lung volume rather than alveolar pressure, because banding the chest prevents the increased permeability. (5) In cases of an abnormal extracellular matrix—for example, Goodpasture's syndrome—the strength of the capillary wall is diminished by the attack by antibodies on the collagen of the basement membrane. Alveolar hemorrhage may occur even at normal vascular pressures.

Pulmonary Vascular Resistance

A variety of approaches have been used to measure changes in pulmonary vascular resistance *in vivo*. These include measurement of pressure-flow curves and the pressure gradient across the pulmonary vascular bed at end-diastole. Pulmonary vascular resistance for the pulmonary circulation is calculated from the following equation:

$$R = (P_{pa} - P_{pv})/\dot{Q}$$

where R is pulmonary vascular resistance; P_{pa} is mean pulmonary arterial pressure (mmHg); P_{pv} is mean pulmonary venous pressure (mmHg; often the pulmonary wedge pressure is used), and $\dot{Q}$ is pulmonary blood flow (L/min). For the normal pulmonary circulation the value for R is approximately 2.0 mmHg/L/min. To express pulmonary vascular resistance in dynes sec^{-1} cm^{-5}, the numerator of the equation is multiplied by 80 (1.332×60 sec); the normal value is then ≈ 160.

Although the resistance equation has the form of Ohm's Law for electrical circuits (voltage difference divided by current flow), the resistance of an electrical resistor does not depend on either the voltage drop or the flow of current. This is not true for the pulmonary vascular resistance, which is affected by both driving pressure and blood flow. For example, in the normal pulmonary circulation, as pulmonary arterial pressure is increased at constant left atrial pressure, pulmonary vascular resistance falls. Of course, this is associated with an increase in pulmonary blood flow (Fig. 6). Also, pulmonary vascular resistance decreases when venous pressure is raised (with pulmonary arterial pressure held constant). In this case, however, pulmonary blood flow decreases (Fig. 6). Thus, it should be apparent that a single value for pulmonary vascular resistance is an incomplete description of the pressure-flow properties of the pulmonary circulation. Nonetheless, pulmonary vascular resistance measurements are useful in clinical practice for the diagnosis of pulmonary vascular diseases and for monitoring therapeutic interventions.

In humans, the pressure drop across the pulmonary

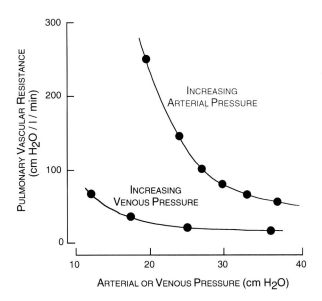

FIG. 6. Relationship between pulmonary vascular resistance and pulmonary arterial or venous pressure. Experiments in a dog lung preparation in which one pressure was changed while the other was held constant. (Reproduced with permission from West JB. *Respiratory Physiology—The Essentials.* 4th ed. Baltimore: Williams & Wilkins; 1990.)

vascular bed is ≈10% of the pressure drop across the systemic circulation. Different approaches have been used to determine the pattern of pressure drop along the pulmonary blood vessels. These include measuring the transudation pressure on the pleural surface of isolated lung; measuring the pressure transient resulting from the injection of a bolus of low- or high-viscosity blood into the pulmonary artery; measuring transient pressure following rapid occlusion of the venous outflow, the arterial inflow, or both; determining pressure-flow curves under zone 2 conditions, and direct puncture of different-sized vessels along with direct measurement of hydrostatic pressure. The values obtained from the various measurements are surprisingly consistent; in the normal lung, precapillary and postcapillary resistances are about equal, favoring a slightly higher precapillary resistance. Morphologically, the major site of pulmonary vascular resistance is in the small muscular arteries (100–1000 μm) and arterioles (<100 μm), because the cross-sectional area of the vascular network expands suddenly at the precapillary level.

Effect of Lung Volume on Vascular Resistance

The pulmonary vascular resistance depends greatly on the degree of inflation of the lung. The relationship between lung volume and pulmonary vascular resistance is shown in Fig. 7. The *solid line* in Fig. 7 indicates the total vascular resistance. *Two dashed lines* denote vascular resistances contributed by alveolar and extra-alveolar vessels. The lung normally operates near the minimal

value of vascular resistance, which occurs at approximately FRC. Both increases and decreases in lung volume from the resting position are associated with increased resistance to blood flow. As shown in Fig. 7, increasing pulmonary vascular resistance with decreasing lung volume results mainly from increases in the resistance of extra-alveolar vessels. This is most likely related to the decrease in caliber of the extra-alveolar vessels caused by decreases in the forces of radial traction exerted by the surrounding parenchyma. At states of high lung inflation, the increase in pulmonary vascular resistance is probably caused by distortion of the pulmonary capillaries. This distortion increases the resistance of blood moving through it. Direct measurements on frozen lungs of dogs show that the average width of the capillaries decreases greatly at high levels of lung inflation.

Active Versus Passive Modulators of Pulmonary Vascular Resistance

Pulmonary vascular resistance is modulated by various factors that can be divided conveniently into "passive" and "active" processes. Passive factors change the caliber of pulmonary blood vessels without a significant response in the tone of vascular smooth muscle. Table 2 summarizes the pertinent passive factors. Of these passive factors, the effect of blood viscosity on pulmonary vascular resistance is the most difficult to quantify, but it ap-

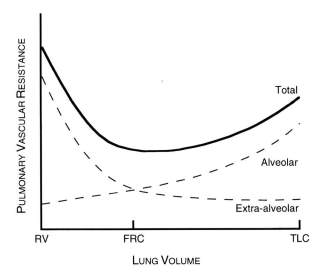

FIG. 7. Relationship between lung volume and pulmonary vascular resistance. The effects of changes in vital capacity on total pulmonary vascular resistance and the contributions to the total afforded by alveolar and extra-alveolar vessels are depicted. Note that changes in total pulmonary vascular resistance form a U-shaped curve during lung inflation, with the nadir at FRC. *RV*, residual volume; *TLC*, total lung capacity. (Reprinted with permission from Murray JF. *The Normal Lung.* 2nd ed. Philadelphia: WB Saunders; 1986.)

TABLE 2. *Factors causing "passive" changes in pulmonary vascular resistance and direction of responses*

Factor	Response
Pulmonary arterial pressure (P_{PA})	Increased P_{PA} causes decreased PVR
Left atrial pressure (P_{LA})	Increased P_{LA} causes decreased PVR
Transpulmonary pressure (P_i)	Increase and decrease of P_i from value at FRC cause increased PVR
Total interstitial pressure (P_{is})	Increased P_{is} causes increased PVR
Pulmonary blood volume	Shift of blood from systemic vessels into lung vessels causes decreased PVR
Whole-blood viscosity	Increase in viscosity causes increased PVR

PVR, pulmonary vascular resistance; FRC, functional residual capacity.

pears to depend on the capillary hematocrit, the physical properties of red blood cells, and the composition of plasma. In the isolated lung, as hematocrit increases, progressively greater pressure is required to overcome the contribution of blood viscosity to resistance and to maintain the blood flow. In contrast, active factors alter pulmonary vascular resistance by contracting or relaxing the smooth muscles of blood vessel walls. These factors can be humoral, neural, or chemical in nature. Some of the important active factors are shown in Table 3.

The pulmonary circulation is exposed constantly to passive influences, making it sometimes difficult to demonstrate that changes in pulmonary vascular resistance are caused by active pulmonary vasoconstriction or dilation. Notable exceptions occur when the vasomotor responses are opposite to and prevail over responses to passive factors. Similarly, changes in pulmonary arterial pressure alone cannot be interpreted as indicating changes in pulmonary vascular resistance unless left atrial pressure and cardiac output are known.

Advanced lung diseases such as pulmonary fibrosis and pulmonary emphysema can cause increases in pulmonary vascular resistance and thus pulmonary hypertension. Pulmonary vasoconstriction is caused by alveolar hypoxia, but distortion of lung architecture by the disease processes and increased interstitial fluid in the perivascular spaces of the extra-alveolar vessels (pulmonary edema) also play important roles. When edema is severe, fluid also may accumulate in the interstitium of the alveolar wall, thus encroaching on alveolar vessels and increasing their vascular resistance.

Distribution of Perfusion

The distribution of pulmonary blood flow can be measured with tracer methods. Radioactive carbon dioxide

($C^{15}O_2$) was the first test substance to be used to study the distribution of pulmonary blood flow. After the tracer gas is breathed into the lung, regional perfusion can be determined by monitoring the disappearance of the gas, whose uptake from alveoli depends on the blood flow to the alveoli. Insoluble tracer gases such as ^{133}Xe also can be dissolved in saline solution and injected into a peripheral vein. When the xenon reaches the pulmonary capillaries, it is transferred into the alveolar gas. The tracer pattern within the lung then reflects the perfusion of gas-filled alveoli in various regions. The distribution of blood flow also can be measured with labeled particles, such as radioactive- or fluorescent-labeled microspheres. These particles are sized appropriately to be trapped within small pulmonary vessels as they pass into the pulmonary circulation.

Each of these procedures has advantages and disadvantages, but all have detected the presence of a vertical gradient of blood flow in a normal upright lung. The vertical gradient is largely the consequence of differences in hydrostatic pressure in the pulmonary circulation associated with gravity. As the adult upright human lung is about 30 cm high, the hydrostatic difference in pressure between the extreme apex and the bottom of the base can be as much as 30 cm of blood (23 mmHg). This means that the intravascular pressure in vessels at the lung base can be higher than that in apical vessels by as much as 23 mmHg. When the pulmonary venous pressure and intra-alveolar pressure are held constant, this translates to

TABLE 3. *Important causes of "active" changes in pulmonary vascular resistance and direction of responses*

Factor	Response
Neurogenic stimuli	
Sympathetic stimulation	Increases PVR in experimental animals; no effect in humans
Parasympathetic stimulation	Decreases PVR in experimental animals with pre-existing vasoconstriction; no effect in humans
Humoral stimuli	
Norepinephrine, serotonin, histamine, angiotensin, fibrinopeptides, prostaglandin $F_{2\alpha}$	Vasoconstriction
Acetylcholine, bradykinin, prostaglandin E_1, prostacyclin (prostaglandin I_2)	Vasodilation; bradykinin affects humans with pulmonary hypertension
Nitric oxide	Vasodilation
Chemical stimuli	
Alveolar hypoxia	Increases PVR
Alveolar hypercarbia	Increases PVR in experimental animals; no effect in humans
Acidemia (decreased pH)	Increases PVR

PVR, pulmonary vascular resistance.

a greater transmural pressure for the vessels at the base. As a result, the diameter of blood vessels at the base of the lung is greater and more blood flows through them. The difference between apical and basal blood flow no longer exists when the lung is supine, but a perfusion gradient can be detected between the independent (uppermost) and dependent (lowermost) regions of the lung. In the upright position, exercise increases apical blood flow more than basal blood flow because of the recruitment of collapsed vessels (West zone 1; see below), and the perfusion gradient is reduced greatly.

Gravity-Dependent Distribution of Blood Flow

The intravascular pressures of the pulmonary circulation are influenced by the hydrostatic pressure created by gravity. As alveolar pressure is relatively independent of gravity, the relationships among pulmonary arterial, pulmonary venous, and alveolar pressures must also influence the distribution of pulmonary blood flow. This principle was predicted by Dock. West subdivided the lung into four zones with differing patterns of blood flow. Figure 8 shows this zonal distribution.

Zone 1 is the region of the lung wherein alveolar pressure exceeds both the pulmonary arterial and venous pressures. In zone 1, the alveolar vessels are collapsed and there is no pulmonary blood flow. In the presence of corner vessels that are protected from alveolar pressure, however, some flow still occurs in this zone.

Zone 2 is the part of the lung in which pulmonary arterial pressure exceeds alveolar pressure, but alveolar pressure exceeds venous pressure. Under these conditions, the resistance to blood flow is determined by the difference between pulmonary arterial and alveolar pressures, rather than by the expected arterial-venous pressure difference. This behavior has been referred to variously as the *waterfall* or *sluice effect* and can be simulated in a Starling resistor model made of rubber tubing. The flow properties of capillaries, however, are very different from those of a Starling resistor. For one thing, capillary flow tends to be laminar. This differs from the Starling resistor, which usually oscillates and creates turbulent flow. In addition, the capillaries contain trains of red blood cells that essentially fill the diameter of the small vessels. These vessels cannot collapse in the same way as a rubber tube. Nevertheless, the lung in zone 2 conditions has essentially the same pressure-flow characteristics as a

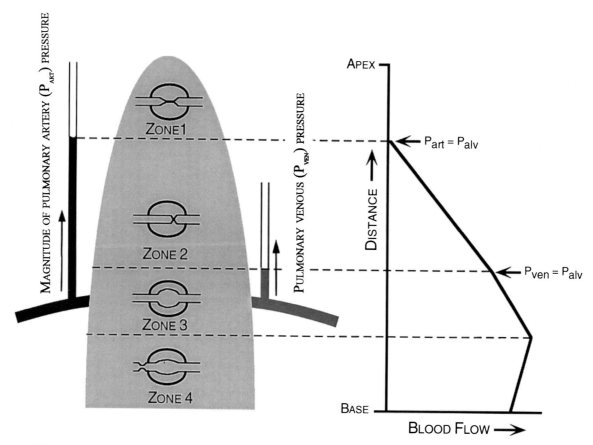

FIG. 8. Schematic representation of the four zones of the lungs in which different hemodynamic conditions govern blood flow. Alveolar pressure (P_{alv}) is assumed to be 0; the heights of the *blue column* and the *red column* represent the magnitude of pulmonary arterial (P_{art}) and pulmonary venous (P_{ven}) pressures, respectively. (Reprinted with permission from Hughes JM, et al. Effect of lung volume on the distribution of pulmonary blood flow in man. *Respir Physiol* 1968;4:58–72.)

Starling resistor. Also in zone 2, blood flow increases progressively down the lung because of the increasing hydrostatic effect on pulmonary arterial pressure, which increases the driving pressure in this region (pulmonary arterial pressure minus alveolar pressure).

Zone 3 is the part of the lung in which pulmonary venous pressure exceeds alveolar pressure. Blood flow also increases down this zone, although the rate of increase in relation to distance is less than in zone 2. Because the arterial-venous pressure difference is responsible for flow and is constant, it is not immediately apparent why blood flow would increase down this zone. Because the transmural pressure across the vessel wall increases with distance down zone 3, however, pulmonary arterial and venous pressures both increase while alveolar pressure remains constant. Thus, if the vessels are distensible, their caliber will increase and their vascular resistance will decrease down the zone. Indeed, micrographs of rapidly frozen lung confirm an increase in vessel caliber down zone 3. It is also possible that retrograde recruitment of capillaries contributes to the increase in blood flow.

In zone 4, the relationships between intravascular and alveolar pressures are the same as in zone 3, but the blood flow decreases. Zone 4 occurs in the lowermost region of the upright human lung and diminishes as lung volume increases. Conversely, as lung volume decreases, this region of reduced blood flow extends farther and farther up the lung, so that at FRC blood flow decreases progressively down the bottom half of the lung. At residual volume, zone 4 extends nearly all the way up the lung, so that blood flow at the apex exceeds that at the base. This condition obviously cannot be explained by the interactions among the pulmonary arterial, venous, and alveolar pressures. Instead, the reduced blood flow in zone 4 can be attributed to narrowing of extra-alveolar vessels at the lung base that results from lower lung inflation. The increased contribution of extra-alveolar vessels to pulmonary vascular resistance results in the presence of a zone of reduced blood flow in that region. This explanation is supported by the observation that vasoconstrictor drugs such as serotonin cause zone 4 to extend farther up the lung. The opposite effect is seen when vasodilator drugs are infused into the pulmonary circulation.

Zone 4 would be expected to increase in the presence of interstitial pulmonary edema, because the edematous fluid increases interstitial pressure in the vascular sheath and thereby narrows the extra-alveolar vessels. This is a plausible mechanism for the inverted distribution of blood flow (cephalization of pulmonary vasculature on chest x-ray) in pulmonary edema. The interaction of interstitial edema with blood flow distribution, however, remains poorly understood.

Gravity-Independent Distribution of Blood Flow

Not all the inhomogeneity of blood flow in the lung can be explained by gravitational effects. In normal people flying Keplerian arcs in aircraft, where periods of up to 25 sec of microgravity are possible, much of the normal topographic inhomogeneity disappears. Indirect measurements of inhomogeneity of pulmonary blood flow have been made in astronauts in space shuttles by monitoring the magnitude of cardiogenic oscillations on the expired carbon dioxide tracing. A striking reduction in inhomogeneity of blood flow was detected during weightlessness compared with that observed in the upright posture before or after the flight. Interestingly, substantial inhomogeneity of blood flow still remained, indicating that some gravity-independent mechanism was also present. Variations in the length of the pathways from the main pulmonary artery to the terminal respiratory units and variations within a single terminal respiratory unit may contribute to this process. The unequal length of pathways leads to different transit times for red blood cells and earlier perfusion of first-order respiratory bronchioles and their alveoli than of the more distal ones. Another suggestion is that regions of intrinsically high resistance (low conductance) exist normally because of differences in caliber or geometric features of the pulmonary vascular bed. Evidence for this has been obtained in isolated dog lungs. It also has been suggested that isogravitational inhomogeneity of blood flow can be explained by fractal geometry. According to this concept, the inhomogeneity is a consequence of a fractal configuration of vascular branching that is replicated from larger to smaller blood vessels. Such a fractal model might also explain the radial gradient of perfusion and the regional differences in conductance mentioned above.

Pulmonary Blood Flow in Cardiopulmonary Diseases

The normal distribution of pulmonary blood flow is altered by many cardiopulmonary diseases. The redistribution of blood flow frequently increases mismatching of ventilation and perfusion and may result in hypoxemia or increases in dead space (see below, Ventilation-Perfusion Distribution and Gas Exchange). For example, localized structural lung disease resulting in the formation of bullae or cysts usually causes local reductions in flow. The same is also true of pulmonary embolism, in which the local blood flow is obstructed by the presence of clots. Such abnormalities of perfusion are usually coupled with normal ventilation and hence increase the dead space. This pattern of ventilation-perfusion abnormality provides an important diagnostic clue on ventilation-perfusion scan. The blood flow to the lung on the side of a pneumothorax may be compromised because of compression or kinking of large or small pulmonary vessels. Blood flow may be reduced to some parts of the lung because of destruction of the pulmonary vasculature or distortion of pulmonary vascular geometry in diffuse lung diseases such as pulmonary fibrosis or chronic obstructive pulmonary disease.

In patients with pulmonary hypertension or increased blood flow secondary to left-to-right shunts, the blood flow is usually distributed more uniformly. During severe hypotension and circulatory shock, perfusion to the lung apices is reduced significantly. Increased pulmonary venous pressure, as in mitral stenosis, initially causes a more uniform distribution than normal. In more advanced disease, inversion of the normal distribution of blood flow is frequently seen, with more perfusion to the upper than to the lower lung zones. The mechanism for this shift is not understood fully, but, as indicated earlier, it may be related to perivascular edema causing an increased resistance within the extra-alveolar vessels.

Control of the Pulmonary Circulation

The distribution of pulmonary blood flow and the pressure-flow relations of the pulmonary circulation are highly influenced by the ''passive'' factors shown in Table 2. Thus, gravity and the mechanisms of recruitment and distention can account for most of the behavior of the normal circulation. By contrast, when the amount of smooth muscle is increased—for example, in the lungs of fetuses, of long-term residents of high altitudes, or of patients with prolonged pulmonary hypertension—''active'' regulatory factors begin to play a more significant role in the control of the pulmonary circulation.

One example of active control of the pulmonary circulation is hypoxic pulmonary vasoconstriction. The precise mechanism of this response is unknown. It clearly does not depend on central nervous system input, as it occurs in excised isolated lungs. Furthermore, the local action of hypoxia on the artery itself is important, because excised segments of pulmonary artery can be shown to constrict in hypoxic environments. It is also known that hypoxic pulmonary vasoconstriction can be elicited by lowering the partial pressure of oxygen (PO_2) in the alveolar gas or mixed venous blood.

The stimulus-response curve for hypoxic pulmonary vasoconstriction is very nonlinear. When the alveolar PO_2 is altered in the region above 100 mmHg, little change in vascular resistance is seen; however, when alveolar PO_2 is reduced to 60 mmHg, vasoconstriction may occur. At PO_2 values approaching that of mixed venous blood, local blood flow may be almost abolished. The intensity of hypoxic vasoconstriction varies from subject to subject, among different species, and in different parts of the same lung.

The site of hypoxic vasoconstriction is still not certain, but some evidence suggests it occurs in pulmonary pre-capillary vessels (small muscular pulmonary arteries and arterioles). Some studies also suggest alveolar vessels may be, at least in part, responsible for the increased resistance, and contractile cells have been described in the interstitium of the alveolar wall; these cells conceivably could distort capillaries and increase their resistance.

The cellular mechanisms of hypoxic pulmonary vasoconstriction remain obscure despite a great deal of research. Some chemical modulators of the response, including catecholamines, histamine, angiotensin, and prostaglandins, have been studied extensively. None of these substances, however, meets all the necessary criteria for the mediator of hypoxic pulmonary vasoconstriction. Recently, it has been suggested that inhibition of endothelium-derived relaxing factor (EDRF) or nitric oxide may be involved. As the biosynthesis of nitric oxide requires molecular oxygen, hypoxic vasoconstriction may in part represent loss of vasodilator effects normally provided by nitric oxide.

Hypoxic pulmonary vasoconstriction has the effect of directing blood flow away from hypoxic regions of lung. This tends to reduce the extent of ventilation-perfusion mismatching in diseased lungs and limits the decline in the arterial PO_2. A good illustration of this effect is seen in patients with pulmonary hypertension who are treated with systemic vasodilators, such as calcium channel blockers, in an attempt to reduce pulmonary arterial pressure. This treatment can be associated with nonspecific vasodilation that causes an increase in blood flow to poorly ventilated areas. The process may lead to a reduction in arterial PO_2. Hypoxic pulmonary vasoconstriction also occurs in both newcomers and in permanent residents of high altitudes. At altitude, the increase in pulmonary arterial pressure is especially marked during exercise. These responses result in improvement in gas exchange.

GAS EXCHANGE

The composition of normal gas changes in various lung compartments during inspiration (Fig. 9). As can be seen, the partial pressure of oxygen (PO_2) decreases as soon as the ambient gas reaches conducting airways. This is caused by warming of the inhaled air and its saturation with water vapor. These processes dilute the inspired mixture of N_2 and O_2. At body temperature of 37°C, water

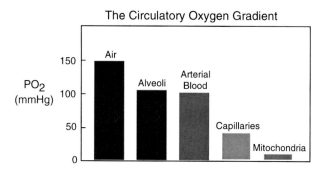

FIG. 9. The O_2 gradient from the alveolar space to the mitochondria. Note that there is a stepwise decrement in PO_2 from 100 mmHg in the alveolar space to values of a few mmHg at the mitochondria, where most of the O_2 is consumed.

vapor pressure adds 47 mmHg of pressure to dry gas. Once the inspired gas reaches the terminal respiratory units, gas exchange takes place. Slightly more O_2 is removed than carbon dioxide (CO_2) is added (at a normal respiratory exchange ratio of 0.8), which causes the volume of each gas exchange unit to diminish slightly and raises the concentration of N_2 within the alveoli slightly. The gas composition of the blood in the pulmonary capillaries leaving the alveoli is approximately the same as the gas phase of the terminal units. The PO_2 in the arterial blood is slightly lower because local matching of ventilation and perfusion in normal lungs is imperfect and unoxygenated blood is added to capillary blood from postpulmonary shunt.

Ventilation-Perfusion Distribution and Gas Exchange

Exchange of O_2 and CO_2 between blood in the pulmonary arterial system and alveolar gas occurs continuously in more than 100,000 terminal respiratory units of the lungs. The adequacy of function of each gas exchange unit is determined by local matching of ventilation and perfusion ($\dot{V}_A/\dot{Q}$). In general, inadequate ventilation relative to perfusion (i.e., low $\dot{V}_A/\dot{Q}$ regions and shunt) has the greatest effect on O_2 uptake by the lung and thus may result in hypoxemia. On the other hand, excessive ventilation relative to perfusion (i.e., high $\dot{V}_A/\dot{Q}$ regions and dead space) has more influence on CO_2 elimination by the lung and predisposes to hypercapnea.

The effects of $\dot{V}_A/\dot{Q}$ matching on the efficiency of gas exchange in the lung can be understood using the two-compartment lung model. In an ideal lung consisting of two alveolar units (A and B), each receiving 2.0 L/min of alveolar ventilation and 2.5 L/min of blood flow, the $\dot{V}_A/\dot{Q}$ ratio is 0.8 for the individual units A and B, and 0.8 for the entire lung. Assuming no barrier to diffusion of O_2 and a normal PO_2 in the pulmonary artery, the PO_2 of alveolar gas is the same as the PO_2 of end-capillary and arterial blood. There is no O_2 gradient from alveolus to capillary (alveolar-arterial PO_2 difference). A "normal" lung has a slight degree of $\dot{V}_A/\dot{Q}$ mismatch, which is caused primarily by the greater effects of gravity on the distribution of perfusion than on ventilation (Fig. 10). Thus, in the "normal" lung, while the $\dot{V}_A/\dot{Q}$ ratio for the whole lung remains at 0.8, the $\dot{V}_A/\dot{Q}$ ratios for the two units A and B are 1.0 and 0.6, respectively. This causes the mean PO_2 in the blood leaving the lung to decrease slightly and produces an alveolar-arterial PO_2 difference of 4.4 mmHg. Uneven distribution of blood flow may also result in similar effects, especially in the upright lung.

Assessment of Abnormalities in Gas Exchange

The effectiveness of gas exchange (and thus the distribution of $\dot{V}_A/\dot{Q}$ ratios) can be assessed by several methods. The simplest approach is to sample the composition of arterial blood and alveolar gas. More complicated approaches rely on tracer gases and modeling of gas exchange—for example, the multiple inert gas elimination technique. No measurement technique, however, allows an exact description of the complex behavior of gas exchange in the lung.

Arterial PO_2

The arterial PO_2 certainly provides some information about the degree of ventilation-perfusion matching. The major advantage of the measurement is its simplicity. In general, a low PO_2 almost always indicates the presence of $\dot{V}_A/\dot{Q}$ mismatch or shunt, but a normal PO_2 (greater than 80 mmHg) does not necessarily imply that the $\dot{V}_A/\dot{Q}$ distribution of the lung is "normal."

Alveolar-Arterial PO_2 Difference

The alveolar-arterial PO_2 difference ($A-aDO_2$) is calculated readily from the alveolar PO_2 (PAO_2) and the arterial PO_2 (PaO_2). The alveolar PO_2 is computed from the alveolar gas equation:

$$PAO_2 = F_IO_2 (PB - PH_2O) - (PACO_2/R)$$

where PB is barometric pressure; PH_2O is water vapor pressure at body temperature (47 mmHg at 37°C); FIO_2 is the fractional concentration of O_2 in inspired gas (0.21 in air); and R is the respiratory exchange ratio. The equation simplifies to

$$PAO_2 = FIO_2 (713) - 1.25 PaCO_2$$

by substituting the arterial for alveolar PCO_2 and 0.8 for the respiratory exchange ratio. The alveolar-arterial PO_2 difference is more informative than the arterial PO_2 alone because it takes into account the level of ventilation.

The alveolar-arterial PO_2 difference in healthy adults breathing room air increases with age. As a general rule, the alveolar-arterial PO_2 difference for an individual should be no more than half of the chronologic age, with a maximum of 25 mmHg. The alveolar-arterial PO_2 difference is caused by the combination of $\dot{V}_A/\dot{Q}$ mismatch and right-to-left postpulmonary shunting of blood. Each of these mechanisms is responsible for about half of the total alveolar-arterial PO_2 difference in normal adults. None of the alveolar-arterial PO_2 difference at normal barometric pressure is caused by failure of diffusion equilibrium to occur, even during heavy exercise. Diffusion disequilibrium may occur during exercise at high altitudes.

The alveolar-arterial PO_2 difference increases with increasing alveolar PO_2, in part because the upper part of the oxygen-hemoglobin dissociation curve is concave. The alveolar-arterial PO_2 difference reaches a maximum

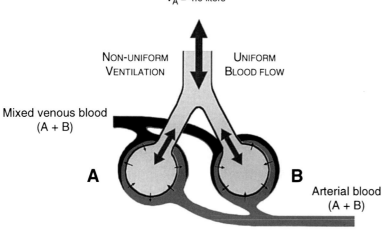

NORMAL LUNG

$\dot{V}_E$ = 6.0 liters

$\dot{V}_A$ = 4.0 liters

NON-UNIFORM VENTILATION

UNIFORM BLOOD FLOW

Mixed venous blood (A + B)

A

B

Arterial blood (A + B)

	A	B	A+B
Alveolar Ventilation (L/min)	2.5	1.5	4.0
Pulmonary Blood Flow (L/min)	2.5	2.5	5.0
Ventilation / Blood Flow Ratio	1.0	0.6	0.8
Mixed Venous O2 Saturation (%)	75.0	75.0	75.0
Arterial O2 Saturation (%)	97.8	96.4	97.1
Mixed Venous O2 Tension (mm Hg)	40.0	40.0	40.0
Alveolar O2 Tension (mm Hg)	111.0	94.0	104.6
Arterial O2 Tension (mm Hg)	111.0	94.0	100.2

FIG. 10. Ventilation-perfusion relationship of a normal lung is illustrated using a two-compartment model. Note that the ventilation-perfusion maldistribution is responsible for an alveolar-arterial PO_2 difference of about 4.4 mmHg; the remainder of the normal PO_2 difference is caused by postpulmonary shunts (ignored in this illustration). (Reproduced with permission from Forster RE, et al., eds. *The Normal Lung: Physiological Basis of Pulmonary Function Tests.* 3rd ed. Chicago: Year Book; 1986.)

and then decreases at higher PO_2. The decline in the alveolar-arterial PO_2 difference occurs when inspired PO_2 exceeds 350 to 450 mmHg, because alveolar PO_2 rises to more uniform levels despite the nonuniform distribution of $\dot{V}_A/\dot{Q}$ ratios.

Physiologic Shunt

The presence of right-to-left shunt can be differentiated from low $\dot{V}_A/\dot{Q}$ causes of hypoxemia by having the patient breathe 100% O_2. While the patient is breathing pure O_2, the alveolar PO_2 in different lung units differs according to differences in alveolar PCO_2. Lung units with low $\dot{V}_A/\dot{Q}$ ratios, even though they may be ventilated only poorly via collateral pathways or intermittently at high lung volumes, will show an increase in PO_2 nearly maximally with elevation of the inspired PO_2. This response also occurs with impairment of diffusion for O_2 between alveolar gas and capillary blood. This maneuver usually increases the arterial PO_2 to >600 mmHg. The size of the shunt can be calculated using the following equation:

$$Q_s/Q_T = (CcO_2 - CaO_2)/(CcO_2 - C\overline{v}O_2)$$

where Q_s/Q_T is the shunt as a fraction of cardiac output; CcO_2 is end-capillary O_2 content; CaO_2 is arterial O_2 content; and $C\overline{v}O_2$ is mixed venous O_2 content. End-capillary blood is assumed to have a PO_2 equal to that in the alveolar gas. The O_2 contents are measured in samples of arterial and mixed venous blood. Alternatively, a value for the arterial-mixed venous difference in O_2 content, which is relatively constant among patients, normally can be assumed to be 5 mL/dL. Healthy individuals have a small "anatomic shunt" that amounts to 2%–5% of the cardiac output. This shunt occurs because some venous blood normally drains into pulmonary veins, left atrium, or left ventricle from bronchial and myocardial (thebesian) circulation.

The use of 100% O_2 to measure Q_s/Q_T can exclude shunt as a cause of hypoxemia. The procedure does not determine the location of a shunt, which may be intracardiac or intrapulmonary. Alveoli with low $\dot{V}_A/\dot{Q}$ ratios (<0.1) also may collapse completely during O_2 breathing if O_2 diffuses into the blood faster than fresh gas is added by ventilation. These collapsed alveoli can lead to overestimation of the true shunt fraction, as they allow pulmonary arterial blood to bypass the alveoli.

Physiologic Dead Space

Whereas physiologic shunt reflects the amount of blood flow going to lung units with near-zero ventilation-perfusion ratios ($\dot{V}_A/\dot{Q} = 0$), physiologic dead space is a measure of the amount of ventilation going to units with unusually high ventilation-perfusion ratios ($\dot{V}_A/\dot{Q} \approx \infty$). The physiologic dead space can be computed from the Bohr equation:

$$V_D/V_T = (P_{A}CO_2 - P_{E}CO_2)/P_{A}CO_2$$

where V_D is physiologic dead space, V_T is tidal volume, $P_{E}CO_2$ is expired PCO_2, and $P_{A}CO_2$ is alveolar PCO_2. The $P_{A}CO_2$ is assumed to be equal to the P_aCO_2. The Bohr equation requires a measurement of mixed expired gas, which is not conveniently obtained in many clinical settings. Instead, V_D/V_T can be estimated from the $\dot{V}_E$ and P_aCO_2 using an isopleth nomogram (Fig. 11).

Distribution of Ventilation-Perfusion Ratios

It has long been recognized that the lungs must contain some sort of distribution of ventilation-perfusion ratios.

Major conceptual advances became possible with the introduction of the multiple inert gas elimination technique (MIGET). The MIGET is based on the straightforward principles governing inert gas elimination by the lung. When an inert gas in solution is steadily infused into the venous circulation, the proportion of gas that is eliminated by ventilation from the blood by a unit of the lung depends only on the solubility of the gas and the ventilation-perfusion ratio. The relationship is given by the following equation:

$$\frac{Pc'}{P\bar{v}} = \frac{\lambda}{\lambda + \dot{V}_A/\dot{Q}}$$

where Pc' is the partial pressure of the gas in end-capillary blood and λ is the blood-gas partition coefficient. The end-capillary partial pressure divided by the mixed venous partial pressure ($P\bar{v}$) is known as the *retention*.

In practice, a saline solution containing low concentrations of six gases (such as sulfur hexafluoride, ethane,

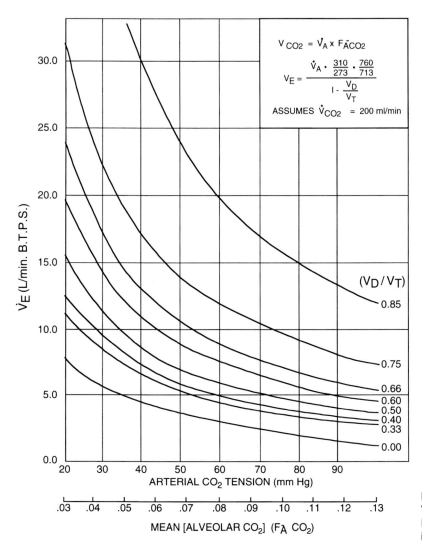

FIG. 11. An isopleth nomogram for estimating V_D/V_T from minute ventilation ($\dot{V}_E$) and arterial PCO_2. Assumptions and calculations are given in the *box in the right upper corner.*

cyclopropane, halothane or isoflurane, diethyl ether, and acetone) of differing solubilities is infused slowly into a peripheral vein until a steady state is reached (about 20 min). During measurements, simultaneous samples of arterial and mixed venous gases and expired gas are collected and analyzed for the inert gases by gas chromatography. Retention and excretion values for the inert gases are graphed against their solubility in blood, as shown in Fig. 12. The data for inert gas retention plotted against solubility are joined by a *broken line* in the upper panel of Fig. 12. Below this are the data points for excretion against solubility, also joined by the *broken line*. The *two solid lines* show how retention and excretion would behave for an ideal lung with no ventilation-perfusion maldistribution but with the same overall ventilation and

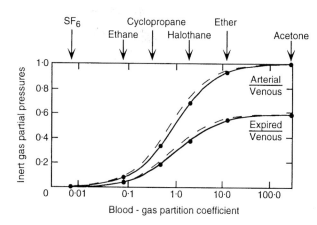

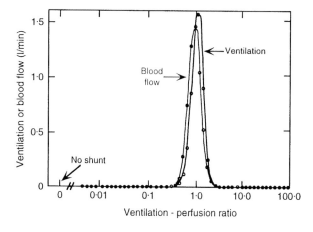

FIG. 12. Distribution of ventilation-perfusion ratios determined by the multiple inert gas elimination technique. Data from a 22-year-old normal subject are illustrated. **Upper panel:** Data points for inert gas retention (*upper curve*) and excretion (*lower curve*). Broken lines join the points. The *two solid lines* show the values of retention and excretion for a lung with no ventilation-perfusion inequality. **Lower panel:** Recovered distribution of ventilation-perfusion ratios. SF$_6$, sulfur hexafluoride. (Reproduced with permission from Wagner PD, Laravuso RB, Uhl RR, West JB. Continuous distributions of ventilation-perfusion ratios in normal subjects breathing air and 100% O$_2$. *J Clin Invest* 1974;54:53–68.)

blood flow. The *broken* and *solid lines* are very close together in normal lung (Fig. 12).

The retention-solubility plots from the MIGET contain information about the distribution of $\dot{V}A/\dot{Q}$ ratios in the lung. For example, a lung containing units that are perfused but not ventilated (shunt) will show increased retention of the least soluble gas, sulfur hexafluoride. Conversely, a lung having large amounts of ventilation to lung units with very high $\dot{V}A/\dot{Q}$ ratios will show increased retention of the high-solubility gases, ether and acetone. In practice, the distribution of ventilation-perfusion ratios that best fits the pattern of inert gas retention and excretion based on a 50-compartment model can be obtained by an iterative process using a computer.

The use of the multiple gas elimination technique requires certain assumptions about the behavior of the lung. The method assumes no diffusion barrier for O$_2$ and negligible O$_2$ consumption by the lung. The fitted $\dot{V}A/\dot{Q}$ distribution from a set of measurements is not unique, but in most cases the range of possible distributions compatible with the data is small. Also, more than three modes of a distribution can be recovered, and only smooth distributions can be obtained. Despite these limitations, the technique provides much more information about the distribution of $\dot{V}A/\dot{Q}$ ratios in patients with lung disease than was previously available. In addition, the MIGET is very sensitive. A shunt of only 0.5% of the cardiac output approximately doubles the arterial concentration of sulfur hexafluoride.

The retention and excretion solubility curves and the derived distribution of ventilation-perfusion ratios from a 22-year-old normal volunteer is shown in Fig. 12. It is apparent from Fig. 12 that the recovered distributions for both ventilation and blood flow (*lower panel*) are narrow and span only one log of ventilation-perfusion ratios. Essentially no ventilation or blood flow occurs outside the range of approximately 0.3 to 3.0 on the ventilation-perfusion ratio scale, and no significant intrapulmonary shunt (i.e., regions with blood flow but no ventilation) is detected.

In older normal subjects, the dispersion of the $\dot{V}A/\dot{Q}$ distribution has been found to increase. For example, some older people with apparently normal lungs have a ''shoulder'' to the left of the main blood flow distribution, with some 10% of the total blood flow going to lung units with ventilation-perfusion ratios of <0.1. Despite this region of low $\dot{V}A/\dot{Q}$, there may still be no shunt. The cause of such age-related $\dot{V}A/\dot{Q}$ mismatch is believed to be degenerative processes in the small airways with aging.

Ventilation-Perfusion Distributions in Lung Disease

The distribution of ventilation-perfusion ratios from a patient with chronic obstructive lung disease is shown in Fig. 13. The $\dot{V}A/\dot{Q}$ distribution is typical of that seen in

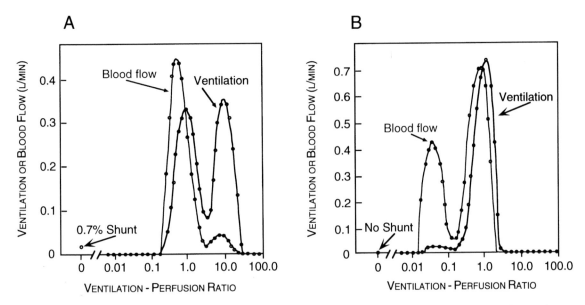

FIG. 13. Examples of the distribution of ventilation-perfusion ratios in patients with chronic obstructive pulmonary disease. **A:** Type A (patients with predominantly emphysema) tends to have areas of very high $\dot{V}_A/\dot{Q}$. **B:** Type B (patients with predominantly chronic bronchitis) often has areas of very low $\dot{V}_A/\dot{Q}$. Shunt ($\dot{V}_A/\dot{Q}$ = 0) is rarely seen in either type. (Reproduced with permission from Wagner PD, Dantzker DR, Dueck R, Clausen JL, West JB. Ventilation-perfusion inequality in chronic obstructive pulmonary disease. *J Clin Invest* 1977;59:203–216.)

patients believed to have predominantly emphysema. The $\dot{V}_A/\dot{Q}$ distribution is bimodal, and large amounts of ventilation go to lung units with extremely high $\dot{V}_A/\dot{Q}$ ratios (alveolar dead space) (Fig. 13A). Presumably, the high $\dot{V}_A/\dot{Q}$ regions reflect ventilation to lung units in which many capillaries have been destroyed by the emphysematous process. The presence of a small shunt (3.1%) and slight shift to the left of the main mode of blood flow can explain mild arterial hypoxemia found in this patient (PaO_2 of 63 mmHg).

Patients with chronic obstructive lung disease who have predominantly bronchitis generally show a different pattern of $\dot{V}_A/\dot{Q}$ distribution (Fig. 13B). The main abnormality in these patients is the large amount of blood flow distributed to lung units with very low $\dot{V}_A/\dot{Q}$ ratios, between 0.003 and 0.1, explaining the more severe hypoxemia generally found in this type of patient. Presumably, the low ventilation-perfusion ratios in chronic bronchitis are the result of diseased airways blocked by retained secretions. It also should be emphasized that the $\dot{V}_A/\dot{Q}$ distributions found in severe chronic bronchitis show considerable variability.

Ventilation-Perfusion Mismatch and Carbon Dioxide Retention

It is important to appreciate that ventilation-perfusion mismatch interferes with the efficiency of CO_2 elimination by the lung, although patients with ventilation-perfusion mismatch often have a normal or even low $PaCO_2$. The reason for this is that the regulatory chemoreceptors increase the ventilatory drive whenever they sense a rising $PaCO_2$. Such patients can maintain a normal PCO_2 by increasing the total ventilation at a cost of increasing the work of breathing. A significant portion of this increased ventilation, however, goes to lung units with high $\dot{V}_A/\dot{Q}$ ratios, which are inefficient at eliminating CO_2 (physiologic dead space).

When high $\dot{V}_A/\dot{Q}$ areas predominate in diseased lungs, the capacity to hyperventilate is readily exceeded and CO_2 retention may ensue. Patients with CO_2 retention are sometimes said to be "hypoventilating" as a result of the hypercapnia. Such patients with chronic lung disease and ventilation-perfusion mismatch, however, actually have "relative" hypoventilation, because the total ventilation is almost always increased.

Regulatory Control of Ventilation-Perfusion Matching

The alveolar PO_2 appears to be the most important factor involved in regulating the distribution of ventilation-perfusion within the lung. In this respect, hypoxic pulmonary vasoconstriction can be considered as part of a negative feedback loop. For example, in lung units with low $\dot{V}_A/\dot{Q}$ ratios, there is a fall in the local alveolar PO_2, and constriction of the associated microvessels reduces the local pulmonary blood flow. This tends to restore the local $\dot{V}_A/\dot{Q}$ ratio toward its normal value. This effect can be appreciated in residents of high altitudes, who are exposed constantly to lower ambient O_2 concentrations. Residents of high altitudes have better $\dot{V}A/\dot{Q}$ matching than sea level residents, as reflected by a smaller alveolar-arterial PO_2 difference. The intensity of hypoxic pulmonary vasoconstriction varies among different lung regions, and probably depends on the smooth muscle tone in different vessels. The effectiveness of hypoxic pulmonary vasoconstriction on preserving $\dot{V}A/\dot{Q}$ ratios also depends on the type of inhomogeneity. For example, when collateral ventilation is present, the regulatory effectiveness of hypoxic vasoconstriction may be greater than it would be if there were a parallel ventilatory arrangement between lung units. More recently, a role for nitric oxide in regulating local ventilation-perfusion matching has been suggested. The hypothesis is reasonable for the following reasons: (1) Nitric oxide is produced endogenously by endothelial cells and may regulate the local blood flow through its vasodilating effect, and (2) nitric oxide inhibits hypoxic pulmonary vasoconstriction. The nitric oxide-mediated mechanism may be especially important in patients with inflammatory lung diseases, in whom production of nitric oxide is increased. The loss of local hypoxic vasoconstriction would worsen ventilation-perfusion mismatch.

DIFFUSION CAPACITY

O_2 from the ambient air is carried into the lungs by two physical processes: bulk flow, which occurs in the conducting airways, and molecular diffusion, which is the main mechanism of gas transfer in the distal alveolar units. From the alveolar region, O_2 must diffuse across the alveolar-capillary membrane and enter the plasma and red cell membrane before it reacts with hemoglobin. The diffusion gradient for O_2 is determined by the PO_2 difference between alveolar gas and mixed venous blood at the entry to the pulmonary capillaries. Because of the high affinity of hemoglobin for O_2, the PO_2 in the capillary blood quickly rises to that in the alveolar gas, and the diffusion gradient for O_2 falls from approximately 60 mmHg to almost nil. At rest, this diffusion process is virtually complete in the first third of the mean capillary transit time of 0.75 sec.

The physical process of diffusion of gases across the alveolar capillary membrane behaves according to Fick's Law of Diffusion. Fick's Law states that for a given gas, the amount of gas transferred across a tissue sheet ($\dot{V}_{gas}$) is proportional to the area (A), a diffusion constant, and the difference in partial pressure ($P_1 - P_2$), and is inversely proportional to the thickness of the barrier (T):

$$\dot{V}_{gas} = \frac{A}{T} \times D(P_1 - P_2)$$

where D is a diffusion constant that depends on the properties of the tissue and the particular gas.

The lung is too complex to determine the area and thickness of the blood-gas barrier during life. Instead, the diffusion equation is written to combine the factors A, T, and D into one constant, D_L, as follows:

$$\dot{V}_{gas} = D_L \times (P_1 - P_2)$$

where D_L is called the *diffusing capacity of the lung*. The diffusing capacity includes the area, thickness, and diffusion properties of the membrane as well as the properties of the diffusing gas. Thus, the diffusing capacity for a gas is given by the following equation:

$$D_L = \frac{\dot{V}_{gas}}{(PA - Pc)}$$

where PA and Pc are the partial pressures of the gas in alveolar space and capillary blood, respectively.

Carbon monoxide (CO) is usually the gas of choice for measuring the diffusion properties of the lung, because its transfer is limited almost entirely by diffusion. The partial pressure of CO in capillary blood is very low because of its high affinity for hemoglobin (200 times greater than that of O_2), so that Pc in the above equation can generally be neglected. In this case, the above equation can be simplified as follows:

$$D_LCO = \frac{\dot{V}CO}{PACO}$$

The diffusing capacity of the lung for carbon monoxide (D_LCO) is thus expressed in units of milliliters of CO transferred per minute per millimeter of mercury of alveolar partial pressure. Of note, this unit is analogous to that for conductance. Some people—heavy cigarette smokers, for example—have sufficient carboxyhemoglobin in their blood that the partial pressure of CO in the pulmonary capillaries cannot be neglected. In this case, the partial pressure of CO can be measured in alveolar gas using a rebreathing technique and a correction made for back-diffusion of CO during the D_LCO maneuver.

The capacity for O_2 diffusion in the lungs can be estimated by multiplying the diffusing capacity for CO by 1.25. The uptake of O_2 by the lung is typically limited by perfusion under normal conditions. This process becomes limited partly by perfusion and partly by diffusion under hypoxic conditions. For this reason, measurements of diffusion using O_2 are often difficult to interpret.

The diffusing capacity of the lung can be separated into two components: (1) the alveolar-capillary membrane plus the erythrocyte cell membrane and (2) the reaction with hemoglobin (Fig. 14A). These components can be regarded as "resistances" in series to the transfer of O_2. This type of analysis was carried out by Roughton and Forster, who showed that the following relationship exists:

$$1/D_L = 1/D_M - 1/\theta Vc$$

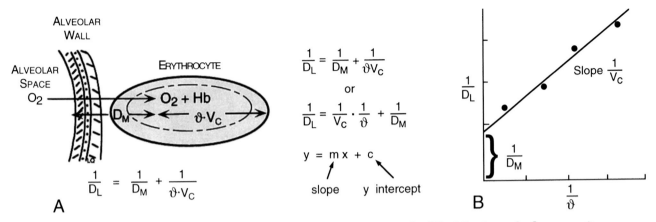

FIG. 14. The two components of the measured diffusing capacity (D) of the lung. **A:** Components attributable to the diffusion process itself and the time taken for O_2 (or CO) to react with hemoglobin. **B:** The graphic solution of D_M and V_c according to the Roughton and Forster analysis. D_M and V_c are derived by plotting against $1/D_L$. (Reproduced with permission from West JB. *Textbook of Respiratory Medicine.* 2nd ed. Philadelphia: WB Saunders; 1994.)

where D_L refers to the diffusing capacity of the lung, D_M is the diffusing capacity of the membrane (which includes the plasma and red cell membrane), θ is the rate of reaction of O_2 (or CO) with hemoglobin, and V_c is the volume of blood in the pulmonary capillaries. In the equation, values for D_M and V_c can be obtained graphically by measuring the diffusing capacity for CO at both high and normal alveolar PO_2 values (Fig. 14). Increasing the alveolar PO_2 reduces the value of θ for CO, because the CO has to compete with a higher pressure of O_2 for the hemoglobin. When the values of $1/D_L$ obtained at two different values of PO_2 are plotted against $1/\theta$, as shown in Fig. 15, the slope of the line is $1/V_c$ and the intercept on the vertical axis is $1/D_M$.

The Roughton-Forster equation is useful to demonstrate the factors that influence the diffusing capacity of the lung. Thus, the diffusing capacity can be reduced if D_M is increased, as when the thickness is increased or the area is reduced. The diffusing capacity also can be altered if the rate at which CO combines with blood (θ) is reduced (e.g., in anemia) or if capillary blood volume (V_c) is reduced (e.g., in pulmonary embolism).

According to the Roughton-Forster equation, the term D_M should be just as important as θV_c in determining the diffusing capacity of the lung. In clinical practice, however, the most important factor affecting the diffusing capacity is V_c; this is true in normal subjects as well as in many patients with pulmonary diseases. Changes in D_M are much less significant. It can be shown that raising the pulmonary arterial pressure when left atrial pressure is low increases the D_L substantially. This occurs because higher perfusion pressure recruits and distends pulmonary capillaries, and thus increases V_c. This effect is diminished if left atrial pressure is already elevated. Capillary recruitment and thus increased V_c probably also account for the increase in D_L measured during exercise and dur-

ing changes from the upright to the supine position. Similarly, changes in D_L induced by certain drugs can be explained best by their effects on V_c. This is also true in diseases associated with increased thickness of the alveolar membrane (e.g., idiopathic pulmonary fibrosis). The reduced diffusing capacity under these conditions usually can be attributed to decreased V_c that results from decreased lung volume caused by destruction and distortion of lung parenchyma. In addition to desaturation of the test gas, a decreased D_L is seen in emphysema, partly because destruction of pulmonary capillaries decreases the V_c.

Measurements of Diffusing Capacity

Single-Breath Method

The single-breath method was first described by Marie Krogh in 1914. The patient performs a single inhalation of a dilute mixture (about 0.3% each) of CO and an inert tracer gas (e.g., helium or methane), followed by a 10-sec breath-hold. The rate of disappearance of CO from the alveolar gas during the 10-second breath-hold is calculated. At the end of the breath-holding period, a sample of alveolar gas is obtained after discarding the dead space. The exhaled sample is then analyzed for CO using an infrared analyzer. The inert tracer gas is used to measure alveolar volume by dilution. The single-breath equation is as follows:

$$D_LCO_{sb} = K \times V_A \times \ln\left(\frac{F_ACO_i/F_ACO_s}{F_AHe_i/F_AHe_s}\right)\{(P_B - 47) \times t\}$$

where V_A is the alveolar volume in liters, t is breath-

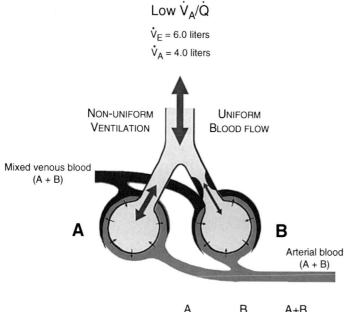

Low $\dot{V}_A/\dot{Q}$

$\dot{V}_E$ = 6.0 liters

$\dot{V}_A$ = 4.0 liters

	A	B	A+B
Alveolar Ventilation (L/min)	3.2	0.8	4.0
Pulmonary Blood Flow (L/min)	2.5	2.5	5.0
Ventilation / Blood Flow Ratio	1.3	0.3	0.8
Mixed Venous O2 Saturation (%)	75.0	75.0	75.0
Arterial O2 Saturation (%)	98.2	91.7	95.0
Mixed Venous O2 Tension (mm Hg)	40.0	40.0	40.0
Alveolar O2 Tension (mm Hg)	116.0	66.0	106.0
Arterial O2 Tension (mm Hg)	116.0	66.0	84.0

FIG. 15. Effects of nonuniform distribution of ventilation with uniform blood flow on gas exchange in a two-compartment lung model. Note that uneven ventilation produces a low $\dot{V}_A/\dot{Q}$ unit (*unit B*) and results in an alveolar-arterial PO_2 difference of 22 mmHg. (Reproduced with permission from Forster RE, et al., eds. *The Normal Lung: Physiological Basis of Pulmonary Function Tests.* 3rd ed. Chicago: Year Book; 1986.)

holding time in sec, and K is a constant. The fractional concentrations of CO and helium in inspired and sample gas ($FACO_i/FACO_s$ and $FAHe_i/FAHe_s$, respectively) are indicated by the appropriate terms.

The analysis of data based on the single-breath method involves several assumptions. The inhalation is assumed to be instantaneous, although in reality it is not. As the alveolar concentration of CO continues to decrease during breath-hold period, calculation of DL can be affected by the breath-hold time. Alternative methods have been proposed to circumvent these problems. For example, equations for changes in the alveolar concentrations of CO can be developed to fit each of the three phases of the single-breath maneuver (inhalation, breath-hold, and exhalation). The three-equation method appears to give a more accurate measurement of the diffusing capacity.

In many patients with lung diseases, the single-breath diffusing capacity is reduced. The decrease in $DLCO$ is usually caused by uneven ventilation-perfusion distribution and diffusion-perfusion properties in diseased lungs rather than by true changes in diffusion across the alveolar-capillary membrane. Such diseased lungs tend to empty unevenly, and the post-dead space sample of expired gas that is analyzed for CO is not representative of the whole lung. For this reason, the diffusing capacity is

sometimes referred to as the *transfer factor* (especially in Europe), to emphasize that it is more a measure of the lung's overall ability to transfer gas into the blood than a specific test of diffusion. Nevertheless, the test gives considerable information about gas exchange in the normal lung. Even in patients with severe disease, the results are useful for assessing the severity and type of lung disease in the pulmonary function laboratory.

Steady-state Method

In this method, the subject breathes a low concentration of CO (about 0.1%) for about 30 sec, until a steady state of gas exchange has been reached. The constant rate of disappearance of CO from alveolar gas is then measured for a further short period, along with the alveolar concentration of the gas. This technique is better suited for measurements during exercise, when breath-hold becomes a problem. The normal value of the diffusing capacity for CO depends on age, sex, and height (as is the case for most pulmonary function tests), and appropriate regression equations are available.

Intrabreath Method

More recently, with the development of rapidly responding infrared analyzers, the diffusing capacity can be measured using a single-breath–slow exhalation, or "intrabreath," technique. The gas concentrations are monitored continuously during slow inhalation and exhalation. Multiple estimates of DL can be made during a single exhalation, giving DL as a function of lung volume. Alternatively, a single estimate of DL can be obtained by applying a linear regression to exhaled CO concentration continuously measured during slow exhalation. Regression equations for the "intrabreath" diffusing capacity for CO based on age and height have been published.

Distribution of Diffusing Capacity

The Roughton-Forster approach to analyzing diffusing capacity assumes a homogeneous pulmonary system. The interpretation of the results is affected by heterogeneity in alveolar ventilation, alveolar lung volume, alveolar perfusion, and pulmonary diffusing capacity. The relative importance of heterogeneity in each of these factors and their interactions vary according to individual characteristics and the particular method chosen to measure DL.

A single acinus is sufficiently small so that ventilation and perfusion within such units can be assumed to be homogeneous. In the whole lung, however, perfusion depends on gravity as well as other regional stress factors. The higher perfusion pressure in the bottom of the lung results in greater recruitment of capillaries and therefore a larger capillary volume and capillary surface area for diffusion. In addition, larger regional differences in lung volume and alveolar ventilation are known to occur. These variations may result in significant local variations in diffusing capacity. This was demonstrated experimentally by Hamer, who showed, using a breath-hold technique, that overall DL, DM, and Vc vary as a function of lung volume. Using a single-exhalation technique, Denison et al. measured regional $\dot{V}A$, $DL/\dot{V}A$, and $\dot{Q}/\dot{V}A$ through a bronchoscope within individual lobes of the lungs of normal human subjects. They found a vertical gradient for $DL/\dot{V}A$ in the sitting position. $DL/\dot{V}A$ ranged from 0.86 in the upper lobe to 1.13 in the lower lobe. Clinically, diffusing capacity measured by the breath-hold method gives little information about its distribution in the lung. Since use of the rapid infrared analyzer has been combined with the single-exhalation method, the regional distribution of diffusing capacity can be measured in the lung.

MECHANISMS OF HYPOXEMIA

An arterial PO$_2$ value below the range for normal subjects of the same age establishes the presence of hypox-

emia. In general, arterial hypoxemia is defined by PO$_2$ values of <80 mmHg in adults breathing room air at sea level.

Hypoventilation as a Cause of Hypoxemia

The simplest derangement of gas exchange occurs when insufficient fresh air is breathed. Such hypoventilation decreases the arterial PO$_2$ and increases the arterial PCO$_2$. If $\dot{V}A/\dot{Q}$ distribution remains uniform, no alveolar-arterial difference develops for either O$_2$ or CO$_2$. The common causes of hypoventilation-associated hypoxemia are anesthetics or narcotics that depress the central nervous system, and neuromuscular diseases that affect respiratory muscle function.

Ventilation-Perfusion Mismatch as a Cause of Hypoxemia

Ventilation-perfusion mismatch (low $\dot{V}A/\dot{Q}$ regions) is the most common cause of hypoxemia in lung disease. Figure 15 illustrates the effects of $\dot{V}A/\dot{Q}$ mismatch on hypoxemia using a two-compartment lung model. If the total ventilation remains constant at 4 L/min but unit A receives four times as much ventilation as unit B (3.2 L/min vs. 0.8 L/min), and if the distribution of perfusion is uniform (2.5 L/min for each unit), the $\dot{V}A/\dot{Q}$ ratio for unit A becomes 1.3, whereas that for unit B is 0.3. O$_2$ tension and saturation must decrease in blood leaving the hypoventilated unit B; O$_2$ saturation must rise in blood leaving the hyperventilated unit A. Because of the nearly linear nature of the hemoglobin dissociation curve, the final PO$_2$ in the pulmonary venous blood, which is derived from the blood flow-weighted average of O$_2$ content, has to decrease. Thus, the high PO$_2$ in the blood leaving high $\dot{V}A/\dot{Q}$ unit A is not sufficient to compensate for the low PO$_2$ contributed by low $\dot{V}A/\dot{Q}$ unit B. The arterial blood would then have a PO$_2$ of 84 mmHg instead of 100 mmHg, as in the normal lung.

Right-to-Left Shunt as a Cause of Hypoxemia

A shunt is defined as a region where there is blood flow from the right side of the heart to the left, but no ventilation ($\dot{V}A/\dot{Q} = 0$). The effects of a right-to-left shunt on gas exchange are shown schematically in Fig. 16. In this example, 33% of the total blood flow (2.0 L/min) is shunt. Although gas exchange in units A and B is unimpaired, the net result from mixing of blood from these two units and the shunt pathway is a reduction of arterial PO$_2$ and the creation of the alveolar-arterial O$_2$ gradient. This effect on PO$_2$ is similar to that caused by $\dot{V}A/\dot{Q}$ mismatch. In fact, a shunt in mathematical terms is the ultimate ventilation-perfusion mismatch, one in which

Right-to-left-shunt

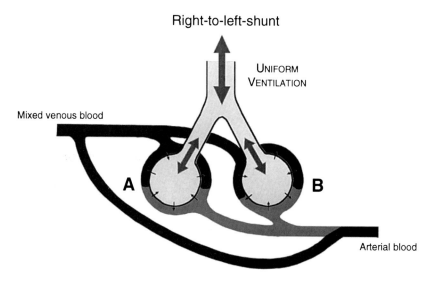

	A+B	Shunt	A+B+ Shunt
Alveolar Ventilation (L/min)	4.8	0.0	4.8
Pulmonary Blood Flow (L/min)	4.0	2.0	6.0
Ventilation - Perfusion Ratio	1.2	0.0	0.8
Mixed Venous P_{O_2} (mmHg)	40.0	40.0	40.0
Mixed Venous S_{O_2} (mmHg)	75.0	75.0	75.0
Mixed Venous P_{CO_2} (mmHg)	46.0	46.0	46.0
Alveolar P_{O_2} (mmHg)	114.0	--	114.0
Arterial P_{O_2} (mmHg)	114.0	--	59.0
Arterial S_{O_2} (%)	98.2	--	90.5
Arterial P_{CO_2} (mmHg)	36.0	--	39.0
A-a P_{O_2} difference (mmHg)	0.0	--	55.0

FIG. 16. Effects of right-to-left shunt on gas exchange in a two-compartment lung model. (Reproduced with permission from Forster RE, et al., eds. *The Normal Lung: Physiological Basis of Pulmonary Function Tests.* 3rd ed. Chicago: Year Book; 1986.)

there is perfusion but no ventilation. Because of the absence of ventilation, hypoxemia resulting from shunt cannot be corrected by breathing 100% O_2. This technique allows $\dot{V}_A/\dot{Q}$ mismatch to be differentiated from shunt as the cause of hypoxemia.

When a normal, healthy person breathes 100% O_2, an alveolar-arterial P_{O_2} difference of between 30 and 50 mmHg can usually be detected. This is consistent with the presence of a right-to-left shunt of approximately 2%–3% of the cardiac output. The multiple inert gas method, which measures only intrapulmonary shunt, indicates virtually no right-to-left shunt through the normal lung. These two results, taken together, imply that most of the shunt in normal subjects occurs distally to the gas exchange units (i.e., "postpulmonary shunt"). The main sources of the normal postpulmonary shunt are bronchial and mediastinal veins that empty into pulmonary veins and the Thebesian vessels of the left ventricle, which empty directly into the left ventricular cavity. When shunt occurs in patients with lung disease, it is usually accounted for by the perfusion of nonventilated lung regions through relatively normal vascular channels. Sometimes, shunt flow may occur through intracardiac communications, as in patent foramen ovale, when pressure in the

right atrium is increased—for example, from pulmonary hypertension.

Diffusion Impairment as a Cause of Hypoxemia

In normal subjects at rest, O_2 equilibrates quickly between the blood and gas phases in the alveolar region of the lung, and there is no diffusion limitation. This is true for healthy persons at sea level and at low altitude. During exercise at higher altitudes (>10,000 ft), the alveolar-arterial P_{O_2} difference can increase due to diffusion disequilibrium (Fig. 17).

Many patients with lung disease have abnormal diffusing capacity measured by the single-breath CO method. A diffusion impairment causing an increased alveolar-arterial P_{O_2} difference is unusual in these patients while at rest. As mentioned earlier, the major reason for a decreased diffusion capacity measured in the pulmonary function laboratory in patients with lung disease is maldistribution of ventilation-perfusion. Abnormal diffusion as a cause of an increased alveolar-arterial P_{O_2} difference is much more likely during exercise in these patients. Exercise-induced diffusion abnormalities result from

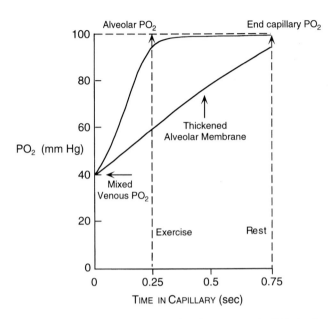

FIG. 17. Typical time courses for the change in PO₂ in the pulmonary capillary when diffusion is normal and the blood-gas barrier is abnormally thick. The time course for CO uptake is also shown.

lengthening of the diffusion pathway across the alveolar-capillary membranes or, more commonly, from a decrease in pulmonary blood volume in combination with an increase in the rate of blood flow, thus shortening the capillary transit time for the erythrocytes. Similar to hypoxemia caused by $\dot{V}A/\dot{Q}$ mismatch, hypoxemia caused by diffusion impairment can be corrected by having the patient breathe 100% O_2.

Decreased Mixed Venous Oxygen Content as a Cause of Hypoxemia

The O_2 content of pulmonary arterial (mixed venous) blood usually has little effect on arterial PO₂ in persons with normal lungs. In patients with very low cardiac output (e.g., patients in cardiogenic shock), a decrease in $C\bar{v}O_2$ contributes substantially to hypoxemia provided the amount of venous admixture is small. In the presence of lung disease with a substantial amount of venous admixture, resulting from either ventilation-perfusion abnormality, a large right-to-left shunt, or both, the O_2 content in the mixed venous blood has a considerable effect on arterial PO₂. For a given amount of ventilation-perfusion mismatch, the lower the mixed venous O_2 content, the lower the arterial PO₂. This mechanism of hypoxemia is particularly important in critically ill patients with serious cardiopulmonary diseases.

MECHANISMS OF HYPERCAPNIA

Ideally, CO_2 exchange should be characterized by (1) complete equilibration between aqueous and gaseous phases before blood leaves the pulmonary capillary, (2) identical PCO₂ in mixed alveolar gas and arterial blood, and (3) an inverse relationship between these gas tensions and the amount of ventilation of the alveolar spaces. Although it is not likely that all three postulates are ever achieved completely, CO_2 exchange is so close to the ideal that for practical purposes they can be assumed to hold true in the normal lung. This situation is certainly not the case for the abnormal lung.

Increased Dead Space as a Cause of Hypercapnia

As ventilation in the lung is cyclical—that is, gas enters and leaves by the same conduit—a portion of the inhaled gas never reaches the exchange surface. The last portion of each inspired breath remains in the tracheobronchial tree and is exhaled without its participating in either O_2 or CO_2 exchange. This portion of each tidal volume, VD/VT, is calculated from the difference between the PCO₂ of arterial blood and mixed expired gas and is expressed by the Bohr equation (see above). If tidal volume itself is measured, physiologic dead space can be described as a volume rather than a ratio. The *anatomic dead space* varies little in disease but does vary moderately with tidal volume, as airway volume increases slightly at higher lung volumes. The volume of anatomic dead space is important to consider when assessing ventilation, particularly during mechanical ventilation, but it does not need to be measured, because its size is not affected by disease.

Alveolar dead space for the most part is a conceptual space rather than an actual anatomic volume. A complete lack of gas exchange is present only in alveoli in which $\dot{V}A/\dot{Q}$ equals infinity (i.e., ventilated but not perfused at all). This situation is relatively rare. Far more commonly, alveoli have an excess of ventilation in relation to blood flow, and all the ventilation to such alveoli participates in gas exchange, but with lower efficiency than normal. This decrease in efficiency, measured in terms of its effect on CO_2 exchange, contributes to the alveolar dead space.

It is difficult to separate alveolar from anatomic dead space because of the difficulty of obtaining an expired gas sample that represents alveolar gas. Nor is it important, because both are factors in gas exchange and must be taken into consideration. Physiologic dead space (VD/VT) represents the sum of the anatomic dead space and the alveolar dead space, the latter usually resulting from ventilation-perfusion imbalance. The VD/VT describes CO_2 exchange as if the tidal volume were divided into a portion that does not participate at all in CO_2 exchange (physiologic dead space) and a remaining volume that exchanges CO_2 in a completely normal fashion. In reality, almost all the tidal volume, exclusive of the anatomic dead space, participates in CO_2 exchange, but to a degree that varies with the local $\dot{V}A/\dot{Q}$. In the sitting position, VD/VT is about 30% and varies little with age. It can increase to 60% or more in disease, reflecting gas exchange units with elevated $\dot{V}_A/\dot{Q}$. In the normal individual, V_D/V_T decreases with exercise, because changes in the physiologic dead space volume are small compared with the increases in tidal volume accompanying exercise. The responses of V_D/V_T to exercise in disease are variable, but usually V_D/V_T decreases, although not generally to normal levels.

Because physiologic dead space is a clearance index, it is affected by any factor that influences the efficiency of CO_2 exchange. It is useful in assessing $\dot{V}_A/\dot{Q}$ inequality only because this abnormality has a far greater effect on CO_2 exchange than all other factors combined.

Ventilation-Perfusion Mismatch as a Cause of Hypercapnia

Although maldistribution of ventilation and blood flow is not usually characterized by hypercapnia, there is no question that CO_2 exchange is affected by $\dot{V}_A/\dot{Q}$ imbalance. As $\dot{V}_A/\dot{Q}$ falls, local PCO_2 rises, reaching the value of the mixed venous PCO_2 when $\dot{V}_A/\dot{Q}$ equals zero. The maximum increase is slight in terms of gas tension but represents a considerable change in content because of the steep slope of the CO_2 dissociation curve. Besides the direct effect of the decrease in ventilation on CO_2 excretion, the simultaneous failure to oxygenate blood completely further hinders CO_2 exchange. With oxygenation, the carrying capacity of blood for CO_2 decreases, facilitating CO_2 excretion (Haldane effect). A quantity of CO_2 equal to that retained in alveoli with low $\dot{V}_A/\dot{Q}$ must be excreted in other gas exchange units to avoid hypercapnia. As noted previously, this can be accomplished in alveoli in which $\dot{V}_A/\dot{Q}$ is higher than normal. Because CO_2 is excreted less efficiently in these alveoli, alveolar dead space is increased, and the total ventilation must be increased to keep the alveolar exchange at a normal level. The incremental ventilation is achieved rapidly because of the sensitivity of central chemoreceptors to altered levels of PCO_2.

The ventilatory work required for this compensation is usually small, as can be illustrated by an extreme example. If one-half the cardiac output went to alveoli that were no longer ventilated, the remaining alveoli would have to excrete twice the normal amount of CO_2 to prevent hypercapnia. This could be accomplished by maintaining a PCO_2 in the low 30s in these units, and it would require an increase in ventilation of 25%–30% over that needed to exchange the same quantity of CO_2 with an ideal ventilation-perfusion distribution. This is only a small fraction of the normal ventilatory reserve. The ease of this compensation and the magnitude of normal ventilatory reserve account for the low incidence of hypercapnia in patients with $\dot{V}_A/\dot{Q}$ disturbances. As the disparity of $\dot{V}_A/\dot{Q}$ throughout the lung becomes greater, however,

compensation becomes more difficult to achieve. In the previous example, if retained CO_2 was excreted in only 10% rather than 50% of the alveoli, a much higher $\dot{V}_A/\dot{Q}$ would be present in the compensating alveoli, and alveolar dead space would increase correspondingly. In this circumstance, a 200% increase in ventilation would be required to maintain normocapnia. Although it is unlikely that normal ventilatory reserve would be exceeded except in an extreme $\dot{V}_A/\dot{Q}$ disturbance, the reserve may be minimal in disease. Moreover, the work of breathing can be increased substantially in disease. CO_2 produced by respiratory muscles may place an undue burden on the lungs when increments in ventilation require high levels of muscular work. Thus, a decreased ventilatory reserve combined with a high work of breathing and severe $\dot{V}_A/\dot{Q}$ imbalance can lead to an increase in alveolar dead space that cannot be overcome easily. These processes result in hypercapnia.

Hypoventilation as a Cause of Hypercapnia

In the homogeneous lung, the definition of alveolar ventilation is quite simple. Under these conditions, alveolar dead space does not exist, because early inspired gas in the anatomic dead space does not exchange CO_2. A discussed earlier in this chapter, alveolar ventilation can be defined as follows:

$$\dot{V}_A = \dot{V}CO_2/P_ACO_2 \times 0.863$$

where $\dot{V}CO_2$ is CO_2 output and P_ACO_2 is alveolar PCO_2 (assumed to be the same as arterial PCO_2). The definition of alveolar ventilation becomes more difficult when the lung is not ventilated uniformly. Alveolar and arterial PCO_2 are then no longer identical, and it is not possible to obtain an expired sample that is known to represent alveolar gas. Indeed, the term *alveolar gas* is misleading, as the composition of gas in the alveoli varies widely depending on local $\dot{V}_A/\dot{Q}$ relationships. Classically, the response to this problem has been to define alveolar ventilation in a functional manner by using the right side of the above equation. Hence, if arterial PCO_2 is elevated, alveolar ventilation is decreased and insufficient to excrete CO_2 in a normal fashion. Likewise, hyperventilation is signaled by a less-than-normal arterial PCO_2. With this approach, alveolar ventilation is equal to the difference between total expired ventilation and the physiologic dead space. In this context, there are two reasons for alveolar hypoventilation (i.e., arterial hypercapnia). First, if total minute ventilation is decreased, the alveolar component decreases and arterial PCO_2 rises. Second, alveolar hypoventilation occurs if physiologic dead space increases because of ventilation-perfusion imbalance and the necessary increase in total ventilation cannot be sustained to compensate for the change in dead space. In the latter circumstance, the $\dot{V}_A/\dot{Q}$ disturbance can be so severe that hypercapnia may be present, even though the total minute ventilation measured at the mouth is greater than normal. This is the result of defining alveolar ventilation in terms of alveolar PCO_2.

West has challenged this functional definition, arguing that the quantity of ventilation of the alveolar space is normal in $\dot{V}A/\dot{Q}$ mismatch and that the approach based on arterial PCO_2 overlooks the underlying problem. This viewpoint defines alveolar ventilation in an anatomic rather than a functional manner by making use of the concept of *effective ventilation* when the arterial PCO_2 is used as an index of ventilation. The term *alveolar ventilation* has a long tradition and is unlikely to be changed, although it would be more useful to identify the precise mechanisms involved in producing hypercapnia. No simple bedside techniques are available, however, to sort out accurately the degree of hypercapnia resulting from inadequate ventilation and that caused by severe ventilation-perfusion mismatch.

BLOOD GAS TRANSPORT

In air-breathing vertebrates, the metabolic processes of the body are supported by the integrated functions of the heart, lungs, and blood. Atmospheric oxygen, brought into proximity with the blood in the alveolar capillaries of the lungs, diffuses into the erythrocyte and is bound reversibly to hemoglobin. The erythrocyte circulates to the tissue capillaries, where oxygen dissociates from hemoglobin and diffuses down its concentration gradient into the cells to be consumed by mitochondria. The erythrocyte then carries carbon dioxide generated in the mitochondria to the alveolar capillaries, where it diffuses down its concentration gradient into the air spaces of the lung. These physiologic processes make use of the physical processes of diffusion, chemical reaction, convection, and diffusion again. This portion of the chapter describes the remarkable properties of the blood that enable it to carry oxygen and carbon dioxide and maintain acid-base homeostasis. It also summarizes the processes of convective oxygen transport to the microcirculation, diffusion of oxygen into the tissues, and cellular respiration. Examples have been selected to describe the effects of disease processes such as anemia, hypoxemia, ischemia, and heterogeneity of blood flow on oxygen delivery and cellular metabolism.

The Metabolic Milieu of the Body

The gas transport mechanisms in the blood are designed primarily to handle large quantities of the metabolic gases O_2 and CO_2, although soluble inert gases, such as N_2, also are transported in dissolved form. The circulation supports a basal metabolic rate for O_2 of about 3.0 mL/min and a CO_2 production rate of 2.4 mL/min per kilo-

gram of body weight for the adult human. The demands on the circulation, however, can increase as much as 20-fold under conditions of extreme exercise. The large size and high metabolic requirements of vertebrate animals for molecular O_2 confounds diffusion as a transport mechanism, because the distances and the rates of O_2 consumption become too great. These requirements can be met only by an efficient convective transport system to deliver O_2 to more dense regions of the circulation, where diffusion again becomes an effective process for its distribution. In addition, having a carrier molecule for O_2 is adaptive, because the amount of the gas that can be dissolved in the blood at normal barometric pressures is not adequate to meet the metabolic requirements of higher organisms.

When the plasma comes in contact with a gas such as O_2, its concentration rises to a value determined by the partial pressure of the gas and the solubility coefficient of plasma for O_2. As the solubility of O_2 in plasma is quite low (0.0224 mL O_2 per milliliter of plasma at body temperature), the amount of O_2 dissolved in plasma at normal barometric pressure is quite low. The number of milliliters of dissolved O_2 in a liter of blood plasma at STPD (standard temperature and pressure, dry) is given by the following simple relationship:

$$Dissolved\ O_2 = [0.0224\ PO_2\ (PB - PH_2O)] \times 100\ mL$$

$$= [0.0224\ PO_2\ (760 - 47)] \times 100\ mL$$

$$= 0.0031\ PO_2$$

where PB is the barometric pressure, PH_2O is water vapor pressure, and PO_2 is the partial pressure of O_2 in the blood. Hence, for a PO_2 in the blood of 100 mmHg, the dissolved O_2 content is only 0.3 mL/dL or 3.0 mL/L of blood. To meet a basal requirement for O_2 of 3 mL/kg/min, the minimum cardiac output would have to be 1.0 L/kg/min, or, for an adult of normal size, about 70 L/min. During exercise at an O_2 consumption rate of 3.0 L/min, the cardiac output would have to increase to an amazing 1000 L/min. To circumvent this problem, hemoproteins capable of carrying large quantities of O_2 have evolved in higher animals. These hemoproteins are the hemocyanins of invertebrates and the hemoglobins of vertebrates.

Structural Biology and Molecular Properties of Hemoglobin

Hemoglobin is the major protein of erythrocytes. It allows vertebrates to transport molecular O_2 from the lungs to the tissues and CO_2 from the tissues to the lungs. Human hemoglobin is a tetramer of two α and two β polypeptides, each containing a heme moiety. The tetramer consists of 547 amino acids and has a molecular weight of 64,800 Da. The heme and the globin interact with each other in a way that determines the O_2-binding characteristics of hemoglobin. The heme groups to which the O_2 binds are harbored within the protein parts of the molecule. Heme is the complex of chelated iron in a cyclic tetrapyrrole (porphyrin) ring. The porphyrin of hemoglobin is called *protoporphyrin IX*. The iron atom is kept in the center of the porphyrin ring between four nitrogen atoms. The porphyrin carries side chains that maintain the heme group in the proper orientation within the protein portion of the hemoglobin molecule. Double bonds in the heme moiety cause hemoglobin to have a bright red color when oxygenated and a purple color when deoxygenated.

The location of the heme group in the globin portion of the molecule is important for maintaining the iron in a ferrous valence state (Fe^{2+}). Normally, when iron reacts with O_2, the iron valence state changes to ferric (Fe^{3+}) and an oxide (rust) is formed. In the folds of the globin chain, ferrous iron is protected and its reaction with O_2 is reversible. One important part of this mechanism is the linkage of the heme iron to the amino acid histidine, which supplies a negative charge and enables the iron to form a weak bond with O_2. Thus, the interactions between heme and globin in the molecule are responsible for the reversible linkage of O_2 with the heme group. The basic features of the molecular physiology of hemoglobin, including the interactions of heme with globin, are summarized below, along with the chemical mechanisms for inducing conformational changes in hemoglobin in the presence of O_2, organic phosphates, protons, and CO_2.

Hemoglobin consists of four globin molecules: two identical α subunits and two identical β subunits. In the evolution of the globin molecule in higher vertebrates, the amino acids responsible for proper heme orientation and cooperative O_2 binding have been conserved. The secondary structure of α and β subunits of hemoglobin is characterized by a high content of α helices (about 75%), which vary in length between 7 and 23 amino acids. The surfaces of the α and β subunits have nonpolar regions that allow them to form an $\alpha_2\beta_2$ tetramer. The four subunits make a total of six contacts and are held together by hydrophobic interactions, by hydrogen bonds, and by electrostatic interactions of salt bridges. These noncovalent interactions allow the subunits to move easily during reversible binding of O_2 with the heme group. Among the contacts between the subunits, only the most extensive one, the $\alpha_1\beta_1$ contact, remains the same on O_2 binding. The surface of the hemoglobin molecule contains many polar groups that are all hydrated and therefore contribute to the high water solubility of hemoglobin. This feature allows dense packing of hemoglobin within erythrocytes, each of which contains about 3 trillion molecules of tetrameric hemoglobin.

The binding of O_2 to the heme iron provides the crucial triggering mechanism for the conformational change of the globin part of hemoglobin (Fig. 18). Molecular O_2 is bound to the iron atom by an end-on geometry with an Fe-O-O angle of 155°. Iron in deoxyhemoglobin is five-coordinated with the four pyrrole nitrogens of porphyrin and the imidazole nitrogen of the proximal histidine, resulting in four unpaired electrons in the iron atom. In oxyhemoglobin, the iron is six-coordinated, leading to a state in which all the electrons are paired. This pairing of electrons leads to a reduction of magnetic moment in oxyhemoglobin compared with that in deoxyhemoglobin. The magnetic changes in iron accompanying the binding of O_2 give rise to stereochemical changes in the heme that produce the conformational changes in globin responsible for cooperative O_2 binding and allosteric effects, such as the Bohr effect. The mechanism that triggers the changes in the structure of the hemoglobin molecule when O_2 is bound or released is the movement of the heme iron. When heme iron reacts with O_2, it reorients the iron in the porphyrin ring. The bond between the imidazole nitrogen is shortened in deoxyhemoglobin by about 0.6 Å compared with that of oxyhemoglobin. In addition, the porphyrin structure is flexed in deoxyhemoglobin but not in oxyhemoglobin. These changes in electronic configuration are transmitted to the globin part of the molecule.

A standard terminology is used for the different properties of deoxyhemoglobin and oxyhemoglobin to describe how changes in the heme structural affect the globin. Deoxyhemoglobin is said to be in the T or tense state, and oxyhemoglobin is said to be in the R or relaxed state. The T state of hemoglobin has a low O_2 affinity, whereas the R state has an O_2 affinity about 150 times greater than that of the T state. The transition between these conformational states is induced by the shift of the heme iron when O_2 is bound or released. The most important changes that occur in hemoglobin on binding or release of O_2 occur in the $\alpha_1\beta_2$ and $\alpha_2\beta_1$ contacts. These contacts fit together, and the respective hydrogen donor and acceptor sites are constructed so that only two positions of the two subunits are stable. This is the structural basis for the two-state model that explains most of the physiologic properties of hemoglobin. The cooperativity of O_2 binding is also a direct consequence of the fact that hemoglobin assumes only these two stable structures: the R structure whose O_2 affinity is high and the T structure whose O_2 affinity is lowered by molecular interactions such as salt bridges and the binding of organic phosphates.

Diphosphoglycerate

The erythrocytes of humans and most other mammals contain high concentrations of the glycolytic intermediate 2,3-diphosphoglycerate (DPG). Its concentration within human erythrocytes is normally about 5 mmol/L of erythrocytes, equivalent to the concentration of tetrameric hemoglobin. DPG is negatively charged at physiologic pH values and binds to deoxyhemoglobin in a 1:1 molar ratio.

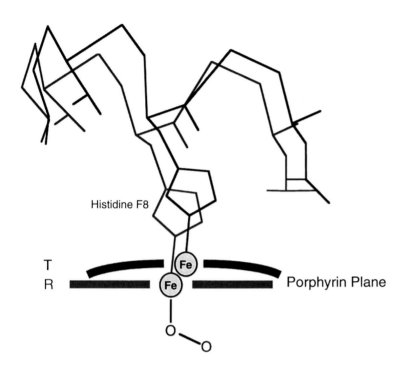

Histidine F8

T

R

Porphyrin Plane

FIG. 18. Schematic illustration of the hemoglobin molecule. Changes in globin structure with O_2 binding to heme in hemoglobin are shown for the R (oxy) and T (deoxy) states.

It binds to deoxyhemoglobin much more tightly than to oxyhemoglobin. The overall reaction is as follows:

$$Hb_4(DPG) + 4O_2 \rightleftharpoons Hb_4(O_2)_4 + DPG$$

Deoxyhemoglobin has a DPG binding site that is complementary in shape and charge to the phosphate that is able to stabilize the T structure of hemoglobin. The binding of O_2 results in a loss of complementarity and expulsion of the DPG molecule. The presence of O_2 decreases the binding constant of DPG and hemoglobin by two orders of magnitude at physiologic pH, temperature, and salt concentrations. O_2 binding changes the quaternary structure of deoxyhemoglobin by increasing the distance between the partners of the salt bridges, causing them to break. When a salt bridge is broken, the apparent pK value of the two partners falls. Therefore, protons tend to be set free by oxyhemoglobin and taken up by deoxyhemoglobin. This difference in proton binding between oxyhemoglobin and deoxyhemoglobin is the basis for the dependence of the O_2 affinity of hemoglobin on pH, also known as the *Bohr effect*. Quantitatively, about 2.0 H^+ are set free on oxygenation at neutral pH in the absence of DPG according to the following reaction:

$$Hb_4(H)_2 + 4O_2 \rightleftharpoons Hb_4(O_2)_4 + 2H^+$$

Protons are released from four pairs of salt bridges on O_2 binding. The sum of the changes in the apparent pK of these groups gives rise to the Bohr effect (effect of pH on O_2 affinity) and to the difference in proton binding between oxyhemoglobin and deoxyhemoglobin (Haldane effect).

Carbon Dioxide

The hemoglobin molecule, like other proteins, directly binds CO_2. The chemical interaction of CO_2 with the unprotonated forms of protein amino groups occurs according to the following reactions:

$$Hb—NH_2 + H^+ \rightleftharpoons Hb—NH_3$$
$$Hb—NH_2 + CO_2 \rightleftharpoons Hb—NHCOO^- + H^+$$

The carbon atom of CO_2 and the amino group of hemoglobin form a complex known as a *carbamate*. Carbamate formation proceeds only when the amino group is unprotonated; therefore, 50% of the N-terminal α-amino groups but less than 1% of the ϵ-amino groups within the protein can bind with CO_2 in the physiologic pH range. Deoxyhemoglobin binds more CO_2 as carbamate than does oxyhemoglobin, and about 80% of this oxygen-labile carbamate is confined to the β subunits at physiologic pH. The pK value of the α-amino groups of the α subunits increases with deoxygenation from 7.0 to 7.8, thereby inhibiting carbamate formation. The pK value of the N-terminal α-amino groups of the β subunits remains nearly constant at around 7.0, regardless of oxygenation. Carbamates formed at the N-terminal α-amino group of the β subunits is stabilized by positively charged groups near the N-termini of the β subunits in deoxyhemoglobin. During the process of oxygenation, these positively charged groups move apart, destabilizing the carbamate and releasing CO_2 from the binding sites. This process is discussed in more detail in the section on CO_2 transport.

The Oxygen Equilibrium Curve of Hemoglobin

The relationship between the fractional saturation of hemoglobin with O_2 and the PO_2 under equilibrium conditions is the sigmoid O_2 equilibrium curve (OEC) of hemoglobin (Fig. 19). The sigmoid shape of the hemoglobin OEC determines the loading and unloading of O_2 under physiologic conditions. Its position is often expressed by the PO_2 at half-saturation (P_{50}). The normal P_{50} for human hemoglobin is approximately 27 mmHg. When the O_2 affinity increases, the OEC shifts to the left (reduced P_{50}). When the O_2 affinity decreases, the OEC shifts to the right (increased P_{50}). The principal physiologic determinants of the functional OEC within erythrocytes are H^+, 2,3,-DPG, and CO_2. Other effectors, such as Cl^- and adenosine triphosphate (ATP), also decrease O_2 affinity, but their physiologic roles are minor. One of the most powerful ways to decrease O_2 affinity is to bind CO to hemoglobin. CO has 200 times the affinity for heme as does O_2, and when CO binds to one heme site, it increases the O_2 affinity of the other binding sites. The OEC is also very sensitive to changes in temperature; hypothermia decreases the P_{50} approximately 2 mmHg per degree centigrade.

The first physiologists to observe the sigmoid nature of the OEC concluded that O_2 affinity increased during progressive oxygenation. They called this phenomenon *cooperativity*. This cooperativity was described mathematically by Hill using an equation that empirically relates hemoglobin saturation to O_2 tension. The Hill plot for the OEC falls on a straight line with a slope determined by the degree of cooperativity. This empiric description of the OEC, however, provides no information about the mechanism of O_2 binding. A more general approach to the quantitation of the oxygenation of hemoglobin was made by Adair, who recognized that hemoglobin was made up of four subunits, each of which could bind

a single O_2 molecule. Adair derived equations for the stepwise oxygenation of hemoglobin:

$$Hb(O_2)i + O_2 \rightarrow Hb(O_2)i + 1$$

where i ranges from 0 to 3. The association constants for the sequence of equilibrium reactions are difficult to determine experimentally because of the interdependence among the parameters. In addition, the approach says nothing of molecular structure; thus, it is not useful for understanding structure-function relationships.

The two-state model provides a better functional description of the physiologic behavior of hemoglobin, because each of the two states of hemoglobin, R (relaxed) and T (tense), has its own unique O_2 affinity. The equilibrium constants for their reactions with O_2 are K_R and K_T. The ratio of these constants,

$$C = K_T/K_R$$

is less than 0.01 for human hemoglobin A; that is, the affinity of molecules in the R state for O_2 is much greater than the affinity of those in the T state. The constant C is characteristic of a given hemoglobin structure. The equilibrium between the two conformations is given by the allosteric constant:

$$L = [Hb]_T/[Hb]_R$$

This is influenced by mutations in the globin chains and by several small allosteric molecules. These small molecules react with hemoglobin at nonheme sites in such a way as to stabilize the T conformation. Thus, a mixture of R and T hemoglobin molecules will show a reactivity with O_2 related to the position of the T-R equilibrium. For deoxyhemoglobin, the equilibrium is almost entirely on the T side. The T (deoxygenated) state is constrained by salt and hydrogen bonds to a much greater degree than the R state. Successive oxygenation of the heme groups

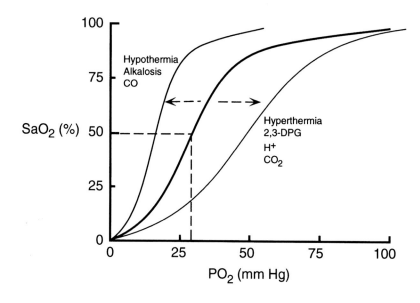

FIG. 19. OEC of hemoglobin. The normal P_{50} value is indicated by the *dashed lines*. The changes in position of the OEC associated with various effector molecules are indicated by the *dashed arrows*.

causes some of these bonds to break, decreasing the stability of the T structure. When the molecules transit from the T to the R state, the constraints are released and the oxygen affinity increases. The shift from T to R during oxygenation accounts for cooperativity of O_2 binding. For normal hemoglobin, the shift from T to R occurs primarily between binding of the second and third O_2 molecules; hence, the OEC is steepest in the middle part of the curve.

The behavior of the OEC can affect O_2 transport to tissues. For instance, certain genetic alterations in the hemoglobin molecule may lead to polycythemia. A reduced O_2 affinity may improve O_2 delivery to tissues when arterial oxygenation is inadequate. In animals, chemical modifications of hemoglobin that shift the OEC to the right will increase PO_2 in the tissues during normoxia. During CO poisoning, the OEC is shifted to the left by CO binding to hemoglobin. This leftward shift exacerbates the tissue hypoxia resulting from the CO-mediated decrease in O_2 carrying capacity. An extreme leftward shift in the OEC caused by respiratory alkalosis is also a feature of O_2 transport in humans at high altitude. The effects of other changes in the position or shape of the OEC on O_2 transport, however, have been difficult to demonstrate in humans.

The actual shape and position of the OEC in vivo is influenced most strongly by hydrogen ion concentration, although O_2 and CO_2 also interact with hemoglobin in a very complex way to regulate the position and shape of the OEC. Hydrogen ion effects are regulated by PCO_2 and the buffering capacity of hemoglobin. Buffering by hemoglobin, in turn, is determined by hemoglobin concentration and the degree of O_2 saturation. The O_2 saturation is determined by the PO_2 and O_2 affinity of hemoglobin. These complex interactions are difficult to sort out in the efficiency of gas exchange by blood. Other properties of erythrocytes that affect O_2 transport include the rates of binding of physiologic ligands (O_2, CO_2, H^+, 2,3-DPG), buffering capacity, the barrier to diffusion of the red blood cell membrane, the unstirred plasma layer immediately surrounding the cell, and the blood viscosity.

An increase in 2,3-DPG normally augments tissue oxygenation by shifting the OEC to the right. At high altitude, if O_2 uptake by the lung is limited by diffusion, a lower O_2 affinity of hemoglobin would limit O_2 loading of hemoglobin, whereas a higher O_2 affinity would augment it. Whether or not the latter effect would be offset by lower tissue unloading remains unclear, because few measurements of venous PO_2 are available under severely hypoxic conditions. The 2,3-DPG effect does not seem well suited to O_2 delivery at high altitude, but the traditional view that shifting the OEC to the right facilitates O_2 unloading in tissue sites also may not be appropriate under certain conditions. Barcroft et al. first proposed that increased O_2 affinity was an important adaptation to high altitude based on analogy with the placental circulation, in which fetal blood has a higher affinity than that of the mother. Chemical modification of hemoglobin to increase its O_2 affinity confers better survival in hypoxic rats, and mutant hemoglobins with increased O_2 affinity may protect against the effects of hypoxia. On the summit of Mt. Everest, respiratory alkalosis decreases the P_{50} of whole blood to about 19 torr, a value that would help maintain the O_2 saturation of arterial blood. The arterial desaturation during exercise in extreme hypoxia might be ameliorated by the increase in the O_2 affinity of hemoglobin, although its effects on O_2 release to the tissues are uncertain.

Carbon Dioxide Transport and the Carbon Dioxide Dissociation Curve

The CO_2 dissociation curve of hemoglobin describes overall CO_2 transport as a function of CO_2 tension. The CO_2 dissociation curve is relatively steep in comparison with the O_2 equilibrium curve (Fig. 20). Consequently, large volumes of CO_2 can be exchanged by the lungs with relatively small changes in blood PCO_2. These small changes in blood PCO_2 minimize oscillations in blood pH, and the hydrogen ion concentration of blood at rest varies only 10% between arterial and mixed venous values. The steepness of the CO_2 dissociation curve also permits continued excretion of CO_2 even in the presence of significant mismatching of pulmonary ventilation and blood flow.

Most of the CO_2 in blood exists in the form of bicarbonate ion. CO_2 also is transported in a physically dissolved state in blood, and it is bound to amino groups of proteins as carbamate compounds. Although CO_2 has an aqueous solubility approximately 20 times that of O_2, CO_2 dissolved in physical solution accounts for only 5% of the CO_2 content of arterial or venous blood. Dissolved CO_2, however, is important for CO_2 transport and exchange because the bicarbonate and carbamate pools are linked through dissolved CO_2. Molecular CO_2 is highly lipid-soluble and diffuses rapidly across cell membranes. Exchange of CO_2 in both the lung and peripheral tissues occurs via diffusion of molecular CO_2 across the vascular endothelium. CO_2 diffuses across the alveolar capillary membrane so rapidly that limitation of the process cannot be measured in vivo.

Hydration of CO_2 produces carbonic acid (H_2CO_3), which is almost completely ionized to hydrogen and bicarbonate in blood because the pK of carbonic acid (≈ 3.8) is much lower than the pH of blood:

$$CO_2 + H_2O \rightarrow H_2CO_3 \rightarrow H^+ + HCO_3^- \qquad (1)$$

This process involves two steps. The first step is the hydration of CO_2 to carbonic acid, and the second step is the ionization of carbonic acid to bicarbonate. Bicarbonate ion can further dissociate into hydrogen and carbonate ions; however, little carbonate is formed in the

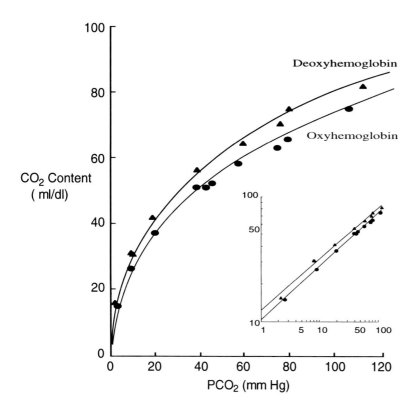

FIG. 20. CO_2 dissociation curve of blood. *Inset* shows log arithmetic transformation of the curve that linearizes the relationship between CO_2 content and PCO_2.

body, because the pK of this reaction is greater than 10.0. CO_2 is hydrated to H_2CO_3 inside erythrocytes at a very slow rate. This reaction when catalyzed by carbonic anhydrase in the erythrocyte, however, occurs so quickly that the process is completed during the passage of the red cell through the peripheral capillaries. The reverse reaction, the dehydration of H_2CO_3 to CO_2, occurs during pulmonary excretion of CO_2 and similarly requires enzymatic catalysis. Carbonic anhydrase is present within the erythrocyte in high concentrations but is virtually absent from plasma. Carbonic anhydrase also is found in the capillary endothelium of the lung and other organs, but the quantity of enzyme there is small.

Human erythrocytes contain two isoforms of carbonic anhydrase. Carbonic anhydrase I is a low-activity enzyme that is inhibited by anions such as chloride. This isoform probably does not catalyze reactions of CO_2 in vivo. The other isoform, carbonic anhydrase II, has high catalytic activity and is resistant to anion inhibition. Human carbonic anhydrase II is comprised of 259 amino acids and has modest homology with carbonic anhydrase I. All isoforms of carbonic anhydrase contain a zinc atom that is essential for enzymatic activity. Activity is lost with binding of an unsubstituted—SO_2 NH_2 group of aromatic sulfonamides to the zinc ion. Acetazolamide is the most widely known of these inhibitors.

CO_2 and hydrogen ions reversibly bind to uncharged amino groups of proteins as described for hemoglobin:

$$R—NH_2 + H^+ \rightarrow R—NH_3^+$$

$$R—NH_2 + CO_2 \rightarrow R—NHCOOH$$

where R represents the protein moiety and R—NHCOOH is the carbamic acid. Under physiologic conditions, carbamic acids release protons and form carbamate ions, R—NHCOO$^-$. Because both molecular CO_2 and protons compete for uncharged amino groups, carbamate formation is pH-dependent and increases with alkalinity. Transport of CO_2 as carbamates is also influenced by PCO_2 and by the pK of the amino groups on the protein. The pK values of α-amino groups of the N-termini of blood proteins lie within the physiologic range of pH. Therefore, these frequently exist in the uncharged R—NH$_2$ form and are available to bind CO_2. In contrast, ϵ-amino groups, which are located throughout the protein chains, have a pK well above the physiologic pH range. This means that most ϵ-amino groups are bound to hydrogen ions and cannot bind CO_2. The concentration of carbamates in plasma is approximately 0.6 mM, and binding of CO_2 to α-amino groups accounts for 60% of this quantity. Plasma carbamates, however, do not participate in CO_2 exchange, because the steep slope of the CO_2 dissociation curve minimizes changes in pH and PCO_2 between arterial and venous blood. This effect in turn minimizes changes in plasma carbamate concentration in the lung and systemic capillaries.

Under physiologic conditions, binding of CO_2 to α-amino groups of hemoglobin is an important factor in CO_2 exchange. The total concentration of hemoglobin-carbamates in blood is relatively low, but as pointed out earlier, deoxyhemoglobin binds more CO_2 as carbamate than does oxyhemoglobin. The difference in bound CO_2 between the deoxygenated and oxygenated hemoglobin, or "oxylabile carbamate," has a role in CO_2 exchange. When O_2 is released by hemoglobin in the tissues, it is accompanied by increased binding of CO_2 to α-amino groups. Conversely, oxygenation of hemoglobin in the lung promotes release of CO_2 bound as carbamate. The presence of 2,3-DPG decreases the total CO_2 content, and binding of oxylabile carbamate to hemoglobin relates inversely to 2,3-DPG concentration. The interaction between 2,3-DPG and CO_2 binding involves inhibition of carbamate formation when 2,3-DPG is bound to the N-terminal amino groups of the β chains of hemoglobin. Because the α chains of hemoglobin do not bind 2,3-DPG, organic phosphates do not affect carbamate formation in these subunits of the molecule. Carbamate binding measurements indicate that both the α and β chains of hemoglobin participate equally in oxylabile carbamate formation at physiologic PCO_2 in the presence of 2,3-DPG. This effect of organic phosphates on oxylabile carbamate formation decreases the role of this pathway in CO_2 exchange. The oxylabile carbamate accounts for perhaps 10% of total CO_2 exchange.

The CO_2 content of deoxygenated blood is greater than that of oxygenated blood at any PCO_2. This feature of CO_2 transport is referred to as the *Haldane effect*. The CO_2 dissociation curve of blood is nonlinear, but when plotted on logarithmic axes it becomes linear (Fig. 20). The slope of the line depends on the hemoglobin concentration of blood. The logarithmic expression of the CO_2 dissociation curve also permits definition of the curve by measuring a single experimental point and the hemoglobin concentration. The most important physiologic value is the slope of the CO_2 dissociation curve, as this determines the efficiency of CO_2 exchange. The slope of the CO_2 dissociation curve is essentially constant at a constant hemoglobin concentration. Thus, calculations of arterial-venous content differences and other parameters of gas exchange from CO_2 dissociation curves are correct as long as the appropriate slope and hemoglobin concentration are used.

Two thirds of the total CO_2 contained in whole blood is distributed in the plasma, and one third in erythrocytes at equilibrium. The CO_2 in circulating blood is increased by the large internal buffering capacity of erythrocytes, the presence of cellular carbonic anhydrase, and the exchange of bicarbonate and chloride ions across the erythrocyte membrane. Similarly, two thirds of the bicarbonate in blood is distributed in the plasma and one third in the erythrocytes. The plasma volume is about 55% and the erythrocyte volume about 45% of whole blood, and bicarbonate ion is transported primarily in the aqueous phase. Plasma also has a greater fraction of water than do the erythrocytes, owing to the high concentration of hemoglobin inside the red cells. The Donnan effect, a consequence of charge restriction by negatively charged hemoglobin molecules inside the erythrocyte, also leads to a lower intracellular concentration of diffusible anions, such as bicarbonate.

Despite the lower bicarbonate content of erythrocytes, they are essential for almost all bicarbonate transport. CO_2 entering the blood from the tissues diffuses into the erythrocytes, where the large buffering capacity favors bicarbonate formation. Formation of bicarbonate from CO_2 is catalyzed rapidly by carbonic anhydrase within the erythrocytes, and CO_2 in minimal amounts remains hydrated as carbonic acid during the short period of capillary transit. The erythrocyte membrane facilitates the rapid exchange of intracellular bicarbonate ions for extracellular chloride ions, thereby shuttling bicarbonate ions produced within the erythrocyte into the plasma. Coupling of bicarbonate and chloride in the exchange process is accomplished via a transport protein, so that transmembrane potential is not altered and electrical potentials are not established that would prevent bicarbonate from moving out of the erythrocyte. This facilitated transport permits rapid exchange of bicarbonate across the cell membrane during the short period of capillary transit. Thus, even though the majority of bicarbonate is carried within the plasma, it is almost exclusively formed within the red cells. The entire process is reversed in the lungs as bicarbonate is converted to molecular CO_2, which is able to cross the alveolar-capillary membrane.

The facilitated exchange of bicarbonate and chloride across the erythrocyte membrane is mediated by an anion exchange protein (AE1, formerly band 3 protein). There are approximately 10^6 molecules of AE1 in each erythrocyte membrane. A variety of anions are transported by this carrier transmembrane, but bicarbonate and chloride ions exhibit the fastest rates of exchange. The actual mechanism of the exchange is characterized by 1:1 bidirectional anion flux associated with a conformational change in the protein structure.

The influence of O_2 on the CO_2 dissociation curve, the Haldane effect, has received less attention than the converse relationship, the effect of CO_2 on the O_2 dissociation curve of blood, the Bohr effect. The Bohr effect is responsible for only 2% of total O_2 exchange in the tissues, whereas the Haldane effect accounts for nearly half of resting CO_2 exchange. Oxygen-dependent exchange of CO_2 occurs via both the carbamate and bicarbonate pathways and is a function of pH, PCO_2, and the concentration of 2,3-DPG. With normal 2,3-DPG concentrations, the Haldane effect increases with increasing pH, reaching its maximal value under normal acid-base conditions. The importance of the carbamates in this process increases as the pH increases, because carbamate formation is promoted by the lack of protons and by less 2,3-DPG binding at higher pH. The contribution of the bicarbonate pathway to CO_2 transport peaks in the physiologic range of pH, but it decreases at higher pH as a result of increasing prominence of carbamates. When protons are released from deoxyhemoglobin on O_2 binding, some are consumed by the carbamate reaction, thereby leaving fewer protons to combine with bicarbonate ion to form CO_2. CO_2 exchange would occur without a functioning Haldane effect despite the fact that half of CO_2 excretion normally occurs by this mechanism. The cost of such a loss would be greater changes in arterial-venous CO_2 content, increased tissue hypercarbia, and altered acid-base status.

ACID-BASE PHYSIOLOGY

A discussion of respiratory acid-base problems requires a basic understanding of the chemical behavior of acids and bases in aqueous solution. Chemical reactions proceed at a velocity that is proportional to the active concentrations, or "activities," of the reactants. In a reaction that may proceed in either direction, the Law of Mass Action may be written as follows:

$$[A] + [B] \rightleftharpoons [C] + [D]$$

Rate constants of the reactions in both the forward (k_1, $[A] + [B] \rightarrow [C] + [D]$) and reverse ($k_2$, $[C] + [D] \rightarrow [A] + [B]$) directions determine the concentrations of reactants until chemical equilibrium is reached, when

$$k_1/k_2 = [C][D]/[A][B]$$

The term k_1/k_2 is the equilibrium constant, K_e. For an acid in solution, the equilibrium constant is known as the dissociation constant:

$$K_a = [H^+][A^-]/[HA]$$

K_a determines the concentration of hydrogen ion, $[H^+]$. If the acid is "strong," K_a is large and $[H^+]$ and $[A^-]$ are much higher than $[HA]$.

In 1909, L. J. Henderson used the Law of Mass Action to express the hydrogen ion equilibrium for carbonic acid:

$$[H^+] = K \times [CO_2]/[HCO_3^-]$$

Using the convention in which $[H^+]$ is expressed as pH, in which p is the negative power of 10, Hasselbalch rearranged Henderson's equation and applied it to the carbonic acid buffer system to obtain the following:

$$pH = pK + \log([HCO_3^-]/[CO_2])$$

When methods for the measurement of PCO_2 became available, $[CO_2]$ was replaced by PCO_2 and the equation written as follows:

$$[H^+] = 24 \, PCO_2/[HCO_3^-]$$

where $[H^+]$ is in nEq/L, PCO_2 is in mmHg, and $[HCO_3^-]$ is in mEq/L. The familiar form of the Henderson-Hasselbalch equation is obtained by substituting 6.1, the pK_a of the system, and 0.0301, the solubility constant for CO_2 in plasma, into the equation:

$$pH = 6.1 + \log([HCO_3^-]/0.0301 \, PCO_2)$$

As the PCO_2 of arterial plasma is regulated by alveolar ventilation, it is used to indicate the respiratory component of the acid-base state. The $[HCO_3^-]$ is an estimate of the nonrespiratory, or "metabolic," contribution to $[H^+]$. Although the Henderson-Hasselbalch equation accurately describes the equilibrium relationships between these variables, it does not describe how acid-base balance is regulated. The regulation of acid-base balance could be described by the Henderson-Hasselbalch equation only if both PCO_2 and $[HCO_3^-]$ acted independently without influencing each other significantly or being affected by the other systems involved in acid-base control. This assumption is not valid, because the bicarbonate buffer system is influenced by the independent and direct effect of PCO_2 on $[HCO_3^-]$. Hence, changes in $[HCO_3^-]$ do not indicate "metabolic" changes alone. This difficulty was addressed by titration studies of plasma to produce the Siggaard-Andersen nomogram, along with normalizing the PCO_2 to 40 mmHg. This approach produced the concept of "base excess," the excess $[HCO_3^-]$ in arterial plasma that accounts for changes in ventilation. The concept of the base excess, however, did not hold when applied to whole blood or to plasma changes in which the acid-base adjustments were made *in vivo*. This issue required standardizing in vitro data to whole blood having a constant hemoglobin concentration.

The contribution of strong electrolytes to $[H^+]$ in the blood is another problem that has been approached conventionally by analyzing the difference between the concentrations of anions and cations. In plasma, cations predominate and exert a basic, or alkalizing, effect. The effect of strong ions other than Na^+, K^+, and Cl^- is expressed as the "anion gap," the anion concentration that cannot be explained by the inorganic anions and bicarbonate $([Na^+] + [K^+]) - ([Cl^-] + [HCO_3^-])$. An excessive anion gap represents unmeasured anions, such as lactate or ketones. The working principle of the strong ion difference ($[SID]$) is similar to that of the anion gap, but it has the advantage of functioning as an independent variable in acid-base regulation.

The Physicochemical Approach to Acid-Base Interpretation

Acid-base problems are best approached by identifying and assessing changes in the buffer systems that contribute to changes in $[H^+]$. The recognition of both independent variables (those not altered by changes outside the system) and dependent variables (those influenced by the independent variables and by changes in other systems) can be described in a series of equations in which the independent variables are specified. This physicochemical approach identifies the dependent and independent variables that determine the acid-base status of plasma, cells, and body fluids.

Because body fluids are dilute aqueous solutions, the chemical behavior of water underlies all acid-base physiology. There is a small dissociation in pure water expressed in the following reaction:

$$2H_2O \rightleftharpoons H_3O^+ + OH^-$$

The extent of the dissociation defined by the Law of Mass Action is as follows:

$$K_W = [H^+][OH^-]/[H_2O]$$

In this equation, $[H_2O]$ in pure water is 55 mol/L, and because $[H^+]$ and $[OH^-]$ are 10^{-7} Eq/L or less, the $[H_2O]$ is effectively a large constant, and

$$K'_W = [H^+][OH^-]$$

where K'_W, the ion product for water, is $K_W \times [H_2O]$. In pure water, H^+ and OH^- are the only ions and are equal in concentration (neutral pH). At 25°C, K'_W has a value of 1.008×10^{-14} Eq²·L⁻². This value is usually rounded off to 1.0×10^{-14}; thus,

$$K'_W = [H^+][OH^-] = 10^{-14}$$

and

$$[H^+] = [OH^-] = 10^{-7}$$

Neutral $[H^+]$ is 10^{-7} (pH = 7.0) at 25°C. At body temperature (37°C), however, neutral $[H^+]$ is not be 10^{-7} Eq/L because

$$K'_W = 4.4 \times 10^{-14}$$

and

$$[H^+] = (4.4 \times 10^{-14})/[OH^-] \text{ Eq/L} \qquad (1)$$

Thus, neutral $[H^+]$ is the square root of 4.4×10^{-14}, or 2.1×10^{-7} (pH = 6.68).

In aqueous solutions, strong electrolytes are dissociated completely, and they are defined as having K values that are greater than 10^{-4} (strong acids) or less than 10^{-12} (strong bases). In blood and body fluids, K can be ignored for strong electrolytes because they are dissociated; that is, strong acids (HA) exist only as H^+ and A^-, and strong bases (BOH) exist only as B^+ and OH^-. In physiologic fluids, the main strong electrolytes are Na^+, K^+ and Cl^-. These strong ions influence $[H^+]$ by the Law of Electrical Neutrality and the dissociation of water. This means that in any system at equilibrium the net charge must be zero; thus, in a solution of Na^+, K^+, and Cl^- in water,

$$[Na^+] + [K^+] + [H^+] - [Cl^-] - [OH^-] = 0$$

The effect of strong ions may be lumped into a single term that expresses the net negative or positive charge that they exert. This is the "strong ion difference" ([SID]), which in plasma is normally $[Na^+] + [K^+] -$ $[Cl^-]$. Strong organic ions, such as lactate or ketones, also contribute to [SID], as they may be present in high concentrations. Other strong inorganic ions are usually ignored, as they are present in low concentrations. Therefore,

$$[SID] + [H^+] - [OH^-] = 0$$

where the independent variable is the [SID] and the dependent variables are $[H^+]$ and $[OH^-]$. In normal plasma, $[Na^+]$ is 140 mEq/L, $[K^+]$ is 4 mEq/L, and $[Cl^-]$ is 104 mEq/L. Thus, the normal [SID] is approximately 40 mEq/L. Without bicarbonate or other basic electrolytes in plasma, $[OH^-]$ would have to be close to 40 mEq/L (4×10^{-2} Eq/liter). If true, then

$$[H^+] = 4.4 \times 10^{-14}/4 \times 10^{-2} \text{ Eq/L}$$
$$= 1.1 \times 10^{-12} \text{ Eq/L}$$

or a pH of nearly 12. This calculation shows how important strong ions, weak acids, and the HCO_3^- buffer system are for the control of $[H^+]$ in body fluids. With these systems in plasma, the $[H^+]$ is 4×10^{-8} (pH = 7.4).

Total weak acids (A_{tot}) are the buffers present in a partially dissociated state in the physiologic pH range. These acids have dissociation constant (K_a) values between 10^{-4} and 10^{-12}; however, only weak acids with a K_a close to pH 7.4 are effective buffers. Buffer systems include plasma proteins ($K_a = 3 \times 10^{-7}$), proteins and phosphates in cells ($K_a = 5.5 \times 10^{-7}$), and hemoglobin in red cells. The K_a of the imidazole group of the histidine residues in proteins is virtually identical to the neutral $[H^+]$ of water, while in hemoglobin, the imidazole groups are associated closely with the heme, and the imidazole groups become less acidic when the heme structure tenses on the release of O_2. For oxyhemoglobin, K_a is 2.5×10^{-7}, and for deoxyhemoglobin, it is 6.3×10^{-9}. For plasma proteins at 37°C:

$$[H^+] \times [A^-] = (3 \times 10^{-7}) \times [HA] \text{ Eq/L} \qquad (2)$$

The effectiveness of weak acids as buffers depends not only on the dissociation constant, but also on total concentration ([A_{tot}]) of the acid. The sum of the dissociated (A^-) and undissociated (HA) forms of any weak acid remains constant:

$$[HA] + [A^-] = [A_{tot}] \text{ Eq/L} \qquad (3)$$

where [A_{tot}] is an independent variable and [HA] and [A^-] are dependent variables. In plasma, [A_{tot}] represents the ionic equivalent of the plasma proteins and may be estimated by multiplying the protein content by 0.24. Thus, at a normal total protein levels of 70 g/L, [A_{tot}] is 17 mEq/L. This value is comprised of [A^-] of 15 mEq/L and [HA] of 2 mEq/L at pH 7.4. Hence, even though plasma proteins behave as weak acids, they are mostly dissociated (15/17) at normal arterial pH.

Carbon Dioxide and the Bicarbonate Buffer System

The CO_2 buffer system acts mainly through variations in total CO_2 content brought about by variations in PCO_2 and $[H^+]$. As indicated earlier, the two components of the system are hydration of CO_2 and the dissociation of carbonic acid into HCO_3^- and H^+. These two equations can be combined and solved for $[H^+]$ to yield an equation containing two constants and $[H_2O]$. These constants may all be incorporated into a single overall ionization constant (K'_a) to obtain:

$$[H^+] = K'_a[CO_2]/[HCO_3^-]$$

where $[CO_2]$ is the concentration of dissolved CO_2 and is related to the PCO_2 by the solubility constant for CO_2 (3.01×10^{-5} Eq/L/mmHg). Substituting the solubility constant into the equation:

$$[H^+] = K'_a (3.01 \times 10^{-5} PCO_2)/[HCO_3^-] \text{ Eq/L}$$

For K'_a of 7.94×10^{-7} the single constant can be used:

$$K_c = (7.94 \times 10^{-7}) \times (3.01 \times 10^{-5})$$

$$= 2.4 \times 10^{-11}$$

Thus,

$$[H^+] = (2.4 \times 10^{-11}) \times PCO_2/[HCO_3^-] \text{ Eq/L} \quad (4)$$

For PCO_2 expressed in torr and $[HCO_3^-]$ in mEq/L,

$$[H^+] = 24 \times PCO_2/[HCO_3^-] \text{ nEq/L}$$

This is Henderson's equation. PCO_2 is the independent variable of the CO_2 system, whereas $[H^+]$ and $[HCO_3^-]$ are both dependent variables. Using the pK_a of the bicarbonate system in the expression yields the Henderson-Hasselbalch equation. At a normal $PaCO_2$ of 40 mmHg, if $[H^+]$ is 40 mEq/L, then $[HCO_3^-]$ is 24 mEq/L.

The hydration of CO_2 to carbonic acid in aqueous solution is a slow process, but as noted earlier, it is accelerated greatly by carbonic anhydrase. Carbonic acid dissociates into H^+ and bicarbonate, and bicarbonate itself dissociates into H^+ and carbonate ion. The equilibrium equation is as follows:

$$[H^+] = (6 \times 10^{-11})[HCO_3^-]/[CO_3^{2-}] \text{ Eq/L} \quad (5)$$

where 6×10^{-11} is the K_a for the reaction. All three variables in this equation depend on changes in the CO_2 and other systems.

The interactions between the different buffer systems in the body must satisfy the Law of Electrical Neutrality when the systems are in equilibrium. Hence, all the charges of ions in the systems must be summed, including $[H^+]$ and $[OH^-]$ for water, the net positive charge of $[SID]$ for strong electrolytes, $[A^-]$ for weak electrolytes, and CO_2, $[HCO_3^-]$, and $[CO_3^{2-}]$. Thus,

$$[SID] + [H^+] - [HCO_3^-]$$
$$- [CO_3^{2-}] - [A^-] - [OH^-] = 0 \quad (6)$$

The $[H^+]$ and $[OH^-]$ in plasma cannot be computed from this equation because the $[SID]$, $[HCO_3^-]$, and $[A^-]$ are orders of magnitude greater than $[H^+]$ and $[OH^-]$ in body fluids. The equation must be satisfied, however, to quantify the effects of the variables governing electrolyte physiology. The calculated $[H^+]$ and $[OH^-]$ also have to satisfy each equation in which they appear as dependent variables. Because the relationships between the variables are complicated, the six numbered equations (Eqs. 1–6) must be solved simultaneously to account fully for all the interactions. The three independent variables only appear once in the series: $[A_{tot}]$ (Eq. 3), PCO_2 (Eq. 4), and $[SID]$ (Eq. 6). The dependent variables appear in more than one equation: $[H^+]$, $[OH^-]$, $[HCO_3^-]$, $[CO_3^{2-}]$, and $[A^-]$.

The equations can be solved simultaneously for any values of $[SID]$, $[A_{tot}]$, and PCO_2 in plasma, or by changing parameters to fit the acid-base status of any other body fluid or any other conditions. Also, the equations may be combined into a single fourth-order polynomial from which $[H^+]$ can be computed. This computation has no practical role in the assessment of the acid-base status of plasma, in which pH can be measured directly, but the measured $[H^+]$ and calculated $[H^+]$ generally agree because the acid-base systems have been defined rigorously in terms of their dependent and independent components. This enables identification of the mechanisms that lead to changes in $[H^+]$ in plasma, cells, and interstitial fluid. Calculations of "base excess" and the "anion gap" are replaced by the variables $[SID]$ and $[A^-]$. This approach also clarifies some fuzzy concepts, including the use of the Henderson-Hasselbalch equation to imply that $[H^+]$ is controlled by changes in $[HCO_3^-]$, the concept of protons being produced or eliminated, and concepts implying that $[HCO_3^-]$ may be produced, removed, or retained (by the kidneys), or administered as a useful therapy.

The use of graphs or solutions of the equations to obtain the variables that satisfy the measured arterial $[H^+]$ and PCO_2 are useful clinically. Also, plasma electrolyte measurements yield a measured inorganic $[SID]$ ($[Na^+] + [K^+] - [Cl^-]$) that may be compared with the value of $[SID]$ that satisfies $[H^+]$ and PCO_2 for possible effects of other strong ions. A difference between the inorganic $[SID]$ and total $[SID]$ indicates the presence of unmeasured ions, such as lactate or ketoacids. This exercise is similar to the calculation of the anion gap, except that $[A^-]$ is a variable rather than a constant. Because $[H^+]$, $[OH^-]$, and $[CO_3^{2-}]$ are in micromolar concentrations or less, Eq. 6 may be simplified as follows:

$$[SID] - [HCO_3^-] - [A^-] = 0$$

This simplification makes it possible to evaluate the effects of the three independent variables ($[SID]$, PCO_2, and protein) and to determine whether unmeasured strong anions are contributing to the acid-basis status.

Variations in the relative magnitude of the independent

variables involved in control of acid-base status produce differing effects in different fluid compartments and different tissues (Fig. 21). In intracellular fluid, [SID] is large and dominated by a high [K$^+$]. Large protein and phosphate concentrations (A$_{tot}$) also minimize the effects of reductions in [SID] resulting from falls in [K$^+$] or accumulation of strong organic ions such as lactate. In tissues, PCO$_2$ is high and increased by metabolism, but [HCO$_3^-$] is low. Changes in PCO$_2$ in tissue influence [H$^+$] much less than in plasma. Control of intracellular [H$^+$] is achieved through buffering by A$_{tot}$ and exchange of strong ions with extracellular fluid, thereby changing the [SID], and by diffusion of CO$_2$ out of the cell. In interstitial fluid and other ultrafiltrates of plasma, such as lymph or cerebrospinal fluid, [H$^+$] is influenced only by changes in [SID] and PCO$_2$, because protein is virtually absent and there is no role for the weak acid system. In plasma, the [SID] also tends to regulate the pH, but variations in PCO$_2$ may bring about large and rapid changes in arterial [H$^+$].

Inside erythrocytes, all three systems have similar values, because [SID] and [A$_{tot}$] are high and PCO$_2$ is in equilibrium with the PCO$_2$ of the surrounding plasma. The situation is also complicated because the state of oxygenation influences the dissociation constant. These considerations emphasize the importance to acid-base balance of fluid, strong ion, and CO$_2$ shifts between the different body compartments, because the molecules making up A$_{tot}$ (e.g., proteins) do not move readily.

Intracellular pH and the Alphastat Hypothesis

For many years, partly because of the difficulty in studying pH changes within tissues, acid-base physiology

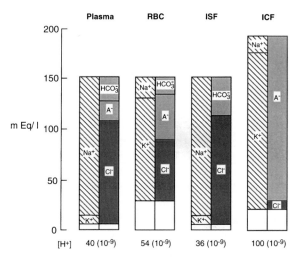

FIG. 21. Diagrams of ionic status of various body fluid compartments: *RBC*, red blood cell; *ISF*, interstitial fluid, *ICF*, intracellular fluid. Electrical neutrality is shown by equal heights of the two panels in each plot. The strong ion difference [SID] is occupied by the [A$^-$] and [HCO$_3^-$]. The [H$^+$] is shown beneath each plot.

has dealt primarily with the status of the blood. Marked changes in biochemical and physiologic function, however, accompany alkalosis and acidosis in the systemic organs. For example, alkalosis stimulates glycolysis, whereas increases in [H$^+$] impair membrane function, blunt hormonal responses, and inhibit enzyme activity. Such effects appeal to the concept of control of the intracellular [H$^+$]; however, good evidence in living systems suggests that regulatory mechanisms are attempting to keep a constant state of protein ionization. This concept is based on the parallel effects of temperature on tissue pH and on the pK of the imidazole group of histidine in proteins, which is very close to neutral pH. This principle was first pointed out by Rahn et al., who suggested that regulation protected the fractional dissociation of the cellular imidazole—NH groups. They termed the fractional dissociation *alpha,* and they called the control mechanism the *alphastat.* The close involvement of imidazole groups in enzyme regulation, receptor function, and the operation of membrane pores and ion exchangers explains many physiologic effects of acid-base perturbations previously explained by changes in [H$^+$].

In clinical circumstances, intracellular acid-base measurements are not usually available; however, intracellular [H$^+$] is important because of its influence on cellular metabolic processes. Large variations clearly exist in pH in different tissues in different clinical situations. Experimental studies in animals and humans have attempted to establish the magnitude of intracellular fluid (ICF) changes relative to those of extracellular fluid (ECF). Studies in which arterial PCO$_2$ has been raised or lowered have shown that ICF [H$^+$] is well defended in a range of arterial PCO$_2$ between 40 and 80 mmHg. This can be explained in terms of the differences in [SID] and [A$_{tot}$] between ICF and ECF. Studies of metabolic acidosis and alkalosis have similarly shown good control of [H$^+$] in ICF, but the defense against alkalosis appears to be less effective than that against acidosis. The reasons for this difference probably lie in the different extent to which ECF changes in [SID] are capable of influencing the [SID] in the ICF.

Erythrocytes and Acid-Base Control

Erythrocytes buffer sudden changes in ions or PCO$_2$ and help maintain relatively constant conditions in plasma and thus in the ECF. The ICF composition of the erythrocyte lies between that of ICF and plasma. The [K$^+$] is not as high as in ICF, but [Na$^+$] and [Cl$^-$] are higher, although still well below plasma values. The erythrocyte [SID] is 60 mEq/L, compared with 130 mEq/L in ICF. Hemoglobin also provides an [A$_{tot}$] of 60 mEq/L, which compares with 20 mEq/L in plasma and 200 mEq/L in ICF. The R and T forms of hemoglobin also provide a variable K$_a$, which enables deoxyhemoglobin to buffer venous acidity more effectively. The carbonic anhydrase in the erythrocyte enables the hydration of CO_2 to proceed rapidly, and carbonate formation enhances CO_2 content without a comparable increase in $[H^+]$. Cell membrane transport systems also facilitate ion exchange between the plasma and erythrocyte while controlling erythrocyte volume.

When O_2 dissociates from hemoglobin, $[H^+]$ inside the erythrocyte tends to decrease. As CO_2 enters the erythrocyte, this decrease in $[H^+]$ is offset by the ionization of carbonic acid. Bicarbonate moves out of the cell, and Cl^- moves into the cell. This tends to increase plasma $[SID]$ and leads to a rise in plasma $[HCO_3^-]$. At the same time, CO_2 forms carbamates very rapidly. This reaction is facilitated by deoxygenation, which allows the α-amino groups of the β chain of deoxyhemoglobin to form carbamates. In addition to these reactions associated with the deoxygenation of hemoglobin and CO_2 content of venous blood, the erythrocyte can modulate rapid changes in plasma ion concentration.

Ventilation and Acid-Base Control

The PCO_2 in arterial plasma is controlled mainly by changes in ventilation, as shown in the alveolar ventilation equation, which expresses the simple inverse relationship between $PaCO_2$ and $\dot{V}A$. The equation is useful because neither metabolic rate nor ventilation needs to be measured to assess the adequacy of breathing in relation to metabolic demand. Arterial PCO_2 represents the balance between metabolic CO_2 production and ventilation. In tissues and venous blood, PCO_2 is regulated primarily by the balance between metabolism and blood flow. The extent to which arterial PCO_2 reflects the adequacy of ventilation also depends on the activity of carbonic anhydrase in allowing rapid equilibration of PCO_2 between pulmonary capillary blood and alveolar gas. Thus, it is affected by carbonic anhydrase inhibition.

The alveolar ventilation equation expresses the combined effects of changes in $\dot{V}A$ and $\dot{V}CO_2$ on $PaCO_2$. In patients with severely impaired ventilatory capacity, respiratory failure may be worsened by changes in $\dot{V}CO_2$. In patients with an increase in PCO_2, several factors may contribute to underventilation, including inefficient gas exchange leading to dead space ventilation ($\dot{V}D$), increased work of breathing, impaired respiratory muscle strength and endurance, and disorders of respiratory control. The ventilatory responses to acid-base disorders of nonrespiratory origin are extremely important for regulating $[H^+]$, because they may change rapidly. In long-term responses to acid-base disturbances, the response of the central medullary chemoreceptors is the most important factor in the ventilatory set point. The major effector is the $[H^+]$ in cerebrospinal fluid, and because cerebrospinal fluid is protein-free, the PCO_2 and $[SID]$ are the two important independent variables in central control of ventilation.

The Kidneys and Acid-Base Control

The kidneys influence acid-base status mainly by changing the $[SID]$ of the plasma. In the glomerulus, Na^+ reabsorption from plasma ultrafiltrate in the tubules is an active process that lowers both $[Na^+]$ and osmolality in the tubules, leading to water reabsorption. This process in the distal tubule is under the control of antidiuretic hormone. Chloride reabsorption is mediated in part electrically and in part by an active process related to ATPase-driven membrane pumps on renal tubular cells. If Cl^- is reabsorbed less rapidly than Na^+, urinary $[Cl^-]$ increases relative to $[Na^+]$ and urinary $[SID]$ falls and increases urinary $[H^+]$. If Na^+ is less rapidly reabsorbed than Cl^-, the opposite occurs. In the tubular lumen, a fall in $[SID]$ and an increase in $[H^+]$ tend to increase PCO_2. The increase in PCO_2 occurs because the tubule is partly closed to the circulation and the removal of CO_2 by the renal capillary blood flow may not keep pace with its production. The $[HCO_3^-]$ tends to fall with the increase in $[Cl^-]$, and when urinary pH has fallen to <6, urinary $[HCO_3^-]$ is very low. In this way, the excretion of Cl^- in excess of Na^+ and K^+ contributes to control of plasma $[SID]$ and $[H^+]$. When $[H^+]$ has increased because of accumulation of organic anions such as lactate, the renal tubular cells can excrete the lactate, Cl^-, or both. Because the reabsorption of strong organic anions is less efficient, Cl^- is reabsorbed in preference to lactate, resulting in a very high urinary $[La^-]$ and low $[Cl^-]$. In this situation, the kidney prevents urinary pH from becoming too low by excreting more water and Na^+, if they are available, and by excreting ammonia and phosphates. This allows reabsorption of Na^+ or excretion of Cl^- without an increase in urinary $[H^+]$. Both effects tend to increase plasma $[SID]$ and decrease plasma $[H^+]$. As ammonia and phosphate excretion have limited capacities, adequate Na^+ and water delivery to the distal tubule in an organic acidosis is very important. The kidneys normally are able to adjust to ranges of water excretion between 0.5 and 25 L/d and to ranges of Na^+ excretion between 0.05 and 25 g/d.

Disorders of Acid-Base Physiology

The primary acid-base disorders may be thought about in terms of abnormalities in the three acid-base variables capable of independent action: the $[SID]$, $[A_{tot}]$, and PCO_2 in arterial blood. Primary acid-base changes are modified by "compensatory" changes that, to be effective, have to involve independent variables—for example, changes in ventilation leading to changes in PCO_2, or movement of strong ions into cells or urine to modify $[SID]$.

Primary Metabolic Acidosis and Alkalosis

Processes that reduce [SID] (e.g., an increase in [Cl$^-$]) tend to increase [H$^+$], leading to a primary metabolic acidosis (Table 4). A number of compensatory responses take place to minimize this effect. Reductions in [SID] may be offset by responses to increase [SID]; for example, in diabetic acidosis, dehydration may increase [Na$^+$], and more Cl$^-$ excretion in urine may help to reduce plasma [Cl$^-$]. These two changes help compensate for the effects of the increase in plasma ketoacid concentration. In disease states (e.g., uremic acidosis), these adaptive responses may not be available. Measurement of urinary electrolyte excretion may be helpful in assessing the role of the kidneys in an acidosis. A tendency for [H$^+$] to increase also leads to an association of weak acids (plasma proteins, A$_{tot}$) and thus to a reduction in [A$^-$], which may amount to 3 to 4 mEq/L (slightly more in very severe acidosis). Increases in [H$^+$] also stimulate

TABLE 4. *Causes of primary metabolic acidosis and alkalosis*

Metabolic acidosis: decreases in SID
- Reduction in Na$^+$. Hyponatremia often presents without a fall in SID because loss of Na$^+$ is paralleled by a loss of Cl$^-$. The fall in Na$^+$ rarely exceeds the reduction in Cl$^-$, and SID is reduced. This may occur in diarrhea, water intoxication, syndrome of inappropriate secretion of antidiuretic hormone, and renal tubular defects.
- Increase in Cl$^-$. This occurs in renal failure, in ureterosigmoidostomy, and with administration of chloride solutions.
- Metabolic production of strong anions. This occurs in lactic acidosis and in diabetic ketoacidosis.
- Ingestion of strong anions. This occurs with salicylates, glycolate in ethylene glycol poisoning, and formate in methanol poisoning.
- Accumulation of strong ions that are normally excreted by the kidney. This occurs with sulfate retention in renal failure.

Metabolic alkalosis: increases in SID
- Increase in Na$^+$. This is a rare cause of alkalosis, because most conditions tending to increase Na$^+$ also increase Cl$^-$ without much of a change in SID. Alkali ingestion, transfusions, penicillin and carbenicillin therapy, and dehydration with urinary loss of chloride (contraction alkalosis) predispose to this state.
- Increases in K$^+$ are self-limiting, because the toxic effects of hyperkalemia occur before an important increase in SID can occur.
- Reductions in Cl$^-$ underlie most increases in SID. Losses of Cl$^-$ may be from the kidneys and identified by a high urine Cl$^-$ excretion ("saline unresponsive"), or from the gut ("saline responsive"). This occurs in vomiting, gastric suction, in diarrhea caused by villous adenoma of the colon, in diuretic therapy with severe K$^+$ depletion, and in Bartter's syndrome. It also occurs with mineralocorticoid excess in primary aldosteronism and in Cushing's syndrome, and can be caused by ingested mineralocorticoid, such as licorice and carbenoxolone.

SID, strong ion difference.

ventilation, leading to a decrease in PaCO$_2$. The effectiveness of this response depends on the ventilatory capacity, the efficiency of pulmonary gas exchange, and ventilatory control mechanisms. If none of these physiologic mechanisms is impaired, the increase in [H$^+$] expected for a given reduction in [SID] may be used to identify the adequacy of the responses.

An increase in [SID] (e.g., a decrease in [Cl$^-$]) tends to reduce [H$^+$], producing a metabolic alkalosis. The causes of primary metabolic alkalosis are given in Table 4. The compensatory responses to an increase in [SID] may be considered in terms similar to those seen in low [SID] states. These are retention of Cl$^-$ by the kidneys in patients with normal renal function, and sometimes movement of Na$^+$ into ICF. Although [H$^+$] may be defended by dissociation of weak acids with an increase in [A$^-$], this effect usually amounts to 1 mEq/L or less. Decreases in plasma [H$^+$] are usually accompanied by a reduction in ventilatory responsiveness, and PaCO$_2$ rises by about 1.0 mmHg for each increase in [SID] of 10 mEq/L. In some cases of metabolic alkalosis, severe loss of K$^+$ may accompany Cl$^-$ in the kidneys, leading to depletion of intracellular [K$^+$] and a fall in ICF [SID]—an intracellular acidosis complicating the extracellular alkalosis. This effect may lead to respiratory muscle weakness.

Plasma Proteins and Total Weak Acid Concentration

Normally, the weak acid concentration [A$_{tot}$] is determined by the plasma protein concentration alone. The [A$_{tot}$] may increase if plasma proteins or other weak acids (such as phosphate) increase. Increases of more than 2 or 3 mEq/L in [A$_{tot}$] are uncommon, but because they act as weak acids, the effect of increasing [A$_{tot}$] is similar to a reduction in [SID]—a metabolic acidosis. The effects of increases in plasma proteins, as in multiple myeloma, vary depending on the isoelectric points of the class of globulin involved. Most globulins have isoelectric points similar to that of albumin, a pK of around 6.5, and thus act as weak acids. The IgG class has an isoelectric point that is close to pH 9.0.

When plasma protein concentration is reduced, the [A$_{tot}$] is reduced, leading to a fall in [A$^-$]. The effects are similar to increases in [SID] of equimolar size—a metabolic alkalosis. Quantitatively, the effect may be assessed by multiplying the total protein concentration in grams per liter by 0.24 [A$_{tot}$] and by taking 0.9 of this value as [A$^-$], as A$_{tot}$ is about 90% dissociated in most situations. This value may then be added to [Cl$^-$] and [HCO$_3^-$] to identify the presence of any unmeasured anions. The major exception is an increase in IgG paraproteins in myeloma; these act as weak bases because of the basic amino acids lysine and arginine, whose isoelectric points are close to pH 9.0. They have a weak positive charge in the physiologic pH range, and $[A_{tot}]$ and $[A^-]$ appear falsely low their presence.

Primary Respiratory Acidosis and Alkalosis

An elevated $PaCO_2$ indicates alveolar hypoventilation, and when it is not a response to a metabolic alkalosis, it is termed a *primary respiratory acidosis*. The common causes of alveolar hypoventilation are shown in Table 5. The potential effect of an increase in $PaCO_2$ on plasma $[H^+]$ may be seen by moving to the right along the normal $[SID]$ isopleth in a plot of $[H^+]$ versus $PaCO_2$ (Fig. 22). Similarly, it may be seen that the effect of an increase in $PaCO_2$ may be minimized by an increase in $[SID]$. Virtually the only compensatory mechanism that is effective and well tolerated is a reduction in plasma $[Cl^-]$. Acutely, this occurs through a shift of Cl^- into erythrocytes; over a longer time, excretion of Cl^- in excess of Na^+ and K^+ in urine leads to a fall in plasma $[Cl^-]$. In general, $[Cl^-]$ falls acutely by 1 mEq/L and in chronic states by 3 to 4 mEq/L for each increase of 10 mmHg in $PaCO_2$. These changes in $[Cl^-]$ are accompanied by increases in $[HCO_3^-]$ of similar magnitude.

The effectiveness of increases in $[SID]$ in limiting increases in $[H^+]$ also may be appreciated by looking at Fig. 22. The figure may be used to assess the presence

TABLE 5. *Causes of primary respiratory acidosis and alkalosis*

Causes of CO₂ retention and respiratory acidosis
With normal lungs
  Anesthesia
  Sedative drugs
  Neuromuscular disease (e.g., poliomyelitis, myasthenia gravis, Guillain-Barré syndrome)
  Obesity-hypoventilation syndrome
  Brain injury
With abnormal lungs
  Chronic obstructive pulmonary disease (e.g., chronic bronchitis, emphysema)
  Diffuse interstitial pulmonary disease (late)
  Severe kyphoscoliosis
Causes of excess CO₂ elimination and respiratory alkalosis
With normal lungs
  Anxiety
  Fever
  Drugs (e.g., salicylates)
  Hypoxemia (e.g., high altitude)
  Central nervous system lesions (e.g., tumors, meningitis)
  Sepsis
  Hormonal excess (e.g., progesterone, thyroxine)
With abnormal lungs
  Pneumonia
  Diffuse interstitial pulmonary disease (early)
  Acute bronchial asthma
  Pulmonary vascular disease
  Congestive heart failure

of superimposed metabolic acidosis, in which $[SID]$ increases are less than expected for the rise in $PaCO_2$, or metabolic alkalosis, in which $[SID]$ increases are more than expected. In recovery from ventilatory failure, resolution of the changes in $[SID]$ is also time-dependent. If the reduction in $PaCO_2$ toward normal occurs rapidly, there is a delay in the increase in $[Cl^-]$ (*posthypercapnic metabolic alkalosis*).

Reductions in $PaCO_2$ are caused by hyperventilation. When the reduction in $PaCO_2$ is the primary disturbance, the condition is termed *primary respiratory alkalosis*. Conditions that give rise to this situation are shown in Table 5. Reductions in $PaCO_2$ tend to reduce $[HCO_3^-]$ in plasma, but unless a decrease occurs in $[SID]$, this reduction is quite limited and a marked fall in $[H^+]$ results, especially in acute hyperventilation. Reductions in $[SID]$ minimize the fall in $[H^+]$, and they are the result of two compensatory responses. These are retention of Cl^- through a fall in its renal excretion and a small accumulation of lactate resulting from the stimulation of glycolysis in erythrocytes and liver. Retention of Cl^- tends to characterize chronic states of hyperventilation, but increases in $[La^-]$ may occur very rapidly. These compensatory changes are associated with increases in $[H^+]$ toward normal and a fall in $[HCO_3^-]$. The usual reduction in total $[SID]$ that results from an increase in both $[Cl^-]$ and $[La^-]$ accompanying an acute fall in $PaCO_2$ amounts to only 1 to 2 mEq/L for each fall of 10 mmHg in $PaCO_2$; this increases to 3 to 4 mEq/L when hyperventilation is sustained for several days. The reductions in $PaCO_2$ and $[H^+]$ in hyperventilation are accompanied by a surprisingly large increase in $[CO_3^{2-}]$, predisposing to hypocalcemia and tetany.

Complicated Acid-Base Disorders

Complicated acid-base disturbances are those disorders defined as either mixed (acidosis plus alkalosis) or combined (respiratory plus metabolic acidosis, or respiratory plus metabolic alkalosis). Not infrequently, complicated problems occurs in which the expected compensatory responses are inefficient or absent because of coexisting impairment of function. The most common functional impairments are the presence of renal disease or ventilatory failure. Usually, such situations have to be considered within the clinical context and need to be identified by the response to the primary disorder. For example, a patient with a metabolic acidosis resulting from poor control of diabetes may have a $PaCO_2$ that is higher than expected in response to the accumulation of ketoacids that reduces the $[SID]$. The poor ventilatory response may be caused by impaired ventilatory capacity resulting from air flow obstruction or respiratory muscle weakness. Poor renal function also may lead to an inappropriate compensatory response. For example, in chronic respiratory failure, the

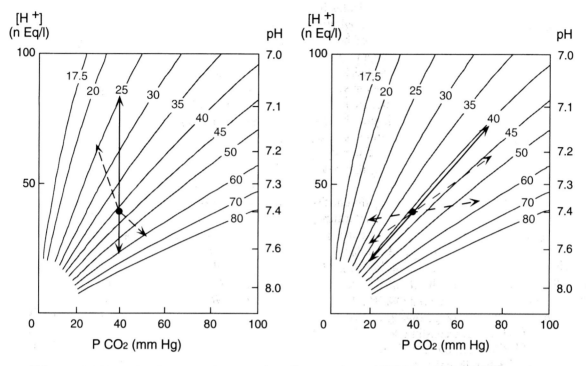

FIG. 22. Acid-base isopleths. Isopleths are for different values of [SID] in mEq/L at a normal weak acid concentration. **Left panel:** Changes in [H⁺] accompanying changes in [SID] without respiratory compensation (*solid black arrow*) and with respiratory compensation (*dashed red arrow*). **Right panel:** Changes in $PaCO_2$. *Solid arrow* shows [H⁺] changes with $PaCO_2$ in absence of changes in [SID]. *Dashed arrows* show changes in [SID] with acute (*red*) and chronic (*blue*) respiratory acidosis and alkalosis.

kidneys may be unable to excrete Cl^-, adding a metabolic acidosis to the respiratory acidosis. Urinalysis, including measurement of electrolytes and pH, may be valuable in assessing these situations.

OXYGEN TRANSFER FROM BLOOD TO MITOCHONDRIA

Convective Oxygen Delivery

The net uptake of O_2 from the lungs to the body tissues is determined by the blood flow rate multiplied by the difference between the O_2 contents of arterial and venous blood ($avDO_2$). This relationship is expressed as Fick's First Principle:

$$\dot{V}O_2 = \dot{Q}_T [CaO_2 - C\bar{v}O_2]$$

where $\dot{V}O_2$ is the O_2 consumption of the body, $\dot{Q}_T$ is the cardiac output, and CaO_2 and $C\bar{v}O_2$ are the values for arterial and mixed venous O_2 content, respectively. The O_2 content (CO_2) of blood is determined as follows:

$$CO_2 = [Hb] (1.34) (SO_2) + 0.0031 \times PO_2$$

where [Hb] is hemoglobin concentration in grams per deciliter, 1.34 is the binding capacity of hemoglobin for

O_2 in mL (O_2) per gram (Hb), and SaO_2 is the O_2 saturation of hemoglobin as a fraction of 1.0. The term 0.0031 PO_2 represents the dissolved O_2 per mmHg of O_2 partial pressure. At the resting metabolic rate with a cardiac output of 5 L/min (50 dL/min) and an arterial-venous difference in O_2 content of 5 mL/dL,

$$\dot{V}O_2 = 50 \text{ dL/min} \times 5 \text{ mL } O_2/\text{dL}$$

$$= 250 \text{ mL/min}$$

The convective delivery of O_2 to the body tissues ($\dot{D}O_2$) is defined as $\dot{Q}_T \times CaO_2$. Solving the Fick equation, this is normally

$$(50 \text{ dL/min}) (15 \text{ g/dL}) (1.34 \text{ mL } O_2/\text{dL}) (1.0)$$

$$= 50 \times 20 \text{ mL } O_2/\text{min}$$

$$= 1000 \text{ mL } O_2/\text{min}$$

At an $avDO_2$ of 5 mL/dL, approximately 250 mL O_2 is extracted by the body per minute. This results in a mixed venous hemoglobin saturation of 75% and an O_2 extraction ratio of 250 mL O_2/1000 mL O_2, or 0.25. In other words, only one fourth of the O_2 delivered to the tissues is utilized by the body at rest. During work, increased metabolic demands by the tissues for O_2 can be met by increasing $\dot{D}O_2$, the O_2 extraction ratio, or both.

$\dot{D}O_2$ can be altered by changes in any of the variables in the Fick equation, including cardiac output, hemoglobin concentration, changes in O_2 binding capacity of hemoglobin, and hemoglobin O_2 saturation. In general, alterations in one of these parameters is compensated for by adjustments in one or more of the others to maintain "adequate" $\dot{D}O_2$ to the tissues. For example, anemia is compensated for by increases in cardiac output, whereas chronic hypoxia causes increases in both cardiac output and hemoglobin concentration. At extremes of exercise, the $\dot{D}O_2$ can increase as much as sixfold and the O_2 extraction ratio as much as threefold.

The distribution of cardiac output to the different tissues of the body under normal conditions is determined by the local metabolic needs. Normally, the O_2 consumption of tissues is independent of $\dot{D}O_2$ provided that more than the critical amount of O_2 is delivered. For example, the human brain receives approximately 20% of the cardiac output to support its normal O_2 requirement. Increasing $\dot{D}O_2$ to the normal brain (e.g., during hypercapnia) does not increase the metabolic consumption of O_2 by the brain. Under pathologic conditions such as hypovolemia, however, the cardiac output is redistributed by autonomic mechanisms to tissues with high obligatory needs for O_2. This response preserves the functions of the heart and brain at the expense of blood flow to skin, skeletal muscle, and splanchnic organs.

In some diseases, such as adult respiratory distress syndrome (ARDS) and sepsis, concerns have been raised about whether at a particular $\dot{D}O_2$ the body can extract O_2 adequately to meet the needs of the tissues. If not, O_2 consumption will fall if O_2 delivery falls. This situation is called *pathologic supply dependence of O_2 consumption.* It is distinguished from physiologic supply dependence, which occurs when O_2 delivery falls below the point at which normal O_2 extraction has reached its maximal limit of approximately 75% (Fig. 23). Pathologic O_2 supply dependence has been reported in a variety of clinical conditions; however, the finding is difficult to interpret under most circumstances. It is difficult to determine the clinical significance of small changes in systemic $\dot{V}O_2$ without sensitive methods for measuring the adequacy of oxidative metabolism in individual tissues. Therapeutic attempts to improve systemic O_2 consumption by increasing O_2 delivery in septic shock and ARDS have met with limited success once the circulatory blood volume has been restored adequately. The pathophysiologic mechanisms that may contribute to pathologic O_2 supply dependence are discussed later in this chapter.

In the intensive care unit, measurements of cardiac output by thermodilution, mixed venous oxygen content, and systemic O_2 consumption are made routinely using a flow-directed, balloon-tipped pulmonary arterial catheter (Swan-Ganz catheter). Alternatively, the $\dot{V}O_2$ can be measured by respiratory gas analysis. The $\dot{V}O_2$ represents the sum and venous O_2 content represents the flow-weighted average of all the tissues of the body. The measurements contain a number of potentially serious pitfalls in regard to interpretation, and misconceptions are common about the clinical utility of the information obtained from them. This is particularly true for an increase in the mixed venous O_2 saturation, which cannot be interpreted as an improvement in the hemodynamic status of a critically ill patient.

The coefficient of variation for the measurement of cardiac output by thermodilution is approximately 15%. Very few tissues of the body require 15% of the cardiac output to meet their normal O_2 requirements (the brain being a notable exception). As shown from the Fick equation, the cardiac output and $avDO_2$ can both be used to compute the systemic O_2 consumption. When pulmonary arterial catheter measurements are used to compute the $\dot{V}O_2$, then the $\dot{D}O_2$ measurement and $\dot{V}O_2$ measurement are linked mathematically, and errors in the measurement of cardiac output can produce systematic errors in $\dot{V}O_2$. This is the source of some of the association between

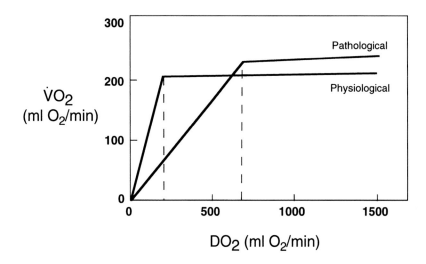

FIG. 23. Relationship between O_2 delivery and O_2 consumption for the body. Physiologic O_2 supply dependence shows a lower critical delivery than pathologic O_2 supply dependence. $\dot{D}O_2$, delivery; $\dot{V}O_2$, consumption.

decreased $\dot{D}O_2$ and decreased $\dot{V}O_2$ in critically ill patients (O_2 supply dependence).

As systemic $\dot{D}O_2$ falls, mixed venous O_2 saturation also falls, because normal organ systems attempt to maintain $\dot{V}O_2$ by increasing O_2 extraction. If the organ system fails to extract O_2, systemic measurements show a fall only in the systemic $\dot{V}O_2$. If the $\dot{V}O_2$ of the organ system is low (e.g., for the kidney), then the change in systemic $\dot{V}O_2$ will be within the measurement error by thermodilution for the cardiac output. If an organ system with failing blood flow had been extracting O_2 nearly maximally, the complete loss of its perfusion will cause the mixed venous O_2 saturation to rise, not fall (Fig. 24). In this circumstance, the increase in venous O_2 saturation reflects the loss of the perfusion to the organ and not an improvement in tissue oxygenation. In other words, the mixed venous O_2 saturation is useful only as a measure of the degree of stress on the O_2 extraction mechanism; it cannot be used as a means to determine adequacy of tissue oxygenation. Thus, under most clinical circumstances in critically ill patients, a low mixed venous O_2 saturation indicates inadequate $\dot{D}O_2$ to some vascular bed(s); a normal mixed venous O_2 saturation means only a normal average O_2 extraction for tissues that are using O_2 at the time the measurement is taken. Tissues that are no longer extracting oxygen (e.g., because of ischemia or anoxia) are no longer represented in the mixed venous O_2 saturation value.

The Partial Pressure of Oxygen in Tissues

The convective delivery of O_2 from the lungs to the other body tissues produces a measurable PO_2 in the tissues. Measurements of PO_2 in living tissue, however, are difficult to make and difficult to interpret because of variability of the results. Predictions of tissue PO_2 from theoretical calculations also have led to conclusions that are sometimes inconsistent with experimental measurements. There is controversy concerning the effects of the serial resistances to O_2 transport from the erythrocyte to the mitochondria, and in particular concerning the question of whether the primary resistance resides at the capillary level or within the tissue. Although many aspects of this problem have been investigated, our understanding of tissue oxygenation is still quite incomplete, particularly for disease states.

The diffusion of O_2 from the capillaries into the tissues produces an O_2 distribution profile in the tissues. Tissue measurements of PO_2 with surface electrodes or indwelling microelectrodes usually yield very irregular PO_2 profiles. When various PO_2 values are plotted as percentages of their frequencies, a PO_2 histogram is obtained; the range and the peak PO_2 values provide an estimate of the dispersion of PO_2 values in the tissue. An example of a PO_2 histogram is provided in Fig. 25. The implications of the distribution of PO_2 values within a tissue are discussed below.

Before experimental measurements of tissue PO_2 became possible, the theoretical approach of Krogh, with his model of a tissue cylinder around a central capillary running parallel to resting muscle fibers, was used to calculate the PO_2 in an ideal tissue. Although it is quite simple, the Krogh model has been conceptually useful to describe the principles of tissue O_2 transport. In the Krogh tissue cylinder, the critical location for O_2 supply is at the periphery of the venous end of the cylinder. This is called the *lethal corner* (Fig. 26). Other models have been devised, in which O_2 is supplied to a solid cylinder from

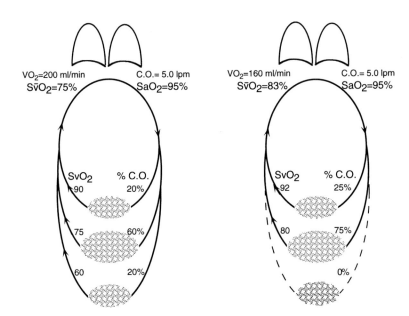

FIG. 24. Effects of loss of tissue perfusion on the mixed venous SaO_2 and O_2 consumption by the body. Note that SaO_2 increases when loss of perfusion occurs in a tissue previously extracting a large amount of O_2.

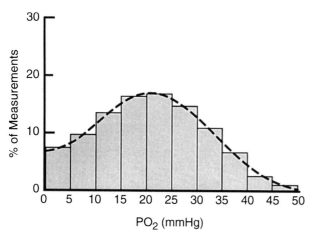

FIG. 25. PO_2 histogram of brain tissue. Measurements made in the brain of an anesthetized cat using platinum needle electrodes.

a homogeneous peripheral sheet of blood (Hill model) or, more realistically, from a number of peripheral capillaries. Most models assume an ideal cylindrical geometry and, for the most part, the delivery of O_2 from a uniform source of capillaries. In the Krogh cylinder, a single cylinder and capillary are considered assuming homogeneity of the tissue and its microcirculation; more complex models admit the possibility of differing numbers, distributions, and types of capillaries.

The PO_2 gradient from capillary blood to tissue depends on the sum of convective and diffusive resistances to O_2 transport. The Krogh and Hill models stipulate a limitation by diffusion; however, there are circumstances in which $\dot{V}O_2$ may be limited not by diffusion but by O_2 delivery. The Krogh model also does not predict O_2 supply dependence because of its assumptions or its inherent limitations. The ideal $\dot{D}O_2/\dot{V}O_2$ relationship appears to be similar for anemic, hypoxic, and stagnant hypoxia as

long as the intercapillary distance (ICD) is small (below 80 μm). The calculated O_2 extraction ratio, however, is too high. The high O_2 extraction predicted by the Krogh model may be caused by the assumption of tissue homogeneity and can be made more realistic by including an O_2 shunt of about 30%. Such precapillary O_2 loss has been demonstrated experimentally; however, its true magnitude is unknown. The O_2 extractions predicted by the Krogh model improve when ICD is increased (above 80 μm), but the critical point becomes higher for hypoxic hypoxia, indicating an effect of diffusion at large distance.

Support for the Krogh diffusion theory of capillary exchange has been found in controlled animal experiments suggesting that $\dot{V}O_{2max}$ is limited by O_2 diffusion during normoxia. It is not possible, however, to determine the location of the limiting resistance to diffusion from such experiments. Intracellular PO_2 values in working muscle also have been deduced from the myoglobin (MbO_2) dissociation curve in animal experiments. The MbO_2 saturation measured by cryomicrospectroscopy *ex vivo* suggests that the intracellular PO_2 is only a few torr and evenly distributed at $\dot{V}O_{2max}$. This finding has been ascribed to Mb-facilitated O_2 and a low apparent K_m for O_2 (PO_2 for half-maximal O_2 consumption) similar to that of isolated mitochondria. These findings suggest there is no lethal corner—that is, the muscle is "well stirred," tissue PO_2 is much lower than $P\bar{v}O_2$, and the main PO_2 gradient occurs across the capillary endothelium. In contrast, measurements of oxidized cytochrome a,a_3 in mitochondria in situ versus MbO_2 saturation diverge as $\dot{V}O_2$ increases *in vivo*, indicating the PO_2 gradient between cytosol and mitochondria increases with increasing $\dot{V}O_2$. Thus, the apparent behavior of the tissue PO_2 differs greatly between normal, isolated and *ex vivo* experiments. Isolated cells and tissues also differ from intact tissue, in which $\dot{V}O_2$ varies with the metabolic needs of the tissue. In

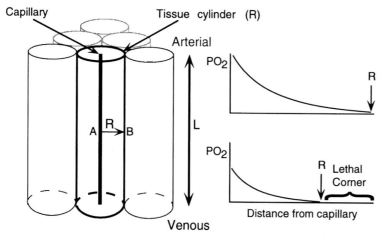

$$MO_2(R) = G(R)\,[PO_2(A) - PO_2(B)]$$

FIG. 26. Model of tissue oxygenation based on the Krogh cylinder. The predicted O_2 gradient in two regions of a single capillary and tissue cylinder are shown. The model assumes constant and uniform $\dot{V}O_2$ throughout the tissue cylinder. The diffusion of O_2 is given by the O_2 conductance (G) of the tissue and the difference in O_2 partial pressures between points A and B on the model.

living tissues, the functional microcirculation regulates many of the factors influencing the O_2 supply of tissues. These features of the microcirculation are summarized briefly in the following sections.

Effect of Oxygen Equilibrium Curve

Normally, only one fourth of the O_2 carried by oxyhemoglobin is unloaded in the tissues; however, because of countercurrent exchange of O_2 in precapillary vessels, hemoglobin in the capillaries probably operates closer to the steep, middle portion of the OEC. The effect of a shift of the OEC on O_2 unloading in tissues depends on the level of oxygenation. High P_{50} increases and low P_{50} decreases venous saturation in normoxia and mild hypoxia, whereas the opposite occurs in severe alveolar hypoxia. It is the steepness of the OEC that determines this difference. A P_{50} inadequate for a particular O_2 requirement can be compensated for by an increase in blood flow. The effect of a shift of the OEC on tissue oxygenation has been confirmed in many studies, but the significance of moderate shifts is often questioned. At normoxia, an increase in P_{50} (e.g., from the Bohr effect) makes the capillary blood maintain a higher PO_2 toward the venous end of the capillary.

Capillary Transit Time and Oxygen Shunting

Heterogeneous capillary geometry (e.g., variable spacing) leads to variable volume of perfused tissue, and variability of capillary transit time results in differing PO_2 patterns in various volumes of tissue. Capillaries with long transit times (low flow) are vulnerable to stagnant conditions with rapid depletion of O_2; capillaries with very short transit time (high flow) are prone to O_2 shunting. There must be optimal transit times for gas exchange somewhere in between these extremes for various tissues. There is also significant countercurrent exchange of O_2 between small arterioles and venules in some tissues (precapillary O_2 loss).

Heterogeneity of Perfusion

Many of the relevant variables that determine the adequacy of tissue O_2 availability are distributed inhomogeneously in the tissues. These variables include capillary density, capillary length and diameter, blood flow, transit time of erythrocytes through the capillary, $\dot{V}O_2$, and hemoglobin and myoglobin O_2 saturation values. The following example illustrates the problem. In resting skeletal muscle, most of the capillaries are perfused; however, blood flow rates in individual capillaries are inhomogeneous and often intermittent. This provides a physiologic reserve of capillaries in which the distribution of blood

flow regulates tissue PO_2 over a range of changes in O_2 supply and/or $\dot{V}O_2$. In normal skeletal muscle, perfusion inhomogeneity may even increase during contraction and relaxation. Under conditions of submaximal exercise, however, all capillaries are open and flow is more homogeneous. Capillary heterogeneity during exercise, however, may decrease or increase at very high workloads. Heterogeneity also may markedly affect the O_2 supply at high $\dot{V}O_2$. On the other hand, local heterogeneity in O_2 delivery may be reduced by diffusion of O_2 between adjacent capillaries, particularly under conditions of high blood flow.

Capillary Hematocrit

The role of the capillary hematocrit in tissue gas exchange remains poorly understood. It is generally accepted, however, that capillary hematocrit is much lower than systemic hematocrit (perhaps as low as 10%), and it bears little relation to systemic hematocrit. Capillary hematocrit fluctuates in parallel with $\dot{V}O_2$ and the contractile state of the arterioles, which suggests it is a regulated variable in the maintenance of tissue oxygenation.

Venous PO_2 Versus Tissue PO_2

The venous PO_2 and mean tissue PO_2 generally agree for an organ under normal conditions, but there are significant deviations when changes occur in capillary density, $\dot{V}O_2$, hemoglobin concentration, and cardiac output. The change in venous PO_2 after an increase in capillary density provides a good estimate of mean tissue PO_2, even in conditions deviating from normal resting conditions. Misleadingly high venous PO_2 values, however, occur in the presence of functional arteriovenous O_2 shunting resulting from countercurrent blood flow, very short capillary transit times, preferential flow channels, or shock. Some of these problems have been discussed earlier in the context of clinical interpretation of the mixed venous O_2 saturation.

Oxygen Supply Dependence of Respiration

One of the simplifying concepts often used in thinking about tissue oxygenation is that cellular O_2 uptake has zero-order kinetics—that is, it is independent of PO_2 throughout the tissue. This assumption is based on the observation that the Michaelis-Menton constant (K_m) for O_2 is very low in well-stirred mitochondrial suspensions (order of 0.1 torr). Longmuir first showed that $\dot{V}O_2$ of cells depends on PO_2 up to considerably higher values than expected from zero-order kinetics; he ascribed this to intracellular resistance to O_2 diffusion. Slices of liver follow Michaelis-Menten kinetics rather than zero-order kinetics, with an apparent K_m about 100 times higher than that for mitochondrial suspensions. Thus, the difference between "true" mitochondrial K_m and "apparent" K_m for O_2 in cells and tissues must be appreciated.

In intact tissues, the mitochondrial oxidation-reduction state depends on PO_2 over a physiologic range of PO_2; thus, metabolic adjustment ensures a reasonably constant ATP supply and $\dot{V}O_2$ with decreasing PO_2. These findings imply that the critical PO_2 in intact cells is very low, and they diminish the potential effect of O_2 gradients on respiration rate. O_2 diffusion would be expected to limit $\dot{V}O_2$ only during an extreme lack of O_2 (e.g., ischemia or profound hypoxemia) or at extremes of $\dot{V}O_2$ with mild to moderate hypoxemia. Isolated small muscles and muscle slices in vitro show O_2 supply dependency, presumably caused by very low PO_2 values in the center of the tissue.

As discussed earlier, physiologic O_2 supply dependence is defined as a condition in which $\dot{V}O_2$ decreases with diminishing O_2 delivery below a low critical threshold. The slope below the critical threshold indicates optimal O_2 extraction. Above the critical threshold there is a horizontal plateau; decreases in O_2 delivery do not lower $\dot{V}O_2$ in the plateau region because O_2 extraction increases proportionately. When O_2 supply is reduced below the critical threshold, $\dot{V}O_2$ falls because O_2 extraction no longer increases proportionately and cannot compensate for the reduction in O_2 delivery (Fig. 23).

Pathologic O_2 supply dependence of $\dot{V}O_2$ has been reported over a wide range of O_2 delivery values in ARDS patients. This form of O_2 supply dependence is characterized by a higher critical O_2 supply, a lower slope below the critical PO_2, and a higher supercritical plateau or no plateau at all (Fig. 23). The lower slope indicates a deficiency in O_2 extraction from the blood with an increase in mixed venous PO_2. The underlying mechanisms that can contribute to this deficiency are complex and multifactorial. They include vascular microembolization, disruption of endothelial function resulting in a protein-rich permeability edema, microvascular dysregulation, and loss of mitochondrial function. Experimental injuries that produce O_2 supply dependency are characterized by a decrease in capillary reserve, an increase in capillary distances (loss of open capillaries and edema), heterogeneity of capillary distribution and flow, and an increase in capillary shunts. These problems contribute to derangements of the microvascular function and impaired O_2 extraction from the blood, with compromise of O_2 supply to the tissue.

CELLULAR ENERGY METABOLISM

Cellular Energy Requirements

The immediate energy source for practically all the energy-requiring processes in the cell is the hydrolysis of adenosine triphosphate (ATP) to adenosine diphosphate (ADP) and inorganic phosphate (P_i). ATP is replenished continuously by the cell through the processes of glycolysis and oxidative phosphorylation. In these processes, sequences of chemical reactions partially trap changes in chemical free energy in the synthesis of ATP. The ATP-ADP cycle (Fig. 27) constitutes a basic feature of energy metabolism in all cells and functions as the link between the energy-utilizing and the energy-consuming processes. The rate of ATP utilization can increase more than 100 times during exercise, utilizing the whole muscle store of ATP in about 3 seconds. For cellular homeostasis, the rate of ATP regeneration generally equals the rate of ATP utilization, and the cellular ATP content remains approximately constant. Of all the tissues of the body, cardiac and skeletal muscle are faced with the most intricate problems of metabolic regulation because of their unique need to change metabolic rate.

The ultimate and most efficient process for ATP formation in aerobic cells is the intramitochondrial oxidation of substrates by the citric acid cycle, with conservation of free energy by the coupled processes of electron transport and oxidative phosphorylation. In the final process, molecular O_2, the ultimate electron acceptor, is reduced to water. For a limited period of time, however, ATP can be produced through processes that do not require O_2 (e.g., glycolysis). Some species have evolved with a special ability to survive for a prolonged period under anaerobic conditions. The physiologic relationship between aerobic and anaerobic energy production is well illustrated by a discussion of exercise metabolism.

Metabolism During Exercise

Progressive muscular exercise is accompanied by proportional increases in $\dot{V}O_2$ until the maximal aerobic capacity is reached ($\dot{V}O_{2max}$). Workloads beyond those required to reach $\dot{V}O_{2max}$ produce no further increase in O_2 consumption. A major determinant of the $\dot{V}O_{2max}$ during exercise under normoxic conditions is the cardiac output. The cardiac output sets an upper limit of the capacity to deliver O_2 to the tissues. Heavy exercise with only 10 kg of muscle may be sufficient to elicit an average person's maximal O_2 uptake; however, the system for convective O_2 delivery also can be seen as being well matched to the ability of the muscle to consume O_2. At high muscle blood flow rates and extraction ratios, the availability of O_2 to the mitochondria may be limited by diffusion.

The type of fuel utilized during physical activity is determined by work intensity, duration, training status, and substrate availability. The major part of the energy demand during low-intensity exercise is supplied by oxidation of fat, whereas oxidation of carbohydrates is required during exercise at higher intensities. The amount of ATP that can be produced by glycolysis corresponds

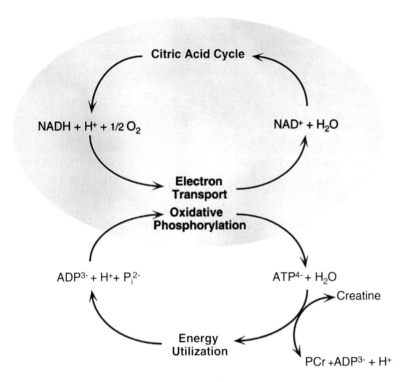

FIG. 27. The ATP-ADP cycle. The major means of conserving energy in the cell is oxidative phosphorylation, which is coupled to electron transport in the mitochondrion (*shaded area*). Oxidative phosphorylation generates ATP from ADP and P_i to support the energy needs of the cell. Additional energy can be stored in the form of PCr, which can be used later to phosphorylate ADP and regenerate ATP.

to about 20 seconds of maximal work. This limitation is caused by depletion of the store of creatine phosphate (PCr) and the accumulation of lactic acid in the muscles. ATP formed by glycolysis is therefore important during short bursts of high-intensity exercise or during ischemic conditions, but it is negligible in terms of energy provision for sustained exercise. During sustained exercise at low or moderate intensities, the rate of pyruvate oxidation is similar to the rate of glycolysis, but at higher intensities the entry of pyruvate into the mitochondrion is incomplete and lactic acid is formed and accumulates in the body fluids. Accumulation of lactate in muscle and blood begins at about 50%–70% of $\dot{V}O_{2max}$. At 100% of $\dot{V}O_{2max}$, 10%–20% of the total energy production is provided by glycolysis with lactate formation. Accumulation of lactate in blood is accompanied by an increased ventilation and CO_2 exchange. The exercise intensity when blood lactate and ventilation increase more than the increase in intensity and $\dot{V}O_2$ has been termed the *anaerobic threshold* or *lactate threshold*. This value is widely used in exercise physiology to define the training status of subjects.

During muscular work, the major store of high-energy phosphates in the cell is PCr. PCr can maintain the cellular ATP concentration approximately constant despite fluctuating energy demands. During maximal short-term exercise, the muscle content of PCr can become depleted, and the amount of energy provided corresponds to about 0.3 mol of ATP. The classic view of PCr is that it serves as a high-energy phosphate buffer during periods of high demand for energy. The concept is valid, but changes occur in the PCr level under other conditions. It has been shown that PCr decreases during submaximal exercise in

relation to the intensity of the exercise. The decline in PCr occurs at the onset of exercise, and its value remains practically constant during the exercise.

The relative concentrations of ATP, ADP, and the other adenine nucleotides are important for the control of bioenergetic processes. Their concentrations are determined by the energy potential of the system and the adenylate kinase (AK) reaction. AK is considered to be close to equilibrium:

$$\overset{\text{AK}}{2\ \text{ADP} \leftrightarrow \text{AMP} + \text{ATP}}$$

The total cellular concentrations (including both the free and bound nucleotides) of AMP, ADP, and ATP are related to each other in a ratio of roughly 1:10:100. The cellular concentration of ATP remains fairly constant during most physiologic conditions, but because it is present in much greater concentrations than the other adenine nucleotides, a small decrease in ATP results in a large relative increase in ADP and in an even more pronounced increase in the relative concentration of AMP. The availability of ADP is a primary determinant of the mitochondrial respiratory rate.

Breakdown of PCr is catalyzed by creatine kinase, and because the enzymatic activity in muscle is high, the reaction appears to be close to equilibrium under most conditions. An increase in free ADP and H^+, both of which are products of ATP hydrolysis, promotes breakdown of PCr. Aerobic energy production through an increase in free ADP will therefore, through the creatine kinase equilibrium, result in a breakdown of PCr. Thus, depletion of PCr is not necessarily a sign of anaerobiosis but may reflect increased energy turnover and activation of aerobic metabolism.

In addition to ADP, signals of major importance for the control of the energetic processes are intracellular concentrations of Ca^{2+}, AMP, P_i, and the mitochondrial redox state. Increases in Ca^{2+}, ADP, AMP, and P_i are linked to the contraction process and the energy demand and ensure that the rate of ATP formation equals the rate of ATP utilization. Further control of the different pathways is achieved through substrate activation, feedback inhibition, and allosteric regulation. At low metabolic rates, the rate of glycolysis is balanced by an equal rate of pyruvate oxidation, and there is no accumulation of pyruvate or lactate in the tissues despite a large increase in the rate of glycolysis. At higher metabolic rates, when either the availability of O_2 is limited or the maximal aerobic capacity of the tissue is approached, formation of pyruvate exceeds pyruvate oxidation and lactate accumulates. The metabolic signals to turn on pyruvate formation (glycogenolysis and glycolysis) and pyruvate oxidation (citric acid cycle and mitochondrial respiration) are similar: increases in ADP, P_i, and Ca^{2+}. An imbalance between these processes shown by lactate formation at higher exercise intensity or during hypoxia may be related to a change in the oxidation-reduction state of the NAD^+/NADH couple, which regulates pyruvate entry into the citric acid cycle.

As lactate formation and PCr breakdown during exercise are not necessarily related to anaerobiosis, the term *anaerobic threshold* is misleading. The term *lactate threshold* better describes the condition related to work intensity, when ATP synthesis occurs to a greater extent through glycolysis. Therefore, the lactate threshold does indicate an important functional point in metabolism. Experimental evidence suggests that a decrease in tissue O_2 availability has metabolic consequences (e.g., PCr breakdown and enhanced glycolysis) before cellular respiration is limited by hypoxia. These metabolic changes reflect the adaptation of the tissue to an increased metabolic rate relative to the availability of O_2.

Cellular Respiration and the Mitochondrion

As noted in the previous section, the primary role of cellular respiration is to produce ATP from O_2 consumption during the process of oxidative phosphorylation (Fig. 28). This fundamental process and its regulation occur within the mitochondria. In mitochondria, various nutrients are converted by intermediary metabolism to CO_2 and NADH for oxidation. This oxidation provides the energy to establish an electrochemical proton gradient (Δp) across the mitochondrial inner membrane. The Δp drives the influx of precursors for substrate oxidation, synthesis of ATP, export of products, and maintenance of osmotic stability. The cell depends on mitochondrial

provision of ATP because glycolysis, the only other metabolic process to produce significant amounts of ATP, yields just four ATP molecules, compared with 26 from oxidative phosphorylation.

Supply of Oxidizable Substrates

Most of the substrates for cellular energy production are supplied by dietary fats, proteins, and carbohydrates. Carbohydrates and some amino acids are converted to three-carbon acids (e.g., pyruvate), whereas fats and other amino acids are converted to two-carbon acetyl compounds. Mitochondria convert pyruvate and hydrocarbon chains to acetyl-CoA and oxidize acetyl-CoA to CO_2. The systems involved in these processes directly supply the reducing equivalents (electrons) to the mitochondrial electron transport chain and are essential for mitochondrial ATP production.

Oxidation of acetyl-CoA to CO_2 is catalyzed by the enzymes of the citric acid cycle. The electrons from this oxidation are handled by three dehydrogenases that reduce NAD^+ to NADH, and one that reduces ubiquinone to ubiquinol. The enzymes involved in the production of NADH are isocitrate, α-ketoglutarate, and malate dehydrogenases. Succinate dehydrogenase contains a flavin coenzyme (FAD) and does not require NAD^+. Several other dehydrogenases transfer electrons to the electron transport chain through NADH and ubiquinone; however, these reactions contribute little relative to the citric acid cycle. The most important factors affecting turnover in the citric acid cycle are the availability of NAD^+, the rate of acetyl-CoA production, mitochondrial ADP concentration, and loss of tricarboxylic acid for other biosynthetic function. Under some conditions, the rate of flux through the cycle is limited by formation of citrate by condensation of acetyl-CoA and oxaloacetate. Because oxidation of NADH and ubiquinol are coupled to synthesis of ATP, regulation of respiration also occurs at the level of the dehydrogenases.

Mitochondrial Electron Transport

The electrons from NADH formed in the reactions of the citric acid cycle are transported to O_2 through a series of respiratory complexes in the mitochondrial inner membrane. These complexes catalyze three successive redox reactions in which the mobile carrier ubiquinone and cytochrome c catalytically oxidize NADH to NAD^+, culminating in the four-electron reduction of molecular O_2 to water. Each of the respiratory complexes also transports protons out of the mitochondrial matrix in response to the flow of electrons, thereby capturing the energy available from the oxidation-reduction process in the form of the electrochemical proton gradient (Δp) across the inner membrane. This Δp provides the energy to drive ATP

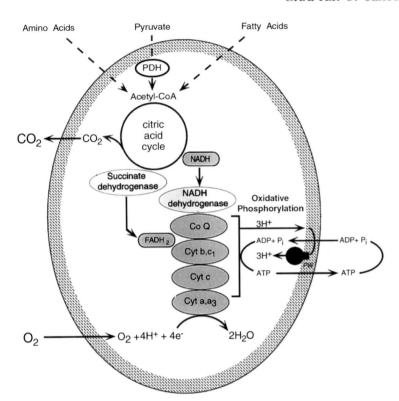

FIG. 28. Schematic drawing of mitochondrial respiration. CO_2 is produced from the oxidation of carboxylic acids in the citric acid cycle. Reducing equivalents in the form of NADH and $FADH_2$ are generated and supplied to the respiratory chain from the citric acid cycle. Molecular O_2 is reduced by cytochrome c oxidase as NADH and $FADH_2$ are reoxidized for use in the citric acid cycle. Energy in the form of ATP is generated from ADP by oxidative phosphorylation.

synthesis from ADP and P_i by coupling the reaction to the movement of protons.

The electrochemical proton gradient has two components: a chemical gradient (ΔpH) and an electrical potential ($\Delta\psi$). The chemical gradient is the difference in the concentration of protons between the matrix space and the cytoplasm. The concentration of protons is expressed as pH, so that the chemical gradient is given as ΔpH. The matrix pH is about 7.6, whereas the cytoplasmic pH is approximately 7.0. The energy available from ΔpH is insufficient to drive ATP synthesis under normal conditions in the cell. Multiple transport systems enable the energy available from oxidation to maintain a large electrical potential across the inner membrane. This potential is about -160 mV inside the mitochondrion. It drives positively charged molecules into the matrix and supplies much of the energy needed for ATP synthesis.

ATP Synthesis

The synthesis of ATP from ADP and P_i during oxidative phosphorylation is catalyzed by an ATP synthase. This enzyme is an electrogenic proton transporter that utilizes energy from the Δp. Under most conditions, the Δp formed by electron transport is sufficient to support ATP synthesis. Without electron transport, as occurs during anoxia and with mitochondrial inhibitors, the ATPase can generate Δp by hydrolyzing ATP from glycolysis. The ATPase also can hydrolyze ATP when the membrane

cannot maintain the pH gradient, as occurs in the presence of uncouplers of oxidative phosphorylation. The physiologic significance of the latter two modes of operation of the enzyme is unknown.

Mitochondrial Metabolite and Ion Transport Systems

Compartmentation of metabolites and ions across the inner mitochondrial membrane is tightly regulated and plays an integral part in respiratory control. The entry of carbon substrates into the mitochondrial compartment, along with extrusion of products (e.g., ATP) is achieved by specific transporter systems driven by components of the Δp. Electroneutral ΔpH-dependent transport systems for pyruvate and Pi effect the accumulation of pyruvate and P_i in the matrix according to the ΔpH across the inner membrane. The dicarboxylate and tricarboxylate carriers catalyze electroneutral exchange of P_i for citric acid cycle intermediates. Hence, the mitochondrial distribution of these anions depends indirectly on ΔpH. Some mitochondrial systems catalyze transport that is dependent on $\Delta\psi$ and results in a net charge movement across the inner membrane. These systems can establish a potential (electrogenic movement) or can move charged species according to an existing potential (electrophoretic movement). The adenine nucleotide transporter catalyzes the exchange of matrix ATP^{4-} for cytosolic ADP^{3-}, allowing electrophoretic movement of a negative charge out of the matrix. This is the major mechanism for supplying ADP to the ATP synthase, and subsequently ATP to the cytoplasm.

Heterogeneity of Mitochondrial Distribution and Function

Although aerobic respiration occurs in all mammalian tissues, the maximal O_2 consumption rate, respiratory control characteristics, mitochondrial morphology, and mitochondrial distribution vary among tissues. In most cell types, the need for a continuous supply of energy to support function is met by specific associations of mitochondria with energy-requiring systems. Because energy demand varies with workload, there is no ''normal'' O_2 consumption rate; instead, cellular function determines the O_2 consumption rate. Changes in function can markedly alter the relative contributions of different tissues to the total O_2 consumption by the body.

Variations in energy needs and other functional demands are associated with differences in mitochondrial respiratory components and their regulation. In muscle, cycles of contraction require cyclical changes in mitochondrial shape and cellular oxygenation. Myocytes have features to accommodate these demands. Muscle mitochondria are found as networks, or reticula, and myocytes contain myoglobin to facilitate cellular transfer. Other types of cells also have highly specialized adaptations to function.

Mitochondria from various tissues also differ in protein composition. The contents of some enzymes and transporters vary qualitatively, whereas indispensable enzymes and transporters vary quantitatively. Molecular studies show that tissue-specific isoenzymes exist for essential components such as the adenine nucleotide transporter, cytochrome c, and cytochrome c oxidase. Mitochondrial function may be optimized by regulation of enzyme contents and activities per volume of mitochondria, volume percent of mitochondria in cells, and spatial distribution of mitochondria in cells. In various cells, the distribution of mitochondria is different at the morphologic level. The volume of mitochondria per cell (volume density) also varies up to 100-fold in different human tissues. Furthermore, mitochondria differ between tissues in size and shape, inner membrane folding, and buoyant density. Differences in mitochondrial structure and composition also occur in different cells of the same cell type.

Regulation of mitochondrial function occurs at several sites, especially those involving generation and utilization of Δp and volume regulation. Regulation of Δp involves control of electron flow into the electron transport complexes at the NAD^+-linked dehydrogenases and at cytochrome c oxidase. Several of the important NAD^+-linked dehydrogenases are regulated by Ca^{2+}, and cytochrome c oxidase contains regulatory subunits. Electrophoretic transport systems, including the adenine nucleotide trans-

porter, also regulate the Δp. Variations at different sites could result in significant differences in regulation of respiratory function without changes in overall mitochondrial structure.

Adaptive changes in mitochondria can occur in response to physiologic challenges. These mitochondrial changes serve to adapt function to the prevailing conditions, and they include changes in volume density, adjustment of enzymatic and transport activities per unit mass, and spatial distribution of the organelles within cells. Changes in volume density are associated with altered aerobic work capacity; greater mitochondrial density provides a greater maximal ATP production under these conditions. This principle does not hold in disease, as impaired mitochondrial function can necessitate increased density to maintain function. Change in mitochondrial volume density also occurs in response to development and differentiation, exercise, conditioning, starvation, chronic hypoxia, changes in diet, and pharmacologic agents.

Altered expression of enzyme and transport activities per unit of mitochondrial volume occurs with adaptation to different physiologic states. For instance, thyroxine administration and recovery from hyperthyroidism result in changes in cytochrome c oxidase and citrate synthase. Urea cycle enzymes are increased by high-protein diets and by starvation. Chronic hypoxia causes a decrease in mitochondrial enzymes, whereas physical conditioning increases the concentrations of these enzymes. Thus, alterations in the composition of enzymes and transport systems provide another mechanism for cells to optimize ATP production.

At the cellular level, mitochondrial density and distribution are important determinants of the O_2 concentration required to maintain cellular ATP production. The distribution of mitochondria appears to represent a balance between the need to have a high capacity for ATP production at sites of high ATP demand and the need to oxygenate the cells adequately at physiologic blood PO_2. Most cells and tissues have a functional reserve that allows enhanced activity under physiologic or pathologic challenge. For tissues with high energy requirements, the metabolic demand is met by high volume density of mitochondria and, in some tissues, by clustering of mitochondria. The higher volume density and clustering can increase the O_2 concentrations required for function. Tissues with high mitochondrial volume density and clustering are inherently more susceptible to O_2 deficiency, and this susceptibility is increased by higher metabolic needs.

The effects of hypoxia on mitochondrial function indicate that different metabolic pathways are selectively vulnerable to tissue hypoxia. The apparent K_m of cytochrome c oxidase in many adult mammalian cells occurs at a PO_2 10 to 160 times greater than the isolated oxidase, which has a K_m of less than 0.1 mmHg. This means that failure of mitochondrial function can occur at a relatively high

O_2 concentration compared with that of isolated mitochondria. Many reactions that depend indirectly on O_2 (i.e., those dependent on ATP) are vulnerable over the same O_2 concentration range. Studies of activities of different ATP-requiring systems in cells show that some are much more sensitive to ATP depletion, and hence to tissue hypoxia, than others. The order of these sensitivities is determined both by the K_m values of the enzymes for ATP and by the location of the enzymes in the cell relative to the mitochondria. Depending on whether changes in enzymatic activities cause irreversible injury, the different sensitivities of the O_2- and ATP-dependent enzymes to O_2 availability can affect cell viability directly.

All mammalian cells can survive some period of severe O_2 deficiency without irreversible injury. Such nonlethal hypoxic periods occur when cells function with reduced metabolic and respiratory capacity. These conditions are distinct from both normal and irreversible hypoxic or anoxic states. During brief anoxia, the mitochondrial Δp is maintained despite substantial decreases in cellular ATP concentrations. The energy required for maintenance of Δp is made available when specific ion transport systems are inhibited that drive ATP synthase activity. Such selective inhibition of ion transport allows cells to preserve the mitochondrial milieu and facilitates their recovery on reoxygenation. Similar metabolic suppression may occur in other tissues, such as the kidneys, where inhibition of transport functions protects against anoxic injury. The myocardium exhibits a response termed *stunning,* in which an ischemic episode results in inhibition of mitochondrial respiratory functions and reversible cessation of contractile activity. Suppression of synaptic function (*idling*) protects neurons from anoxic injury, and postanoxic suppression of cellular respiratory rate in the brain also may be the consequence of an endogenous mechanism to preserve viability. Whether such conditions occur in critically ill patients during ARDS, sepsis, or other shock states is unknown. The precise mechanisms regulating respiratory function in these diseases also are not clear, but the existence of such mechanisms clearly would influence cellular O_2 demand and the amount of O_2 that must be delivered to the tissues by the circulation.

BIBLIOGRAPHY

Astrup P, Severinghaus JW. *History of Acid-Base Physiology.* Stockholm: Munksgaard; 1986. *Excellent review of the history of acid-base physiology.*

Benesch R, Benesch RE. Intracellular organic phosphates as regulators of oxygen release by haemoglobin. *Nature* 1969;221:618–622. *A biochemical summary of the relationship between 2,3-diphosphoglycerate and O_2 affinity of hemoglobin.*

Dawson CA, Linehan JH, Bronikowski TA. Pressure and flow in the pulmonary vascular bed. In: Will JA, Dawson CA, Weir EK, Buckner CK, eds. In: *Lung Biology in Health and Disease.* Vol. 38. Weir EK, Reeves JT, eds. Marcel Dekker: New York; 1989;51–105. *A comprehensive review on the pressure-flow relationship of pulmonary vasculatures.*

Forster RE. Diffusion of gases across the alveolar membrane. *Handbook of Physiology,* Section 3. 1987. *Detailed discussion of principles of gas diffusion at the levels of the acinus.*

Forster RE, Dubois AB, Briscoe WA, Fisher AB, eds. *The Normal Lung. Physiological Basis of Pulmonary Function Tests.* 3nd ed. Chicago: Year Book; 1986. *A textbook with emphasis on mechanical behavior and gas exchange and transport of the lung.*

Glazier JB, Hughes JMB, Maloney, JE, West JB. Measurements of capillary dimensions and blood volume in rapidly frozen lungs. *J Appl Physiol* 1969;26:65–76. *An original observation on different dimensions of pulmonary capillaries in different regions of the lung.*

Hochachka PW, Somero GN. *Biochemical Adaptation.* Princeton, NJ: Princeton University Press; 1984. *Wonderful summary of studies in biochemical adaption using a comparative physiological approach.*

Howell JBL, Permutt S, Proctor DF, Riley RL. Effect of inflation of the lung on different parts of pulmonary vascular bed. *J Appl Physiol* 1961;16:71–76. *An original study that evaluates the effect of lung volume on vascular resistances of alveolar and extra-alveolar vessels.*

Jones DP. Intracellular respiration. In: Crystal RG, West JB, et al, eds. *The Lung: Scientific Foundation.* New York: Raven Press; 1991: 1445–1454 (vol 2). *Excellent summary of the factors that govern respiration at the cellular level.*

Jones, NL. Acid-base physiology. In: Crystal RG, West JB, et al, eds. *The Lung: Scientific Foundation.* New York: Raven Press; 1991: 1251–1265 (vol 2). *Complete description of the physicochemical approach to acid-base problems.*

Kadenbach B, Reinmann A, Stroh A, Huther F-J. Evolution of cytochrome *c* oxidase. In: King TE, Mason HS, Morrision M, eds. *Oxidases and Related Redox Systems.* New York: Alan R Liss; 1988:654–668. *Summary of principles involved in conservation of the oxygen-consuming function of mitochondria.*

Kayar SR, Hoppeler H, Mermod L, Weibel ER. Mitochondrial size and shape in equine skeletal muscle: a three-dimensional reconstruction study. *Anat Rec* 1988;222:333–339. *Description of the morphological distribution of mitochondria in skeletal muscles.*

Klocke RA. Carbon dioxide transport. In: Farhi LE, Tenney SM, eds. *Gas Exchange (The Respiratory System;* vol 4). Bethesda, MD: American Physiological Society; 1987:173–197 (*Handbook of Physiology*; section 3). *Comprehensive description of CO_2 transport by the blood.*

Krogh A. The number and distribution of capillaries in muscles with calculations of the oxygen pressure head necessary for supplying the tissue. *J Physiol* 1919;52:409–415. *An original paper on the exchange of oxygen in tissue.*

Milic-Emili J, Henderson JAM, Dolovich MB, Trop D, Kaneko K. Regional distribution of inspired gas in the lung. *J Appl Physiol* 1966; 21:719–759. *A comprehensive discussion of the regional distribution of ventilation.*

Mitzner WA. Collateral ventilation. In: Crystal RG, West B, et al, eds. *The Lung: Scientific Foundations.* New York: Raven Press; 1991: 1053–1063. *A comprehensive review of collateral ventilation with extensive references.*

Monod J, Wyman J, Changeux JP. On the nature of allosteric transition: a plausible model. *J Mol Biol* 1965;12:88–118. *Classic paper on biochemical function and two-state allosteric transitions.*

Nunn JF. Distribution of pulmonary ventilation and perfusion. In: *Nunn's Applied Respiratory Physiology.* Oxford: Butterworth-Heinemann; 1993:156–197. *A clear and concise summary of $\dot{V}_A/\dot{Q}$ relationships in the lung.*

Perrella M, Bresciani D, Rossi-Bernardi L. The binding of CO_2 to human hemoglobin. *J Biol Chem* 1975;250:5413–5418. *A basic description of the interaction of CO_2 with hemoglobin.*

Perutz MF. Molecular anatomy, physiology, and pathology of hemoglobin. In: Stamatoyannopoulos G, Nienhuis AW, Leder P, Majerus PW, eds. *The Molecular Basis of Blood Disease.* Philadelphia: WB Saunders; 1987:127–178. *Basic review of the molecular behavior and physiological rule of hemoglobin in the body.*

Perutz MF, Muirhaed H, Mazzarella L, Crowther RA, Greer J, Kilmartin JV. Identification of residues responsible for the alkaline Bohr effect in haemoglobin. *Nature* 1969;222:1240–1243. *Molecular localization of the amino acids involved in the Bohr effect.*

Rahn H, Reeves RB, Howell BJ. Hydrogen ion regulation, temperature, and evolution. *Am Rev Respir Dis* 1975;112:165–172. *A description of the "alphastat" hypothesis by the original authors.*

Rodman DM, Voelkel NF. Regulation of vascular tone. In: Crystal RG,

West JB, et al, eds. *The Lung: Scientific Foundations.* New York: Raven Press; 1991:1105–1120. *A summary of the factors involved in regulatory control of pulmonary vascular tone.*

Russell JA, Phang PT. The oxygen delivery-consumption controversy. *Am J Respir Crit Care Med* 1994;149:433–437. *Summary of the debate about the relationship between systemic O₂ delivery and O₂ consumption.*

Sahlin K. Aerobic and anaerobic mechanisms. In: Crystal RG, West JB, et al, eds. *The Lung: Scientific Foundations.* New York: Raven Press; 1991:1455–1465 (vol 2). *Basics of cellular metabolism during exercise.*

Saltin B, Gollnick PD. Skeletal muscle adaptability: significance of metabolism and performance. In: Peachey LD, Adrian RH, eds. *Skeletal Muscle.* Washington, DC: American Physiological Society; 1987: 555–631 (*Handbook of Physiology,* Section 10). *Description of the link between muscle metabolism and function during exercise.*

Tenney SM. A theoretical analysis of the relationship between venous blood and mean tissue oxygen pressures. *Respir Physiol* 1974;20: 283–296. *A classic paper on the interpretation of the venous PO₂.*

Voelkel NF. Mechanisms of hypoxic pulmonary vasoconstriction. *Am Rev Respir Dis* 1986;133:1186–1195. *An extensive overview of the nature of hypoxic pulmonary vasoconstriction.*

Wagner PD, Saltzman HA, West JB. Measurement of continuous distributions of ventilation-perfusion ratios: theory. *J Appl Physiol* 1974; 36:588–599. *The original description of the theory and application of the multiple inert gas elimination technique for measuring ventilation/perfusion distribution of the lung.*

Ward JP, Robertson TP. The role of the endothelium in hyperoxic pulmonary vasoconstriction. *Exp Physiol* 1995;80:793–801. *A review of hypoxic pulmonary vasoconstriction, with emphasis on the role of endothelium and endothelium-derived vasoactive factors.*

Weibel ER. *Morphometry of the Human Lung.* Berlin: Springer-Verlag; 1963. *A classic textbook on quantitative lung morphology.*

Weibel ER. *The Pathway of Oxygen.* Cambridge, MA: Harvard University Press; 1984. *Elegant monograph on the physiologic and biochemical factors responsible for the transfer of O2 from the lungs to the mitochondria.*

West JB. Causes of carbon dioxide retention in lung diseases. *N Engl J Med* 1971;284:1232–1236. *A comprehensive discussion of the exchange of carbon dioxide in the diseased lungs.*

West JB. Life in space. *J Appl Physiol* 1992;72:1623–1630. *A review of the effects of weightlessness on various aspects of human physiology.*

West JB, Dollery CT, Naimark A. Distribution of blood flow in isolated lung: relation to vascular and alveolar pressure. *J Appl Physiol* 1964; 19:713–724. *An original description of the interplay of alveolar pressure, flow rate and pulmonary vascular resistance caused by gravity that led to the "West zone" model.*

West JB, Mathieu-Costello O. Stress failure of pulmonary capillaries: role in lung and heart disease. *Lancet* 1992;340:762–767. *A concise summary of cardiopulmonary disease in which stress fracture of pulmonary vessels plays an important role in pathogenesis.*

Textbook of Pulmonary Diseases, 6th ed.
edited by G.L. Baum, J.D. Crapo, B.R. Celli, and J.B. Karlinsky,
Lippincott–Raven Publishers, Philadelphia, © 1998.

CHAPTER

4

Respiratory Mechanics

F. Dennis McCool · Frederic G. Hoppin, Jr.

INTRODUCTION

For effective respiration, air must be drawn through the airways and distributed among approximately 400,000,000 alveolar compartments within the lung parenchyma. Respiratory mechanics is the study of the forces involved in this task and how these forces govern the volumes and flows of gases, blood, and interstitial fluids in the lung. Abnormalities of respiratory mechanics are central to the pathophysiology of most disorders of the respiratory system. An understanding of respiratory mechanics is essential for the rational assessment and treatment of these disorders, and the purpose of this chapter is to provide a basis for such understanding.

We emphasize the mechanical properties of the lung and passive chest wall. Intersecting topics, such as the function of the respiratory muscles, gas exchange with the pulmonary circulation, and the control of ventilation, are developed in detail in other chapters. We start by describing the passive respiratory system as a simple *viscoelastic* system, which means that the forces developed can be resolved into those in phase with flow (viscous forces) and those in phase with volume (elastic forces). This approach is useful, because these viscoelastic properties and their derangements in disease can be clearly assigned to specific structures (e.g., lung versus chest wall, airway caliber, loss of surfactant) and easily evaluated.

We then turn to a very different mechanical phenomenon—namely, expiratory flow limitation. This operates only at high rates of ventilation in normal subjects but is responsible for the ventilatory disability of patients with obstructive lung diseases. Next, we discuss the mechanical basis governing the distributions of volume and ventilation among the gas-exchanging air spaces of the lung. In health, there is a degree of nonuniformity of volume and of ventilation that is ordinarily of little physiologic consequence. In disease, however, there may be sufficient nonuniformity to impair gas exchange. We also discuss the impact of lung mechanics on blood flow and interstitial fluid balance in the lung. This becomes particularly important during mechanical ventilation. Finally, we deal with the energetics of breathing, describing the mechanical loads placed on the respiratory muscles in terms of work of breathing, and the physiologic costs incurred in terms of oxygen consumption by the respiratory muscles.

MECHANICAL PROPERTIES OF THE PASSIVE RESPIRATORY SYSTEM

The mechanical loads that the muscles of respiration must overcome to ventilate the lungs are imposed by the passive components of the respiratory system—the airways, lungs, and chest wall. To assess these passive loads, measurements must be made with the muscles relaxed; the assumption is made that the properties of the passive components remain the same in the presence or absence of respiratory muscle activity.

Respiratory mechanics deals primarily with the *flows, velocities, volumes,* and *pressures* developed by the respiratory system and the gas contained within it. Flow is a

F. D. McCool: Department of Medicine, Brown University Medical School, Providence, Rhode Island 02906.

F. G. Hoppin, Jr.: Departments of Medicine and Physiology, Brown University Medical School, Providence, Rhode Island 02906.

117

measurement of the volume of gas per unit time (e.g., peak expiratory flow of 10 L/s). It is different from velocity, which is a measurement of the distance per unit time (e.g., a mean of 15 m/s, for a peak flow of 10 L/s in a trachea with a cross-sectional area of 6.7 cm^2). Volume generally refers to the gas contained in a space (e.g., a volume of gas in the lung at ordinary end-expiration, or functional residual capacity, of 3.5 L). Pressure is the force per unit area applied perpendicularly to a surface (i.e., no shear force). Generally, the absolute pressure (e.g., ambient pressure of 1000 cm H_2O) is of no interest in respiratory mechanics, and the pressure in a given location is reported relative to the ambient air pressure (e.g., a pleural pressure of -5 implies a pressure 5 cm H_2O below the ambient pressure). More often than not, the pressure *difference* across the wall of a structure (transmural pressure) is of more importance than the absolute pressures, because it is the pressure differences that have mechanical effects. For example, the pressure difference between the alveolar gas and the pleural space is the same at a given lung volume during a maximal inspiratory effort against a closed glottis (Müller's maneuver) as it is during a maximal expiratory effort against a closed glottis (Valsalva's maneuver), because that difference depends only on the elastic tensions in the lung parenchyma, which in turn depend on lung volume.

Viscoelastic Properties

Viscoelastic Model

Elasticity is the property of matter that causes it to return to its resting shape after deformation by an external force. The passive components of the respiratory system exhibit elastic properties, storing energy during inspiration as would a steel spring. That stored energy is the source of the pressure difference across the relaxed respiratory system. It is available to return the respiratory system to its original volume when the inspiratory muscles relax during expiration. *Viscosity* is the frictional property of fluids (gaseous or liquid). It is the major source of the flow-related pressure differences across the respiratory system.

In quiet breathing, the passive respiratory system behaves very much like a simple viscoelastic structure. The viscoelastic properties of the respiratory system may be modeled by two passive elements arranged in series, so that the airways contribute the pressure difference between the airway opening and the alveolar gas, $P_{ao} - P_{alv}$, and the alveolar parenchyma and passive chest wall contribute the pressure difference between the alveolar gas and the body surface, $P_{alv} - P_{bs}$. Their sum, measured during relaxation of the respiratory muscles, is the pressure difference across the passive respiratory system:

$$P_{rel,rs} = P_{ao} - P_{bs} = (P_{ao} - P_{alv}) + (P_{alv} - P_{bs}) \quad (1)$$

The first term in parentheses is the viscous, flow-related pressure difference, and the second mostly represents the elastic, volume-related pressure difference. The behavior of such a model during a volume excursion can be described by the equation of motion:

$$P_{rel,rs} = P_{rel,rs,o} + (1/C_{rs}) \, \Delta V + R_{rs} \, \dot{V} \quad (2)$$

where $P_{rel,rs,o}$ is the initial passive transrespiratory system pressure, ΔV is the volume excursion, $\dot{V}$ is instantaneous flow, and C_{rs} and R_{rs} are characteristic moduli of the elastic (compliance) and viscous (resistance) components, respectively. This behavior can be displayed as a plot of passive transrespiratory system pressure against lung volume (Fig. 1). When the volume is cycled very slowly to minimize the viscous contribution, the plot describes a narrow loop (*solid tracing*). The overall slope of this loop reflects the elastic properties, $1/C_{rs}$. When volume is cycled more rapidly, the loop widens (*interrupted tracings*). The width of the loop divided by the difference of flow reflects the viscous properties, R_{rs}. In addition to the elastic and viscous contributions to the transrespiratory system pressure equation, an additional pressure component is sometimes added to represent the inertial effects of the gas and chest wall structures as they accelerate and decelerate. At ordinary breathing frequencies, however, inertial factors are small and are usually ignored.

Elastic Recoil Properties of the Respiratory System

Typical elastic properties of the relaxed respiratory system are shown in Fig. 2. Over the range of about 20%–80% of the vital capacity (VC), the curve is reasonably linear, and the elastic properties can be characterized simply by specifying the recoil pressure and slope at a specified volume. In the example illustrated, the curve crosses the zero pressure axis at about 3 L of lung gas volume and has a slope (elastance or its inverse, compliance) of about 100 mL for every 1 cm H_2O. Away from this volume in either direction, the elastic forces act to return the respiratory system toward this zero pressure point. Thus, a normal subject at rest expires passively to this zero elastic recoil position by the end of each breath, and under these conditions, the end-expiratory lung volume, or functional residual capacity (FRC), is elastically determined.

The pressure at any given volume on the passive curve indicates the elastic load, that is, the inspiratory or expiratory forces that would be required to hold the respiratory system at that volume. The elastic load increases as volume increases, reaching about 40 cm H_2O at total lung capacity (TLC) in the example shown. Note that the slope of the curve decreases at high and low lung volumes, that is, the positive and negative elastic loads increase sharply. At these extremes of volume, the strength that the muscles

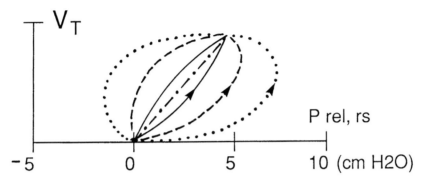

FIG. 1. Idealized viscoelastic behavior during passive ventilation in a normal subject, showing the pressure difference across the relaxed respiratory system, $P_{rel,rs}$, as a function of tidal volume, V_T, during very slow flow (*solid curve*) and sequentially higher flows (*dashed and dotted curves*). The viscoelastic model envisions an elastic component, represented by the *thin line* drawn between the points of no flow, with a slope of $1/C_{rs}$, and a viscous component, represented by the flow-related departures from the thin line, adding to the elastic pressure during inflation and subtracting from it during deflation, and accounting for the counterclockwise looping.

can apply with a maximal inspiratory or expiratory effort also wanes sharply. The volume at which the elastic load and the maximal inspiratory strength available to overcome that load converge is the limit to further inspiration (e.g., TLC). For this reason, a decrease of TLC (restriction) signifies an increase in elastic recoil, a decrease in the effective strength of the inspiratory muscles, or both. The converse mechanism sets the limit to expiration in healthy young subjects, the residual volume (RV). (The dynamic mechanism that sets RV in older subjects and patients with obstructive airways disease is discussed later.)

The separate contributions of the lung and chest wall to the elastic properties of the respiratory system can be readily distinguished. That of the lung is the pressure difference across the visceral pleura, $P_{alv} - P_{pl}$, and that of the relaxed chest wall is the pressure difference between the parietal pleura and the external surface of the body, $P_{pl} - P_{bs}$. Although direct measurements of alveolar and pleural pressures are difficult, they can be inferred

from relatively noninvasive measurements. P_{alv} is the same as P_{ao} when measured statically, and P_{pl} is the same as esophageal pressure, P_{es}, which is easily measured with a thin-walled balloon introduced *per nares*. Thus, a plot of lung volume versus the static transpulmonary pressure difference ($P_{st,L} = P_{ao} - P_{es}$) characterizes the elastic properties of the lung (*dashed curve*, Fig. 3), and a plot versus the pressure difference across the relaxed chest wall ($P_{rel,cw} = P_{es} - P_{bs}$) characterizes the elastic properties of the chest wall (*dotted curve*). The latter measurement requires complete relaxation of the respiratory muscles, which is difficult to ensure in the awake subject. Surface electromyograms have been helpful by providing a feedback reference for adequacy of voluntary relaxation, and reliable data have been obtained in subjects who are anesthetized and paralyzed.

Elastic Properties of the Lung

A typical normal curve is shown in Fig. 3. Elastic recoil is about 4 cm H_2O at FRC, and compliance, C_L, is about 200 mL/cm H_2O over most of the volume range, but elastic recoil increases and compliance decreases markedly near TLC. The recoil pressure is positive over the full range of attainable volumes, reflecting the remarkable fact the lung is under tension, inflated above its resting volume, for its entire life.

Elastic tensions in the lung are borne mainly by two components: (1) the fibrous network of collagen and elastin that supports the alveolar septa, airways, and pleura, and (2) the air-liquid interface of the alveolar septa. Elastin fibers have the requisite extensibility to sustain tensile force, F, over the full range of operating lung volumes. The elastic fiber network of the lung elastically increases tension when the network is stretched during inflation. Collagen fibers, by contrast, are very stiff and produce

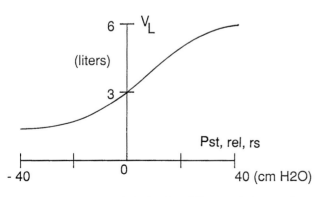

FIG. 2. Idealized elastic behavior of the respiratory system, as shown by the pressure at the airway opening measured statically (no flow) in the relaxed subject, $P_{st,rel,rs}$, as a function of lung gas volume.

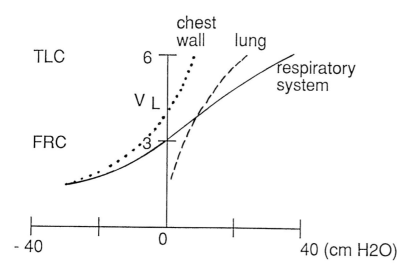

FIG. 3. Similar display to Fig. 2, showing the elastic contributions of the lung, P_L (*dashed curve*), and of the relaxed chest wall, $P_{rel,cw}$ (*dotted curve*). Note that the curves sum to the transrespiratory system pressure, $P_{rel,rs}$.

large increases in tension when stretched by only a small amount. The collagenous component of the fibrous network has been thought to serve as a safety net against overdistension, coming under tension at high lung volume and accounting for the pronounced stiffening (decrease in C_L) seen near TLC. The complex anatomic relationship of collagen fibers with elastin fibers suggests that collagen also participates at lower volumes. The energy stored as a result of elastic work during inspiration by the increase in length of the fibrous components, dl, under tension, F, is the integral $\int F\, dl$ and is equal to the area under the inspiratory limb of the static volume-pressure curve.

Surface or interfacial tension, τ, provides a second force that contributes to the elastic recoil of the lung. Evidence for this is the substantial reduction of recoil that occurs when the air-liquid interface is obliterated by filling the lung with saline solution. The physical basis for interfacial tension is the attraction between the molecules of the liquid phase, which far exceeds the attraction between the liquid and gas molecules. As a result, the forces acting on each liquid molecule at the interface are unbalanced, with a net force directed into the liquid phase, away from the gas phase. With every such molecule being pulled down out of the interface, the favored, least-energy configuration is that with the smallest surface area—that is, the surface is always "trying" to get smaller. For this reason, fine drops of water, as in a fog, are nearly spherical, the shape with the smallest surface area for a given volume. The elastic energy stored by the increase in area, dA, of the interface under tension, τ, is the integral $\int \tau\, dA$. In the lung, interfacial tension is substantially reduced by the presence at the interface of pulmonary surfactant, produced by the type II alveolar cells. (The biology and biochemistry of pulmonary surfactant are treated in detail in Chapter 17; only its mechanical effects are dealt with here.)

The manner in which these tension-bearing structures interact with each other can be inferred from their ana-

tomic relationships. First, the pseudoplanar alveolar septum connects along most of its edges to other alveolar septa, forming a continuously interconnected network, suggesting that septal elastic tension is directly transmitted from one septum to the next throughout the alveolar parenchyma. The alveolar parenchyma attaches to the inner aspect of the visceral pleura, so that its elastic tensions pull inward on the visceral pleura, lowering pleural pressure, P_{pl}, relative to alveolar gas pressure, P_{alv}, and accounting for the measurable $P_{st,L}$. Second, the alveolar septum is constructed like a sandwich, with a pseudoplanar fibrous network placed between two air-liquid interfaces. The mechanical consequence of this parallel physical arrangement is that the elastic tensions of the fibrous network and air-liquid interfaces are additive, so that elimination of the two air-liquid interfaces when the lung is filled with saline solution eliminates a substantial portion of lung recoil.

On the other hand, a series relationship exists at the point where alveoli open onto alveolar ducts. Here, tensions are transmitted directly from the septum to a structure of very different composition, the curved "cables" of the alveolar entrance rings, composed of relatively heavy, elastin-rich connective tissue and smooth muscle. The mechanical consequence of such a series relationship is that although the tensions in the two components must be in equilibrium, changes in the mechanical state of either structure cause distortion. For example, constriction of the smooth muscle of the entrance ring narrows the duct and pulls the radial septa inward toward the lumen of the duct. Conversely, increased tension in the septum, as with a deficiency of surfactant, draws the radial septa away from the center of the duct, dilating it. Despite the very different shapes and compositions of the duct and its surrounding alveolar tissues, their elastic properties are relatively well-matched, such that they expand and contract nearly proportionally with inflation and deflation.

Third, peribronchial and perivascular pressures, $P_{p\text{-}br}$

and P_{p-vasc}, can be considered to be nearly the same as pleural pressure, because the elastic elements of the alveolar parenchyma surround the bronchovascular structures, and elastic recoil at that site lowers P_{p-br} and P_{p-vasc} relative to P_{alv}, just as it lowers P_{pl} relative to P_{alv} at the visceral pleura.

The effects of disease on these tension-bearing components have predictable functional effects. Emphysema, by damaging the elastin fibers and destroying alveolar septa, reduces lung recoil, shifting the volume-pressure curves of the lung and respiratory system to the left and increasing compliance. This reduction of elastic recoil permits inspiration to higher volumes, accounting in part for the increase in TLC seen in emphysema. It also reduces the tethering forces applied to the airways, which causes them to be narrower at a given lung volume. This results in increased resistance and allows them to obstruct more readily at low lung volumes, thereby leading to a markedly decreased expiratory flow limit (see below). Conversely, the increase of collagenous fibers seen in pulmonary fibrosis restricts the lung by increasing lung recoil. This reduces TLC and FRC and tends to keep the airways open, thereby decreasing airways resistance and allowing them to remain open at lower lung volumes. Most significantly, the increase in elastic recoil increases the elastic load on the inspiratory muscles.

Reduced levels of surfactant or surfactant with an abnormal composition has similar ''restrictive'' effects, increasing lung recoil. The most significant functional consequences, however, are a decrease in end-expiratory lung volume (FRC) and a marked increase in the tendency of regions of the parenchyma to collapse at low lung volumes. This mechanism is responsible for the microatelectasis found in the adult respiratory distress syndrome (ARDS) and the respiratory distress syndrome of premature neonates.

There are two important additional mechanical effects of impaired surfactant, both a consequence of the pressure difference across the curved air-liquid interface. The first is the effect on the ''critical opening pressure'' of collapsed portions of lung. When portions of lung deflate during expiration to the point that the airways serving them close, gas is trapped in the distal alveolar regions; a plug of liquid may be found in the lumen of the closed airway. At both ends of the plug are air-liquid interfaces, concave to the air phase. Surface tension in these interfaces lowers the pressure in the fluid of the plug relative to that in the gas, and this pressure difference is described by the Laplace relationship:

$$P_{alv} - P_{liq} = \tau/r_1 + \tau/r_2 \qquad (3)$$

where r_1 and r_2 are the radii of curvature of the surface. This negative pressure holds the airway walls together until distending pressure is applied at a level great enough to open the airway (critical opening pressure). As long as the airway remains shut, the compliance of the region

is zero. This mechanism operates where and when distending pressures are low: at end-expiration at the bases of lungs of elderly subjects, in obese subjects, or in patients with diaphragmatic paralysis in the supine position. Critical opening pressures may be increased further in areas of the lung in which the distal air spaces are gas-free (e.g. microatelectasis of ARDS). In such cases, airway opening pressures may be as high as 10 to 20 cm H_2O.

The second effect is on lung fluid balance. Although the air-liquid interface is relatively flat over much of the surface of the alveolar septum, it is concave in the corners of the alveolus, and consequently the pressure in the liquid phase in the corner is lower than that in the gas phase. Interfacial tension, then, becomes important in determining the Starling equilibrium governing fluid balance in the lung. High τ favors pulmonary edema, drawing liquid from the capillaries into the interstitial space and into the alveolar spaces. Conversely, pulmonary surfactant, by reducing τ, permits the alveoli to remain dry despite their small size.

Elastic Properties of the Chest Wall

A typical chest wall volume-pressure curve is shown in Fig. 3. The recoil pressure of the relaxed chest wall is about -4 cm H_2O at FRC. The curve for the chest wall, like that of the lung, is quite linear over most of the range of lung volumes, and it has a similar compliance, $C_{rel,cw}$, of about 200 mL/cm H_2O. In contrast to the lung, which stiffens near TLC, the chest wall stiffens near RV.

Elastic energy is stored in and released from the passive chest wall by bending, stretching, and raising the abdominal wall, diaphragm, rib cage, and spine during inspiration and expiration. In particular, the marked stiffening of the chest wall near RV is caused by inward bending of the ribs and stretching of the diaphragm up into the thoracic cavity.

The elastic properties of the chest wall may be adversely affected by specific disease processes. The chest wall may be restricted by skeletal changes, such as ankylosing spondylitis or kyphoscoliosis, or by abdominal changes, as in massive ascites, pregnancy, or morbid obesity. Each of these conditions increases the recoil pressure of the passive chest wall, displacing the volume-pressure curves of the passive chest wall and respiratory system to the left, increasing the passive load on the inspiratory muscles, and decreasing the maximal end-inspiratory lung volume, TLC, and the relaxed end-expiratory lung volume, FRC.

Viscous Properties of the Respiratory System

The major source of the pressure differences in phase with flow is frictional pressure losses along the conducting airways. These losses produce a pressure difference between the airway opening and the alveolus, $P_{ao} - P_{alv}$, that depends on the dimensions of the airways, the physical properties of the gas, the flow rate itself, and the flow regime or velocity profile (streamlines) of gas movement. In quiet breathing, the streamlines are parallel and straight (*laminar flow*). The physics of this flow regime is expressed by Poiseuille's Law, which relates the pressure loss between the inlet, P_i, and outlet, P_o, of a cylindrical tube to its length, l, its radius, r, the viscosity of the gas, μ, and the flow rate, $\dot{V}$:

$$P_i - P_o = (8/\pi) \mu \, l \, r^{-4} \, \dot{V} \tag{4}$$

With laminar flow, then, the pressure loss increases directly with the flow rate (Eq. 4 and the *solid portion of the curve* in Fig. 4). Under these conditions, the ratio of the frictional pressure loss to the flow rate, $(P_i - P_o)/\dot{V}$, is a constant, the *flow resistance*, R. This ratio is often expressed as its reciprocal, the *conductance*, G.

When flows are increased, as during exercise, or when the airways are much narrowed, the streamlines do not remain straight and parallel. Eddies develop; laminar flow becomes *turbulent flow*. The velocity at which this changeover occurs can be predicted by the ratio of the inertial forces to the viscous forces, Reynold's number:

$$N_R = (2 \, \rho \, u^2)/(\mu \, u \, r^{-1}) \tag{5}$$

where ρ is gas density, u is mean velocity, and μ is gas viscosity. The conditions that lead to turbulent flow (N_R

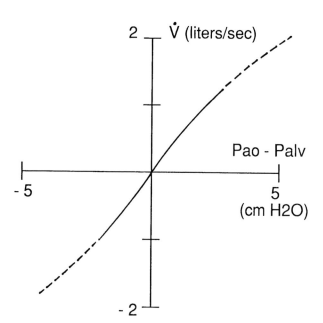

FIG. 4. Expiratory flow as a function of the pressure difference between the airway opening, P_{ao}, and the alveolar gas, P_{alv}, for a given volume. The resistance at a given point on the curve is the inverse slope of a line drawn between the origin and that point. The *solid portion of the curve* is linear, indicating constant airways resistance, consistent with laminar flow, but bends over, indicating higher resistance, at higher inspiratory or expiratory flow rates as turbulent flow begins.

2000) generally do not occur in the distal airways, where the velocity of gas, u, is relatively low. In the proximal airways, however, where u is higher, conditions for a high Reynold's number occur more readily, and flow becomes turbulent when ventilatory rates are high. The pressure loss under a turbulent flow regime is as follows:

$$P_i - P_o = (1/\pi^2) \, f \, l \, r^{-5} \, \dot{V}^2 \tag{6}$$

where f is a friction factor that depends on wall roughness and N_R.

A critical insight from Eqs. 4 and 6 is the importance (fourth and fifth powers!) of airway caliber. This is the basis for the increases in airways resistance seen when the airways are narrowed by mucus, smooth-muscle constriction, or remodeling in asthma, or by reduced tethering of the airways resulting from reduced elastic recoil in emphysema. A second critical insight is the dependence of turbulent flow on the density of the gas, ρ, rather than on its viscosity, μ, as in laminar flow. This is the basis for the sometimes dramatic clinical reduction in upper airway obstruction caused by local narrowing (tracheal tumor) observed when the low-density gas helium ("heliox") is substituted for the nitrogen in inspired gas.

Resistance in turbulent and orifice flow is higher than in laminar flow and is not constant, but increases with increasing flow and is characterized by curvilinearity of the overall pressure-flow relationship at higher flows (*dashed portion*, Fig. 4). This relationship may be approximated by the empiric Rohrer equation:

$$P_{ao} - P_{alv} = K_1 \, \dot{V} + K_2 \, \dot{V}^2 \tag{7}$$

where the constant K_1 reflects primarily the behavior under low flow and laminar conditions, and K_2 the additional costs of turbulent flow.

To measure the viscous pressure losses down the airways, it is necessary to know the gas pressure in the alveoli, P_{alv}. This cannot be measured directly in the intact chest, but it can be inferred by body plethysmography. The difference between P_{ao} and P_{alv} divided by the flow rate recorded with a pneumotachograph during a panting maneuver (to open the glottis as much as possible) yields airway resistance, R_{aw}. Another approach is to analyze volume-pressure loops (Fig. 1) and simultaneously measure flow rates; R may be obtained by dividing the width of the loop at a given volume by the difference in flow rates at that volume. A third approach, which may be used to estimate airway resistance in an intubated patient on a mechanical ventilator, takes advantage of the abrupt equilibration of the pressure at the mouth (P_{ao}) with the alveolar gas pressure (P_{alv}) when the distal end of the breathing circuit is briefly occluded at the end of inspiration. The abrupt decrement in pressure observed when the circuit is occluded may be attributed to the flow-related pressure drop along the airways. This observed pressure drop, divided by the preocclusion flow rate, gives R_{aw}.

At the distal end of the conducting airway tree, individual airways are very small and therefore each has a high resistance. Nevertheless, the flow through any one airway is very small because of the very large number of airways arranged in parallel, and consequently, the pressure drop across any one of these airways is quite small. Indeed, the greatest part of the total airway frictional pressure loss is incurred in the upper airways (nose, pharynx, and larynx); the loss is smaller in the trachea and proximal bronchi, and least in the distal airways. The overall airways resistance decreases with increasing lung volume because of the effect of lung recoil on airway caliber. Because their lengths and radii vary nearly as $V_L^{1/3}$, airways resistance, as can be derived after inserting such values in Eq. 4, is inversely related to lung volume. For this reason, R_{aw} is often multiplied by lung volume to obtain *specific airways resistance*, SR_{aw}, a parameter that is nearly independent of the lung volume at which it is measured. Its reciprocal is the *specific airways conductance*, SG_{aw}.

Frictional Pressure Differences Across the Lung Tissues

The solid structures of the respiratory system also incur frictional energy loss during breathing. This is the source of the openness of the very slow loop in Fig. 1. In contrast to the energy loss associated with gas flow in the airways, however, the frictional energy loss across the lung tissue is relatively independent of flow rate. Instead, it is a nearly constant fraction, η, of the tidal volume, V_T, multiplied by the overall tidal pressure excursion, V_T^2/C_L. The mechanism for this behavior has not as yet been worked out, but there is some appeal in relating the observed energy losses to a parameter η, that is relatively constant, rather than to resistance, a parameter that is an inverse function of frequency and compliance. These tissue frictional losses are small. Nonetheless, in quiet breathing the airway pressure losses are also small, and the tissue frictional losses then represent a large fraction of the total.

Expiratory Flow Limitation

A very different phenomenon supersedes viscoelastic behavior at high rates of ventilation in normal subjects, or at lower rates of ventilation and even at resting ventilation in subjects with obstructive lung disorders. This phenomenon is expiratory flow limitation. Up to a certain relatively modest expiratory effort, flow increases linearly with increasing effort (*solid portion of the lines*, Figs. 4 and 5). Beyond this effort, however, flow is *effort-independent*, and for a given lung volume, flow does not increase even if more effort is applied (*dashed lines*, Fig. 5).

Maximal expiratory flow is also *volume-dependent*. This is readily seen by comparing the three curves in Fig. 5, each of which shows the flow-pressure relationship for a given lung volume. The limiting flow is higher for the higher volumes. This positive volume-dependence is directly demonstrated when maximal expiratory flow is plotted against lung volume (maximal expiratory flow-volume curve, or MEFVC) (Fig. 6).

The example shown is of a normal subject performing a maximal forced expiratory maneuver followed by a maximal inspiratory maneuver. Having first inspired as deeply as possible, the subject makes a vigorous, sustained expiratory effort. The initial, rising portion of the MEFVC (roughly the first 20% of the VC) varies somewhat with effort, but the rest of expiration is flow-limited (i.e., effort-independent). In this flow-limited region, flow falls progressively during expiration and approaches zero flow at RV. This maximal forced expiratory maneuver has been dubbed an ''unnatural act,'' because it is not performed except in the laboratory and in certain individuals with severe obstructive lung disease during normal breathing. The concept of flow limitation and its indices, derived from the MEFVC, are useful in understanding and assessing ventilatory limitation and failure in obstructive airways disease.

In obstructive lung disease, maximal expiratory flow is reduced at all lung volumes (Fig. 6B). One consequence

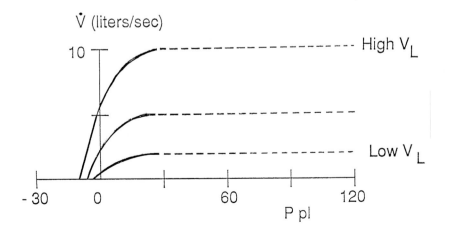

FIG. 5. Expiratory flow as a function of transpulmonary pressure for three different lung volumes. At each lung volume, the relationship is linear at low driving pressures, as in Fig. 4 (*solid portion of each curve*). At relatively modest expiratory efforts, however, flow reaches an absolute maximum; in other words, maximal flow is *effort-independent*. The maximal flow, however, is very much lower at lower lung volumes, showing that maximal flow is *volume-dependent*.

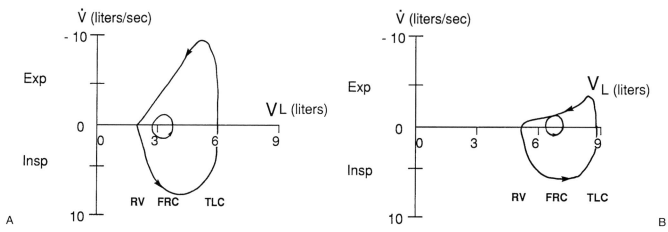

FIG. 6. A: Flow as a function of volume in a normal subject. The *outer loop* shows a forced expiration followed by a forced inspiration. The maneuver starts from a maximal inspiratory position, TLC. The expiratory flow rate peaks when about 20% of the VC has been expired and through the rest of expiration falls inexorably toward zero at maximal expiration, RV. Over this lower 80% of the forced expiratory VC, the curve is effort-independent and is extraordinarily reproducible in an individual *unless* there is a change in airway caliber (e.g., asthma) or lung recoil (e.g., emphysema). Flow during forced inspiration depends on airways resistance and the force/length/velocity properties of the inspiratory muscles. The *inner loop* shows quiet breathing, well within the outer (limiting) loop. As ventilation is increased, the loop increases its vertical dimensions (higher inspiratory and expiratory flows) and usually its horizontal dimensions (increased tidal volume) as well. At high levels of ventilation, however, the loop encounters the expiratory flow limit. Higher flows are then possible only if the curve moves to the right (to higher operating volumes), where the flow limit is higher. **B:** Similar plots in a subject with severe emphysema. Maximal expiratory flow at all volumes is severely decreased. This dynamically increases RV. Furthermore, the loop representing quiet breathing has been forced by the slope of the flow-limiting curve to move to the right. This increases FRC (hyperinflation). TLC is increased mainly because of the loss of elastic recoil. The increase of TLC is typically less than the increase of RV, and therefore the difference between TLC and RV (the VC) is decreased. Maximal *inspiratory* flow is decreased because of higher airways resistance and impaired inspiratory function at high chest wall volumes, but is less pronounced than is the decrease of maximal *expiratory* flow.

of this is an increase in the RV. A young, healthy subject can expire down to a statically determined volume at which the elastic recoil of the respiratory system and the available strength of the expiratory muscles are matched but oppositely directed (see above), but in obstructive lung disease the maximal expiratory flow is reduced, preventing the subject from expiring down to the statically determined RV; RV becomes dynamically determined.

With more severe disease, flow limitation may also increase FRC ("hyperinflation"). In the normal subject, quiet breathing follows a small inspiratory-expiratory flow-volume loop contained within the maximal loop. In obstructive lung disease, however, expiratory flow may encounter the flow limit even at rest. Passive expiration then may be interrupted by the next inspiration before the pressure difference across the passive respiratory system reaches zero (Fig. 2). FRC then also becomes dynamically increased above the elastically determined volume. The increase in volume may permit the ventilatory needs to be met, because of the positive volume-dependence of maximal expiratory flow.

One consequence of hyperinflation is elevation of end-expiratory alveolar gas pressure, as can be predicted from Fig. 2. This is readily measured in intubated patients when

the airway is momentarily occluded at the end of passive expiration, and it provides a useful indication ("auto-PEEP") of hyperinflation. With very severe disease, the expiratory flow limitation may be so extreme that resting FRC may end up higher than the premorbid TLC (Fig. 6B)! For hyperinflated patients to increase their ventilation above resting levels, they must breathe at even higher volumes. Although this increase in operating volumes permits a higher level of ventilation, it also impairs inspiratory muscle function by requiring the muscles to operate at shorter lengths and with less favorable mechanical purchase on the chest wall (e.g., flat diaphragm). Ironically, *expiratory* limitation burdens the *inspiratory* muscles! This mechanism (*expiratory* flow limitation → *increased* operating volumes → decreased *inspiratory* muscle reserve) is in fact the main cause of exercise limitation, fatigue, and ventilatory failure in acute and chronic obstructive lung diseases. Note that ventilatory capacity in obstructive lung disease is improved by improvement of inspiratory function (e.g., the ability of the chronically hyperinflated patient to inspire to very high lung volumes), and not by strengthening of the expiratory muscles.

It is not useful to think of expiratory flow limitation in terms of a flow resistance. Resistance is the inverse slope of the chord connecting a particular point on the expiratory flow/P_{pl} curve to the zero flow point (Fig. 5). R, as we have seen, is a very useful parameter at lower flows, predicting how much flow can be achieved for a given effort and explaining that prediction in terms of structure and physical properties. All of that significance is lost, however, when excess expiratory pressure is applied to the respiratory system (*dashed portions of the curves*, Fig. 5), and the slope of the chord, R, then varies with the expiratory effort.

The mechanism of expiratory flow limitation involves an interplay between the mechanical properties of the airways, the lung parenchyma, and the characteristics of the respired gas. Consider that in the absence of flow, the airways are effectively distended by lung recoil, P_{alv} − P_{pl}. The pressure difference across their walls is the intra-airway pressure, P_{aw}, less the peribronchial pressure, P_{p-br}. P_{aw} is the same as P_{alv} in the absence of flow, and P_{p-br} is approximately the same as P_{pl}. In expiration, however, P_{aw} is lower than P_{alv} because of frictional viscous losses and the Bernoulli effect. The Bernoulli effect is the lowering of pressure associated with an increase of velocity, and it becomes important in the proximal airways because of convective acceleration, resulting from a substantial increase in the velocity (Δv) of the expired gas as it enters the much smaller net cross-sectional area of the large airways and trachea. A lower intrabronchial pressure produces a lower bronchial transmural pressure difference, which in turn produces a narrower airway, which in turn requires a higher velocity because of convective acceleration, which in turn produces a lower intra-bronchial pressure because of the Bernoulli effect. And so on. This cycle of effects has an equilibrium at low expiratory flows solution at all points in the airway. But at some particular higher expiratory flow rate, the cycle of effects reaches the point at some location along the airways at which any higher flow rate would be impossible because it would be incompatible with the airway remaining open! This location is called the aerodynamic ''choke point,'' and the flow at which it develops is the maximal expiratory flow rate. This maximal flow depends (positively) on three conditions: (1) cross-sectional area and stiffness of the airway at the choke point, (2) elastic recoil (because it provides the driving pressure for flow in the airways upstream of the choke point and because its tethering action increases the cross-sectional area and stiffness of the airway), and (3) low resistance of the airways upstream of the choke point. The features of expiratory flow limits in health and disease can be understood in this framework. None of these three conditions depends on expiratory effort—hence the *effort-independence* of maximal expiratory flow. The second and third conditions are increased by higher lung volumes—hence the positive *volume-dependence* of maximal flow. Asthma lowers maximal expiratory flow by reducing the caliber of the airways (the first and third

mechanisms), and emphysema largely by reducing lung elastic recoil (the second mechanism).

The principles of flow limitation are also relevant to cough. Immediately upstream of the choke point, the airways are dynamically compressed during a cough and the velocity of the air stream is high. As the kinetic energy of the air stream is proportional to the square of its velocity, the energy available to shear mucus from the airway walls is markedly enhanced by this dynamic compression. The choke point moves peripherally as lung volume decreases, and for this reason serial coughs at lower volumes clear progressively more peripheral airways.

DISTRIBUTIONS OF VOLUME AND VENTILATION

The lung parenchyma, consisting largely of interconnected alveolar septa, divides the gas in the human lung into an estimated 400,000,000 gas-exchanging alveolar spaces. What governs the distribution of gas volume within the parenchyma? What mechanisms ensure that inspired gas distributes itself so that there is a reasonable turnover of the resident gas throughout the parenchyma?

Distribution of Volume

The alveolar septa and the alveoli exhibit a degree of variability in size and shape but generally appear to be made of the same structural components. There is no evidence of nonuniformity of elastic properties at a scale larger than about 0.5 cm. Furthermore, at a local level the parenchyma is stable in the sense that one small region is constrained from enlarging or shrinking at the expense of its neighbors. This stability, ''mechanical interdependence,'' is an inherent property of a network constructed of elastic elements with positive length-tension compliances.

At a regional level, however, there is significant nonuniformity of inflation, primarily because of gravity. The weight of the lung tissue (including blood) makes it sag. As a result, the alveoli in the upper regions are relatively inflated and those in the dependent regions relatively deflated. In the upright position, this gradient of inflation applies from apex to base. In the left lateral decubitus position, it applies from right to left. A vertical gradient of inflation reflects a vertical gradient of elastic tensions, the septal tensions being greater in the upper region from which the lung is ''hung'' and lesser in the dependent region on which the lung is ''sitting.'' Although the details of the distribution of pleural pressure remain somewhat controversial, a reasonable starting assumption is that pleural pressure and the associated elastic tensions within the parenchyma maintain a vertical gradient (in centimeters of water per centimeter of vertical distance) equal to lung density (in grams per cubic centimeter), such that the difference in lung recoil between the apex and base of a lung 30 cm in height might be on the order of 6 cm H_2O.

Distribution of Ventilation

In the healthy lung, there is both local and regional nonuniformity of ventilation. At a scale of about 0.5 cm, the nonuniformity of ventilation is modest. At FRC, the variability of the distribution of ventilation has been quantitatively estimated (in terms of the variability of the volume of regions as fractions of their volumes at full expansion) as being on the order of 0.013. The source of the variability presumably is local nonuniformity of elastic tensions. A much greater nonuniformity, however, results from the systematic vertical gradient of ventilation. With quiet breathing in a sitting position, the ventilation of the dependent regions of the lung is about twice that of the apical regions. The generally accepted mechanism for this is that the more distended apical regions of the lung are less compliant than the less distended basilar regions.

Figure 7 shows the specific compliance to be a decreasing function of elastic recoil. Specific compliance is the inverse slope of the $V/P_{el,L}$ curve *divided by V*. It represents the volume change for a given volume of gas rather than for a given anatomic entity, such as an alveolus, and is useful for calculating the fractional turnover of resident gas. Given the assumption that the amplitudes of the pressure swings during the breathing cycle are reasonably uniform, the specific compliance predicts that the turnover of resident alveolar gas volume will be less where the

distending pressure is greater, at the apices in the vertical lung, and greater where the distending pressure is very low, in the more dependent regions. An additional nonuniformity of ventilation is seen when portions of lung deflate so far during the breathing cycle that the airways serving them close, trapping gas in the alveolar regions they serve, until a deep inspiration increases the local inflating pressures above the critical opening pressures of the regions.

Finally, viscous properties may cause nonuniformity of ventilation at higher levels of ventilation or with narrowing of the airways. Consider a model in which a number of viscoelastic units ventilate in parallel (e.g., lobes, lobules, or smaller units). Each ventilating unit consists of a flow-resistive element (airway) and an elastic element (distensible parenchyma) in series. The passive emptying of such a unit follows an exponential time course:

$$V = e^{-t/(RC)} \tag{8}$$

where t is the time from the onset of the passive expiration, R is the flow-resistance of the airway of the unit, and C is its compliance. The product, RC, is the *time constant* of the exponential decay and is the time when emptying is 1/e, or about half completed. When regional time constants are short compared with the time of expiration, as they are in the healthy lung during quiet breathing, all units expire to their elastically determined volume. However, when breathing is rapid, and particularly when time constants are longer (higher airway resistance, higher compliance, or both), passive emptying is not completed in all lung units; those units with higher time constants

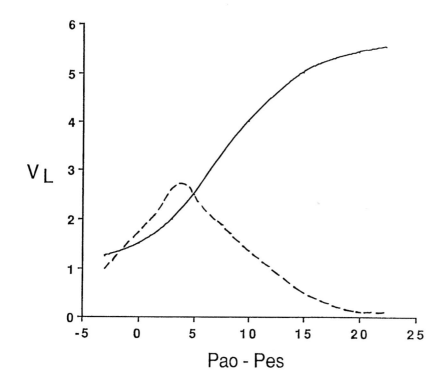

FIG. 7. Regional ventilation depends on regional specific compliance. Lung volume (V_L) (*solid curve*) and specific compliance (SC_L) (*dashed curve*) as functions of lung recoil pressure ($P_{ao} - P_{es}$) obtained during a slow expiration. In the upright chest, the recoil pressure is greater at the apex of the lung ($P_{ao} - P_{es} \sim 8$) than at the base ($P_{ao} - P_{es} \sim 2$). Because SC_L is less at 8 than at 2, the apical region is correspondingly less ventilated.

lag behind those with lower time constants. Units with lower time constant are preferentially ventilated.

In disease states, volumes may be very unevenly distributed because of local changes in elastic properties, either from altered connective tissue properties or impaired surfactant. Ventilation may also become unevenly distributed because of uneven time constants, as in asthma, in which the R of small airways is (unevenly) increased, and in emphysema, in which both the R and the C (because of the loss of elastic structure) are increased.

Different patterns of respiratory muscle recruitment may also result in uneven distribution of ventilation, although the effect is small relative to that produced by inequalities of unit time constants. Inhalations deriving from contractions of rib rather diaphragmatic muscle result in preferential distribution of ventilation to the upper lung units, as does active expiration to RV followed by a passive inspiration.

LUNG MECHANICS AND PULMONARY HEMODYNAMICS

Respiratory mechanics directly affect the right ventricular preload, the right ventricular afterload, the left ventricular afterload, and the volume of the intrapulmonary extracapillary vessels. These effects become particularly important during mechanical ventilation.

Lung mechanics affect pulmonary hemodynamics by three distinct mechanisms.

The first mechanism is a consequence of the effects of intrathoracic pressure on right ventricular preload and left ventricular afterload. Intrathoracic pressure varies during spontaneous breathing, voluntary inspiratory or expiratory efforts, and mechanical ventilation. Such changes alter the relationships between the intrathoracic and extrathoracic vascular pressures; in particular, the intravascular pressure gradients at the thoracic inlet and at the level of the diaphragm may be affected. For example, during normal breathing, inspiration *decreases* all intrathoracic pressures relative to extrathoracic pressures. The fall of pressure in the intrathoracic vena cava relative to that in the extrathoracic great veins momentarily aids return of venous blood from the abdomen, head, and limbs. Similarly, the fall of blood pressure in the thoracic aorta relative to that in the arteries of the upper extremities, neck, and abdomen momentarily impedes arterial outflow. A spontaneous inspiration, then, has the effects of momentarily *increasing* right ventricular preload and left ventricular afterload.

Opposite effects occur when the inspiration is passively delivered by mechanical ventilation, because it passively *increases* all intrathoracic pressures relative to extrathoracic pressures. This impedes filling of the right side of the heart and aids emptying of the left side of the heart (i.e., it momentarily *decreases* both the right ventricular

preload and the left ventricular afterload). Greater effects are seen when pressure changes affect the full breathing cycle, as in continuous positive airway pressure (CPAP) or positive end-expiratory pressure (PEEP). The increase in intrathoracic pressure under these circumstances is predictably the increase of chest wall volume achieved by the CPAP or PEEP divided by the compliance of the passive chest wall (Fig. 3). Although the changes of pressure may be small, the effects on right ventricular preload may be large, because the right ventricle in diastole is highly compliant. This reduction of right ventricular preload and left ventricular afterload explains the immediate benefit of CPAP or PEEP in acute pulmonary edema, and also the reduction of cardiac output that may ensue when CPAP or PEEP is applied in patients whose intravascular volumes are low or applied pressures are high.

No hemodynamic effects are *directly* attributable to changes of intrathoracic pressure on structures that lie completely *within* the thorax. Consider, as an example, the rise in pulmonary capillary wedge pressure, PCWP, seen when PEEP or CPAP is applied to the airway. The PCWP tracing provides an estimate of left atrial pressure and, in the absence of mitral disease, of left ventricular end-diastolic pressure. The increases of these pressures associated with PEEP or CPAP, however, do not quantitatively reflect increases in the transmural pressure differences across the atrium or ventricle (the measurements with functional meaning because they indicate the degree of filling of the chambers and their compliance) except in the unlikely event that the intrathoracic pressure is unchanged. Fortunately, the relevant transmural pressure differences can be estimated from $PCWP - P_{es}$.

The second mechanism operates through effects of lung elastic recoil, $P_{alv} - P_{pl}$, on right ventricular afterload. Consider the relationships among the pressures in the alveoli, P_{alv}, the pleural space, P_{pl}, the pericardial space, P_{pc}, and the cavity of the right ventricle, P_{RV}. The contractile tension of the right ventricular myocardium during systole creates a transmural pressure difference between the right ventricular cavity and its pericardial (equivalent of pleural) surface, $P_{RV} - P_{pl}$. Pressure in the right ventricle exceeds that in the pulmonary capillary because of frictional losses, $P_{RV} - P_{pc}$. The distending pressure of the pulmonary capillary must be positive for it to remain open, $P_{pc} - P_{alv}$. Pressure in the alveolus exceeds pleural pressure because of lung elastic recoil, $P_{alv} - P_{pl}$. These serial pressure differences can be related in the algebraic identity as follows:

$$(P_{RV} - P_{pl}) = (P_{RV} - P_{pc}) + (P_{pc} - P_{alv}) + (P_{alv} - P_{pl}) \tag{9}$$

which shows that the right ventricular transmural pressure difference equals the sum of the frictional pressure drop in the pulmonary arteries, the distending pressure of the capillaries, and lung recoil. The latter is generally the largest of the three, and it becomes particularly important when high inflating pressures are imposed by mechanical ventilation.

A third mechanism, probably of little clinical significance other than that it contributes to tamponade physiology, links lung distention to the blood volumes of the intrapulmonary, extra-alveolar arteries and veins. Lung distention *per se* distends all but the smallest intrapulmonary arteries and veins, as was demonstrated in the 1920s by C. C. Macklin, who found that positive-pressure inflation of an excised lung paradoxically sucked fluid into these vessels! The explanation of this phenomenon is that these vessels, lying within the bronchovascular compartments, exhibit "mechanical interdependence" with the elastic structure of the surrounding lung. The result of this mechanism is that the volumes of both vascular compartments increase and decrease cyclically as the lung inflates and deflates.

ENERGETICS: WORK RATE AND COSTS OF BREATHING

Spontaneous ventilation reaches its limit and respiratory failure may ensue when respiratory muscles, usually the muscles of inspiration, are overloaded. Up to this point, we have characterized only the *pressure* loads presented by the passive respiratory system. The ability of the muscles to accomplish a given ventilatory task, however, depends not only on the forces they must develop to overcome the pressure loads of the task, but also on the required *velocity* of shortening, on the *duration* of activation, and, most importantly, on their *operating lengths.* These factors may be linked through consideration of the energetics of breathing, first by calculating the *viscoelastic work rate,* which is the rate of *physical* energy required by the passive respiratory system to carry out a given ventilatory task in a given time, and second by measuring the *oxygen consumption,* which is the *chemical* energy actually expended by the muscles in carrying out the task. As the inspiratory muscles are far more critical to ventilation than are the expiratory muscles, we focus on the *inspiratory* work load.

Viscoelastic Work of Breathing

The physical work, W, performed by a muscle in carrying out a given task is the integral of force it develops, F, times the incremental distance it shortens, dl—that is, $\int F \, dl$, or equivalently the integral of pressure times the incremental volume displaced, $\int P \, dV$. The mean inspiratory work *rate,* $\dot{W}_{insp}$, is the work of a single inspiration times the frequency, f. The integral can be depicted graph-

ically (Fig. 8), so that the work performed on the passive respiratory system in a single inspiration is the area between the $V_L/P_{rel,rs}$ curve and the volume axis.

Work performed on the respiratory system can be partitioned into two components. That expended on the lung can be distinguished from that expended on the chest wall by integrating the transpulmonary pressure difference, $P_L = P_{ao} - P_{es}$ (lung component), and the pressure difference across the chest wall, $P_{rel,cw} = P_{es} - P_{bs}$ (chest wall component). Work can be further partitioned between elastic and viscous sources based on the assumption that the elastic component (Fig. 9) is linear between the end-inspiratory and end-expiratory points. A line drawn between these two points separates the work expended to overcome elastic forces (*horizontal shading*) from that expended to overcome the viscous forces (*vertical shading*).

The effects of increasing ventilation, of changing the pattern of breathing, or of changes in the mechanical properties of the respiratory system can be analyzed graphically or mathematically. Graphically, the elastic work of a single inspiration (area) is increased when tidal volume, V_T, is increased (extending the line representing the elastic component), when compliance, C_{rs}, is decreased (lowering the slope of the V/P_L curve), or when there is hyperinflation (sliding the operating volumes up the elastic line), and the elastic work rate is that area times the frequency, f. Mathematically, these relationships can be expressed in the following equation:

$$\dot{W}_{el} = (V_T/C_{rs})(V_T/2 + \Delta FRC) \, f \qquad (10)$$

where ΔFRC is the increment above FRC determined elastically, and $\dot{W}_{el}$ is the rate of elastic work performed.

Graphically, the viscous work is increased when the volume-pressure loop is widened by increase of inspiratory flow, $\dot{V}$, or resistance, R_{rs}. Mathematically, these

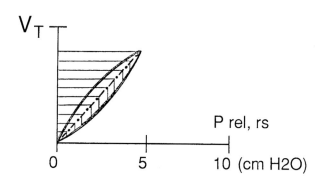

FIG. 8. The pressure difference across the passive respiratory system, $P_{rel,rs}$, as a function of displaced volume, as in Fig. 1. The work of a single inspiration is the integral $\int P_{rel,rs} \, dV$ and can be partitioned into elastic (*horizontal shading*) and viscous (*vertical shading*) work with the assumption of linearity of elastic recoil between end-inspiration and end-expiration.

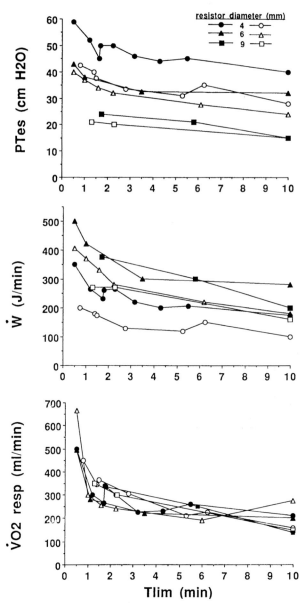

FIG. 9. Endurance in a variety of strenuous ventilatory tasks. A normal subject was assigned a variety of tasks, each of which entailed breathing an assigned tidal volume at an assigned frequency from spontaneous or increased FRC (*closed and open symbols*), through a range of inspiratory resistors (*circles, triangles, squares*), until he could no longer maintain the task. **A:** Plot of the esophageal pressure-time product, PT_{es}, against time to task failure, T_{lim}. **B:** Data replotted to show the work rate, $\dot{W}$. **C:** Data replotted to show the incremental oxygen consumption incurred in carrying out the assigned task. The ability of the inspiratory muscles to sustain a specific ventilatory task is reduced as the pressure, flow, duty cycle, or lung volume is increased. There are trade-offs among the four variables such that, for example, the same time to task failure, T_{lim}, is seen in high-pressure, low-flow tasks and low-pressure, high-flow tasks. Neither pressure nor work rate of an imposed breathing task predicts endurance well when volume or flow is varied. The incremental oxygen cost of the task is the best predictor.

effects on viscous work rate can be seen from the following relationship:

$$\dot{W}_{res} = (\pi^2/4) \, R_{rs} \, V_T^2 \, f^2 \qquad (11)$$

where $\dot{W}_{res}$ is the rate of resistive work performed.

Note the interactions between frequency, tidal volume, and ventilation. For example, at a given ventilation, an increase in frequency requires a decrease in tidal volume. These changes have opposing effects on work rate. More rapid, shallower breaths increase overall ventilation for a given alveolar ventilation, increasing the inspiratory flow rates, $\dot{V}$, and therefore the viscous load, but decreasing the elastic load. The net effect on $\dot{W}$ is relatively small over the usual breathing rates, but the effect may become significant at very high or very low frequencies. Usually with increases in ventilation, both frequency and tidal volume increase and $\dot{W}$ increases on both counts. Finally, the work of decompressing intrathoracic gas during inspiration against airway resistance can also be calculated; it can become significant when inspiratory resistance is high, as in asthma.

Energy Costs of Breathing

More relevant to the ability of the respiratory muscles to accomplish a given ventilatory task is the (metabolic) energy cost of that task, and this may differ substantially from the energy actually converted into viscoelastic work. First, it is possible for metabolic costs to be considerable even when no viscoelastic work is accomplished, as during inspiratory effort against a closed glottis, in which chemical energy (adenosine triphosphate) is expended but no work is done. Second, the purpose of muscular contraction is to displace the chest wall against a pressure load, accomplished by shortening of the muscle against a force load. However, the displacement and pressure effected by a given muscle depend on its mechanical coupling to the respiratory system and on the coordination of its contraction with the contraction of the other respiratory muscles. For these reasons, the viscoelastic work of a particular breathing task may be a very misleading index of the difficulty of actually accomplishing the task. Furthermore, the ability of a muscle to develop force depends on its length. For this reason, inspiratory muscles are weak at high lung volumes and cannot perform as they can at lower lung volumes. These three conditions (expenditure of energy without accomplishing work, operating at unfavorable mechanical advantage or with suboptimal coordination, and operating at unfavorable sarcomere lengths) particularly impair inspiratory muscle function at high lung volumes.

The energy costs of a breathing task turn out to be a much better predictor of the ability of the respiratory muscles to perform a task than is the viscoelastic work. Time to task failure has been studied for a variety of sustained tasks. It is shortened by tasks in which inspiration is elastically loaded, resistively loaded, or performed at increased lung volumes. The incremental energy cost (oxygen consumption) is not simply related to the physical work accomplished (viscoelastic work rate in the loaded breathing task); the efficiency of the system is variable among different tasks. Oxygen consumption has been found to be the parameter that best predicts the time to task failure (Fig. 9). This suggests that the limit to sustainable performance of the respiratory muscles is the rate at which they can aerobically generate adenosine triphosphate. This in turn depends on the pattern of pressure and flow loads rather than the external work accomplished. More critically, it depends on the operating lung volume, which is so critical to respiratory failure and to the ability of a hyperinflated patient to be weaned from mechanical ventilation.

BIBLIOGRAPHY

Agostoni E, D'Angelo E. Topography of pleural surface pressure during simulation of gravity effect on abdomen. *Respir Physiol* 1971;12: 102. *In-depth description of the effects of gravity on the pleural pressure gradient.*

Cherniack RM. *Pulmonary Function Testing.* 2nd ed. Philadelphia: WB Saunders; 1992. *Concise presentation of pulmonary mechanics.*

Dawson SV, Elliott EA. Wave-speed limitation on expiratory flow—a unifying concept. *J Appl Physiol* 1977;43:498. *An original work applying the principles of fluid dynamics to explain expiratory flow limitations by the "choke point" mechanisms.*

Dubois AB, Botelho SY, Comroe JH Jr. A new method for measuring airway resistance in man using a body plethysmograph. Values in normal subjects and in patients with respiratory disease. *J Clin Invest* 1956;35:327. *Details the use of body plethysmography to measure airways resistance.*

Fry DL, Hyatt RE. Pulmonary mechanics. A unified analysis of the relationship between pressure, volume, and gas flow in the lungs of normal and diseased human subjects. *Am J Med* 1960;29:672. *Reviews the effects of effort on expiratory flow.*

Hoppin FG Jr, Stothert JC Jr, Greaves IA, Lai YL, Hildebrandt J. Lung recoil: elastic and rheological properties. In: Macklem PT, Mead J, eds. *Handbook of Physiology;* section 3. *The Respiratory System;* vol 3, part 1. Bethesda, MD: American Physiological Society; 1986;195–216. *In-depth review of factors contributing to lung recoil.*

McCool FD, Tzelepis GT, Leith DE, Hoppin FG Jr. Oxygen cost of breathing during fatiguing inspiratory resistive loads. *J Appl Physiol* 1989;66:2045–2055. *Original work describing the relationships among inspiratory work, inspiratory muscle fatigue, and oxygen consumption.*

Mead J. Mechanical properties of lungs. *Physiol Rev* 1961;41;281. *Classical exposition of lung mechanics.*

Mead J, Whittenberger JL. Physical properties of human lungs measured during spontaneous respiration. *J Appl Physiol* 1953;5:779. *Classic description of the viscoelastic-elastic properties of the respiratory system.*

Mead J, Whittenberger JL. Evaluation of airway interruption technique as a method for measuring pulmonary air-flow resistance. *J Appl Physiol* 1956;6:408–416. *Details the use of airway interruption to measure airways resistance.*

Topulos GP, Butler JP. Correction of a recurrent error. *Anesthesiology* 1985;63:563–564. *Correct resistance formulas and references.*

West JB. Distribution of mechanical stress in the lung. A probable factor in localization of pulmonary disease. *Lancet* 1971;1:839. *General review of pulmonary mechanics in health and disease.*

Textbook of Pulmonary Diseases, 6th ed.
edited by G.L. Baum, J.D. Crapo, B.R. Celli, and J.B. Karlinsky,
Lippincott–Raven Publishers, Philadelphia, © 1998.

CHAPTER

5

Nonrespiratory Functions of the Lung

John W. Swisher · D. Eugene Rannels

INTRODUCTION

The human respiratory tract is a complex organ system specialized for exchange of gases between environmental air and blood circulating through the pulmonary vascular bed. The respiratory system also performs a spectrum of important nonrespiratory functions (Table 1). Certain of these lung functions, such as speech, heat and water conservation, host defense, and filtration of systemic blood, are a consequence of unique anatomic features of the respiratory system. Functional diversity of the lungs also arises from a heterogeneous population of constituent cells that participate in water and electrolyte transfer, air space defense, local neuroendocrine regulation, xenobiotic metabolism, and excretion of volatile substances. This chapter reviews the nonrespiratory functions of human respiratory tract cell populations as they relate to morphologic organization within functionally distinct compartments, including the conducting airways, alveolar region, and vascular structures. The important role of the lung in host defense is reviewed elsewhere in this volume; therefore, only a summary table of lung host defenses is provided for reference (Table 2).

J. W. Swisher: Department of Medicine, The Pennsylvania State University College of Medicine, Hershey, Pennsylvania 17033, and Department of Medicine, the Veterans Administration Medical Center, Lebanon, Pennsylvania.

D. E. Rannels: Departments of Cellular & Molecular Physiology and Anesthesia, The Pennsylvania State University College of Medicine, Hershey, Pennsylvania 17033.

FUNCTIONS RELATED TO CONDUCTING AIRWAYS

Speech

Speech and language are uniquely human characteristics generated by coordinated activity of the cerebral cortex, the brain stem respiratory drive center, and structural components of the upper airway. Phonation, or creation of sound, results from purposeful expiration of air through the vocal cords located within the larynx. Changes in the pitch of sound emitted by the larynx are achieved by stretching or relaxing the vocal cords and by altering the shape and mass of vocal cord edges. Resonance is added by several structures, including the mouth, nose and paranasal sinuses, pharynx, and chest cavity. Final articulation of sound into language is accomplished with the lips, tongue, and soft palate.

Heat and Water Conservation

During normal spontaneous respiration, inspired air is fully saturated with water vapor at body temperature (Fig. 1). Incoming ambient air is warmed by conduction and convection as it passes through the nasopharynx and tracheobronchial tree. As inspired air is warmed, it is also humidified by evaporation of water from the airway lining. Evaporation of water from the mucosal surface during inspiration transfers thermal energy to the passing air stream and results in net cooling of the airway surface.

During expiration, temperature and vapor pressure gradients are reversed, and air loses thermal energy to the

TABLE 1. *Nonrespiratory functions of the lung*

Speech
Heat and water conservation
Electrolyte transport
Host defense
Neuroendocrine secretion
Xenobiotic metabolism
Surfactant synthesis and turnover
Antioxidant defense
Excretion of volatile substances
Filtration
Hemofluidity

cooler airway surface. As air cools during expiration, its ability to hold water decreases, and water condenses along the airway surface. Countercurrent exchange of heat and water during normal tidal respiration allows conditioning of inspired air while thermal energy and water are conserved during expiration. Under normal circumstances, tidal respiration results in a net loss of only about 250 mL of water and 350 kcal of heat from the airways in a 24-hr period.

Countercurrent heat and water exchange is influenced by environmental factors and air flow velocity. Net transfer of heat and water depend on temperature and vapor pressure gradients between the airway surface and passing air stream. Low environmental temperatures increase convective cooling of the airway surface; low humidity enhances evaporative cooling of the airways. The additional heat and water required to condition inspired air raise caloric requirements in cold climates.

Transfer of heat and water from the mucosal surface to inspired air is also related to linear velocity of air flow.

TABLE 2. *Lung host defense*

Irritant reflexes
Cough
Sneeze
Bronchoconstriction
Mechanical barriers
Nasal vibrissae
Nasal turbinates
Nasopharyngeal and oropharyngeal walls
Airway carinae
Lymphoid tissues
Waldeyer's tonsillar ring surrounding orifice to lower airways
Bronchus-associated lymphoid tissue (BALT)
Mucociliary escalator
Humoral immunity
IgA—predominant in upper airways
IgG—predominant in lower airways
IgM and IgE also present
Cellular defenses
Lymphocytes—individual or aggregates
Natural killer cells
Macrophages—intravascular, interstitial, or alveolar
Polymorphonuclear leukocytes

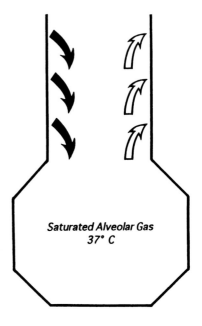

Unsatured Ambient Air
< 37° C

Saturated Alveolar Gas
37° C

➤ *Direction of heat and water transfer during inspiration*

⇨ *Direction of heat and water transfer during expiration*

FIG. 1. Countercurrent heat and water exchange in conducting airways.

Higher flow velocities are associated with lower rates of heat and water transfer to the air stream during inspiration and reduced condensation during expiration. Increases in ventilation during physical activity or other stresses thereby augment the net loss of heat and water from the mucosal surface.

Temperature of the internal milieu can also affect net heat and water transfer. The reduction in temperature gradient between air leaving the lungs and the mucosal surface that occurs at elevated body temperatures facilitates water loss. Net water loss in the setting of fever or physical exertion may actually serve as a mechanism for temperature regulation. The respiratory tract has a major role in temperature control in fur-bearing animals; however, it is not thought to affect core temperature regulation significantly in humans under normal circumstances.

Airway heat and water exchange may have important clinical implications in asthmatic patients, in whom airway cooling caused by low ambient temperatures or increased minute ventilation may provoke bronchospasm. Bronchoconstriction in cooler environments may result from acute stimulation of thermally sensitive body surface and mucosal receptors; however, airway constriction in some asthmatic patients may outlast the duration of thermal receptor stimulation. In this setting, bronchoconstriction is thought to relate to enhanced heat and water loss from the mucosal surface. Ambient temperature-induced bronchoconstriction may be mimicked in asthmatic subjects by increasing minute ventilation at any level of ambient temperature and humidity.

Heat and water exchange in the conducting airways may affect the mucociliary transport mechanism. Effective ciliary action depends on the volume and composition of the overlying mucus layer. Although characteristics of this fluid layer are largely determined by active ion transport across the epithelium and by autonomic control of submucosal gland secretion, evaporative losses and thermally regulated secretion and reabsorption may also contribute to fluid characteristics at the mucosal surface.

Electrolyte Transport

Airway epithelial cells actively transport electrolytes between the airway lumen and the interstitial compartment of the alveolar wall (Fig. 2). Water absorption passively follows net Na^+ transfer from the mucosal surface to the interstitial compartment. In contrast, net fluid secretion is a function of active epithelial cell Cl^- transport from the interstitium to the airway lumen; water passively follows Cl^- movement into the lumen. The balance between Na^+ absorption and Cl^- secretion, and hence net water movement, depends on airway region, pharmacologic intervention, and neurohumoral influences.

The predominant direction of fluid movement under basal conditions is from airway lumen to interstitium. Fluid accumulates in the proximal airways as secretions converge from distal regions of greater cross-sectional area via mucociliary transport. Fluid homeostasis is maintained primarily by absorption of Na^+ from the airway lumen down an electrochemical gradient. Cl^- and water follow Na^+ through permeable paracellular pathways. Net Cl^- secretion by epithelial cells is unusual under basal circumstances. However, inhibition of Na^+ absorption, with amiloride, for example, may shift the electrochemical gradient in favor of Cl^- secretion. Furthermore, Cl^- secretion may be stimulated by several neurohumoral agents. Prostaglandins E_2 and $F_{2\alpha}$, β-adrenergic agents, leukotrienes, adenosine, vasoactive intestinal peptide (VIP), and bradykinin stimulate epithelial Cl^- and water secretion; these mediators activate intracellular second messengers (cAMP, diacylglycerol, Ca^{2+}) that in turn activate apical Cl^- channels and lead to net water secretion.

As previously noted, effective mucociliary clearance depends on mucosal epithelial cell electrolyte and fluid transport. Mucociliary transport forms an important defense against foreign material that comes in contact with the mucosal surface of the airway. The fluid component of the mucociliary transport system is produced by secretory epithelial cells and submucosal glands. Two layers of fluid cover the airway mucosa (Fig. 3). A thin, watery sol layer of low viscosity is in direct contact with epithe-

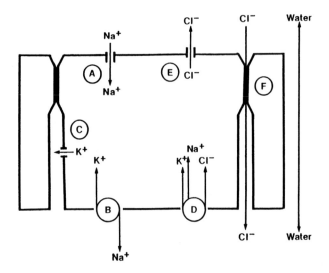

Airway Lumen

Interstitium

FIG. 2. Electrolyte transport by lung epithelial cells. Na^+ moves passively from the airway lumen into the epithelial cell through a selective Na^+ channel (**A**) down an electrochemical gradient. Na^+, K^+-ATPase (**B**) located in basolateral membranes actively pumps Na^+ from the cell into the interstitium in exchange for K^+, thereby maintaining an intracellular Na^+ concentration that favors passive Na^+ diffusion from the lumen. The accumulation of K^+ within the cell creates an electrochemical disequilibrium that favors passive movement of K^+ out of the cell through basolateral K^+ channels (**C**). Movement of K^+ into the interstitial compartment maintains an intracellular electrochemical gradient that is favorable for Na^+ entry and Cl^- secretion. Cl^- enters the cell from the interstitial space on the Cl^--Na^+-K^+ cotransporter (**D**). Cl^- is then secreted by passive movement down an electrochemical gradient through selective apical membrane Cl^- channels (**E**). Under normal basal conditions, Na^+ is absorbed from the lumen down its electrochemical gradient. Cl^- and water are passively absorbed through a permeable paracellular pathway (**F**) secondary to net Na^+ movement toward the interstitium. Water secretion occurs when the electrochemical gradient favors Cl^- movement into the airway lumen. Cl^- secretion requires activation of apical Cl^- channels.

lial cells and allows free movement of cilia. A slightly thicker and more viscous gel layer rests above the sol layer and traps particulate matter for removal by rhythmic ciliary beating. The sol layer is produced by secretory epithelial cells, whereas the more viscous gel layer arises from submucosal glands.

Epithelial secretory cells of the conducting airways are generally of three varieties. Goblet cells produce a complex mixture of glycoprotein, lipid, immunoglobulin, salt, and water. Serous epithelial cells contribute neutral glycoproteins, lysozyme, and an epithelial transport component of IgA to the sol layer. Clara cells are nonciliated epithelial cells found in highest density in the bronchioles. These cells demonstrate secretory granules containing

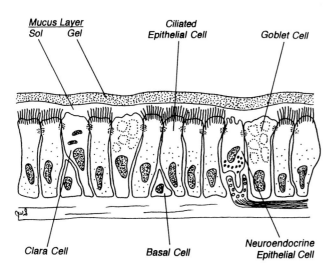

FIG. 3. Histology of conducting airway epithelium.

lipid, protein, and neutral glycoprotein. It has been suggested that Clara cells secrete the hypophase of the surfactant layer.

The clinical impact of epithelial secretory function is demonstrated in cystic fibrosis. In cystic fibrosis, abnormally increased epithelial Na^+ absorption and decreased Cl^- secretion result in relatively dehydrated mucus and defective mucociliary transport. As a result, individuals with cystic fibrosis frequently have severe respiratory infections.

Metabolism

Epithelial cells of the conducting airways are generally metabolically active cells engaged in production of mucoid secretions, electrolyte transport, and xenobiotic metabolism. Synthesis and release of soluble mediators, such as the eicosanoids prostacyclin (PGI_2) and PGE_2, have been reported. Lung epithelial cells demonstrate antioxidant defense mechanisms against free radical oxygen species that may arise from endogenous oxidative metabolism; high concentrations of inspired oxygen, ozone, or airborne chemicals; and circulating xenobiotic compounds.

Xenobiotic Metabolism

Xenobiotic metabolism is largely a function of the liver; however, the presence of xenobiotic metabolizing enzymes in the human lung is well documented. These pathways generally involve both metabolic (phase I) and conjugative (phase II) reactions. Phase I reactions include oxidation, reduction, or hydrolysis; they generate metabolites that may or may not retain pharmacologic activity of the original xenobiotic. Oxidative reactions most often involve metabolism via the cytochrome P_{450} enzyme system. Phase II reactions involve glucuronidation, sulfation, acetylation, or con-

jugation with glutathione or amino acids. These reactions render the parent xenobiotic, or its metabolite, water-soluble and devoid of pharmacologic activity.

Relatively low concentrations of several xenobiotic deactivating enzymes have been identified in the lung (Table 3). The fact that the distribution of xenobiotic metabolizing enzymes is limited to Clara cells and type II alveolar epithelial cells may account for the relatively low levels of these enzymes in the lung as a whole. Cytochrome P_{450} mono-oxygenase activity has been localized within Clara cells of the conducting airways. Other phase I enzymes, including ethoxycoumarin-O-de-ethylase, a microsomal enzyme that catalyzes O-demethylation, and epoxide hydrolase, which catalyzes hydrolysis of epoxides arising from oxidative metabolism, have been identified in the lung. Their cellular distribution is less well defined. Activity of several conjugative enzymes has also been demonstrated in the lung; these enzymes include glutathione-S-transferases, acetyltransferase, and sulfotransferases.

Many circulating basic lipophilic amines undergo first-pass retention in the lung as a result of endothelial metabolism. Significant first-pass removal has been demonstrated for propranolol, meperidine, fentanyl, and sufentanil, as examples. Retention and extraction of drugs is a function of diffusion or active transport of the substance into the intracellular compartment, followed by enzymatic modification. First-pass retention appears to be a partially saturable phenomenon, whereas overall extraction occurs independently of substance concentration.

Antioxidant Defense

By virtue of its large surface area that is continuously exposed to environmental air, the respiratory epithelium is at risk for damage caused by free radical oxygen metabolites. Generation of free radicals from exogenous sources may be achieved by direct interaction between inhaled agents and epithelial cells, and indirectly via activation

TABLE 3. *Relative activities of deactivating enzymes in major organ systems[a]*

	Lung	Liver	Intestine	Kidney
Phase I activity				
ECOD	1.0	20.6	0.5	1.2
mEH	0.1	2.1	<0.1	<0.1
Phase II activity				
GST	0.1	0.2	0.1	0.2
AT	0.1	0.7	0.3	0.2
P-ST	<0.1	0.1	<0.1	<0.1

ECOD, ethoxycoumarin-O-de-ethylase; mEH, microsomal epoxide hydrolase; GST, glutathione-S-transferases; AT, acetyltransferases; P-ST, phenol sulfotransferases.

[a] The table shows relative activities of five enzymes in lung, liver, intestine, and kidney. All activities, which are expressed relative to ECOD in lung, were derived from data presented by Krishna and Klotz.

of airway inflammatory cells that generate large quantities of reactive oxygen species. Endogenous oxidative metabolism also generates oxygen-derived free radical species that may interact with cell membrane phospholipid moieties and glycoproteins and thereby disrupt their structural integrity. Reaction of oxygen-derived free radicals with cellular components is thought to contribute to the pathogenesis of many disease processes, including bronchopulmonary dysplasia, asthma, emphysema, pulmonary fibrosis, and ARDS (adult respiratory disease syndrome).

The most biologically active oxygen species include superoxide, hydrogen peroxide, hydroxyl radical, and nitric oxide, although several other species have been identified. Superoxide is generated as a by-product of mitochondrial respiration or by interaction of microsomal and nuclear membrane cytochromes with oxygen; it subsequently spontaneously dismutates or is scavenged by superoxide dismutase. Hydrogen peroxide is formed indirectly from enzymatic and nonenzymatic dismutation of superoxide or directly by a cytoplasmic reaction catalyzed by xanthine oxidase. Hydrogen peroxide decomposes into water and oxygen in the presence of catalase. Hydrogen peroxide and alkylhydroperoxides are also scavenged by glutathione redox reactions. Superoxide and hydrogen peroxide react to generate hydroxyl radicals. Hydroxyl radicals also arise from Haber-Weiss and Fenton reactions, which are catalyzed by trace levels of transition metals such as Fe^{2+}. Nitric oxide is formed from the terminal guanidine nitrogen atom of L-arginine by NADPH-dependent oxidation; the reaction is catalyzed by nitric oxide synthase. Although nitric oxide has become well-known for its favorable vasodilatory properties, it can react with superoxide to form peroxynitrite, which degenerates into other very potent mediators of oxidant injury. Free radicals may be released into the extracellular environment if they are produced in quantities that exceed intracellular scavenging mechanisms.

Lung antioxidant defense mechanisms protect airway epithelial and other cell types from harmful effects of reactive oxygen species generated by endogenous metabolism and inhaled chemicals. The major intracellular defense mechanisms against reactive oxygen species include superoxide dismutase, catalase, and glutathione redox enzymes. Different cell populations within the lung vary in their resistance to oxidative injury. Although knowledge of antioxidant enzyme distribution in the human respiratory tract is limited, most antioxidant enzymes in the respiratory tract appear to be localized in the airways. Lower relative concentrations of mitochondrial superoxide dismutase and catalase are present in the bronchial epithelium. Extracellular superoxide dismutase is found in high concentrations in areas rich in type I collagen, in connective tissues surrounding smooth muscle, and in the junctions between epithelial cells. Antioxidant enzymes that have been identified in other cell populations of the lung are discussed below with other functions involving those cell types.

Neuroendocrine Function

Cells with neuroendocrine characteristics have been identified in the respiratory tract of humans and several other animals. Sensitive immunocytochemical and radio-labeling techniques have localized a wide variety of peptide mediators in the lung (Table 4). Although many of these mediators have been localized in association with autonomic nerve fibers, the present discussion is limited to their association with neuroendocrine epithelial cells and pulmonary vascular endothelial cells.

Neuroendocrine Epithelial Cells

Epithelial cells that produce peptide mediators have been identified throughout the tracheobronchial tree. These neuroendocrine epithelial cells are demonstrated with silver impregnation staining or antibodies to general endocrine markers, such as chromogranin. Neuroendocrine epithelial cells of the airways share many characteristics with APUD (amine precursor uptake and decarboxylation) cells of the diffuse neuroendocrine system. In humans, pulmonary neuroendocrine epithelial cells are identified by expression of peptide mediators, such as gastrin-releasing peptide (bombesin) and serotonin. In human fetal bronchi, neuroendocrine epithelial cells appear as early as at 8 weeks' gestation and may be involved

TABLE 4. *Peptide mediators identified within the lung*

Peptides associated with parasympathetic nerves
Vasoactive intestinal peptide (VIP)
Peptide histidine isoleucine (PHI)
Galanin
Peptides associated with sympathetic nerves
Neuropeptide Y (NPY)
Peptides associated with sensory nerves
Calcitonin gene-related peptide (CGRP)
Substance P
Peptides associated with endocrine cells
Calcitonin gene-related peptide
Calcitonin
Gastrin-releasing peptide or bombesin (GRP)
Endothelin
Enkephalin
Serotonin (5-HT)
Somatostatin
Cholecystokinin
Substance P
Human chorionic gonadotropin (HCG)
Pancreatic secretory trypsin inhibitor
Pituitary adenylate cyclase-activating peptide
Peptides associated with pulmonary endothelium
Prostacyclin
Endothelial-derived relaxant factor (EDRF/nitric oxide)
Acetylcholine
Endothelin
Peptide associated with large pulmonary vessels
Atrial natriuretic peptide (ANP)

in regulation of normal lung development. Peptides are expressed in a differential pattern during human airway development. Gastrin-releasing peptide is the primary peptide produced during early human fetal development, whereas calcitonin predominates later in development.

Limited evidence suggests that tracheobronchial neuroendocrine epithelial cells communicate with nonadrenergic, noncholinergic neurons located within the airways. The significance of this communication is unclear. Large numbers of neuroendocrine epithelial cells develop in the airways of animals subjected to experimental hypoxia and in humans who live at high altitudes. From these observations, it has been postulated that neuroendocrine epithelial cells serve a chemosensitive function and relay information about air oxygen content to the central nervous system.

FUNCTIONS RELATED TO THE ALVEOLAR SPACE

Metabolism

The alveolar surface is lined by two distinct populations of epithelial cells (Fig. 4). Type I alveolar epithelial cells

are thin, flattened cells that cover approximately 95% of the alveolar surface; they are thought to be relatively quiescent metabolically and form the epithelial surface of the gas diffusion barrier. Type II alveolar cells, in contrast, are cuboidal, metabolically active epithelial cells that cover the remainder of the alveolar surface.

Type II alveolar epithelial cells are the source of pulmonary surfactant, as discussed below. They also demonstrate a capacity for xenobiotic metabolism, as well as enzyme activities that protect against oxidant stress. Type II cells secrete soluble factors that act locally to modulate functions of other lung cells, such as fibroblasts. These regulatory mediators may be important in the coordination of normal lung development, as well as in repair of a damaged alveolar region. Among soluble factors produced by type II cells are several eicosanoids (PGI_2, PGE_2, TXB_2, LTB_4, and LTC_4). The functions of type II cell-derived eicosanoids are poorly defined but may be important in regulation of regional blood flow and ventilation-perfusion matching.

Several investigators have shown that type II alveolar cells synthesize and secrete extracellular matrix components in vitro. Moreover, cultured type II cells participate

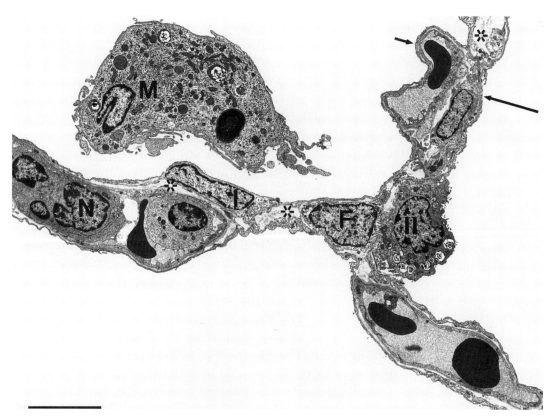

FIG. 4. Morphology of alveolar septum from a normal human lung. *M*, macrophage; *I*, type I alveolar epithelial cell; *II*, type II alveolar epithelial cell; *F*, interstitial fibroblast; *N*, intravascular neutrophil. *Bar* = 5 μm. Note the relatively thin air-blood barrier (*short arrow*) along at least one side of most capillaries. In the region of the *small arrow*, the thickness of the air-blood barrier is less than 0.5 μm. The diameter of the alveolar capillaries is less than 5 μm in most regions. The thick portions of the alveolar septal blood-gas barrier (*long arrow*) commonly range from 3 to 5 μm in thickness and contain connective tissues (*asterisk*) and fibroblasts within the interstitium.

in the turnover of their underlying substratum. It has been postulated that type II cell matrix synthesis and turnover may be important in repairing damaged substratum such that it will support restoration of differentiated alveolar epithelial cell function.

Surfactant Turnover

Pulmonary surfactant is a complex lipoprotein substance forming a thin fluid film over the alveolar surface. Surfactant is a heterogeneous substance composed of lipid (primarily phospholipid) and specific surfactant-associated proteins (SP-A, SP-B, SP-C, and SP-D). Surfactant is best known for its role in lowering surface tension at the alveolar air-liquid interface; more recent evidence suggests that surfactant is also important in host defense against invading organisms, and that it contains antioxidant enzyme activity.

Type II alveolar epithelial cells synthesize and secrete the lipid and apoprotein components (SP-A, SP-B, SP-C, and SP-D), as demonstrated schematically in Fig. 5. Surfactant is stored in cytoplasmic lamellar bodies that fuse with the cell membrane to release surfactant components into the alveolar space by exocytosis. Surfactant secretion is regulated by soluble mediators, such as glucocorticoids and β-adrenergic agonists, as well as by intracellular second messenger signals generated by mechanical strain in the type II cell.

Following secretion, surfactant components transform into a three-dimensional, latticelike structure, tubular myelin. Tubular myelin is thought to be a precursor to the surface tension-lowering film of dipalmitoylphosphatidyl-

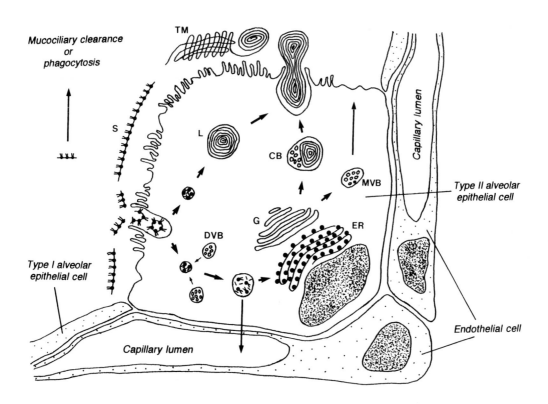

FIG. 5. Pathways of blood coagulation. Surfactant phospholipid and apoproteins are synthesized in the endoplasmic reticulum (*ER*). Phospholipid components are released from the Golgi (*G*) as lamellar bodies (*L*) or combination bodies (*CB*) containing both phospholipid and apoprotein moieties. Surfactant apoproteins may also be released from the Golgi packaged as multivesicular bodies (*MVB*). Lamellar bodies are secreted from the type II alveolar epithelial cell by exocytosis. Surfactant apoproteins A, B, and C are thought to be secreted with lamellar body phospholipids; it has also been suggested that surfactant apoprotein A may be secreted directly from multivesicular bodies. Following exocytosis, the lamellar body uncoils into a lattice structure designated as tubular myelin (*TM*), which subsequently forms the phospholipid-rich surfactant monolayer (*S*) at the air-liquid interface. Surfactant components are cleared from the alveolar space by several mechanisms. A small amount of surfactant may be removed by mucociliary clearance or alveolar macrophage phagocytosis. The type II cell actively clears surfactant components by endocytosis. Some surfactant that has undergone endocytosis is recycled directly into lamellar bodies and resecreted; other surfactant components are metabolized by enzymes contained within dense microvesicular bodies (*DVB*). Metabolized surfactant components may then be recycled for synthesis of new surfactant or released into the circulation for elimination.

choline. Alveolar surfactant is in a constant state of flux; it turns over every 5 to 10 hrs. The quantity of surfactant in the alveolar space is adjusted with changes in alveolar volume, so that an adequate reduction in surface tension is provided at all times. Adjustments in the surfactant pool occur rapidly; alveolar surfactant can increase by 60% during exercise and quickly return to pre-exercise levels with rest.

Clearance of surfactant from the alveolus may involve uptake and resecretion, degradation and incorporation into new surfactant, or complete removal from the surfactant pool. Turnover studies *in vivo* demonstrate that surfactant components are internalized by type II cells and resecreted. Other investigations suggest that surfactant is degraded by type II cells, alveolar macrophages, or within the surfactant fluid layer, and its degradation products are incorporated into newly synthesized surfactant components. Removal of surfactant from the lung may also occur by movement up the mucociliary escalator and swallowing, transfer across the alveolar endothelial-epithelial barrier into the lymph and blood, or degradation and transfer of breakdown products to other organs.

Excretion of Volatile Substances

The importance of human lung in excretion is readily demonstrated by its ability to eliminate the equivalent of more than 10,000 mEq of carbonic acid each day. Details of this important respiratory function have been discussed elsewhere in this volume. Several nonrespiratory metabolites that are volatile at body temperature are also excreted from the alveolar surface. A large number of volatile compounds arise from normal endogenous metabolism; they may also arise from pathologic metabolic pathways characteristic of certain disease states. Measurement of volatile substances in expired air can provide useful diagnostic information relating to abnormal metabolic processes or ingestion of toxic substances. Measurement of breath alcohol concentration, for instance, is used commonly to determine the degree of intoxication.

More than 300 volatile organic compounds have been detected in exhaled air from humans. Most of these substances are hydrocarbons that are either aliphatic (alkanes, alkenes, alkynes) or aromatic (benzene) in nature. The source of exhaled hydrocarbons is often uncertain. A significant number of aliphatic and aromatic hydrocarbons are detectable in expired air by virtue of their prevalence in ambient air. Cigarette smoking is a source of hydrocarbons such as ethene, propene, and propane. A variety of normal and pathophysiologic metabolic processes give rise to volatile carbohydrates that may be excreted from the lung. Hydrocarbons are primarily eliminated by cytochrome P_{450} metabolism in the liver; a smaller number are excreted as volatile gas from the alveolar surface. Lung hydrocarbon excretion assumes a more important

role in conditions associated with decreased hepatic cytochrome P_{450} activity.

Certain volatile constituents of exhaled air reflect specific underlying disorders of metabolism. For instance, elevated breath levels of isoprene have been reported in hypercholesterolemia. Isoprene is a breakdown product of dimethylallylpyrophosphate and thereby is linked to the synthesis of the cholesterol precursor, mevalonic acid. The presence of acetone in exhaled breath during ketoacidosis is a well-known phenomenon. Limited glucose availability in conditions such as diabetes mellitus and starvation results in increased mobilization and oxidation of fatty acids. In turn, the production of acetoacetate, acetone, and/or β-hydroxybutyrate increases, and consequently acetone can be detected in urine and exhaled breath. Methylmercaptan, a derivative of methionine metabolism, is excreted from the alveolar surface in hepatic failure and imparts a distinctive odor (fetor hepatis) to exhaled air.

Measurement of breath hydrogen concentration has been employed as an indicator of carbohydrate malabsorption; bacterial breakdown of unabsorbed carbohydrate in the intestine releases hydrogen. Methane is also released by bacterial metabolism in the intestine in some individuals. Furthermore, bacteria in the intestinal tract of methane excretors may convert hydrogen to methane. Combined measurement of breath hydrogen and methane levels has been advocated as a useful indicator of carbohydrate malabsorption in methane excretors.

A large group of volatile hydrocarbons is generated by oxygen radical-induced peroxidation of cellular lipids and proteins. Free radicals generated by ionizing radiation, chemical exposure, physical stress, and other factors may overwhelm endogenous antioxidant defenses and react with polyunsaturated fatty acids and cell glycoproteins to disrupt cell membranes and other structures. The major end products of lipid peroxidation in humans are ethane (arising from degradation of the 3-carbon family of polyunsaturated fatty acids, e.g., linolenic acid) and pentane (arising from degradation of the 6-carbon family of polyunsaturated fatty acids, e.g., linoleic acid and arachidonic acid). Aldehydes and ketones (acetaldehyde, propanal, pentanal, hexanal, and acetone among others) also arise from n-3 and n-6 polyunsaturated fatty acid metabolism and are detectable in human breath. Several investigations have produced data that suggest measurement of breath ethane and pentane concentrations is a useful noninvasive means of evaluating lipid peroxidation in humans.

Lipid peroxidation has been implicated in the pathobiology of aging and a multitude of other pathophysiologic processes. Measurement of breath hydrocarbon levels may have diagnostic potential in disease processes that involve lipid peroxidation. In fact, elevated breath levels of hydrocarbons have been reported after acute myocardial infarction, in relation to lung malignancy, in cirrhosis, and in neurologic illnesses, including multiple sclerosis and schizophrenia.

FUNCTIONS RELATED TO THE VASCULAR COMPARTMENT

Filtration

The pulmonary capillary bed serves as a filter that detains formed blood elements and particulate matter larger than the average capillary diameter of 8 to 10 μm. Pulmonary arterioles may remove larger particles as they taper distally into the capillary network. Filtration in the lung protects other, more sensitive organs, such as the brain and heart, from disabling, or even fatal, effects of particulate embolism.

The lungs commonly remove thrombi that migrate from the peripheral venous circulation. Most of these thrombi are small and do not significantly compromise gas exchange function of the lung. Pulmonary thromboembolism has been identified in as many as two thirds of consecutive patients undergoing autopsy. These observations may provide an underestimate of the true incidence of pulmonary thromboembolism, as intrinsic thrombolysis may remove clot in many instances.

Filtration of cellular elements in the lung may provide a mechanism for modifying the cellular composition of circulating blood. Studies of venous and arterial blood demonstrate higher numbers of megakaryocytes in venous blood and greater numbers of platelets in arterial blood. These findings suggest that megakaryocytes released from the bone marrow are detained and fragmented in the pulmonary circulation. Autopsy observations confirm the presence of significant numbers of megakaryocytes within the lung.

Both white and red blood cells are removed from circulating blood as it traverses the lungs. Lymphocytes and leukocytes may be detained in the pulmonary vascular bed. Limited evidence from transfusion of leukemic blood suggests that the lungs may serve to maintain a preset level of circulating leukocytes. The lung also removes damaged or lysed erythrocytes.

The lung traps a number of other physiologic emboli, including air, fat, bone marrow, and fragments of placental tissue or amniotic fluid during pregnancy. Malignant cells that have migrated from other tissues may be captured by the lung and establish pulmonary metastases. Infectious organisms can also migrate from other sites and establish infection in the lung. Pulmonary complications of infectious emboli most commonly result from tricuspid or pulmonic valve endocarditis. Foreign materials, such as talc, may be filtered from the venous circulation in intravenous drug users.

Although gas exchange can be disrupted by detention of certain blood particulates, embolic events are often physiologically insignificant or completely reversible if limited to the lung. Enzymatic destruction or phagocytosis of particulate material in lung may prevent fatal embolic events in more sensitive organs, such as the brain.

Metabolism

The pulmonary vascular endothelium forms an expansive blood-tissue barrier that is exposed to the entire volume of cardiac output and, thereby, is uniquely positioned for metabolic functions. Products of endothelial metabolism can be released directly into the circulation; moreover, a number of circulating peptide mediators, lipids, and nucleotides undergo processing by pulmonary endothelial cells (Table 5).

Several peptide mediators arise from pulmonary vascular structures. Atrial natriuretic peptide (ANP) is produced, stored, and released from specialized myocardial cells that extend into the pulmonary veins. ANP mediates pulmonary blood vessel and airway smooth muscle relaxation. Pulmonary vascular endothelium produces a number of vasoactive and bronchoactive mediators. Prostacyclin and endothelial-derived relaxant factor (EDRF/ nitric oxide) have vasodilator properties, whereas endothelin produces vasoconstriction and bronchoconstriction. Endothelin has been shown to have trophic effects on smooth muscle cells and fibroblasts that may be important in repair of damaged lung.

Some circulating substances are processed by lung endothelial cells after being transported from the circulation to the intracellular compartment. The best-known example of intracellular metabolism of circulating compounds is serotonin. Serotonin, or 5-hydroxytryptamine (5-HT), is primarily synthesized from tryptophan in endocrine cells of the gastrointestinal tract. 5-HT serves as a central nervous system neurotransmitter; its release from circulating platelets promotes platelet aggregation. After secretion by the gastrointestinal tract, 5-HT is taken up and stored by nerve endings and platelets, or removed from the circulation by liver and lung.

The lungs remove serotonin from the circulation by a sodium-dependent, carrier-mediated process. After 5-HT is taken up by endothelial cells, it is rapidly metabolized by monoamine oxidase and aldehyde dehydrogenase to physiologically inactive 5-hydroxyindole acetic acid (5-HIAA). Elevated urinary excretion of 5-HIAA is noted in patients with carcinoid syndrome, a neoplasm of endocrine argentaffin cells (APUD cells) characterized by oversecretion of 5-HT. Pulmonary endothelial cells also

TABLE 5. *Vascular endothelial metabolism in the lung*

Substances metabolized after endothelial uptake
  Serotonin
  Prostaglandins E and F
  Leukotrienes
  Norepinephrine
Substances metabolized at the endothelial surface
  Bradykinin
  Angiotensin
  Adenine nucleotides

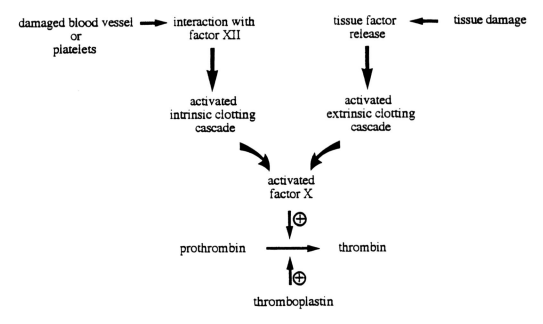

FIG. 6. Schematic representation of surfactant turnover.

remove norepinephrine and prostaglandins of the E and F series from the circulation via an active transport process.

Metabolic processing of other substances occurs at the cell surface without intracellular uptake. Perhaps the best-known example of a substance that undergoes metabolism at the cell surface is angiotensin. Angiotensin-converting enzyme, a carboxypeptidase, activates the vasoconstrictor, angiotensin II, from a decapeptide precursor molecule, angiotensin I. Angiotensin I is produced by the enzymatic action of renin on circulating angiotensinogen secreted by the liver. Bradykinin and adenine nucleotides also are inactivated at the pulmonary endothelial cell surface.

Hemofluidity

Normal respiratory functions of the lung depend on continuous blood flow through the pulmonary vascular bed. The entire cardiac output passes through the pulmo-

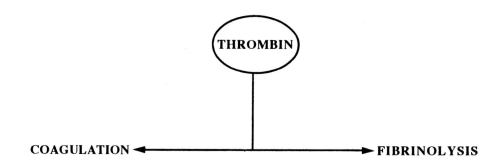

FIG. 7. Modulation of clotting and fibrinolysis by thrombin-dependent mechanisms.

nary vascular system, making these vessels vulnerable to damage by circulating organisms, toxins, and embolic material. Whereas injured pulmonary vessels may provide a nidus for bleeding or clot formation, intrinsic mechanisms that determine hemostasis and anticoagulation are modulated by the pulmonary vascular endothelium.

Clotting results from the generation of thrombin by either intrinsic or extrinsic pathways of coagulation (Fig. 6). The intrinsic pathway is initiated by interaction between clotting factors and injured vessel wall or platelets; activation of the extrinsic pathway requires release of lipoprotein activity (tissue factor) from damaged tissue. Coagulation by either pathway involves controlled interaction of several clotting factors that converge with the activation of factor X. Activated factor X catalyzes the conversion of prothrombin to thrombin; thrombin in turn cleaves soluble fibrinogen to create a meshwork of insoluble fibrin strands. Platelets and red cells are trapped among the fibrin strands to form a stable clot. In addition to cleaving fibrinogen to fibrin, thrombin also cleaves factor XIII to stabilize the fibrin clot.

Generation of thrombin in the lung is also mediated by thromboplastin. Thromboplastin is a phosphatide-protein complex, found in abundance in the lung, that augments conversion of prothrombin to thrombin.

Thrombin is involved in limitation, as well as initiation, of clot formation (Fig. 7). Thrombin interacts with the endothelium via thrombomodulin to activate protein C, which inhibits clotting factors V and VIII and activates fibrinolysis. In addition to activating protein C, thrombin also initiates release of plasminogen activator from endothelial cells. Plasminogen activator in turn cleaves circulating plasminogen to plasmin, which digests fibrin. The vascular endothelium can also bind and inactivate thrombin; furthermore, it can modify coagulation by releasing the vasodilator prostacyclin in response to thrombin.

CONCLUSION

Although the respiratory system is specialized for gas exchange, it also performs many important nonrespiratory functions. The functional diversity of the lung arises from its unique organization of heterogeneous constituent cells into branching airways ending in an expansive gas exchange surface intimately surrounded by an extensive capillary network through which the entire cardiac output flows. Structural features of the conducting airway system provide important functions in nonrespiratory activities such as speech, heat and water conservation, and host defense against inhaled foreign material or organisms. Cells of the conducting airways, alveolar region, and pulmonary vascular system participate in many nonrespiratory functions, including electrolyte and water transport, xenobiotic metabolism, antioxidant defense, surfactant production and turnover, neuroendocrine secretion, excre-

tion of volatile substances, and maintenance of hemofluidity. Many nonrespiratory activities of the lung serve to maintain the gas exchange integrity of the respiratory system. Other nonrespiratory activities are important in maintaining physiologic homeostasis overall.

ACKNOWLEDGMENTS

The authors thank Dr. David Phelps for advice in the preparation of Fig. 5 and Dr. James Crapo for providing Fig. 4. We also acknowledge research support from grants HL-20344 and HL-31560 from the National Institutes of Health, as well as from the American Lung Association of Central Pennsylvania.

BIBLIOGRAPHY

Adriaensen D, Scheuermann DW. Neuroendocrine cells and nerves of the lung. *Anat Rec* 1993;236:70–85. *Review of peptide mediators associated with neuroendocrine epithelial cells of the lung. Includes a review of techniques that are available for the study of neuroendocrine cells in the respiratory tract.*

Batenburg JJ. Biosynthesis, secretion, and recycling of surfactant components. In: Lenfant C, ed. *Lung Biology in Health and Disease.* New York: Marcel Dekker; 1995:47–73 (vol 84). *Review of type II alveolar epithelial synthesis, secretion, and recycling of surfactant.*

Berger HA, Welsh MJ. Electrolyte transport in the lungs. *Hosp Pract* 1991;26:53–59. *Electrolyte transport in human respiratory epithelium is reviewed, with emphasis on clinical implications of abnormal electrolyte transport in cystic fibrosis.*

Dahl AR, Lewis JL. Respiratory tract uptake of inhalants and metabolism of xenobiotics. *Annu Rev Pharmacol Toxicol* 1993;32:383–407. *Review of the metabolic clearance of xenobiotic compounds at all levels of the respiratory tract in several species, including humans.*

Dunsmore SE, Rannels DE. Extracellular matrix biology in the lung. *Am J Physiol* 1996;270:L3–L27. *Comprehensive review of extracellular matrix composition and biologic activity in the alveolar region of the lung.*

Gail DB, Lenfant CJM. Cells of the lung: biology and clinical implications. *Am Rev Resp Dis* 1983;127:366–387. *In-depth review of the structural and physiologic features of major cell types in the respiratory tract.*

Gordon SM, Szidon JP, Krotoszynski BK, Gibbons RD, O'Neill HJ. Volatile organic compounds in exhaled air from patients with lung cancer. *Clin Chem* 1985;31:1278–1282. *Gas chromatography/mass spectrometry investigation of volatile organic compounds in the breath of patients with lung cancer.*

Hart CM, Block ER. Lung serotonin metabolism. *Clin Chest Med* 1989; 10:59–70. *Serotonin metabolism by pulmonary endothelium is reviewed in the context of normal and pathophysiologic lung functions.*

Kelley J. Cytokines of the lung. *Am Rev Resp Dis* 1990;141:765–788. *Comprehensive review of cytokines produced in the lung and their role in lung biology and disease.*

Kinnula VL, Crapo JD, Raivio KO. Generation and disposal of reactive oxygen metabolites in the lung. *Lab Invest* 1995;73:3–19. *Detailed review of free radical oxygen metabolite generation and cellular defense mechanisms against free radicals in the lung. Includes clinical correlation of free radical biology and pathophysiology of lung disease.*

Kneepkens CMF, Lepage G, Roy CC. The potential of the hydrocarbon breath test as a measure of lipid peroxidation. *Free Radic Biol Med* 1994;17:127–160. *A comprehensive review of lipid peroxidation and detection of its hydrocarbon by-products in exhaled air; includes discussion of the clinical relevance of lipid peroxidation and breath hydrocarbon measurement in a variety of disease states.*

Krishna DR, Klotz U. Extrahepatic metabolism of drugs in humans. *Clin Pharmacokinet* 1994;26:144–160. *Comparison of xenobiotic metabolism in several extrahepatic sites, including the lung.*

Luchtman-Jones L, Broze GJ. The current status of coagulation. *Ann Med* 1995;27:47–52. *Brief review presenting evidence for a revised hypothesis of blood coagulation.*

McFadden ER Jr. Respiratory heat and water exchange: physiological and clinical implications. *J Appl Physiol* 1983;54:331–336. *Brief review of the mechanism and clinical importance of heat and water exchange in the conducting airways.*

Noone PG, Olivier KN, Knowles MD. Modulation of the ionic milieu of the airway in health and disease. *Annu Rev Med* 1994;45:421–434. *Ion transport by airway epithelia is discussed in the context of normal and pathologic states, including cystic fibrosis and other airway diseases that may involve disordered ion transport mechanisms.*

Phillips M, Erickson GA, Sabas M, Smith JP, Greenberg J. Volatile organic compounds in the breath of patients with schizophrenia. *J Clin Pathol* 1995;48:466–469. *Case comparison study distinguishing schizophrenic patients from controls on the basis of patterns of volatile organic compound excretion in the breath.*

Phillips M, Greenberg J, Awad J. Metabolic and environmental origins of volatile organic compounds in breath. *J Clin Pathol* 1994;47:1052–1053. *Brief report of several volatile organic compounds identified in a group of normal patients, with emphasis on determination of endogenous or environmental origin.*

Robinson GR III, Canto RG, Reynolds HY. Host defense mechanisms in respiratory infection. *Immunol Allergy Clin North Am* 1993;13:1–25. *Discussion of integrated respiratory tract defenses against inhaled pathogens.*

Rooney SA, Young SL, Mendelson CR. Molecular and cellular processing of lung surfactant. *FASEB J* 1994;8:957–967. *Detailed review of surfactant synthesis and its regulation at the molecular level. Additional consideration is given to the mechanism of surfactant secretion and reuptake.*

Rumessen JJ, Nordgaard-Andersen I, Gudmand-Hoyer E. Carbohydrate malabsorption: quantification by methane and hydrogen breath tests. *Scand J Gastroenterol* 1994;29:826–832. *This investigation considers the relative value of breath hydrogen and methane levels as indicators of carbohydrate malabsorption.*

Ryan US, Ryan JW, Crutchley DJ. The pulmonary endothelial surface. *Fed Proc* 1985;44:2603–2609. *Concise review of the structure and metabolic activities of the pulmonary endothelium.*

Springall DR, Polak JM. Localization of peptides in the lung. *Ann N Y Acad Sci* 1991;629:288–304. *Description of methods for localization of peptide mediators in the lung; the histologic localization of major peptide mediators in the lung is also described. Histologic localization is correlated with potential roles in the pathophysiology of lung diseases.*

Toews GB. Pulmonary defense mechanisms. *Semin Respir Infect* 1993;8:160–167. *Pulmonary defense mechanisms against inhaled organisms and particulate matter are reviewed, with emphasis on specific cellular inflammatory and immune responses.*

Voelkel NF, Stenmark KR, Westcott JY, Chang S-W. Lung eicosanoid metabolism. *Clin Chest Med* 1989;10:95–105. *Localization of eicosanoid production in the lung is related to potential roles in normal and pathophysiologic lung function.*

West JB. *Respiratory Physiology.* Baltimore: Williams and Wilkins; 1995. *Textbook of basic pulmonary physiology.*

Wright JR, Dobbs LG. Regulation of pulmonary surfactant secretion and clearance. *Ann Rev Physiol* 1991;53:395–414. *In-depth review of factors that regulate surfactant secretion; mechanisms of surfactant clearance from the alveolar space and their regulation are also discussed.*

Textbook of Pulmonary Diseases, 6th ed.
edited by G.L. Baum, J.D. Crapo, B.R. Celli, and J.B. Karlinsky,
Lippincott–Raven Publishers, Philadelphia, © 1998.

CHAPTER

6

The Respiratory Muscles

Bartolome Celli · Alejandro Grassino

INTRODUCTION

The worldwide poliomyelitis epidemic in the 1950s affected millions of people. The polio virus targeted many motor neuron pools, amongst which were those in charge of ventilation control causing, in many cases, clinical ventilatory failure. An ingenious, albeit palliative, answer to this type of ventilatory failure was the development of the iron lung, an external negative pressure ventilator that saved the lives of countless patients infected during the epidemic. The purpose of assisted ventilation was not to restore the function of the motor neurons, but to take over the work of the failing muscles. Even though polio is now very infrequent in the developed parts of the world, the use of ventilators has increased and the machines have evolved in sophistication and capability. Close to half of all patients admitted to intensive care units require mechanically assisted ventilatory support. Almost all the ventilatory support currently provided uses positive rather than negative pressure, but the overall aims and principles remain the same: to replace the flailing chest. This book has several chapters devoted to mechanical ventilation. In this introduction we point out how, under a variety of clinical conditions, the ventilatory control lapses, and muscles fail to ventilate the lungs, whose final result is ventilatory failure with hypoxia and, frequently, hypercapnia.

Basically, ventilation depends upon the ability of the respiratory pump to move air in and out of the gas exchange portion of the lung. The respiratory muscles serve as the vital link between the different components of the pump: the respiratory centers, the conducting nerves and, ultimately, the lung itself.

The respiratory muscles contract during the breathing cycle, thereby changing the anatomical configurations of the chest wall by displacing its components, so that air can move in and out of the lungs. This chapter systematically analyzes the overall anatomical and physiological arrangements of the respiratory muscles. It specifically addresses the clinical application of these concepts, and familiarizes the reader with the different clinical conditions that are described in other portions of this textbook.

ANATOMICAL CONSIDERATIONS

There are many muscles that participate in ventilation, and they can be divided into those that are inspiratory in action and those that, by their anatomical arrangement, are predominantly expiratory in function. In turn, the inspiratory muscles are divided into ones that actively contribute to inspiratory pressure generation during regular tidal breathing (the so-called primary muscles of respiration) and the accessory muscles, which are activated to participate in ventilation under conditions of increased ventilatory demands.

There are also muscles that participate in breathing whose function is not primarily to displace the ribcage or abdomen. These muscles, located in the upper airways, act to prevent the collapse of the conduits and, in this way, facilitate airflow. The pharyngeal constrictor muscles, genioglossus, and neck strap muscles all increase

B. R. Celli, M.D., Division of Pulmonary and Critical Care, St. Elizabeth's Medical Center, Tufts University, Boston, Massachusetts 02135.

A. Grassino, M.D., Hopital Notre-Dame. McGill University. Montreal. Quebec. Canada.

patency of the pharynx, while the laryngeal abductor muscles open the vocal cords. The activation of these muscles must be synchronized, and actually precede the contraction of the inspiratory muscles.

The diaphragm is the most important muscle of inspiration. As shown in Figure 1, it has a central noncontractile tendon, from which muscles fibers radiate down and outwards to fit into the lower ribcage, and in the first 3 lumbar vertebrae. During contraction, it assists lung inflation through three mechanisms. The diaphragm uses the abdomen as a fulcrum against which it leans, thereby expanding the rib cage. During contraction, the diaphragm also helps inflation because of the cephalocaudal orientation of its fibers, and the curvature of its shape. This anatomical arrangement will expand the ribcage as the fibers shorten. The curvature of the diaphragm approximates the shape of a hemisphere with a radius r. Laplace's law for a sphere states that $P = 2T/r$, where P is the pressure inside the sphere, and T is the tension in the wall. If T is maintained constant and the diaphragm flattens, its curvature will decrease, r will increase and, by definition, P must decrease. Finally, the diaphragm transmits the increase in abdominal pressure during contraction to the rib cage, through its zone of apposition. This action also has an expansive action on the ribcage.

Patients with COPD characteristically develop lung hyperinflation, causing an increase in the resting volume of the ribcage. It is believed that hyperinflation reduces diaphragmatic strength by shortening of the diaphragmatic fibers, which places the muscle at a suboptimal point on its length tension curve. However, recent studies have demonstrated that when diaphragmatic fibers are experimentally shortened, the muscles adapt by dropping sarcomeres and achieving a new optimal length, so that each bundle is capable of generating its maximal tension for that new length. It can therefore be implied that the decreased diaphragmatic pressure generating capacity in COPD patients is either due to anatomical and mechanical derangement, or to contractile dysfunction, and not to simple length-tension changes.

The other primary inspiratory muscles (some of them also shown in Fig. 1) are the external intercostals, the parasternal part of the internal intercostals, the triangularis sterni and the scalene. They are activated during tidal breathing in normal individuals, but significantly increase their participation in ventilation during increased ventilatory demand. They play a particularly important role in diseases characterized by hyperinflation such as in COPD because they undergo less anatomic shortening, and therefore operate at a lesser mechanical disadvantage than the diaphragm. On the other hand, the true "accessory muscles", i.e. the sternomastoid, subclavian, pectoralis minor and major, serratus anterior, upper and lower trapezius, and latissimus dorsi, which are usually inactive during normal breathing may become increasingly important under special circumstances, like in strenuous exercise and in cases of severe ventilatory load. They are also active in patients with severe COPD.

There are other muscles that are not thought to be respiratory in nature such as the muscles of the shoulder girdle. These muscles have dual actions that include fixing the upper ribcage, partaking in upper torso positioning and elevating the upper extremity. They may also exert a pulling action on the rib cage, when they contract and are fixed at their extrathoracic anchoring point. Because of this, patients with severe COPD will often find relief to their dyspnea when they lean on a surface and fix their shoulder girdle.

The respiratory muscles have functions other than breathing. They also participate in very complex functions, like speaking and singing. This requires the simultaneous activation of the inspiratory and expiratory muscles. In other instances synchronous expulsive maneuvers will be needed to achieve other functions such as sneezing, vomiting, and defecating. They may also need to act in concert to facilitate parturition and micturition. A

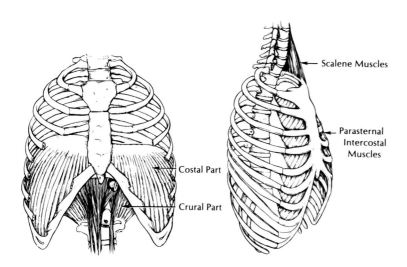

FIG. 1. The left panel shows the human diaphragm in situ at the full expiratory position. Notice the non-contractile central tendon, the radical cephalocaudal orientation of its fibers, and how it is opposed the inner aspect of the lower ribcage. The right panel shows the parasternal intercostal and scalene muscles. Only the left scalene muscles are shown, to illustrate their origin on the spine and their insertion on the first rib.

unique aspect of to the respiratory system is the sneezing and coughing reflex. These maneuvers require an initial deep inspiratory effort, followed by the closure of the glottis and a forceful contraction of the diaphragm and the abdominal muscles. When the upper airways are suddenly opened, the increased intra-abdominal pressure results in an explosive expiratory effort. This sudden increase in peak flow helps clear airways, and is very important for the management of secretions. Conditions that result in impaired coughing frequently results in the accumulation of secretions in the lungs, leading to development of atelectasis.

Physiologic Principles

There are two basic principles that control the behavior of muscles when subjected to physiologic stimuli. They are applicable to muscles in general and also include the respiratory muscles. The first is the relationship between the length of a muscle and its capacity to generate force (Fig. 2). The muscle generates more force as it lengthens until it reaches an optimal length. Stretching the muscle beyond that point is associated with decreased strength, until the muscle fibre brakes. More importantly, as the resting length of a muscle shortens (which occurs in diseases that cause lung hyperinflation) the force generating capacity for a given electrical stimuli decreases. In the case of the respiratory muscles, if a similar pressure is required to maintain ventilation then the only possible compensatory mechanism is the recruitment of more muscle fibers, i.e. increasing the motor output of the central

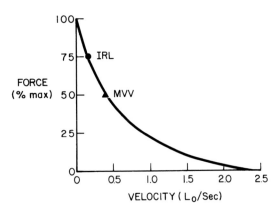

FIG. 3. Idealized representation of the relationship between contractile force(% of maximum) and velocity of shortening (Lo/s) of the human diaphragm. Maximum shortening velocity, measured in vitro, is about 2.5 Lo/s. The points identified as IRL and MVV are estimates of the shortening velocity when measured through a resistance (IRL) and during unencumbered maximal voluntary ventilation (MVV). As shortening velocity increase, force output falls. Force output during the MVV maneuver is estimated to be half that during the maximal static contraction of the diaphragm (Reproduced from Fishman A (ED), Update: Pulmonary diseases and disorders. New York : McGraw-Hill, 1992:88).

nervous system, and then increase the firing rate to the muscle.

The second principle is that of the inverse relationship between the velocity of muscle contraction, and force generation capacity (Fig. 3). As the velocity of contraction increases (as in increased respiratory rate), the capacity to generate forces decreases. Although of limited clinical importance because of the usually relatively low speed of contraction of the respiratory muscles, it may become important at very fast breathing rates, or in patients whose respiratory ailment is associated with very short inspiratory times. Under resting breathing conditions the velocity of contraction and the inspiratory muscle force generated is about 5% of their maximal capacity. Up to 50% of maximal force or velocity can be sustained for prolonged periods of time (hrs).

Skeletal Muscle Cell Types

Skeletal muscles are composed of different types of muscle fibers. Based upon histochemical staining they have been divided into types I, IIa, and IIb. Type I fibers have a high oxidative capacity and a low concentration of glycolytic enzymes. When activated, they develop a slow rise in force. Physiologically, they are the first to be recruited during muscle activation, because they generate low levels of force and are fatigue resistant. Type IIb fibers which have a low oxidative capacity and a high concentration of glycolytic enzymes, are the last to be recruited, and generate the optimal level of force quickly and may also fatigue rapidly. Type IIa has moderate en-

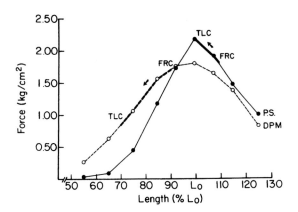

FIG. 2. The relationship between contractile force(kg/cm2) and resting length (%lo) for isolated, perfused strips of canine diaphragm (DPM) and parasternal (PS). Contractile force of both muscles is greatest at optimum resting length(LO). In situ, at functional residual capacity (FRC), the diaphragm is shorter and the parasternal muscles are longer than Lo, and loses force generating capacity. In contrast, the parasternal muscles shorten less. Towards their Lo, and gain force generating capacity. (Reproduced from Farkas G et al. J Appl Physiol 1985;59:528).

zyme concentrations, and is intermediate with respect to fatigability. The diaphragm is composed of approximately 50% Type I and 50% type II fibers, enabling it to withstand the enduring work it has to perform over an individual's lifetime. These properties of the skeletal muscle bear an important relevance to their response to training. In the case of the respiratory muscles, an increasing number of motor units are recruited with increased ventilatory loads, with the type I, IIa, and IIb fibers being recruited in a sequential fashion.

The effects of training on fiber composition vary, depending on the method of training utilized. Endurance training increases the myoglobin content, the capillary density, the mitochondrial density, and the oxidative enzyme capacity of type I fibers. In contrast, strength training increases fiber size (i.e. muscle hypertrophy); with little or no effect on enzyme concentration. Animal studies using biopsy specimens of the ventilatory muscles before and after different forms of training have shown the aforementioned training effects of the diaphragm and other inspiratory muscles. It is now becoming evident that these are a continuum on the fiber composition of type II cells, rather than two distant groups.

METABOLIC AND ENERGY DEMANDS OF THE RESPIRATORY MUSCLES

The concept that muscles behave in the same way as mechanical devices do by consuming energy and producing work, both of which are measurable, was developed in the early part of the twentieth century. Skeletal muscle efficiency was, in fact, reported to be about 25%, while respiratory muscle efficiency was noted to vary from 2% to 24%. The idea that a lack of energy supply, manifested in the form of insufficient oxygen and substrate, result in muscle failure is also well established. Because of these assertions, the role of blood perfusion has been widely explored; hyperpnea is equated to an increase in the blood flow of the diaphragm, as well as other respiratory muscles. Blood flow to the diaphragm, increases by up to 260 mL/100gr min in maximally exercised ponies. This value which is similar to other skeletal muscles, is achieved by dilatation of the diaphragm vasculature.

Blood flow to the diaphragm has been studied during phrenic nerve stimulation. As opposed to limb muscles, where the duty cycle is relatively constant, the respiratory muscle's duty cycle can vary. The duty cycle is considered to be important because during contraction, the blood flow is either partially or completely interrupted, with flow restitution occurring during the relaxation phase. The first comprehensive study quantifying the relationship between diaphragmatic blood flow (Qdi) and the duty cycle was published by Bellemare et. al. In that study perfusion was related to the product of Pdi multiplied by the duty cycle. The mathematical product was called the tension

(or pressure) time index, and has been very useful for defining the physiological behavior of the loaded diaphragm. The authors described a parabolic relation between TTdi and Qdi. Diaphragmatic perfusion rises up to a TTdi value of .20, then declines. Post contraction hyperpnea begins to increase, which is suggestive of blood flow limitation (Fig. 4). Earlier studies have, in fact, shown that the endurance time of the diaphragm when breathing against resistance was also related to the product of force developed and the duty cycle, and that time to task failure was predictable. If breathing was held at a TTdi of .20 or lower, that time is about one hour. In contrast, time to task failure will be about 15 min at TTdi of 0.30. Interestingly, a much higher Pdi (70% of Pdi max) can be also sustained for 1h, provided that the duty cycle in decreased to .30, which gives more perfusion time (TTdi remains at 0.21). The effect of high tension is offset by the shorter duty cycle. The concept of a pressure threshold is, in reality, valid only if Ti/Ttot is 0.40 -0.45. A duty cycle of 0.30 is common among severe COPD patients. The concept of a threshold TTdi, below which task failure does not develop, and above which it will eventually occur, was proposed by Bellemare and Grassino and is graphically shown in Fig. 5. It should be noted that these results apply to the prevailing experimental conditions from which the data was obtained (constant perfusion pressure and square pressure wave). Regardless of the conditions, the results emphasize the relevance of

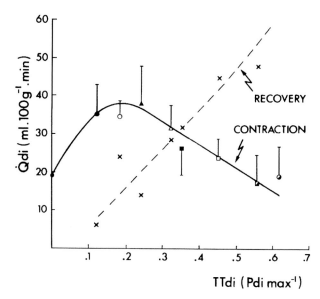

FIG. 4. Relationship between the diaphragmatic blood flow (Qdi) and the Tension Time index (Ttdi). Resting breathing values are the first point to the left. All subsequent data points were obtained with higher inspiratory resistances until a steady state was reached; bilateral phrenic stimulation was used. Peak values of Qdi were obtained at a Ttdi of .15 to .20. Higher Ttdi resulted in decreased flows. The dashed line represents the values of a post-stimulation Qdi. It increases linearly with the amount of Ttdi achieved by stimulation. This is an expression of O2 debt incurred.

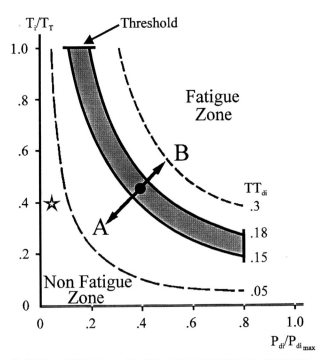

FIG. 5. The Tension Time (or Pressure Time) Index. It is the product of the inspiratory time expressed as a percentage of the total duration of the breathing cycle (Ti/Ttot), multiplied by the Pdi/Pdi max. (Mean trandiaphragmatic pressure developed expressed as a percentage of the Pdi maximal). Each point on the diagram defines a unique breathing pattern. Threshold: all breathing patterns in this zone can be sustained for 45 min or longer in normal human subjects breathing against inspiratory levels (Ttdi of .15 to .20). Fatigue zone: breathing patterns in this zone will result in a failure to sustain the pressure in less than 45 minutes. Muscle fatigue was the main cause of failure in the well motivated subjects. The main mechanism was insufficient blood flow as shown in fig. A. The fatigue threshold can be achieved at smaller Ttdi (arrow A) if the mean blood pressure is lower than normal. The threshold can be higher (B0 if the tension is higher (hyperfusion). The star in this figure is the Ttdi of a normal subject breathing at rest. The Ttdi in normal subjects exercising at 80% of their VO2 max is about .15, but the mechanisms of fatigue may be more complex than in resistive breathing.

blood perfusion to the maintenance of diaphragm contractility.

Respiratory muscle endurance can be shorter or longer (for a given TTdi), depending on perfusion pressure. If perfusion pressure is increased, endurance is prolonged. In shock, TTdi task failure develops at a TTdi lower than 0.15 to 0.20. Respiratory rate can also affect respiratory muscle perfusion. Faster frequencies increase Qdi for a given TTdi, since Qdi is linearly related to the respiratory muscle's oxygen consumption in normal humans. Other conditions may also influence diaphragmatic perfusion. For example, hypoxemia also increases blood to the diaphragm. The aforementioned mechanisms seem to be adaptive in COPD, where both a fast respiratory rate and a lower tidal volume (faster, shallow breathing) may help preserve muscle performance.

The cellular mechanisms through which blood flow regulates muscle contractibility are not only related to the delivery of oxygen and other substrates, but also to the washout of the catabolites. Limitations of the aerobic metabolism lead to a dependence on creatinine kinase and myokinase for ATP synthesis from ADP only, with the accumulations of Pi and H^+, both of which are deleterious to muscle contractibility.

NEURAL CONTROL AND COORDINATION

The diaphragm and the other respiratory muscles are controlled by central motor neurons which normally maintain rhythmic breathing. The muscles of the upper airways are innervated by lower cranial nerves (ninth, tenth, eleventh and twelfth). The innervation of the other muscles depend on their anatomical location, and in descending order include: the sternocleidomastoid supplied by the spinal accessory nerve (eleventh cranial nerve) with roots from cervical 1 and 2 levels, the diaphragm, supplied by the phrenic nerves with roots from C3 to C5, the parasternal intercostal, supplied by the intercostal nerves. The abdominal muscles, which are mainly expiratory in action, are supplied by motorneurons arising from T8 to L2 levels.

It is evident that given the wide array of neurons that may participate in ventilation, a great degree of coordination is needed to maintain efficient and appropriate ventilation. Unique to the respiratory system is the fact that the natural rhythmic automatic breathing can be voluntarily overridden by the cortex. The system usually functions smoothly, because during quiet breathing we use primarily the diaphragm, the scalene, and some intercostals. With increased ventilatory loads, "accessory muscles" increase their participation in ventilation. Apart from their potential role in respiration, some of these muscles participate in other functions. For example, the upper torso and shoulder girdle muscles assist in positioning the upper extremities, abdominal muscles help with speech, defecation and parturition. Therefore, in situations where these muscles are being used for nonventilatory work, it is important that they maintain a high degree of coordination. When incoordination occurs, either because of an increased load or because of competing control integration, the resulting dysfunction can compromise the patient with underlying lung disease. It has been shown that when patients with severe COPD perform unsupported arm exercise, they develop early thoracoabdominal dyscoordination and fatigue. This type of exercise causes dyssynchrony between the rib cage the and diaphragm-abdomen, because of the competing output of the centers controlling respiratory and tonic activities of the accessory ventilatory muscles and the diaphragm.

Clinical evaluation of Respiratory Muscle Function

The most frequent symptom of respiratory muscle dysfunction is dyspnea. This symptom can be described with different degrees of exercise in many different conditions, including heart conditions. Indeed, dyspnea, which is caused by respiratory muscle dysfunction, is frequently confused with heart ailments. Characteristically, patients with diaphragmatic dysfunction will complain of dyspnea when supine (like cardiac patients), and sometimes have extensive workup including catheterization, before the exact nature of the problem is elucidated. Patients with bilateral diaphragmatic paralysis report an immediate onset of dyspnea when supine as opposed to patients with heart failure who will complain of dyspnea after a variable time in the supine position. A physical exam can help sort out the nature of the problem. Measurement of the breathing frequency is helpful, because patients with respiratory muscle dysfunction will breathe at a faster rate. Similarly, the patients will adopt a shallow breathing pattern, irrespective of the reason of the muscle dysfunction. Close observation may reveal use of the accessory muscle, and paradoxical inward retraction of the abdomen during inspiration, because the diaphragm is unable to generate pressure to displace the abdominal wall.

Under certain circumstances special considerations apply. In patients with central nervous depression (drug overdoses), the breathing pattern tends to be shallow and slow irrespective of the degree of ventilatory failure. Likewise, patients with hypothyroidism can develop slow shallow breathing which will reverse with thyroid replacement. Patients with severe COPD will not develop the very fast rate seen in patients with interstitial lung disease because of the expiratory obstruction to airflow which tends to prolong the expiratory phase. On the other hand those patients will ineffectively contract the diaphragm and this will retract the lower ribcage (Hoover's sign). They will also contract the abdominal muscles during expiration. This pattern can be easily detected on the physical exam in the most severe cases but not be quite so visible in the milder stages.

During the evaluation, it may be helpful to induce coughing as patients with global respiratory muscle weakness will not be able to generate effective cough. A summary symptoms and signs, and their correlates to disease states and mechanisms is shown in Table 1.

Laboratory Evaluation of Respiratory Muscle Function

The most accurate source of information on respiratory muscle function is provided by measuring muscle specific physiological properties, like their level of neural activation, force generation, operational length, velocity of shortening, electrophysiological properties, and pattern of recruitment.

In practice, evaluation of the collective function of all the inspiratory and expiratory muscles is the most convenient way for their clinical assessment. It is remarkable that the lung volume-intrathoracic pressure relationship of all the muscles forming the chest wall strongly resembles the force-length characteristic function of a single skeletal muscle fiber. It is, in fact, near functional residual capacity that all inspiratory muscles combined are at their optimal length, and provide the highest intrathoracic inspiratory force. In contrast, all the expiratory muscles develop their maximal force near total lung capacity, where their length is optimal. Their force decreases as lung volume decreases.

The causes of respiratory muscle dysfunction can be found within the neuromuscular activation pathway, as shown in Fig. 6. Upon nerve stimulation, acetylcholine (Ach) is liberated at the neuromuscular junction, where it binds to Ach receptors postsynaptically, thereby causing changes in the muscle fiber membrane potential, and leading to the propagation of membrane depolarization along the surface of the fiber, a signal that is clinically measurable as the electromyogram (EMG). This depolarization also travels towards the center of the muscle fiber via the transversal tubules, which triggers the release of Ca^{++} ions from the sarcoplasmic reticulum into the cytoplasm. In the presence of ATP, CA^{++} links to troponin and triggers the sliding of myosin on actin, thereby generating force (clinically measured as intrathoracic pressure) and velocity of shortening (estimated by mouth flow). The magnitude of intrathoracic pressure developed depends on the initial degree of overlapping between thick and thin filaments within the muscle sarcomere. The magnitude of the shortening depends on the load the muscle encounters, as well as on the number of muscle fibers recruited, and the motorneurones firing rate. The overall degree of muscle activation can be estimated from the recorded EMG signal. Appropriate analysis of the signal, such as the root mean square value (RMS), can be used to quantify muscle activation.

The ultimate consequence of respiratory muscle dysfunction is ventilatory failure. There are several pathways that can lead to ventilatory failure. One is a lack of central drive (usually due to an overdose of neural depressants such as barbiturates or opiates). This results in lack of muscle activation, and overall hypoventilation. Another path is an alteration in the natural inactivation of acetylcholine or its rate of liberation. This also leads to hypoventilation due, to failure at the neuro muscular junction (myasthenia gravis, curare or curare like muscle relaxants). If respiratory muscle activation occurs, the muscle may still fail to generate adequate pressure through failure of the excitation contraction coupling mechanism. This is a complex step. Dysfunction can happen when the membrane Na^+/K^+ channels are blocked, when lactic acid

TABLE 1. *Clinical evaluation of respiratory muscle dysfunction*

Symptom/sign	Disease	Putative mechanism
Dyspnea on exertion. Tachypnea.	Chronic heart failure	Weak respiratory muscles, disused because of sedentary life. Low blood perfusion to the muscles.
Abdominal paradoxing during inspiration. Shortness of breath.	Diaphragm paresia. Paralysis of the diaphragm. Post upper abdominal surgery.	Weak muscle that cannot generate the force to overcome the pleural pressure swing.
Intercostals and supraclavicular space are indrawn during inspiration.	Increase in the pleural pressure swing, because of airway obstruction and/or low lung compliance.	Subatmospheric pleural pressure overcome the compliance of tissues.
Alternans, i.e. shifts from predominant rib cage to predominant abdominal breathing.	Elastically or resistively loaded breathing.	It may be a central mechanism whose purpose is to unload either group of muscles. It can be done voluntarily.
Hiccups.	Neurological: CNS local lesion. Mediastinal infection or tumor.	A sudden discharge of phrenic nerve activation.
Paradoxical movements of the rib cage during an inspiration without air flow.	Sleep apnea during REM stage.	Closing of the upper airway with a predominantly active Diaphragm.
Small VC, tachypnea. SOB.	Obesity, lung fibrosis, neuromuscular disease, OAP, steroid treatment, polymitosis, malnourishment, post polio syndrome.	Any form of muscle weakness relative to respiratory system compliance.
Cheyne Stokes breathing.	Neurological, stroke. CHF.	Unknown. Effect on patterns of breathing generation (CNS).
Weak, ineffective cough to clear bronchial secretions.	Chest pain, flail chest, Kyphoscoliosis, COPD, Quadriplegia. Guillian Barre. Central airway obstruction.	Insufficient expiratory muscle force to create a peak expiratory flow above 5 l/sec.
Rapid loss of ventilation during MVV. Sensations of fatigue. Weakness	Myasthenia Gravis	Lack of acetyl choline receptors on the muscles. NM junction fatigue.
Hypercapnea with normal lungs	Neuromuscular weakness caused by disease. Ex.: muscular distrophy, post polio syndrome.	Loss of muscle fibers; the remaining ones cannot generate enough force, even if activation is high. They could be derecruited.
Muscle stiffness. Slow relaxation rigor.	After heavy exercise. Severe acidosis.	Lack of ATP to bring Ca^{++} back to the SR.
A saw-toothed pattern in a flow volume curve.	Parkinson's. Upper airway weakness.	Instability of the upper airway's dynamics. Starling resistor effect.
EMG and pleural pressure swings preceding mouth flow.	Intrinsic Peep. In COPD. high threshold load in a ventilator.	Neural output builds up pressure over 50–250 ms before overcoming PEEP. The same for overcoming threshold pressure in a ventilator.

or inorganic phosphates accumulate in muscle fibers, or when CA^{++} does not recycle fast enough in and out of the sarcoplasmic reticulum. Excitation-contraction coupling failure leads to loss of muscle force in spite of neuronal activation. This step can be assessed in several ways:

1) Loss of force upon maximal stimulation of the phrenic nerve, which then reverses with muscle rest (fatigue),

2) a slowing down of the relaxation rate of the diaphragm (measured as the rate of decay of transdiaphragmatic pressure), and

3) a change in the central frequency of the power spectrum of the EMG signal.

This is an indicator of the membrane's reduction in the velocity of conduction of myopotentials. A final pathway

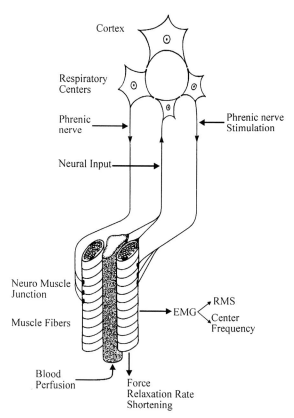

FIG. 6. The diagram shows the different levels of central control of breathing, the afferent and efferent neural pathways. Muscle failure or fatigue can happen A) at the central level (i.e. derecruitment) because of nerve lesions. B) At the nuero muscular junction (transmission failure) C) at the fiber level, being caused by insufficient perfusion, leading to excitation failure or contraction failure . On the right side, there are indications about how to test failure, a maximal phrenic stimulation, which can increase the max. Voluntary force, is an indication of Central Fatigue . EMG Centroid Frequency is an indicator of the muscle membranes conduction velocity. EMG Root Mean Square is an indicator of activation levels reached at the muscle cell. Force is the final mechanical output. Relaxation rate is an index of sarcomere function. Spontaneous shortening is an index of the respiratory center output and muscle force for a given breath.

relates to phenomena independent of adequate intrinsic muscle function. It may be that the activation and contraction are normal, but the muscles are highly preloaded (COPD, obesity, ribcage deformity, interstitial lung disease), so an inordinate amount of muscle force is used to overcome the load before air actually moves onto the lung. Clinical observation of how the chest wall moves, measurements of ribcage and abdomen movements or relative changes in the simultaneously determined pleural (esophageal) and abdominal (gastric) pressures swings may help define the degree of respiratory muscle dysfunction.

Respiratory Muscle Strength

The oldest, simplest and most useful test of respiratory muscle strength is the maximal inspiratory (PI max) and expiratory (PEmax) pressures. There is a significant literature reporting values in normal subjects, patients with COPD, lung fibrosis, and obesity. There are acceptable instruments and techniques adaptable to clinical practice. The pressures are measured during maximal static efforts against a partially closed airway. A small airleak is created during the efforts, in order to avoid the suction effect of the mouth muscles if the glottis is allowed to close. The test has also been expanded to determine mouth pressure over a range of lung volumes over the vital capacity. Like many tests in pulmonary research, the maximal PI and PE are dependent on subject's cooperation, and the value obtained may underestimate the true strength of the respiratory muscles. Nevertheless, there are several practical uses for the measurement of PI max. Its serial evaluation over time can provide insight as to the progression or regression of muscle weakness (as in Guillain-Landry-Barrett syndrome, and weaning from mechanical ventilation) or fatigue. Patients with a maximal inspiratory force of <25 cmH$_2$O are at high risk of developing ventilatory failure. Similarly, maximal expiratory force of <30 cmH$_2$O at FRC is seen in patients with ineffective cough, which forecasts an accumulation of bronchial secretions and possible atelectasis, pneumonia and ventilatory failure.

Knowledge of the pressure swing required to sustain ventilation and the value of maximal inspiratory pressure (PImax) allows the calculation of the ''force reserve'' (Fig. 7). Pressure swings of higher than 50% of maximal inspiratory pressure are associated with rapid (within 15 min) fatigue and task failure. This may occur during some clinical conditions, and could be a reason for ventilatory failure.

The direct measurement of PI and PE max can be complemented by the determination of the force exerted by the elastic recoil of the lungs and the chest wall. At FRC, the outward recoil of the chest wall and the inward recoil of the lung are balanced, so the PI and PE max represent the true force of the respiratory muscles. At total lung capacity and residual volume, the values of PI are under or overestimated by about 25%. At TLC, PI max at the mouth is in fact 0, because the muscles have to overcome the elastic recoil of the lungs and the chest wall, which is approximately 30 cmH$_2$O. Intrathoracic pressure measured with an esophageal balloon would provides the correct value of the respiratory muscle force.

Maximal Transdiaphragmatic Pressure (Pdi)

This test requires the simultaneous measurement of esophageal (to represent pleural) and gastric (to represent abdominal) pressure, using balloon catheters placed in the mid-esophagus and in the stomach, respectively. Pdi is calculated as the difference between Pga and Pes, measured at isotime during a maximal voluntary effort. Pdi

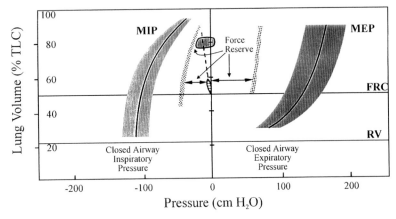

FIG. 7. Force reserve: the values of the MIP (Maximal Inspiratory Pressure) or PI max measured at the mouth against an occluded airway and MEP (pressure at the mouth during a maximal expiratory effort) or PE max. On the ordinate is lung volume, expressed as a percentage of total lung capacity. Predicted MIP-MEP values are shown in the shade areas. The dotted area represents pressures of about 40% of max, levels beyond which a sustains breathing pattern will result in failure. The dashed line is the elastic recoil of the lungs. The loop at FRC is the plural pressure swing required during resting breathing. Notice the margin of force reserve . The upper loop simulated the COPD patient. Hyperinflation and COPD result in lower forces and higher resistances decreasing considerably the force reserve margin.

can also be estimated by using the difference between Pga and occluded mouth pressure (P mouth). The pressure needed to overcome elastic recoil of the lungs is added to mouth pressure (-5 cms H_2O at FRC and -25 cmH$_2$O at TLC in normals). The measurement of PdI max is performed while maintaining a small air leak, whose purpose is to help keep the glottis open. With all its caveats, Pdi max is the best index of intramuscular tension and the pressure developed across the diaphragm. There should be a negative pressure in the thorax with simultaneous positive pressure in the abdomen. Pdi should be recorded at known lung volume, keeping the chest wall configuration constant. Values from normal subjects and patients with different lung diseases, as well as details about the technique, have been published. There is considerable variability in the Pdi values obtained in humans, depending on the technique and the subject's capacity to complete the maneuvers. At Pdi values higher than 50% of maximum, blood flow is interrupted altogether. Blood flow is, however, partially reestablished during expiration. This physiological phenomenon is the basis for the explanation about how fatigue develops while breathing against high inspiratory resistance. A Pdi max value higher than 100 cmH$_2$O is not associated with muscle weakness, and cannot be the cause of ventilatory failure. A low Pdi max value can, however, be the consequence of many different factors, such as a lack of muscle mass, malnutrition, neurological disorder, neuromuscular junction disorder, and intrinsic muscle disease.

Another method of measuring the pressure generating capacity of the diaphragm is the so-called Sniff Test. This test is done by having the person perform a brisk maximal voluntary inspiratory effort through one of the nostrils. The pressure is measured at the nostril or the mouth. The major advantage of this test is that it can be successfully completed by most people with very little training, and it can be easier to perform than a Pdi max maneuver. Its main disadvantage is that it is a dynamic maneuver, where force is affected by the velocity and degree of muscle shortening. This tends to underestimate the value of the force, with respect to those obtained during static maneuvers. A sniff pressure value higher than 80 cmH$_2$O is likely to represent a good force, and respiratory muscle weakness is unlikely to be present. Low sniff pressure values provide less certainty regarding the presence of weakness. This test is being perfected and, as more experience is gained, it might be better standardized.

Phrenic Nerve Stimulation Techniques

This consists of supramaximal bilateral stimulation of the phrenic nerves at the neck using surface electrodes, resulting in a single brisk diaphragmatic contraction (twitch) pressure. Esophageal and gastric pressures are measured simultaneously with the double balloon technique. This allows the determination of Pdi. Adequate stimulation can be achieved with the use of an electric current, or through magnetic depolarization coils. The former stimulates the phrenic nerves specifically, while the latter is more likely to stimulate several nerve groups as the coils are relatively large. This problem may be solved with the development of smaller coils. Magnetic phrenic nerve stimulation can be done in either the sitting or supine position, and does not require abdominal binding. Cervical magnetic stimulation allows for prospective studies of the respiratory muscles of supine patients. It is nevertheless important to note that magnetic stimulation can interfere with the function of pacemakers and should never be used in patients with these devices in place.

Electrical stimulation should be done in the sitting position, with control of the diaphragm's compound muscle action potential, in order to achieve "supramaximal" nerve stimulus. Changes in the distance between the electrode and the nerve can change the stimulating current intensity, and thereby influence the test's outcome. In some instances, wires have been implanted close to the nerve and left in place to repeat the test, as well as document the changes in force as a function of time. Cutaneous stimulation can be painful, can cause ballistic movement of the arm and is difficult to perform in obese persons. There are numerous studies that provide comparative values from normals and patients with lung disease. The electrically induced twitch pressure values range from 25 to 35 cmH$_2$O, whereas they range from 30 to 35 cmH$_2$O for magnetic stimulation. Measurement of the time interval from nerve stimulation until the beginning of the action potential (CMAP) provides the phrenic nerve velocity of conduction. Absence of CMAP indicates phrenic nerve transection, or neuro muscle junction failure.

Respiratory Muscle Endurance

These are important and relevant tests of respiratory muscle function. This should provide more relevant information than tests of respiratory muscle force. There are a few techniques that have both broad acceptance and recognized clinical value; these results are shown in Fig. 8. The first one is the measurement of endurance while breathing at high levels of ventilation. Under these conditions, the respiratory muscles develop high velocity of

shortening at relatively low forces, as seen in bicycle exercise. Maximal voluntary ventilation (MVV) is sustainable for about 10 to 15 sec by a normal subject. At this point ventilation decreases, because tidal volume and breathing frequency cannot be sustained. This is fatigue of the respiratory muscles. Maximal voluntary sustainable ventilation is about 50% to 60% of the MVV in normal subjects. It is also the level of VE observed during heavy aerobic exercise (competitive cross country skiing, and marathon running). Maximal sustainable ventilation for 1 to 2 hrs is not a practical clinical test, but has been used in research. Shorter versions using step increases of 10% in the VE every three minutes, starting at 20% of maximum MVV, and going on until the subject cannot sustain the load, have proven to be useful. In patients with airflow limitations, the load increase is limited by the airflow limitation and progressive hyperinflation, which leads to chest wall configuration changes and muscle shortening. Similarly, its applicability for other patients with different respiratory diseases is limited.

Evaluation of Endurance While Breathing Against Inspiratory Loads

Under these conditions, the respiratory muscles develop high force and slow velocity of shortening. In essence, the subject tested has to breathe against an inspiratory threshold load, which must be overcome before air can flow into the lungs. Mouth flow can be maintained at comparable value, despite the range of load. The load is increased periodically (i.e: every 3 minutes), until the subject cannot overcome it, and consequentially has to stop the test. The highest load value tolerated for a total

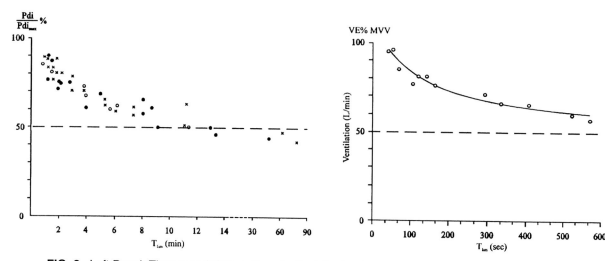

FIG. 8. Left Panel: Time to task failure (time limit) of the inspiratory muscle during resistive breathing in normal subjects. A Pdi of about 50% of max. Can be sustained for about 1h. Right Panel: Time to task failure (Time limit) of the various levels of voluntary ventilation (expressed as a percentage of maximal voluntary ventilation). Ventilation of about 55% max can be sustained for about 10 min or longer. This test was extended to 1 h. In subsequent studies. Sustainable ventilation value is about 50-60% of MVV.

period (3 minutes, in this case) is then recorded. This test has gained some acceptance, but requires some learning before it yields reproducible results. In the initial reported tests, the breathing pattern was controlled. Subsequent tests conducted in COPD patients resulted in varying breathing patterns, because the patients adopted different breathing strategies when faced with the load. To avoid the influence of force and timing, the pressure time index, or breathing pattern, can be monitored during the test.

One of the most widely accepted methods of measuring respiratory muscle endurance consists of letting the subjects or patients breathe at a level that is a known fraction of the maximal force (PI max). For example, beginning at 30% of PI max, while keeping the CO_2 constant. The load is then increased every 2 minutes by 10%, until the person can no longer sustain the pressure for a full period (2 minutes, in this case). The value of the load causing task failure or the tension time index value achieved at that time, can be used to quantify endurance.

Electrophysiological Evaluation of Respiratory Muscles

The EMG is the electrical signal recorded during muscle activation. The muscle is activated by the depolarization and repolarization of the muscle membrane, caused by neural stimulation at a rate of 5 to 50 pulses/sec. If the phrenic nerve is electrically stimulated with a short pulse (0.2 msc), it induces a biphasic muscle action potential on the diaphragm. This can be measured at the surface of the thorax with two electrodes placed along the diaphragm. This is called the compound muscle action potential. During voluntary contractions, motor units are recruited and the firing rate increases resulting, in increasing force production. The spatial and temporal summation of individual motor unit action potentials generate the interference pattern signal. As mentioned previously, the signal can be analyzed by calculating the root mean square (RMS or time domain analysis), which is then expressed as a percentage of a maximal RMS value previously obtained by sustaining an active TLC. Either the RMS peak value (at the end of each inspiration), or the average RMS during a breath is reported. This signal is proportional to the number of fibers recruited, as well as the frequency of motor unit firing rate. RMS is also proportional to muscle force for any given muscle length.

Another form of EMG analysis is to calculate the power spectrum in the frequency domain. This EMG domain is measured in periods (windows) of 20 to 200 msc, where heart PQRST signals are excluded (gated). The index Pdi/RMSdi is an expression of diaphragm effectiveness, because it provides an indirect indication of the ability of the muscle to convert an electrical signal into force. This index is low at FRC (lengthened muscle), and high at TLC (shortened muscle). The power spectrum can be quantified by calculating its moments, one of which is the center frequency. Values of center frequency have been shown to be related to the velocity of propagation of the potential along the membrane. When the EMG of the crural diaphragm is measured with a 10 mm bipolar esophageal electrode, the normal value for CF is 100 ± 4 Hz. During fatigue, CF progressively decreases to values around 60 Hz, at which point it tends to stabilize. A decrease of 15% to 20% of the resting CF is thought to represent a value associated with the development of fatigue. Center frequency returns to baseline values within 5 min after withdrawing the load. Experimental evidence obtained in animals shows that fatiguing loads sustained for periods close to 2 hrs considerably prolongs the recovery time of the center frequency, which can now take several hours. Under these conditions, there is evidence of membrane injury and sarcomere disruption. Whether this occurs in humans is unknown, but is theoretically possible. Muscle injury can explain the prolonged recovery of force observed in some cases of respiratory muscle fatigue.

Electromyographic quality recording of the diaphragm has recently been standardized by Sinderby et. al. It is expected that the standardization of methods and automatization of data recording and analysis will allow for a wider applicability of this important signal. Fig. 9 shows an example of uncoordinated EMG RMS (the patient's neural drive) while ventilated in the assist mode.

Evaluation of Respiratory Muscle Coordination

The use of respiratory inductance plethysmography bands or magnetometers on the ribcage and abdomen, is a noninvasive tool that allows simultaneous recording of the volume displacement of each of the two compartments. Plotting each signal against the other (Konno-Mead plots) provides qualitative and quantitative evaluation of respiratory muscle coordination. Normally, inspiration increases the diameter of both the ribcage and abdomen. Simultaneous calibration against a known lung volume (spirometer) allows for the continuous noninvasive evaluation of tidal volume, and course of breathing. It is very useful because it can help monitor occurrence of apnea, hyperpnea, irregular, and rapid shallow patterns of breathing. Dyssynchronous and paradoxical thoracoabdominal movements can be identified under a variety of experimental and clinical conditions as shown in Figure 10. When well calibrated, tidal volume and minute ventilation can be measured within 5% to 10% of the values obtained via measurements at the mouth. Time based recording of EMG, pressure swings, thoracoabdominal displacements, and airflow allows inferences about the time course of muscle recruitment and their interaction. Application of these techniques to real clinical situations will provide us with a better understanding of the

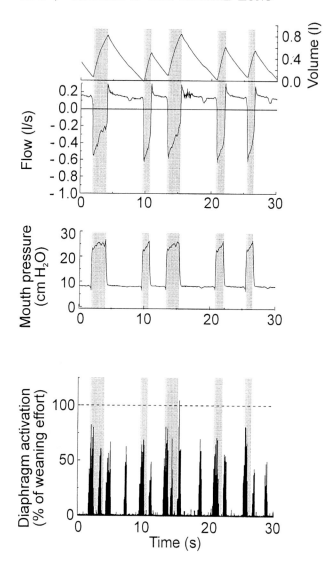

of shortening of the muscle). The causes are many, and can concurrently develop from the motor cortex to the sarcomere microfibers. Loss of the capacity to generate maximal force due to exertion, recoverable during rest, is defined as *muscle fatigue*. Since the concept of fatigue is a temporary loss of force, maximal force must be mea-

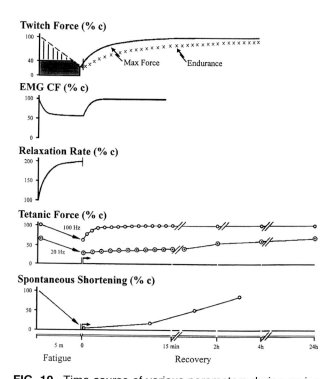

FIG. 9. Neuro mechanical coupling: The panels show 30 seconds of breathing in a patient ventilated on the demand mode. The top panel shows tidal volume and flow, indices of mechanical performance. The lower panel shows the firing of the diaphragm (EMG s RMS from the crural portion). Notice the discrepancy in breathing frequency between the ventilator (10 / min) and patient (30 / min). A considerable number of inspiratory efforts are out of phase with the ventilator. The middle panel shows the simultaneously monitored airway pressure.

respiratory system, and its behavior during different conditions, such as patient ventilator interaction, prediction of weaning failure, and the complex interrelation between sleep and respiration.

Respiratory Muscle Fatigue

Definitions

It is now widely accepted that sustained muscular activity causes a reduction in the maximal force (or velocity

FIG. 10. Time course of various parameters during an isometric contractions held at 40% of maximal force (task) until failure. Panel from the top: Maximal force: voluntary contraction is held at 40% of the force obtained during maximal voluntary effort or during maximal electrical supramaximal pulses of the nerve. The vertical lines are pressure swings obtained by electrical stimulation, showing a progressive loss of maximal force. Task failure occurs when maximal force is equal to task force. The time elapsed from the start until task failure is known as the time limit, or endurance. The exercise is defined as a fatiguing task, because there was loss of maximal force. Regaining the ability to develop maximal force takes a few minutes. Regaining the ability to perform the same task again, however, takes hours. This panel shows the time course of the central frequency (CF) of the EMG obtained via surface electrodes and Fast Fourier transforms in the same exercise. Decay of CF is fast, and is a forewarning of task failure. This parameter is an expression of membrane potential conduction velocity. Relaxation rate shows the time course of relaxation time (if the contraction if interrupted). Control values are the same as in a rested muscle. This parameter is linked to a failure at the sarcomere level, mainly related to calcium coupling and release from troponin. Tetanic force shows the decrease in force during an electrical stimulation at 100Hz or 20Hz, and its ensuing rate of recovery. Recovery from fatigue is faster when the muscle is probed with 100Hz than with 20Hz; the former is proposed to be caused by conduction mechanisms, while the latter is done by contraction mechanisms. Spontaneous shortening of the diaphragm before (100%) and after task failure, and time of recovery.

sured two or more times during the trial period. *Task failure* is defined as the inability of the muscle to continue to perform a given prefixed target (work, force, tidal volume, ventilation). Although fatigue precedes task failure, task failure does not necessarily follow fatigue. Task failure of the respiratory muscles occurs when they lose the capacity to generate the force required to sustain normal alveolar ventilation. Muscle injury can be defined as a structural change in the sarcolemma or sarcoplasm, and is usually induced by fatiguing contractions, sustained for long periods of time (several hours), as may happen to the respiratory muscles during airway obstruction. Recovery from injury takes several days, giving place to muscular remodeling where, in addition to muscle repair, there are changes in the quality of the muscle's structural or contractile proteins. Muscle weakness is a permanent loss of force, regardless of its origin.

Mechanisms of Respiratory Muscle Fatigue and the Rationale for Diagnostic Tests

Breathing tasks that are "sustainable" will be held mainly by recruitment of fatigue resistant fibers (type I), requiring oxygen to generate ATP. By themselves, type I fibers will not generate more than 30% of the maximal force, but will be able to sustain force for prolonged periods of time. High force (about 40%–50% of max) limits muscle perfusion and may deprive all cells of adequate oxygen supplies and catabolite removal. Low force will allow adequate perfusion of type I fibers, which are fatigue resistant and sustain breathing for life. The chemical composition of the muscles' interstitial space (e.g. K^+ concentration, low pH) provides neural feedback to the respiratory center.

Fatigue, which can be thought of as a regulatory mechanism through which a temporary hypoventilation is allowed to avoid muscle injury, may happen at the central level by derecruitment of fibers, at the neuro muscular junction (failure of transmission), and at the muscle levels (failure of the membrane to conduct potentials, or sarcomere to shorten or relax). Muscle force is the conventional parameter used to determine the level of muscle activity, and is dependent on length and the velocity of shortening. We can now measure parameters other than force that are known to change as fatigue develops. The challenge is to determine how they contribute or how they are related to force, and how they can be used as diagnostic tools for muscle dysfunction.

Figure 10 shows the parameters that help evaluate neuro muscular function and the techniques available for measuring fatigue. A nerve stimulation test can be performed by giving short pulses (.2 msec) of electrical or magnetic currents applied to the nerves during contraction (upper pannel). The resulting twitch force produces a maximal muscle force output. A decrease in twitch force

is an indication of muscle fatigue. Presence of twitch force while the muscle is developing maximal voluntary effort is an indication of "central" fatigue or submaximal activation. Techniques for stimulating abdominal muscles through percutaneous low dorsal nerve stimulation is now under development.

Partial mechanisms of muscle fiber function relevant to fatigue can be monitored by several other techniques Membrane excitability due to changes in the sarcolemma polarity induced by nerve stimulation can be measured using the EMG. When the index force/RMS decreases during sustained contractions at constant length, it is an indication of failure of the muscle contraction mechanism, relative to the neural command (fatigue). The frequency domain analysis of EMG provides information about the velocity of propagation of potentials along the fibers, through calculation of the frequency power spectrum. Fatiguing muscle fibers while exerting high force shows a shift towards an increased power in the low frequency component of the spectrum. Membrane excitation is a relevant function because it is the key mechanism to liberate Ca^{++} from the sarcoplasmic reticulum, which is necessary to induce contraction of the sarcomere.

Shifts in the frequency power spectrum occur early in a fatiguing contraction (within a minute of loading), and may serve as a marker for the prediction of task failure (second panel). Fatigue is not, however, the only factor that changes the velocity of propagation of potentials. An alternative to measuring EMG generated by voluntary contraction is to measure the compound muscle action potential resulting from a single .2ms electrical stimulation given to the nerve of a relaxed muscle. Here, all fibers are recruited at once resulting in a biphasic potential, the length and shape of which permits to distinguish neuro muscular abnormalities and/or fatigue.

Velocity of muscle contraction. Once the muscle contracts, its velocity of shortening and velocity of relaxation have been used as an expression of the sarcomere function. Inadequate Ca^{++} binding to and release from troponin (mainly due to lack of ATP) results in a slowing of the sarcomere velocity of relaxation (the muscle becomes stiffer during fatigue). The relaxation rate of the diaphragm during fatiguing contractions is slower than in the fresh diaphragms of normal subjects. When the muscle is subjected to fatiguing contractions, changes in relaxation rates are seen well before task failure occurs, and so the test can be used to herald task failure. Figure 10 also shows the time course of recovery of after low and high frequency stimulation.

Muscle Metabolism

Muscle biopsies and nuclear magnetic resonance spectroscopy (NMR) are the techniques most frequently used to monitor metabolic changes in the contracting muscle.

While these techniques have been of great value to study limb muscles, their use in respiratory muscles is much more limited. Phosphorous was the earliest and most frequently used atom to measure high energy phosphates (ATP, ADP, P2r or Ph). The carbon atom (CMRS) has been used to label substrates such as glucose, acetate and pyruvate.

The use of atoms of sodium and potassium (Na^+ and K^+ MRS) permits the monitoring of the intracellular ionic compositions, both of which have great significance in the propagation of membrane potential, and intracellular and extracellular water movement in muscle tissue. Cine MRI is a recent technological development, which has been applied to visualize dynamic internal events such as the beating of the heart or displacement of the diaphragm. Intense muscle exercise results in an accumulation of Pi and an increase in H^+, both affecting pH and the enzyme's capacity to generate ATP. Metabolic changes leading to muscle fatigue may soon be amenable to *in vivo* measurements.

Documentation of Respiratory Muscle Fatigue in Human Subjects. Some of the experimental studies of respiratory muscle fatigue were, in reality, measurements of the total duration during which a given force could be sustained, i.e. time to task failure, or endurance. Once task failure is established, we can assert that fatigue preceded (fatiguing contraction pattern). The evolution of maximal force as a function of time has been well documented in fatiguing contractions. Two major types of tasks have been used to elicit fatigue of the respiratory muscles: a) breathing against high inspiratory (or expiratory) resistance, and b) performing maximal voluntary ventilation under isocapnic conditions (Fig. 7). The resistive breathing protocol consists of setting a target Pdi, duty cycle, and frequency of breathing, or mouth pressure. The target is held until failure; with PaCO2 remaining at a normal level. Fewer studies offered breathing resistance without instructions about how to breathe (i.e. the subject chooses his/her own pattern of breathing). Under these conditions, PaCO2 tended to increase or decrease; in general, it increases considerably when resistances are high, and decreased when resistances were low. Overall, the results of resistive breathing experiments have shown that a pressure swing of about 50% of maximum force sustained at a duty cycle of .4 could be endured for one hour or longer. A few studies have evaluated fatigue in accessory respiratory muscles or abdominal muscles. Task failure was well documented, and we can therefore infer that fatigue did occur. In resistive breathing, the pattern of contraction consists of slow velocity, high force, small shortening, and high intramuscular pressure. Presence of muscle fatigue has been documented by measuring the force frequency curves in the diaphragm before and after task failure. All have shown decreases in maximal pressure following resistive breathing which ended in task failure. It is possible to conclude that fatigue of the respiratory

muscles in human subjects does happen during experimental loaded breathing.

The model of fatigue caused by inspiratory resistance breathing may apply to some clinical conditions like heavy snoring or sleep apnea, where peak plural pressures of 40 to 60 cm H_2O have been reported. Such conditions are, however, prevalent for short periods (minutes), followed by unloading (airway opening), and are not expected to cause fatigue.

Expiratory resistive breathing was shown to result in fatigue of abdominal muscles, and can happen in severe expiratory airway disease. Patients with COPD represent a unique situation. Their mean Pdi swing is in the range of 10 to 15cm H_2O (rest), and can increase to 20 cm during exercise; these values are close to 50% of their maximum. It is well documented that high intramuscular tension limits muscle blood perfusion leading to failure. In COPD it is likely that the relatively low Pdi measured may underestimate the intramuscular tension, since the flat diaphragm is far less effective in developing intrathoracic pressure, due to a defective coupling with the rib cage. It is not known if diaphragm perfusion is impaired in COPD. There are, in fact, studies that report a lack of increase in diaphragm perfusion in animals whose lungs were hyperinflated via PEEP: despite a threefold increase in work of breathing and pressure time index. It is known that the degree of activation of the diaphragm in COPD during resting breathing is about three times higher than in normal subjects. Recent studies show that activation of the diaphragm in COPD can rise to 85% of maximal during moderate exercise, and support the hypothesis of a high intramuscular tension in the diaphragm, which is not evident from Pdi measurements.

The second method used to induce respiratory muscle fatigue is to ask normal subjects to sustain the maximal voluntary ventilation (MVV) as long as they can, which is usually a very short period of time (about 30 sec.). Normal subjects can sustain a VE of about 55%-60% of their MVV for periods of 20 min or longer. Such levels of ventilation are seen in aerobic sports such as the marathon, skiing, and biking. During MVV the muscles contract at high speed, relatively low force, and undergo large changes in length with every breath.

In order to measure fatigue of the diaphragm at high levels of minute ventilation, the Pdi generated has been measured by applying a single electrical pulse and short trend stimulations of 10 and 20 Hz. to the phrenic nerves of normal subjects before and after exercise at 85% or 95% of their VO2 max (ventilation in the range of 80 and 120 L/min, respectively). A decrease in the value of the Pdi twitch, volitional Pdi max, and a reduction in the relaxation rate was observed during the test exercising at 95% of VO2 max. No difference was found after exercising at 85% VO2 max. Studies of Pdi max following a marathon run resulted in decreases in volitional Pdi max. It is therefore reasonable to assume that fatigue of the diaphragm develops when VE is held at 50% to 60% levels of MVV or higher. This is of relevance in sports medicine, where the limitations of body performance can be attributed to limitations in ventilation. Fatigue of the respiratory muscle in aerobic exercise may be a more relevant issue in well trained athletes than in sedentary people.

In summary, the loss of force of the respiratory muscles leading to fatigue does happen in human subjects. This becomes evident when subjects are sustaining either 50% of their maximal force or 50% of their maximal voluntary ventilation. Losses in force at lower rates have not been well documented. The monitoring of parameters showing more subtle evidence of muscle dysfunction than a loss of maximal force during loading in both normal and diseased subjects remains an exiting challenge.

Respiratory Muscles Training

In patients with COPD, as the diaphragm becomes functionally impaired, the accessory muscle contribution to ventilation progressively increases. Patients with symptomatic lung disease like COPD are limited in their capacity to exercise, because of dyspnea. Evidence suggests that the dyspnea relates more to respiratory control and muscle function than to airflow obstruction. As the ratio between the pressure needed to ventilate and the maximal pressure that the muscles can generate (Pdi/Pdimax or PI/PImax) increases, there is a proportional increase in dyspnea. Dyspnea also increases with increases in the duration of the contraction (Ti/Ttot) cycle and respiratory frequency. Because these factors have been shown to correlate with EMG evidence of respiratory muscle fatigue, changes in any of them may help explain the observed increase or decrease in exercise performance after training.

Based upon these principles one may postulate the following treatment goals:

1) Decrease in inspiratory force,
2) Shortening of inspiratory time,
3) Increases in maximal inspiratory pressures,
4) Decrease in respiratory frequency, and
5) Improved coordination among the different respiratory muscles.

Data suggests that it is primarily through the last three mechanisms that systematic training in COPD may result in improved exercise endurance.

Exercise Conditioning

Lower Extremity Exercise

Patients with underlying lung disease are restricted in their ability to perform exercise. This leads to a progres-sive reduction in their physical activity. This, in turn, deconditions the muscles further, perpetuating physical inactivity and a sedentary lifestyle. This is depicted as the downward spiral of patients with COPD. A major goal of exercise training in pulmonary rehabilitation is to interrupt the downward spiral by enabling patients to tolerate a higher level of activity. It is clear that exercise conditioning improves exercise endurance.

In the mostly uncontrolled studies that have evaluated the effect of rehabilitation on exercise performance, the results are clear. Most patients included had moderate to severe airway obstruction with hypoxemia, without carbon dioxide retention. In most studies, the subjects exercised an average of 3 days per week for a total duration of 6 weeks. Walking, with or without treadmill and bicycle ergometry, were the more commonly used exercise modalities. Irrespective of the training mode, exercise endurance increased, without measurable changes in pulmonary function. In none of these studies were ventilatory muscles adequately studied, but the lack of change in vital capacity or lung volume suggest minimal if any effect of general exercise on respiratory muscle function.

Data obtained from several randomized studies with control groups in patients with underlying COPD is now available. The results revealed a significant increase in the 12-minute walking test and peak oxygen uptake with important decreases in the perception of dyspnea and improvement in health related qality of life. Based upon a review of the existing literature, increased VO_2 following exercise training as demonstrated in a few studies, can be interpreted as an enhanced physiological response to exercise. Some studies have demonstrated a decrease in the heart rate, VCO_2, and VE following exercise training. Recent data suggest that the changes are due to true physiological changes, because there have been documented increases in the enzyme content of the mitochondria of peripheral muscle biopsy in trained patients. On the other hand, most evidence indicate that ventilatory muscle function per se is not significantly affected by aerobic leg exercise, although this hypothesis has not been well studied.

Arm Exercise Conditioning

It has been demonstrated that eight weeks of 3 times weekly unsupported arm exercise results in a significant decrease in VE, VO_2 and VCO_2 for simple arm elevation. Several studies have looked at both arm and leg training, and have demonstrated improved task specific performance. Although theoretically possible, arm training has not resulted in significant changes in respiratory muscle function. Its beneficial effects are probably related to the decreased ventilatory demands, because the ''efficiency'' of the shoulder girdle and arm muscles improve with the training.

Methods of Specific Respiratory Muscle Training

As discussed above, whole body exercise fails to improve ventilatory muscle endurance in patients with COPD, whereas normal subjects and patients with cystic fibrosis may increase ventilatory muscle strength with intense aerobic exercise. It is possible that the levels of ventilation achieved during exercise in COPD is inadequate to generate the appropriate increase in ventilatory endurance. Since reduced inspiratory muscle strength is evident in patients with COPD, considerable efforts have been made to define the role of respiratory muscle training in these patients.

Training has been achieved using two different strategies: strength training and endurance training.

Strength Training. This is achieved through the application of a high intensity low frequency stimulus. This is done by performing repeated inspiratory effort maneuvers against a closed glottis or shutter. Studies have determined an increase in PImax with respiratory muscle strength training. In one study, the Pi max increased by 53% in patients with COPD after 5 weeks of training. Another demonstrated a 50% increase in PImax in 9 patients after 4 weeks of training. The extent to which strength training contributes to clinical improvement is debatable, but it is not unreasonable to assume that some of the observed benefits reported after respiratory muscle endurance training may relate to the increased strength achieved.

Endurance Training. Achieved through the application of low intensity, high frequency stimulus, the following three methodologies have been explored: flow resistive loading, threshold loading and ventilatory isocapnic hyperpnea.

Flow Resistive Loading: The goal is achieved by having the patient breathe through orifices of progressively smaller diameters. Although it is tempting to attribute the ability to breathe through smaller orifices as improved endurance, this may very well just represent an adaptive breathing strategy. It has, indeed, been shown in patients that just by changing the breathing pattern to one of slow long breaths, there was an improvement in resistive breathing endurance, despite the use of a smaller orifice.

In studies where attention was given to the breathing pattern, the results have been encouraging. One first group demonstrated improved ventilatory muscle strength, endurance and exercise capacity in COPD patients who underwent ventilatory muscle training in addition to rehabilitation versus rehabilitation alone. Another study demonstrated improved respiratory muscle strength and endurance in a treated group, as compared to controls. The treatment group reached progressively higher target pressures, whereas the control group breathed through an unloaded system. It is of interest that a significant reduction of dyspnea was observed in the treatment group.

Threshold Loading: The principle of this training mode

is to ensure an adequate inspired pressure to ensure training independent of inspiratory flow rate. The results of the controlled studies that have evaluated threshold load training, have shown an increase in respiratory muscle strength, increased endurance to a ventilatory load and a decrease in dyspnea during this maneuver. Those studies which evaluated other important outcomes, such as health related quality of life and exercise capacity, unfortunately demonstrated only minimal improvements. In conclusion, although threshold loading improves ventilatory muscle strength and endurance for resistive breathing; it also seems to decrease dyspnea with exercise, there are minimal systemic benefits from these changes. Other outcomes have not been examined, and require further studies.

Ventilatory Isocapnic Hyperpnea: In this form of training, the patient maintains a high level of minute ventilation for 10 to 15 minutes 2 or 3 times daily while CO_2 is kept constant. This concept simulates whole body exercise such as running, by subjecting the diaphragm and other inspiratory muscles to low tension, high levels of repetitive activity. The level of hyperpnea is measured as the maximum sustained ventilatory capacity (MSVC), defined as the maximum level of ventilation that can be sustained under isocapnic conditions for 15 minutes. The few studies that used this training mode showed that muscle endurance improved in the range of 20% to 50%. Controlled studies by 2 groups have demonstrated that although MSVC improves in COPD patients trained for 6 weeks, exercise endurance is no better than the control groups. Because it is difficult to implement and with no demonstrable change in outcomes other than the improved respiratory muscle endurance, isocapneic hyperventilation is not used as a from of ventilatory muscle training.

Breathing Retraining. There are other less conventional forms of training that are open to critical review, but are conceptually solid and may offer new avenues of treatment. Patients with COPD manifest a higher ventilatory drive than normal patients. In fact, patients on mechanical ventilation who cannot wean have a higher ventilatory drive than those patients who successfully wean. If we could decrease this drive, it would become possible to decrease the consequences of such a high drive: increased work of breathing, respiratory rate and perhaps dyspnea. Although it is scant, there is some available data that supports the study and application of these therapeutic tools.

Feedback: In a recent study, 40 patients were evaluated after at least 7 days of mechanical ventilation. They were randomized to conventional weaning or weaning with the use of electromyographic feedback training using the frontalis signal as an indication of tension and to induce relaxation. They also used the surface EMG of intercostals and diaphragm as indicators of respiratory muscle activity. Using feedback signals to encourage relaxation and larger tidal volumes, there were differences between treated and untreated patients. The results indicate a reduction in mean ventilator days for the biofeedback group. Tidal volume and mean inspiratory flow increased significantly for this group. The increase was also significant when corrected by diaphragmatic EMG amplitude. This was interpreted as improved diaphragmatic efficiency. The authors concluded that breathing retraining resulted in a more efficient breathing pattern which, in turn, decreased dyspnea and anxiety, and allowed for quicker weaning time in the treated patients.

Postural Changes: It is known that musculoskeletal tone and contraction may be determined by habitual positioning. Over the last few years, increasing attention has been given to the voluntary inhibition of those patterns. This has been particularly useful for artists. A recent study demonstrated improved peak expiratory flow rate, maximal voluntary ventilation and maximal inspiratory and expiratory pressures in normal subjects who underwent lessons in proprioceptive musculoskeletal education, compared to controls. This method has not, per-se, been systematically evaluated in patients with lung disease, but breathing retraining (pursed lip breathing and diaphragmatic breathing) constitutes a form of therapy that resembles the above discussed techniques.

Pursed Lip Breathing: Indeed, pursed lip breathing results in a slowing of the breathing rate with increases in tidal volume. PLB will result in a shift in the pattern of recruitment of the ventilatory muscles from one that is predominantly diaphragmatic to one that recruits more the accessory muscles of the ribcage and abdominal muscles of exhalation. Perhaps this shift may contribute to the relief dyspnea that has been reported by patients when this breathing technique is adopted. Patients on ventilators cannot purse lip breath, but it has been shown that the administration of respiratory retard, or PEEP, improves oxygenation, decreases respiratory rate, augments ventilation, and improves work of breathing in weaning patients. Pursed lip prevalence in COPD is related to the degree of airway obstruction.

CONCLUSION

Over the last two decades, numerous studies of ventilatory muscle training on patients with chronic airflow limitations have been reported. Uniformly, they indicate that VMT results in either increased strength or endurance for the specific task for which they were trained. Several questions have been answered regarding the acceptable methods of training. However, based upon the existing literature, we still cannot recommend routine ventilatory muscle training to all patients with COPD, since there is limited evidence that it improves outcomes such as quality of life, or activities of daily living. Future research will attempt to evaluate the role of VMT as an adjunct to other well proven training strategies, such as aerobic leg

training. The scientific evaluation of less accepted techniques, such as breathing retraining, yoga, and biofeedback deserve interest and efforts.

Surgery and Respiratory Muscle Function

By removing the most abnormal emphysematous lung and decreasing resting lung volume, lung pneumoplasty allows the respiratory muscles and especifically the diaphragm to regain length and/or mechanical coupling advantage. Recent data shows improved respiratory muscle performance at rest and during exercise and decreased dyspnea. The latter may happen because of a reduction in the neural drive, as overall mechanics and impedance improve after LVR. As more experience is gained with this procedure, it will become a therapeutic option for selected patients with severe COPD.

BIBLIOGRAPHY

Aubier, M., G. Farkas, A. deTroyer, C. Roussos. Detection of Diaphragmatic Fatigue in Man by Phrenic Stimulation. *J. Appl. Physiol.* 1981; 50:538–44. *This experimentally difficult work shows a loss of diaphragm force following resistive breathing. It documents the presence of muscular, rather than central, fatigue.*

Beck, J. C. Sinderby, J. Weinberg and A. Grassino. Effects of Muscle To Electrode Distance on the human Diaphragm EMG. *J. Appl. Physiol.* 1995; 79:975–85. *Through the use of ring electrodes, this work sets a new standard of EMG recording. It helps the reader understand the complexities of EMG analysis.*

Begin, P., A. Grassino. Inspiratory Muscle Dysfunction and Chronic Hypercapnia. *Am. Rev. Resp. Dis.* 1991; 143:905–12. *This is a study of over 300 stable COPD, where the role of the respiratory muscles and other variables on chronic hypercapnia was explored. It contais a wealth of information regarding the pattern of breathing in COPD.*

Bellemare, F., B. Bigland Ritchie. Central Components of Diaphragm Fatigue Assessed by Phrenic Nerve Stimulation. *J. Appl. Physiol.* 1987; 62:263–77. *First work measuring the partition of loss of diaphragm force into a central component and a peripheral muscular component. Elegant technique that may be used in humans.*

Bellemare, F., and A. Grassino. Effect of Pressure and Timing of Contraction on Human Diaphragmatic Fatigue. *J. Appl. Physiol.* 1982; 53(5):1190–95. *The concept of tension-time as a factor limiting respiratory muscle endurance is derived from experimental data in humans. This work expands upon and complements the concept of force being an endurance limiting parameter.*

Bellemare, F., D. Wight, C. Lavigne and A. Grassino. Effect of Tension and Timing of Contraction on the Blood Flow of the Diaphragm. *J. Appl. Physiol.* 1983; 54:1597–1606. *This work extends the observation that relate force and duration of contraction to respiratory muscle endurance. In this work, both factors are shown to influence diaphragmatic blood flow, and hence energy supply to the working muscle.*

Bertocci, L. A. *Emerging Opportunities with Nuclear Magnetic Resonance: Fatigue.* S. Gandevia, et. al., eds. 1995. New York, London: Plenum Press, 211–240. *An updated and extensive description of the applications of MNR to the in vivo study of muscle cell metabolism. This work shows how repetitive breathing against inspiratory resistances soliciting pressure. The time close to fatigue threshold results in muscle membrane and sarcomere injury in the in vivo dog.*

Black, L. and R. Hyatt. Maximal Respiratory Pressure: Normal Values and Relationship to Age and Sex. *Am. Rev. Resp. Dis.* 1969; 99: 696–702. *This was the first work to establish standard techniques to measure the pressure generated by the respiratory muscles. It established the differences between inspiratory and expiratory stength and the effect of lung volume on their magnitude.*

Celli BR, Rassulo J, Make B. Dyssynchronous breathing during arm but not leg exercise in patients with chronic airflow obstruction. *N Engl J Med.* 1986;314:1485–1490. *This work adreeses the issue of coordination of the shoulder girdle accessory muscles of respiration and the diaphragm. It also points out the dual function of some of the muscles of respiration.*

Chokoverty, S., S. Shah, M. Chokoverty, A. Deutch, and A. Belsh. Percutaneous Magnetic Coil Stimulation of the Phrenic Nerve and Roots and Trunk. *Electr. Clin. Neurophys* 1995;97:369–74. *This paper recapitulates data on pressure swings in normal subjects via the magnetic stimulation technique. Provides values for normal subject.*

Clanton, T. L. *Respiratory Muscle Endurance in Humans. The Thorax,* 1996 part B. Roussos, C., ed. Marcel Recker, Inc. pp. 1199–1230. *An excellent review on muscle endurance, methods of evaluation, physiology and applications. It provides the reader with an update of a difficult area.*

DeTroyer A, Estenne. Coordination between ribcage muscles and diaphragm during quiet breathing in humans. *J Appl Physiol* 1984;57(3):899–906. *Excellent work devoted to evaluate the contribution of the ribcage muscles to breathing. It determined that some of the until then called accessory muscles such as the scalene are in reality primary ventilatory muscles.*

DeTroyer A, Sampson M, Sigrist S, et al. How the abdominal muscles act on the ribcage. *J Appl Physiol* 1983;54(2):465–469. *This work determined the priamry function of the abdominal muscles as being that of helping exhalation.*

DeVito, E., A. Grassino. *Respiratory Muscle Failure. Rationale For Diagnostic Tests. The Thorax.* 1996 C. Roussos ed. M. Dekker, Inc. pp. 1857–1880. *This review explores in detail most of the techniques used for the evaluation of the respiratory muscle in humans, and their biological meaning.*

Eastwood, P. R., D. Hillman, K. Finucaine. Ventilatory Responses to Inspiratory Threshold Loading and Rate of Muscle Fatigue in Task Failure. *J. Appl. Physiol* 1994;76(1):185–95. *A theoretical paper on signal analysis. Includes mathematical models. A good review for those interested in a deeper understanding of analysis of signals.*

Epstein S. An overview of Respiratory Muscle Function. *Chest Clin N.A.* 1994;15:619–639. *A solid review of muscle anatomy and function. A special emphasis was made of their importance in neuromuscular diseases.*

Esau, S., F. Bellemare, A. Grassino, S. Permutt, C. Roussos. Changes in Relaxation Rate With Diaphragmatic Fatigue in Humans. *J. Appl. Physiol* 1983;54:1353–60. *This work examines the relation of relaxation rate of a post contraction muscle and muscle fatigue. This study shows that a slower muscle relaxation rate serves as an early marker of fatigue, matching the time course of EMG frequency changes.*

Grassino A., C. Roussos . *Static Properties of the Chest Wall in Crystal,* R. and J. B. West, eds. The Lung 1991. Vol. I. New York: Raven Press, pp. 855–67. *This Chapter describes the evaluation of the understanding of chest wall physiology from the one compartment model through two compartments and their micro-mechanics.*

Gross, D., A. Grassino, W. Ross, P. Macklem. EMG Pattern of Diaphragmatic Fatigue. *J Appl Physiol* 1979;46:1–7. *The first work describing a shift to lower frequencies of the power spectrum of the EMG of the diaphragm during resistive breathing.*

Holliday JE, Hyers TM. The reduction of weaning time from mechanical ventilation using tidal volume and relaxation feedback. *Am Rev Respir Dis* 1990;141:1214–1220. *Interesting experiments in ventilated patients in the ICU. Through feedback training it was possible to shorten ventilator dependency time. It raises the possibility of using the cortex to influence ventilatory pattern.*

Hussain, S. Regulation of Ventilatory Muscle Blood Flow. *J. Appl. Physiol* 1996;81(4):1455–68. *A sharp, updated, and lucid description of respiratory muscle blood flow from physiology to molecular mechanisms.*

Johnson, B., M. Babcock, E. Suman., J. Dempsey . Exercise Induced Diaphragmatic Fatigue in Healthy Humans. *J. Physiol (Lond)* 1993;460:385–405. *This experiment proves that diaphragm fatigue can be present (low pressure twitch, Pdi volitional and relaxation rate) following exercises at 95% VO2 max in normal subjects, but not so at 85% of VO2 max. Relevant to athletics.*

Laporta, D., A. Grassino. Assessment of Transdiaphragmatic Pressure in Humans. *J. Appl. Physiol* 1985;58:1469–1476. *The paper analyses different maneuvers to obtain maximal transdiaphragmatic pressure (Pdi max) , and also provides values in normals.*

Martinez F, Couser J, Celli B. Factors influencing ventilatory muscle recruitment in patients with chronic airflow obstruction. *Am Rev Respir Dis* 1990;142:276–282. *This work on a large number of patients describes the progressive use of accessory muscles as the hyperinflation of COPD increases. It also showed that patients with COPD utilize the muscles of exhalation even during tidal breathing.*

Martinez F, Montes de Oca M, Whyte R, Stetz J, Gay S, Celli B. Lung volume reduction improves dyspnea, dynamic hyperinflation and respiratory muscle function. *Am J Respir Crit Care Med* 1997;155:1984–1990. *This study documents the effect of lung volume reduction surgery in several aspects of respiratory physiology. Amongst them, there was a significant improvement in respiratory muscle strength, and a normalization of the recruitment pattern of the respiratory muscles after surgery.*

Martyn, J., R. Moreno, P. Pare, R.L. Pardy . Measurement of Inspiratory Muscle Performance with Incremental Threshold Loading. *Am. Rev. Resp. Dis* 1987;135:919–923. *One of the few papers proposing a practical technique to measure respiratory muscle endurance in patients.*

Mead J. Functional significance of the area of apposition of diaphragm to ribcage. *Am Rev Respir Dis* 1979;119:31–32. *Landmark work that descrbed the way in which the diaphragm moves the ribcage. It comes from the laboratory that established the role of respiratory muscles in breathing.*

Miller, J.M., J. Moxham, M. Green. The Maximal Sniff in the Assessment of Diaphragmic Function in Man. *Clin. Sci* 1985;69:91–96. *This work provides an alternative form of assessing diaphrgamatic function in humans. The sniff technique may be easier to perform and provides excellent valid information. This concise review by its supporters is important for those measuring respiratory muscle performance.*

Moxham, J., C. Wiles, D. Newman, R. H. T. Edwards. Sternomastoid Function and Fatigue in Man. *Clin. Sci* 1980;5:433–468. *This work underscores the importance of accessory muscles of respiration. It was the first to show thar fatiguecan also occur in the sternocleidomastoid muscle in humans.*

NHLBI Workshop on Respiratory Muscle Fatigue: Report of the Respiratory Muscle Fatigue Workshop Group. *Am. Rev. Resp. Dis* 1990;142:474–480. *Excellent review of the state of the art of respiratory mucle and their function until 1990. It provides a framework which includes definitions, applications and future areas for research. Good source of general information.*

Ninane V, Rypens F, Yernault JC, DeTroyer A. Abdominal muscle using during breathing in patients with chronic airflow obstruction. *Am Rev Respir Dis* 1992;146:16–21. *Confirms the use of abdominal muscles during respiration in patients with COPD. This needs to be taken into account when evaluating positive pressure at the end of exhalation in patients with the disease.*

Rochester DF. The diaphragm: contractile properties and fatigue. *J Clin Invest* 1985;75:1397–1402. *Excellent overall review of diaphragmatic anatomy and physiology. Good summary of all the important aspects of this muscle.*

Roussos, C., P. Macklem. Diaphragmatic Fatigue in Man. *J. Appl. Physiol* 1977;43:189–197. *Excellent review that helped rekindle the interest in the function of the respiratory muscles.*

Roussos CH, Macklem PT. The respiratory muscles. *N Engl J Med* 1982;307:786–797. *Landmark review of respiratory muscles and their importance. Besides its theoretical contents it is also a practical compendium of the issues related to respiratory muscle function.*

Sinderby, C., L. Lindstrom, A. Grassino. Automatic assessment of Electromyogram Quality. *J. Appl. Physiol* 1995;79:1803–1815. *This paper starts with a basic model of an electrical potential conductivity on a fiber and builds up to many fibers, thereby developing a rationale about how and why EMG can be analyzed. It provides a basis on how to obtain quality EMG in humans.*

Smith K, Cook D, Guyatt GH, Madhavan J, Oxman A. Respiratory Muscle Training in Chronic Airflow Limitation: A meta-analysis. *Am Rev Respir Dis* 1992;145:533–539. *This study summarized our knowledge about the changes in outcomes that have been shown to occur after ventilatory muscle training in COPD. It confirms that even though strength and endurance imporve after VMT, its clinical significance remains to be explored.*

Sorli, J., A. Grassino, A. Lorange, G. J. Milic Emili. Control of Breathing in Patients With COPD. *Clin Sci Mol Med* 1978;54:295–304.

The first paper showing that respiratory neural output in resting COPD was 3 to 5 times higher than in normal individuals.

Supinsky GS, Kelsen SG. Effects of elastase-induced emphysema on the force-generating ability of the diaphragm. *J Clin Invest* 1982;70: 978-988. *This experimental work in animals proved that the diaphragm may adapt to changes in length by adding or substracting sarcomeres. This would imply that patients with chronic shortening of muscle fibers may be functioning at a new optimal lenght and that the decreased forces that are generated are due to overall geometrical changes and not to length-tension changes perse.*

Tenney, S., R. E. Reese. The Ability To Sustain Great Breathing Efforts. *Resp Phsysiol* 1968;5:187–201. *A classic paper measuring how long diferent levels of ventilation can be sustained by normal subjects. It brings up the concept of an endurance threshold, but the paper was was focused on energetics.*

Tobin M. The respiratory muscles in disease. *Clin Chest Med* 1988;9: 263-286. *Good clinical review of the changes in respiratory muscle function in disease states. Easy to read and very informative.*

Vinken, W., C. Guilleminault, M. Cosio, A. Grassino. Onset of Diaphragmatic Fatigue. *Am Rev Resp Dis* 1985;135:372–377. *The paper explores the possible relation of fatigue to Obstructive Sleep Apnea and found no evidence of fatigue.*

Vollestad, N. *Changes in Activation, Contractile Speed, and Electrolite Balances During Fatigue.* The Thorax. 1996. C. Roussos, ed. M. Dekker, Inc. Part A: pp. 235–253. *This is a lucid description of the main patterns leading to muscle cell fatigue.*

Zhu, E., B. Petrof, J. Gea, N. Comptois, and A. Grassino. Diaphragm Muscle Fiber Injury After Inspiratory Resistive Breathing. *Am J Respir Crit Care Med* 1997;155:1110–1116. *Experimental work that proves that resistance breathing may induce damage of the muscle fibers. This is very important as the load level may be close to that seen by humans in respiratory distress.*

Textbook of Pulmonary Diseases, 6th ed.
edited by G.L. Baum, J.D. Crapo, B.R. Celli, and J.B. Karlinsky,
Lippincott–Raven Publishers, Philadelphia, © 1998.

CHAPTER

7

Molecular Biology of Lung Disease

N. Tony Eissa · Shan C. Chu · Joel Moss

INTRODUCTION

In the past two decades, the techniques of molecular biology have been used increasingly, not only in basic science but also in clinical research. Today, clinicians, including specialists in pulmonary medicine, are confronted frequently with reports of studies in which the techniques of molecular biology are employed. This chapter is intended to help readers understand the information and techniques that are the basis of molecular biology. The concepts of genomic deoxyribonucleic acid (DNA), primary messenger ribonucleic acid (pre-mRNA) processing, including alternative splicing, and translation of mRNA into protein are introduced first. The common techniques of molecular biology are presented next, followed by examples of recent advances in pulmonary research in which these techniques have been used.

BASIC CONCEPTS

Genomic DNA

The nucleus of each normal human somatic cell contains 46 chromosomes—44 somatic chromosomes and two sex chromosomes, which are either XX in a female or XY in a male. Each chromosome contains a single, linear, compacted, double-stranded DNA molecule, which is the genetic material, plus associated proteins, such as histones. The structure of DNA consists of two long complementary polynucleotide chains that wind around each other to form a double helix. The basic building block of the polynucleotide chain is a mononucleo-

N. T. Eissa, S. C. Chu, and J. Moss: Pulmonary-Critical Care Medicine Branch, National Heart, Lung, and Blood Institute, National Institutes of Health, Bethesda, Maryland 20892.

tide, comprised of a phosphate group, a sugar ring (deoxyribose), and a base moiety, either a purine (adenine, *A,* or guanine, *G*) or a pyrimidine (cytosine, *C,* or thymine, *T*). The backbone of the helix consists of deoxyribose-phosphate groups. Except at the 5' end of the DNA strand, each phosphate group forms a 5'-3' phosphodiester bond between the fifth carbon of one deoxyribose ring and the third carbon of the adjacent deoxyribose ring. The nucleotide base (G, A, T, or C) attached to each deoxyribose moiety is in the center of helix, oriented perpendicularly to its axis. The two strands of the DNA helix are held together by hydrogen bonds between complementary base pairs (two bonds between adenine and thymine, three between guanine and cytosine). The strands are antiparallel, one running in the 5' to 3' direction and the other in the 3' to 5' direction. Because adenine pairs only with thymine and guanine only with cytosine, the sequence of nucleotides in one strand of the double helix determines the sequence of the other.

The complete DNA sequence, comprising the total genetic information carried on all chromosomes in a cell, is called *genomic DNA*. It is estimated that haploid human genomic DNA contains 3×10^9 base pairs (bp), representing 100,000 to 500,000 genes. A gene, which consists of the entire DNA sequence necessary for the synthesis of a functional polypeptide or RNA molecule, such as transfer RNA (tRNA) or ribosomal RNA (rRNA), is the smallest functional physical unit of inheritance. A gene contains not only the nucleotides that encode the amino acids of a protein (coding sequences) or the sequence of a functional RNA, but also all the other DNA sequences needed to produce the primary RNA transcript (Fig. 1). In the eukaryotic genome, critical noncoding sequences include (1) transcription regulatory sequences with promoter, promoter-proximal elements, and enhancers, (2) a sequence at the 3' end of a gene that signals the position for 3' cleavage and polyadenylation, and (3) intervening se-

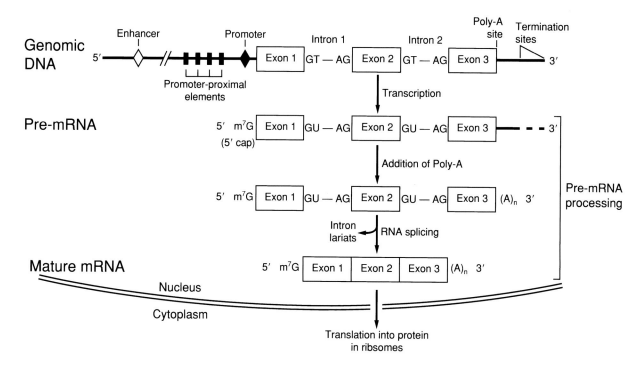

FIG. 1. Gene expression in mammals. Shown at the top is the basic structure of a gene in genomic DNA. Exons (sequences preserved in the mature mRNA), introns (intervening noncoding sequences), and important elements of gene regulation, including the promoter, promoter-proximal elements, enhancer, poly(A) site, and the universally conserved dinucleotides (GU and AG) at the 5' and 3' ends of each intron, are indicated. The gene is first transcribed into pre-mRNA transcripts. After several steps of pre-mRNA processing, including 5' capping with 7-methylguanylate (m^7G), polyadenylation at the 3' end, and RNA splicing to excise introns and ligate exons, mature mRNA is ready to be transported to the cytoplasm for translation into protein in ribosomes. See text for details.

quences (introns) that are later removed by splicing of primary RNA transcripts.

The promoter contains a sequence that determines the site of transcription initiation by an RNA polymerase. Promoter-proximal elements, usually adjacent to the promoter, bind specific factors (transcription factors) to regulate the rate of transcription of the gene into pre-mRNA. An enhancer consists of sequence, located either upstream or downstream at a distance from the transcription initiation site, that can increase or decrease the rate of transcription of the gene by binding to a specific factor(s).

Primary Messenger RNA Processing and Alternative Splicing

Although the genetic information is stored in DNA in the nucleus, the protein (gene product) is synthesized on ribosomes in the cytoplasm. The mRNA, an edited copy of the gene, carries the genetic information from the nucleus to the cytoplasm. The structure of RNA is slightly different from that of DNA, in that uracil replaces thymine and ribose replaces deoxyribose.

As the first step in transferring genetic information from DNA to protein in eukaryotic cells, a protein-encoding gene is transcribed by RNA polymerase II into pre-mRNA (Fig. 1). The pre-mRNA includes exons (sequences preserved in the mature mRNA) and introns (intervening sequences). RNA polymerase II initiates transcription at the first nucleotide of the first exon (the transcription initiation site) of a gene and stops at any one of multiple sites 0.5 to 2 kilobases (kb) downstream from the 3' end of the last exon (termination sites). To yield a functional mature mRNA, the pre-mRNA undergoes several processing steps in the nucleus, including capping at the 5' end, cleavage and polyadenylation at the 3' end, and ligation of exons with concomitant excision of introns (RNA splicing). Shortly after transcription of pre-mRNA begins, the 5' end of the newly formed RNA is capped with 7-methylguanylate. In addition, in vertebrate cells, the 2' hydroxyls of the ribose of the first and second nucleotides at the 5' end are methylated. This 5' cap facilitates ribosome binding to RNA and increases the efficiency of translation of mRNA into protein. At the 3' end, an endonuclease cleaves the pre-mRNA at the 3' end of the last exon [poly(A) site], usually 10 to 30 bp downstream from the poly(A) signal, which often includes an AAUAAA sequence. Then, a sequence of 100 to 250 adenylate residues [poly(A) tail] is added by a polymerase. Finally, introns are excised by RNA splicing before the mature mRNA is transported to the cytoplasm, where it can be translated.

Pre-mRNA splicing is a tightly regulated process in which introns must be accurately and efficiently removed and exons spliced together to yield mature mRNA. In each mammalian intron, the nucleotides GT are at the 5' end and AG at the 3' end. Important *cis*-acting elements are required for accurate and efficient splicing, including highly conserved consensus sequences at the 5' and 3' splice sites. In addition, many *trans*-acting elements are involved in forming the complex spliceosome for pre-mRNA splicing. These include small nuclear ribonucleoproteins (snRNPs) U1, U2, U4, U5, and U6, and many non-snRNP factors. During pre-mRNA splicing, the 5' splice junction is cleaved first, and the most 5' nucleotide of the intron (G) is joined in a 2'-5' phosphodiester bond to a specific point nucleotide (A) to generate a lariat intermediate. Then, cleavage at the 3' splice junction releases the lariat intron and the two exons are ligated. Mature mRNA is formed in this manner, ready to be transported to the cytoplasm for translation.

Different exons in a given pre-mRNA can be included in the final mature mRNA. This is termed *alternative splicing,* which greatly increases the diversity of proteins that can be derived from a single pre-mRNA. Alternative splicing usually is regulated in a tissue- or development-specific manner. For example, fibronectin (a large extracellular matrix protein) mRNA in fibroblasts contains EIIIA and EIIIB exons, whereas the fibronectin mRNA in hepatocytes does not. Alternative splicing can occur because of differences in sequences at critical splice sites. For example, there is a variable in-frame skipping of exon 9 in cystic fibrosis transmembrane conductance regulator (CFTR) mRNA transcripts. From 0%–92% of CFTR mRNA transcripts in the respiratory epithelium may have a deletion of exon 9 sequences (exon 9⁻). This is mainly because of differences among individuals in the length of a polythymidine tract close to the 3' splice site of exon 9. An inverse relationship exists between the length of the polythymidine tract (5T, 7T, or 9T) and the proportion of exon 9⁻ CFTR mRNA transcripts in respiratory epithelium.

Protein Synthesis: Translation of mRNA into Protein

In the cytoplasm, protein synthesis occurs on ribosomes, where the nucleic acid sequence of mRNA (A, U, G, C) is translated into an amino acid sequence to form a polypeptide by the combined action of tRNAs and ribosomes. From the starting point of translation of mRNA, each triplet of bases forms a ''codon'' that specifies which amino acid is to be incorporated into the growing polypeptide chain by interaction with a specific tRNA, which contains a unique complementary three-base ''anticodon.'' There are 64 (4^3) possible codons. Of these, 61 are used to specify 20 different amino acids, and three are stop signals to indicate the end of a polypeptide chain. With the exception of methionine and tryptophan, each amino acid is encoded by more than one codon. Remarkably, every cell of every organism, from bacteria to humans, uses the same three-base genetic code to designate the amino acid that is to be incorporated into the growing polypeptide chain. Ribosomes consisting of rRNAs and many associated ribosomal proteins provide binding sites for all the accessory molecules of protein synthesis. Ribosomes and bound tRNAs move along an mRNA transcript to translate its genetic information into a protein.

COMMON TECHNIQUES OF MOLECULAR BIOLOGY

Isolation of Samples

The lung provides the molecular biologist with a relatively convenient source of samples for evaluation of gene expression and function. Whereas obtaining tissue samples from most organs may require a surgical procedure, the lung is readily accessible via fiberoptic bronchoscopy, which is a less invasive procedure. During bronchoscopy, sampling of respiratory epithelium is performed by brushing with a cytology brush, whereas bronchoalveolar lavage (BAL) allows sampling of the epithelial lining fluid and inflammatory cells in the bronchoalveolar space. Evaluation of sputum or cells from the lining of the nasal passages may be accomplished without bronchoscopy.

Sputum

Sputum can yield information about the cellular and biochemical composition of the lung. Expectorated sputum can be collected easily and analyzed repeatedly. Induction of sputum by inhalation of hypertonic saline aerosol has been used successfully to diagnose lung infections (e.g., *Pneumocystis carinii* pneumonia in patients infected with HIV). Analysis of the cellular constituents of sputum has been used as a less invasive method than bronchoscopy to evaluate and monitor airway inflammation in asthmatic patients. Sputum consists of soluble (SSP) and gel (SGP) phases, which can be separated by centrifugation. Like BAL fluid, SSP can be analyzed to give information about exudation of plasma protein into the airway lumen of patients with lung disease. The amount of protein in SSP is reported to be elevated in several lung diseases, including asthma, chronic bronchitis, and cystic fibrosis (CF), and is reduced by therapy. To assess proteins in SGP, it is necessary to solubilize the SGP with dithiothreitol, a reducing agent that cleaves disulfide bridges in the mucin molecules. Analysis of proteins in sputum with specific antibodies is a valuable tool for studying inflammatory processes in the lung. Analysis of sputum from patients with CF revealed the presence of excess DNA from desquamated epithelial cells, neutrophils, and eosinophils, resulting in increased viscosity and impaired clearance and thereby playing a significant role in airway disease in these patients. This finding led to the development of a specific therapy using recombinant human deoxyribonuclease I, an enzyme that acts as a "molecular scissors" to cleave DNA in purulent lung secretions, making them easier to expectorate.

Bronchoalveolar Lavage

BAL is an invaluable means of evaluating inflammatory and immune processes in the lung. Lavage recovers cells resident in the bronchoalveolar space; these can be used for a variety of morphologic and functional studies after separation from fluid by simple centrifugation. A sample of cells is evaluated by light microscopy for total cell number, differential cell count, cell morphology, and the presence of any abnormal substances (e.g., asbestos bodies). In normal subjects, lavage yields macrophages (90%), lymphocytes (10%), and <1% neutrophils, eosinophils, and/or basophils. A high lymphocyte count is frequently found in hypersensitivity pneumonitis and sarcoidosis. Elevated numbers of neutrophils are common in CF, idiopathic pulmonary fibrosis (IPF), connective tissue disorders, and adult respiratory distress syndrome.

Depending on the cells needed, an array of techniques can be used to isolate specific types of cells from lavage fluids for further characterization. These techniques include the following: adherence to plastic, band-density-gradient centrifugation, and the use of cell-specific antibodies immobilized on the surface of superparamagnetic microspheres (Dynabeads). Dynabeads coated with a specific ligand can be added to a heterogeneous suspension to bind the desired target molecule, forming a complex that is removed from the suspension using a magnet. This technology allows for further subdivision of cell populations (e.g., separation of lymphocytes into B cells and T cells and further categorization of T cells into CD4$^+$ and CD8$^+$ populations). In sarcoidosis, for instance, the lymphocytes in BAL fluid are predominantly CD4$^+$, whereas CD8$^+$ T lymphocytes predominate in hypersensitivity pneumonitis.

Inflammatory cells from BAL fluid can also be evaluated for gene expression at the mRNA or protein level or for the presence of a specific DNA sequence. As gene expression can be altered when cells are removed from the body, it is important that they be processed promptly. When the cells are lysed, released RNases and proteases degrade RNA and proteins, respectively. Cells should be lysed, therefore, in a "protective buffer" appropriate for their intended use. Cells destined for RNA analysis should

be handled in an RNase-free environment and lysed in a buffer containing guanidium thiocyanate, a powerful inactivator of RNases. Cells processed for protein analysis need to be lysed in the presence of antiproteases. An alternative approach is to freeze cells as a pellet to be thawed in a specific buffer, depending on the intended use. The latter approach, however, carries a risk for degradation if samples are accidentally thawed.

It may be important to define changes in gene expression in cells after their removal to an *ex vivo* environment. This can be done by maintaining the isolated cells in culture while the desired studies are performed. For instance, one may ask whether bronchial epithelial cells continue to express high levels of inducible nitric oxide synthase after their removal from the lung.

Evaluation of proteins, cytokines, and other mediators in BAL fluid can yield useful information regarding the inflammatory status of the lung. Results of analysis of BAL fluid are usually expressed relative to the volume of epithelial lining fluid. The latter is estimated by comparing concentrations of urea in samples of lavage fluid and plasma obtained simultaneously.

Brushing Techniques

Brushing of the nose and/or main bronchi is useful to obtain samples of respiratory epithelium. Nasal epithelial cells are obtained from the inferior turbinate under direct visualization using a cytology brush. Bronchial epithelial cells are obtained from the trachea and main bronchi during bronchoscopy using a cytology brush. Samples obtained by brushing can be processed in a fashion similar to that described for lavage cells.

Blood

Genomic DNA, purified from blood cells, can be used to correlate pulmonary findings with genetic information (e.g., polymorphism in a specific gene to be related to airway hyperreactivity). It is often useful to compare levels of a component in sputum or lavage fluid with systemic levels in plasma or serum. In addition, estimation of quantities of epithelial lining fluid requires that levels of urea in BAL fluid be compared with levels of urea simultaneously measured in plasma.

Polymerase Chain Reaction

The polymerase chain reaction (PCR) has revolutionized molecular genetic analysis by allowing the exponential amplification of DNA. PCR can produce an enormous number of copies of a single DNA molecule, enough DNA for most molecular biology procedures. DNA polymerase, the enzyme that normally is responsible for DNA replication, is used to synthesize a complementary strand of DNA with the four nucleotides as substrates and a single DNA strand as a template. Because DNA polymerase is not able to initiate DNA synthesis *de novo,* PCR requires a short piece of complementary polynucleotide that acts as a primer. PCR, therefore, mimics the in vivo process of DNA replication.

The particular sequence of DNA to be amplified is defined by a specific pair of DNA primers. The latter are added, in excess, to a tube that contains a mixture of all four deoxynucleotide precursors, the DNA to be amplified, and DNA polymerase. The mixture is heated to 95°C to denature the template DNA (denaturing step). At this temperature, double-stranded DNA molecules separate, forming single strands that become templates for the production of copies with the primers and DNA polymerase. The temperature is then lowered to allow primers to anneal to the complementary sequences in the DNA molecules (annealing step), generating the primed templates for DNA polymerase. This annealing temperature is a key variable in determining the specificity of the PCR and differs depending on the sequence of the primers. The temperature is then raised to 72°C, the optimal temperature for activity of heat-stable *Taq* DNA polymerase, which was isolated from bacteria that live in thermal springs. The temperature is held at 72°C, allowing DNA synthesis to proceed (extension step). At the end of this period, the temperature is raised again to 95°C, so that double-stranded DNA (the original strand and the newly synthesized complementary strand) separates. These single strands become templates for another round of DNA synthesis, and the cycle of denaturation, annealing of primers, and synthesis of new strands by DNA polymerase is repeated for 20 to 50 cycles. PCR does not require a highly purified DNA as a template and can therefore be performed directly on cell lysates from virtually any source.

"RNA" Polymerase Chain Reaction (Reverse Transcription-Polymerase Chain Reaction)

The adaptation of PCR for the analysis of specific mRNA molecules provided a breakthrough. In this technique, short oligonucleotides are annealed to mRNA to act as primers for reverse transcriptase. This enzyme, isolated from certain RNA viruses, uses RNA as a template to synthesize a complementary DNA (cDNA) strand, which then becomes a template for PCR amplification. The exquisite sensitivity of this simple modification of PCR makes possible the detection and sequence analysis of mRNAs that are extremely rare. Because RNA must be reverse transcribed to cDNA before amplification can take place, this technique has become widely known as *reverse transcription-polymerase chain reaction (RT-PCR).* Given the proclivity of enzymatic amplification

to reveal rare molecules, one must consider whether the amplified products arise from RNA or from contaminating DNA. Whenever possible, PCR primers should be chosen from different exons. Inadvertent amplification of DNA can then be recognized by the size of the products resulting from amplification of the intervening introns. It may be avoided by enzymatic treatment of samples with DNase before RT-PCR. DNA amplification may also be detected by amplification of a control sample without prior reverse transcriptase treatment.

"Hot-Start" Polymerase Chain Reaction

The specificity of PCR can be further enhanced using the "hot-start" technique, which minimizes nonspecific binding of primer to template during preparation of PCR reactions at room temperature. All reagents except one (usually DNA polymerase) are mixed and kept at 70° to 95°C. Just before cycling, the missing component is added to initiate the reaction at the elevated temperature. The method can be automated by interposing a physical barrier of wax between the reaction mixture and the component to be added last. Mixing occurs only at high temperature, when the wax melts. A recent innovation is the use of a neutralizing monoclonal antibody to block DNA polymerase activity during the mixing of PCR components. When the temperature is raised above 70°C during the first PCR cycle, the enzyme-antibody complex dissociates, the antibody is inactivated, and the DNA polymerase becomes active. Typical applications of hot-start PCR include reactions involving complex genomic or cDNA templates, very-low-copy-number targets, "multiplex" PCR (i.e., multiple primer pairs in the same tube), and "long" PCR (see below).

"Touchdown" Polymerase Chain Reaction

"Touchdown" PCR involves gradually decreasing the annealing temperature (e.g., by 1°C every other cycle) to a "touchdown" annealing temperature, which is then used for approximately 10 cycles. The approach takes advantage of the exponential nature of PCR to favor products resulting from correct matches between primers and template rather than incorrect intermediates. In the above example, a difference of 1°C between specific and spurious annealing temperatures will give a twofold difference in favor of the specific product per cycle.

"High-Fidelity" Polymerase Chain Reaction

DNA replication in vivo is extraordinarily accurate. Most bacterial DNA polymerases possess an exonucleolytic activity that scrutinizes DNA synthesis and removes mismatched nucleotides. *Taq* polymerase, however, does not have this "proofreading" capability and incorporates one incorrect nucleotide per approximately every 2×10^4 nucleotides. When an exact sequence is required, such as when PCR is being used for cloning, high-fidelity enzymes with "proofreading" exonuclease activity are required (e.g., *Pfu* polymerase, which has an error rate of one per approximately 2×10^6 nucleotides).

"Long" Polymerase Chain Reaction

This is one of the most important recent advances in PCR technology and is likely to have revolutionary effects on molecular biology. Until recently, it has been difficult to amplify more than 5 kb of DNA, probably because of premature termination of synthesis at sites of mismatched base pairs. Although DNA polymerases with "proofreading" exonuclease activity can remove mismatches and extend the chain, they can not overcome this length limitation, probably because their exonuclease activity eventually degrades the PCR primers. The solution was to use a mixture of *Taq* polymerase and a small amount of polymerase that possesses a "proofreading" exonuclease activity. Evidently, very little exonuclease activity is sufficient for removal of the mismatches, permitting the predominant polymerase activity to complete strand synthesis. The capability of "long" PCR to amplify DNA sequences of up to 42 kb will make it possible for the speed and simplicity of PCR to facilitate and complement many techniques in molecular genetics.

Rapid Amplification of cDNA Ends

Conventional approaches to the characterization and sequencing of mRNA rely on the preparation and screening of a cDNA library. Frequent problems, however, include loss of rare messages during library preparation and failure to produce complete cDNA molecules because of premature termination of reverse transcription. Rapid amplification of cDNA ends (RACE) offers an opportunity to isolate a message of interest directly by amplification of full-length mRNA. Unlike conventional PCR, which requires knowledge of the sequences flanking the region of interest to design PCR primers, an anchored PCR can be performed when only a small amount of sequence information is available (40 to 50 nucleotides). Amplification is carried out between a defined site (known sequence) and unknown sequences at either the 3' or 5' end of the mRNA. 3' RACE takes advantage of the natural poly(A)$^+$ tail present in virtually every mRNA. In this procedure, mRNAs are converted to cDNA using reverse transcriptase with an oligo(dT) adapter primer. Specific cDNA is then directly amplified by PCR using a gene-specific primer that anneals to the region of known sequence and an adapter primer that targets the poly(A) tail region. 5' RACE uses a sequence-specific primer to initi-

ate the synthesis of the cDNA strand. By means of terminal transferase, cDNA is modified by the addition of a poly(A) tail to flank the 5' end. PCR amplification is then carried out with a sequence-specific primer and an oligo(dT) primer complementary to the newly synthesized tail. Reamplification using a second, internal (nested) sequence-specific primer greatly reduces spurious amplification products. It is advisable to monitor PCR products by Southern blot hybridization using a specific oligomer, to confirm that the desired product has been amplified. After amplification, 5' and 3' RACE products can be combined by ligation to produce an intact, full-length cDNA that can be sequenced directly or cloned into an appropriate vector for further analysis.

Limitations of Polymerase Chain Reaction

The great sensitivity of PCR, although a major advantage, is also its major limitation. Because of the enormous amplification attainable by PCR, small amounts of DNA contamination, either from previous PCR amplification, positive control templates, or samples with large amounts of DNA, can result in product formation even in the absence of added template DNA. Aerosol droplets from a pipette tip may contain amplifiable molecules after prior handling of a positive sample. The use of dedicated equipment and pipette tips with hydrophobic filters is recommended to minimize the incidence of false-positives. All reaction mixtures should be prepared in an area separate from that where PCR products are analyzed. Irradiation of PCR solutions with ultraviolet (254 nm) light before adding DNA template "sterilizes" or renders nonamplifiable any contaminant DNA by causing thymine dimers to form. Another approach is to use uridine triphosphate (UTP) instead of deoxythymidine in the PCR reaction mixture and include the enzyme uracil-*N*-glycosylase (UNG). UNG will degrade any DNA from a former PCR because it contains UTP. UNG is then inactivated by the high temperature initiating the new PCR, so that desired products of the amplification can accumulate.

A second limitation that poses a major hurdle to the concept of quantitative PCR stems from the nonlinear nature of the amplification process. Because of the exponential nature of PCR, an early error can be amplified exponentially and in an unpredictable manner, preventing accurate quantitative results. Two approaches can circumvent this problem: (1) During reverse transcription of mRNA, a known quantity of synthetic mRNA, which can be easily differentiated from the endogenous message, is added, and the two cDNAs are amplified simultaneously in the same reaction mixture with the same sets of primers. The amplified unknown is then compared with the amplified standards. (2) During PCR amplification, a known amount of modified cDNA is added to the PCR medium to compete with the target sequence for the same primers. If the competitor were present at the same concentration as the unknown, both DNAs would be amplified to the same extent. By using several different percentages of the competing DNA, the amount of endogenous DNA can be estimated.

Differential Gene Expression

Paramount to understanding the molecular biology of lung disease is a knowledge of genes that are differentially expressed during physiologic and pathologic processes. Differentially expressed genes can be identified by detecting differences in levels of mRNAs in different types of cells or under different conditions in the same cell. This may be important, for example, to an investigator who would like to identify genes involved in the pathogenesis of IPF. After a group of patients fitting the diagnostic criteria and a group of normal subjects to be used as controls have been screened, and with the knowledge that the alveolar macrophage is important in the pathogenesis of this disease, samples may be obtained by BAL from both groups. Differential cDNA library screening, subtracted cDNA libraries, or PCR-based differential display can be used to identify genes expressed differently in alveolar macrophages from the two groups.

Differential Screening

Differential screening allows a gene-by-gene comparison of mRNA populations in the two samples. For this purpose, a cDNA library is prepared using mRNA isolated from the alveolar macrophages of patients with IPF, plated on agar, and transferred to duplicate sets of filters. Filter A is hybridized to a cDNA probe prepared from alveolar macrophage mRNA of normal subjects. Filter B is hybridized to a cDNA probe prepared in a similar fashion from alveolar macrophage mRNA of patients with IPF. Unlike Southern or Northern hybridization, differential screening must be performed under conditions of limiting (rather than excess) probe to detect differences in the concentrations of mRNA from the two populations. cDNA clones (as plaques) that demonstrate different levels of hybridization with the two probes represent mRNAs that are differentially expressed and can be isolated and screened to confirm their differential expression. This method is straightforward and works well for genes that are highly expressed. It is difficult, however, to isolate mRNAs of low abundance, because of variable signal intensity and relatively high background. The use of subtracted libraries and/or subtracted probes improves the chances of cloning rare cDNAs (see below).

Subtractive Hybridization

Subtractive cloning can be used to construct a cDNA library that is enriched in transcripts of genes specifically expressed in cells of patients with IPF. Single-stranded cDNA is synthesized using mRNA from these cells and then hybridized to an excess of biotinylated mRNA from cells of normal subjects. The cDNA sequences representing mRNAs expressed in normal cells will hybridize, whereas those unique to the cells of patients with IPF will remain single-stranded. By adding streptavidin, a protein that binds to biotin, the biotinylated sequences and cDNA hybridized to them can be removed. Nonbiotinylated single-stranded cDNAs from patients with IPF remaining in the solution can then be used to create a subtracted cDNA library enriched in clones that are unique to patients with IPF. This library is then screened using a probe made from RNA of normal subjects. To enhance specificity, a subtracted probe can be used. Subtracted cDNA probes can be prepared using the same principle as for subtracted cDNA libraries. A major problem with subtracted libraries is the very small number of colonies sometimes obtained, in part as a result of the loss of mRNA during the two or more rounds of hybridization that may be needed to remove shared sequences. This can be overcome by using PCR amplification of both the original and the subtracted DNAs. With very limited amounts of starting RNA, multiple rounds of subtraction and amplification may be needed.

Differential Display Reverse Transcription-Polymerase Chain Reaction

Differential display combines the power of PCR amplification and the high resolution of polyacrylamide gel electrophoresis. Each RNA is transcribed to a cDNA by means of a set of four oligo(dT) primers that anneals to the poly(A) tails, each with an anchored two bases at the 3' end, $T_{12}XA$, $T_{12}XC$, $T_{12}XG$ and $T_{12}XT$ (where X is a degenerate mixture of A, G, and C). Each degenerate anchored oligo(dT) primer will, in theory, reverse transcribe one fourth of the total mRNA population. In combination with a set of 5' random 10-mer oligonucleotide primers, which should anneal to arbitrary subsets of mRNA present in the cell, the cDNA population is amplified by PCR. Each of the random 10-mers anneals to a complementary sequence located at a different distance from the 3' terminus, yielding PCR products of different sizes. By varying primer combinations, most of the RNA species in a cell can be represented. PCR reaction products (labeled with a radioactive isotope, such as sulfur 35 or phosphorus 33, or fluorescein) are separated by electrophoresis in a polyacrylamide gel for side-by-side comparison of RNA samples from different cells, allowing recognition of differentially expressed genes. Differential expression is detected by inspection of autoradiograms to identify bands present in only one group, such as patients with IPF. Fluorescent products can be analyzed using an automated DNA sequencer. Although band intensity may correlate with mRNA abundance, the method is not believed to be quantitative.

Further analysis of differentially displayed sequences requires excision of the band from the gel and elution of the DNA, followed by repeated amplification and gel purification. The DNA is then subcloned, so that it can be sequenced and used to make probes for analysis of Northern blots. High-efficiency cloning can be carried out by taking advantage of the single additional A residues at the 3' ends of PCR products; single T residues are added at the 3' ends of a vector to facilitate ligation to the PCR product (TA cloning). The chosen DNA is then directly used as a probe in Northern blot analysis, utilizing the pools of mRNA from the two groups to confirm differential expression and provide information about the molecular weight of the identified transcripts. Once differential expression of a band is confirmed and sequence is known, it should be determined whether the sequence is part of a true open reading frame (i.e., encodes a protein sequence). The identified sequence can be compared with a gene database to determine if it is part of a novel gene and if it bears sequence similarities to other gene families, which may provide clues to function. The same cDNA can then be used to obtain a full-length clone of the novel gene by screening a cDNA library.

Although differential display provides a rather simple and rapid way of identifying differentially expressed genes, several problems are inherent to the technique. Because of its great sensitivity, it can potentially detect a very large number of genes. Screening and confirmation of differential expression of all these could be very time-consuming. Differential amplification, display, and confirmation should therefore be carried out with multiple identical samples before proceeding. Every experiment requires appropriate controls (e.g., samples without reverse transcriptase paired with reverse transcribed PCR samples to detect amplification of products from contaminating DNA not removed by DNase treatment of RNA samples), as well as confirmation of differential expression by Northern analysis before further cloning or sequencing procedures.

Screening for Members of Common Family Genes

The methods considered above illustrate a rather random approach to identifying novel genes. This may not always be the best strategy. When looking for related genes, which presumes prior knowledge of amino acid sequence of the proteins analogous to the one that is sought, degenerate pools of oligonucleotide primers can be designed for PCR amplification, usually performed at a low annealing temperature to permit several possible mismatches. This, however, can result in an enormous number of irrelevant PCR products. If enough sequence is known, it is advisable to screen PCR products by hybridization with a specific probe before further analysis. An alternative approach is to use a degenerate oligonucleotide probe to screen a cDNA library for the desired gene. For instance, a conserved sequence of seven or more contiguous amino acids provides enough information to design a degenerate oligonucleotide probe to select and clone cDNAs encoding related proteins. If the sequence of another conserved region of the desired gene is known, screening can be simplified by using a second probe to evaluate clones positive on initial screening.

Screening for a Specific Protein or Specific Function

If the nucleotide sequence is not known, functional assays or specific antibodies that recognize the desired gene product can be used. This is accomplished by constructing and screening an expression library of cDNAs with an open reading frame that encodes the desired protein fused to a bacterial protein inserted adjacent to bacterial promoters. Fusion proteins may be more stable than native proteins in bacteria and are therefore likely to yield more product. The cDNA library is screened by incubation with an antibody specific for the protein of interest (primary antibody); then, following removal of unbound antibody, a second antibody is added to react with the primary antibody. The second antibody can be labeled with radioactive isotope, coupled to biotin, or conjugated with an enzyme such as alkaline phosphatase; each provides a means to detect the clone expressing the desired protein. The clone is then isolated and the cDNA sequence determined. Similar principles apply in screening with a functional assay (e.g., ADP-ribosyltransferase activity) instead of antibodies.

Identifying a Protein by Western Blotting

Western blotting is a simple, sensitive, and powerful method for immunologic detection of particular proteins of interest in a complex mixture of proteins. This commonly used technique combines the resolving power of gel electrophoresis, the specificity of antibodies, and the sensitivity of enzyme assays. Proteins are first denatured in the presence of sodium dodecyl sulfate and separated according to molecular weight by polyacrylamide gel electrophoresis. Then, an electric field is applied to drive the separated protein molecules out of the gel and onto a paper-thin nitrocellulose membrane or its equivalent, where they are immobilized. In the second step, the specific protein of interest is identified by soaking the membrane in a solution containing an antibody (primary antibody) specific for that protein (antigen). Then, the antibody bound to the antigen is reacted with a second antibody, which is covalently linked to alkaline phosphatase or horseradish peroxidase. After washing the membrane, the enzyme linked to the second antibody is detected by reaction with a chromogenic substrate to yield a visible product or with a substrate that yields a luminescent product,, which can be detected by autoradiography. Alternatively, the antigen-antibody complex can be detected using protein A labeled with iodine 125, which binds to the antibody.

RECENT ADVANCES IN PULMONARY RESEARCH

Polymerase Chain Reaction in the Diagnosis of Pulmonary Infections

Standard diagnostic procedures for pulmonary infections are based on the ability to grow organisms in culture or to detect their presence in serum using antibodies. These tests can be relatively insensitive and time-consuming. Because of its high sensitivity, PCR may facilitate the early diagnosis of many infectious diseases.

Mycobacterium tuberculosis *Infection*

The diagnosis of *M. tuberculosis* infection requires growth of organisms in culture, a procedure that takes several weeks. More rapid diagnosis of pulmonary tuberculosis can be made by detection of acid-fast organisms in sputum smears. The results of smears are positive, however, in only 50%–75% of cases. Prompt and sensitive diagnosis by PCR is feasible using specific primers for a sequence within a gene that is highly conserved in all mycobacterial species. The amplified fragment is then hybridized with species-specific oligonucleotide probes to identify the specific strain. As few as 10 bacilli in 10^6 cells can be detected by PCR, which has also been used to identify *M. tuberculosis* in blood samples. With the inherent potential for false-positives owing to its great sensitivity, positive PCR results must be interpreted in conjunction with clinical information. In contrast, a negative PCR result rules out the diagnosis. Although at present PCR has not totally replaced established procedures for the diagnosis of *M. tuberculosis* infection, it may be particularly useful in certain categories of patients. In a patient with negative smear results and positive culture results, PCR could provide an early diagnosis on which to base initial therapy. In addition, by the amplification of bacterial DNA sequences that contain mutations associated with antibiotic resistance, PCR may play an important role in the rapid identification of multidrug-resistant strains of *M. tuberculosis*. PCR may be used to diagnose primary tuberculosis in children, which is sometimes difficult to diagnose by conventional means. The results of direct examination of sputum or gastric aspirates are usually negative, and the results of culture are positive in only 20% of cases. Tuberculin skin tests are difficult to interpret in children who are immunosup-

pressed or have received Calmette-Guérin vaccination. *M. tuberculosis* has been detected by PCR in gastric aspirates from many children with primary tuberculosis and cultures negative for bacteria.

Cytomegalovirus Pneumonitis

The diagnosis of cytomegalovirus (CMV) pneumonitis in immunocompromised patients may be difficult, because of its clinical similarity to diffuse lung injury of other causes. Immunofluorescent staining of alveolar macrophages and epithelial cells for CMV antigens with specific monoclonal antibodies has been used, in combination with clinical findings, to make the diagnosis. PCR provides a very sensitive assay for the detection of CMV in bronchoalveolar lavage fluid. For rapid diagnosis of CMV infection, the combination of PCR and immunofluorescence is an optimal strategy that provides almost 100% sensitivity and specificity. PCR is also useful as a rapid assay to exclude the diagnosis of CMV pneumonitis. In addition, detection of CMV in blood by PCR has been used to predict in which patients CMV pneumonitis is likely to develop or, after completion of initial therapy, which patients are likely to relapse.

Pneumocystis carinii *Pneumonia*

PCR is a highly sensitive technique for the identification of *P. carinii* in BAL fluid or induced sputum; it detects the gene that encodes the mitochondrial rRNA of *P. carinii*. Diagnostic PCR is more sensitive for detecting *P. carinii* than are traditional silver staining and immunofluorescent procedures. The specificity of PCR detection can be enhanced by hybridizing PCR products to specific oligonucleotide probes on Southern blots. Detection by PCR of *P. carinii* in serum has been proposed as a simple test for the diagnosis of disseminated pneumocystosis.

Other Pulmonary Infections

Candida albicans, Mycoplasma pneumoniae, Bordetella pertussis, Aspergillus fumigatus, Legionella pneumophila, respiratory syncytial virus, and influenza virus are examples of other organisms that have been identified using PCR.

Latent Infections

In several studies, the results of PCR in diagnosis of *Mycoplasma* infections were discordant with serologic findings, consistent with the observation that *Mycoplasma* can persist in tissues long after clinical disease has resolved. Although PCR can be useful for detection of persisting sequences of an infectious agent, the clinical interpretation of the finding depends on establishing whether it represents continuing or latent infection. There are situations, however, in which the mere presence of the sequences in a host may have important clinical implications, as in the case of gene therapy protocols utilizing adenovirus (AV) vectors in the lung. In this approach, the normal gene is directly delivered to the respiratory epithelium using AV vectors that have been rendered replication-defective by deletion of a region, E1a, that is critical for viral replication. There is the possibility, however, of a replication-defective AV vector replicating as a result of recombination or complementation with viral E1a sequences present in the host cells from prior infections. Using specific primers to amplify E1a by PCR and evaluating PCR products with a probe specific for that region, it is possible to identify individuals who harbor that viral sequence in their cells. Special precautions in these individuals may be warranted, such as frequent monitoring for evidence of viral replication.

Gene Therapy

Gene therapy is a medical intervention designed to alter the genetic program of cells with therapeutic intent. The goal is to modify specific cells to express, temporarily or permanently, a specific set of new genetic information in a fashion that will be beneficial in the treatment of hereditary or acquired disease. There are two basic strategies of gene therapy. First, cells may be genetically modified ex vivo for subsequent implantation in the host target tissue or organ. This can be carried out using either autologous cells derived from the intended recipient of the therapy or cells from other individuals or species. Alternatively, cells may be modified in vivo. Viral or nonviral vectors can be used for gene therapy (Table 1).

Vectors

Retrovirus (RV) is an RNA virus that enters the cell through specific viral receptors on the cell surface. Once inside the cell, RNA is converted to DNA by the reverse transcriptase activity of the virus itself. The double-stranded DNA provirus is then randomly integrated into the host genome, if the cell is actively dividing. In most RV vectors, the *gag, pol,* and *env* genes are replaced with the gene of interest, so that vectors are capable of entering cells and inserting the new genes into the genomes but cannot direct cells to produce infectious RVs. Theoretically, the newly integrated exogenous gene will be passed on to progeny of the cell when it divides. RV is, thus far, the most widely used vector in gene transfer protocols approved by the Recombinant DNA Advisory Committee (RAC) of the National Institutes of Health. A major disadvantage of RV as a vector for use in vivo, however, is that it cannot be used to express genes in nondividing cells.

The AV vector is more efficient than RV for in vivo gene therapy. AV is a double-stranded DNA virus that provides several major advantages. Replication of host cells is not required for expression of a gene transferred by AV, and there is no known association of human malignancies with AV infection despite its high incidence. In most AV vectors currently used, the E1 region, which is important for viral replication, is deleted. Disadvantages of the AV vector are that (1) many AV genes included in the presently used vectors induce an immune reaction, and (2) gene expression is not stable, as the vector does not integrate into the host genome.

Adeno-associated virus (AAV) is a 4.7-kb, single-stranded DNA virus of the parvovirus family. The AAV genome consists of two genes, *rep* and *cap,* flanked by inverted terminal repeats that serve as signals for origin

TABLE 1. *Methods of gene transfer to mammalian cells*

Method	Applicability		Integration
	In vivo	Ex vivo	
Viral			
Retrovirus	+	+++	yes
Adenovirus	+++	+	no
Adeno-associated virus	+++	++	yes
Herpes virus	+++	+	no
Other viruses (e.g., vaccinia)	+++	+	no
Nonviral			
Naked plasmid	+++	+	no
Liposome-plasmid complex	+++	+	no
Ligand-plasmid complex	+++	+	no
Particle bombardment	++	++	?
Combination system			
Co-internalization	+++	+	no

+++, High applicability; ++, medium applicability; +, low applicability; ?, integration results not definitive.

of DNA replication and packaging. AAV is nonpathogenic and appears not to alter the clinical course of AV infection. AAV cannot naturally replicate and requires coinfection with AV or herpesvirus, which provide helper functions. AAV has the ability to integrate into the DNA of nondividing cells. In the absence of helper virus, AAV infection results in high-frequency, stable DNA integration, usually into a specific site on human chromosome 19 at q13.4. In AAV vectors, the *rep* and *env* genes are usually deleted and replaced with the gene of interest to minimize the possibility of inducing immunity by the expression of viral genes. AAV can be produced to titers of $>10^{10}$ plaque-forming units (pfu) per milliliter. All these features make AAV vectors attractive for human gene therapy. Their disadvantages, however, include the inability to accommodate large genes (packaging limit of 4.5 kb) and the potential risk for contamination by helper viruses, as production of AAV vector requires coinfection with AV or herpesvirus.

Liposomes

Liposome-plasmid complexes are the most frequently used nonviral vectors for human gene therapy. Liposomes are lipid model membranes that can form a complex with DNA and facilitate its transfer into cells, probably through nonspecific fusion of the liposome-plasmid complex with cell membranes.

Gene Transfer Protocols

To date, >100 human gene transfer protocols have been approved by RAC. Of these, 18 are aimed at treating individuals with lung diseases: 13 for CF, one for α_1-antitrypsin deficiency, and four for primary lung cancer (Table 2).

For CF, AV vectors are used in nine protocols, AAV vectors in two, and liposome-plasmid complexes in two. In five protocols, vectors are delivered to both nasal epithelium and lung respiratory epithelium, in two to respiratory epithelium only, and in six to nasal and/or maxillary sinus epithelium. In twelve protocols, the vector is instilled in the lung via bronchoscopy or delivered to the nasal and/or maxillary sinus epithelium through a rhinoscope or catheter under direct visualization. In one protocol, the AV vector is administered by aerosol to the lung.

It has been observed that about 30% of adenocarcinomas of the lung have a mutated K-*ras* oncogene, and 50% of non–small-cell lung cancers have mutations or deletions of the p53 tumor-suppressor gene. In two protocols for lung cancer, an RV or AV vector containing wild-type p53 cDNA (for tumors with mutated or deleted p53) or antisense K-*ras* (for tumors with mutated K-*ras*) is injected into a residual endobronchial lesion of non–small-cell lung cancer. Immunotherapy was proposed in two other protocols. In one protocol, intradermal injection of recombinant carcinoembryonic antigen (CEA) vaccinia virus is followed by subcutaneous injection of CEA peptide to induce a host immune response. In the other, autologous tumor cells, irradiated to prevent proliferation, are transduced ex vivo with a liposome-plasmid complex containing an interleukin-2 cDNA and then injected subcutaneously.

Of protocols for gene therapy of human lung diseases, data from four studies of patients with CF have been reported in detail. An AV vector was used in three and a liposome-plasmid complex in one. In all studies, suc-

TABLE 2. *Summary of approved protocols for gene therapy of human lung diseases*[a]

Disease	Gene	Vector	Tissue transduced	Number[b]
Hereditary				
Cystic fibrosis	CFTR	Adenovirus	Nasal and respiratory epithelium	4
	CFTR	Adenovirus	Nasal epithelium and/or maxillary sinus	3
	CFTR	Adenovirus	Respiratory epithelium	2
	CFTR	Adeno-associated virus	Nasal and respiratory epithelium	1
	CFTR	Adeno-associated virus	Maxillary sinus	1
	CFTR	Liposome-plasmid complex	Nasal epithelium	2
α_1-Antitrypsin deficiency	α_1-AT	Liposome-plasmid complex	Nasal and respiratory epithelium	1
Lung cancer				
Non–small-cell lung cancer	p53 K-*ras* (AS)	Retrovirus	Tumor	1
	p53	Adenovirus	Tumor	1
Small-cell lung cancer	IL-2	Liposome-plasmid complex	Skin	1
Adenocarcinoma	CEA	Vaccinia virus	Skin	1

CFTR, cystic fibrosis transmembrane conductance regulator; α_1-AT, α_1-antitrypsin; p53, p53 tumor suppressor gene; K-*ras* (AS), antisense sequence of K-*ras* oncogene; IL-2, interleukin-2; CEA, carcinoembryonic antigen.
[a] Only protocols approved by the Recombinant DNA Advisory Committee (RAC) of the National Institutes of Health by December 1995 are included.
[b] Number of protocols approved.

cessful gene transfer to a small fraction (<1%–14%) of nasal or respiratory epithelial cells was demonstrated, and CFTR protein or mRNA was detected for at least 9 days. In three studies, two with AV vectors and one with a liposome-plasmid complex, partial correction of abnormalities of potential difference across nasal epithelium was noted. One controlled study using an AV vector, however, failed to demonstrate correction of functional defects in nasal epithelium. In one study, the AV vector caused the level of interleukin-6 in serum to increase, and pneumonia developed in one person who received 2 x 10^9 pfu of AV vector into a large airway. Parameters of pulmonary function and chest roentgenographic and computed tomographic findings in this patient returned to baseline after 1 month.

Although the technologies are still far from ideal, data relevant to human gene therapy are encouraging; after further refinement, it seems likely that gene therapy will become an increasingly useful therapeutic option.

Transgenic Mouse Model

Transgenic mice have recently been used as models for the study of many human diseases, not only because mice are relatively closely related to the human species but also because their genetic manipulation and propagation are relatively rapid.

Transgenic mice are produced by the permanent alteration of a small part of the genome, which is achieved by at least two different strategies. In the first, a cloned DNA construct is delivered into the male pronucleus of the newly fertilized mouse egg by microinjection. The introduced foreign DNA randomly integrates into the mouse genome, without preference for a particular chromosomal location, and the injected eggs are implanted into a foster mother. Of the 10%–30% of those that develop to term, up to 40% may contain integrated foreign DNA. They are heterozygous and can be bred to homozygosity. Mice that carry the foreign gene are termed *transgenic,* and the integrated DNA is the transgene. Because the foreign DNA is randomly integrated into the mouse genome, there are several potential problems, such as insertion of the transgene into an essential gene or differential expression of the transgene resulting from differences in sites of integration or differences in the number of gene copies introduced.

In contrast to random integration of transgenes, the second strategy modifies a selected gene at a precise location within the genome of a mouse embryonic stem (ES) cell by homologous recombination. Mouse ES cells are derived from the inner cell mass, which corresponds to the future embryo, of a mouse blastocyst. Under suitable culture conditions, the ES cells can proliferate in vitro, remain undifferentiated, and be subcultured repeatedly. Usually, ES cells are grown on a monolayer of fibroblasts

that have been treated so that they cannot divide. A cloned DNA construct is then delivered into the ES cells by electroporation. The foreign DNA becomes integrated into the homologous gene locus of the mouse genome by homologous recombination and disrupts or mutates the endogenous gene. ES cells with integrated foreign DNA can be identified by PCR and/or Southern analysis. They can be positively and/or negatively selected, taking advantage of properties of specific, simultaneously introduced genes. Recombinant ES cells are then microinjected into blastocysts derived from mice with a coat color different from that of the donor of ES cells and implanted in a foster mother. From the coat color of the chimeric offspring, the contribution of recombinant ES cells can be easily evaluated.

Examples of transgenic mouse models for human pulmonary diseases are described below.

Idiopathic Pulmonary Fibrosis

Tumor necrosis factor-α (TNF-α) produces both fibrogenic and inflammatory effects. Expresssion of TNF-α mRNA and protein is increased in type II pneumocytes of individuals with IPF. Surfactant protein C (SP-C) is synthesized and secreted by type II pneumocytes. By microinjecting a construct containing a mouse TNF-α gene, including the entire 3' untranslated region directed by a 3.7-kb fragment of the 5'-flanking region of the human SP-C gene (SP-C/TNF-α), into the male pronucleus of mouse fertilized eggs, Miyazaki et al. generated transgenic mice with elevated expression of TNF-α in alveolar epithelium, mainly in type II pneumocytes. Five of thirteen founder mice died at birth or after 1 month with severe lung lesions. Surviving mice transmitted a pulmonary disease to their offspring, the severity of which was correlated with levels of TNF-α mRNA in the lung. At 1 to 2 months of age, leukocytic alveolitis, with a predominance of T lymphocytes, was extensive within the interlobular septa, beneath the pleurae, and around extra-alveolar small vessels. The extent of fibrosis was minimal at this stage. However, at 6 months of age, the alveolar septa were markedly thickened, resulting in large part from the accumulation of desmin-containing fibroblasts. Alveolar spaces were enlarged and contained desquamated epithelial cells. Alveolar surfaces were lined by hyperplastic type II pneumocytes. Increased levels of vascular cell adhesion molecule-1 (VCAM-1) mRNA, enlargement of the endothelial cytoplasm, and increased platelet trapping in alveolar capillaries were also observed. In general, the numerous pulmonary lesions in the SP-C/TNF-α mice were very similar to those in individuals with IPF.

Transgenic mice in which human transforming growth factor-α (hTGF-α) was expressed under the control of a 3.7-kb fragment of the 5'-flanking region of the human

SP-C gene also exhibited pulmonary fibrosis. The fibrosis was prominent in subpleural, peribronchiolar, peribronchial, and perihilar regions. There was, however, no apparent fibrosis or thickening of the alveolar interstitium. The severity of fibrosis differed with the founder line and the abundance of transgene product in the lungs. In addition, greater than normal mitotic activity and numbers of epidermal growth factor (EGF) receptors in the interstitial cells of the fibrotic lesions were observed. These findings support the hypothesis that hTGF-α produced by respiratory epithelial cells stimulates the growth of mesenchymal components of the lung.

These kinds of transgenic mice provide valuable models for evaluating the molecular mechanisms that contribute to the pathogenesis of pulmonary fibrosis and for testing therapeutic strategies in vivo.

Pulmonary Alveolar Proteinosis

Granulocyte-macrophage colony-stimulating factor (GM-CSF), a 23-kd (kilodalton) glycoprotein, stimulates the proliferation of hematopoietic progenitor cells, as well as their differentiation to monocytes/macrophages, neutrophils, and eosinophils. To delineate the *in vivo* function of GM-CSF, Dranoff et al. generated mice carrying a null allele of the GM-CSF gene by homologous recombination in embryonic stem cells. Unexpectedly, the homozygous transgenic mice had normal numbers of peripheral bloods cells, bone marrow progenitors, and tissue hematopoietic populations, including splenic dendritic cells. However, in all homozygous mutant mice, but not in heterozygous or wild-type mice, a progressive accumulation of surfactant lipids and proteins developed in the alveolar space, characteristic of human pulmonary alveolar proteinosis. In mutant mice, levels of surfactant proteins SP-A, SP-B, and SP-C were markedly increased in BAL fluid, although the abundance of surfactant mRNA was indistinguishable from that in wild-type mice. Moreover, the alveolar macrophages of mice deficient in GM-CSF were filled with surfactant protein and lipid, although no accumulation of SP-A was observed in type II pneumocytes. It appeared that alveolar macrophages were defective in processing pulmonary surfactants, as a result of the absence of GM-CSF in the mutant mice, leading to pulmonary alveolar proteinosis. In addition, extensive pulmonary lymphoid hyperplasia surrounding the airways and veins, developed in mutant mice, which could have been the result of an excessive response to otherwise innocuous inhaled antigens.

ACKNOWLEDGMENT

We thank Dr. Martha Vaughan and Dr. Vincent C. Manganiello for critical reviews of the manuscript.

BIBLIOGRAPHY

Alberts B, Bray D, Lewis J, Raff M, Roberts K, Watson JD. *Molecular Biology of the Cell.* 3rd ed. New York: Garland Publishing; 1994. *A popular comprehensive textbook of molecular and cellular biology.*

Ausubel FM, Brent R, Kingston RE, Moore DD, Seidman JG, Smith JA, Struhl K. *Current Protocols in Molecular Biology.* New York: John Wiley; 1996. *A continuously evolving manual of state-of-the-art technical protocols in molecular biology, with new protocols added as quarterly supplements.*

Barnes WM. PCR amplification of up to 35-kb DNA with high fidelity and high yield from λ bacteriophage templates. *Proc Natl Acad Sci U S A* 1994;91:2216–2220. *Critical evaluation of amplification of long targets by PCR.*

Bronson SK, Smithies O. Altering mice by homologous recombination using embryonic stem cells. *J Biol Chem* 1994;269:27155–27158. *Concise review of techniques to generate transgenic mice with modification at a precise locus in the genome, using homologous recombination in mouse embryonic stem cells.*

Caplen NJ, Alton EWFW, Middleton PG, Dorin JR, Stevenson BJ, Gao X, Durham SR, Jeffery PK, Hodson ME, Coutelle C, Huang L, Porteous DJ, Williamson R, Geddes DM. Liposome-mediated CFTR gene transfer to the nasal epithelium of patients with cystic fibrosis. *Nat Med* 1995;1:39–46. *Double-blind, placebo-controlled study, in which the ion transport abnormality in nasal epithelia of some individuals with cystic fibrosis was transiently, partially corrected by liposome-mediated CFTR gene transfer.*

Cathomas G, Morris P, Pekle K, Cunningham I, Emanuel D. Rapid diagnosis of cytomegalovirus pneumonia in marrow transplant recipients by bronchoalveolar lavage using the polymerase chain reaction, virus culture, and the direct immunostaining of alveolar cells. *Blood* 1993;81:1909–1914. *Comparison of PCR, viral culture, and immunostaining of alveolar cells used alone and in combination as diagnostic methods.*

Chu CS, Trapnell BC, Curristin SM, Cutting GR, Crystal RG. Extensive post-transcriptional deletion of the coding sequences for part of nucleotide-binding fold 1 in respiratory epithelial mRNA transcripts of the cystic fibrosis transmembrane conductance regulator gene is not associated with the clinical manifestations of cystic fibrosis. *J Clin Invest* 1992;90:785–790. *Description of four individuals with a normal cystic fibrosis phenotype although 73%–92% of cystic fibrosis transmembrane conductance regulator (CFTR) mRNA in bronchial epithelial cells lacks exon 9.*

Chu CS, Trapnell BC, Curristin SM, Cutting GR, Crystal RG. Genetic basis for variable exon 9 skipping in cystic fibrosis transmembrane conductance regulator mRNA. *Nat Genet* 1993;3:151–156. *First demonstration ex vivo of an inverse relationship between the length of the polythymidine tract at the 3' splice site of a human gene and the relative amount of mRNA transcripts lacking the exon following the polythymidine tract.*

Crystal RG. Transfer of genes to humans: early lessons and obstacles to success. *Science* 1995;270:404–410. *Excellent review of the clinical status of human gene therapy, including hurdles still to be overcome before gene therapy can become an established therapeutic intervention, by a scientist who pioneered adenovirus-mediated human gene therapy.*

Crystal RG, McElvaney NG, Rosenfeld MA, Chu C-S, Mastrangeli A, Hay JG, Brody SL, Jaffe HA, Eissa NT, Danel C. Administration of an adenovirus containing the human CFTR cDNA to the respiratory tract of individuals with cystic fibrosis. *Nat Genet* 1994;8:42–51. *First report of adenovirus-mediated gene transfer to the lungs of individuals with cystic fibrosis, with successful transfer and expression of CFTR cDNA and development of transient systemic and pulmonary signs and symptoms, including headache, fever, hypotension, and pulmonary infiltrates, by recipient of the highest dose of recombinant adenovirus vector.*

D'Aquila RT, Bechtel LJ, Videler JA, Eron JJ, Gorczyca P, Kaplan JC. Maximizing sensitivity and specificity of PCR by pre-amplification heating. *Nucleic Acids Res* 1991;19:3749. *Description of "hot-start" PCR.*

Don RH, Cox PT, Wainwright BJ, Baker K, Mattick JS. "Touchdown" PCR to circumvent spurious priming during gene amplification. *Nucleic Acids Res* 1991;19:4008. *Description of the "touchdown" method.*

Dranoff G, Crawford AD, Sadelain M, Ream B, Rashid A, Bronson RT, Dickersin GR, Bachurski CJ, Mark EL, Whitsett JA, Mulligan RC. Involvement of granulocyte-macrophage colony-stimulating factor in pulmonary homeostasis. *Science* 1994;264:713–716. *Description of homozygous mutant mice carrying null alleles of the GM-CSF gene with unexpected characteristics of human idiopathic pulmonary alveolar proteinosis.*

Eissa NT, Chu C-S, Danel C, Crystal RG. Evaluation of normals and individuals with cystic fibrosis for the presence of adenovirus E1a sequences relevant to the use of E1a⁻ adenovirus vectors for gene therapy for the respiratory manifestations of cystic fibrosis. *Hum Gene Ther* 1994;5:1105–1114. *Comprehensive evaluation of the presence of adenovirus sequences in respiratory epithelial cells, inflammatory cells of BAL fluid, and blood cells. Comparison of conventional methods for virus detection by culture and antibody assays, and implications for gene therapy protocols.*

Eriksson B-M, Brytting M, Zweygberg-Wirgart B, Hillerdal G, Olding-Stenkvist E, Linde A. Diagnosis of cytomegalovirus in bronchoalveolar lavage by polymerase chain reaction, in comparison with virus isolation and detection of viral antigen. *Scand J Infect Dis* 1993;25:421–427. *Examination of BAL products from 52 immunocompromised patients with symptoms of pulmonary infection for CMV by virus isolation, PCR, and immunofluorescent staining.*

Fahy JV, Liu J, Wong H, Boushey HA. Analysis of cellular and biochemical constituents of induced sputum after allergen challenge: a method for studying allergic airway inflammation. *J Allergy Clin Immunol* 1994;93:1031–1039. *Analysis of inflammatory cells and markers in induced sputum after aerosolized allergen challenge.*

Glasser SW, Korfhagen TR, Wert SE, Whitsett JA. Transgenic models for study of pulmonary development and disease. *Am J Physiol* 1994;267:L489–L497. *Review of application of transgenic mouse technology to study of lung development and diseases, such as analysis of cis-acting elements controlling lung epithelial cell gene expression and models of cystic fibrosis and pulmonary adenocarcinoma.*

Harlow E, Lane D. *Antibodies—a Laboratory Manual.* Cold Spring Harbor, NY: Cold Spring Harbor Laboratory Press; 1988. *Useful laboratory manual providing a practical guide to most immunochemical methods.*

Hubbard RC, McElvaney NG, Birrer P, Shak S, Robinson WW, Jolley C, Wu M, Chernick MS, Crystal RG. A preliminary study of aerosolized recombinant human deoxyribonuclease I in the treatment of cystic fibrosis. *N Engl J Med* 1992;326:812–815. *The first human clinical trial to demonstrate that rhDNase acts in vivo to cleave high-molecular-weight DNA in purulent lung secretions and improves lung function in patients with cystic fibrosis.*

Innis MA, Gelfand DH, Sninsky JJ, White TJ, eds. *PCR Protocols: a Guide to Methods and Applications.* New York: Academic Press; 1990. *A technical manual for various PCR applications.*

Kai M, Kamiya S, Yabe H, Takakura I, Shiozawa K, Ozawa A. Rapid detection of *Mycoplasma pneumoniae* in clinical samples by the polymerase chain reaction. *J Med Microbiol* 1993;38:166–170. *PCR amplification of 16S ribosomal RNA gene sequences used to detect M. pneumoniae in throat swab samples.*

Knowles MR, Hohneker KW, Zhou Z, Olsen JC, Noah TL, Hu P-C, Leigh MW, Engelhardt JF, Edwards LJ, Jones KR, Grossman M, Wilson JM, Johnson LG, Boucher RC. A controlled study of adenoviral vector-mediated gene transfer in the nasal epithelium of patients with cystic fibrosis. *N Engl J Med* 1995;333:823–831. *Randomized, double-blind, vehicle-controlled study of adenoviral vector-mediated CFTR gene transfer, with no correction of functional defects in nasal epithelia of individuals with cystic fibrosis, and development of mucosal inflammation in two of three patients who received the highest dose of vector.*

Korfhagen TR, Swantz RJ, Wert SE, McCarty JM, Kerlakian CB, Glasser SW, Whitsett JA. Respiratory epithelial cell expression of human transforming growth factor-α induces lung fibrosis in transgenic mice. *J Clin Invest* 1994;93:1691–1699. *Report of the development of fibrotic lesions in the peribronchial, peribronchiolar, perivascular, and juxtapleural regions of transgenic mice expressing hTGF-α under the control of the human SP-C promoter.*

Lewis B. *Genes V.* Oxford: Oxford University Press; 1994. *A popular book providing an integrated introduction to the structure and function of genes in both prokaryotic and eukaryotic cells.*

Lipschik GY, Gill VJ, Lundgren JD, Andrawis VA, Nelson NA, Nielsen JO, Ognibene FP, Kovacs JA. Improved diagnosis of *Pneumocystis carinii* infection by polymerase chain reaction on induced sputum and blood. *Lancet* 1992;340:203–206. *Comparison of the sensitivity and specificity of two PCR methods with those of conventional staining for detection of P. carinii in induced sputum, BAL fluid, and blood.*

Lodish H, Baltimore D, Berk A, Zipursky SL, Matsudaira P, Darnell J. *Molecular Cell Biology.* 3rd ed. New York: Scientific American Books; 1995. *An excellent comprehensive textbook of molecular and cellular biology.*

Lundberg KS, Shoemaker DD, Adams MW, Short JM, Sorge JA, Mathur EJ. High-fidelity amplification using a thermostable DNA polymerase isolated from *Pyrococcus furiosus. Gene* 1991;108:1–6. *Error rates for Pfu DNA polymerase compared with those of Taq polymerase.*

Ma TS. Applications and limitations of polymerase chain reaction amplification. *Chest* 1995;108:1393–1404. *Discussion of the theory, application, and limitations of PCR technology in basic research and clinical medicine.*

Maser RL, Calvet JP. Analysis of differential gene expression in the kidney by differential cDNA screening, subtractive cloning, and mRNA differential display. *Semin Nephrol* 1995;15:29–42. *A summary of some current approaches to identifying and analyzing differentially expressed genes, with emphasis on cDNA library construction and differential screening.*

Miyazaki Y, Araki K, Vesin C, Garcia I, Kapanci Y, Whitsett JA, Piguet P-F, Vassalli P. Expression of a tumor necrosis factor-α transgene in murine lung causes lymphocytic and fibrosing alveolitis. *J Clin Invest* 1995;96:250–259. *Description of a transgenic mouse model of human idiopathic pulmonary fibrosis generated by inserting the TNF-α gene, controlled by the human surfactant protein C promoter, into the mouse genome.*

Mulligan RC. The basic science of gene therapy. *Science* 1993;260:926–932. *Concise review of methods of gene transfer and preclinical models of gene therapy.*

Mullis KB. The unusual origin of the polymerase chain reaction. *Sci Am* 1990;262:56–65. *A historical perspective of the subject.*

Paton AW, Paton JC, Lawrence AJ, Goldwater PN, Harris RJ. Rapid detection of respiratory syncytial virus in nasopharyngeal aspirates by reverse transcription and polymerase chain reaction amplification. *J Clin Microbiol* 1992;30:901–904. *A rapid method for detection of respiratory syncytial virus in nasopharyngeal aspirates involving a combination of reverse transcription and PCR amplification.*

Pierre C, Olivier C, Lecossier D, Boussougant Y, Yeni P, Hance AJ. Diagnosis of primary tuberculosis in children by amplification and detection of mycobacterial DNA. *Am Rev Respir Dis* 1993;147:420–424. *Comparison of standard microbiologic techniques with a rapid diagnostic method based on amplification by PCR.*

Plikaytis BB, Marden JL, Crawford JT, Woodley CL, Butler WR, Shinnick TM. Multiplex PCR assay specific for the multidrug-resistant strain W of *Mycobacterium tuberculosis. J Clin Microbiol* 1994;32:1542–1546. *Identification of 48 samples of multidrug-resistant strains among 193 isolates of M. tuberculosis using multiplex PCR.*

Rennard SI, Basset G, Lecossier D, O Donnell KM, Pinkston P, Martin PG, Crystal RG. Estimation of volume of epithelial lining fluid recovered by lavage using urea as marker of dilution. *J Appl Physiol* 1986;60:532–538. *Description of a method of estimating the volume of epithelial lining fluid by comparing urea concentrations in samples of lavage fluid and plasma obtained simultaneously; comparison with other techniques.*

Rosenthal N. DNA and the genetic code. *N Engl J Med* 1994;331:39–41. *Concise review of DNA structure and the genetic code.*

Rosenthal N. Regulation of gene expression. *N Engl J Med* 1994;331:931–933. *Concise review of gene expression, including the steps of transcription and pre-mRNA processing.*

Saltini C, Hance AJ, Ferrans VJ, Basset F, Bitterman PB, Crystal RG. Accurate quantification of cells recovered by bronchoalveolar lavage. *Am Rev Respir Dis* 1984;130:650–658. *Description of methods for assessing the types and numbers of cells recovered by BAL, based on >2000 lavage procedures.*

Sambrook J, Fritsch EF, Maniatis T. *Molecular Cloning—a Laboratory Manual.* 2nd ed. Cold Spring Harbor, NY: Cold Spring Harbor Laboratory Press; 1989. *A popular, useful, and comprehensive manual that is a practical guide to most procedures used in a molecular biology laboratory.*

Schaefer BC. Revolutions in rapid amplification of cDNA ends: new strategies for polymerase chain reaction cloning of full-length cDNA ends. *Anal Biochem* 1995;227:255–273. *A comprehensive review that focuses on the application of PCR to cloning unknown flanking cDNA sequences 5' or 3' to a known sequence.*

Schluger NW, Condos R, Lewis S, Rom WN. Amplification of DNA of *Mycobacterium tuberculosis* from peripheral blood of patients with pulmonary tuberculosis. *Lancet* 1994;344:232–233. *Identification by PCR of* M. tuberculosis *DNA in the lymphocyte fraction of peripheral blood in patients with positive sputum cultures indicating active pulmonary tuberculosis.*

Schluger NW, Kinney D, Harkin TJ, Rom WN. Clinical utility of the polymerase chain reaction in the diagnosis of infections due to *Mycobacterium tuberculosis*. *Chest* 1994;105:1116–1121. *Comparison of diagnostic results obtained by PCR with those obtained by acid-fast bacilli smears, culture, pathology, and clinical histories.*

Schluger NW, Rom WN. The polymerase chain reaction in the diagnosis and evaluation of pulmonary infections. *Am J Respir Crit Care Med* 1995;152:11–16. *Review of the application of PCR to the diagnosis and evaluation of respiratory infections, including a comparison with conventional diagnostic techniques.*

Schoonbrood DFM, Lutter R, Habets FJM, Roos CM, Jansen HM, Out TA. Analysis of plasma protein leakage and local secretion in sputum from patients with asthma and chronic obstructive pulmonary disease. *Am J Respir Crit Care Med* 1994;150:1519–1527. *Assessment of the usefulness of sputum analysis in studying plasma protein exudation and local secretion of proteins in the airways; methodology for measurements of specific proteins in soluble and gel phases of sputum.*

Sharp PA. Split genes and RNA splicing. *Cell* 1994;77:805–815. *Excellent review of RNA splicing, adapted from a Nobel Prize lecture.*

Sunday ME. Differential display RT-PCR for identifying novel gene expression in the lung. *Am J Physiol* 1995;269:L273–L284. *A description of the basic concepts, specific methodologies, caveats, and potential applications of PCR-mediated differential display for identifying genes differentially expressed in lung cells.*

Tang CM, Holden DW, Aufauvre-Brown A, Cohen J. The detection of *Aspergillus* spp by the polymerase chain reaction and its evaluation in bronchoalveolar lavage fluid. *Am Rev Respir Dis* 1993;148:1313–1317. *PCR amplification of fragments of genes encoding alkaline proteases from* Aspergillus fumigatus *and* A. flavus *in BAL specimens, with a discussion of active infection versus colonization.*

Watson JD, Gilman M, Witkowski J, Zoller M. *Recombinant DNA.* 2nd ed. New York: Scientific American Books; 1992. *Excellent text introducing the concepts and techniques of molecular genetics and recombinant DNA research. Appropriate for all readers, from novices to professionals.*

Zabner J, Couture LA, Gregory RJ, Graham SM, Smith AE, Welsh MJ. Adenovirus-mediated gene transfer transiently corrects the chloride transport defect in nasal epithelia of patients with cystic fibrosis. *Cell* 1993;75:207–216. *First report of adenovirus-mediated human gene therapy, demonstrating transient correction of the chloride transport defect in nasal epithelia of three individuals with cystic fibrosis by adenovirus-mediated CFTR gene transfer.*

II DIAGNOSTIC METHODS

Textbook of Pulmonary Diseases, 6th ed.
edited by G.L. Baum, J.D. Crapo, B.R. Celli, and J.B. Karlinsky,
Lippincott–Raven Publishers, Philadelphia, © 1998.

CHAPTER

8 ◆ Pulmonary Imaging

Daniel R. Gale · M. Elon Gale

INTRODUCTION

Despite the introduction of many technologically advanced imaging modalities, a conventional chest radiograph remains the initial, and sometimes only, diagnostic image necessary to evaluate patients with suspected chest abnormalities. Typically, observations derived from chest radiography, in combination with the clinical history, suggest at least a differential, if not a definitive, diagnosis. Only after complete characterization and assessment of a chest radiographic abnormality are additional diagnostic imaging studies indicated; these can range from low-technology examinations, such as decubitus chest radiographs, to sophisticated technologic examinations, such as computed tomography (CT), magnetic resonance imaging (MRI), nuclear imaging, pulmonary and bronchial artery angiography, and ultrasonography. At this time, the most important of these additional diagnostic imaging studies is CT of the chest. Chest CT has done more to revolutionize the radiologic evaluation and subsequent care of patients with thoracic abnormalities than any other radiographic technique since the invention of conventional chest x-ray imaging.

In addition to conventional radiography and CT, three other broad categories of radiographic examinations can potentially be used to evaluate chest abnormalities. These include angiography, nuclear imaging, and MRI. Although much less frequently performed than chest radiography or CT, these other examinations listed are essential

tools in the diagnosis and management of patients with specific medical problems, such as hemoptysis, pulmonary embolus, or brachial plexus involvement by neoplasm. It is now routine practice to use images for accurate staging of a thoracic neoplasm, percutaneous biopsy of a mediastinal mass, drainage of a collection of fluid, or quick assessment of the response of a chest abnormality to therapy. The older imaging techniques (plain tomography and bronchography) have generally been supplanted by one of these newer techniques that in conjunction with other procedures, such as fiberoptic bronchoscopy, provide more reliable anatomic and physiologic information with less patient discomfort. Ideally, the pulmonologist and the radiologist should work together to plan a cost-effective diagnostic and therapeutic imaging workup.

In this chapter, the relevant technical principles of common radiologic examinations are described, and the clinical indications, advantages, and limitations of each examination type are reviewed. A comprehensive review of the myriad diagnostic and interpretative findings found on routine chest radiography or the more specialized examinations is beyond the scope of this chapter; however, clinically pertinent signs are illustrated. A systematic, simplified approach to interpreting any imaging study and organizing a relevant differential diagnosis is presented at the conclusion of the chapter.

STANDARD PLANE CHEST RADIOGRAPHY

Radiographic Technique

Two distinct radiographic techniques are used to obtain a conventional chest radiograph (posteranterior and

D. R. Gale and M. E. Gale: Department of Radiology, Veterans Affairs Medical Center, Boston, Massachusetts 02130.

lateral); the high-kilovoltage (>100 kV) and low-kilovoltage (<90 kV) techniques. The principal advantage of the high-kilovoltage technique is better display of the lung parenchyma without interference from overlying ribs, clavicles, or heart. The principal advantage of the low-kilovoltage technique is the enhancement of the contrast between pulmonary vessels and parenchyma and the identification of calcium. Pulmonary nodules are more easily detected on high-kilovoltage films (100 to 130 kV).

The standard chest radiograph is taken at full inspiration with the patient approximately 72 inches from the plane of the x-ray film. This minimizes geometric magnification of the heart and enhances visualization of the pulmonary vasculature. The optimal density of a conventional posteroanterior or lateral chest x-ray film is a matter of individual preference. In general, the mediastinal structures should be easily discernible from the lung parenchyma and the bones. The intervertebral disk spaces and ribs should be identifiable on a routine posteroanterior film, but not at the expense of an optimal view of the lung parenchyma.

After conventional chest radiographs, portable chest radiographs are the next most frequently used radiographic examination of the chest. No commonly accepted standards or techniques are available for performing portable chest radiographs, as they are for standard posteroanterior and lateral chest radiographs. Further, these films are obtained in the anteroposterior direction, so that magnification artifacts occur. Consequently, the quality and reproducibility of a portable chest x-ray film is extremely variable. The rates for repeated portable chest radiographs are two to four times greater than those for repeated conventional radiographs. Portable chest x-ray films are often obtained in the sickest and most unstable patients. The variabilities of exposure, penetration, and positioning make interpretation of these films more problematic. Standard protocols that maximize consistent and reproducible high-quality portable films should be used.

The most commonly employed portable chest x-ray technique uses manually selected low kilovoltages and exposure times, without a grid. This technique results in portable films of relatively high contrast that are often degraded by scatter radiation. The mediastinal structures or lung parenchyma may not be optimally visualized because the films are either underexposed or overexposed. Overexposure may be done intentionally, to improve visualization of a monitoring line or tube. However, this is an unnecessary practice that contributes to poor overall film quality.

Portable chest x-ray films should be obtained using a fixed high-kilovoltage technique (approximately 110 kV) with a grid and phototiming. Phototiming devices are unavailable in many hospitals, and manually selected exposure times are then required. The high-kilovoltage technique is preferred because portable films can be produced that consistently approximate the quality of a conven-

tional chest x-ray film. An important added benefit is decreased radiation exposure to the patient and hospital personnel. The decrease in exposure time more than compensates for the higher kilovoltage used.

Indications

The American College of Radiology Thoracic Expert Panel has developed a set of indications for chest films that includes signs and symptoms referable to the pulmonary or cardiovascular systems, suspicion of pulmonary or cardiovascular involvement by systemic or extrathoracic diseases, and monitoring of progression or regression of previously identified thoracic abnormalities. Chest radiographs are generally indicated in individuals presenting with the following symptoms: hoarseness, dyspnea, productive or nonproductive cough, hemoptysis, or pleuritic pain (Fig. 1). These symptoms suggest abnormalities in the following anatomic structures: trachea and small and large airways (Fig. 2); lung parenchyma; pleural space; mediastinum, including the heart; and the bony thorax. All these structures may be visualized on a high-quality chest radiograph.

Routine/Screening Radiography

The utility of chest radiography in routine, periodic, or screening situations (e.g., routine, daily portable chest radiographs in the intensive care unit setting, periodic screening chest films in asymptomatic ambulatory patients, and screening chest radiographs in asymptomatic HIV-infected adults) remains controversial. Routine/screening radiography may be indicated in high-risk populations, but they have not been found to be of use even in the prospective evaluation of persons who smoke, who have a higher risk for the development of lung carcinoma. Chest radiographs that were formerly taken routinely in various clinical situations but are no longer indicated include routine prenatal chest radiographs, routine admission chest radiographs of asymptomatic individuals, routine chest radiographs of geriatric patients in long-term facilities or of patients in psychiatric facilities, periodic examinations unrelated to occupational exposures, mandated chest radiographs for detection of tuberculosis as a condition of initial or continuing employment, and routine preoperative radiographs of patients under the age of 20. Lateral projections should be eliminated from the routine screening examination in patients between the ages of 20 and 39 years.

Portable Radiography

Portable chest radiographs should be routinely obtained in critically ill patients in the intensive care unit setting,

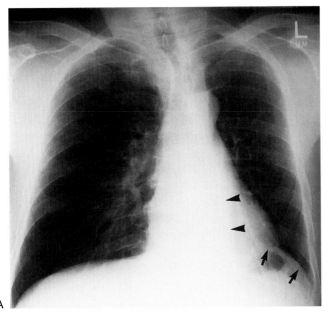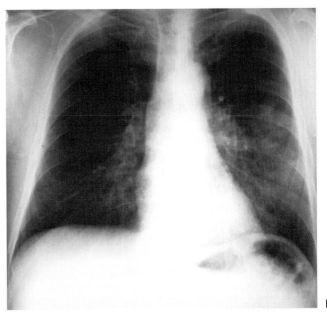

A

B

FIG. 1. A: Classic radiographic findings of left lower lobe collapse. These include volume loss (demonstrated by a shift of the mediastinum, heart, and trachea to the left), a triangular opacity in a retrocardiac location (*black arrowheads*), and silhouetting of the medial portions of the left hemidiaphragm. Only the lateral portion of the hemidiaphragm (*black arrows*) is delineated. **B:** In a radiograph obtained after chest physical therapy, the left lower lobe collapse has resolved. The shift of the mediastinum and the triangular retrocardiac opacity are no longer present. The left hemidiaphragm is identified medially.

as they have been shown to demonstrate unexpected findings or provide an indication for altering therapy in 37%–65% of a population of intubated patients. The American College of Radiology Expert Panel agrees with this opinion and has stated that daily, portable chest radiographs are indicated in patients who are receiving mechanical ventilation, who have acute cardiopulmonary problems to assess lung water, or in whom a new monitoring device or tube has been placed (Fig. 3). Portable chest radiography is indicated only during the initial evaluation of patients who receive just cardiac monitoring.

In settings other than the intensive care unit, the most frequent indications for portable chest radiographs include assessment of a nonambulatory patient for pneumonia or congestive heart failure, or following placement of a monitoring device (Fig. 3). Because of the limitations of the portable technique, it may be difficult to identify or distinguish between atelectasis, pneumonia, adult respiratory distress syndrome (ARDS), pleural effusions, and typical or atypical cardiogenic or noncardiogenic edema.

Utility of the Baseline (Old) Chest Radiograph

A baseline or old chest x-ray film is one of the most important resources in the diagnostic process for two reasons. First, it serves as a baseline examination with which comparisons may be made, so that detection of changes is possible. Second, with the aid of an old film, an assess-

ment of the relative acuity or chronicity of an observation is possible; this is an invaluable aid in the development of a differential diagnosis. Old films should be obtained for comparison whenever possible. Costs are minimized because the need for additional imaging is reduced, and quality of care is improved because the evaluation is expedited.

Decubitus and Oblique Films

On occasion, decubitus and oblique chest views may be indicated to answer or clarify specific diagnostic questions raised by interpretation of the initial chest radiograph. Decubitus views can delineate the presence and quantity of a free-flowing pleural effusion before performance of a diagnostic or therapeutic thoracentesis. Views are obtained with the patient lying in a recumbent position; each hemithorax should be alternatively visualized in the dependent position. An important advantage of obtaining bilateral decubitus views is that as fluid shifts, the underlying lung parenchyma can more adequately be evaluated for potential abnormalities that may have been hidden by the pleural fluid. In unusual circumstances, a decubitus view of the chest can demonstrate a tiny pneumothorax not necessarily seen on an expiratory upright chest film.

Oblique films of the chest, obtained by rotating the patient with respect to the film, are used to ascertain whether an opacity in the lung represents a parenchymal

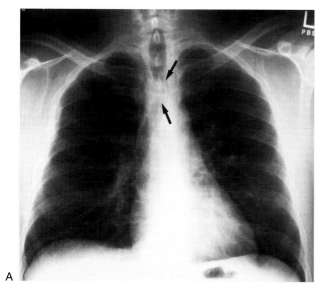

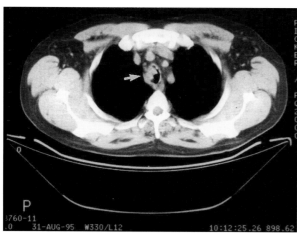

FIG. 2. A: Chest radiograph demonstrating a subtle mass (*black arrows*) projecting into the tracheal air column. **B:** Chest CT confirms the presence of a large fungating mass (*white arrowhead*) within the trachea. The vast majority of tracheal neoplasms are either of squamous cell or minor salivary gland origin. The pathologic specimen revealed adenoid cystic carcinoma.

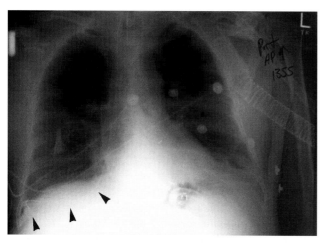

FIG. 3. A portable chest film demonstrating abnormal placement of a nasogastric tube (*black arrowheads*) into the right costophrenic angle. Feeding tubes are much more likely than nasogastric tubes to be inappropriately placed, because they are smaller in diameter and composed of more pliable material.

abnormality versus an overlap of bronchial vascular markings or an abnormality originating in the ribs. These views are usually requested by a radiologist when the level of suspicion is not particularly high that an abnormality seen on a chest x-ray film represents a true parenchymal abnormality or when the availability of CT scanning is limited. Oblique chest radiographs have been used to improve the identification, documentation, and characterization of pleural abnormalities, such as pleural plaques; these functions have now largely been replaced by CT scanning, diagnostic ultrasonography, and MRI.

Rib films, also obtained with the patient positioned obliquely with respect to the film, differ from oblique chest films in that the radiographic techniques used for a rib series are designed to improve the identification of bone abnormalities, such as fractures and metastatic disease, at the expense of visualization of lung parenchyma.

Apical Lordotic Films

Apical lordotic views, obtained with patient standing erect and the x-ray film angled 15° cephalad to the chest, are of limited utility. These views, along with apical kyphotic views, were previously used to improve visualization of the lung apices, thoracic inlet, and superior mediastinum. However, these views rarely provide sufficient additional information to make a diagnosis unequivocal. Questionable parenchymal, thoracic inlet, or mediastinal abnormalities that previously were evaluated by apical lordotic views should now be imaged with chest CT or MRI.

Chest Fluoroscopy

The utilization of chest fluoroscopy has declined in the evaluation of thoracic abnormalities with the advent of chest CT. Unlike routine chest radiography, fluoroscopy of the chest is usually performed at about 70 kV. The low-kilovoltage technique enhances the ability to detect calcium within a thoracic lesion. Current indications for chest fluoroscopy include diagnosis of diaphragmatic paralysis; discrimation between a possible rib or pleural abnormality and a parenchymal lung abnormality (pleural plaques versus a pleura-associated small parenchymal lung nodule); guidance of needle placement during percutaneous needle biopsies of lung, pleural, rib, and mediastinal masses and during percutaneous drainage of fluid collections within the chest; and guidance of bronchoscope and needle placement and confirmation of correct positioning before transbronchoscopic biopsy.

Digital Chest Radiography

The ability to acquire and display radiographs, including chest films, in a digital format should improve efficiency and decrease radiation exposure to patients and medical personnel. This technique is now becoming widely available.

COMPUTED TOMOGRAPHY

CT scans of the chest have two very significant advantages over routine chest radiographs: superior contrast sensitivity, which aids in differentiating fat, water, air, and calcium; and the ability to display cross-sectional anatomy, thereby eliminating superimposition of adjacent anatomic structures. Although images are usually obtained and displayed in a transverse fashion, multiplanar displays now allow sagittal and/or coronal reconstructions. With the advent of spiral CT scans, three-dimensional displays and holographic images may be obtained. All reconstructed display formats are designed to aid in the presentation of complex anatomic relationships. Decreased spatial resolution is the one significant disadvantage of CT in comparison with conventional chest radiography. The identification of small pulmonary nodules is easier on a chest CT scan, not because spatial resolution is enhanced, but rather because contrast sensitivity is enhanced between essentially black normal lung parenchyma and the soft-tissue density characteristic of pulmonary nodules, and also because relevant anatomy is displayed without superimposition of normal structures.

Technique

CT scans are usually obtained at end-inspiration with the patient lying supine. Two basic designs of commercial CT scanners are currently available. In one design, the x-ray tube and detectors rotate simultaneously around the patient, and in the other, the detector wing is stationary and the x-ray tube rotates. Either design produces high-quality images. Routine scanning of the chest is usually done in 8- to 10-mm-thick slices obtained contiguously from the lung apex to base through the diaphragm; the adrenal glands are often imaged as well. This basic scanning protocol may be modified depending on the specific clinical problem.

In general, the use of intravenous contrast material should be limited to evaluations in which vascular lesions (pulmonary arteriovenous malformation, pseudoaneurysm) are suspected, or in which precise vascular anatomy is needed (invasion of a pulmonary artery by a lung neoplasm). Intravenous contrast material can also be used to resolve a central lung mass from associated lung collapse or to identify a pleural effusion as transudative or exudative.

Indications

A compete list of indications for chest CT are too numerous to review here. Some of the more common indications are staging of common primary malignancies of the thorax (bronchogenic carcinoma, esophageal carcinoma); staging of intrathoracic lymphoma; evaluation of suspected vascular abnormalities (arteriovenous malformation, venous varices, pseudoaneurysms, aneurysms with or without dissection); and evaluation or staging of extrapulmonary processes, which include the following:

1. Pleural lesions (mesothelioma) (Fig. 4)
2. Rib lesions (primary bone tumor, Ewing's sarcoma)
3. Pleural space processes (empyema)
4. Lesions of the chest wall
5. Diaphragmatic lesions (diaphragmatic hernias, congenital or posttraumatic)
6. Abnormalities arising from hilar and mediastinal structures, including thymic neoplasms (thymolipoma, thymoma); esophageal abnormalities (duplication cysts); pericardial or cardiac abnormalities (pericardial effusions, pericardial cysts); tracheal neoplasms (primary squamous cell carcinoma, salivary gland tumors); mediastinal or

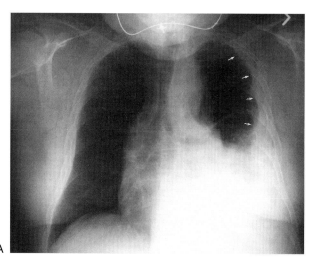
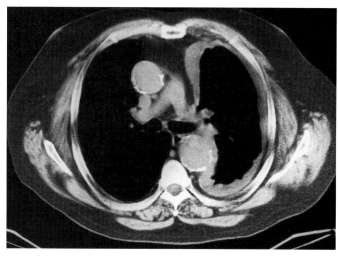

A   B

FIG. 4. A: A chest radiograph reveals a blunted costophrenic angle with a lobular configuration (*white arrowheads*) along the lateral pleural surface. This is atypical for a simple transudative pleural effusion, which would exhibit a smooth interface between the lung and pleura and not surround the entire lung. The chest radiographic appearance is very suggestive of a mesothelioma, which was confirmed on chest CT. **B:** A single image from a chest CT scan shows an encased left lung with associated contraction of the hemithorax.

hilar adenopathy; and neoplasms originating in or invading the mediastinum (germ cell tumors, goiter)

7. Malignant neoplasms with a propensity to metastasize to the lung (melanoma, renal cell carcinoma)

Chest CT may also be indicated to characterize more completely an abnormality of uncertain etiology detected on a chest radiograph (Fig. 5).

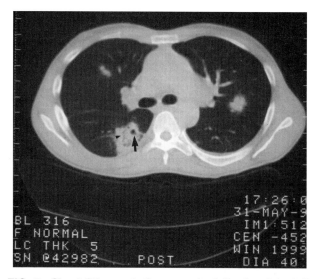

FIG. 5. Chest CT reveals three poorly defined nodular infiltrates. In one of the nodular opacities, air bronchograms (*black arrowhead*) and cavitation (*black arrow*) are visible. The differential diagnosis is broad and includes a diverse clinical conditions such as non-Hodgkins lymphoma, bronchoalveolar cell carcinoma, and Wegner's granulomatosis. With an appropriate clinical history (e.g., a patient with fever and a new systolic murmur), the differential diagnosis is narrowed to septic emboli.

High-resolution chest CT scans employ a modification of the standard acquisition and display protocol to produce thin-section (1.0 to 1.5 mm) cuts that enhance the spatial resolution of lung parenchyma. Edges are sharper and scan times are shorter with this technique. High-resolution CT can detect abnormal lung when the findings on chest x-ray film and conventional CT scan are normal. This modality is used in the evaluation of early interstitial lung disease; active disease is characterized by ground-glass opacities and interstitial or air space nodules, and inactive disease is characterized by scarring. Biopsy specimens can be obtained from areas of lung that appear active on high-resolution CT, or such areas can be followed during therapy.

In the appropriate clinical setting, certain specific diagnoses may be made by high-resolution CT without need of lung biopsy. The entities most confidently diagnosed by high-resolution CT include lymphangiomyomatosis, histiocytosis X, lymphangitic carcinomatosis, sarcoidosis, silicosis, and idiopathic pulmonary fibrosis.

Helical CT scanning is an important recent technologic innovation in which the patient is continuously fed through the scanner gantry as the x-ray images are being taken. This technique generates volumetric information that can be displayed in a conventional axial plane or in a variety of orthogonal planes. Helical CT offers three significant advantages over conventional scans. First, scan times are reduced to 30 to 60 seconds, which increases productivity. Second, less intravenous contrast is required to achieve high-quality scans, and misregistration artifacts are significantly reduced. Third, multiplanar reformation is possible with less degradation of the image. Clinically, helical CT scanning enhances detection and quantification of suspected pulmonary nodules in comparison with conventional CT scans. Vascular imaging is vastly improved, so that helical CT can replace angiography in the evaluation of aortic dissection and trauma and may eventually replace coronary angiography and pulmonary arteriography. Multiplanar reformatting has been used to display complex mediastinal and tracheobronchial anatomy.

NUCLEAR IMAGING OF THE THORAX

Nuclear imaging of the thorax is performed for a variety of clinical indications. The most common and important use of nuclear imaging is in the workup of suspected pulmonary embolus (ventilation-perfusion scans).

Technique

Technetium 99m is the most commonly used radionuclide in diagnostic imaging because it has no particulate emission, has a relatively short half-life (6 hours), and emits almost entirely 40-keV (kiloelectron volt) photons. This makes it a relatively ideal nuclear imaging agent. After intravenous administration, the relevant organ or organs are imaged with a gamma camera. The gamma camera measures the number of photons emitted by the radionuclide and displays these counts as dots; the intensity of the display (number of dots) is proportional to the amount of activity.

The choice of the particular radionuclide or radiopharmaceutical to be used for a particular study is guided by pharmacologic considerations. For example, the radionuclide xenon 133 gas is used almost exclusively for lung ventilation studies because it is not soluble in blood, whereas the radiopharmaceutical agent Tc 99 microaggregated albumin (MAA) is used for multiple indications, but primarily to detect pulmonary emboli or right-to-left shunting. It is extremely soluble in blood and does not appear in exhaled gas.

Pulmonary Embolus

Both ventilation and perfusion nuclear scans are required to assess the likelihood of pulmonary embolism. For these studies, to assess pulmonary ventilation and perfusion simultaneously, a radionuclide is inhaled (xenon 133 gas) and a radiopharmaceutical agent (Tc 99 MAA) is injected intravenously. Images obtained during inhalation, steady-state breathing, and exhalation provide information about regional and overall ventilatory dynamics. Radiolabeled aerosols are sometimes used instead of radioactive gases. Studies using these radioactive aerosols are technically more difficult to perform and may not detect small ventilation defects, but they do provide the important advantage of providing images in views corresponding to the perfusion abnormalities.

The majority of Tc 99 MAA particles injected to assess perfusion are in the 10- to 30-μm range; they mix in the right atrium and ventricle. The particles then enter the pulmonary circulation and become trapped in the pulmonary capillary vascular bed. Because of the relatively small numbers of particles compared with the number of pulmonary capillaries, further vascular obstruction does not occur. Nevertheless, in patients with known pulmonary hypertension or suspected right-to-left shunts, the quantity of Tc 99 MAA injected is usually reduced.

At this time, ventilation and perfusion images are interpreted using criteria and guidelines developed from the Prospective Investigation of Pulmonary Embolus Diagnosis (PIOPED) study. Small but important modifications and refinements to the criteria have been recently made. The size and number of matched and mismatched defects, relative to the concurrent chest x-ray image, are assessed to determine the relative probability of pulmonary embolus. Scans are rated as highly probable for the diagnosis, of intermediate, low, or very low probability, or normal. In the revised PIOPED criteria, four categories have been arbitrarily assigned numeric values: high (80%–100%, probable for the diagnosis), intermediate (20%–79%), low (<19%), and normal. A normal ventilation-perfusion scan essentially rules out the diagnosis of pulmonary embolus.

The classic nuclear imaging characteristics of pulmonary embolus are a high-probability ventilation-perfusion scan, defined as a normal ventilation scan with multiple peripheral perfusion defects corresponding to lobar or segmental anatomy, and a normal chest radiograph. High-probability ventilation-perfusion scans have a specificity for pulmonary embolus of approximately 97%, but a low sensitivity. Only about 41% of the patients demonstrated to have pulmonary embolus by angiography also have a high-probability ventilation-perfusion scan. Angiography studies have shown that a clinically high index of suspicion for pulmonary embolus and a high-probability ventilation-perfusion scan strongly correlate with the presence of pulmonary embolus, and likewise a clinically low index of suspicion for pulmonary embolus and a low-probability ventilation-perfusion scan correlate strongly with the absence of pulmonary embolus.

Other Indications

Perfusion lung scans are also used preoperatively to estimate the amount of lung function that will remain in patients with poor lung function after lobectomy or pneumonectomy (Chapter 13) and to detect and quantify right-to-left shunting (hepatopulmonary syndrome). To document right-to-left shunting, images of the brain or kidney are usually obtained to identify the abnormal location of radioactivity and document the arteriovenous shunt. By measuring the amount of activity in these organs and comparing it with the amount of activity in the lungs, the percentage of shunting can be calculated.

Nuclear imaging may also be used to evaluate occult or suspected pulmonary infection, to assess hilar and mediastinal adenopathy secondary to metastatic disease or lymphoma, and to detect inflammation in the lung parenchyma secondary to adverse drug reactions or alveolitis. Gallium 67 can detect lung injury caused by drugs such as bleomycin before any abnormality can be visualized on chest x-ray films; it can also detect occult lymphoma in mediastinal lymph nodes that appear to be of normal size on CT and occult infections of the interstitium, such as *Pneumocystis* infection. Gallium 67 scanning has been used in conjunction with determination of angiotensin-converting enzyme (ACE) levels to estimate the degree of activity of pulmonary sarcoidosis.

Gallium 67 and thallium 201 scans in combination have been shown to be extremely useful in distinguishing between Kaposi's sarcoma, mycobacterial infection, and lymphoma. This is a common problem in patients with the acquired immune deficiency syndrome (AIDS). Matched patterns of uptake on gallium 67 and thallium 201 scans are suggestive of non-Hodgkin's lymphoma, whereas a gallium-negative and thallium-positive pattern indicates Kaposi's sarcoma. Finally, a gallium-positive and thallium-negative scan is highly suggestive of mycobacterial infection, although other granulomatous infections, such as cryptococcosis, histoplasmosis, or coccidioidomycosis, cannot be completely ruled out by this technique.

PULMONARY ANGIOGRAPHY

Angiography is the least frequently used radiographic study to investigate chest abnormalities. Nevertheless, it is an important diagnostic and potentially therapeutic tool used in the evaluation of specific pulmonary abnormalities.

Technique

Access to the arterial or venous system is gained by catheterization through the groin or upper extremity using the Seldinger technique or one of its variations. Contrast material is injected into the vascular system and rapid-sequence films are obtained. Angiography is associated with low rates of complications, which may be categorized as systemic, local, or catheter-related occurrences.

Systemic complications include the development of contrast-induced nephropathy or severe allergic reaction with cardiovascular collapse. Examples of local complications related to the puncture site are development of a groin hematoma or a pseudoaneurysm. Examples of

catheter-related complications are distal embolization or intimal dissection. Before any interventional procedure is undertaken, the relative benefits versus risks need to be understood clearly by the radiologist, referring clinician, and patient. To prevent complications and assess risk, a complete history should be taken (diabetes, contrast allergy, previous bleeding diathesis), and the coagulation status (platelet count, prothrombin time, partial thromboplastin time) and serum creatinine level should be determined before the procedure is performed.

Indications

Pulmonary arteriography is the most common angiographic procedure involving the thorax and is usually performed to rule out pulmonary embolus. Pulmonary angiography is also indicated in the assessment of chronic thromboembolic disease as a suspected cause of pulmonary hypertension, and as part of the evaluation of small pulmonary arteriovenous malformations. Large malfor-

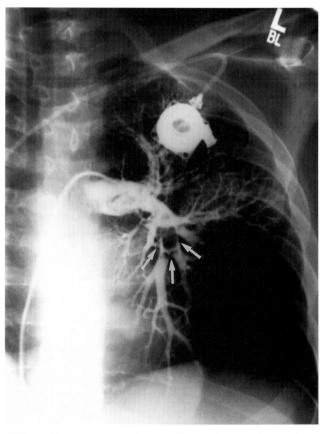

FIG. 6. Pulmonary arteriogram illustrating multiple pulmonary emboli. A large filling defect (*white arrows*), clot, is depicted in the left lower lobe pulmonary artery. Anticoagulation therapy does not immediately take effect to prevent the formation of additional emboli. The indications for fibrinolytic therapy are limited in the treatment of pulmonary embolus.

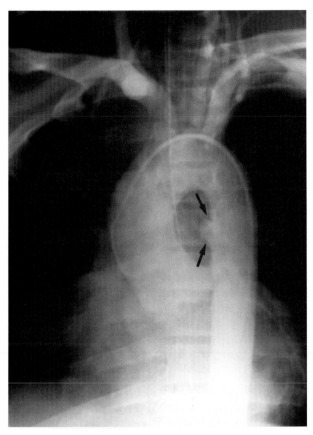

FIG. 7. Thoracic aortogram demonstrating an abnormal collection of contrast (*black arrows*) outside the normal wall of the descending thoracic aorta at the level of the ligament of the ductus arteriosus, diagnostic of an aortic laceration. Aortic lacerations are almost always associated with a deceleration injury, especially in automobile accidents.

mations are more easily diagnosed using contrast-enhanced chest CT.

In the workup of pulmonary embolus, pulmonary arteriography is almost always preceded by ventilation-perfusion scanning. Abnormal findings on the scan can be used to guide the subsequent catheterization of the pulmonary arteries. If the ventilation-perfusion scan demonstrates a segmental defect in the left lower lobe, then the left lower lobe pulmonary artery is catheterized first so as to expedite the diagnosis and obviate the need for additional angiographic runs. However, negative results from the study of the left lower lobe pulmonary artery do not in turn obviate the need to image the entire pulmonary arterial system, as pulmonary emboli do not necessarily correspond to defects observed on a ventilation-perfusion scan.

The classic angiographic findings of pulmonary embolic disease include intraluminal filling defects and abrupt arterial cutoffs (Fig. 6). Because intraluminal clot begins to dissolve after 24 hours and 80% of the clot has lysed by 7 days, pulmonary arteriography should be performed as close in time to the suspected clinical event as possible.

Elevated pulmonary arterial pressure and left bundle branch block are relative contraindications for pulmonary arteriography. An increase in mortality (<0.5%) is associated with right ventricular end-diastolic pressures of >20 mm Hg, and a left bundle branch block may progress to complete heart block during the procedure. These relative contraindications can be addressed by modifying the angiographic technique and placing a temporary transvenous pacing wire.

Angiography is also used to evaluate the systemic circulation, the thoracic aorta (thoracic aortography), and the bronchial circulation (Fig. 7). The indications for thoracic aortography vary from institution to institution, but generally the procedure is performed to evaluate the possibility of thoracic aortic aneurysm, thoracic aortic dissection, and traumatic injury to the thoracic aorta. At the present time, CT and MRI have begun to replace thoracic aortography for these indications, as they are noninvasive, less labor-intensive, and more cost-effective than angiography. Bronchial arterial arteriography is usually performed to identify the site of bronchial arterial bleeding in patients with life-threatening hemoptysis of known cause who cannot undergo surgical resection (Fig. 8). After identification of the site of bleeding, embolization of the vessel may be performed to reduce hemorrhage. Bronchiectasis, aspergillosis, or cystic fibrosis are the most frequent causes of this type of hemoptysis.

Venography of the central veins in the chest, such as the superior vena cava, left and right innominate veins, and the azygos vein, is performed rarely. Thrombosis of these vessels, which may be caused by mediastinal neoplasm, mediastinitis, or iatrogenic instrumentation, is more easily investigated noninvasively with either CT or MRI, or an ultrasonographic examination. Occasionally,

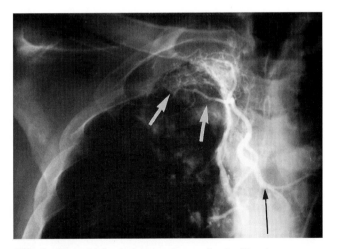

FIG. 8. Bronchial arteriogram in a patient with a known mycetoma who presented with severe recurrent hemoptysis. A bronchial artery is cannulated by a catheter (*black arrow*) before embolization. The abnormal vascularity associated with the mycetoma is visualized in the apex of the right lung (*white arrow*).

vascular stents have been deployed in the treatment of superior vena cava syndrome.

MAGNETIC RESONANCE IMAGING

Principle

MRI is a relatively new imaging technique that produces images without the use of ionizing radiation. In an MR image, each voxel is a gray scale representation of the relative intensity of a radio wave signal emanating from tissue that has been perturbed by a characteristic radio frequency (RF pulse). The radio wave signal emanating from each tissue depends on several factors, the most important of which is time. T_1 and T_2 relaxation times originate from this principle. Cardiac gating and suppression of respiratory motion are essential to produce chest images of diagnostic quality. At the time of this writing, poor spatial resolution, respiratory motion, and the lack of sufficient hydrogen protons in lung make MRI of the lung parenchyma impractical for most indications.

Whereas the information in CT scans is acquired in a transverse plane through the chest, MRI is capable of imaging the chest in any plane. Another advantage of MRI in comparison with CT is its ability to identify vascular structures without the use of intravenous iodinated contrast. If contrast is necessary, gadolinium-based contrast agents have a better safety profile than iodinated contrast and can be used to delineate vascular structures. Although neither CT nor MRI can detect neoplastic invasion of tissues at the microscopic level, the superior contrast resolution of MRI offers an advantage in the diagnosis of subtle invasion of fat or soft tissues by tumor.

Current applications of MRI include evaluation of both the central venous and central pulmonary vasculature. Suspected superior vena cava syndrome, resulting from either malignancy or mediastinitis, may be diagnosed using MRI, as can invasion of pulmonary arteries or even the heart by a large central mass. Thoracic aneurysms and pseudoaneurysms, as well as aortic dissections, are readily identified by MRI (Fig. 9). Mediastinal masses, originating from any compartment, may be imaged.

The ability to study anatomic structures in sagittal or coronal planes and the excellent contrast resolution make MRI the modality of choice in the investigation of abnormalities related to the diaphragm, lung apex, chest wall, and mediastinum (Fig. 10). Diaphragmatic abnormalities, such as posttraumatic or congenital hernias, are displayed to advantage. Similarly, abnormalities originating within the lung apex, such as a superior sulcus neoplasm, are optimally staged with MRI as either confined to the thorax or invading the brachial plexus. Chest-wall or mediastinal masses originating in any lung compartment may also be imaged.

MRI is also extremely useful in evaluating perihilar and pericardial abnormalities. However, MRI is presently used only as an adjunct to CT in the evaluation of nonvascular abnormalities of the mediastinum and hilar regions, primarily because of expense. Unfortunately, MR signal characteristics cannot reliably distinguish between benign and malignant adenopathy in patients with lung carcinoma. However, residual fibrosis can be distinguished

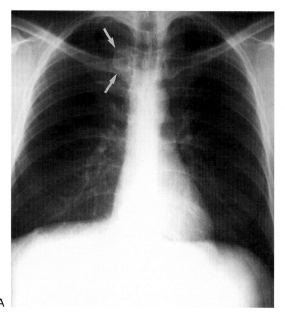

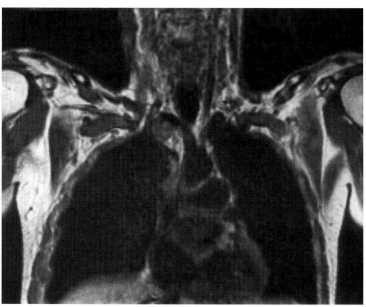

A B

FIG. 9. A: Chest radiograph demonstrating a 2-cm peripherally calcified mass in a right paratracheal location. A vascular origin should be suspected in any chest lesion with peripheral curvilinear calcification. **B:** A coronal MRI displaying a pseudoaneurysm of the right subclavian artery in a patient with a remote history of a penetrating knife wound.

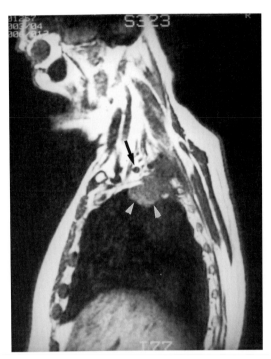

FIG. 10. A superior sulcus neoplasm (*white arrowheads*) extending through the parietal pleura into the supraclavicular fossa is depicted on a sagittal MRI. The cancer spares the subclavian artery (*black arrow*) and brachial plexus, immediately cephalad to the artery.

from active neoplastic disease following radiation therapy for lymphoma. Likewise, MRI is capable of distinguishing between rebound thymic hyperplasia and recurrent disease.

INTERVENTIONAL PROCEDURES

Nonangiographic interventional procedures of the chest that require imaging guidance fall into two general categories: percutaneous biopsy (parenchymal lesions, mediastinal masses, or pleural abnormalities) in which either a skinny or cutting needle is used, and percutaneous aspirations and/or drainage of fluid collections located within the pleural space or lung parenchyma and the mediastinum. Imaging guidance for interventional procedures is provided by fluoroscopy, CT, or ultrasonography. The choice of imaging guidance depends on the availability of equipment and the expertise and experience of the operator.

Significant intrathoracic hemorrhage is an avoidable complication associated with interventional procedures. If the number of adequately functioning platelets is >75,000/mm^3 and the INR (International Normalized Ratio) is normal, then the risk for significant hemorrhage is greatly reduced. Patients with known bleeding disorders or abnormal coagulation parameters require a detailed hemostatic evaluation to avoid morbidity associated with these procedures.

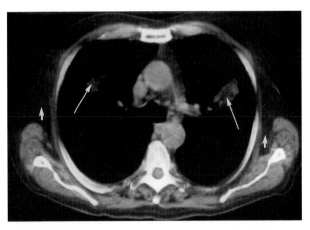

FIG. 11. Chest CT in a patient whose chest radiograph demonstrated multiple, poorly defined nodular opacities that waxed and waned shows bilateral opacities (*long white arrows*) with internal attenuation, similar to that of subcutaneous fat (*short white arrows*). A diagnosis of lipid pneumonia was made.

Also, the needle route should be chosen to avoid larger vessels, such as the internal mammary, intercostal, central hilar, and mediastinal vessels. Significant morbidity has occurred when these vessels have been punctured.

Pneumothorax is the most common complication of percutaneous biopsy of the chest, with a reported rate of 5%–60% of all biopsies (average rate, ~25%–30%). The risk for pneumothorax is related to several factors: the extent of underlying lung disease, especially when adjacent to the lesion from which biopsy samples are being taken (emphysema), and the number of needle passes, especially when passes are made through multiple pleural surfaces or cross a fissure or lung parenchyma during biopsy of the mediastinum.

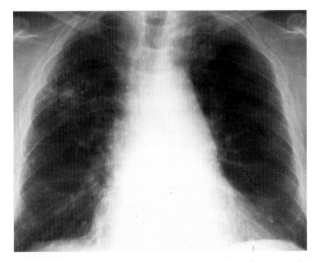

FIG. 12. A chest radiograph demonstrating innumerable pulmonary nodules <1 cm in diameter. Some of the nodules are calcified, and in the right upper lobe the nodules are more confluent. This area represents a developing conglomerate mass in a patient with silicosis.

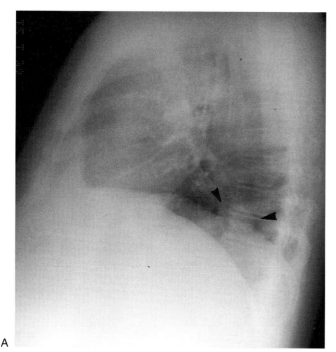
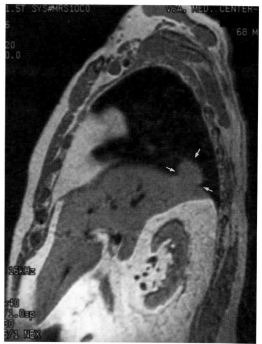

FIG. 13. A: A lateral chest radiograph demonstrating an approximately 2-cm rounded opacity (*black arrowheads*) adjacent to the right hemidiaphragm. Because the inferior margin of the lesion was silhouetted by the diaphragm, it was suspected that the abnormality originated from or below the diaphragm. **B:** A sagittal MRI of the chest shows the liver (*white arrowheads*) herniating through the diaphragm.

The percutaneous biopsy route should therefore be planned to avoid crossing multiple pleural surfaces. Up to half the patients who experience a pneumothorax as a result of a percutaneous biopsy require chest tube drainage. A small pneumothorax that does not affect hemodynamics or respiration may be treated with a small catheter and Heimlich valve. If the pneumothorax is large and affects hemodynamics and/or respiration, a large-bore chest tube should be placed.

Frank hemoptysis is almost always self-limiting.

Percutaneous Lung Biosy

Percutaneous lung biopsy has a relatively high safety profile and is usually performed with needles under 19 gauge, although larger needles are required for core biopsies. The diagnostic yield for malignant lesions is approximately 95%. The diagnostic yield is not as high for nonmalignant lesions. The appropriate handling of a specimen is crucial to ensure an accurate diagnosis and requires cooperation between the radiology, laboratory, and clinical services. For example, malignant cytologies are more likely to be obtained from a percutaneous biopsy specimen directly prepared by the cytopathologist or pathologist. Some specimens require special handling (flow cytometry), which necessitates special preparation of the aspirate.

Percutaneous Drainage of Fluid Collections

Although large pleural effusions are usually managed without image-guided drainage procedures, percutaneous drainage of smaller pleural, parenchymal, or mediastinal fluid collections requires imaging for optimal placement of drainage catheters. Small and loculated pleural effusions are most conveniently aspirated under ultrasonic guidance. Uncomplicated empyema is characterized by early clinical presentation, lack of loculations, relatively nonviscous purulent material, and the absence of a thick pleural peel, and may be drained successfully with a percutaneously placed catheter. Postoperative or loculated empyema, or empyema associated with bronchopleural fistula, is less likely to be drained successfully by the percutaneous technique. Fibrinolytic agents have been introduced into the pleural space to aid in the drainage of loculated empyemas. Percutaneous drainage of lung abscesses and mediastinal abscesses has a limited role.

APPROACH TO INTERPRETATION OF RADIOGRAPHIC STUDIES

There are many approaches to the interpretation of a radiographic study. Some approaches are unique to a particular diagnostic imaging modality, and others are unique to a specific clinical problem. The approach to the interpretation of radiographic studies discussed here utilizes a series of simple but informative questions applicable to simple and sophisticated radiologic techniques and most clinical problems. The answers to these questions assist in characterizing an abnormality identified on a radiographic examination and thereby help to build a differential diagnosis. After a radiologic differential diagnosis has been constructed, a clinical decision can be made as to further diagnostic workup.

In the interpretative process, the answers to a set of specific questions that more clearly define the radiologic abnormality can aid in forming a diagnosis. The order in which these questions are asked is not necessarily critical. Although each individual question may seem simple and not likely to elicit important information, the combination of questions and their subsequent answers are extremely enlightening.

An accurate clinical history is a critical component in the diagnostic process of identifying and characterizing an observed radiologic abnormality and developing a differential diagnosis. Whereas a clinical history aids in the interpretation of an examination, the radiologic history (previous film) is also an important tool that improves and contributes to the accuracy of observations. For example, a clinical history of dyspnea, cough, wheezing, pedal edema, and jugular venous distension would suggest the likelihood of finding signs of congestive heart failure on a chest radiograph. Or, a prominent hilum that might otherwise be dismissed as a normal variant would be re-evaluated as a probable mass in the light of an old film showing a normal hilum.

The *temporal history* of the abnormality should be assessed. A widened mediastinum on a chest radiograph has a large differential diagnosis, but knowing the chronicity or acuity of the finding limits the differential diagnosis. A chronically widened superior mediastinum unchanged over many years suggests a benign etiology, such as mediastinal lipomatosis. A newly widened superior mediastinum suggests a more acute process, such as lymphoma or metastatic adenopathy. An acutely widened mediastinum indicates a probable mediastinal hematoma, especially with the confirmatory clinical history of a recent line placement or an automobile accident.

Is the abnormality *solitary, multifocal,* or *diffuse?* For example, a solitary pulmonary nodule on a chest x-ray film has a vast differential diagnosis, but in a specific clinical situation (e.g., in a patient with a long smoking history and occupational exposure to asbestos), a primary lung carcinoma is very likely. However, if subsequent chest CT shows this solitary pulmonary opacity to be one of three pulmonary nodules, the differential diagnosis now suggests metastatic disease to the lung. Similarly, if a follow-up chest radiograph in 3 days demonstrates multiple nodular opacities and cavitation, the differential diagnosis would change again to include multiple septic emboli or granulomatous disease with cavitation.

What is the *density* (composition) of an abnormality? Although the internal composition of a lesion can sometimes be determined on a chest radiograph, chest CT or MRI can accomplish this task more accurately and is therefore indicated for this purpose. Five important internal tissue types may be easily identified on CT or MR scans:

1. Gas (cavitation)
2. Low-density material (lipid) (Fig. 11)
3. High-density material (hemorrhage)
4. Intermediate-density material (soft tissue)
5. Calcification

A lesion that exhibits *cavitation* may represent a lung abscess, a carcinoma with cavitation, or mycetoma. A lesion that is calcified might represent a calcified granuloma, if located centrally, or a lung carcinoma engulfing an adjacent calcified granuloma, if located eccentrically. A solitary lesion containing material of several types of density by CT suggests a hamartoma.

What are the *shape, size,* and *margins* of the lesion? For example, a defect that conforms to the shape of a segment of lung on a perfusion scan has considerably more significance than a perfusion defect with a shape that is either subsegmental or round in appearance. An earlier principle (solitary vs. multiple) is combined with the principle of shape and size, and the presence of multi-

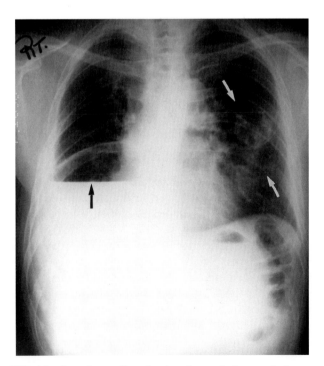

FIG. 14. A postoperative chest radiograph demonstrates an air-fluid level (*black arrow*) in the right pleural space following an open lung biopsy. In the left lung, two cavitary masses (*white arrows*) are identified. The masses, which waxed and waned during a period of months, were pathologically proved to be Wegner's granulomatosis.

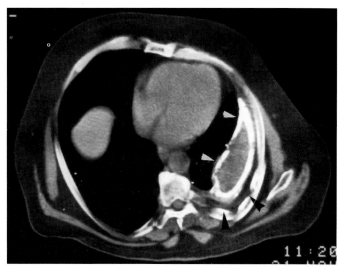

FIG. 15. A: A chest radiograph depicts a relatively small left hemithorax, pleural thickening, and extensive pleural calcification. **B:** Subsequent chest CT reveals calcification of the visceral (*white arrowheads*) and parietal pleura surrounding a high-density pleural effusion. The apparent pleural thickening on the chest radiograph is shown to be extensive subpleural fat (*black arrowheads*). Increased asymmetric subpleural fat associated with a pleural effusion is almost always indicative of an empyema, in this case a tuberculous empyema.

ple segmental defects on a perfusion lung scan without corresponding matches on a ventilation scan then changes the interpretation of the examination to a high probability for pulmonary embolus.

Similarly, the differential diagnosis for multiple bilateral rounded opacities is vastly different depending on the size of the opacities. When the radiologic differential diagnosis is broad, the clinical history becomes very important. A fine nodular pattern on a chest radiograph in a febrile patient suggests a differential diagnosis that includes fungal, tuberculous, nocardial, and viral infection, whereas in an afebrile patient the differential diagnosis includes sarcoidosis, inhalational disease, metastasis, and less common entities, such as eosinophilic pneumonia (Fig. 12).

It is also important to determine whether the margins of a lesion are sharply or poorly demarcated. A sharply demarcated lesion suggests encapsulation, whereas indistinct and fuzzy margins suggest a lesion that may be infiltrating into adjacent structures (Fig. 13). For example, multiple bilateral rounded opacities with poorly defined margins on a chest x-ray film suggest a differential diagnosis that includes inflammatory, neoplastic, connective tissue, vascular, occupational, iatrogenic, and idiopathic entities. Additional information, such as whether the opacities wax and wane, occasionally show cavitation, or are associated with febrile episodes, restricts the differential diagnosis to etiologies such as Wegener's or lymphomatoid granulomatosis (Fig. 14). Violation of anatomic boundaries usually suggests an aggressive process, although not necessarily a neoplasm. An abnormality located in the periphery of the lung with evidence of pleural

reaction and rib destruction might be caused by actinomycosis rather than carcinoma of the lung.

From what tissue does the abnormality originate? Specifically, does the lesion arise from the rib or pleura, or from the lung parenchyma, or from within a mediastinal structure? The characteristics of the margin of the lesion also yield important information. For example, a peripherally situated mass forming acute angles with the pleural surface suggests that the mass originates within the lung parenchyma, whereas the same mass forming obtuse angles suggests an origin in the pleura or chest wall.

Sometimes the anatomic location of an abnormality is easily determined from the chest radiograph, as in the case of rib destruction (implying that the abnormality is located in part in the pleural space and also in the chest wall). CT or MRI is usually required to obtain such information (Fig. 15).

Localizing an abnormality within a specific anatomic compartment is also extremely valuable when constructing a differential diagnosis. For example, if a mediastinal mass can be localized to the posterior mediastinum, or if interstitial lung disease is confined to the lung bases, then the differential diagnosis is further narrowed.

BIBLIOGRAPHY

Acquino SL, Webb WR, Gushiken BJ. Pleural exudates and transudates: diagnosis with contrast-enhanced CT. *Radiology* 1994;192: 803–808. *Parietal pleural thickening usually indicates the presence of a pleural exudate. In this study, all cases of empyema and approximately half the cases of parapneumonic effusion demonstrated pleural thickening.*
Benacerraf BR, McLoud TC, Rhea JT, Tritschler V, Libby P. An

assessment of the contribution of chest radiography in outpatients with acute chest complaints: a prospective study. *Radiology* 1981; 138:293–299. *A prospective study designed to identify selective indications, including symptoms, physical findings, and demographics, for adult chest radiography in an ambulatory clinic and an emergency room setting.*

Bessis L, Callard P, Gotheil C, Biaggi A, Grenier P. High-resolution CT of parenchymal lung disease: precise correlation with histologic findings. *Radiographics* 1992; 12:45–58. *A review illustrating and correlating high-resolution chest CT and histologic specimens obtained at autopsy.*

Brown LR, Aughenbaugh GL. Masses of the anterior mediastinum: CT and MR imaging. *AJR Am J Roentgenol* 1991; 157:1171–1180. *A review article discussing the indications, techniques, and findings as well as the relative merits of CT and MRI in the evaluation of anterior mediastinal masses.*

Brown MJ, Miller RR, Muller NL. Acute lung disease in the immunocompromised host: CT and pathologic examination findings. *Radiology* 1994; 190:247–254. *CT pattern of parenchymal abnormalities closely resembles the gross morphologic features identified on pathologic specimens. A nodular pattern is very suggestive of an infectious etiology in immunocompromised patients. The same etiology can appear as a nodular, ground-glass, and/or consolidative pattern.*

Buckley JA, Scott WW Jr, Siegelman SS, Kuhlman JE, Urban BA, Bluemke DA, Fishman EK. Pulmonary nodules: effect of increased data sampling on detection with spiral CT and confidence in diagnosis. *Radiology* 1995; 196:395–400. *A study demonstrating one of several advantages of spiral over conventional chest CT. The rate of detection of pulmonary nodules was increased and the false-positive detection rate was decreased in less experienced interpreters.*

Butcher BL, Nichol KL, Parenti CM. High yield of chest radiography in walk-in clinic patients with chest symptoms. *J Gen Intern Med* 1993; 8:114–119. *A prospective study of adult men in an ambulatory care setting with chief symptoms of cough, dyspnea, or pleuritic chest pain demonstrating clinically important new radiographic abnormalities in approximately 35% of patients regardless of past medical history, vital signs, or smoking history.*

Corcoran HL, Renner WR, Milstein MJ. Review of high-resolution CT of the lung. *Radiographics* 1992; 12:917. *The anatomy of the secondary pulmonary lobule is detailed and the patterns of findings on high-resolution chest CT are illustrated.*

Erdman WA, Peshock RM, Redman HC, Bonte F, Meyerson M, Jayson HT, Miller GL, Clarke GD, Parkey RW. Pulmonary embolism: comparison of MR images with radionuclide and angiographic studies. *Radiology* 1994; 190:499–508. *An investigation demonstrating accurate detection of large and medium-sized pulmonary emboli using MRI.*

Forman HP, Fox LA, Glazer HS, McClennan BL, Anderson DC, Sagel SS. Chest radiography in patients with early-stage prostatic carcinoma. *Chest* 1994; 106:1036–1041. *A retrospective study of routine preoperative chest radiographs in patients with prostate carcinoma, demonstrating a significant medical impact in a small number of patients. Cost effectiveness could not be confirmed because of, among other factors, sample size.*

Fortier M, Mayo JR, Swensen SJ, Munk PL, Vellet DA, Muller NL. MR imaging of chest wall lesions. *Radiographics* 1994; 14:597–606. *The appearance of both benign and malignant lesions of the chest wall is illustrated.*

Friedman PJ. Lung cancer staging: efficacy of CT. *Radiology* 1992; 182:307–309. *A recent editorial discussing the current role of chest CT in the management of mediastinal disease in patients with non-small-cell lung cancer.*

Grover FL. The role of CT and MRI in staging of the mediastinum. *Chest* 1994; 106:391S–396S. *A recent review of the literature discussing the sensitivity and specificity of CT and MRI in staging non-small-cell lung cancer in the mediastinum and the implications for surgical management.*

Harris JH (report from the chairman of the board). Referral criteria for routine screening chest x-ray examinations. *Am Coll Radiol Bull* 1982; 38:17. *A useful review.*

Hayabuchi N, Russell WJ, Murakami J. Problems in radiographic detection and diagnosis of lung cancer. *Acta Radiol* 1989; 30:163–167. *Errors in detecting lung cancer within a screening population (an abnormality was identified but thought to be some disease other than cancer) were related equally to perception and decision making. A higher index of suspicion would reduce decision-making errors.*

Heckerling PS, Tape TG, Wigton RS, Hissong KK, Leikin JB, Ornato JP, Cameron JL, Racht EM. Clinical prediction rule for pulmonary infiltrates. *Ann Intern Med* 1990; 113:664–670. *A study demonstrating that a prediction rule based on clinical findings accurately discriminates between patients with and without radiographic pneumonia.*

Heiken JP, Brink JA, Vannier MW. Spiral (helical) CT. *Radiology* 1993; 189:647–656. *The technical details of helical CT and their application to clinical CT scanning are reviewed.*

Henschke CI, Yankelevitz DF, Wand A, Davis SD, Shiau M. Accuracy and efficacy of chest radiography in the intensive care unit. *Radiol Clin North Am* 1996; 34:21–31. *A review of the technical aspects as well as the accuracy and efficacy of portable chest radiography in intensive care units. The diagnosis of specific conditions, such as pneumonia and pulmonary edema, and the utility of radiographic monitoring and therapeutic devices are considered.*

Hubbell FA, Greenfield S, Tyler JL, Chetty K, Wyle FA. The impact of routine admission chest x-ray films on patient care. *N Engl J Med* 1985; 312:209–213. *In a population with a high prevalence of cardiopulmonary disease, routine admission chest radiography had a very small impact on patient care.*

Jochelson MS, Altschuler J, Stomper PC. The yield of chest radiography in febrile and neutropenic patients. *Ann Intern Med* 1986; 105: 708–709. *A helpful review.*

Klein JS, Schultz S, Heffner JE. Interventional radiology of the chest: image-guided percutaneous drainage of pleural effusions, lung abscess, and pneumothorax. *AJR Am J Roentgenol* 1995; 164:581–588. *The role of percutaneous interventional procedures in a variety of chest abnormalities is reviewed.*

Kuhlman JE, Bouchard LM, Fishman EK, Zerhouni EA. CT and MR imaging evaluation of chest wall disorders. *Radiographics* 1994; 14:571. *The advantages of each modality in detecting and characterizing abnormalities of the chest wall is addressed. CT more readily demonstrates small calcifications and cortical bone destruction. MRI more accurately depicts bone marrow invasion and infiltration of soft tissues by masses.*

Leung AN, Staples CA, Muller NL. Chronic diffuse infiltrative lung disease: comparison of diagnostic accuracy of high-resolution and conventional CT. *AJR Am J Roentgenol* 1991; 157:693–696. *Only a few high-resolution CT scans obtained at three different levels are necessary to arrive at a level of accuracy comparable with that of complete conventional CT scans in evaluating chronic diffuse infiltrative disease.*

Line BR. Scintigraphic studies of inflammation in diffuse lung disease. *Radiol Clin North Am* 1991; 29:1095–1114. *Review of the mechanism of uptake and selective use of gallium 67 in the evaluation of diffuse lung disease.*

Link KM, Samuels LJ, Reed JC, Loehr SP, Lesko NM. Magnetic resonance imaging of the mediastinum. *J Thorac Imaging* 1993; 8:34–53. *A review of the applications of MRI in the mediastinum, including evaluation of solid and cystic masses, vascular applications, and assessment of lymphadenopathy.*

Mayo JR. Magnetic resonance imaging of the chest. *Radiol Clin North Am* 1994; 32:795–809. *A review of the indications for MRI, not only in the mediastinum but also in the cardiovascular system, chest wall, and lung parenchyma.*

McLoud TC, Bourgouin PM, Greenberg RW, Kosiuk JP, Templeton PA, Shepard JO, Moore EH, Wain JC, Mathisen DJ, Grillo HC. Bronchogenic carcinoma: analysis of staging in the mediastinum with CT by correlative lymph node mapping and sampling. *Radiology* 1992; 182:319–323. *A prospective study demonstrating that chest CT is an important adjunct in staging non-small-cell lung cancer in the mediastinum but does not eliminate the use of mediastinoscopy or thoracotomy.*

McLoud TC, Flower CDR. Imaging the pleura: sonography, CT, and MR imaging. *AJR Am J Roentgenol* 1991; 156:1145–1153. *Use of the three different imaging modalities in evaluating pleural abnormalities is reviewed.*

Mirvis SE, Bidwell JK, Buddemeyer EU, Diaconis JN, Pais SO,

Whitley JE, Goldstein LD. Value of chest radiography in excluding traumatic aortic rupture. *Radiology* 1987;163:487–493. *A retrospective review of 205 patients with blunt chest trauma, 45 of whom had proven aortic rupture. Although certain findings on conventional chest radiography were suggestive of aortic rupture, no single sign or combination of signs had a very high positive predictive value, but normal findings on examination did have a high negative predictive value.*

Muller NL. Differential diagnosis of chronic diffuse infiltrative lung disease on high-resolution computed tomography. *Semin Roentgenol* 1991;26:132–142. *A review describing and illustrating the basic radiologic features and signs used in interpreting high-resolution CT.*

Muller NL. Computed tomography in chronic interstitial lung disease. *Radiol Clin North Am* 1991;29:1085–1093. *A review discussing the CT appearance of a variety of common chronic interstitial lung diseases.*

Muller NL. Imaging of the pleura. *Radiology* 1993;186:297–309. *A review article summarizing the typical appearances of clinically important pleural abnormalities and the role of interventional radiology in their diagnosis and management.*

Naidich DP. Helical computed tomography of the thorax. *Radiol Clin North Am* 1994;32:759–774. *A review and illustration of the important applications of helical chest CT.*

Naidich DP, Marshall CH, Gribbin C, Arams RS, McCauley DI. Low-dose CT of the lungs: preliminary observations. *Radiology* 1990;175:729–731. *A preliminary study suggesting that low-dose CT of the lung parenchyma provides images of diagnostic quality.*

Padley SG, Brendan A, Muller NL. High-resolution computed tomography of the chest: current indications. *J Thorac Imaging* 1993;8: 189–199. *The current indications for high-resolution CT, including acute and chronic lung disease, pneumoconiosis, emphysema, and bronchiectasis, are addressed.*

Padovani B, Mouroux J, Seksik L, Chanalet S, Sedat J, Rotomondo C, Richelme H, Serres JJ. Chest wall invasion by bronchogenic carcinoma: evaluation with MR imaging. *Radiology* 1993;187:33–38. *The sensitivity of MRI was 90% and the specificity was 86% to detect invasion of the chest wall by bronchogenic lung cancer.*

PIOPED Investigators. Value of the ventilation-perfusion scan in acute pulmonary embolism. *JAMA* 1990;263:2753–2759. *Classic article reporting the findings of a multicenter trial to determine the sensitivity and specificity of ventilation-perfusion lung scans in the detection of pulmonary embolus.*

Potchen EJ, Bisesi MA. When is it malpractice to miss lung cancer on chest radiographs? *Radiology* 1990;175:29–32. *A commentary examining the elements of negligence, sources of errors, and observer performance.*

Quint LE, Francis IR, Wahl RL, Gross BH, Glazer GM. Preoperative staging of non-small-cell carcinoma of the lung: imaging methods. *AJR Am J Roengenol* 1995;164:1349–1359. *A review of the use of CT, MRI, and nuclear medicine in staging non-small-cell lung cancer, not only in the mediastinum and hilum but also in the chest wall and pleural space.*

Ralph DD. Pulmonary embolism. The implications of prospective investigation of pulmonary embolism diagnosis. *Radiol Clin North Am* 1994;32:679–687. *A coherent and thoughtful review of the PIOPED results and a cogent consideration of the implications for the diagnostic and therapeutic management of a patient with suspected pulmonary embolus.*

Remy-Jardin M, Duyck P, Remy J, Petyt L, Wurtz A, Mensier E, Copin MC, Riquet M. Hilar lymph nodes: identification with spiral CT and histologic correlation. *Radiology* 1995;196:387–394. *Review of the location and varying appearance of hilar lymphadenopathy and possible causes of misinterpretation of CT images.*

Rucker L, Frye EB, Staten MA. Usefulness of screening chest roentgenograms in preoperative patients. *JAMA* 1983;250:3209–3211. *In a retrospective study, a routine preoperative chest radiograph was not indicated for a select population <60 years of age having no significant risk factors and essentially negative findings on medical history, review of symptoms, and physical examination. However, 60% of the study population had at least one risk factor.*

Sagel SS, Evens RG, Forrest JV, Bramson RT. Efficacy of routine screening and lateral chest radiographs in a hospital-based population. *N Engl J Med* 1974;291:1001–1004. *A prospective study analyzing >10,000 examinations identified a lack of efficacy of routine (chest disease not considered associated with the patient's clinical condition) screening chest radiographs before hospital admission or scheduled surgery in patients <20 years of age and a lack of utility of the lateral projection in patients between 20 and 39 years of age.*

Samuel S, Kundel HL, Nodine CF, Toto LC. Mechanism of satisfaction of search: eye position recordings in the reading of chest radiographs. *Radiology* 1995;194:895–902. *A very intriguing investigation into the psychology of perception. Among the important conclusions is that obvious abnormalities capture visual attention and that their presence decreases the rate of detection of more subtle abnormalities.*

Shepard JO. Complications of percutaneous needle aspiration biopsy of the chest. *Semin Intervent Radiol* 1994;11:181–186. *A review discussing the variety of complications associated with percutaneous chest biopsy as well as possible techniques to reduce complication rates.*

Sostman HD, Coleman RE, DeLong DM, Newman GE, Paine S. Evaluation of revised criteria for ventilation-perfusion scintigraphy in patients with suspected pulmonary embolism. *Radiology* 1994;193:103–107. *With the more accurate, revised PIOPED criteria, experienced interpreters of ventilation-perfusion lung scans can increase their accuracy by using subjective judgment after applying formal criteria.*

Su WJ, Lee PY, Perng RP. Chest roentgenographic guidelines in the selection of patients for fiberoptic bronchoscopy. *Chest* 1993;103: 1198–1201. *The positive diagnostic yield of fiberoptic bronchoscopy in patients with abnormal chest radiographic findings demonstrating lobar collapse, hilar abnormalities, pericardial effusion, pleural effusion, or a mass lesion >4 cm was significantly greater than in patients with a mass lesion <4 cm, suggesting that a diagnosis should be made by percutaneous biopsy in these subjects.*

Swenson SJ, Aughenbaugh GL, Douglas WW, Myers JL. High-resolution CT of the lungs: findings in various pulmonary diseases. *AJR Am J Roentgenol* 1992;158:971–979. *The technical aspects of high-resolution CT and the appearances of commonly identified pulmonary diseases are reviewed.*

Touliopoulos P, Costello P. Helical (spiral) CT of the thorax. *Radiol Clin North Am* 1995;33:843–861. *A current review discussing the important advances provided by helical chest CT in the evaluation of solitary pulmonary nodules, metastatic lung disease, aortic dissection, pulmonary embolus, and the airways.*

Trerotola SO. Can helical CT replace aortography in thoracic trauma? *Radiology* 1994;197:13–15. *An editorial discussing the diagnostic controversies related to traumatic thoracic aortic injury.*

Tsai TW, Gallagher EJ, Lombardi G, Gennis P, Carter W. Guidelines for the selective ordering of admission chest radiography in adult obstructive airway disease. *Ann Emerg Med* 1993;22:1854–1858. *An unselected, nonconsecutive study population of patients requiring admission for exacerbation of chronic obstructive pulmonary disease classified as uncomplicated did not benefit from routine admission chest radiography.*

vanSonnenberg E, Casola G, Ho M, Neff CC, Varney RR, Wittich GR, Christensen R, Friedman PJ. Difficult thoracic lesions: CT-guided biopsy experience in 150 subjects. *Radiology* 1988;167: 457–461. *The authors obtained diagnostic material in approximately 83% of their patients, with a pneumothorax complication rate of approximately 43%.*

vanSonnenberg E, D'Agostino HB, Casola G, Wittich GR, Varney RR, Harker C. Lung abscess: CT-guided drainage. *Radiology* 1991;178:347–351. *The clinical indications for percutaneous drainage of lung abscess are addressed, along with technical considerations.*

Wandtke JC. Bedside chest radiography. *Radiology* 1994;190:1–10. *The issues of efficacy, film quality, standards of practice, and potential for improvement through the use of computed radiology (CR) are considered.*

Webb WR. High-resolution lung computed tomography. *Radiol Clin North Am* 1991;29:1051–1063. *An analysis of normal lung anatomy and abnormal lung pathology, with emphasis on their appearance on high-resolution CT.*

Wernly JA, Kirchner PT, Oxford DE. Clinical value of quantitative ventilation-perfusion lung scans in the surgical management of bronchogenic carcinoma. *J Thorac Cardiovasc Surg* 1980;80: 535–543. *The importance of preoperative (pneumonectomy) quantification of expected postoperative pulmonary function values in patients with marginal (1-second forced expiratory volume <2.0L) preoperative pulmonary function values is addressed, and the ability of perfusion lung imaging to predict postoperative pulmonary function accurately is demonstrated.*

Worsley DF, Alvai A, Aronchick JM, Chen JTT, Greenspan RH, Ravin CE. Chest radiographic findings in patients with acute pulmonary embolism: observations from the PIOPED study. *Radiology* 1993;189:133–136. *Westermark's sign, Fleischner's sign, Hampton hump, and a variety of other findings on conventional chest radiographs were all poor predictors of pulmonary embolus.*

Zerbey AL, Dawson SL, Mueller PR. Pleural interventions and complications. *Semin Intervent Radiol* 1994;11:187–197. *A discussion of the management of pleural disorders using interventional techniques.*

Zerhouni EA, Boukadoum M, Siddiky MA, Newbold JM, Stone DC, Shirey MP, Spivey JF, Hesselman CW, Leo FP, Stitik, Siegelman SS. A standard phantom for quantitative CT analysis of pulmonary nodules. *Radiology* 1983;149:767–773. *The ability to distinguish between benign and malignant solitary pulmonary nodules is enhanced with use of a phantom.*

Textbook of Pulmonary Diseases, 6th ed.
edited by G.L. Baum, J.D. Crapo, B.R. Celli, and J.B. Karlinsky,
Lippincott–Raven Publishers, Philadelphia, © 1998.

CHAPTER

9 ◆ Pulmonary Function Testing

Robert O. Crapo

INTRODUCTION

Pulmonary function tests are widely used to provide objective measures of lung function for (1) detecting and quantifying pulmonary impairment in cardiopulmonary diseases; (2) following the evolution of diseases and monitoring response to therapy; (3) monitoring the effects of environmental, occupational, and drug exposures associated with lung injury; (4) assessing preoperative risk; and (5) assessing disability and impairment. This chapter focuses on the practical pulmonary function tests that are of most use in day-to-day clinical medicine.

The steps in gas exchange from ambient air to cell (Table 1) help put pulmonary function testing in perspective. As respiratory gases move by passive diffusion, optimal concentrations of oxygen (O_2) and carbon dioxide (CO_2) in alveolar gas are necessary to transfer them to and from pulmonary capillary blood. The alveolar environment for gas transfer is established by alveolar ventilation, a function of the bellows action of the lung. Many lung function tests (static lung volumes, spirometry, airways resistance, and respiratory muscle function) characterize the mechanical aspects of the air pump. By themselves, they do not prove that gas exchange is either normal or abnormal. The second step in gas exchange, gas transfer from the alveolar air to blood, is traditionally assessed with carbon monoxide (CO) diffusing capacity (transfer factor) and arterial blood gas measurements. Diffusing capacity is an indirect test, whereas arterial blood

R. O. Crapo: Department of Medicine, University of Utah School of Medicine, and Pulmonary Laboratory, LDS Hospital, Salt Lake City, Utah 84143.

gases allow a more direct assessment of O_2 loading and CO_2 removal from blood. Assessing gas transport and gas transfer from blood to cells involves evaluation of arterial and mixed venous blood gases, cardiac output, and end-organ function (usually brain and kidney function). These aspects of gas transfer are usually the focus of the intensive care unit and are not directly assessed in traditional pulmonary function laboratories.

Control of breathing can be assessed by measuring the ventilatory response to progressive hypercarbia or hypoxemia, but these tests are uncommonly used in clinical practice. The final element in practical lung function testing is measuring cardiac and respiratory responses to exercise. Because exercise stresses the entire heart, lung, and blood system, exercise testing provides an opportunity to tease out the factors leading to dyspnea and impaired exercise capacity. Exercise testing is covered in Chapter 10. Reference sources for exercise are also included in this chapter's reference list.

Lung function tests are different from most other medical tests in that many of them require patients to participate actively and vigorously. Test quality depends on coaching every patient to an acceptable, vigorous effort. My own experience in evaluating pulmonary function laboratories suggests that it is not uncommon to find poor test quality in more than half of the studies at an initial evaluation. It is also not uncommon to see dramatic improvement in test quality after the staff has been trained to recognize quality tests and encouraged to coach more vigorous effort. Even when test quality is carefully controlled, some patients are unable to perform the tests. In a general population study, in which test quality was carefully controlled, Hankinson and colleagues found

TABLE 1. *Gas exchange between the atmosphere and body cells: gas transport system steps*

Step	Purpose	Structure(s)	Tests to characterize structure or function
Ventilation	Maintain normal alveolar O_2 and CO_2 pressures (PaO_2 and $PaCO_2$)	Air pump (lungs, chest wall, and neuromuscular apparatus)	$PaCO_2$, spirometry, lung volumes, airways resistance, respiratory muscle strength
Gas transfer (lungs)	Transfer of gases between alveolar air and pulmonary capillary blood	Alveolar capillary membrane	Arterial blood gases (PaO_2 and $PaCO_2$), alveolar-arterial PO_2 gradient [$P(A-a)O_2$], oxygen content, carbon monoxide diffusing capacity
Circulation	Delivery of O_2 from the lungs to the systemic capillaries and CO_2 from the systemic capillaries to the lungs	Blood pump (heart and blood)	Heart function (e.g., cardiac output, oxygen content, oxygen delivery)
Gas transfer (periphery)	Transfer of gases between systemic capillaries and metabolizing cells	Systemic capillary membranes and metabolizing cells	Difficult to assess. Tests of end-organ function (e.g., central nervous system and renal function) provide regional information and are the best clinical indicators. Lactic acidosis may occur with tissue hypoxemia but is not a definite indicator of its presence.

about 85% of more than 6000 spirometry studies met American Thoracic Society (ATS) standards of quality. Individual pulmonary laboratories can institute quality control measures and, with modest effort, bring their test quality to these standards.

STATIC LUNG VOLUMES

The static lung volume subdivisions, illustrated in Fig. 1, are grouped into volumes and capacities. Volumes, the primary subdivisions, cannot be subdivided. Capacities contain two or more volumes and, therefore, can be subdivided. Total lung capacity (TLC), the volume of air in the lungs at the end of a maximal inspiration, is attained when maximal inspiratory muscle force is counterbalanced by the recoil forces of the lung and chest wall. The

maximal volume of air that can be exhaled after a maximal inhalation is vital capacity (VC). Vital capacity can be measured with either an inspiratory or an expiratory maneuver and with either an unforced, slow exhalation (SVC) or a nearly maximally forced maneuver (FVC). The volume of air remaining in the lungs after a maximal exhalation is residual volume (RV). RV is determined by the balance of the forces tending to reduce lung volume (maximal expiratory muscle force and inward lung recoil) against the force tending to increase lung volume (outward recoil of the chest wall). Tidal volume (VT) is the volume of air moved with each breath during normal breathing. Functional residual capacity (FRC) is usually defined as the volume of air in the lungs at the end of a quiet, relaxed exhalation, although it is sometimes used to indicate the volume of air in the lungs at the end of a

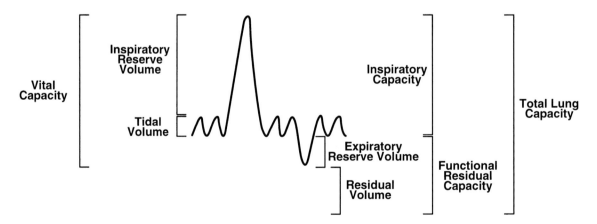

FIG. 1. Lung volumes and capacities. Volumes cannot be subdivided. Capacities contain two or more volumes. (Reproduced with permission from Aldose MD. Practical aspects of pulmonary function testing. In: Baum GL, Wolinsky E, eds. *Textbook of Pulmonary Diseases.* Boston: Little, Brown; 1993.)

tidal breath regardless of whether exhalation is active or passive. Inspiratory capacity (IC) is the maximal volume of air that can be inhaled from FRC. Expiratory reserve volume (ERV) is the maximal volume of air that can be exhaled from FRC. IC and ERV have little role in diagnostic testing, although ERV is the most commonly reduced lung volume in the morbidly obese.

The displaceable lung volumes—those that can be inhaled and exhaled from the mouth—are measured with a spirometer. Two types of spirometer are schematically illustrated and described in Fig. 2. The parameters measurable with a spirometer are vital capacity, tidal volume, inspiratory capacity, and expiratory reserve volume (Fig. 1). The remaining volumes and capacities contain residual volume, which cannot be measured with a spirometer. Plethysmographic, gas dilution, and radiographic techniques each measure one of the capacities that contains residual volume. Once measured, this capacity can be combined with the appropriate displaceable volumes to calculate all the remaining lung volumes and capacities. The following descriptions are brief overviews. The reader is directed to the reference list for more detailed descriptions of the tests and how they are performed.

A

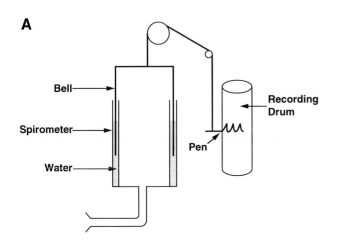

B

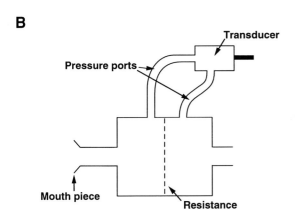

FIG. 2. Two types of spirometers. **A:** Volume-based spirometer that uses water as a seal. Air blown into the spirometer causes the bell to rise, inscribing the height of a cylinder and, therefore, volume. Time is also recorded to allow measurement of volumes as a function of time. As volume is the primary measurement, flows are derived by differentiating the volume-time information. **B:** Flow-based spirometer. Air is blown across a resistor; differential pressures measured across the resistor are related to flow. As flow (volume/time) is the primary measurement, it must be integrated to get volumes. (Reproduced with permission from Aldose MD. Practical aspects of pulmonary function testing. In: Baum GL, Wolinsky E, eds. *Textbook of Pulmonary Diseases.* Boston: Little, Brown; 1993.)

Gas Dilution Techniques

Gas dilution techniques measure the gas volume in the lungs that communicates via the airways. Although the techniques vary in details, all use a mass balance approach to calculate lung volume. The most common approach is schematically illustrated in Fig. 3. The patient is allowed to breathe from a known volume and concentration of a relatively insoluble and inert tracer gas [e.g., helium (He)]. Mixing is allowed to occur for a variable length of time, and the final mixed concentration of tracer gas is measured. A mass balance equation uses the initial volume and tracer gas concentration and the final tracer gas concentration to calculate the volume present in the patient's lungs at the moment tracer gas breathing began. The assumptions that the tracer gas is relatively insoluble and inert and is well mixed in lung air are critical. Use of a relatively soluble gas would cause lung volumes to be overestimated; incomplete gas mixing would cause them to be underestimated. In the case of the He rebreathing method, the patient quietly rebreathes from the test circuit for 4 to 7 min, with occasional deep breaths, until gas measurements demonstrate the concentration of He in the circuit is stable, indicating complete mixing in lung air. The long rebreathing time (up to 7 min) allows complete mixing of He in the circuit, but it also means that CO_2 has to be removed from and O_2 added to the circuit to ensure patient safety and comfort.

A gas dilution measurement of TLC (usually reported as alveolar volume, or V_A) accompanies every measurement of the single-breath CO diffusing capacity test. In this test, subjects inhale a VC-sized volume of gas that contains about 10% He, 0.3% CO, and 17%–21% O_2, hold their breath for 10 sec, and then exhale. An alveolar gas sample is analyzed to get the diluted alveolar He concentration. The assumption that He is completely mixed during the 10-sec breath-hold is reasonably acceptable in healthy individuals; for healthy people, TLC is only minimally underestimated compared with the multibreath technique. In patients with airway obstruction, mixing becomes less complete as obstruction worsens, and TLC is progressively underestimated. Therefore,

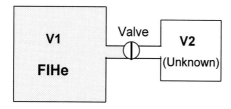 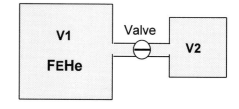

V1, FIHe, and FEHe are measured   VTotal = V1 + V2

$$FIHe \times V1 = FEHe \times VTotal$$

$$\frac{FIHe}{FEHe} \times V1 = VTotal$$

$$V2 = VTotal - V1$$

FIG. 3. Schematic illustration of the basic theory of gas dilution measurement of lung volume. Air in a subject's lungs is allowed to come into equilibrium with a known mass of a relatively insoluble and inert gas, such as He. Initial volume (V_1) and He concentration (FIHe) are known. The diluted, final He concentration (FEHe) is used to calculate the unknown volume (V_2).

in patients with airway obstruction, the single-breath technique has little utility as a technique for measuring TLC.

Nitrogen (N_2) washout techniques also use a mass balance approach to estimate TLC. In the multibreath N_2 washout method, the subject begins breathing 100% O_2 at FRC. O_2 is breathed until N_2 is displaced from the lungs, and the mass of displaced N_2 is measured. FRC is calculated assuming (1) that the mass of displaced N_2 is equal to the mass of N_2 in the lungs at the beginning of the test, and (2) that the initial concentration of N_2 in the lungs was 80%. TLC is estimated as FRC + IC (Fig. 1). N_2 washout techniques also underestimate TLC when airway obstruction is present.

Plethysmography

Plethysmography is used to measure lung volumes and airway resistances. For lung volumes, plethysmography measures the compressible gas volume in the chest using Boyle's Law: the product of gas volume and pressure is a constant ($V_1 \times P_1 = k$) when temperature is held constant. The test is performed by having the patient sit in a sealed box and pant gently against a closed shutter located at the mouth. During the inspiratory phase of the panting maneuver, the thoracic volume increases, slightly decompressing the volume of air in the lungs while compressing the air in the box. In the expiratory phase of the panting maneuver, thoracic gas volume decreases slightly, compressing the air in the lungs and decompressing box air. By Boyle's Law,

$$V_1 \times P_1 = V_2 \times P_2$$

The initial pressure and volume at FRC (the beginning volume before panting) are P_1 and V_1. Pressure and volume at the end of the inspiratory phase of the pant are P_2 and V_2, which can be rewritten as $(P_1 + \Delta P) \times (V_1 + \Delta V)$. P_1 and ΔP are measured at the mouth, assuming that mouth pressure is equal to alveolar pressure, and ΔV is measured using the change in box pressure. The equation can then be solved for V_1.

Body plethysmography is still considered the "gold standard" of techniques used to measure static lung volumes. It is, however, sensitive to technical and procedural errors and, like all other lung volume techniques, requires exquisite attention to quality control. For example, the assumption that mouth pressure equals box pressures tends to fail when panting frequency exceeds one pant/sec, because there is inadequate time for the pressure changes at the mouth to equilibrate with alveolar pressure. This is a particular problem in patients with airway obstruction, in whom rapid panting causes a significant overestimation of TLC.

When plethysmographic and single-breath gas dilution measurements of TLC are made during the same test session, the difference between the two ($TLC_{PL} - TLC_{GAS}$) can be used as an estimate of the poorly ventilated gas volume in the lungs, commonly referred to as trapped gas. The volume of trapped gas is increased in the presence of airway obstruction.

Radiographic Total Lung Capacity

TLC can also be estimated from standard posteroanterior and lateral chest radiographs. A radiographic TLC measurement starts with a calculation of total intrathoracic gas volume, from which estimated volumes for the mediastinum, heart, blood, and diaphragm are subtracted. Several studies show excellent correlation between radiographic TLC and plethysmographic TLC in healthy individuals and those with airway obstruction. The advantages of radiographic measurement of TLC are that the methodology is simple, requires no special equipment, and takes little time. However, chest radiographs solely for measuring TLC cannot be justified, even though the radiation exposure is small. Luckily, chest radiographs are often available because they are commonly included in evaluations for respiratory diseases. In addition, the radiographic method can be used to re-create a history of TLC. Old chest radiographs often provide the only source of lung volume information from a patient's past. They can provide evidence of change in a patient whose loss of lung volume would otherwise not have been detectable. This advantage is being compromised by the current trend to destroy radiographs earlier.

The radiographic TLC method has not yet been proved accurate in patients with interstitial lung diseases, and test variability is larger than for other methods. Chest structures are magnified slightly on chest radiographs. Published methods usually use a magnification factor based on a target-film distance of 72 inches (183 cm). For other target-film distances, the magnification factors differ and must be computed by the reader.

Pathophysiologic Correlates with Lung Volumes

The three basic patterns of lung volumes illustrated in Fig. 4 are normal, overinflation (too large), and restriction (too small). In the normal pattern, TLC, VC, and RV fall within a reference range based on healthy people. RV in the young constitutes about 25% of TLC, and FRC about 40%. With aging, lung recoil decreases causing a slight shift in the pattern of air flow toward one of obstruction. With aging, TLC remains essentially unchanged, RV increases, and FRC either increases slightly or does not change. RV increases with aging primarily because the slight shift toward an obstructive pattern makes it impossible for a true expiratory plateau to be reached and RV becomes a dynamic measurement, dependent on expiratory time.

Diseases that alter the elastic properties of either the chest wall or lungs may alter lung volumes. Diseases such as emphysema reduce lung recoil and may cause TLC, FRC, and RV to be increased, even when minimal airflow obstruction is present. In emphysema, airway obstruction commonly accompanies decreased lung recoil, and both contribute to overinflation. Mechanically, airway obstruction leads to the initiation of inspiration before expiration is complete; overinflation follows. The process is exacerbated when respiratory rate increases, causing expiratory time to be shortened. Asthma is a classic illustration of a disease with overinflation secondary to airflow obstruction. There is also evidence in asthma that inspiratory muscle activity persists throughout expiration, contributing to overinflation.

Overinflation is primarily determined by an elevated TLC. Other patterns may be used to suggest the presence of overinflation, but one should be cautious in calling overinflation when TLC is within the normal range. The suggestive patterns are an elevated RV or the presence of significant gas trapping.

Lung volumes may be reduced (restriction) in any disease process that increases lung recoil (e.g., pulmonary

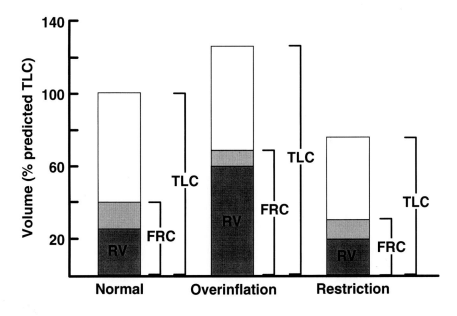

FIG. 4. The three basic lung volume patterns: normal, overinflation (too large), and restriction (too small). (Reproduced with permission from Aldose MD. Practical aspects of pulmonary function testing. In: Baum GL, Wolinsky E, eds. *Textbook of Pulmonary Diseases.* Boston: Little, Brown; 1993.)

fibrosis), compresses the lungs (pleural effusion), decreases chest wall compliance (kyphoscoliosis, morbid obesity), alters the shape of the chest (kyphoscoliosis), or decreases respiratory muscle function (neuromuscular diseases, diaphragmatic paralysis).

TLC is also the primary variable used to determine the presence of restriction. Technically, the presence of restriction can be determined only by a reduction in TLC. From a practical standpoint, however, a reduced VC in the absence of airway obstruction has proved to be an excellent predictor of restriction and is an inexpensive, simple parameter to monitor change in patients with restrictive diseases. When both TLC and VC are measured and one is low and the other normal, decisions to classify the presence of restriction should default to TLC. The default to TLC assumes there is no evidence that TLC is underestimated because of technical problems.

DYNAMIC TESTS OF LUNG FUNCTION

Spirometry

Spirometry, which can include both quiet and forced VC maneuvers, is the most common and useful of the lung function tests. Its clinical utility has been proved extensively, it is the least expensive test to perform, and it should be the test most widely available in doctors' offices, clinics, and hospitals. The FVC test is performed by having a patient inhale to TLC and then make a maximally forced exhalation into a spirometer. Classically, exhaled volume is measured as a function of time. Flow may also be measured and displayed as a function of

exhaled volume. The three primary spirometric indices in the forced test are FVC, forced expiratory volume in 1 second (FEV_1), and their ratio, FEV_1/FVC. Numerous other spirometric measures are available, but their clinical utility is less well established. Typical volume-time and flow-volume spirographic displays for a healthy individual are shown in Fig. 5.

Test quality depends on achieving a maximal inhalation, a nearly maximal effort during the initial few seconds of exhalation, and a complete exhalation. A complete exhalation is indicated by a plateau in the volume-time tracing; a minimum expiratory time of 6 sec is recommended. A plateau is rarely reached in individuals with airflow obstruction or in healthy older people who have reduced airflow at low lung volumes because of the normal age-related loss of lung recoil. Because expiratory flow never truly reaches a plateau in these individuals, VC increases and FEV_1/VC falls with increased expiratory time. The effect of expiratory time on the FEV_1/VC ratio is minimized if expiratory time lasts at least 10 seconds or if SVC is used rather than FVC.

Syncope may occur, even in healthy subjects, when maximal expiratory force is exerted throughout the entire maneuver. Recent evidence suggests that spirogram quality is not be altered if patients are allowed to reduce their expiratory effort after about 3 seconds and continue to exhale without squeezing hard.

Detailed standards for quality control published by the ATS and the European Respiratory Society (ERS) are outlined in Fig. 6. The first step is to acquire a spirometer that has been demonstrated to meet accuracy standards. Although this statement seems flagrantly obvious, a study

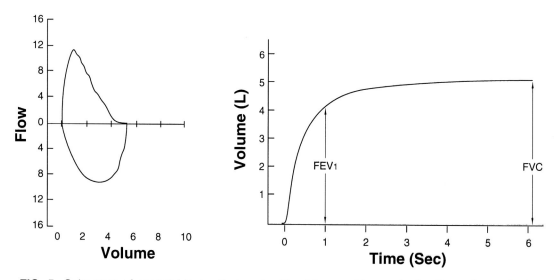

FIG. 5. Spirogram of acceptable quality in a healthy 54-year-old man. In the flow-volume display, markers of good quality include a quick start with a rapid rise in expiratory flow, a well-defined peak flow, the absence of a cough or hesitation in the early portion of the spirogram, and an exhalation that exceeds 6 seconds. The slight tail at the end of exhalation and the continued increase in volume even after 6 seconds of exhalation (volume-time tracing) reflect normal age-related changes.

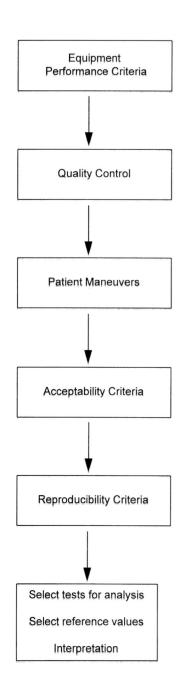

Measure volumes within ±3% or 50 ml whichever is greater; flows within ± 5% or 200 ml/s using standard waveforms. Validate accuracy.

Check accuracy and linearity daily with a calibrated 3.0 liter syringe. Test a technician weekly as a biologic control.

Explain and demonstrate the maneuver
Position the patient properly
Repeat tests with additional coaching until 3 acceptable tests are obtained or the patient has made 8 attempts

Good, quick start with vigorous effort
No cough or pause in the first second
A satisfactory end of test - 6 second minimum or a good plateau without a glottic closure

From 3 acceptable tests, the difference between the largest two FVC's and the largest two FEV1's should be within 200 ml of each other

Analyze largest FVC and FEV1 from among the acceptable tests.
Select reference values appropriate for your patient clientele
Use established guidelines for interpretation

FIG. 6. Summary of ATS recommended steps to assure good-quality spirometric measurements. The same steps can be modified slightly to ensure good quality of all other pulmonary function tests. (Modified and reproduced with permission from Crapo RO, Chair. Standardization of spirometry: 1994 update. Official statement of the ATS. *Am J Respir Crit Care Med* 1995;152:1107−1136).

of more than 50 instruments on the market in the early 1980s found that only about half met ATS accuracy standards. The problems have largely been corrected, and most but not all commercially marketed spirometers now meet accuracy standards. Care should still be taken to be certain of the accuracy of a spirometer before purchase. Once in use, spirometers need regular quality control checks to ensure proper performance. Such checks are especially important after an instrument has been serviced or upgraded.

As instrumentation has improved, the major quality issues now have to do with how the tests are performed. Test quality includes acceptability criteria for each effort and reproducibility criteria for the series of tests per-

formed (Fig. 6). Current standards require that at least three acceptable quality spirograms be obtained. The reproducibility criteria are then applied to the acceptable spirograms to ensure that the data are representative of the patient (Fig. 6). If spirograms of acceptable quality do not meet reproducibility criteria, the patient should be asked to perform the test again. If both the acceptability and reproducibility criteria are not met in eight tries, it is unlikely that they will be with further tests, and the study may be terminated. Efforts to improve the procedural aspects of spirometry include immediate computerized analysis of each test waveform with feedback to the technician about test quality, often with a statement about how to correct problems. Computer displays have also been created to help motivate patients to make good efforts.

Acceptability and reproducibility criteria are ideal targets for the quality of test performance. Even suboptimal tests may provide some useful information, and patient data should not be discarded only because of failure to meet acceptability and reproducibility criteria. The best data available should be submitted for interpretation, and the interpretation should deal with the limitations. Often, partial information can be gleaned from a less-than-optimal test. For example, a test with completely inadequate initial effort still may yield a VC if a reasonable end of test is achieved. Failure to meet acceptability criteria in an individual test occurs for a variety of reasons, including inability or unwillingness of a patient to perform the test, even with vigorous coaching. Failure to meet reproducibility criteria in an individual test may also indicate the presence of hyperreactive airways. Frequent test failures in a laboratory indicate the presence of quality control problems.

Most quality issues are the responsibility of the laboratory and its director, but clinicians who use pulmonary function tests in their medical practice should be able to recognize good-quality tests as well as various disease patterns. Spirograms should be analyzed for quality by visually inspecting both flow-volume and volume-time displays. Typical good-quality spirograms along with several faulty spirogram patterns are illustrated in Figs. 5, 7, and 8.

Full spirometry should include both FVC (forced) and SVC (unforced) maneuvers. SVC is often larger than FVC, especially in older persons and those with airway obstruction, in whom the forced maneuver effectively causes some air trapping. If the unforced maneuver is excessively slow, VC will be underestimated. The largest VC found during testing, whether from the forced or the unforced maneuver, should be used to calculate the FEV_1/VC ratio.

For studies that meet acceptability and reproducibility standards, the next question is choosing which measurements to use for interpretation. In general, selecting only from acceptable tests, the largest FVC, FEV_1, and peak flow are used for interpretative purposes; they need not come from the same trial. If midflows (e.g., $FEF_{25\%-75\%}$) or instantaneous flows (e.g., $V_{max50\%}$) are used for interpretation, they should be selected from the single, acceptable-quality spirogram that has the largest sum of FVC and FEV_1. Average ($FEF_{25\%-75\%}$) and instantaneous flow ($V_{max50\%}$) variables should be used only to assist in decision making when the primary indices (FVC, FEV_1, FEV_1/VC) are close to the lower limits of their normal ranges. Average and instantaneous flows have limited clinical utility and are not discussed further here.

Pathophysiologic Correlations with Spirometry

From a diagnostic standpoint, spirometry is used only to classify patients as having one of three patterns: nor-

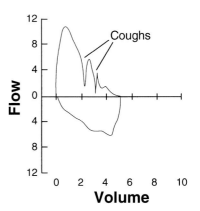

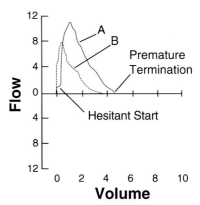

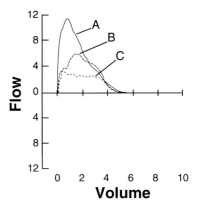

FIG. 7. Several types of faulty spirograms. **Top panel:** Multiple coughs begin early in exhalation (before 1 second). Coughs are characterized by sudden falls in flow followed by quick restoration of flow. Early coughs may cause FEV_1 to be underestimated. **Middle panel:** A hesitant start (waveform A) could cause FEV_1 to be overestimated, and a premature termination of exhalation would cause FVC to be underestimated. Waveform B, from the same patient, illustrates an inadequate inhalation followed by a good expiratory effort. Alone, the curve would be graded acceptable; it is unacceptable when compared with waveform A. **Bottom panel:** Nonreproducible tracings. Waveform A is an acceptable tracing. Waveforms B and C show two different but submaximal initial efforts. FEV_1 may be underestimated with the submaximal efforts; FVC may be acceptable in all tracings depending on the presence of an adequate inhalation and end of test.

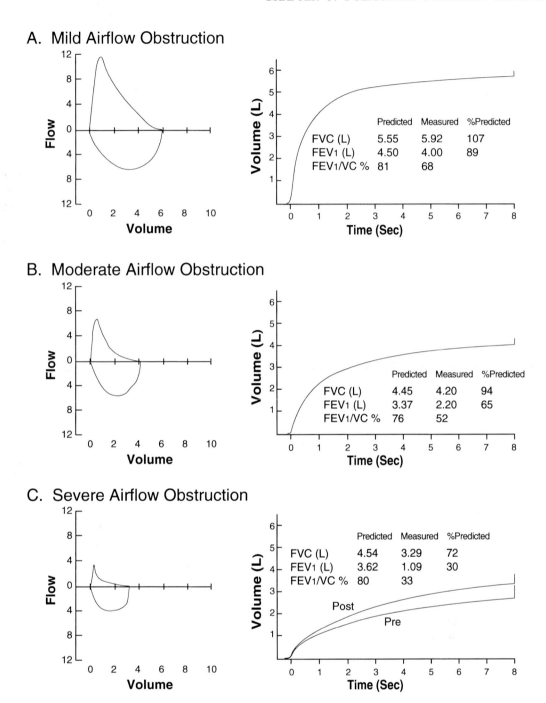

FIG. 8. Typical spirograms for mild, moderate, and severe airway obstruction. Note that with increasing obstruction, the flow-volume tracings show increasing concavity toward the horizontal axis. The *bottom panel* contains prebronchodilator and postbronchodilator tracings, illustrating a good response to administration of an inhaled bronchodilator.

mal, airflow obstruction, and restriction. Specific diagnoses cannot be made with spirometry alone; spirometry patterns must be interpreted according to the clinical questions being asked. The interpretation of spirometry is discussed in detail in the section below on interpretation.

Maximum Voluntary Ventilation

Maximum voluntary ventilation (MVV) is the maximum amount of air that a person can exhale while breathing as fast and deep as possible with vigorous coaching. It is measured over 12 to 15 sec and expressed as L/min at BTPS (body temperature, ambient pressure, and saturated with water vapor) conditions. Test duration is short, because people cannot sustain the MVV maneuver much beyond 15 sec. It is often estimated rather than measured by multiplying the FEV_1 by 35 or the $FEV_{0.75}$ by 40. An optimal test is somewhat hard to describe, because V_T decreases as respiratory rate increases. As a general rule, the peak MVV in healthy subjects occurs at a respiratory rate close to 100 breaths/min with a V_T about 35% of VC. There is, however, not much variation in MVV for respiratory frequencies from 70 to 120/min.

The MVV is a nonspecific test. Reductions in MVV occur in the presence of airway obstruction and chest restriction associated with neuromuscular diseases, loss of coordination, and diminished cognitive function. It may also be reduced because the subject is unwilling to work maximally during the test, as may occur in elderly patients, those with chronic illness, and individuals for whom a poor test result promises secondary gain. Because it is so nonspecific, the clinical utility of MVV is limited. One could, however, argue that the nonspecific nature of the test might also be an advantage in some instances. Reductions in MVV correlate well with postoperative risks for respiratory complications and with dyspnea from any cause. If measured MVV is significantly below calculated MVV, one can tentatively speculate that nonpulmonary factors are involved in the reduction.

The MVV is often used in exercise studies to estimate ventilatory reserve. The common practice of using an estimated MVV for this purpose is problematic, because the normal between-individual variation in measured MVV is large and because there are so many variables besides FEV_1 that affect MVV.

Peak Expiratory Flow and Peak Flow Meters

Peak expiratory flow (PEF) is the maximum flow achieved during an FVC maneuver. It occurs very early in the FVC maneuver (usually within the first 0.2 sec if the maneuver is well performed). This places the measurement in the most effort-dependent portion of the FVC maneuver. Thus, PEF is significantly more effort-dependent than FEV_1, and of less clinical utility from that aspect. The value of PEF in clinical medicine derives from the availability of small, easily portable, highly reproducible, inexpensive peak flow meters. The meters are acceptably accurate but are less accurate than good spirometers. Reproducibility is excellent for individual PEF meters, but there is less reproducibility between meters and there can be marked differences among different PEF meter models. The low cost and reproducibility of PEF meters makes them a practical monitoring device for patients with asthma. Because asthma symptoms and physical findings are imperfect indicators of the severity of asthma, the addition of a relatively inexpensive, objective assessment of lung function is attractive. Monitoring information from PEF meters is of two basic types: (1) trending over days to months, and (2) trending across a day. Increased variability across a day (>20%) indicates airway hyperreactivity and may be an indication of diminished asthma control or a reaction to a provocative stimulus (asthma trigger). At the present time, PEF meters should not be used diagnostically to define normal or abnormal function, because there are no reference values that are applicable to all PEF meter models.

Peak flow meters can be used to track response to medication, monitor the course of asthma, and quantify the effects of exposures to potential triggers or other environmental factors. In numerous national and international guidelines, peak flow meters are used to structure individualized asthma management plans. In the midst of all the enthusiasm for PEF meters, a small note of caution must be sounded. At present, the role of PEF meters in the management of asthma is largely based on reasonable suppositions; there is little science to document exactly what their benefits are and who should be using them.

Bronchodilator Administration and Testing

In patients with airway obstruction, it is common practice to perform spirometry before and after the administration of an inhaled, rapidly acting β_2-selective agonist. The test is performed by obtaining baseline spirometry, administering the bronchodilator medication, waiting a brief period (usually about 15 min), and then repeating the spirometry. The 15-min wait is conservative; some studies suggest 5 min is enough. The test is best performed with a spirometer but can be done with a peak flow meter. An improvement in FEV_1 of 12% and 200 mL is considered an unequivocally positive response. There is, however, some controversy on how to calculate the percentage of change. The ATS statement calculates it as percentage of change from the baseline study, and the ERS publication as a percentage of the reference value for FEV_1. An increase in peak flow of 60 L/min is considered a positive response.

A positive response is considered strong evidence that the patient will benefit from bronchodilator therapy. The converse, however, is not true. The absence of a bronchodilator response in a single laboratory setting does not predict whether bronchodilator therapy will benefit an individual patient. The laboratory outcome can be affected by several technical issues, including the dose and method of administration of the bronchodilator, the wait time, and the quality of the spirogram efforts. In addition, patient response is variable from one day to the next and may vary with the choice of β-adrenergic agonist. Finally, the obstructive effect of mucous plugging and mucosal edema might be large enough to mask a smooth muscle response to bronchodilator medication. Often, a several-week trial of regular bronchodilator therapy is required to decide whether a patient is benefitting or not. The decision to use bronchodilator medication in a patient is therefore a clinical decision. Bronchodilator response in a laboratory setting contributes to the decision but should not be the sole determinant.

Bronchial Reactivity Testing

Airway hyperresponsiveness, an index of the degree of airway narrowing on exposure to provocative stimuli, is one of the primary characteristics of asthma. On average, the airways of asthmatic patients are far more sensitive to provocative stimuli than those of nonasthmatic subjects. Airway hyperreactivity can usually be suggested by simple tests, such as documenting a response to a bronchodilator or documenting excessive variation in peak flow during a day (most nonasthmatic subjects have a within-day variation in peak flow of <20%). Specific tests measuring response to provocative stimuli are, however, sometimes needed to document the presence of airway hyperresponsiveness.

Two broad categories of stimuli are used to provoke airway narrowing: (1) exposure to aeroallergens like ragweed antigen or chemicals like toluene diisocyanate (specific stimuli), or (2) exposure to methacholine, histamine, exercise, hyperventilation, or cold dry air (nonspecific stimuli). However, the bronchoconstrictive response will vary with the individual stimulus regardless of category.

The most common nonspecific bronchoprovocation test uses methacholine, a parasympathomimetic analogue of acetylcholine, as the bronchoconstricting agent. Methacholine chloride is prepared in several dilutions and administered as a nebulized aerosol in progressively increasing doses. The test begins with baseline measurements of FEV_1 and/or airway resistance. If airway resistance is measured, changes are usually expressed as specific conductance (1/resistance/thoracic gas volume). A second set of measurements follows administration of the diluent alone. Each methacholine dose is followed, after a brief wait, by measurement of FEV_1. A response is considered positive if a sustained 20% fall (calculated from the post-diluent value) in FEV_1 is observed within the prescribed dosage schedule (Fig. 9). The dose of methacholine that elicits a 20% fall in FEV_1 is designated as the PC_{20}, the provocative concentration that causes a 20% fall in FEV_1. As the study is performed in steps, the PC_{20} is calculated either mathematically or graphically from the stepwise changes in FEV_1 (Fig. 9). The response is a continuum; the lower the PC_{20}, the more reactive the airways. Most asthmatic patients have a PC_{20} of ≤ 8 mg/mL. If specific conductance is used as the measure of response, a positive response is indicated by a 35% fall (PC_{35}) during the test. Methacholine challenge testing deals with complex issues and requires rigid standardization to ensure that proper doses of active drug are administered on a proper schedule, that timing of spirometry relative to the dose is controlled, and that spirometry quality and patient safety are properly addressed. Details of these issues and protocols are provided in articles in the reference list. Standard protocols for methacholine challenge that include seven dosage steps are time-consuming; abbreviated protocols with fewer steps have been found to produce acceptable results for clinical testing.

Methacholine challenge studies are common in research protocols involving asthma because they allow bronchial hyperreactivity to be quantified and monitored. In most clinical settings, it is not necessary to document or quantify airway hyperreactivity with formal challenge tests. However, when the diagnosis of asthma is uncertain, bronchoprovocation studies may be clinically useful, as in a patient who has normal spirometry results but also has chest symptoms, such as cough or chest tightness, that suggest asthma. A positive methacholine challenge test result in this setting is highly suggestive of asthma. Clinical monitoring airway hyperreactivity during therapy as a means of quantifying response to treatment is controversial. Currently, such monitoring would be indicated only in selected patients under special circumstances.

Methacholine challenge testing is a safe procedure, but when methacholine is administered in large doses to asth-

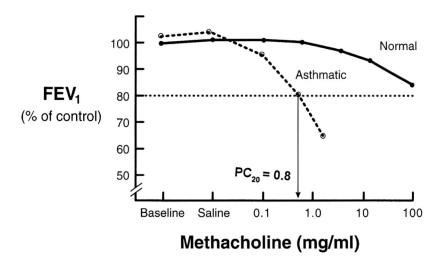

FIG. 9. Graphic display of normal and asthmatic responses to a methacholine challenge test. FEV_1 expressed as a percentage of the control (diluent value) is graphed against the methacholine dose. The point at which the fall in FEV_1 exceeds 20% is used to calculate the provocative concentration, PC_{20}. (Figure courtesy of Charles Irvin, Ph.D.)

matic patients it can provoke severe attacks. Excessive salivation, abdominal cramping, diarrhea, and sweating can occur if the systemic dose is excessive. Atropine is a specific antidote. Contraindications and precautions are well described in standard references. Bronchoprovocation with sensitizing agents like antigens or occupational sensitizers is associated with higher risks, and more caution is warranted. Testing with sensitizing agents should be limited to laboratories specializing in such studies.

Exercise Bronchoprovocation

Exercise provokes bronchospasm in 60%–90% of asthmatics. The level of ventilation obtained during exercise is probably the most important determinant of this response to exercise. For testing outside a laboratory, a fall in FEV_1 of 15% or more in response to modest amounts of exercise (achieving ventilation at 40%–50% of predicted MVV) is considered a positive test result. With formal testing in a laboratory, a 10% fall in FEV_1 with exercise may be significant. Standardized protocols are available.

DIFFUSION

After arterial blood gas measurement, the most common test of gas transfer across the lungs is the CO diffusing capacity ($DLCO$), also called *transfer factor* ($TLCO$). The test measures the rate of transfer of CO from the lungs to the blood. Units of measurement are expressed in two ways. In North America, $DLCO$ is expressed as mL CO/min/mmHg driving pressure; in Europe, $TLCO$ is expressed as mmol CO/min/kPa. CO, rather than O_2, is used as the gas of interest because in the lungs it behaves similarly to O_2, with the advantage that $DLCO$ can be measured, whereas DLO_2 cannot. The pathway for the movement of CO or O_2 from alveolus to hemoglobin (Hb) molecule is illustrated in Fig. 10. Diffusion across the alveolar-capillary membrane is only a small portion of the pathway. In fact, accumulating evidence suggests that mixing within the red cell and the chemical reaction rate are far more important limiting factors in healthy individuals than is diffusion across the alveolar-capillary membrane. This supports the European community's decision to describe the test as transfer factor rather than diffusing capacity.

Diffusing capacity can be measured with single-breath, steady-state, and rebreathing techniques. The single-breath technique is by far the most common, best-standardized, and readily available technique. It also is the method on which most of our clinical information relating $DLCO$ to disease states is based. The single-breath test is performed as follows: The patient exhales to RV, a valve is opened, and the patient inhales to full VC the test gas, which in addition to N_2 contains 0.3% CO, an inert, insoluble tracer gas (e.g., He), and 18%–

21% O_2. The patient relaxes into a breath-hold at TLC for 10 sec and then exhales rapidly. An alveolar sample is collected for analysis after anatomic and mechanical dead space is flushed out by exhaled air. The test is safe and easy to perform. Details of the technique and the computations involved are well described in current ATS and ERS standards documents.

Several important technical and physiologic issues must be considered to avoid interpretive errors. The first is that the selection of reference values for $DLCO$ is confounded by the fact that in early studies, $DLCO$ measured in the same person in different laboratories could vary by as much as 90%. These differences occur because test results are affected by variations in procedural and computational techniques. Although recent testing has demonstrated that standardizing the performance and calculation procedures reduces this large interlaboratory variability, there are still differences of 15%–20% between well-standardized laboratories. Thus, reference data must be carefully selected, or interpretative errors will be frequent.

The remaining issues center on physiologic variables that can influence $DLCO$ without indicating the presence of an abnormality in lung function. CO competes with O_2 for the same Hb sites, and the number of binding sites available influences $DLCO$. Anemia decreases and polycythemia increases $DLCO$. Interpreting $DLCO$ in patients without knowing their Hb concentration is potentially misleading, especially in settings in which Hb is likely to be altered. In patients being monitored for pulmonary injury while receiving chemotherapy, for exam-

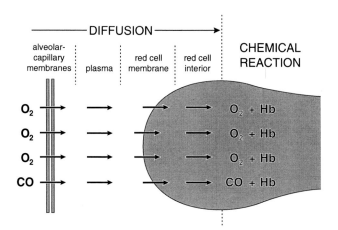

FIG. 10. The diffusion pathway for O_2. Pathway lengths in this figure do not reflect true pathway distances. The pathway is identical for CO, the gas used in the diffusing capacity test. O_2 and CO move across the alveolar-capillary membrane, traverse a very thin plasma layer, cross the red cell membrane, diffuse within the red cell interior, and chemically react, binding with Hb. O_2 and CO compete for the same binding sites on the Hb molecule (Reproduced with permission from Forster RE, DuBois AB, Brisco WA, Fisher AB. *The Lung: Physiologic Basis of Pulmonary Function Tests.* 3rd ed. Chicago: Year Book; 1986).

ple, a fall in DLCO could reflect lung injury, the development of anemia, or both. If carboxyhemoglobin (COHb) is elevated, as in smokers, the COHb effectively reduces the available binding sites while at the same time creating a small CO back pressure in the plasma. These effects combine to lower DLCO artifactually about 1% for each 1% increase in COHb. The best (although, not the easiest) method of avoiding problems with COHb is to have patients refrain from smoking overnight before testing. An optimal procedure is to also measure Hb and COHb once during each DLCO testing session and adjust measured DLCO accordingly. The small back pressure created by CO is another factor to keep in mind during testing. The test gas itself will raise the COHb level about 0.5% for each trial.

Because CO and O_2 compete for the same Hb binding site, changes in O_2 pressure that give one or the other a competitive advantage also artifactually alter DLCO. For example, administration of supplemental O_2 increases the inspired O_2 concentration (FIO_2), gives the advantage to O_2, and lowers DLCO. As individuals move from sea level to higher altitudes, the decreased barometric pressure lowers FIO_2 and gives the advantage to CO, causing DLCO to increase about 0.35% for each decrease of 1 mmHg in alveolar partial pressure of O_2 (PAO_2). Using a correction factor in the computation or simulating the FIO_2 at sea level (150 mmHg) by adding O_2 to the test gas mixture will compensate for the effect of altitude.

Pathophysiologic Correlations

Diseases associated with decreased DLCO include those that (1) reduce lung surface area (emphysema and pulmonary fibrosis), (2) thicken or alter the structural components of the alveolar-capillary membrane (pulmonary fibrosis), or (3) obstruct or obliterate pulmonary capillaries (pulmonary embolism, fibrosis, emphysema, pulmonary hypertension). Although the combination of airway obstruction, overinflation, and a reduced DLCO are the best physiologic markers for emphysema, this entire constellation of findings does not usually occur until later stages of the disease. Isolated reductions in DLCO have been reported to be early indicators of the presence of both emphysema and interstitial fibrosis. For example, in one report of patients with dyspnea, normal chest radiographs, and pathologically demonstrated pulmonary fibrosis, a reduced DLCO was the among the most common functional abnormalities. However, the sensitivity and specificity of an isolated reduction in DLCO, even in the presence of dyspnea, are still unknown.

Reductions in DLCO are thought to predict exercise-associated arterial O_2 desaturation. In patients with chronic obstructive lung disease and restrictive lung diseases, DLCO values that are <50% of predicted have been shown to correlate with exercise hypoxemia. Reports

are not entirely consistent, however. One should view the 50% threshold with some suspicion because of the known large interlaboratory variability in percentage of predicted values for DLCO.

Increases in DLCO are not commonly encountered clinically. They occur in the presence of polycythemia and with intrapulmonary hemorrhage (e.g., Goodpasture's syndrome). They may also represent a technical problem, as DLCO can be dramatically increased when an individual continues to try to inhale during the breath-hold part of the test (Mueller maneuver).

RESPIRATORY MUSCLE STRENGTH

Routine pulmonary function tests may be useful in suggesting the presence of respiratory muscle dysfunction. Typically, individuals who cannot generate normal respiratory muscle force have a reduced VC. In patients with bilateral diaphragmatic paralysis, VC is usually smaller in a supine than in an upright position. VC may also be a useful tool to follow patients with respiratory muscle dysfunction. MVV is commonly reduced in the presence of respiratory muscle dysfunction, but its use is limited because so many different factors reduce it.

Overall respiratory muscle strength is usually assessed by measurement of maximum inspiratory (MIP) and expiratory (MEP) pressures at the mouth. These pressures can be easily measured with portable pressure meters in most clinical settings. MIP is usually measured from RV, and MEP from TLC. Patients should be coached to make the maneuver from their lungs and not use their cheek muscles, which can generate falsely high pressures. The measurements are made against a closed valve; a small, 1-mm fixed air leak is introduced to reduce the effect of using the cheek muscles to generate pressure. Mouth pressures well within a normal range (MIP >80 cm H_2O) can be used to exclude clinically significant respiratory muscle weakness. Lower values are more problematic, because they can represent disease or inadequate effort.

In patients for whom measurements of MIP and MEP do not resolve the question being asked, more sophisticated assessment of respiratory muscle function can be performed with measurement of transdiaphragmatic pressures and with nerve stimulation tests. These tests have the disadvantage that they are more technically demanding and therefore are usually limited to specialty laboratories.

Tests of respiratory muscle strength are useful when neurogenic and myopathic processes are known or suspected. They are also useful when diaphragmatic weakness, fatigue, or paralysis are suspected. Diaphragmatic weakness, when severe, can cause dyspnea and tachypnea and can, even when mild, contribute to dyspnea resulting from other disease processes.

TESTS OF ELASTIC PROPERTIES

These tests are used to characterize the elastic properties of the lung and chest wall. They require the measurement of transmural pressures across the lung (lung elastic recoil pressure, or P_{el}) and across the chest wall (chest wall elastic recoil pressure, or P_{th}). The chest wall includes the abdomen. Measurement of these transmural pressures requires estimates of pleural pressure (P_{pl}) and alveolar pressure (P_{alv}). A small esophageal balloon is inserted into the lower third of the esophagus; esophageal pressure is used to approximate pleural pressure. Mouth pressure under static conditions (no air flow in a relaxed patient with an open glottis) is used to approximate alveolar pressure. Under static conditions, esophageal and mouth pressures are measured at several lung volumes between TLC and RV. Curves relating transmural pressures to lung volume (pressure-volume curves) are calculated separately for the lungs and chest wall and for the respiratory system (lung and chest wall combined). Compliance is calculated as change in lung volume divided by change in pressure ($\Delta V/\Delta P$).

Normal aging and diseases like pulmonary emphysema, which involve disruption of the alveolar walls, are associated with decreased lung recoil pressures for a given lung volume and, consequently, increased lung compliance. Diseases like pulmonary fibrosis increase lung elastic recoil pressures and reduce lung compliance. Aging and chest wall disorders are associated with decreased chest wall compliance.

Although these tests are critical for clarifying the pathophysiology of lung function in various diseases, their clinical utility in routine patient care has never been proved. Interested readers should consult pulmonary physiology texts for further information.

ARTERIAL BLOOD GASES

Thus far, the discussion has been concerned with tests of the mechanical properties of the lung—the bellows action that moves air into and out of the lungs. The mechanical studies, including spirometry, lung volumes, and respiratory muscle testing, characterize the function of the lung but do not provide any estimate of how adequately the lung is performing its primary function. Measurement of arterial blood gases provides direct evidence about the adequacy of gas transfer across the lungs.

It is important to understand both what information is provided by arterial blood gases and what is not. Arterial blood gases define how well the lung is loading O_2 into and removing CO_2 from blood. However, they characterize only the initial steps in the gas transport system (Table 1). They do not allow an overall assessment of the adequacy of delivery of O_2 to cells or of the adequacy of cellular function.

Blood gas technology is advancing rapidly. Blood gas machines are now highly automated. They calibrate and monitor themselves for errors. They wash and rinse themselves and provide numerous alert messages when conditions are not properly controlled. They measure temperature and barometric pressure and compensate for electrode nonlinearity with empirically derived mathematical algorithms. Because they do so much and the technician needs to do so little, laboratory physicians and technicians may become less knowledgeable about the details of blood gas analysis. The increased accuracy of modern blood gas machines partially compensates for this lack of knowledge while at the same time exacerbating it.

The field of noninvasive monitoring of blood gas parameters is also advancing rapidly. Pulse oximeters are widely used, and other techniques for continuously monitoring blood gas parameters are being developed. In the managed care environment, blood gas analysis, along with most other laboratory measurements, is under increasing scrutiny. Documentation for the efficacy of these measurements is being required.

Details of blood gas measurement and interpretation are available in several of the references listed. Briefly, analysis of arterial blood gases involves three separate issues: (1) acid-base status, (2) ventilation status, and (3) oxygenation status. The importance of the lungs in maintaining acid-base balance is illustrated by the fact that the lungs excrete approximately 13,000 mEq of CO_2 per day. In contrast, the kidneys excrete 40 to 80 mEq of fixed acid per day. In a blood gas report, pH and $PaCO_2$ are the two measured elements relating to acid-base balance. The pH and arterial pressure of CO_2 ($PaCO_2$) are used to calculate bicarbonate concentration using the Henderson-Hasselbalch equation. Calculated bicarbonate may provide quick insight into the metabolic component of acid-base derangements.

The adequacy of ventilation is assessed with the $PaCO_2$, according to Eq. 1:

$$PaCO_2 \propto \frac{\dot{V}CO_2}{\dot{V}_A} \propto \frac{\dot{V}CO_2}{\dot{V}_E - \dot{V}_D} \qquad (1)$$

where $\dot{V}CO_2$ is CO_2 production, $\dot{V}_A$ is alveolar ventilation, $\dot{V}_E$ is minute ventilation, and $\dot{V}_D$ is dead space ventilation.

Equation 1 illustrates that $PaCO_2$ is determined by the matching of $\dot{V}_A$ to $\dot{V}CO_2$. An elevated $PaCO_2$ indicates hypoventilation; that is, $\dot{V}_A$ is inadequate relative to $\dot{V}CO_2$. Inadequate $\dot{V}_A$ can occur because $\dot{V}_E$ is reduced and/or $\dot{V}_D$ is increased. If $PaCO_2$ is low, hyperventilation is present. A normal $PaCO_2$ implies adequate matching of $\dot{V}_A$ to $\dot{V}CO_2$, but it is not the sole determinate of the efficiency of ventilation. Efficiency of ventilation must be interpreted in light of the clinical setting, including breathing parameters and $\dot{V}CO_2$. Problems with $\dot{V}CO_2$ can usually be diagnosed simply by looking for markers associated with increased $\dot{V}CO_2$ that may be driving the metabolic processes. In the intensive care unit, these markers include fever and overfeeding with parenteral nutrition. Increases in $\dot{V}CO_2$ are rarely reflected directly as increases in $PaCO_2$ because the ventilatory reserve is so large.

Evaluation of oxygenation parameters includes assessment of the PaO_2 and arterial O_2 content. The PaO_2 provides a valuable—but incomplete—estimate of the adequacy of O_2 loading in the pulmonary capillary blood. It is useful to think of PaO_2 as an intensive rather than a quantitative variable. Although very useful, PaO_2 by itself gives no information about the volume of O_2 contained in the blood (O_2 content). Analyzing both PaO_2 and O_2 content enhances blood gas information.

CO-oximeters are available for accurate measurement of Hb concentration, arterial O_2 saturation (SaO_2), COHb concentration, and methemoglobin (Met-Hb) concentration. Their availability improves the accuracy of estimations of SaO_2 and simplifies the diagnosis of CO poisoning. Blood gas reports should now routinely include a calculation of arterial O_2 content (CaO_2) using CO-oximeter measurements (Eq. 2). Its components include Hb concentration, SaO_2, and the volume of O_2 dissolved in plasma, calculated as $0.0031 \times PaO_2$. The amount of O_2 dissolved in the plasma is trivial compared with the amount bound to Hb in most clinical settings.

$$CaO_2 = 1.39\ Hb \times SaO_2 + 0.0031\ PaO_2 \qquad (2)$$

Calculation of the alveolar-to-arterial pressure gradient for O_2, or $P(A\text{-}a)O_2$, when the patient is breathing room air can be useful in separating the physiologic causes of hypoxemia. The method of calculating $P(A\text{-}a)O_2$ is shown in Eq. 3:

$$P(A\text{-}a)O_2 =$$

$$FiO_2(P_B\text{-}47) - PaCO_2\left(FiO_2 + \frac{1\text{-}FiO_2}{R}\right) - PaO_2 \qquad (3)$$

where $P(A\text{-}a)O_2$ is the alveolar-to-arterial pressure gradient for O_2, FiO_2 is the inspired O_2 concentration, (P_B − 47) is the barometric pressure minus water vapor pressure at 37°C, and R is the respiratory quotient (usually assumed to be 0.8). For blood gases obtained at sea level with a patient breathing room air, Eq. 3 can be reduced for rapid clinical use as follows:

$$P(A\text{-}a)O_2 = 150 - 1.2 \times PaCO_2 - PaO_2$$

It is clinically useful to categorize the physiologic causes of hypoxemia. Physiologic causes of hypoxemia are summarized in Table 2, along with corresponding alveolar-to-arterial gradients when appropriate.

The most common noninvasive measurement of oxygenation status is made by pulse oximetry. Pulse oximeters do not directly measure SaO_2 but relate light ab-

TABLE 2. *Physiologic causes of hypoxemia*

Cause	$P(A\text{-}a)O_2$
Low PaO_2	
• Low inspired PO_2 $\quad$ FiO_2 is low $\quad$ Barometric pressure is $\quad$ low	• Normal $\quad$ If inspired PO_2 is $\quad$ incorrectly assumed to $\quad$ be 21%, the A-a gradient $\quad$ may be elevated.
• Hypoventilation $\quad$ (Elevated $PaCO_2$)	• Normal
• $\dot{V}/\dot{Q}$ mismatching	• Elevated
• Diffusion impairment	• Elevated $\quad$ Rarely a cause of $\quad$ hypoxemia
• Right-to-left shunting	• Elevated $\quad$ With large shunt, $\quad$ response to oxygen poor
Low oxygen content (CaO_2)	
• Anemia	
• Low SaO_2 $\quad$ Presence of other $\quad$ hemoglobin species, $\quad$ such as COHb or Met-Hb $\quad$ Shift of oxyhemoglobin $\quad$ curve to right	

COHb, carboxyhemoglobin; Met-Hb, methemoglobin; CaO_2, arterial oxygen content; FiO_2, fraction of inspired oxygen; PO_2, partial pressure for oxygen; PaO_2, arterial partial pressure for oxygen; $P(A\text{-}a)O_2$, alveolar-arterial gradient for oxygen; $PaCO_2$, arterial partial pressure for carbon dioxide; V/Q, ventilation/perfusion.

sorption across the finger to arterial blood gas data from volunteers in whom arterial blood gases and pulse oximeter light absorption are simultaneously obtained. One side of a pulse oximeter probe contains two light-emitting diodes, each emitting light at a different wavelength (one at about 660 nm and one at about 940 nm). The other side contains a photocell to measure light intensity after light has passed through a finger or ear lobe. A clever variation of Beer's Law (the light absorbed by a solute in a solution is related to the concentration of the solute) is used to estimate SaO_2. Light is absorbed in a pulsatile fashion, increasing with each heartbeat. The assumption is that the increased absorption is caused by arterial blood.

It is important to keep in mind the limitations of pulse oximetry. These include the margin of error, the fact that pulse oximetry does not differentiate between different Hb species, and the effect of substances in the body that may affect light absorption. As a general rule, a single isolated measurement of SaO_2 by pulse oximetry will be within ±4% of the saturation measured in blood directly. Therefore, a pulse oximeter reading of 90% could actually be between 86% and 94%. If the device is being used to monitor SaO_2 in a single individual, a 2% change is considered significant. As pulse oximetry only uses two wavelengths of light, it cannot distinguish either COHb or Met-Hb. Pulse oximeters measure COHb as if it were oxyhemoglobin. In a patient with CO poisoning, therefore, the low SaO_2 would not show up on a pulse oximeter reading.

Other conditions that may result in misleading readings include presence of dyes (methylene blue), elevated bilirubin, states of low perfusion, anemia, and presence of strong external light sources, which may interfere with absorbance measurement. On occasion, the assumption that the pulsatile waveform marks arterial blood does not hold. For example, in a patient with tricuspid regurgitation and strong venous pulsations, the pulse oximeter cannot separate arterial from venous pulsations, and an erroneous reading may occur.

REFERENCE VALUES AND INTERPRETATION

Background

The first step in interpreting pulmonary function tests is selecting the best possible reference values. For many tests, the selection is made by a laboratory physician, but as equipment moves into offices and clinics, individual clinicians will be called on more and more often to make that choice. Guidelines for selecting reference values are widely available. For pulmonary function tests, the ATS and ERS provide access to appropriate reference values.

Medical decisions are made after comparing clinical observations with one or more sets of reference data. This is not as simple as defining a normal range. Results of clinical tests that fall within a normal range often imply absence or low risk of disease. This may not be correct when the typical representative comparison is made. For example, a cholesterol value may fall well within an average range from a general population sample but indicate increased risk for coronary disease when compared with reference data based on total risk assessment. In pulmonary function testing, the assumption may also be incorrect. For example, an individual who starts out with an FEV_1 that is 110% of the predicted value could suffer a reduction of 25% or more in FEV_1 and still have a value within the normal range. The loss—and thus the underlying disease process—would not be detected by routine lung function testing.

Interpreting lung function tests may also be based on comparisons of observed values with reference value information, including comparisons with recognized disease patterns or values previously measured in the same patient. Using historical lung function data from the same patient neatly eliminates all the between-individual variability that exists in the representative group comparison; changes as small as 5% can be detected. However, it is not practical to perform baseline studies in every patient against the unlikely chance that a pulmonary disease will

develop. It is practical, however, to track individual lung function in at-risk populations, such as those in occupations with a known tendency to cause lung injury.

The issues involved in reference value selection and comparison have been the subject of many expert panels and are well described by Solberg (1989) and Grasbeck (1990). The general rules, modified slightly for pulmonary applications, are as follows: (1) The reference population must be clearly defined and described. (2) The patient being examined must resemble the reference study subjects as much as possible in regard to the biologic factors known to contribute to lung function variability. For lung function, these factors are sex, age, height, weight, ethnic group, past and present health, socioeconomic status, and environmental exposures, including cigarette smoke, air pollution, and occupational exposures (Fig. 11). (3) Clinical and reference value measurements should be made with adequately standardized methods and appropriate quality control. Technical variability is reduced when a clinical laboratory makes measurements with the same standardized methods as those used in a reference value study. This last issue is the basis for the development of equipment and procedural standards that have been published by many different respiratory societies.

Reference data vary depending on the population being sampled, the method of sampling the population, and the methods of analyzing the data. The data may be gathered from a subset of a population sample in a larger epidemiologic study, or it may come from a study specifically

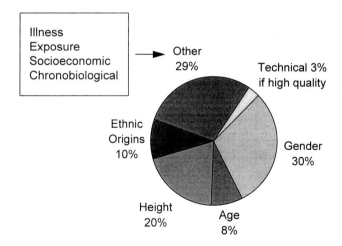

FIG. 11. Schematic illustration of the sources of variability in lung function tests. These sources of variability must be dealt with as part of the performance and interpretation of lung function tests or else the noise encountered in the testing will overwhelm the signal of interest, which in a clinical setting is usually change in lung function with disease. Note that the 3% technical variability assumes high-quality tests. Substandard tests can cause technical variability to exceed all other sources of variability. (Created from data contained in Becklake MR, White N. Sources of variation in spirometric measurements. *Occup Med State of the Art Rev* 1993; 8:241–264.)

designed as a reference value study. Although the optimal method of sampling a population is random sampling, volunteer samples are less expensive and easier to perform and thus more frequently used. Sample size is important. In general, lung function reference studies are better if they include at least 10 subjects of each sex for each decade. The method of analysis also influences reference ranges. In some pulmonary function reference studies, only linear relationships are considered; in others, complex models are used.

Lower Limits for Reference Ranges (Lower Limits of Normal)

Once reference values have been selected, a reference range defines the limits for comparisons. In pulmonary function testing, three sets of limits are commonly used. The most common is also the least desirable. It defines the normal range for FEV_1/VC as >70% or >75% and the normal range for everything else as the predicted value $\pm 20\%$. This method is popular because of its simplicity, but it is statistically incorrect and should be abandoned. The FEV_1/VC ratio falls with aging, so a fixed ratio to define normal is inappropriate. Using ± 20 to define a reference range causes false-negative results in younger and taller patients and false-positive tests in shorter, older patients. It causes large numbers of false-positive errors in the interpretation of midflows and instantaneous flow variables, for which statistically appropriate lower limits of normal approach 50% of the predicted value.

Two statistically acceptable approaches to lower limits of normal are available. One, based on an assumption that the data distribution is Gaussian, uses 95% confidence intervals, usually calculated as 1.645 times the standard error of the estimate in a linear regression equation. The other is based on a calculated lower (or upper) 5th percentile. The percentile calculation is usually based on data expressed as a percentage of the predicted value. Calculation of percentiles avoids the Gaussian distribution assumption. Both are probably acceptable for basic pulmonary function tests that involve FVC and FEV_1. The instantaneous and midflow variables are more likely to have skewed distributions; reference ranges defined with percentiles are preferable for these variables.

Lower limits of normal are variable and should not be treated as arbitrary demarcations. Measured values that lie well within or outside the normal range can be interpreted with confidence. Those that lie close to lower or upper limits should be interpreted with caution. In these borderline cases, clinical information is the best guide to categorizing a test result.

Restricting the Number of Tests Used in an Interpretation

More than 30 parameters can be obtained from spirometry, lung volumes, and diffusing capacity. By chance alone, more than 25% of healthy subjects would have an abnormal result in one or more tests if all 30 were used. The chances for a false-positive test decrease when one is selective about the number of results analyzed. For spirometry, the interpretation should focus on three variables: VC, FEV_1, and FEV_1/VC. For static lung volumes, the interpretation should focus on TLC, and for diffusing capacity, on DLCO. The other results reported may help make decisions in borderline cases, but clinical data are even more useful in those borderline situations.

General Interpretative Guidelines

Spirometry

A simple algorithm for interpreting spirometry using three variables is outlined in Fig. 12. Obstructive lung diseases are characterized by decreased expiratory flows compared with healthy persons. Early airway obstruction, which begins in the small airways, tends to reduce flows at lower lung volumes. Numerous tests for small-airways disease have been studied. Tests, including closing volume, $V_{max50\%}$, and $FEF_{25\%-75\%}$, tend to correlate well with small-airways disease in groups, but there is still no convincing evidence they can be effectively used in a clinical setting to diagnose the presence of small-airways disease in a given individual. The pattern of reduced air flow at lower lung volumes is also seen as part of normal aging, reflecting the loss of elastic recoil of the lungs with age.

As airway obstruction worsens, air flow is reduced at higher lung volumes. The flow-volume display shows progressively more concavity toward the horizontal axis; the volume-time curve shows a slowly rising volume even after 6 to 10 sec. The primary marker for the presence of airway obstruction is the FEV_1/VC ratio. Once airway obstruction has been diagnosed on the basis of FEV_1/VC, severity is classified using the $FEV_1\%$ (FEV_1 as a percentage of the predicted value) (Fig. 12). The characteristic patterns of severe airway obstruction are illustrated in Fig. 8. All expiratory flows are reduced. With good effort, a well-defined but reduced peak flow is seen, followed by a rapid fall in flow to a very low level. At that point flow decreases almost linearly, and the patient never achieves a true expiratory plateau.

Central airway obstruction has a characteristic pattern, depending on the location of the obstruction (Fig. 13). The classic pattern is not seen, however, until the obstruction is rather advanced. The pattern of central airway obstruction can be replicated by submaximal inspiratory and expiratory efforts. Therefore, vigorous patient effort is especially important when central airway obstruction is suspected.

Restrictive patterns in spirometry are characterized by a reduced VC in the absence of airway obstruction (FEV_1/VC is normal). Flows taken from a spirogram are typically

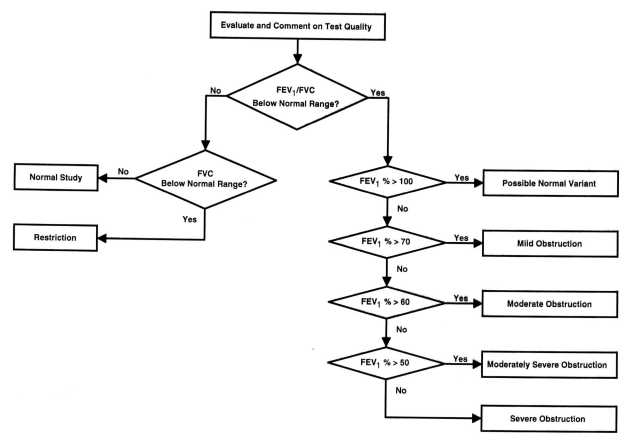

FIG. 12. Simple algorithm for interpretation of spirometry. For simplicity, the severity of restriction based on VC is not diagrammed. Severity of restriction here would use percentage of predicted VC and use a scale similar to that for obstruction. (Adapted from information contained in Becklake MR, Crapo RO, co-chairs. Lung function testing: selection of reference values and interpretative strategies. Official statement of the American Thoracic Society. *Am Rev Respir Dis* 1991;144:1202–1218.)

reduced when restriction is present because of the smaller absolute lung volume, and by themselves they do not indicate the presence of combined obstruction and restriction. Small VCs commonly occur in the presence of obstruction because expiratory time is relatively short. If airway obstruction is present and VC is low, no certain determination of restriction can be made on the basis of spirometry alone. If it is clinically indicated, a measurement of TLC is necessary to confirm the presence of a combined obstructive and restrictive pattern. The presence of restriction can also be determined in most patients who have airway obstruction by simply reviewing the chest radiograph obtained for other clinical reasons.

Static Lung Volumes

The static lung volume variables used for interpretation should be limited to TLC to avoid excessive numbers of false-positive results. Statistically based lower limits of normal should be used. In the classification of restriction,

occasionally TLC and VC findings will conflict. If there are no obvious technical problems, TLC should determine the estimation of restriction. The classic pattern of overinflation includes elevations in TLC, FRC, and RV. Increases in FRC and RV may precede increases in TLC, but one should be cautious in using them to diagnose overinflation, because they also increase the risk for false-positive calls. Overinflation can also be recognized in chest radiographs when classic signs are present.

Diffusing Capacity

The primary variable used for interpretation is DLCO. There is increasing hesitancy to use DL/VA in interpretative schemes, largely because it frequently conflicts with DLCO and the clinical situation. A laboratory can usually categorize DLCO only as within or outside the reference range. The one pattern of findings that suggests a clinical diagnosis is the combination of airway obstruction, evidence of overinflation, and a low DLCO (suggesting em-

Fixed Upper Airway Obstruction

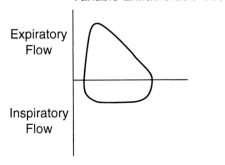

Expiratory
Flow

Inspiratory
Flow

Variable Extrathoracic Obstruction

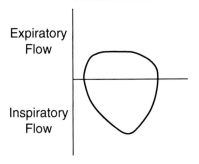

Expiratory
Flow

Inspiratory
Flow

Variable Intrathoracic Obstruction

Expiratory
Flow

Inspiratory
Flow

FIG. 13. Central airway obstruction patterns. Three basic forced expiratory flow-volume patterns seen in the presence of at least moderate upper airway obstruction are schematically illustrated. The basic pattern of airflow obstruction in central airways is constant flow over a significant portion of the inhaled and/or exhaled volumes. In fixed central airway obstruction, the pattern does not vary with inspiration or expiration. Variable extrathoracic obstruction is associated with a relatively normal pattern during expiration, as extrathoracic airways widen during exhalation and narrow during inspiration. Conversely, variable intrathoracic obstruction tends to have a more normal pattern during inspiration, as intrathoracic airways tend to widen during inspiration and narrow during expiration. The patterns may also be seen with submaximal effort. The patterns are present to some degree in patients with milder degrees of obstruction but may be more subtle.

physema). Further interpretation of alterations in DLCO requires knowledge of the clinical question being asked. A common pattern is to find a reduced DLCO as the only abnormality in a battery of pulmonary function tests. In the absence of other clinical or functional information,

an isolated reduction in DLCO does not have clinical significance and need not be pursued further.

Changes in Lung Function Measurements with Time

It is difficult to define precisely a significant change with time. A consistent trend in lung function revealed with multiple measurements will define significant change earlier than will two or three measurements. For changes in VC and FEV$_1$ occurring within a few weeks, a 12% change in healthy subjects and 20% in subjects with obstruction is likely to be significant. Through years, a 15% change (adjusting for age) is probably significant for both. For DLCO and TLC, within-test and between-test variability are increased, and criteria defining change with time are largely absent. When no trending information is available, I tend to consider changes of >15% as significant, but do so with some discomfort.

BIBLIOGRAPHY

Acres JC, Kryger MH. Clinical significance of pulmonary function tests: upper airway obstruction. *Chest* 1981;80:207–211. *Illustrates the various flow-volume patterns of central airway obstruction.*

Becklake MR, Crapo RO, Co-chairs. Lung function testing: selection of reference values and interpretative strategies. Official statement of the American Thoracic Society. *Am Rev Respir Dis* 1991;144:1202–1218. *ATS statement summarizing the issues involved in selecting reference values and interpreting lung function tests. A recognized standard for the interpretation of lung function tests.*

Becklake MR, White N. Sources of variation in spirometric measurements. *Occup Med State of the Art Rev* 1993;8:241–264. *Excellent summary of the sources of variability in lung function tests. This paper is must reading for everyone involved in lung function testing or interpretation.*

Celli BR. Clinical and physiologic evaluation of respiratory muscle function. *Clin Chest Med* 1989;10:199–214. *Good review of the physiology of respiratory muscles and tests used to measure their function.*

Cherniack RM. *Pulmonary Function Testing.* 2nd ed. Philadelphia: WB Saunders; 1992. *A concise, well-written summary of lung physiology and lung function tests. Outstanding figures.*

Clausen JL, ed. *Pulmonary Function Testing Guidelines and Controversies: Equipment, Methods, and Normal Values.* New York: Academic Press; 1982. *Still an excellent source of information on lung function tests. The controversies have not changed much since 1982.*

Cotes JE. *Lung Function. Assessment and Application in Medicine.* 4th ed. Oxford: Blackwell Scientific Publications; 1979. *A comprehensive textbook covering the physiology of lung function in detail.*

Crapo RO, Chair. Standardization of spirometry: 1994 update. Official statement of the American Thoracic Society. *Am J Respir Crit Care Med* 1995;152:1107–1136. *Update of the ATS standards for spirometry. Contains the details and justifications for technical and procedural standards. Does not deal with interpretation.*

Crapo RO, Forster RE. Carbon monoxide diffusing capacity. *Clin Chest Med* 1989;10:187–198. *A review paper discussing the clinical and technical aspects of DLCO.*

Forster RE, DuBois AB, Brisco WA, Fisher AB. *The Lung: Physiologic Basis of Pulmonary Function Tests.* 3rd ed. Chicago: Year Book; 1986. *Basic review of pulmonary physiology.*

Grasbeck R. Reference values, why and how. *Scand J Clin Lab Invest* 1990;50(Suppl 201):45–53. *Reviews the use of reference values in detail. Should be mandatory reading for physicians who use reference values daily but may not understand the details and pitfalls in the comparisons they make.*

Hankinson JL, Bank KM. Acceptability and reproducibility criteria of the American Thoracic Society as observed in a sample of the general population. *Am Rev Respir Dis* 1991;143:516–521, *An analysis of the acceptability and reproducibility criteria for spirometry in 6486 persons from a general population sample.*

Malley WJ. *Clinical Blood Gases.* Philadelphia: WB Saunders; 1990. *Text covering the measurement, physiology, and interpretation of blood gases.*

Nunn AJ, Gregg I. New regression equations for predicting peak expiratory flow in adults. *Br Med J* 1989; 298:1068–1070. *The most recent large reference value study for peak expiratory flow measured with peak flow meters.*

Polkey MI, Green M, Moxham J. Measurement of respiratory muscle strength. *Thorax* 1995;50:1131–1135. *Reviews the evaluation of respiratory muscle strength, with discussions of the more recent advances.*

Rosenthal RR. Approved methodology for methacholine challenge. *Allergy Proc* 1989;10:301–312. *Details on standard methods for performing methacholine challenges.*

Rotman, HH, Liss HP, Weg JG. Diagnosis of upper airway obstruction by pulmonary function testing. *Chest* 1975;68:796–799. *Upper airway obstruction is characterized by typical reductions in both inspiratory and expiratory flows.*

Scanlon PD, Beck KC. Laboratory medicine and pathology: methacholine inhalation challenge. *Mayo Clin Proc* 1994;69:1118–1119. *A good review of methacholine challenge testing.*

Shapiro BA, Harrison RA, Cane RD, Templin R. *Clinical Application of Blood Gases.* 4th ed. Chicago, Year Book; 1989. *Textbook covering the measurement and analysis of blood gases.*

Solberg HE, Grasbeck R. Reference values. *Adv Clin Chem* 1989;27: 1–79. *An excellent review of reference values—their flaws, measurement, and utility.*

Stoller JK, Basheda S, Laskowski D, Goormastic M, McCarthy K. Trial of standard versus modified expiration to achieve end-of-test spirometry criteria. *Am Rev Respir Dis* 1993;148:275–280. *Points out that you don't have to make the patient exert maximal effort throughout the entire spirogram.*

Wanger J. *Pulmonary Function Testing: A Practical Approach.* Baltimore; Williams and Wilkins; 1992. *This is a good how-to-do-it book—very practical and well illustrated.*

Wasserman K, et al. *Principles of Exercise Testing and Interpretation.* Philadelphia: Lea and Febiger; 1993. *One of the classic texts on exercise testing.*

Working Party of European Community for Steel and Coal. Standardized lung function testing. Official statement of the European Respiratory Society. *Eur Respir J* 1993;6(Suppl 16). *A standardization document from the ERS. It covers almost all aspects of lung function testing. The reference value section is excellent.*

Zavala DC. *Manual on Exercise Testing: A Training Handbook.* 3rd ed. Iowa City, IA: University of Iowa; 1993. *A good how-to manual for exercise testing.*

Textbook of Pulmonary Diseases, 6th ed.
edited by G.L. Baum, J.D. Crapo, B.R. Celli, and J.B. Karlinsky,
Lippincott–Raven Publishers, Philadelphia, © 1998.

CHAPTER

10 ⟩ Exercise Testing

Issahar Ben-Dov

THE INTEGRATIVE CARDIORESPIRATORY EXERCISE TEST

The essence of clinical integrative cardiorespiratory exercise testing is the ability to assess oxygen uptake ($\dot{V}O_2$) from measurements of ventilation and respired gas concentrations. When considered together, these parameters (ventilation, gas exchange, $\dot{V}O_2$, and others) allow for extended conclusions to be made regarding diverse cardiovascular, respiratory, and metabolic adaptations to the stress of exercise. Normal peak O_2 uptake indicates adequate (although not necessarily optimal) gas transport from the atmosphere to the mitochondria of muscle and effective utilization of molecular O_2 by the cellular enzymatic machinery. Fick's relationship portrays the factors governing O_2 consumption:

$$\dot{V}O_2 = \dot{Q} \times C(a\text{-}\bar{v})O_2 \qquad (1)$$

where $\dot{Q}$ is cardiac output, C is content, a denotes arterial blood, and $\bar{v}$ denotes mixed venous blood. The determinants of O_2 uptake, as delineated by Fick's relationship, are presented in Table 1. O_2 utilization depends on a synchronized response of many supporting systems to the metabolic load. However, normal values for peak $\dot{V}O_2$ do not ensure that each element of the O_2 transport chain is normal, as not all are rate-limiting. Exercise capacity can be normal for age despite certain loss of heart, lung, or hemoglobin structure and/or function. On the other hand, when peak $\dot{V}O_2$ is reduced (if this is not caused by poor effort), one (or more) of the components of the O_2 transport/utilization chain is evidently abnormal.

When exercise capacity is restricted, it is a challenge for the clinical physiologist to identify the organ(s) or system(s) whose malfunction is causing the limitation. This goal is approached by a thorough analysis of the response to exercise, including symptoms, electrocardiographic pattern, blood pressure, ventilation, gas exchange, O_2 uptake, partial pressure of arterial blood gases, and blood pH and lactic acid concentrations. These are assessed at submaximal and/or at the highest tolerable work rate. More than one protocol may be used for exercise testing. In this review, we concentrate (unless otherwise stated) on data collected during incremental maximal studies (on a cycle ergometer or a treadmill). Various aspects of exercise physiology are addressed only briefly, and the reader is referred to recent editions of comprehensive textbooks and review articles for the details of physiology, muscle fiber type, bioenergetics, cardiovascular and ventilatory control issues, and clinical applications. As is discussed later, it is usually possible to differentiate between ventilatory and cardiovascular mechanisms leading to exercise limitation. However, discrimination among potentially limiting constituents within the O_2 transport chain (mainly cardiovascular factors) and between cardiovascular limitation and poor fitness is more subtle (poor fitness may be considered a reversible form of cardiovascular dysfunction).

WHY PERFORM AN INTEGRATIVE EXERCISE STUDY?

Metabolic exercise challenge is not performed to arrive at a specific pathophysiologic diagnosis, even though, on

I. Ben-Dov: The Pulmonary Institute, Chaim Sheba Medical Center, Sackler Medical School, Tel-Aviv University, Israel.

TABLE 1. *Determinants of O₂ uptake, as described by Fick's relationship*

Variable	Determinants
Cardiac output	Heart function, normality of peripheral and pulmonary vascular beds, volume status, blood viscosity, and drugs
Arterial O₂ content	Hemoglobin concentration, P_{50}, poisonous gases (CO), lung function, pulmonary vascular bed, central ventilatory control, and inspired O₂ pressure
Mixed venous O₂ content	Cardiac output, status of peripheral vascular bed and oxidative cellular machinery, including poisonous gases (CO)

P_{50}, oxygen half-saturation pressure of hemoglobin; CO, carbon monoxide.

occasion, such diagnosis is feasible (i.e., myocardial ischemia or asthma induced by exercise). Exercise is performed to evaluate how an individual (with normal or diseased organs) adapts to physical stress, and/or to answer specific, quantitative physiologic questions. Examples of such questions are shown in Table 2. They are often difficult or impossible to settle based on resting pulmonary functions or resting hemodynamic data. Marked discrepancy often exists between resting measurements and the actual peak exercise O₂ uptake. For example, in patients with severe heart or lung disease, such as a left ventricular ejection fraction of <20%, or a forced expiratory volume in 1 sec (FEV_1) of <1 L, exercise capacity varies; it may be nearly normal or severely reduced.

The pattern of response to the exercise challenge should direct any subsequent diagnostic workup (if needed). At that stage, workup should be targeted to arrive at a specific diagnosis (e.g., pulmonary angiography for an apparent pulmonary embolic disease, or specific muscle enzyme assay for an apparent metabolic myopathy). The algorithms used for interpretation of the exercise data are based on recognition of distinctive patterns. These algorithms are founded on known physiologic principles, but their predictive power in some specific disease categories needs further clarification.

NORMAL AND ABNORMAL CARDIOVASCULAR, VENTILATORY, AND GAS EXCHANGE RESPONSES TO AN INCREMENTAL WORK RATE EXERCISE TEST

Cardiovascular Response

Stroke Volume and Heart Rate

Cardiac output ($\dot{Q}$) increases during exercise as a linear function of the metabolic rate at all levels of fitness. How-

ever, heart rate (HR) and stroke volume (SV) react differently. The SV rapidly reaches its highest level at a work rate that is about one third of the maximal. This SV is maintained throughout the range of work rates. In contrast, HR increases linearly with $\dot{V}O_2$ throughout exercise. From rest to peak exercise, SV may double in fit subjects, and HR rises even more.

In heart disease or in unfit subjects (3 weeks of bed rest is sufficient to induce a state of unfitness), SV augmentation during exercise is limited, and SV often actually falls below resting level. In these patients, augmentation of cardiac output is mostly or solely dependent on HR, which is high at rest and rises steeply during exercise. If the chronotropic effect is also depressed, the rise in cardiac output is further limited.

In trained subjects, at rest and at any given work rate, SV is higher, HR is slower, and the slope of the HR response is more shallow. In addition, with training, as $\dot{V}O_2$ rises, the O₂ content of the venous blood ($\bar{v}O_2$) becomes progressively smaller, but maximal HR does not rise. In sedentary subjects, the lowest $\bar{v}O_2$ content, at peak exercise, is 3 to 4 mL/100 mL [$C(a-\bar{v})O_2$ = 16 to 17 mL/100 mL], whereas in athletes, values for $\bar{v}O_2$ can be lower. SV is augmented as a result of higher venous return during exercise (Starling's effect) and of the inotropic, sympathetic effect. The change in HR is brought about by loss of parasympathetic tone at the low range of work rates and by sympathetic stimulation at the higher range of work rates. If the normal response is inhibited by a negative chronotropic process, a pharmacologic agent (e.g., a beta blocker), or by actual denervation (e.g., heart transplantation), the cardiac output response is delayed or limited.

Augmentation of O₂ consumption during physical activity is supported by a rise of O₂ flux ($\dot{Q}$), but also by augmented extraction of the O₂ stored in the arterial blood, which increases the $C(a-\bar{v})O_2$. By using Fick's equation and assigning an estimate to these parameters

TABLE 2. *Examples of questions that can be answered by an integrative cardiorespiratory exercise test*

1. Is exercise capacity reduced, and if yes, to what extent?
2. Which supporting system is limiting exercise or causing exertional dyspnea?
3. Are gas exchange and arterial blood gases normal during exercise, and if not, what is the extent of the abnormality?
4. What is the metabolic cost ($\dot{V}O_2$) of performing a given work rate task?
5. What is the ventilatory requirement for performing a given work rate task?
6. Is there a clue that suggests the presence of metabolic abnormality or myopathy?
7. Does the exercise intolerance represent a behavioral abnormality or an apparent intolerance is being fabricated for a secondary gain?
8. What is the metabolic level ($\dot{V}O_2$) that a subject can sustain?

during exercise, we can calculate peak $\dot{V}O_2$ in a subject. Assuming a peak $\dot{Q}$ of 20 L/min and arterial and mixed venous O_2 concentrations of 20 and 2 mL/100 mL, peak $\dot{V}O_2$ = 20 L/min × 0.18 = 3.6 L/min. This level is characteristic for a relatively fit subject.

Peripheral and Pulmonary Vascular Resistance and Blood Pressure

The elevated O_2 flux during exercise is directed preferentially to the muscles (up to 70%–80% at peak exercise) secondary to a marked fall in peripheral vascular resistance in the vascular bed of the active muscles. Local accumulation of active metabolites (including endothelium-derived relaxing factors, i.e., nitric oxide) contribute to selective vasodilation at the metabolically active tissues. Generalized sympathetic stimulation causes vasoconstriction in nonactive vascular beds. If vascular resistance is relatively fixed, as in peripheral vascular disease, the capacity of the muscle to sustain generation of force will be limited. In systemic hypertension, peripheral vascular resistance at rest is elevated and the fall during exercise is also limited. These factors contribute to exercise limitation in hypertensive patients. Pulmonary vascular resistance also falls considerably during exercise. This is brought about by marked recruitment of capillary bed not perfused at rest. However, even in normal subjects, the increment in blood flow exceeds the capacity of the peripheral resistance to fall, and as a result, systemic blood pressure normally rises during exercise. The systolic pressure rises linearly with exercise intensity, but the peak value and the slope increase with age. A level of 200 mmHg is considered normal for systolic pressure at peak exercise. Diastolic pressure rises to a lesser extent, with a maximum of about 90 mmHg. Despite equal augmentation of flow in the two circuits, the mean pulmonary arterial pressure rises during exercise to an absolute value of 15 mmHg, whereas the mean systemic arterial pressure rises 50 mmHg above the resting level. The rise of the pulmonary pressure during exercise becomes marked if pathologic processes affect the pulmonary vascular bed.

Ventilatory Response

Whereas cardiac output for a given $\dot{V}O_2$ is mostly predictable, ventilation can vary markedly, even at similar metabolic rates. Unfortunately, disease processes affecting the lungs or heart are commonly associated with a higher ventilatory demand, thus placing affected patients at further disadvantage.

Factors Affecting Exercise Ventilation

Ventilation is determined by factors described by the following equation:

$$\dot{V}_E = K \times \dot{V}CO_2/PaCO_2 + \dot{V}_D \qquad (2)$$

where $\dot{V}_E$ is ventilation, K is a constant, $\dot{V}CO_2$ is CO_2 production, and $\dot{V}_D$ is dead space volume flow ($V_D \times$ respiratory rate). The linkage of $\dot{V}CO_2$ and $\dot{V}_D$ to ventilatory demand is clear. These factors represent the metabolic rate and the fraction of wasted ventilation. Ventilation is tightly linked to $\dot{V}CO_2$ rather than to $\dot{V}O_2$. This linkage facilitates the regulation of arterial pH (which changes with fluctuating $PaCO_2$) rather than the regulation of alveolar PO_2 (PAO_2). As the slope of the hemoglobin dissociation curve at nearly normal PaO_2 is shallow, the effect of larger PAO_2 fluctuations on arterial hemoglobin saturation is modest.

The contribution of the third factor, $PaCO_2$, to the ventilatory demand is less clear. For a given metabolic rate, ventilation is higher if resting $PaCO_2$ is lower. This results from the fact that when the concentration of CO_2 in the arterial blood, $PaCO_2$, and hence in the alveolar air, is lower, any ventilated volume eliminates less CO_2 than when CO_2 concentration in the alveolar air is higher. This set-point effect is advantageous to patients with chronic obstructive pulmonary disease (COPD) which is associated with abnormally elevated $PaCO_2$, because the high $PaCO_2$ leads to a reduced ventilatory demand at any given $\dot{V}CO_2$. However, this same set-point effect imposes a larger ventilatory response in healthy or COPD subjects when $PaCO_2$ is low or needs to be lowered, as in chronic metabolic acidosis. As shown by the above relationship (Eq. 2), $\dot{V}_E$ is directly proportional to $\dot{V}CO_2$. Therefore, the higher the $\dot{V}CO_2$, the larger the $\dot{V}_E$ increment for any given decrement of $PaCO_2$. As a result, trained subjects, operating at high metabolic levels, require a progressively larger ventilatory response to compensate for the lactic acidosis produced during exercise.

The integrated effect of these three factors governing exercise ventilation is illustrated in the four-quadrant graph of Fig. 1. It is shown that ventilation in response to exercise at $\dot{V}O_2$ of 1 L/min can vary markedly. This variation is related to the respiratory exchange ratio (R), the CO_2 set point, and the ratio of dead space to tidal volume (V_D/V_T). It can be as low as 20 L/min or as high as 60 L/min. This relationship illustrates why the ventilatory response during exercise may be markedly increased, even in the absence of intrinsic lung disease. With the exception of V_D/V_T, the factors governing ventilation, $\dot{V}CO_2$ and $PaCO_2$, can be abnormal as a result of metabolic causes, such as metabolic acidosis. Even V_D/V_T can vary without any apparent lung disease, as a consequence of the breathing pattern.

In addition to these three factors, ventilation is affected by various other stimuli, such as PaO_2, pH, and temperature, and it can be modified voluntarily.

Periodic Breathing in Heart Failure

In patients with advanced failure of the left side of the heart (and rarely in otherwise healthy subjects), breathing

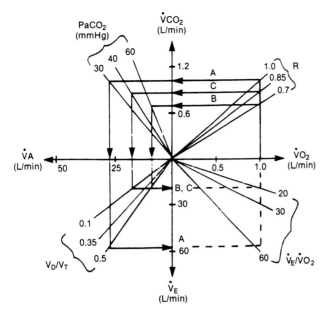

FIG. 1. Schematic representation of the effect of the respiratory exchange ratio (R), the $PaCO_2$ set point, and the dead space fraction of the breath (V_D/V_T) on the ventilatory response to exercise ($\dot{V}_E$) at a metabolic rate of O_2 uptake ($\dot{V}O_2$) of 1.0 L/min. If values for all three determinants are normal [*line B*; the ventilatory equivalent for O_2 ($\dot{V}_E/\dot{V}O_2$)] will be 20], the $\dot{V}_E$ will be 20 L/min. However, if R is elevated, the $PaCO_2$ set point is low (such as if the load is above the subject's anaerobic threshold), and the V_D/V_T is high (*line A*), the ventilatory response will be 60 L/min. [Modified with permission from Whipp BJ. The bioenergetics and gas exchange basis of exercise testing. In: Weisman IM, Zeballos RJ, eds. *Clinical Exercise Testing*. Philadelphia: WB Saunders; 1994 (*Clin Chest Med;* vol 15).]

is oscillatory, with alternating phases of hyperventilation and hypoventilation; each cycle (peak to peak) lasts up to 1 min. This pattern is more distinct during exercise of low to moderate intensity and is attenuated at high intensity. The oscillations are associated with simultaneous oscillations of O_2 uptake. However, as shown in Fig. 2, the $\dot{V}O_2$ oscillations exceed (in amplitude) and precede (in phase) the ventilatory oscillations. True $\dot{V}O_2$ oscillations must result from oscillatory blood flow, not from oscillatory breathing. Therefore, the coexistence of $\dot{V}O_2$ and $\dot{V}_E$ fluctuations suggests that circulatory oscillations (represented by $\dot{V}O_2$ oscillations) play an important or even a primary role in the induction of ventilatory oscillations.

Pattern of Breathing During Exercise

The ventilatory response is brought about by increasing both the tidal volume (V_T) and the respiratory rate. Normally, at low work rates, the change in V_T predominates. V_T reaches its maximal exercise value, which is about 60% of the vital capacity (VC), and this ratio is unchanged across age groups. V_T at peak exercise is, however, 70% of the inspiratory capacity (IC). Respiratory rate, which rises minimally at low work rates, is the predominant variable at the higher range of work rates [above the anaerobic threshold (AT)] and does not reach a plateau during exercise. In disease states, such as COPD, interstitial lung disease, and congestive heart failure, the pattern is similar. However, the contribution of V_T to ventilation is smaller and that of the respiratory rate is larger. In these disease states, the 60% ratio of V_T to VC is maintained, but the ratio of V_T to IC, especially in interstitial lung disease, approaches 100%. The normal and abnormal relationships between V_T, VC, IC, and maximal voluntary

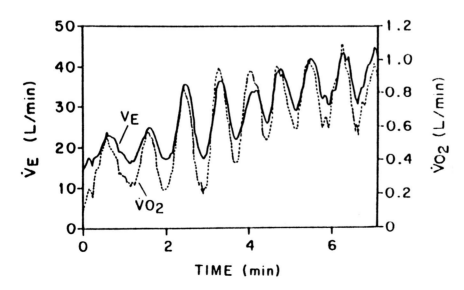

FIG. 2. Ventilation ($\dot{V}_E$) and O_2 uptake ($\dot{V}O_2$) in a subject with heart failure during 2 minutes of rest (time 0 to 2 minutes) and during incremental exercise. Oscillations are present at rest and are augmented as exercise starts. $\dot{V}O_2$ oscillations exceed (in amplitude) and precede (in phase) the $\dot{V}_E$ oscillation. Because hemoglobin is fully saturated, the $\dot{V}_E$ oscillations cannot induce these $\dot{V}O_2$ oscillations. Therefore, pulmonary blood flow must be oscillatory. (Modified with permission from Ben-Dov I, Sietsema KE, Casaburi R, Wasserman K. Evidence that circulatory oscillations accompany ventilatory oscillations during exercise in patients with heart failure. *Am Rev Respir Dis* 1992;145:776–781.)

ventilation (MVV) in healthy subjects and patients with obstructive and restrictive lung disease are schematically illustrated in Fig. 3.

When breathing is periodic, as in congestive heart failure, the fluctuations are brought about predominantly by oscillations of the V_T. Fluctuations in respiratory rate are smaller in magnitude and are opposite in phase to the fluctuations of V_T. Therefore, the respiratory rate fluctuations, if anything, attenuate the amplitude of the $\dot{V}_E$ oscillations.

Gas Exchange During Exercise

Oxygen Cost for Performing Work: Work Efficiency

The O_2 cost for a given increment in work rate is constant. Small, true variations depend on the specific substrate being utilized, and false variations result from differences in motor skills when various tasks are performed. This O_2 cost, which is 10.2 ± 1 mL/min per watt (W) for upright cycling, holds true irrespective of a subject's age, sex, or training status. At high-intensity exercise (above the AT), the contribution of anaerobic metabolism increases. Theoretically therefore, $\Delta\dot{V}O_2/\Delta$work rate is expected to be lower. However, it has been found that if the work rate increments are between 10 and 25 W/min, the normal ratio is sustained. Analysis of the position and shape of the $\dot{V}O_2$-work rate relationship is of clinical importance. Upward displacement of the curve is characteristic of situations of high metabolic cost, such as obesity or thyrotoxicosis. The slope of the relationship is apparently normal in these situations, although small differences in the slope (within the normal range) have been

suggested, at least in hyperthyroidism (Fig. 4). Flattening of the slope is characteristic of low O_2 availability or utilization. The normal value of 10.2 mL/min/watt translates to muscular work efficiency (for that task) of approximately 30%—that is, the caloric equivalent of the work generated is 30% of the caloric equivalent of the energy consumed, as shown in Eq. 3:

$$\text{Efficiency} = \text{Work Done} \times 100/\text{Energy Cost} \quad (3)$$

The work done per unit of time is the work rate in watts. Energy cost for that change in watts is actually measured or calculated by multiplying change in watts (above 0 W) by 10 mL of O_2 per minute per watt. To convert the denominator to calories, the caloric value of 1 mL of O_2/min is 5 cal/min. In the numerator, each 4.186 W = 1 cal/sec [1 cal = 4.186 J (joules)], and 1 W is defined as 1 J/sec, so that 1 W = 14 cal/min. For example, if $\Delta\dot{V}O_2$ from 0 to 100 W = 1000 mL of O_2/min, the efficiency can be calculated as follows:

$$\text{Efficiency} = 100 \times \frac{100 \text{ W} \times 14 \text{ cal/min}}{1000 \text{ mL} \times 5 \text{ cal/min}} =$$

$$100 \times \frac{1400}{5000} = 28\%$$

Anaerobic (Lactate) Threshold

At a certain work intensity, usually about 50% of the individual $\dot{V}O_{2max}$, lactic acid starts to accumulate in the muscles and in the blood at a faster rate, and this metabolic level can be detected from measurements of gas exchange. The first gas exchange criterion used for the

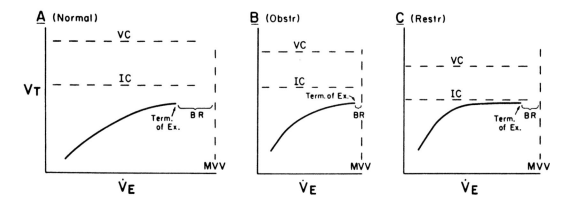

FIG. 3. Tidal volume (V_T) related to the vital capacity (VC), inspiratory capacity (IC), and maximal voluntary ventilation (MVV; *vertical dashed line*), as a function of minute ventilation ($\dot{V}E$), during an incremental exercise. The normal response (**A**), the pattern in obstructive lung disease (**B**; *Obstr*), and the response in restrictive disease (**C**; *Restr*) are shown. V_T as a fraction of the VC is not different. However, in restrictive diseases it approaches the IC at an early stage of exercise. Breathing reserve (BR; MVV minus end-exercise $\dot{V}E$) is low in B and C. (Modified with permission from Wasserman K, Hansen JE, Sue DY, Whipp BJ, Casaburi R, eds. *Principles of Exercise Testing and Interpretation.* 2nd ed. Philadelphia: Lea & Febiger; 1994.)

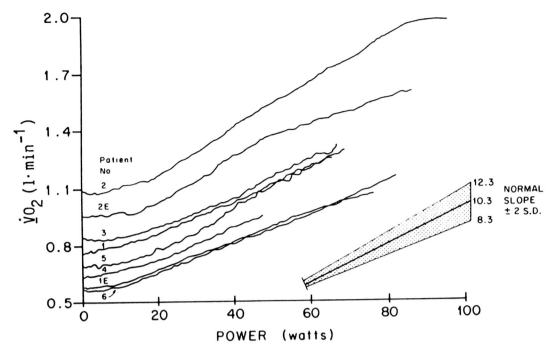

FIG. 4. Relationship of work rate and O_2 uptake in six patients (*1–6*) with hyperthyroidism during an incremental exercise test. Patients 1 and 2 repeated the test at the euthyroid state (*1E* and *2E*). Despite high O_2 uptake during pedaling at 0 W (consistent with hyperthyroidism), the relationship fell within the normal range. The normal range of the slope, 10.2 ± 1 mL/W, is shown by the *dashed area*. In the euthyroid state (*1E* and *2E*), the curves, as expected, are displaced downward. However, the slope is also more shallow relative to the hyperthyroid state (*1* and *2*). This suggests a mild change of work efficiency in hyperthyroidism. (Modified with permission from Ben-Dov I, Sietsema KE, Wasserman K. Oxygen uptake in hyperthyroidism during constant work rate and incremental exercise. *Eur J Appl Physiol* 1991;62:261–267.)

detection of accumulation of lactic acid is the respiratory exchange ratio (R). This accumulation of lactic acid represents a larger contribution of anaerobic metabolism to the energy utilized, as shown in Fig. 5. The metabolic rate ($\dot{V}O_2$) at which this shift occurs is defined as the anaerobic threshold (AT). The lactic acidosis of exercise is crucial for performing at high work intensities. Acid pH facilitates O_2 dissociation from hemoglobin at low capillary PO_2. This is achieved by inducing a shift to the right of the hemoglobin dissociation curve, thereby allowing higher capillary PO_2 (high driving pressure for diffusion) despite lower O_2 content. The shift towards a larger contribution by anaerobic metabolism could result from a limited O_2 supply to the muscle mitochondria at the AT. However, some authors dispute this. In any case, the accumulation of lactic acid is clearly linked to O_2 supply. Situations in which O_2 supply to the muscles rises (such as breathing a high concentration of O_2 and perhaps training) increase the AT, whereas situations in which O_2 supply falls (anemia, heart failure, low inspired O_2, carboxyhemoglobinemia) reduce the AT.

Besides O_2 shortage, other mechanisms have been proposed as explanations for the accumulation of lactic acid. Two alternative mechanisms may account for the lactic acidosis of exercise. The first is the possible role of shifting at the AT to the activation of more glycolytic, type II muscle fibers with lower oxidative capacity. The other is the possible role of rate-limiting mitochondrial oxidative enzymes. There is no evidence, however, that either of these mechanisms is operative. Irrespective of its mechanism, the AT is physiologically important as a metabolic level. It represents the highest work intensity that an individual can endure; higher levels provoke lactic acidosis and rapid fatigue. It also represents the metabolic level above which, even with a constant work rate effort, a steady state for $\dot{V}O_2$ (and for other gas exchange variables) is delayed or not attained.

The AT can reproducibly be determined noninvasively from gas exchange parameters. The criteria used for determination of the AT from an incremental test are summarized in Table 3 and demonstrated in Fig. 6. It has been found that in healthy subjects and in disease states the noninvasive AT corresponds or is close to the AT determined invasively by measuring lactate concentration, lactate-to-pyruvate ratio, blood pH, or blood bicarbonate concentration. If a low normal value for the AT is chosen (e.g., <40% of predicted peak $\dot{V}O_2$), the AT becomes a sensitive index to distinguish normality from various

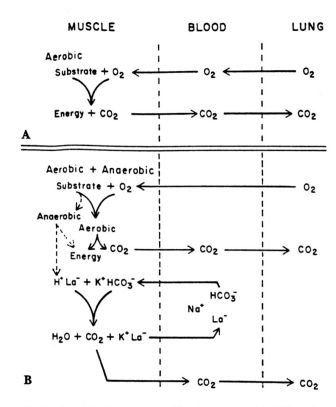

FIG. 5. Aerobic (**A**) and aerobic plus anaerobic (**B**) pathways for energy generation from substrates and molecular O_2. The aerobic pathway produces CO_2 and ATP. The anaerobic pathway produces lactic acid and ATP. The acid is buffered by intracellular bicarbonate ions, a reaction that produces additional CO_2, which is eliminated by ventilation. As lactate accumulates in the cell, part diffuses to the extracellular space and to the blood in exchange for a bicarbonate ion. If the substrate is glucose, 36 ATP molecules are produced by aerobic metabolism, whereas only two ATP molecules are produced by the anaerobic pathway. (Modified with permission from Wasserman K, Hansen JE, Sue DY, Whipp BJ, Casaburi R, eds. *Principles of Exercise Testing and Interpretation.* 2nd ed. Philadelphia: Lea & Febiger; 1994.)

kinds of cardiovascular dysfunction. However, low AT is also found when O_2 flow is reduced, in severe ventilatory diseases, and in deconditioning.

The AT can be determined noninvasively in most normal subjects and in many patients with cardiovascular disease. However, in some normal subjects the data are not discriminative. In moderate to severe COPD, the AT is attained (and can be detected) in approximately two thirds of patients. In general, because of higher noise-to-signal ratio, the lower the peak $\dot{V}O_2$, the less likely it is that a distinct value for the AT can be determined from gas exchange parameters. When the respiratory response is erratic or irregular, as in periodic breathing, it is difficult to discern the AT. However, even in these latter situations, the V-slope method, in which $\dot{V}O_2$ is plotted against $\dot{V}CO_2$, using an appropriate scale (Fig. 7), is often helpful. By this method, determination of the AT is not dependent

on ventilation (control or mechanics). In situations in which the AT cannot be detected from gas exchange data, it can be discerned by invasive measurements after plotting $\dot{V}O_2$ against lactate, bicarbonate, or the lactate-to-pyruvate ratio. In rare situations, when an even more sensitive method is needed, O_2 should be plotted against lactate levels using a log scale for both axes. This method enables discrimination between the early and late slopes of lactic acid accumulation, below and above the AT.

The kinetics of lactic acid accumulation and wash out at the transition from rest to exercise and during recovery is shown for a representative subject in Fig. 8. If a single blood sample is drawn for peak exercise lactic acid, bicarbonate, or pH change, the levels at 2 to 3 min after exercise are representative of the peak exercise values.

The AT can be estimated if needed from a constant work rate test, but this demands repetition of the test at several work rates. At a below-AT intensity, a steady-state $\dot{V}O_2$ is maintained. At an intensity above the threshold, a steady state is delayed or not attained. Therefore, if $\dot{V}O_2$ at minute 3 of a constant work rate exercise is subtracted from $\dot{V}O_2$ at minute 6 ($\Delta\dot{V}O_2$), the proximity to the AT can be estimated (Fig. 9). The larger the difference, the farther the metabolic level is above the AT. If the difference is 0, the metabolic level is below (or at) the individual AT. This method of calculating the AT from a constant work rate test is useful in patients with severe

TABLE 3. *Gas exchange criteria for determination of the anaerobic threshold from incremental exercise testing*

Definition of criterion	Explanations and critique
Slope is steeper for $\dot{V}_E$ and for $\dot{V}CO_2$ response curves.	Reflects excess $\dot{V}CO_2$ and $\dot{V}_E$. The initial small change of the slopes is often obscured. $\dot{V}_E$ is often irregular.
$P_{ET}O_2$ rises while $P_{ET}CO_2$ remains unchanged.	Reflects excess breathing relative to $\dot{V}O_2$. This point is often obscured because of small absolute change of $P_{ET}O_2$ and relatively shallow slope of $P_{ET}CO_2$.
$\dot{V}_E/\dot{V}O_2$ rises while $\dot{V}_E/\dot{V}CO_2$ remains stable.	Ratios between these changes. Using the ratios highlights the turning point.
R ($\dot{V}CO_2/\dot{V}O_2$) rises, usually to >1, CO_2 approaches the value of $\dot{V}O_2$.	Reflects the excess $\dot{V}CO_2$, but practically often obscured by fluctuations resulting from an irregular $\dot{V}_E$.
V-slope, $\dot{V}CO_2$ starts to accelerate faster relative to $\dot{V}O_2$.	Reflects the excess $\dot{V}CO_2$ above $\dot{V}O_2$. Eliminates the dependency on normal ventilatory response to the acid load (normal ventilatory control and mechanics are not required).

$\dot{V}_E$, minute ventilation; $\dot{V}O_2$, O_2 uptake; $\dot{V}CO_2$, CO_2 production; $P_{ET}O_2$ and $P_{ET}CO_2$, end-tidal pressure of O_2 and CO_2, respectively.

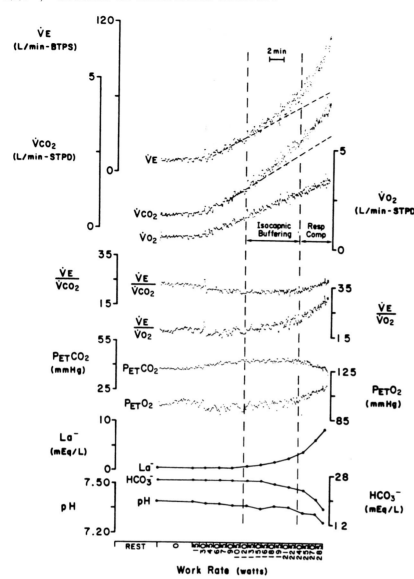

FIG. 6. Parameters used to determine the anaerobic threshold. Gas exchange parameters, lactic acid and bicarbonate concentrations, and blood pH are recorded at rest, during unloaded pedaling, and during an incremental period. The *left vertical dashed line* represents the anaerobic threshold. At this metabolic level, the slopes of the following curves accelerate: lactic acid, PETO₂, ventilatory equivalent for O₂ ($\dot{V}_E/\dot{V}O_2$), O₂ uptake ($\dot{V}O_2$), ventilation ($\dot{V}_E$), and the respiratory exchange ratio (R; not shown). The slopes of the following curves show a fall: pH and bicarbonate. The slopes of the PETCO₂ and the $\dot{V}_E/\dot{V}CO_2$ remain stable at the threshold and change only at a later stage, when respiratory compensation starts. (Modified with permission from Wasserman K, Hansen JE, Sue DY, Whipp BJ, Casaburi R, eds. Principles of Exercise Testing and Interpretation. 2nd ed. Philadelphia: Lea & Febiger; 1994.)

exercise limitation or for whom maximal exercise is considered too risky.

PARAMETERS USED FOR INTERPRETATION OF EXERCISE DATA

Maximal or Peak O₂ Uptake

Maximal $\dot{V}O_2$ ($\dot{V}O_{2max}$) should be related to the mode of exercise—namely, to the mass of the exercising muscles. $\dot{V}O_{2max}$ is different for running on a treadmill or cycling with the legs than for cycling with the upper extremities. Predicted maximum should be based on ideal body weight for a given height. Otherwise, overweight patients will be expected to achieve unusually high values. In underweight individuals, the height may overestimate muscle mass, and therefore the predicted $\dot{V}O_{2max}$. The

maximal $\dot{V}O_2$ is ideally defined as the $\dot{V}O_2$ plateau level (stable $\dot{V}O_2$ despite rising work rate). Our experience has been that true plateau is more often not attained, especially in patients with heart disease. A false plateau is noted when a subject slows the pedaling rate at peak exercise, so that the desired work rate is not maintained. In this situation, the $\dot{V}CO_2$ curve is also relatively flat. If a plateau is not demonstrable, peak $\dot{V}O_2$ rather than $\dot{V}O_{2max}$ should be reported. Peak $\dot{V}O_2$ is meaningful if the patient effort is judged to be adequate and if gas exchange measurements indicate proximity to peak tolerable level (i.e., R >1.2), provided no noncardiovascular mechanism (ventilatory or skeletal) leads to termination of exercise.

Peak Heart Rate and Heart Rate Reserve

HR rises linearly with $\dot{V}O_2$. In heart disease, the rise of cardiac output is more dependent on HR. Therefore,

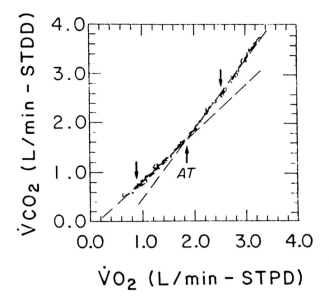

FIG. 7. V-slope method for determination of the anaerobic threshold (AT) from incremental exercise data of a healthy subject. $\dot{V}O_2$ is plotted against $\dot{V}CO_2$. The initial slope of the relationship is linear; at $\dot{V}O_2$ of 1.9 L/min, the slope becomes steeper. The point of deviation of the slope indicates the AT. The *dashed lines* represent the initial and late slopes of the relationship. Determination of AT by this method eliminates dependency on the normality of the ventilatory response. (Modified with permission from Beaver WL, Wasserman K, Whipp BJ. A new method for detecting anaerobic threshold by gas exchange. *J Appl Physiol* 1986;60:2020–2027.)

the relation of HR to work rate shows upward displacement and/or a steeper slope. However, these characteristics of the curve cannot distinguish between heart disease and situations of low O_2 availability and/or deconditioning.

There are limitations to reliance on the HR response. The maximal HR, even in healthy subjects, can deviate markedly from the predicted mean maximum. Furthermore, in patients with heart failure, the predicted maximal HR is typically not attained, and the deviation from the predicted peak value is larger for the more disabled, as shown in Fig. 10. Likewise, HR response can be attenuated by chronotropic dysfunction (ischemia) or by commonly used medications.

Oxygen Pulse

O_2 pulse, the volume of O_2 extracted (or loaded) during one heart beat, is calculated from Fick's relationship ($\dot{V}O_2 = \dot{Q} \times C(a\text{-}\bar{v})O_2$; Eq. 1) by dividing both sides of the equation by HR:

$$\dot{V}O_2/HR = O_2 \text{ Pulse} = SV \times C(a\text{-}\bar{v})O_2 \quad (4)$$

where SV is stroke volume.

The O_2 pulse depends on the product of SV and the $C(a\text{-}\bar{v})O_2$. Therefore, quantitative assessment of each of

these from the O_2 pulse is possible only when the other variable is of a relatively constant value. SV is relatively constant at high levels of exercise or during exercise in the supine position, whereas $\bar{v}O_2$ is temporarily relatively constant (if $\dot{V}O_2$ is measured breath by breath) early in the transition from rest to exercise, when the venous effluent from the exercising muscles has not reached the lung. During this phase, most of the change of pulmonary arterial hemoglobin O_2 saturation is caused by the rise in pulmonary blood flow. Close to peak exercise, when O_2 extraction is near the maximum, $\bar{v}O_2$ is also relatively constant.

O_2 pulse can be reduced in any situation in which $\dot{V}O_2$ is reduced—heart disease, peripheral vascular disease, anemia, and other situations leading to reduced O_2 content or reduced O_2 utilization (including deconditioning).

Ventilatory Equivalents for Oxygen and Carbon Dioxide and the Dead Space-Tidal Volume Ratio

The ventilatory equivalents can be considered as markers of ventilatory efficiency, because they represent the ventilatory demand at a given metabolic rate. Relative to rest, the values of the ventilatory equivalents decline at low- to moderate-intensity exercise, probably because of more optimal matching of ventilation to perfusion. The lowest values are reached around the AT. Above this metabolic rate, the ventilatory equivalents for O_2 and CO_2 diverge. Initially, when excess CO_2 is produced from buffered, newly formed lactic acid, the ventilatory equivalent for O_2 rises. Later, after a short isocapnic period, the ventilatory equivalent for CO_2 also rises, as a result of compensatory hyperventilation (Fig. 6).

The values of the ventilatory equivalents depend on various factors linking ventilation to its metabolic regulators (Eq. 2). The equivalents can also change in response to hyperventilation, either voluntary or secondary to anxiety or discomfort. When the ventilatory equivalents at a given exercise intensity are abnormally elevated, the simultaneous presence of a high $PaCO_2$ indicates (and a high $P_{ET}CO_2$ may suggest) that the abnormality is the result of intrinsic lung disease (poor distribution of ventilation, high $\dot{V}/\dot{Q}$ areas, or an increased dead space). The pattern of change of the ventilatory equivalents during incremental exercise in healthy subjects and in patients with obstructive and restrictive lung disease is schematically shown in Fig. 11. The ventilatory equivalents therefore contribute to our understanding of the ventilatory requirement. However, these parameters do not accurately reflect the dead space volume of the lung, calculation of which should be based on measurement of arterial PCO_2. The V_D/V_T is calculated as shown in Eq. 5.

$$V_D/V_T = (PaCO_2 - P_{ET}CO_2)/PaCO_2 - V_{DV}/V_T \quad (5)$$

MODERATE   **VERY HEAVY**

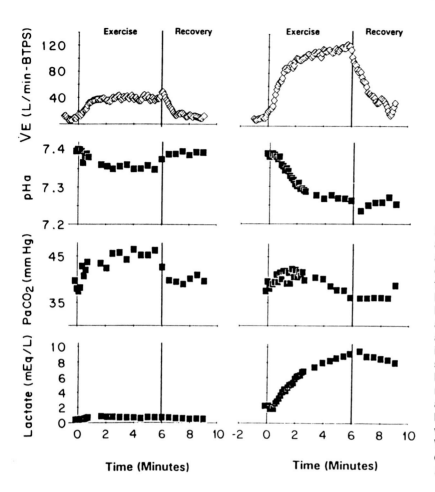

FIG. 8. Ventilation ($\dot{V}_E$), arterial Ph (pHa), arterial PCO2 ($PaCO_2$), and blood lactate in a subject exercising at a constant work rate of moderate intensity (below the anaerobic threshold) and at a constant work rate of very high intensity (close to the highest tolerable level). During the test at moderate intensity, a steady state for $\dot{V}O_2$ during exercise was attained, and lactic acid remained at the resting level. During the test at high intensity, no steady state was attained for the $\dot{V}O_2$ and lactic acid. At the recovery phase, despite a rapid fall of $\dot{V}O_2$, the concentration of lactic acid and the pHa remained at peak exercise levels for at least 2 to 3 minutes. (Modified with permission from Stringer W, Casaburi R, Wasserman K. Acid-base regulation during exercise and recovery in humans. *J Appl Physiol* 1992;72:954–961.)

where $PetCO_2$ is end-tidal partial pressure of CO_2 and V_{DV}/V_T is the dead space volume of the breathing valve apparatus. As noted, the breathing valve volume should be taken into account in this calculation.

The specificity of the ventilatory equivalents as markers of certain diagnoses is low, as high values are seen in lung disease, heart disease, pulmonary vascular disease, and metabolic acidosis. The calculated ratio of dead space to tidal volume (V_D/V_T) is more predictive of an intrinsic lung abnormality. However, the V_D/V_T is high when breathing frequency is high, and its sensitivity is limited even in relatively advanced pulmonary vascular disease, which contradicts previous belief that a lack of fall in V_D/V_T during exercise is sensitive and often the sole detectable abnormality in early pulmonary vascular disease, even at a stage in which it cannot be detected by other clinical modes.

PaO₂ and P(A-a)O₂ Difference

PaO₂ in healthy subjects is normal or increased during exercise, but the P(A-a)O₂ difference usually widens. This behavior is also characteristic of situations of low O_2 carrying capacity that are not caused by lung disease, such as anemia, neuromuscular weakness, and unfitness. In obesity, PaO_2 rises and P(A-a)O₂ narrows early during exercise; subsequently, behavior of the parameters is similar to the normal response. Exceptions to these rules occur in the early phase of exercise, when ventilation lags behind $\dot{V}O_2$ rise, and in trained athletes at peak exercise, when PaO_2 can fall. Interestingly, in uncomplicated heart failure, PaO_2 also remains relatively unchanged throughout exercise.

In patients with COPD, exercise PaO_2 may remain unchanged, slightly improve, or fall. In interstitial and pulmonary vascular disease, an exercise-induced fall (often profound) of PaO_2 is more characteristic, and this fall progresses as exercise intensity increases. Exercise desaturation is a consistent finding in the presence of right-to-left intracardiac shunt, and the degree of desaturation is probably proportional to the magnitude of the shunt. The degree of exercise desaturation cannot be accurately predicted from resting data, such as diffusion capacity for carbon monoxide (D_{LCO}), and needs to be measured directly.

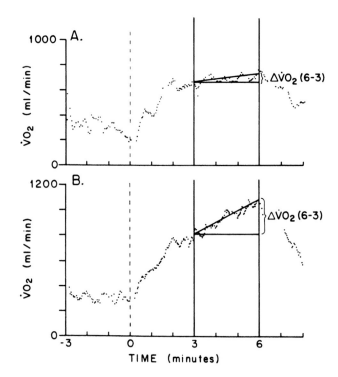

FIG. 9. $\dot{V}O_2$ response to a constant work rate exercise at 25 W (**A**) and 75 W (**B**) of a patient with heart failure. Exercise starts at time 0. The $\Delta\dot{V}O_2$ is calculated from a linear regression of $\dot{V}O_2$ between minutes 3 and 6 of the exercise. In B, the difference is 300 mL. The departure from a steady state for O_2 uptake indicates that this metabolic rate is well above the patient's anaerobic threshold. In A, the difference is 50 mL, indicating that the metabolic rate is just above (or at) the patient's anaerobic threshold. This patient will probably be able to sustain a 25-W task (walking) for long period but will become exhausted after few minutes at a 75-W task. (Modified with permission from Zhang YY, et al. O_2 uptake kinetics in response to exercise: a measure of tissue anaerobiosis in heart failure. *Chest* 1993;103:735–741.)

PaCO$_2$ and P(a-ET)CO$_2$ Difference

In normal subjects exercising at low to moderate intensity, $PaCO_2$ remains at or near the resting level. At higher intensities, $PaCO_2$ progressively falls, as a result of ventilatory compensation for lactic acidosis.

In COPD, $PaCO_2$ may rise slightly during exercise, even in patients in whom the resting value is normal. In interstitial lung disease, $PaCO_2$ is usually normal or slightly reduced.

At rest, the end-tidal partial pressure of CO_2 ($PETCO_2$) is lower by 2 to 3 mm/Hg than $PaCO_2$, so that the P(a-ET)CO_2 is positive. However, during exercise this difference becomes negative. $PaCO_2$ is an average value, measured across several breathing cycles. In contrast, end-tidal partial pressure is obtained during a late stage of a single expiration. During this phase of the breathing cycle, the alveolar partial pressure of CO_2 ($PACO_2$) rises progressively as a result of the CO_2-rich venous blood

reaching the lung. As $\dot{V}CO_2$ rises during exercise, $PACO_2$ during expiration rises at a faster rate, allowing the $PETCO_2$ to surpass the mean $PaCO_2$. In situations in which units of high ventilation-perfusion ratio ($\dot{V}/\dot{Q}$) predominate in the lung (as in pulmonary vascular disease), CO_2 is not being added to the end-tidal gas at a fast rate, and P(a-ET)CO_2 remains positive. In the presence of right-to-left shunt, as venous CO_2 is diverted to the arterial side, even less CO_2 is being added to the alveolar gas, and therefore this difference is consistently positive. The magnitude of the difference is proportional to the fraction of shunted blood.

SYSTEMS LIMITING EXERCISE CAPACITY

The concept of the presence of a supporting system that limits exercise needs clarification. Obviously, the output of every system is restricted, and when a system fails to increase its output to a level required to perform a given task, this system restricts the ability to accomplish that task. However, at peak output of a supporting system (i.e., heart or lung), if the neural stimulus to an exercising muscle to generate force persists, the muscle can respond in two ways. It can either maintain (at least temporarily) the peak or close-to-peak output, or it can cease to generate force (i.e., electromechanical dissociation). If in re-

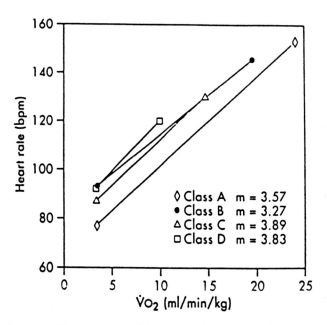

FIG. 10. The response of heart rate (mean) as a function of O_2 uptake ($\dot{V}O_2$) for patients with heart failure of the four functional classes. The higher the functional class, the higher the heart rate at peak exercise. The ability of the sicker patients to increase heart rate (and cardiac output) is more limited. (Modified with permission from Weber KT, et al. *Cardiopulmonary Exercise Testing: Physiological Principles and Clinical Applications.* Philadelphia: WB Saunders; 1986.)

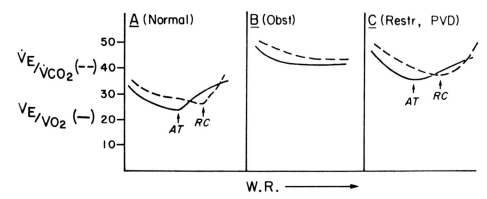

FIG. 11. A: Schematic illustration of the ventilatory equivalents for O_2 ($\dot{V}_E/\dot{V}O_2$) and CO_2 ($\dot{V}_E/\dot{V}CO_2$) as a function of work rate in a normal subject, in obstructive ventilatory (**B**) (*Obst*), restrictive ventilatory (**C**) (*Restr*), and pulmonary vascular disease (*PVD*) states. The anaerobic threshold (AT) at the lowest level of $\dot{V}_E/\dot{V}O_2$ and the respiratory compensation point (RC) at the lowest level of $\dot{V}_E/\dot{V}CO_2$ are marked. The values for the ventilatory equivalents normally fall during light to moderate exercise and rise again when lactic acidosis occurs. **B:** Because of mechanical restraint, the anaerobic threshold is often not attained and/or the respiratory compensation is limited, so that the late rise is not seen. **C:** Pattern is similar, but the absolute values are abnormally elevated. (Modified with permission from Wasserman K, Hansen JE, Sue DY, Whipp BJ, Casaburi R, eds. *Principles of Exercise Testing and Interpretation.* 2nd ed. Philadelphia: Lea & Febiger; 1994.)

sponse to inability of the heart to increase the O_2 flux the muscle ceases to generate force, then the heart obviously limits exercise capacity. However, if despite inadequate O_2 flux the muscle maintains (temporarily) maximal or nearly maximal contractions, then the heart does not directly limit exercise capacity. In this latter situation, the restricted function of the heart induces a deviation from homeostasis (i.e., lactic acidosis), which is perceived as a sensation that cannot be endured.

When a certain intensity of this sensation is reached, it leads to voluntary cessation of muscle contraction. In most situations encountered during clinical exercise testing, there is probably no global failure of force generation, but rather a distasteful sensation, resulting from stimuli such as the ventilatory load or acidosis. According to this description, exercise starts and probably ceases voluntarily. Therefore, the question about a system limiting exercise should be modified. The challenge is to identify the system(s) whose capacity is inferior relative to the load, therefore creating discomfort. To avoid such discomfort, the individual prefers to terminate the effort.

A striking demonstration of the role of intensity of symptoms as a determinant of exercise tolerance is provided by a comparison of responses to work between healthy subjects and patients with moderate to severe COPD. In both groups, the median intensity of dyspnea and of perceived leg exertion at peak exercise were similar (approximately 70% of the maximal intensity on the scales used). This intensity of sensation obviously occurred at a lower work intensity in the patients with COPD.

A partial list of disorders that may limit exercise capac-

ity, including pathophysiology and discriminative findings, is shown in Table 4.

Ventilatory Limitation of Exercise

Ventilatory limitation of exercise is defined on the basis of a limited exercise breathing reserve. The maximal output of the respiratory system is the maximal voluntary ventilation (MVV). It is assumed that the maximal output can be accurately measured or estimated. The 10-sec resting MVV maneuver is the favored method. The estimated MVV is obtained by multiplying the measured forced expiratory volume in 1 second (FEV_1) by a factor of between 35 and 40 (estimated MVV = $FEV_1 \times 40$). It is also assumed that this maximal resting ventilation volume is valid for exercise (a disputable assumption). The actual peak exercise ventilation ($\dot{V}_{Emax}$) is then subtracted from the MVV. The closer the $\dot{V}_{Emax}$ is to the MVV, the closer the subject is to the ventilatory limit. A difference of <15 L/min between MVV and $\dot{V}_{Emax}$ (MVV $- \dot{V}_{Emax}$), or a $\dot{V}_{Emax}$-to-MVV ratio of $>80\%$ ($\dot{V}_{Emax}$/MVV) has been considered diagnostic for the presence of ventilatory limitation to exercise (Fig. 12).

The same principle of breathing reserve can be applied to every tidal breath during exercise (Fig. 13). If the flow rates during exercise approach (or surpass) the boundary of the maximal resting flow volume loop, then a subject is at or close to the ventilatory limit. If the ratio between peak exercise V_T and IC approaches 1 during exercise, this also represents ventilatory limitation (Fig. 3).

Maximal breathing capacity during exercise, however,

TABLE 4. *Pathophysiology and discriminating measurements of some disorders limiting exercise performance (reduced maximum $\dot{V}O_2$)*

Disorders	Pathophysiology	Example of measurements that deviate from normal
Pulmonary		
Airflow obstruction	Mechanical limitation to ventilation; mismatching of $\dot{V}_A/\dot{Q}$, hypoxic stimulation of ventilation; increased work of breathing	↓ Breathing reserve; abnormal expiratory flow pattern; ↑ V_D/V_T; ↑ $\dot{V}_E/\dot{V}O_2$; ↑ $P(A\text{-}a)O_2$; ↑ HR reserve; ↑ $\dot{V}CO_2$
Restriction	Mismatching $\dot{V}_A/\dot{Q}$; hypoxic stimulation of ventilation; V_T increase is limited; increased work of breathing	Arterial hypoxemia during exercise; V_T/IC ratio approaches 1
Alveolar filling	Hypoxic stimulation to breathing	Arterial hypoxemia in response to exercise
Chest wall	Mechanical limitation to ventilation	↓ Breathing reserve; ↑ P_ACO_2 V_D/V_T;
Pulmonary circulation	Nonperfusion of ventilated lung; exercise hypoxemia	work rate-related hypoxemia; ↑ $\dot{V}_E/\dot{V}O_2$; ↑ $P(a\text{-}ET)CO_2$; ↓ O_2 pulse
Cardiac		
Coronary	Coronary insufficiency	ECG: ↓ AT; ↓ $\Delta\dot{V}O_2/\Delta WR$
Valvular	Cardiac output limitation (↓ effective stroke volume)	↓ O_2 pulse; ↓ $\Delta\dot{V}O_2/\Delta WR$
Myocardial	Cardiac output limitation (↓ ejection fraction and stroke volume)	
Anemia	Reduced O_2-carrying capacity	↓ O_2 pulse; ↓ AT; steep $\dot{V}_E/\dot{V}O_2$ relationship
Peripheral circulation	Inadequate O_2 flow to metabolically active muscle	↓ AT; ↓ $\Delta\dot{V}O_2/\Delta WR$; ↑ HR reserve
Obesity	Increased work to move body; if severe, respiratory restriction and pulmonary insufficiency	↑ O_2 cost of work
Psychogenic	Anxiety reaction	Hyperventilation with precisely regular respiratory rate; ↓ PCO_2
Malingering	Secondary gain	Hyper- and hypoventilation with irregular respiratory rate
Deconditioning	Inactivity or prolonged bed rest; loss of capability to effectively redistribute systemic blood flow; muscle atrophy	↓ O_2 pulse; ↓ AT

HR, heart rate; IC, inspiratory capacity; WR, work rate. See text for explanation of other abbreviations.

is not necessarily the same as the resting MVV. There is evidence, at least in COPD, that breathing capacity during exercise often exceeds the resting MVV (Fig. 12), and the calculated reserve may become (absurdly) a negative value. It is likely that in other diseases, such as certain neuromyopathies, and in heart failure, maximal breathing capacity during exercise may be lower than the resting level. Furthermore, when the ventilatory load is profound, subjects often stop exercise because of dyspnea, even before a true physiologic limit has been attained. Factors such as acidosis or hypoxemia enhance the sensation of dyspnea and exaggerate the cessation of effort at a ventilatory level that is lower relative to the resting MVV.

Cardiovascular Limitation to Exercise

In contrast to ventilatory limitation, determination of cardiovascular limitation on the basis of the concept of "cardiac exercise reserve" is difficult to achieve. Measurement (or estimation) of the maximal attainable cardiac output and/or the actual cardiac output at peak exercise is a demanding task. Using the HR reserve (predicted peak exercise HR minus actual peak exercise HR) as a

substitute for cardiac output reserve is not practical. Peak HR is highly variable, and many patients with heart disease do not attain the age-predicted maximal HR, as shown in Fig. 10. Therefore, the diagnosis of cardiovascular limitation (in contrast to diagnosis of ventilatory limitation) is indirect and based on the presence of a combination of gas exchange and other criteria that indicate an exhausted O_2 transport/utilization capacity. These criteria are summarized in Table 5. The criteria are not specific for a distinctive type of cardiovascular dysfunction, but they reveal an exhausted O_2 transport capacity. Therefore, situations such as anemia, certain hemoglobinopathies, carbon monoxide poisoning, or even severe arterial hypoxia, produce similar gas exchange abnormalities.

Different Categories of Cardiovascular Processes Affecting Exercise Capacity

Although many of the gas exchange criteria listed in Table 5 are present in cardiovascular disease of any type (central cardiac, peripheral vascular, or pulmonary vascular disease), certain alterations are more likely to occur with specific abnormalities. For example, exercise desatu-

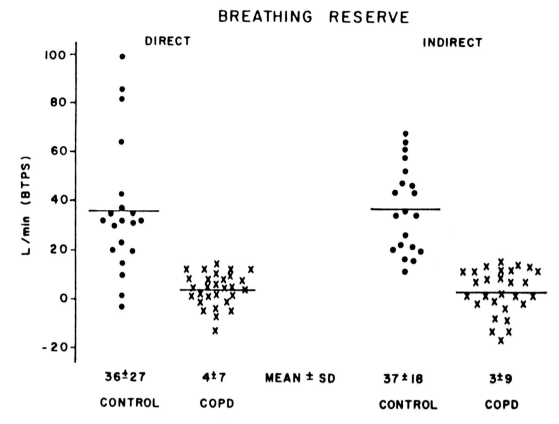

FIG. 12. Breathing reserve (MVV − $\dot{V}_{Emax}$) in patients with COPD and in control subjects. On the *left side,* the MVV was calculated from directly measured MVV. On the *right side,* the MVV was empirically estimated (MVV = $FEV_1 \times 40$). The estimated MVV is slightly higher. In the patients with COPD, the reserve is close to 0, indicating the proximity to the limit of ventilation. Interestingly, the calculated reserve in some patients has a negative value, indicating that breathing during exercise exceeds the resting MVV. (Modified with permission from Wasserman K, Hansen JE, Sue DY, Whipp BJ, Casaburi R, eds. *Principles of Exercise Testing and Interpretation.* 2nd ed. Philadelphia: Lea & Febiger; 1994.)

ration and elevated dead space volume are more likely in pulmonary than in peripheral vascular disease. Elevated ventilatory equivalents are present in failure of the left side of the heart and in pulmonary vascular disease, but are less likely to occur in isolated peripheral vascular disease or anemia. These associated findings are useful to distinguish the specific segment within the cardiovascular circuit that limits exercise.

Clinical Symptoms at Peak Exercise

It is tempting to believe that the subjective complaint at peak exercise is specific for the system leading to exercise limitation. Chest pain, leg pain, fatigue, and lightheadness are suggestive of cardiovascular limitation, whereas shortness of breath suggests ventilatory limitation. However, these symptoms lack specificity and are of low diagnostic value, as the perception of stressful stimuli at peak exercise varies among individuals.

INDICATIONS FOR AN INTEGRATIVE CARDIORESPIRATORY EXERCISE TEST

Exercise study is done primarily to quantitate functional capacity and magnitude of gas exchange abnormalities, and to identify the supporting system(s) limiting exercise. A detailed list of situations in which exercise testing has been recommended, or is potentially valuable, is shown in Table 6. This list includes firmly established indications and also situations in which an exercise test is potentially beneficial, even if its role in these situations has not been systematically evaluated. For exercise to be a useful clinical tool, it should provide sensitive and specific criteria for the diagnosis of diseases, and these should have a high predictive value. However, more remains to be learned concerning the relative merit of various exercise-derived parameters and their combinations. For example, the predictive value of parameters such as low AT or low breathing reserve during exercise (how low is low?) for specific diagnoses (i.e., cardiac or ventilatory limitations) is difficult to ascertain. Because of the lack

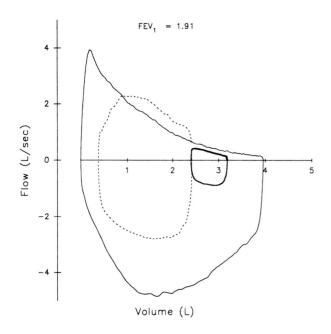

FEV$_1$ = 1.91

FIG. 13. Schematic representation of resting inspiratory and expiratory maximal flow volume loop (*outer solid line*), resting tidal breathing (*inner solid line*), and breathing at peak exercise (*dashed line*) in a patient with COPD. During exercise (but not at rest), the flow rates surpass the boundary of the resting maximal expiratory curve. In addition, the end-expiratory lung volume has increased about 0.75 L (left shift) during exercise relative to rest. This patient is probably close to or at his ventilatory limit during exercise. [Modified with permission from Gallagher CG. Exercise limitation and clinical exercise testing in chronic obstructive pulmonary disease. In: Weisman IM, Zeballos RJ, eds. *Clinical Exercise Testing*. Philadelphia: WB Saunders; 1994 (*Clin Chest Med*; vol 15).]

DATA ANALYSIS

Most commercial exercise systems provide options for data averaging and plotting. For general clinical use, eight breaths, or 15- to 30-second averaging, are acceptable. Despite averaging, however, the data are often obscured by oscillatory noise. Unusually deep or shallow breaths, especially when functional residual capacity (FRC) is oscillating or the breathing pattern is periodic, will predictably obscure the real data. Values are chosen from these averaged time plots or from the tabular report after ensuring that no spurious estimates are selected.

Values for $\dot{V}O_2$, HR, O$_2$ pulse, respiratory exchange ratio, $\dot{V}_E$, work rate, and other parameters are measured at peak exercise. Various parameters, such as the ventilatory

equivalents and AT, are determined at certain submaximal exercise levels. The lowest value should preferably be reported for the ventilatory equivalents. Some parameters, such as VD/VT and blood gases, are recorded repeatedly during exercise, and others, such as $\Delta\dot{V}O_2/\Delta$work rate, are calculated from continuous exercise data. The obtained values are compared with the normal reference values, which should be applicable to the specific population studied, and the percentage deviations from normal means are calculated.

Framework for Interpretation of Cardiorespiratory Exercise Test

Algorithms for interpretation have been published (see Wasserman et al.).

The interpreter should be present during the test. Attention should be paid to patient cooperation—motivation, coordination, and maintenance of the pedaling rate—especially close to peak exercise. Data regarding the course of the test, including symptoms at peak exercise and a note on special events, should be available. Not rarely, a subject stops exercise for a trivial cause (e.g., dry oral mucosa), a situation that does not allow conclusions to be reached regarding the true physiologic maximum. To determine if the measurements are acceptable, it is prudent to allude to the measured metabolic values at rest and during unloaded cycling. Resting $\dot{V}O_2$ should be 200 to 300 mL/min, and R should be 0.8 to 0.9. At unloaded pedaling, $\dot{V}O_2$ roughly doubles (depending on the body

TABLE 5. *Indications that a cardiovascular (or O$_2$ flow) limitation to exercise (a) is present, or that a cardiovascular abnormality (b) is present*

(a)
Chest pain, claudication leg pain or syncope
Ischemic electrocardiographic changes or exercise-induced arrhythmia
Blood pressure fall
High respiratory exchange ratio (R $\geqslant$ 1), in the presence of low $\dot{V}O_2$max, especially when $\dot{V}O_2$-WR relationship becomes shallow
Low and flat O$_2$-pulse-WR relationship
Low HR reserve
Lack of ventilatory limitation (normal or high breathing reserve)
(b)
Tachycardia, steep HR-$\dot{V}O_2$ relationship
Low and relatively shallow O$_2$-pulse-WR relationship, with rise after exercise
Low $\Delta\dot{V}O_2/\Delta$WR ratio
Early lactic acidosis, low anaerobic threshold
Periodic breathing
Low $\dot{V}O_2$max while breathing reserve is normal or high
Abnormally high blood pressure or limited rise of blood pressure during exercise
Limited HR response

of widely accepted and easily obtainable measurements (a "gold standard") for classifying patients according to whether they are limited by cardiac or ventilatory factors, a stringent sensitivity analysis cannot be applied to these exercise-derived gas exchange criteria.

TABLE 6. *Indications for the integrative cardiorespiratory exercise test, and situations in which the test is potentially valuable*

1. Detection of cardiovascular, especially pulmonary vascular, disease at an early stage
2. Evaluation of unexplained effort intolerance/dyspnea
3. Disability/ability evaluation (job qualification)
4. Quantitation of the severity of cardiorespiratory diseases
5. Assessment of relative contributions of ventilatory and cardiovascular dysfunction to functional impairment, when both abnormalities coexist
6. Classification of patients with heart failure according to functional capacity classes, assessing response to therapy in congestive heart failure, determination of prognosis, and determining timing of heart transplantation
7. Evaluation of the progress or regression of a disease process
8. Evaluation of the response to pharmacologic treatment, training, or rehabilitation
9. Estimation of the operative risk associated with thoracotomy and lung resection
10. Selection of work rate to be used for training of an individual subject
11. Evaluation of potentially deleterious effects of medications on exercise tolerance (i.e., beta blockers or carbonic anhydrase inhibitors)
12. Evaluation of need for O_2 during exercise, and evaluation of the effect of O_2 breathing on exercise tolerance
13. Detection of right-to-left shunt during exercise (i.e., patent foramen ovale), and potentially determination of its magnitude
14. Evaluation of the blood pressure response during exercise in patients with hypertension and assessment of the effectiveness of therapy
15. To search for metabolic myopathies affecting exercise tolerance
16. To measure the O_2 cost (work efficiency) and ventilatory requirement (ventilatory efficiency) for a given task
17. To predict the rate of deterioration of gas exchange in interstitial lung disease
18. To assess the contribution of the carotid body to the ventilatory response at a given exercise intensity, by switching to 100% FIO_2, the Dejure maneuver
19. Fitness evaluation and reassurance
20. To evaluate the relative contributions of central cardiac and peripheral vascular disease to functional impairment, when both diseases are present or are suspected
21. To assess severity and response to therapy in primary pulmonary hypertension

weight). $\dot{V}O_2$ at any work rate can be estimated by the following equation:

$$\dot{V}O_2 \text{ (mL/min)} = 5.8 \times \text{weight (kg)} + 10.2$$
$$\times \text{work rate (W)} + 151 \qquad [6]$$

If a value deviates markedly from the expected, the validity of the data should be questioned. After comple-

tion of the test, the following steps are required for data analysis:

1. Assess if exercise capacity, as determined by the $\dot{V}O_{2max}$, is normal. A normal $\dot{V}O_{2max}$ does not in itself indicate normality of either the cardiovascular or ventilatory system. Each or both systems (and others) may be abnormal and yet have sufficient reserve to allow for the age-predicted $\dot{V}O_{2max}$ to be attained. For previously trained subjects, attaining the age-predicted level may actually represent deterioration. Therefore, even if $\dot{V}O_{2max}$ is within the normal range, the cardiovascular and respiratory responses need to be carefully analyzed to prove the normality of the supporting systems.

2. If $\dot{V}O_{2max}$ is reduced, optimal patient cooperation and satisfactory performance of the study should first be ascertained. On occasion, the requested power output is not achieved because of slowing of the pedaling rate at high exercise intensity. This predictably leads to spurious lowering or flattening of the slope of physiologic functions, such as $\dot{V}O_2$ or O_2 pulse. (In this situation, as opposed to true flattening, both $\dot{V}CO_2$ and $\dot{V}O_2$ are level.) The next step is to determine which organ system is limiting exercise, is closer to its maximal capacity, or is inducing the intolerable symptom(s) that are leading to cessation of effort. At first, broad categories, such as respiratory, cardiovascular, metabolic, musculoskeletal, or motivational limitations, should be sought. If breathing reserve is reduced, ventilatory limitation is present. Cardiovascular limitation is suggested by a combination of findings reflecting reduced or exhausted O_2 transport capacity (Table 5). Among these findings, the normality or abnormality of the AT is fundamental. If one system is limiting exercise capacity, it does not mean that the other systems are normal, or even that the other systems are not concomitantly limiting. Cardiovascular and respiratory limitations often coexist at the same metabolic load. On the other hand, when one system is limiting, other supporting systems are not being challenged to their maximal capacity, so that their normality cannot always be ascertained.

3. If exercise capacity is reduced and the major limiting system can be found, the pathophysiology leading to the exercise limitation should be specified. This includes classification according to obstructive versus restrictive lung disease, myocardial (ischemic, valvular, or conductive) versus peripheral or pulmonary vascular disease, or metabolic causes, such as anemia or acidosis. Other contributing factors (especially those that are potentially treatable) to the limitation should be looked for, such as pharmacologic or metabolic causes. This goal is achieved by a detailed analysis of multiple subjective and objective characteristics of the responses, and their comparison with resting subjective and objective data.

4. It should be determined whether information obtained from the exercise test advances understanding of

the patient's symptoms, functional capacity, essential diagnostic workup, and treatment plan. The required complementary diagnostic workup or modes of therapy should be arranged for the patient.

After implementation of this sequential analysis, most patients can be assigned either to a normal exercise tolerance group or to one of the broad diagnostic groups of abnormal exercise tolerance. A certain number of patients remain enigmatic. In our experience, a common dilemma is that of the patient with reduced exercise capacity who, by the cited criteria, is classified with the cardiovascular group but for whom static measurements (e.g., echocardiogram) show no resting cardiovascular abnormality. In some of these individuals, the cause is poor fitness. In others, we believe that heart function, even if normal at rest, may be abnormal during exercise. In some patients, especially hypertensive subjects, diastolic dysfunction may be an important cause of exercise limitation. Another problematic group is comprised of patients with known, often advanced, cardiac and/or ventilatory disease who stop exercise before breathing reserve is exhausted or before significant lactic acidosis (a true physiologic limit) is attained. Some of these patients may be restricted by peripheral causes, such as peripheral and/or respiratory muscle weakness.

BIBLIOGRAPHY

Agusti C, Xaubet A, Agusti AGN, Roca J, Ramirez J, Rodrigez-Roisin R. Clinical and functional assessment of patients with idiopathic pulmonary fibrosis: results of 3 years' follow-up. *Eur Respir J* 1994;7: 643–650. *Only the exercise alveolar-arterial PO₂ difference and the single-breath CO diffusion capacity, measured at presentation, were valuable predictors of the decline of resting arterial oxygenation over 3 years.*

Beaver WL, Wasserman K, Whipp BJ. Improved detection of lactate threshold during exercise using a log-log transformation. *J Appl Physiol* 1985;59:1936–1940. *If O₂-uptake and lactate concentration during incremental exercise are presented on a log-log scale, the threshold behavior is apparent and the anaerobic threshold is readily discriminated.*

Beaver WL, Wasserman K, Whipp BJ. A new method for detecting anaerobic threshold by gas exchange. *J Appl Physiol* 1986;60:2020–2027. *The authors describe a method in which the anaerobic threshold is determined from incremental exercise data by plotting O₂ uptake versus CO₂ output. The threshold is the break point, at which CO₂ output starts to rise faster than O₂ uptake. This method is advantageous, as it does not depend on measurement of ventilation, which is often irregular or abnormally regulated.*

Ben-Dov I, Casaburi R, Sietsema KE, Sullivan C, Wasserman K. Periodic changes of tidal volume and respiratory rate in heart failure during exercise. *Clin J Sport Med* 1992;2:202–207. *Ventilatory oscillations are produced mainly by oscillations of tidal volume and not by oscillations of the respiratory rate.*

Ben-Dov I, Morag B, Farfel Z. The effect of lower extremities venous obstruction on exercise tolerance. *Chest* 1997;111:506–508. *A patient with extensive lower body venous thrombosis had severe exercise intolerance. The authors suggest that the observation that his arm exercise capacity exceeded his leg exercise capacity proves that peripheral venous disease, rather than a central circulatory abnormality, caused the exercise limitation.*

Ben-Dov I, Sietsema KE, Casaburi R, Wasserman K. Evidence that circulatory oscillations accompany ventilatory oscillations during ex-

ercise in patients with heart failure. *Am Rev Respir Dis* 1992;145: 776–781. *The authors analyze the amplitude and phase relationship of the ventilatory and O₂-uptake oscillations. They concluded that to account for these O₂ oscillations, cardiac output must also be oscillatory.*

Ben-Dov I, Sietsema KE, Wasserman K. Oxygen uptake in hyperthyroidism during constant work rate and incremental exercise. *Eur J Appl Physiol* 1991;62:261–267. *The relationship between O₂ uptake and work rate increments in hyperthyroidism falls within the normal range. However, therapy induced a small change in the slope, so that mild changes in work efficiency in this disease are likely.*

Casaburi, Daly J, Hansen JE, Effros RM. Abrupt changes in mixed venous blood gas composition after the onset of exercise. *J Appl Physiol* 1989;67:1106–1112. *The authors tested the hypothesis that mixed venous blood O₂ saturation does not change for 10 to 15 seconds at the onset of exercise (because of circulatory delay from the exercising muscles) by rapid sampling of pulmonary arterial blood. Contrary to the hypothesis, pulmonary arterial blood saturation fell 10% within seconds after the onset of exercise.*

Casaburi R, Patessio A, Ioli F, Zanaboni S, Donner CF, Wasserman K. Reduction in exercise lactic acidosis and ventilation as a result of exercise training in patients with obstructive lung disease. *Am Rev Respir Dis* 1991;143:9–18. *Two groups of patients with moderate to severe COPD were trained at either high or low work intensity (total work done was matched). Both groups gained a training effect. The training effect was significantly larger for the high-work-intensity training group.*

D'Alonzo GE, Gianotti L, Dantzeker DR. Noninvasive measurement of hemodynamic improvement during chronic vasodilator therapy in obliterative pulmonary hypertension. *Am Rev Respir Dis* 1986;133: 380–384. *In 10 patients with obliterative pulmonary hypertension treated with calcium channel blockers, improvement in pulmonary vascular resistance correlated with improvement of peak exercise O₂ uptake and peak exercise O₂ pulse. These noninvasive measurement are valuable for following such patients.*

Davis JA, Vodak P, Wilmore JH, Vodak J, Kurtz P. Anaerobic threshold and maximal aerobic power for three modes of exercise. *J Appl Physiol* 1976;41:544–550. *The authors show that the anaerobic threshold could be determined by gas exchange criteria in 30 subjects performing at three modes of exercise. The gas exchange threshold correlated highly with the threshold determined by measuring venous blood lactate.*

Dempsey JA, Hanson PG, Henderson KS. Exercise-induced alveolar hypoxemia in healthy human subjects at sea level. *J Physiol* 1984;355: 161–175. *In highly fit subjects (peak O₂ uptake = 72 mL/kg/min), arterial hypoxemia was present at peak exercise. PaO₂ at rest was 91 ± 0.9 mmHg, and this fell to 75 ± 2.3 mmHg (lowest value, 60 mmHg) at peak exercise. The authors hypothesize that the hypoxia resulted from diffusion limitation in this high-flow situation.*

Elliot DL, Buist NR, Goldberg L, Kennaway NG, Berkley, Phil D, Powell BR, Kuehl KS. Metabolic myopathies: evaluation by graded exercise testing. *Medicine* 1989;68:163–172. *Case reports of patients with glycogen storage disease, carnitine palmitoyl transferase deficiency, and mitochondrial myopathy. Peak O₂ uptake, anaerobic threshold, and respiratory exchange ratio (R) values during an incremental exercise are presented for the three types of myopathy.*

Franciosa JA, Park M, Levine TB. Lack of correlation between exercise capacity and indexes of resting left ventricular performance in heart failure. *Am J Cardiol* 1981;47:33–39. *Among 21 patients with cardiomyopathy, exercise duration on a treadmill did not correlate with resting ejection fraction. Following therapy, exercise capacity again did not correlate with improvement of resting hemodynamics.*

Green HJ, Hughson GW, Orr GW, Ranney DA. Anaerobic threshold, blood lactate, and muscle metabolites in progressive exercise. *J Appl Physiol* 1983;54:1032–1038. *In 10 healthy subjects, the authors identified the anaerobic threshold from gas exchange criteria, the lactate threshold from blood lactate, and muscle lactate concentration from timed biopsies of the vastus lateralis muscle. They conclude that the gas exchange threshold and the blood lactate threshold do not coincide, and that lactic acid rise in the muscle precedes the former thresholds.*

Hansen JE, Sue DY, Oren A, Wasserman K. Relation of oxygen uptake to work rate in normal men and men with circulatory disorders. *Am J Cardiol* 1887;59:669–674. *The authors describe a method for cal-*

culating the O_2 uptake-work rate relationship during incremental exercise, which takes into account the lag of O_2 rise inherent to this mode of exercise. They demonstrate the usefulness of this ratio, when reduced, as a marker of cardiovascular diseases.

Hansen JE, Sue DY, Wasserman K. Predicted values for clinical exercise testing. *Am Rev Respir Dis* 1984;129(Suppl):49–55. *The study provides a commonly used set of standards for predicting the normal response to exercise among sedentary subjects. This is based on data from 77 male shipyard workers, some of them obese, hypertensive, and smokers, but with no evidence of cardiorespiratory disease.*

Higginbotham MB, Morris KC, Williams RS, McHale PA, Coleman RE, Cobb FR. Regulation of stroke volume during submaximal and maximal upright exercise in normal man. *Circ Res* 1986;58:2281–2291. *An important study in which the hemodynamic (right heart catheterization and nuclear angiography) and gas exchange responses to an upright incremental exercise are measured. The stroke volume attains its maximum at a low level of exercise, whereas the heart rate continues to rise throughout exercise.*

Inbar O, Oren A, Scheinowitz M, Rotstein A, Dalin R, Casaburi R. Normal cardiopulmonary response during incremental exercise in 20- to 70-year-old men. *Med Sci Sports Exerc* 1994;26:538–546. *This is the largest study (to date) describing the normal response to treadmill exercise. The study is based on data from 1,424 male subjects who underwent an incremental exercise study as part of annual medical screening. The authors describe the values of multiple cardiorespiratory parameters at peak exercise and at submaximal work rates.*

Jones NL, ed. *Clinical Exercise Testing.* 3rd edition. Philadelphia: WB Saunders; 1988. *A new edition of a textbook by one of the pioneers in the field. The author addresses exercise physiology, clinical application, interpretation, normal standards, equations, and quality control issues in staged-exercise testing.*

Killian KJ, Leblanc P, Martin DH, Summers E, Jones NL, Campbell EJ. Exercise capacity and ventilatory, circulatory, and symptom limitation in patients with chronic airflow limitation. *Am Rev Respir Dis* 1992;146:935–940. *Dyspnea and leg effort were measured during exercise in 97 patients with COPD and in 320 controls. Unexpectedly, both groups stopped exercise at a similar median level of intensity (on a scale of 0 to 10). The median for dyspnea was 6 (severe), and for leg effort it was 7 (severe to very severe). There was overlapping of the predominant symptom at peak exercise (dyspnea vs. leg effort) between the groups.*

Koike A, Itoh H, Taniguchi K, Hiroe M. Detecting abnormalities in left ventricular function during exercise by respiratory measurements. *Circulation* 1989;80:1737–1746. *The authors measured gas exchange breath by breath and hemodynamics beat by beat, using a radioactive detector, after injecting tagged red cells. At the anaerobic threshold, the ejection fraction, stroke volume, and slope of the cardiac output as related to work rate fell.*

Kremser CB, O'Toole MF, Leff AR. Oscillatory hyperventilation in severe congestive heart failure secondary to dilated cardiomyopathy or to ischemic cardiomyopathy. *Am J Cardiol* 1987;59:900–905. *The first systematic study of periodic breathing (PB) in heart failure during exercise. The authors describe the correlation of PB with severity of heart failure, augmentation of PB with light exercise and its attenuation at heavy exercise, the extremely high wasted ventilation in this mode of breathing, and the oscillation of arterial blood gas tension (the nadir of PaO_2 corresponds to the peak of ventilation).*

Lim PO, MacFadyen RJ, Clarkson PMB, MacDonald TM. Impaired exercise tolerance in hypertensive patients. *Ann Intern Med* 1966;124:41–55. *A review of a large number of exercise studies in hypertensive subjects. Exercise capacity is reduced in these subjects, the blood pressure response during exercise is of prognostic importance, and exercise challenge is potentially helpful in evaluating the adequacy of therapy.*

Mancini DM, Eisen H, Kussmaul W, Mull R, Edmunds LH Jr, Wilson JR. Value of peak exercise oxygen consumption for optimal timing for cardiac transplantation in ambulatory patients with heart failure. *Circulation* 1991;83:778–786. *Ninety-four percent of patients evaluated prospectively with peak O_2 uptake >14 mL/kg/min survived >1 year. Therefore, in this group transplantation could be safely deferred. In contrast, only 70% of patients with peak O_2 uptake <14 mL/kg/min (awaiting transplantation) survived 1 year, and they should be considered in urgent need of transplantation.*

Mohsenifar Z, Tashkin DP, Levy SE, Bjerke RD, Clements PJ, Furst

D. Lack of sensitivity of measurement of V_D/V_T at rest and during exercise in detecting hemodynamically significant pulmonary vascular abnormalities in collagen vascular disease. *Am Rev Respir Dis* 1981;123:508–512. *The authors question the sensitivity of the lack of fall in V_D/V_T during exercise as a marker for significant pulmonary vascular disease. Among eight of nine patients with elevated pulmonary arterial pressure (at rest or during exercise), V_D/V_T fell significantly during exercise.*

Myers JM, Froelicher VF. Hemodynamic determinants of exercise capacity in chronic heart failure. *Ann Intern Med* 1991;115:377–386. *A comprehensive review of published studies in which hemodynamics and exercise capacity were measured simultaneously during exercise in heart failure. The lack of correlation between systolic function and exercise tolerance, biochemical aspects of skeletal muscle metabolism, and β-receptor abnormalities are discussed.*

Nadel AJ, Gold W N, Burgess JH. Early diagnosis of chronic pulmonary vascular obstruction. *Am J Med* 1968;44:16–25. *In a small group of patients with dyspnea and no clinical evidence for pulmonary hypertension, the V_D/V_T rose during exercise (normally it falls). The authors claim that in this group, the change in V_D/V_T during exercise was more sensitive than pulmonary angiography and/or radioisotope scanning for the diagnosis of pulmonary vascular disease.*

Oren A, Sue DY, Hansen JE, Torrance DJ, Wasserman K. The role of exercise testing in impairment evaluation. *Am Rev Respir Dis* 1987;135:230–235. *Among 348 shipyard workers, exercise tolerance could not be accurately predicted from resting clinical data. Therefore, for impairment evaluation, O_2 uptake should be assessed directly during exercise.*

Oren A, Wasserman K, Davis JA, Whipp BJ. Effect of CO_2 set point on ventilatory response to exercise. *J Appl Physiol* 1981;51:185–189. *Resting $PaCO_2$ was altered in healthy subjects by diet-induced changes in the acid-base status. Resting $PaCO_2$ served as a set point, so that ventilation is inversely proportional to the resting $PaCO_2$.*

Robinson BF, Epstein SE, Beiser GD, Braunwald E. Control of heart rate by the autonomic nervous system. *Circ Res* 1966;19:400–411. *In healthy human subjects during exercise, the authors used pharmacologic sympathetic and parasympathetic blocking agents, separately and in combination, to study the role of the autonomic nervous system in regulating heart rate response.*

Saltin B, Henriksson J, Nygaard E, Anderson P, Jansson E. Fiber types and metabolic potentials of skeletal muscles in sedentary man and endurance runners. *Ann NY Acad Sci* 1977;301:3–29. *A relatively old review summarizing our knowledge of muscle fiber types and their metabolic pathways, including changes associated with training. The data are based on muscle biopsies performed by these investigators.*

Sietsema K, Cooper DM, Perloff JK, Child JS, Rosove MH, Wasserman K, Whipp BJ. Control of ventilation during exercise in patients with central venous-to-systemic arterial shunts. *J Appl Physiol* 1988;64:234–242. *Respiratory control in patients with intracardiac right-to-left shunt was studied. Fifteen patients underwent continuous hemoglobin saturation monitoring by ear oximeter. Saturation fell at the onset of exercise, probably because of an increase in the shunt fraction, whereas $PaCO_2$ remained unchanged (measured in six patients).*

Smith TP, Kinasewitz GT, Tucker WY, Spillers WP, George RB. Exercise capacity as a predictor of post-thoracotomy morbidity. *Am Rev Respir Dis* 1984;129:730–734. *Because lung resection exerts stress on the cardiovascular and respiratory systems, the authors investigated an integrative parameter, peak O_2 uptake, as a potential predictor of the ability to tolerate this stress. When normalized for body weight, it was a good predictor of morbidity following thoracotomy.*

Stringer W, Casaburi R, Wasserman K. Acid-base regulation during exercise and recovery in humans. *J Appl Physiol* 1992;72:954–961. *Acid-base and lactic acid were sampled at <10-second intervals during transitions from rest to constant-work-rate exercise (at various intensities) and from exercise to recovery. The kinetics of the acid-base changes and their linkage to lactic acid metabolism are detailed.*

Stringer W, Wasserman K, Cassaburi R, Porszasz J, Maehhara K, French W. Lactic acidosis as a facilitator of oxyhemoglobin dissociation during exercise. *J Appl Physiol* 1994;76:1462–1467. *End-exercise femoral vein PaO_2 did not differ between low- and high-intensity exercise, but femoral vein hemoglobin saturation was lower at the high-intensity test. This shows that the hemoglobin dissociation at high level of exercise (above the anaerobic threshold) is facilitated by the accumulation of lactic acid.*

Sue DY. Exercise testing in the evaluation of impairment and disability. In: Weisman IM, Zeballos RJ, eds. *Clinical Exercise Testing.* Philadelphia: WB Saunders; 1994:369–387 (*Clin Chest Med;* vol 15). *A thorough discussion of the central role of exercise testing in disability evaluation.*

Sue DY, Wasserman K. Impact of integrative cardiopulmonary exercise testing on clinical decision making. *Chest* 1991;99:981–991. *The authors (leaders in the field) review the clinical significance of various gas exchange measurements in understanding the pathophysiology of exercise intolerance. They also address the impact of data obtained from exercise testing, in addition to what can be learned from static measurements at rest in various cardiovascular, pulmonary vascular, and ventilatory disorders.*

Sue DY, Wasserman K, Morica RB, Casaburi R. Metabolic acidosis of exercise in patients with chronic obstructive pulmonary disease. *Chest* 1988;94:931–938. *The anaerobic threshold was determined by the V-slope method and from blood bicarbonate in 22 patients with moderate-severe COPD. In 14, lactic acidosis developed during exercise, and it was possible to identify 10 of the 14 with the gas exchange method.*

Szlachcic J, Massie BM, Kramer BL, Topic N, Tubau J. Correlates and prognostic implication of exercise capacity in chronic congestive heart failure. *Am J Cardiol* 1985;55:1037–1042. *Patients with heart failure underwent exercise testing and hemodynamic monitoring. Only resting pulmonary capillary wedge pressure, peak exercise heart rate, and peak exercise cardiac index correlated with peak O_2 uptake. The patients with low $\dot{V}O_{2max}$ (<10 mL/kg/min) had a high (77%) mortality in 1 year, compared with 21% in the group with a greater $\dot{V}O_{2max}$.*

Tjahja IE, Reddy HK, Janicki JS, Weber KT. Evolving role of cardiopulmonary exercise testing in cardiovascular disease. In: Weisman IM, Zeballos RJ, eds. *Clinical Exercise Testing.* Philadelphia: WB Saunders; 1994:271–285 (*Clin Chest Med;* vol 15). *A summary by authors who have made an important contribution to the field of integrative exercise testing in cardiovascular disease. The review includes data on its role in functional staging, therapy prognostication, and screening for heart transplantation.*

Wasserman K, Hansen JE, Sue DY, Whipp BJ, Casaburi R, eds. *Principles of Exercise Testing and Interpretation.* 2nd ed. Philadelphia: Lea & Febiger; 1994. *A recent edition of the comprehensive book presenting a systematic approach to clinical exercise testing. The authors summarize the classic and the most recent physiologic data, as well as detailed algorithms for interpretation. A large portion of the text is dedicated to case studies, representing many of the known abnormal response patterns to exercise.*

Wasserman K, McIlroy MB. Detecting the threshold of anaerobic metabolism in cardiac patients. *Am J Cardiol* 1964;14:844–852. *That lactate accumulation represents anaerobic metabolism, and that this accumulation leads to excess CO_2 production, was known before this study. However, this study was the first to show the applicability of measuring the respiratory exchange ratio (R) as a noninvasive marker of the onset (threshold) of anaerobic metabolism.*

Wasserman K, Van Kessel AL, Burton GG. Interaction of physiological mechanisms during exercise. *J Appl Physiol* 1967;22:71–85. *A study describing some of the basics of applied aspects in exercise physiology. The ventilatory response was studied in healthy subjects during a 4-min (to allow a steady state to be approached) incremental test. Ventilation is more tightly linked to the rate of CO_2 production, especially at higher work intensities.*

Wasserman K, Whipp BJ. Efficiency of muscular work. *J Appl Physiol* 1966;26:644–648. *The authors describe the basic concepts and methodology for calculating muscular work efficiency. They emphasize the need to eliminate the O_2 cost of moving the legs (unloaded cycling) from the calculation.*

Weber KT, Janicki JS. *Cardiopulmonary Exercise Testing: Physiologic Principles and Clinical Applications.* Philadelphia: WB Saunders; 1986. *A textbook describing basic physiologic aspects and various applications of integrative cardiorespiratory exercise testing in cardiovascular diseases, including hypertension.*

Weisman IM, Zeballos RJ, eds. *Clinical Exercise Testing.* Philadelphia: WB Saunders; 1994 (*Clin Chest Med;* vol 15). *Issue of* Clinics in Chest Medicine *dedicated to clinical aspects of exercise testing, mainly in lung and heart diseases, including aspects of training, transplantation, and dyspnea evaluation. Chapters are written by experts in the fields.*

Whipp BJ. The bioenergetics and gas exchange basis of exercise testing. In: Weisman IM, Zeballos RJ, eds. *Clinical Exercise Testing.* Philadelphia: WB Saunders; 1994: 173–192 (*Clin Chest Med;* vol 15). *A clear, concise, authoritative introduction to exercise bioenergetics, muscle fiber type, and gas exchange kinetics, accompanied by helpful graphic illustrations.*

Whipp BJ, Prady R. Breathing during exercise. In: Macklem P, Mead J, eds. *Handbook of Physiology, Respiration, Pulmonary Mechanics.* Washington, DC: American Physiological Society; 1986:605–629. *A detailed, authoritative critical review of the current understanding of ventilatory control during exercise.*

Textbook of Pulmonary Diseases, 6th ed.
edited by G.L. Baum, J.D. Crapo, B.R. Celli, and J.B. Karlinsky,
Lippincott–Raven Publishers, Philadelphia, © 1998.

Diagnostic Procedures Not Involving the Pleura

II

Austin B. Thompson and Stephen I. Rennard

SPUTUM

The examination of sputum for cytologic and micro-biologic diagnoses continues to be useful despite well-documented shortcomings. Contamination of sputum with oral contents is problematic for the interpretation of bacteriologic findings. However, it is less of a problem for the diagnosis of endobronchial malignancy or infection with organisms, such as *Pneumocystis carinii*, that are not colonizers of the oropharyngeal mucosa.

For cytologic examination, sputum is best collected early in the morning. There are a number of methods for handling sputum before staining for cytologic diagnosis, but in general, the diagnostic yield of the cytologic examination of sputum ranges from 50%–90%. The diagnostic yield for sputum can be increased by examining multiple specimens; improved recovery rates have been demonstrated for up to five samples. The collection of sputum for examination has the advantage of being noninvasive, and adequate samples can be readily obtained on an outpatient basis with a minimal amount of patient instruction. However, obtaining a positive diagnosis from sputum does not always obviate the need for bronchoscopy. In the case of tumors other than the small-cell type, bronchoscopy is often essential for adequate staging when a patient is being considered for surgery. False-positive results from cytologic examination of the sputum are low, ranging from 1%–3% in most series, and tend to occur when acute inflammation is present.

Cytologic examination of sputum in noninfectious, benign disorders is rarely fruitful. Exceptions include the findings of lipid-laden macrophages, suggestive of aspiration, lipoid pneumonia, or fat embolism, or hemosiderin-laden macrophages, suggestive of intrapulmonary hemorrhage associated with Goodpasture's syndrome, idiopathic pulmonary hemorrhage, or diffuse alveolar hemorrhage as a complication of high-dose chemotherapy.

In infectious diseases, attention to detail in sputum collection is essential. The patient must be encouraged to produce secretions from the tracheobronchial tree rather than saliva. Sputum can be induced by inhalation of an aerosolized solution of saline solution, distilled water, propylene glycol, or sulfur dioxide. In any case, observation by trained personnel can greatly aid in the collection of an adequate specimen. Once the sputum specimen has been obtained from the patient, it should be delivered promptly to the microbiology laboratory if bacterial, mycotic, or viral diseases are suspected. Interpretation of sputum Gram stains requires attention to the clinical presentation. Amplification of DNA by polymerase chain reaction can extend the sensitivity of sputum analysis and has been applied in the detection of tuberculosis and infection with *Chlamydia trachomatis* and HIV-1. For the detection of mycobacteria, three fresh, early-morning specimens give the best yield. Because of the hardiness of these organisms, 24- to 72-hr collections of sputum are useful, especially when sputum production is scant and sputum induction is either not available or ineffective.

Cytologic examination of sputum for offending organisms is most clearly diagnostic when organisms are identified that portend significant lung disease in the clinical setting. Thus, isolation of *P. carinii* in patients with AIDS or *Aspergillus fumigatus* in patients with leukemia are indications for specific therapy. In hosts who are not immunocompromised, sputum findings can be diagnostic of pneumonia when the Gram stain demonstrates predomi-

A. B. Thompson and S. I. Rennard: Section of Pulmonary and Critical Care Medicine, Department of Internal Medicine, University of Nebraska Medical Center, Omaha, Nebraska 68198-5300.

nance of a single organism or cultures yield a pure growth of a pathogen. The utility of sputum cytology for diagnosis of pneumonia is maximized by the use of special stains, such as the Grocott-Gomori silver stain for fungi or *P. carinii,* and the use of immunologic and molecular biologic techniques, such as the direct fluorescent antibody stain or polymerase chain reaction for *Legionella.*

TRANSTRACHEAL ASPIRATION

A major limitation of examination of sputum in infectious diseases is contamination by the oropharyngeal contents. Transtracheal aspiration was introduced as a method for bypassing the oropharynx during collection of tracheobronchial secretions. In this technique, the cricothyroid membrane and overlying skin are anesthetized and a large-bore (14-gauge) needle is passed into the trachea with gentle aspiration of air confirming proper placement. A plastic catheter is threaded caudally, and once it is in place, the needle is withdrawn. A small amount of saline solution is infused through the catheter, causing cough, and the secretions that are produced are aspirated into the catheter. False-negative results in transtracheal aspiration are rare, estimated to be <1%. However, false-positive results, resulting from colonization of the lower respiratory tract in association with chronic bronchitis, cigarette smoking, and chronic diseases, are not uncommon, with estimates of a false-positive rate up to 27%. Even in a young, healthy population, Gram stain of a transtracheal aspirate offers no advantage over sputum Gram stain in the initial management of acute pneumonia. Because of these limitations and rare but severe complications, which include mediastinal and subcutaneous emphysema, hypoxemia with complicating cardiac arrhythmias, and hemorrhage (rarely associated with fatality), transtracheal aspiration is not as widely performed as previously. The development of other diagnostic procedures, including bronchoalveolar lavage (BAL), protected specimen brush catheters, and, when more invasive procedures are clinically justified, transthoracic needle aspiration or video-assisted thorascopic lung biopsy, has provided alternatives to transtracheal aspiration that are safer or yield more useful information.

FLEXIBLE FIBEROPTIC BRONCHOSCOPY

Flexible fiberoptic bronchoscopy was introduced by Dr. Ikeda in the late 1960s. By the mid-1970s, the flexible fiberoptic bronchoscope was widely utilized in the United States, and its clinical applications have continued to expand even as limitations of flexible fiberoptic bronchoscopy have become more fully appreciated.

Flexible fiberoptic bronchoscopy can be readily performed in sedated, spontaneously breathing patients following anesthesia of the upper airway mucosa with topically applied agents. The tip of the bronchoscope can be passed through the nose or mouth with the patient sitting or supine. Alternatively, bronchoscopy can be performed in previously intubated patients, or intubation can be performed over the bronchoscope. In intubated patients, a size 7.5-French or larger endotracheal tube assures adequate air flow. Instillation of lidocaine through the bronchoscope effectively suppresses cough. Cough and bronchospasm are minimized by pretreatment with inhaled β-agonists. Atropine is also routinely administered before flexible fiberoptic bronchoscopy to diminish airway secretions and prevent vasovagal reactions. To help ensure safety, patients should have intravenous access established before bronchoscopy. Vital signs should be checked on a regular schedule, cardiac rhythm monitored via electrocardiography, and oxygen saturation monitored continuously.

Flexible fiberoptic bronchoscopy is relatively contraindicated in patients with uncorrected coagulopathies, severe airway obstruction, hypoxia or hypercarbia, or cardiac arrhythmias. It is also contraindicated in patients who are uncooperative. Complications of flexible fiberoptic bronchoscopy are rare but potentially include drug reactions, cardiac arrhythmia, hemorrhage, pneumothorax, pneumonia, and exacerbation of airway diseases.

Flexible fiberoptic bronchoscopy has proved to be an invaluable diagnostic technique for endobronchial lesions. The bronchoscope can be used to visualize the airways directly down to the fourth or fifth generation, allowing for precise localization of endobronchial lesions and visual identification of neoplasms, aspirated foreign bodies, and sites of trauma to the airways, such as tracheal lesions caused by prolonged endotracheal intubation or bronchial wall erosions caused by broncholiths.

In the evaluation of hemoptysis, flexible fiberoptic bronchoscopy has been used to localize anatomic sites of bleeding from peripheral lesions and to visualize directly bleeding from lesions in the central airways.

Direct visualization of the airways by flexible fiberoptic bronchoscopy enables identification of characteristic changes associated with acute inflammation, such as mucosal edema, erythema, friability, and secretion of mucus; thus, it can be used to confirm diagnoses associated with acute inflammation, such as pneumonia or acute bronchitis. Likewise, changes typical of chronic bronchitis may be identified, including hyperemia, thinning and striations of the mucosa, and mucosal pits that represent orifices of enlarged submucosal glands.

Direct visualization of endobronchial lesions is very useful for the staging of lung cancer. The extension of a tumor mass into the trachea, onto the carina or within 2 cm of the carina, implies that the tumor cannot be resected without special techniques to reconstruct the trachea.

Flexible fiberoptic bronchoscopy can also be used for follow-up of chemotherapy or radiation therapy of endobronchial lesions. The ability to sample pulmonary lesions, both endobronchial and extrabronchial, via the flexible fiberoptic bronchoscope greatly extends its clinical utility.

ENDOBRONCHIAL BIOPSY

Endobronchial biopsies are performed with forceps introduced through the suction port of a flexible fiberoptic bronchoscope. A number of instruments can be used for endobronchial biopsy. Biopsy forceps are available in various configurations, all of which can provide adequate samples. Preference for forceps configuration is primarily a function of operator training and experience. If the surface of the endobronchial lesion is smooth and firm, the biopsy forceps may, at times, slide off the lesion. This can be prevented by using a ''spear'' forceps, in which a small knife emerges from the base of the forceps and is encompassed by the forceps. This knife can be plunged into the tumor, anchoring the forceps and allowing biopsy to proceed. If the endobronchial lesion involves an airway wall parallel to the orientation of the bronchoscope, there may not be an adequate surface for the forceps to grab and hold. In this case, a curette designed to flex to 90° can be used to scrape the lesion to obtain a sample for cytologic examination.

The partial occlusion of the suctioning channel by the introduction of the biopsy forceps may limit suctioning of airway secretions, thereby compromising the field of view and increasing the technical difficulty of the biopsy. This problem can be avoided by using a smaller-sized forceps and a larger-sized suctioning channel, or by employing a bronchoscope with two suctioning channels.

Endobronchial biopsies are generally performed following the instillation of lidocaine directly onto the mucosal surface to be sampled. The procedure is typically complicated by small (<5 mL) amounts of bleeding, but with highly vascular lesions, especially endobronchial carcinoid tumors, the resulting bleeding can be massive and life-threatening. Highly vascular endobronchial carcinoid tumors can be recognized by their cherry-red appearance. A flexible fiberoptic bronchoscope should not be used to obtain specimens from endobronchial lesions with this presentation; rather, such lesions should be approached with a rigid bronchoscope and appropriate surgical support.

Endobronchial biopsies have been associated with pneumothorax. However, the incidence of pneumothorax following endobronchial biopsy is exceedingly low and does not justify routine chest roentgenograms following the procedure.

The greatest utility of endobronchial biopsy is in the diagnosis of cancer. Typically, endobronchial malignancies represent bronchogenic carcinoma. However, endobronchial metastases can occur, most frequently from carcinoma of the breast, malignant melanoma, and tumors of the kidney or colon.

Cytologic brushes provide another tool for collection of endobronchial material. Vigorous brushing of the mucosal surface with a stiff brush exfoliates cells that are ideal for cytologic examination. The cytologic brush samples a larger surface area than an endobronchial biopsy forceps. The brush can be used to obtain samples from airways distal to the visual field of the bronchoscope, so that the complications associated with transbronchial biopsy can be avoided (see below). Hemorrhage is rare, but brushing with cytologic brushes is routinely associated with more bleeding than is obtaining samples with a forceps alone. This is especially true if the mucosa is friable, as is often the case when airways inflammation complicates an endobronchial lesion.

The diagnostic yield of direct forceps biopsy of endobronchial lesions is very high. Reported diagnostic yields range from 70%–100%, with most investigators reporting yields of up to 95%. Lesions associated with false-negative results include large necrotic masses from which nondiagnostic, necrotic material is obtained and lesions that are physically difficult to sample because of their shape, surface characteristics, or location.

Brushings also have a high diagnostic yield of up to 93% for directly visualized lesions. However, they do not appear to add significantly to the diagnostic yield of endobronchial forceps biopsy if the lesion is readily visualized. Similarly, cytologic examination of washings gathered through the bronchoscope during the course of the bronchoscopy or expectorated sputum gathered after bronchoscopy has been utilized, but neither of these specimens adds to the diagnostic yield of forceps biopsy.

TRANSBRONCHIAL BIOPSY

Transbronchial biopsy extends the utility of flexible fiberoptic bronchoscopy to include sampling of peripheral masses and pulmonary parenchyma suspected of being diseased or infected. Transbronchial biopsies are performed by extending the biopsy forceps beyond the visual range of the bronchoscope. Patient cooperation is essential. The forceps are opened during deep inhalation and closed during exhalation. This enfolds lung parenchyma into the forceps, increasing the amount of lung parenchyma that is sampled.

The procedure is generally performed under biplanar fluoroscopy to localize sampling of discrete lesions accurately and to prevent extreme peripheral placement of the forceps, which may result in perforation of the lung pleura. Unintentional biopsy of small muscular arteries can lead to bleeding. Instillation of 1 mL of 1:20,000 epinephrine before performing the biopsy and keeping the bronchoscope wedged into the airway at the site of sampling generally controls the bleeding. Thus, it is imperative that the bronchoscope be maintained in a wedged position until hemostasis is ensured. Transbronchial biopsies are also associated with an incidence of pneumothorax as high as 5%. Most of these cases are not serious, but occasionally placement of a chest tube is required.

The diagnostic yield of transbronchial biopsy varies according to the character of the lung lesion being assessed. For peripheral masses, diagnostic yields range from 30%–90%, with a mean of about 60%. Yields have been improved by the use of bronchography to plan the bronchoscopic approach to the peripheral lesion and by the use of bedside cytology with repeated sampling after the procedure. In interstitial lung diseases, transbronchial biopsy can validate clinical diagnoses of sarcoidosis, pulmonary alveolar proteinosis, eosinophilic granuloma, hypersensitivity pneumonitis, and lymphangioleiomyomatosis. Transbronchial biopsies can be diagnostic in each of these diseases because of their distinctive pathologic features. In contrast, transbronchial biopsy is not felt to be diagnostic for idiopathic pulmonary fibrosis or other interstitial pneumonitides. The diagnostic yield for interstitial lung disease has been most extensively studied for sarcoidosis. Sampling errors are minimized by repeated biopsies; for sarcoidosis, four biopsies have been found to produce up to a 90% yield.

Transbronchial biopsy has also been used for the diagnosis of infectious diseases. In most infectious diseases, sampling is best done by BAL (see below), but there are exceptions. The yield of BAL is low in fungal infections, particularly invasive aspergillosis, and such cases should be approached with transbronchial biopsy or transthoracic needle aspiration if clinically feasible. Prophylactic treatment for *P. carinii* in patients with AIDS leads to lower yields with BAL in the diagnosis of *P. carinii* pneumonia. Yields are increased from 60%–80% by the addition of transbronchial biopsy.

TRANSBRONCHIAL NEEDLE ASPIRATION

A variety of needles have been developed for needle aspiration of lesions via the flexible fiberoptic bronchoscope. The choice depends on operator preference and biopsy site. Steel needles are preferred for transbronchial and transtracheal biopsies, whereas flexible plastic needles are better suited for apical biopsies. Needle aspiration is especially useful for the diagnosis of lesions that lie beyond the visual field of the bronchoscope. The technique has been used to sample paratracheal nodes, mediastinal nodes (especially subcarinal nodes), submucosal lesions, extrabronchial lesions, and peripheral masses. Transbronchial needle aspiration can be used to approach peripheral lesions that are, because of airway anatomy, inaccessible to the transbronchial biopsy forceps.

To sample areas contiguous to the large airways, the needle is advanced under direct visualization to the suspected area and pushed through the airway wall, and suction is then applied to aspirate a specimen for cytologic

examination. Following withdrawal of the needle from the bronchoscope, a small amount of saline solution is used to flush the specimen from the needle. To sample peripheral lesions, the needle is advanced under fluoroscopic guidance and plunged transbronchially directly into the lesion. Complications resulting from needle aspiration, which are rare, include pneumothorax and pneumomediastinum with reported rates of <1%.

The diagnostic yield for aspiration of paratracheal and hilar adenopathy, as visualized on chest roentgenograms, is quite high, with a sensitivity of 50% and specificity of 96% in one study. Investigations have suggested that the yield for needle aspiration can be improved by the use of computed tomographic (CT) guidance. The yield for transbronchial needle aspiration of peripheral masses depends on the size of the lesion. The recovery rate is 33% for lesions <2 cm in diameter and 80% for lesions ≥2 cm in diameter. Transbronchial needle aspiration may compliment transbronchial biopsy. In cases in which the transbronchial forceps cannot reach the lesion because of anatomic distortion of the airways, a transbronchial needle can be used to penetrate directly into the lesion through the distorted airway. Transbronchial needle aspiration has not been associated with significant complications.

BRONCHOALVEOLAR LAVAGE

Technique

The lower respiratory tract can also be sampled with the technique of BAL. In this method, a sterile isotonic solution is infused through the biopsy port of the bronchoscope. This fluid fills the intraluminal space of the conducting airways and the alveoli, and it can then be recovered by aspiration. Because the fluid mixes with the intraluminal contents, the resulting lavage fluid effectively samples the intraluminal space of the lower respiratory tract.

A large number of variations of the technique have been developed. In general, however, the procedure is done after wedging the bronchoscope in a segmental or subsegmental bronchus. The wedged position allows the lavage fluid to be infused distally in a controlled manner into a single region of the lung, and more or less prevents the fluid from spreading proximally into other lung regions. The fluid most commonly used is sterile normal saline solution. Warming the fluid to body temperature is felt to reduce cough.

The fluid initially infused reaches the intraluminal space of the more proximal conducting airways more effectively than it reaches the more distal alveolar spaces. As a result, the use of small volumes of fluid can provide a sample enriched for bronchial contents. To have an adequate sampling of alveolar contents, a total volume of at least 100 mL is generally recommended. The fluid is infused in aliquots varying in volume from 20 to 60 mL. Reduced volumes have been successfully used in children. Most bronchoscopists aspirate the fluid immediately after infusion, but some investigators allow the fluid to remain for a period of dwell time. The procedure can be repeated in several subsegments if desired.

Complications

Apart from the procedure of flexible fiberoptic bronchoscopy, BAL itself has some associated risks. The most common complication is fever. The syndrome of post-BAL fever typically develops 4 to 6 hours after the procedure, characterized by the sudden onset of rigors, fever, and malaise. Symptoms generally respond promptly to intravenous meperidine (Demerol) and often to oral acetaminophen. The syndrome is self-limited and generally resolves within 24 hrs. Fever after bronchoscopy is not thought to be caused by infection, but rather by the release of endogenous pyrogens. The occurrence of this complication appears to increase with the volume of fluid used. With a 300-mL lavage, the frequency is felt to be 20%–30%.

Infiltrates on chest roentgenogram are also common, occurring in the majority of individuals studied immediately after the procedure. These infiltrates, which presumably represent retained fluid and atelectasis, generally spontaneously resolve within 24 hrs. True infections may also occur following BAL with a frequency of 1/1000 or less. Patients generally have fever, cough, and often pleuritic chest pain 1 to 3 days following the bronchoscopy. Bleeding, pneumothorax, and bronchospasm have been reported but are rare.

Transient declines in both vital capacity and FEV_1 (forced expiratory volume in 1 second) are frequent, and these can be associated with hypoxemia. They generally are limited to about 10% declines in predicted values. Interestingly, BAL in patients with mild asthma appears to be associated with no statistically significant increased risk for decline in lung function in comparison with normal controls, although bronchospasm has been reported as a complication. These transient declines in lung function are not clinically significant in individuals with normal lung function. However, in individuals with severely compromised lung function, BAL can lead to retention of carbon dioxide or precipitate respiratory failure. Should such individuals require BAL, however, the procedure can still be performed. It is recommended that before BAL is performed, such patients undergo intubation with or without the initiation of mechanical ventilation to support ventilation and gas exchange.

Processing Bronchoalveolar Lavage Specimens

The techniques for handling and processing BAL fluids are varied. It is important that each center have a standardized technique to allow valid interpretation of results from lavage performed by different personnel. Close cooperation between clinicians and pathologists is obviously required.

Indications for Bronchoalveolar Lavage

BAL is often the diagnostic modality of choice in evaluating immunocompromised individuals with suspected pneumonia. Because the lavage fluid effectively samples the peripheral intraluminal space, peripheral intraluminal infections can be diagnosed with a high degree of reliability. For example, the diagnostic yield for *P. carinii* pneumonia in untreated patients is felt to be >95%. Viral infections can also be diagnosed reliably. For cytomegalovirus and herpesvirus, pathognomonic cytopathic changes can be recognized cytologically. The sensitivity for detecting viral material can be increased with the use of special techniques, including monoclonal antibodies, cDNA probes, and the polymerase chain reaction. Samples obtained by BAL can also be cultured for viruses, and the cultures can be analyzed using a variety of diagnostic techniques. Monoclonal antibodies can be used to assist in the diagnosis of other infections, including *Legionella* infection, but the yield is greater when this technique is combined with culture methods. The recent introduction of the analysis of BAL fluid with the polymerase chain reaction provides a very sensitive method for the detection of *Legionella, Mycobacterium, Pneumocystis, Chlamydia, Mycoplasma* organisms, and for an increasing number of viruses.

BAL fluid can also be used for the diagnosis of fungal infection, both cytologically and by culture. Because some fungi, particularly *Mucor-Absidia* and to some extent *Aspergillus,* preferentially invade the vascular spaces, the intraluminal sampling technique of BAL may not be as effective. For this reason, the diagnostic yield of BAL in cases of invasive aspergillosis may only be 50%. Negative results, therefore, must be interpreted with caution.

The sensitivity of BAL for the detection of some microorganisms that are not inevitably associated with disease (e.g., cytomegalovirus and *candida*) creates the problem of distinguishing between infection and colonization. Asymptomatic colonization may precede clinically significant infection in some situations. Thus, although BAL can provide diagnostic information, this information must be used in an appropriate clinical context.

BAL can also provide diagnostic information in individuals who are not immunosuppressed but are suspected of having infections. Not only can unusual organisms be detected, but quantitative cultures can help to confirm the presence of pneumonia when other causes of lower respiratory tract abnormalities are also present. The presence of $>10^5$ organisms on a quantitative BAL culture has a specificity approaching 100% for the diagnosis of bacterial pneumonia. This technique also permits the identification of multiple pathogens, which appear quite frequently in hospital-acquired cases of pneumonia. Quantitative cultures combined with protected BAL, in which a special catheter is used, or with culture of only the last aliquot of fluid infused during BAL appears to have improved specificity. In direct comparisons, the specificity and sensitivity of quantitative BAL appear to be similar to those of the more complex protected brush and protected BAL procedures.

Cytologic examination of BAL fluid for pulmonary malignancy can be performed. Primary and metastatic solid tumors and hematologic malignancies can be readily detected by standard and specialized cytologic techniques. BAL appears to be particularly effective in the diagnosis of lymphangitic carcinomatosis. This is probably because in such cases the tumor involves not only the pulmonary interstitium but also the intraluminal spaces. The diagnostic yield for primary lung cancer by BAL depends on several factors. Most importantly, the appropriate segment must be washed. Diagnostic yields >50% have been reported. In one large series, BAL was felt to have a superior diagnostic yield when compared with transbronchial biopsy for the diagnosis of peripheral lesions not visualized at bronchoscopy. BAL has also been suggested as one means to follow the effectiveness of chemotherapeutic intervention in patients with lung cancer.

Both routine and special cytologic techniques can be used to diagnose pulmonary malignancies in material obtained by BAL. For example, monoclonal antibodies for specific tumor-associated antigens may be helpful in detecting rare cells and determining the type of malignancy. When routine cytologic analysis is used, however, it is essential that material be interpreted by a skilled cytologist and that appropriate clinical correlations be made. In a number of nonmalignant conditions, abnormal cells can be observed that are confused easily with cancer. Infection, cytotoxic therapy, and severe inflammation may all be associated with a range of atypical cells having an appearance that can vary from mildly metaplastic to closely resembling malignancy. Thus, the diagnosis of pulmonary malignancy based on cytologic material obtained by BAL should be made only in an appropriate clinical setting.

It is possible to use BAL to assess inflammatory processes in the lower respiratory tract, such as interstitial lung diseases and lower airways diseases. The BAL findings are not pathognomonic of any particular interstitial disease, but they may be suggestive. For example, increased numbers of neutrophils in BAL fluid are often seen in idiopathic pulmonary fibrosis, whereas increased numbers of T-helper cells are found in pulmonary sarcoidosis and of T-suppressor cells in hypersensitivity pneumonitis. Thus, the analysis of inflammatory cells obtained by BAL, although not specific, can often be helpful in suggesting a diagnosis.

The intensity of alveolitis, as suggested by BAL, may be helpful in making clinical decisions, such as when to proceed to definitive biopsy procedures or when to initiate or change therapy.

Eosinophilia and increased numbers of mast cells, together with increased levels of eosinophil- and mast cell-derived mediators, are commonly found in the airways of patients with asthma. The presence of these cells and their mediators correlates with hyperresponsiveness and clinical symptoms. Increased airways neutrophilia has been reported by some investigators in asthma and has also been reported in chronic bronchitis. Although patients with airways disease have been studied by BAL, at present this technique should be regarded primarily as a research procedure rather than as a clinical tool.

BAL has also been used to obtain material for the analysis of a large number of chemical components present in the lower respiratory tract. These measurements are mainly research activities without current clinical use.

SCALENE NODE BIOPSY

Pulmonary malignancies as well as inflammatory diseases of the lung spread in a somewhat predictable pattern, based on the lymphatic drainage system. The lymphatics of all the lobes of the right lung drain initially into the lymphatic sump of Borrie, a collection of intrapulmonary lymph nodes lying between the upper lobe bronchus and the bronchus medius. From there, the upper lobe drainage enters the lower paratracheal area in the region of the azygos vein. The middle and lower lobes drain to the subcarinal, pulmonary ligament, and paraesophageal nodes. From these locations, all lobes of the right lung drain to the right scalene area. Both lobes of the left lung drain to the lymphatic sump between the upper and lower lobe bronchi and hence to the subcarinal, pulmonary ligament, and paraesophageal nodes. The upper lobe also drains to nodes in the aortopulmonary window, left paratracheal area, and anterior mediastinum. Approximately 25% of left lower lobe drainage crosses over to the right side, whereas 90% of the left upper lobe drainage stays on the left, eventually reaching the left scalene nodes. However, it is important to remember that these drainage patterns are not absolute, and crossover metastases from either side may occur, probably as a result of obstructed lymphatics.

The procedure of scalene node biopsy is well established and is almost always carried out with local anesthesia. A 5-cm transverse incision is made over the lateral border of the sternocleidomastoid muscle, 2 cm superior and parallel to the clavicle. The fat pad containing lymph nodes, located in the space posterior to the sternocleidomastoid muscle and anterior to the anterior scalene muscle, is removed for microscopic study. The most important structures encountered are the subclavian vein inferiorly, the internal jugular vein and carotid artery medially, and the phrenic nerve lying on the anterior surface of the anterior scalene muscle and on the left side the thoracic duct. The operating time for this procedure is short, and postoperative patient discomfort is minimal.

In patients with lung cancer, biopsy of palpable scalene nodes has a positive diagnostic rate of about 80%. In patients with lung cancer but nonpalpable scalene nodes, the positive diagnostic rate is only about 20%. Scalene node biopsy has been used in nonmalignant disease as well. The biopsy of nonpalpable scalene nodes may offer a positive diagnosis in as many as 80% of patients with sarcoidosis and other granulomatous diseases.

Complications of scalene node biopsy include hematoma, seroma, pneumothorax, infection, air embolism, lymph fistula, hoarseness, phrenic nerve palsy, chylothorax, or a Horner's syndrome. These complications are rare, with a total prevalence of all complications of only 1%–2% and a mortality rate of 0.1%. Prior radiation therapy incorporating the scalene nodes in the field of radiation is a relative contraindication, as the resulting fibrosis complicates surgical dissection and healing and may lower the likelihood of a positive biopsy result.

For suspected malignant intrathoracic disease, most authors would recommend that scalene node biopsy be performed first whenever palpable nodes are present. Scalene nodes positive for malignancy are N3 nodes, indicating a stage of IIIB for lung cancer, considered by most to be beyond curative resection. Routine biopsy of nonpalpable scalene nodes in patients with lung cancer has a low diagnostic yield, especially with peripheral lesions and tumors <3 cm in diameter. Although the matter is controversial, most surgeons would forego scalene node biopsy in these patients and proceed with staging using radiologic imaging and mediastinoscopy when indicated. Used judiciously, scalene node biopsy is a simple, valuable procedure that may obviate the need for more invasive staging or even thoracotomy.

MEDIASTINOSCOPY

Technique and Complications

Mediastinoscopy is a surgical procedure performed under general anesthesia with the neck hyperextended and the head turned to the left. A short (4-cm) transverse incision is made centered just above the suprasternal notch. Once the pretracheal fascia is reached, blunt finger dissection is used to open the relatively bloodless plane of loose areolar tissue just anterior to the trachea. The rigid mediastinoscope is introduced into this plane and is advanced down as far as the carina. In this way, right and left paratracheal nodes, anterior subcarinal nodes, and some proximal right hilar nodes may be visualized and sampled. Access to the left hilum is limited by the aortic

arch. In performing this procedure, the surgeon has only monocular vision without depth perception. Expertise is essential, because the pretracheal space entered by the mediastinoscope contains a number of vital structures, including the aortic arch, superior vena cava, brachiocephalic artery, and left atrium. This procedure is relatively brief, and patients require only an overnight hospital stay. Mediastinoscopy requires pliable tissue planes free of adhesions to allow blunt dissection, so that prior mediastinoscopy, other mediastinal surgery, or mediastinal radiation therapy are relative contraindications to this procedure. Prior open heart surgery may fix the mediastinal structures and make mediastinoscopy much more difficult. Superior vena caval obstruction usually causes mediastinal venous engorgement and elevates the risk for bleeding, but it is not an absolute contraindication for mediastinoscopy.

Because the nodes draining the left upper and lower lobes may drain to the subaortic nodes or the anterior mediastinum, they may not be readily accessible to standard cervical mediastinoscopy. To approach these nodes, an extended cervical mediastinoscopy has been described. With this technique, the anterior mediastinum can also be explored through the same neck incision, but this method has not become popular because of its perceived difficulty and higher risks.

Despite the vital structures surrounding the area explored with the mediastinoscope and the limited surgical field, complications from standard cervical mediastinoscopy are infrequent in the hands of an experienced surgeon. The principle risk is hemorrhage from laceration or inadvertent sampling of a blood vessel. Pneumothorax, recurrent laryngeal nerve paralysis, tracheal injury, or wound infection also may occur. The prevalence of all complications is low (1.7%–2.3%), and the rate of emergency thoracotomies required to control serious complications is 0.3%. In two recent clinical series with a combined total of 2259 patients undergoing mediastinoscopy, there were no deaths. A mortality of ≤1% has been reported in most series.

Indications for Cervical Mediastinoscopy

Cervical mediastinoscopy is primarily indicated to evaluate the status of mediastinal lymph nodes in patients with potentially resectable lung cancer who do not have palpable supraclavicular nodes. The technique also provides a tissue diagnosis for any patient whose primary lesion is not accessible or who is not a candidate for resection because of poor pulmonary function or other medical reasons. The diagnostic yield depends largely on patient selection. When routine mediastinoscopy is performed in all patients with presumed operable carcinoma of the lung, 27%–30% of patients have metastatic disease in the excised nodes. The highest yields have been seen in patients with tumors of the right lung, larger central tumors, and small-cell tumors or adenocarcinomas.

An area of considerable interest has been the role of CT of the chest in staging mediastinal metastases in patients with lung carcinoma. Based on studies of CT scans in normal patients and cadavers, nodes up to 1 cm in diameter are generally considered to be normal. Nodes with a diameter of ≥ 1.5 cm are abnormal, and nodes between 1 and 1.5 cm in diameter are indeterminate or suspect. With these criteria, the sensitivity of CT ranges from as low as 61% up to 95%, and specificity from 50%–94%. Magnetic resonance imaging of the chest has not offered any advantages over CT in the assessment of mediastinal nodes.

Recent studies including exhaustive lymph node dissections and meticulous correlation with CT findings have demonstrated that the sensitivity of CT may not be as high as previously thought. Mediastinal metastases were found involving lymph nodes of <1 cm in diameter in as many as 33% of patients. These nodes would have been classified as normal using the CT criterion for normal size of ≤ 1 cm in diameter. Nevertheless, patients with mediastinal micrometastases or minimal N2 disease discovered at the time of thoracotomy have 5-year survival rates of as much as 34% after resection of the tumor and mediastinal metastases followed by postoperative radiation therapy.

CT may be useful in screening for macroscopic metastatic disease indicated by enlarged nodes (>15 mm) or indeterminate nodes (10 to 15 mm) that need to be verified by mediastinoscopy. If CT shows no mediastinal abnormalities and especially if there is a small peripheral lesion, then mediastinoscopy can be bypassed as a surgical staging procedure, and the surgeon can proceed directly to thoracotomy. At thoracotomy, a thorough mediastinal node dissection must be performed in all patients with negative findings at mediastinoscopy or in patients in whom this procedure has not been performed, so as to make an accurate determination of the surgical stage. Meticulous sampling of mediastinal nodes at thoracotomy is also important in all patients with tumors of the left lung, as metastases to some nodal groups may be inaccessible by mediastinoscopy. Thus, a policy of routine mediastinoscopy for all patients is not a reasonable, cost-effective approach in lung cancer.

Mediastinoscopy is also indicated to verify the diagnosis of nonpulmonary malignancies, such as lymphoma, and of granulomatous diseases, such as sarcoidosis, histoplasmosis, and occasionally tuberculosis. The diagnostic yield is high, particularly with CT evidence of mediastinal or hilar adenopathy. Mediastinoscopy is practically 100% accurate in the diagnosis of sarcoidosis in the presence of appropriate CT abnormalities and has become the preferred invasive diagnostic procedure with this disease whenever transbronchoscopic biopsy is unsuccessful and other, more accessible sites are not involved.

Parasternal Anterior Mediastinotomy

Anterior mediastinotomy requires general anesthesia with endotracheal intubation. A short, transverse (''hockey stick'') incision is made over the second or third costal cartilage just adjacent to the sternum on the appropriate side. A segment of cartilage is removed, and through the bed of the resected cartilage an extrapleural plane is bluntly developed toward the hilum of the lung. Use of a headlight and careful retraction allows evaluation of nodes in the anterior mediastinum lying in front of the great vessels, right paratracheal nodes, subaortic nodes on the left, and tracheobronchial angle nodes. Vigorous retraction occasionally permits sampling of paraesophageal nodes, posterior-inferior tracheobronchial nodes, or posterior subcarinal nodes. Entry into the pleural cavity (often done inadvertently) permits direct exposure of hilar masses for biopsy. When the pleura has been entered, a small chest tube is inserted through a separate wound and is left on suction for a short time after wound closure and recovery. Depending on the number of frozen sections obtained and the extent of dissection necessary, most procedures can be completed in a reasonably brief period of time. The in-hospital recovery time is generally 1 to 2 days, depending on whether a chest tube is used or not. Postoperative discomfort is mild but usually greater than that experienced after mediastinoscopy.

Few complications occur with anterior mediastinotomy, although it is more invasive and has a slightly higher complication rate than mediastinoscopy. Bleeding is usually controlled by pressure or suture; if bleeding is severe, the incision can be extended into an anterior thoracotomy for repair of the site of bleeding. Wound infection, pneumothorax from unsuspected pleural entry, pleural effusion, pneumonia, and phrenic nerve damage also have been described. The total rate of all complications is reported at 6.7%–9%, and the mortality rate is 1% or less. Relative contraindications to this procedure include a history of prior median sternotomy or radiation therapy, as adhesions and lack of pliable tissue planes make dissection hazardous through the small mediastinotomy incision.

The indications for anterior mediastinotomy are generally the same as for mediastinoscopy. In patients with nonpalpable supraclavicular nodes who have suspected pulmonary malignancies and evidence of mediastinal adenopathy, anterior mediastinotomy is a good staging alternative to mediastinoscopy. It permits access to nodal areas such as the anterior mediastinum and aortopulmonary window, which are common sites of left lung metastases but are inaccessible by mediastinoscopy. Mediastinotomy is preferred in patients with the superior vena caval syndrome, prior mediastinal radiation therapy, or prior mediastinoscopy. In cases of nonpulmonary neoplasms and inflammatory diseases, mediastinotomy offers the potential for biopsy of enlarged mediastinal nodes seen on CT, and also allows an open lung biopsy to be performed through the same incision should the mediastinal nodes prove nondiagnostic.

Some surgeons prefer anterior mediastinotomy because it provides an open, more accessible surgical field, compared with the limited field provided by mediastinoscopy. However, mediastinoscopy is associated with less morbidity and mortality, a shorter operating time, and less postoperative pain than anterior mediastinotomy. Mediastinotomy and mediastinoscopy can be viewed as complementary rather than competing procedures that have equivalent results in properly selected patients. The procedure to be used is best chosen based on CT and individual patient evaluation, with the goals of minimizing morbidity and maximizing the likelihood of a diagnosis.

PERCUTANEOUS TRANSTHORACIC NEEDLE BIOPSY

Transthoracic needle aspiration or biopsy has several indications, which include the following: (1) diagnosis of parenchymal lung nodules, particularly peripheral lesions, whether solitary or multiple; (2) classification and staging of suspected pulmonary or mediastinal metastasis; (3) diagnosis of suspected infectious diseases (nodules or infiltrates); (4) diagnosis of mediastinal, hilar, and pleural masses; and (5) evaluation of lesions for which bronchoscopic evaluation has failed to provide a definitive diagnosis.

Contraindications include anticoagulation, bleeding dyscrasia, and thrombocytopenia (platelet count <50,000). It is essential that the patient be able to cooperate fully with the procedure. If not, the complication rate rises and adequate specimens may not be obtained. If clinically indicated, coagulation defects can be temporarily corrected, reducing the risk for hemorrhage. Severe chronic obstructive pulmonary disease (COPD) is a relative contraindication. COPD is associated with an increased risk for pneumothorax from percutaneous needle aspiration or biopsy, and such patients are less able to tolerate the effects of a pneumothorax. Other relative contraindications to transthoracic needle aspiration include pulmonary hypertension, positive-pressure mechanical ventilation, and suspected vascular lesions, such as arteriovenous malformations.

Sensitivity of transthoracic needle biopsy ranges from 60%–97%. Diagnostic yield is optimal when adequate samples are provided, and both an experienced surgeon to perform the biopsy and an experienced cytopathologist to interpret the results are required. Transthoracic biopsy of malignant mediastinal and hilar lesions provides an accurate diagnosis in approximately 90% of cases. The positive yield for metastatic pulmonary and mediastinal disease is >80%. Correlation between cytologic and histopathologic diagnoses varies from 77%–82% and depends on sampling error, intraobserver variability in interpretation, and tumor pleomorphism.

Tools and Technique

Several types of needles are available for percutaneous sampling of the lung. These fall into two basic types: aspiration or fine needles and biopsy needles. Aspiration needles for the lung and mediastinum usually range in size from 18 to 23 gauge and are primarily used to aspirate cells for cytologic examination, but they may provide small fragments of tissue for histology as well. Probably the most familiar of the aspiration needles is the Chiba needle, which has a beveled tip angled at 24° and an inner removable stylet. Spinal needles can also be utilized as aspiration needles for the lung and mediastinum. They have a greater bevel angle, possess thicker walls, and hence are stiffer than the Chiba needle.

Biopsy needles also are of two general types: small-gauge biopsy needles and cutting biopsy needles. Small-gauge biopsy needles (e.g., Greene, Turner, Westcott, or Haaga needles) are modified aspiration needles designed to acquire small samples of tissue for histologic examination and preparation of cell blocks. The fine needles are commonly employed for transthoracic needle biopsy of the lung and mediastinum and are superior for obtaining cells for cell block analysis. Cutting needles are designed to obtain adequate amounts of tissue for histology. The sample provided by needle biopsy augments cytologic diagnosis of malignancy, confirming the diagnosis of a specific cell type or supporting a negative cytologic result. However, there is controversy regarding whether histologic sections of tissue obtained with thin needles significantly often lead to a positive diagnostic result when needle cytology specimens have given a negative result. Cutting needles are recommended for the biopsy of an unknown primary or a possible second primary; evaluation of suspected benign disease, especially in the anterior and posterior mediastinum; and for cases in which several passes or prior attempts with an aspiration needle have not revealed a positive cytologic diagnosis. Concerning the question of increased risk for hemorrhage, a recent prospective study demonstrated that the use of large-bore, true-cut needles was not associated with a significantly greater rate of complications than fine-needle aspiration in the evaluation of mediastinal masses, even those situated near major vessels.

Imaging Guidance

Fluoroscopy, CT, and ultrasonography have all proved to be effective guides for transthoracic needle biopsy.

Fluoroscopy has the advantages of low cost and relative ease of operation. Lesions that are at least 1.5 to 2 cm in diameter can be adequately visualized by fluoroscopy. Biplanar fluoroscopy is the most precise fluoroscopic technique. CT of the chest should probably be obtained before fluoroscopically guided needle biopsy to ensure that the suspected lesion is not vascular and to localize the lesion in relation to other vital structures, thus helping to design the optimal pathway for the aspiration or biopsy needle. CT-guided transthoracic needle biopsy should be considered for lung and mediastinal lesions that are not well visualized by fluoroscopy because of small size or other reasons. CT-guided imaging is suggested for lesions between 0.5 and 1.5 cm in diameter that are contiguous to major vascular structures or blebs. CT-guided needle biopsy is limited by the higher cost and longer duration of the procedure.

Complications

The most common complication following transthoracic needle aspiration or biopsy is pneumothorax. The frequency of pneumothorax in most studies ranges from 10%–35% following fluoroscopically guided procedures, and is approximately 37% when CT is the imaging method employed. The increased incidence of pneumothorax in CT-guided needle biopsies is most likely a consequence of the use of this imaging method for more difficult lesions requiring longer biopsy time and multiple passes with the needle. Thoracostomy tubes are required in fewer than half of cases of needle biopsy pneumothorax. In one series of 2421 transthoracic, fine-needle biopsies, a pneumothorax developed in 34% of patients, but only 7.8% required insertion of a thoracostomy tube. Indications for thoracostomy tube treatment of a pneumothorax following biopsy include dyspnea, a pneumothorax >30% in size, or an interval increase in the size of the pneumothorax on repeated x-ray imaging of the chest. A 7-French chest tube with a Heimlich valve is frequently sufficient to treat a pneumothorax following biopsy. Needle size does not appear to affect the incidence of pneumothorax. Factors that do predispose to biopsy-induced pneumothorax include increased number of needle passes, increased depth of the lesion, cavitary lesions, increasing patient age, and the presence of COPD.

Other mild complications include hemoptysis, which occurs in approximately 10% of cases, and subcutaneous emphysema.

Procedure

Transthoracic needle aspiration biopsy is usually an outpatient procedure. Patients who are very anxious may benefit from premedication with short-acting sedatives or benzodiazepines. Atropine has been used to reduce vagal tone and help prevent the possibility of vasovagal reactions. An intravenous line is routinely inserted, and electrocardiogram, arterial saturation, and blood pressure are routinely monitored during and after the procedure. The lesion to be sampled is localized, usually with fluoroscopy, and prior CT radiographs are examined for visualization of the lesion and its relation to vital structures. The patient is placed in the supine, prone, oblique, or lateral decubitus position according to the location of the lesion. The approach for mediastinal and hilar lesions depends on the size and proximity of the lesion to cardiovascular structures. In general, for anterior mediastinal masses, the anterior or parasternal approach is preferred, whereas for posterior mediastinal lesions, a paravertebral approach is often chosen. For biopsy of hilar masses, an anterior or posterior approach is employed, depending on whether the lesion is anterior or posterior to hilar vessels on contrast-enhanced CT of the thorax. Lidocaine (Xylocaine) is used for local anesthesia of the skin, subcutaneous tissue, and parietal pleura. Whenever possible, the needle is advanced over the superior margin of a rib to avoid injury of the intercostal neurovascular bundle. The actual passage of the needle into the lesion should be accomplished during breath-holding at end-expiration. This is particularly important in the biopsy of small nodules.

Techniques have been described that allow for multiple passes of the needle into a suspect lesion without repeated penetration of the pleura. In one method, the coaxial technique, an inner, smaller-gauge needle is used to aspirate samples repeatedly through an outer, larger needle passed just to the outer margin of the lesion. This method can be used with small-gauge biopsy needles and cutting biopsy needles, thereby allowing for histologic as well as cytologic examination. Following the biopsy, some choose to inject 5 to 10 mL of an autologous blood clot to patch the tract of the outer needle. In the second technique (the tandem needle approach), one needle is passed into the lesion to localize or mark the site while the second needle is employed for aspiration and biopsy in tandem to the path of the marker needle. Rapid cytologic processing of the samples can be used both to minimize the number of passes made and to ensure that diagnostic material is obtained. Gram-stained smears and cultures of aspirated materials should be done if indicated. If cores of tissue are obtained, these should be submitted in formalin for histopathologic examination.

A chest radiograph is routinely performed immediately after the procedure, and then 2 to 4 hours later, to detect the presence of a pneumothorax. The patient's vital signs should be monitored after the procedure, and the patient should be observed for symptoms of chest pain, dyspnea, hemoptysis, and cardiovascular instability.

Interpretation and Clinical Application of Results

Difficult clinical decisions must be made when a biopsy result is negative or benign, which occurs in 5%–25% of all transthoracic needle biopsies. Biopsy should be repeated if findings are nonspecific (e.g., inflammation, necrosis, or hemorrhage), as a negative result does not exclude malignancy. Repetition of the procedure with a biopsy needle should be considered if tissue for histology was not obtained, or the surgeon should proceed directly to thoracotomy for a histologic diagnosis. A specifically benign diagnosis, such as hamartoma, granuloma, or infection, is usually reliable. However, if the clinical presentation or radiologic features strongly suggest malignancy, then a thoracotomy should be performed despite specifically benign findings. When the clinical presentation and radiographic features are more consistent with benign disease, the patient can be carefully followed with regular x-ray imaging every 3 months for the first year, then every 4 to 6 months for the second year, and annually thereafter. Subsequent growth of the lesion revealed on chest x-ray films warrants prompt re-evaluation. Conversely, an interval reduction in the size of the suspect lesion lends support to a benign diagnosis, and further observation of the lesion is appropriate.

OPEN LUNG BIOPSY

Technique

When less invasive diagnostic methods fail, or the clinical situation dictates the need for a very rapid definitive diagnosis, open lung biopsy remains the most reliable approach.

Open lung biopsy is performed under general anesthesia with endotracheal intubation. For most diffuse infiltrative or nodular lung disease, a small, 5- to 7-cm incision is made over the fourth or fifth intercostal space anteriorly. The pleural cavity is exposed with a small rib spreader. A portion of the lingula, the anterior portion of the right or left lower lobe, or the right middle lobe is allowed to herniate through the wound. In the inflated state, a transverse or wedge biopsy of lung is excised using lung staplers and is sent fresh for pathologic and bacteriologic examinations. Most importantly, the portion of lung obtained should include adequate amounts of both normal and abnormal tissue. If appropriate, several samples from two lobes may be obtained through the same incision. Lateral and posterior portions of either lung are usually not accessible for biopsy through this anterior incision. A chest tube is left in place in the pleural cavity, usually for 24 to 48 hours. The entire surgical procedure is brief, with minimal blood loss. The small, anterior thoracotomy incision usually does not significantly compromise the mechanics of breathing in a group of patients who usually have serious underlying systemic disease. Localized nodular disease or peripheral nodules, especially in the apical, posterior, and lateral areas of the lung,

generally require a more extensive, full posterolateral thoracotomy for access.

Complications

The reported complications from a small diagnostic anterior thoracotomy include bleeding, wound infections, persistent air leak, pneumonia, or any systemic complication of general anesthesia. In a review of 15 clinical series with a total of 2290 open lung biopsies, the overall complication rate was 7.0% and the mortality was 1.8%, usually related to a patient's underlying disease. The yield of specific diagnoses in this large group was 94%. Relative contraindications to open lung biopsy include patient instability, which can usually be improved by judicious medical management, and coagulopathies, which may be corrected in most cases with blood component therapy.

To minimize the morbidity of an open lung biopsy for diffuse infiltrative disease, the lingula or middle lobe is frequently sampled, as these areas allow for the smallest incision and shortest operating times. The question of the representative accuracy of this approach has been answered by a prospective study, which found a 100% histologic correlation of lingular biopsies with open biopsies of other lung segments obtained at the same thoracotomy. Thus, it appears that lingular biopsies are extremely accurate and representative of the pathologic process occurring in diffuse infiltrative lung disease.

Indications

The indications for an open lung biopsy and its sequence in the diagnostic algorithm depend on the pulmonary process and the patient's systemic condition. Of all patients with chronic infiltrative lung disease, transbronchial biopsy can be expected to provide a definitive diagnosis in only approximately 40%. In contrast, open lung biopsy yields a specific diagnosis in approximately 90%. Transbronchial biopsy findings of interstitial pneumonia, chronic inflammation, nonspecific reaction, and fibrosis are generally regarded as nondiagnostic and should lead to open lung biopsy.

In immunosuppressed patients with pulmonary infiltrates, considerable differences of opinion exist regarding the risk-benefit ratio of an open lung biopsy. In some series, open lung biopsy had a very high (97.5%) diagnostic accuracy rate and determined therapy in 45% of patients. However, the mortality in patients whose biopsy findings dictated a change in treatment was not significantly different from that in patients in whom no change was indicated.

There is much controversy concerning the indications for open lung biopsy in patients with AIDS who have pulmonary infiltrates. In one series, a 70% diagnostic accuracy rate was found in patients in whom transbronchial biopsy was nondiagnostic. In a later, prospective study of AIDS patients with interstitial infiltrates, combined transbronchial lung biopsy and alveolar lavage gave a diagnostic yield of 85% for infections, comparable with that of open lung biopsy (88%), thereby indicating a minimized need for open lung biopsies. An exception to this is an expected diagnosis of Kaposi's sarcoma, for which open biopsy is more frequently diagnostic.

In general, open lung biopsy is accompanied by low morbidity and low mortality with a high diagnostic yield. In properly selected patients, it should not be unduly delayed to perform other, less productive diagnostic techniques when a definitive tissue diagnosis can be readily and safely obtained. Of critical importance is maximal use of the biopsy specimen, including microbiologic examinations in addition to pathologic study and also including chemical and physical examinations when indicated.

VIDEO-ASSISTED THORACOSCOPIC SURGERY

Thoracoscopy has generated a large amount of interest as a newer approach to lung biopsy. When performed with a rigid scope, classic thoracoscopy was a limited procedure that provided the surgeon with poor visualization and access to intrathoracic structures. Application of video-endoscopic technology and percutaneous methods of dissection and exposure developed for abdominal surgery has resulted in a major advance in the diagnosis and treatment of intrathoracic disease.

Technique

Video-assisted thoracic surgery is performed under general anesthesia using a double-lumen endotracheal tube. The patient is positioned in the lateral decubitus position and the skin is antiseptically prepared and draped as for a standard posterolateral thoracotomy. The ipsilateral lung is collapsed and a 2-cm incision is made in the midaxillary line in the seventh intercostal space. After digital entry and palpation of the pleura surrounding the incision to avoid tearing adhesions, a 10-mm operating port is inserted. The video-telescope is inserted through the port to inspect the intrathoracic contents, and images are projected onto a high-resolution video monitor. One to three operating ports are then inserted through small, separate incisions in the anterior and posterior axillary lines, preferably along a line that can be used for a thoracotomy incision should the need arise. The entrance ports need not be sealed, as in laparoscopy, because carbon dioxide insufflation is not required to maintain an operating field. Through the operating ports the surgeon and assistant may dissect, retract, staple, excise, and digitally palpate the lung and intrathoracic structures. Application

of the electrocautery and argon beam electrocoagulator is significant with this method. At the completion of the procedure, one or two small chest tubes are tunneled into the chest and the small thoracoscopy incisions are closed.

The primary reason for the development of thoracoscopy, and now video-assisted thoracic surgical techniques, is to permit invasive intrathoracic diagnostic and therapeutic procedures to be performed with minimal pain and morbidity. Complications of this procedure vary with the actual surgery performed. Pneumothorax, air embolism, bleeding, and inadvertent lung injury are the most common intraoperative complications of the procedure, but these can be controlled easily in most instances with current instrumentation. The results of a large series suggest an overall complication rate of 14% and mortality ranging from 1.5%–9.8%, depending on the underlying clinical condition, indications, and the video-assisted thorascopic surgical procedure performed. Intraoperative complications may lead to urgent thoracotomy in 1%–3% of cases, and patients are draped and prepared for open thoracotomy at the onset of the procedure.

Contraindications to video-assisted thoracic surgery are generally based on limitation of visualization of the intrathoracic space. Absolute contraindications include an obliterated pleural space, an inability to tolerate one-lung anesthesia, the need for high positive-pressure ventilation, and severe chronic or acute respiratory insufficiency, all of which would not allow collapse of the ipsilateral lung for exposure. Thus, when a patient being maintained on a ventilator in the intensive care unit requires open lung biopsy, the standard approach of anterior thoracotomy is generally used. Additionally, the procedure may be ill-advised for patients who have previously undergone thoracoscopy or even tube thoracostomy because of excessive adhesions in the pleural space. The clotting parameters of patients who are receiving anticoagulant medication or who have a coagulopathy must be normalized before video-assisted surgery can be performed.

Indications

The most traditional indication for thoracoscopy is evaluation of pleural effusions and other pleural pathology by visual exploration and directed biopsy. In a series of 102 patients with recurrent pleural effusion in whom all prior studies were nondiagnostic, a definitive diagnosis was obtained in 80.3% with thoracoscopy; there was no procedure-related mortality and a 2% complication rate.

Open lung biopsy an ideal indication for video-assisted surgery. Unlike traditional small anterior thoracotomy and classic lung biopsy, in which sampling is limited, with video-assisted biopsy any segment of any lobe of the lung in which disease has been identified can easily be sampled to make a definitive diagnosis. Small peripheral subpleural lung nodules up to approximately 2 cm in diameter can be resected for diagnosis by means of video-assisted surgery. The expected diagnostic yield with video-assisted open lung biopsy should equal or even exceed that of the standard open procedure. Other specific diagnostic and therapeutic applications of video-assisted thoracic surgery include biopsy of aortopulmonary and other mediastinal nodes; excisional biopsy of a variety of benign and malignant masses of the lung, chest wall, and mediastinum; biopsy and excision of bronchial, pericardial, and mediastinal cysts; evaluation and treatment of recurrent pneumothorax; thoracic sympathectomy; pericardial biopsy and excision; and even lobectomies in selected cases.

Despite the fact that video-assisted thoracic surgery is somewhat more difficult and tedious to perform than surgery done through a traditional open thoracotomy incision, the benefits of lessened postoperative pain, a shortened hospital stay, and quicker recovery have led to increasing use of the technique. As the technology advances, one can expect that the future will bring new diagnostic and therapeutic indications for video-assisted thoracic surgical techniques.

PULMONARY ANGIOSCOPY

Pulmonary vascular diseases present diagnostic dilemmas for which diagnostic and treatment modalities are limited. Direct visualization of vascular structures has been investigated and shows promise for expanding diagnostic capabilities.

The equipment is based on traditional endoscopic designs, except that the fiber bundle is narrow (outer diameter of 2.8 mm) and long (120 cm). Although blood in the peripheral vascular bed and in the very small coronary arterial bed can be flushed from the field of view intraoperatively, visualization in the much larger pulmonary arterial bed is best achieved using an inflatable balloon over the lens to displace blood mechanically from the area to be viewed.

The procedure is very similar to catheterization of the right side of the heart. The angioscope is passed through an introducing catheter, usually in the internal jugular vein, and directed into the right side of the heart and pulmonary arteries using direct visualization and fluoroscopy. The balloon can be inflated or deflated as needed, and distal tip deflection facilitates accurate movement of the angioscope into areas of interest.

Animal studies have established the diagnostic accuracy of angioscopy in detecting acute pulmonary emboli and the hemodynamic safety of the procedure. Safety has been confirmed in subsequent human trials.

To date, angioscopy has been applied to the diagnosis of chronic pulmonary hypertension, particularly to distinguish chronic thromboembolic pulmonary hypertension from other causes of chronic vascular obstruction and hypertension. Chronic thromboembolic pulmonary hypertension was chosen as the initial area of investigation because of significant problems with standard techniques, such as angiography, in establishing the diagnosis or determining operability.

Distinctive endoscopic features of chronic pulmonary emboli can be identified by angioscopy. These include roughening of the intimal lining, presence of bands and webs, irregular vessel contour, vascular obstruction by fibrotic masses of organized emboli, and partial recanalization. Abnormalities associated with other diseases can also be identified, such as atherosclerotic plaques, extrinsic vessel compression, and tumor. Perhaps most importantly, angioscopy has proved useful in determining the proximal extent of the chronic thromboembolic process and is therefore useful in assessing operability, a key issue in this patient population.

With this foundation established in an unusual disease entity, future clinical trials may focus on the more common problem of acute pulmonary emboli, to evaluate the role of angioscopy in relation to lung scanning and angiography. Applications in valvular heart disease will also be an area for future exploration.

BIBLIOGRAPHY

Aronchick JM. CT of mediastinal lymph nodes in patients with non-small cell lung carcinoma. *Radiol Clin North Am* 1990;28:573. *Reviews a large number of investigations of the utility of CT scans for staging mediastinal nodes.*

Baker AM, Bowton DL, Haponick HF. Decision making in nosocomial pneumonia. *Chest* 1995;107:85. *Analysis of quantitative cultures of BAL fluid, compared with protected specimen brush, to provide guidelines for the interpretation of culture results.*

Bartlett JG. Diagnostic accuracy of transtracheal aspiration bacteriologic studies. *Am Rev Respir Dis* 1977;115:777. *Carefully designed study that quantitates the diagnostic accuracy of transtracheal aspiration.*

Bousquet J, Chaenz P, Lacoste JY, et al. Eosinophilic inflammation in asthma. *N Engl J Med* 1990;323:1033. *Correlates the intensity of eosinophilia in the lower respiratory tract, as sampled by BAL and endobronchial biopsies, with the severity of asthma.*

Brantigan JW, Brantigan CO, Brantigan OC. Biopsy of nonpalpable scalene lymph nodes in carcinoma of the lung. *Am Rev Respirs* 1973;107:962. *In patients with known lung cancer, biopsy of palpable scalene nodes had an 83% positive diagnostic rate, whereas biopsy of nonpalpable nodes had a 70% positive rate.*

Carlens E. Mediastinoscopy: a method for inspection and tissue biopsy in the superior mediastinum. *Dis Chest* 1959;36:343. *The original description of mediastinoscopy.*

Crystal RG, Bitterman PB, Rennard SI, Hance AJ, Keogh BA. Interstitial lung diseases of unknown cause. Disorders characterized by chronic inflammation of the lower respiratory tract. *N Engl J Med* 1984;310:154. *Reviews diagnostic procedures for interstitial lung diseases.*

Daniele RP, Elias JA, Epstein PE, Rossman MD. Bronchoalveolar lavage: role in the pathogenesis, diagnosis, and management of interstitial lung disease. *Ann Intern Med* 1985;102:93. *Reviews the role of BAL for the staging and diagnosis of interstitial lung disease and compares the diagnostic accuracy of BAL with diagnostic accuracies of bronchoscopic and open lung biopsy.*

DeCamp MM, Jaklitsch MT, Mentzer SJ, et al. The safety and versatility of video-thoracoscopy: a prospective analysis of 895 consecutive cases. *J Am Coll Surg* 1995;181:113. *Preoperative, intraoperative, postoperative, and outcome considerations of video-assisted thoracoscopic surgery reported for a large, prospectively collected series.*

Fraser RS. Transthoracic needle aspiration. The benign diagnosis. *Arch*

Pathol Lab Med 1991;115:751. *Review of specific benign diagnoses determined by transthoracic needle aspiration and their frequency.*

Gazelle GS, Haaga JR. Biopsy needle characteristics. *Cardiovasc Intervent Radiol* 1991;14:13. *In-depth description of the biopsy needles available for percutaneous transthoracic needle biopsy.*

Hinson KFW, Kuper SWA. The diagnosis of lung cancer by the examination of sputum. *Thorax* 1963;18:350. *Demonstrates low intraobserver variability for interpretation of sputum cytology by experienced pathologists.*

Ikeda S. *Atlas of Flexible Bronchofiberoscopy.* 1st ed. Baltimore: University Park Press; 1974. *Well-illustrated atlas that provides insights from the originator of flexible fiberoptic bronchoscopy.*

Johnston WW. Ten years of respiratory cytopathology at Duke University Medical Center. III. The significance of inconclusive cytopathologic diagnoses during the years 1970 to 1974. *Acta Cytol* 1982;26:759. *Pneumonia, COPD, and granulomatous diseases accounted for about 75% of the inconclusive cytopathologic specimens.*

Johnston WW, Bossen EH. Ten years of respiratory cytopathology at Duke University Medical Center. I. The cytopathologic diagnosis of lung cancer during the years 1970 to 1974, noting the significance of specimen number and type. *Acta Cytol* 1981;25:103. *Multiple specimens were necessary to maximize diagnostic yield for sputum cytology. Five specimens was the optimal number.*

Jules-Elysee KM, Stover DE, Zaman MB, Bernard EM, White DA. Aerosolized pentamidine: effect on diagnosis and presentation of *Pneumocystis carinii* pneumonia. *Ann Intern Med* 1990;112:750. *Prophylactic treatment with aerosolized pentamidine was shown to decrease the diagnostic accuracy of BAL for* Pneumocystis carinii *pneumonia in patients with AIDS. Addition of transbronchial biopsy to BAL largely restored the diagnostic yield.*

Kahn FW, Jones JW. Diagnosing bacterial respiratory infection by bronchoalveolar lavage. *J Infect Dis* 1987;155:862. *This is one of the original descriptions (see also Thorpe et al., below) of quantitative culture of BAL. A cutoff of 105 organisms per milliliter identified patients with pneumonia.*

Kahn FW, Jones JM, England DM. The role of bronchoalveolar lavage in the diagnosis of invasive pulmonary aspergillosis. *Am J Clin Pathol* 1986;86:518. *The authors demonstrate a disappointingly low yield for aspergillosis by BAL alone, underscoring the need for biopsy.*

Kalinske RW, Parker RH, Brandt D, Heoprich PD. Diagnostic usefulness and safety of transtracheal aspiration. *N Engl J Med* 1967;276:604. *Original description of transtracheal aspiration.*

Klech H, Hutter C. Clinical guidelines and indications for bronchoalveolar lavage (BAL): report of the European Society of Pneumology Task Group on BAL. *Eur Respir J* 1990;3:937.

Klech H, Pohl W. Technical recommendations and guidelines for bronchoalveolar lavage (BAL). *Eur Respir J* 1989;2:561. *These two articles report the consensus of a European task force on methods of performing BAL, clinical applications, and the processing and interpretation of BAL fluid.*

Lewis RJ, Caccavale RJ, Sisler GE. Imaged thorascopic lung biopsy. *Chest* 1992;102:60. *Video-assisted thorascopic surgery provides an alternative to open lung biopsy, with similar diagnostic yield and reduced morbidity.*

Libshitz HI, McKenna RJ. Mediastinal lymph node size in lung cancer. *Am J Radiol* 1984;143:715. *Careful correlation of surgical dissection and CT scans demonstrated carcinomatous involvement in nodes <1 cm in size in 33% of patients.*

LoCicero J. Mediastinotomy. In: Shields TW, ed. *Mediastinal Surgery.* Philadelphia: Lea & Febiger; 1991. *Provides a comprehensive review of mediastinotomy, including historical perspective, methods, and complications.*

Luke WP, Pearson FG, Todd TRJ, Patterson GA, Cooper JD. Prospective evaluation of mediastinoscopy for assessment of carcinoma of the lung. *J Thorac Cardiovasc Surg* 1986;91:53. *Reports the results and low complication rate of mediastinoscopy.*

Martini N, Flehinger BJ, Zaman MB, Beattie EJ. Prospective study of 445 lung carcinomas with mediastinal lymph node metastases. *J Thorac Cardiovasc Surg* 1980;80:390. *Micrometastatic disease in mediastinal lymph nodes carries a much better prognosis (34% 5-year survival) than do metastases in mediastinal nodes >1.5 cm.*

McKenna RJ, Campbell A, McMurtrey MJ, Mountain CF. Diagnosis for interstitial lung disease in patients with acquired immunodeficiency syndrome (AIDS): a prospective comparison of bronchial washing,

alveolar lavage, transbronchial lung biopsy and open lung biopsy. *Ann Thorac Surg* 1986;41:318. *Use of BAL and transbronchial biopsy obviates the need for open lung biopsy.*

Meduri GU, Beals DH, Mijub AG, Baselski V. Protected bronchoalveolar lavage. A new bronchoscopic technique to retrieve uncontaminated distal airway secretions. *Am Rev Respir Dis* 1991;143:855. *Describes a catheter for sampling the lower respiratory tract; it includes a balloon that isolates the sampling port of the catheter from other airways. Specificity and sensitivity were very similar to specificity and sensitivity with quantitative culture of BAL fluid.*

Moser KM, Shure D, Harrell JH, Tulumello J. Angioscopic visualization of pulmonary emboli. *Chest* 1980;77:198. *Describes the use of angioscopy in the pulmonary arteries.*

Newmann SL, Michel RP, Wang N. Lingular lung biopsy: is it representative? *Am Rev Respir Dis* 1985;132:1084. *Biopsies of the distal portion of the lingula were found to be inaccurate. (See Westein below for a contrary conclusion.)*

Ng ABP, Horak GC. Factors significant in the diagnostic accuracy of lung cytology in bronchial washing and sputum samples. II. Sputum samples. *Acta Cytol* 1983;27:397. *Reports the specificity and sensitivity of these cytologic techniques for each cell type of lung cancer in a large series.*

Ng VL, Gartner I, Weymouth LA, Goodman CD, Hopewell PC, Hadley WK. The use of mucosylated induced sputum for the identification of pulmonary pathogens associated with human immunodeficiency virus infection. *Arch Pathol Lab Med* 1989;113:488. *Induced sputum was found to be useful for the diagnosis of pneumonia in patients with AIDS.*

Pass HI, Potter D, Shelhammer J, et al. Indications for and diagnostic efficacy of open lung biopsy in the acquired immunodeficiency syndrome (AIDS). *Ann Thorac Surg* 1986;41:307. *A classic article supporting the use of open lung biopsy for the diagnosis of pulmonary diseases in patients with AIDS.*

Prakash UB, Offord KP, Stubbs SE. Bronchoscopy in North America: the ACCP Survey. *Chest* 1991;100:1668. *The results of this survey from the American College of Chest Physicians provide information concerning bronchoscopic methods in widespread use in North America.*

Shelhamer JH, moderator; NIH Conference. The laboratory evaluation of opportunistic pulmonary infections. *Ann Intern Med* 1996;124:585. *State-of-the-art review of immunologic and molecular biologic techniques for identifying pathogens in sputum, BAL fluid, and other secretions.*

Shure D. Fiberoptic bronchoscopy—diagnostic applications. *Clin Chest Med* 1987;8:1. *A complete review of the applications of flexible fiberoptic bronchoscopy for the diagnosis of lung lesions. Provides methods and reported diagnostic accuracy for endobronchial cytology brushing, endobronchial biopsy, transbronchial biopsy, and transbronchial needle aspiration.*

Shure D. Pulmonary angioscopy. In: White GH, White RA, eds. *Angioscopy: Vascular and Coronary Applications.* Chicago: Year Book; 1989;177. *Review of the methods, diagnostic yield, and complications of pulmonary angioscopy for the diagnosis of pulmonary embolism.*

Stover DE, Zaman MB, Hajdu SI, Lange M, Gold J, Armstrong D. Bronchoalveolar lavage in the diagnosis of diffuse pulmonary infiltrates in the immunocompromised host. *Ann Intern Med* 1984;101:1. *Reports on the diagnostic accuracy of BAL in immunocompromised patients, especially those with AIDS. The results demonstrate a very high yield for* Pneumocystis carinii *pneumonia.*

Thermann M, Bluemm R, Schroeder U, Wassmuth E, Dohmann R. Efficacy and benefit of mediastinal computed tomography as a selection method for mediastinoscopy. *Ann Thorac Surg* 1989;48:565. *Routine mediastinoscopy is not a cost-effective approach for staging lung cancer, according to this article.*

Thompson AB, Daughton D, Robbins RA, Ghafouri MA, Oehlerking M, Rennard SI. Intraluminal airway inflammation in chronic bronchitis: characterization and correlation with clinical parameters. *Am Rev Respir Dis* 1989;140:1527. *Quantitates airway inflammation associated with chronic bronchitis by means of BAL.*

Thompson AB, Rennard SI. Clinical applications of bronchoalveolar lavage. *Curr Pulmonol* 1994;15:209. *Critical review of the literature supporting the clinical use of BAL in selected clinical settings. Techniques and methods of BAL are reviewed as well.*

Thompson AB, Teschler H, Rennard SI. Pathogenesis, evaluation, and therapy for massive hemoptysis. *Clin Chest Med* 1992;13:69. *Reviews the evaluation of hemoptysis, including the use of bronchoscopy, both flexible and rigid.*

Thorpe JE, Baughman RP, Frame PI, Wesseler TA, Staneck JL. Bronchoalveolar lavage for diagnosing acute bacterial pneumonia. *J Infect Dis* 1987;155:855. *This report, along with that of Kahn and Jones (see above), is one of the original descriptions of quantitative culture of BAL fluid for the diagnosis of pneumonia. A cutoff of 10^5 organisms per milliliter was found to be diagnostic of pneumonia.*

Wall CP, Gaensler EA, Carrington CB, Hayes JA. Comparison of transbronchial and open biopsies in chronic infiltrative lung diseases. *Am Rev Respir Dis* 1981;123:280. *A large series comparing the indications, diagnostic yield, and complication rates for the two methods. Establishes the importance of open lung biopsy for the diagnosis of interstitial lung disease.*

Wang KP, Haponik EF, Gupta PK, et al. Flexible transbronchial needle aspiration. Technical considerations. *Ann Otol Rhinol Laryngol* 1984;93:233. *A description of methods for transbronchial needle aspiration by the developer of the technique.*

Weisbrod GL. Transthoracic percutaneous lung biopsy. *Radiol Clin North Am* 1990;28:647. *Reviews the methods, results, and complications of the procedure.*

Westein L. Sensitivity and specificity of lingular segmental biopsies of the lung. *Chest* 1986;90:383. *Lingular biopsy results were found to be 100% congruent with biopsy results from other lung segments. (See Newman, et al. above for a contrary view.)*

Yu VL, Muder RR, Poorsattar A. Significance of isolation of *Aspergillus* from the respiratory tract in the diagnosis of invasive pulmonary aspergillosis: results from a three-year prospective study. *Am J Med* 1986;81:249. *Although* Aspergillus *species may be isolated as a contaminant from the sputum of nonimmunocompromised individuals, this study demonstrates that the isolation of* Aspergillus *from the sputum of patients with leukemia is clinically significant and that such patients should be treated.*

Zavala DC. Diagnostic fiberoptic bronchoscopy: techniques and results of biopsy in 600 patients. *Chest* 1975;68:12. *Review of an extensive experience from a single institution with flexible fiberoptic bronchoscopy for the diagnosis of endobronchial lesions.*

Zavala DC. Transbronchial biopsy in diffuse lung disease. *Chest* 1978;73:727. *A sentinel paper describing the author's methods and outcomes and the diagnostic accuracy in a large series.*

Textbook of Pulmonary Diseases, 6th ed.
edited by G.L. Baum, J.D. Crapo, B.R. Celli, and J.B. Karlinsky,
Lippincott–Raven Publishers, Philadelphia, © 1998.

12

Pleural Anatomy, Physiology, and Diagnostic Procedures

Steven A. Sahn

ANATOMY

The pleural space is real, approximately 10 to 20 μm in width and situated between the mesothelium of the parietal and visceral pleurae. The parietal and visceral pleurae are continuous at the hilum, where they are penetrated by the pulmonary and bronchial vessels and the two main bronchi with their accompanying nerves and lymphatic vessels. The areas of the two pleural surfaces are approximately equal (2000 cm^2 in a person weighing 70 kg) if the interlobar fissures of the visceral pleura and the costophrenic recesses of the parietal pleura are included. Both the visceral and parietal pleurae consist of a single layer of pleomorphic mesothelial cells, a basement membrane, and layers of collagen and elastic tissue in addition to the microvessels and lymphatics.

The mesothelial cells vary in shape from flattened with an elongated nucleus and minimally discernible cytoplasm to cuboidal or columnar with a round nucleus and an indistinct luminal surface. Despite differences in morphology, mesothelial cells remain a single layer at all sites. Mesothelial cells vary in thickness from 1 to 4 μm and in surface diameter from 16 to 40 μm. Mesothelial cells contain surface microvilli that are approximately 0.1 μm in diameter and up to 3 μm in length. The density of microvilli is higher on the visceral than on the parietal mesothelial cells, possibly to trap hyaluronic acid-rich glycoprotein, particularly in the lower portion of the thorax, to decrease friction between the lung and chest wall.

Openings between mesothelial cells, called *stomata*, range in size from 2 to 12 μm and are found only on the parietal pleural surface by scanning electron microscopy.

These stomata communicate directly with lymphatic lacunae, the roofs of which contain bundles of collagen. Stomata are the usual exit point for pleural liquid, protein, and cells that are removed from the pleural space.

In humans, the visceral pleura is supplied by branches of the bronchial circulation. The venous return from the subpleural capillaries drains largely into the pulmonary veins. The human parietal pleura is supplied by branches of the arteries that flow to the adjacent chest wall. The costal pleura is supplied by branches of the intercostal and internal mammary arteries; the mediastinal parietal pleura by branches of the bronchial and upper diaphragmatic, internal mammary, and mediastinal arteries; and the apical pleura by branches of the subclavian artery. The venous system of the parietal pleura drains into the bronchial veins. The diaphragmatic pleura is supplied by branches of the internal mammary artery, thoracic and abdominal aorta, and celiac arteries; drainage is into the inferior vena cava and brachiocephalic trunk.

The lymph drainage of the pleural space has a major impact on the accumulation of pleural fluid in normal and disease states. Lymphatic drainage of the pleural space begins at the stomata that are located mainly in the mediastinum caudally and on the intercostal and diaphragmatic pleurae. The stomata connect with lymphatic lacunae situated immediately below the mesothelial layer and appear to be closed at their end by the endothelium of lymphatics to form valves. The lymphatic lacunae drain into larger lymphatic channels that course along the intercostal space and drain into the mediastinum. The origin of lymphatic vessels in the parietal pleura determines the node into which the fluid drains. The pleura of the anterior thoracic wall and anterior portion of the diaphragm drains to the sternal lymph nodes; the middle portion of the diaphragmatic pleura drains to the middle mediastinal lymph nodes; the anterior portion of the diaphragmatic and medi-

S. A. Sahn: Division of Pulmonary and Critical Care Medicine, Medical University of South Carolina, Charleston, South Carolina 29425.

255

astinal pleura drains into the anterior mediastinal lymph nodes; the posterior portion of the diaphragmatic pleura drains to the posterior mediastinal lymph nodes; and the costal parietal pleura drains to the intercostal lymph nodes. The majority of the visceral pleura drains to the middle mediastinal lymph nodes, whereas the visceral pleural drainage of the lower lobes flows into the posterior mediastinal lymph nodes.

PHYSIOLOGY

Most of what is known about normal pleural fluid turnover is derived from noninvasive studies of pleural fluid formation in the sheep, an animal with a pleural anatomy similar to that of humans. The assumption is made that in the steady-state condition, pleural fluid absorption is equivalent to pleural fluid formation. The normal pleural fluid-to-plasma protein ratio is approximately 0.15, and the pleural fluid volume is about 0.1 to 0.2 mL/kg. Studies from sheep show that pleural fluid is formed at an hourly rate of 0.01 mL/kg, the equivalent of 0.6 mL/h in a 60-kg person.

Pleural fluid is essentially an ultrafiltrate of the systemic pleural microvessels. Because the parietal pleural microvessels are closer to the pleural space than are the visceral pleural microvessels, the interstitial fluid in the parietal pleura moves between mesothelial cells into the pleural space along a pressure gradient; most or all of the interstitial liquid that moves out of the visceral pleural microvessels is removed by lung lymphatics because the fluid would have to travel a greater distance to enter the pleural space. Therefore, in normal humans, the parietal pleura is responsible for most or all pleural fluid formation. Pleural fluid exits the pleural space via the lymphatic stomata of the parietal pleura. Most pleural fluid exits the pleural space by bulk flow, not by diffusion. In addition to the pleural liquid being removed through the stomata, cells and protein exit by this route. The lymphatic flow from the pleural space is influenced by both the contractility of the lymph vessels and respiratory movements. The circulation of fluid in the pleural space enabling liquid to move into stomata may be driven by respiratory movements.

The lymphatic drainage of the pleural space appears to have a large reserve, so that when an abnormal amount of pleural fluid accumulates in disease states, it must represent increased formation, decreased absorption, or both. Most probably both mechanisms contribute to pleural fluid formation. An increase in pleural fluid formation is unlikely to cause a pleural effusion clinically, as the pleural lymphatics have an extensive reserve to handle excess fluid formation. Furthermore, a decrease in pleural fluid absorption is unlikely to cause a pleural effusion clinically because the normal entry rate is slow.

Mechanisms of increased formation of pleural fluid include the following: (1) an increase in microvascular pressure (as occurs in congestive heart failure); (2) a decrease in pleural pressure (as in atelectasis), which decreases the pressure surrounding the nearby microvessels and increases the gradient of pressures driving fluid across the microvascular barrier; and (3) a decrease in plasma oncotic pressure (as in hypoalbuminemia), which increases the forces for filtration until the balance is restored.

When the lymphatic system is involved by disease at any point from the stomata of the parietal pleura to the mediastinal lymph nodes, a decrease in absorption rate can occur. Factors that may affect lymphatic flow include the following: (1) inhibition of lymphatic contractility during infiltration by malignancy or anatomic abnormalities (as in yellow nail syndrome); (2) limitation of respiratory movement (as in lung collapse); (3) blockage of lymphatic stoma by malignancy or fibrin; (4) acute increases in systemic venous pressure; and (5) decreased fluid availability to the stoma after pneumothorax.

Pleural fluid can form when fluid moves across the diaphragm from the peritoneal cavity, either because of congenital diaphragmatic defects or by convection across the two mesothelial layers. Inflammation may also be a factor, as in acute pancreatitis and increased pleural capillary filtration. There is no evidence for the existence of direct lymphatic channels connecting the peritoneal and pleural spaces across the diaphragm. Lastly, mediastinal inflammation, as seen in esophageal sclerotherapy and esophageal perforation, can lead to a pleural effusion. When fluid from a pancreatic pseudocyst or rupture of the thoracic duct (chyle) collects in the mediastinum, a pleural effusion can form when the mediastinal pleura ruptures.

DIAGNOSTIC PROCEDURES

Thoracentesis

Diagnostic Yield

The discovery of a pleural effusion provides an opportunity for the clinician to verify the disease, procedure, or drug that has caused the effusion. With a simple bedside procedure, thoracentesis, the fluid can be rapidly sampled and observed, its constituents observed microscopically, and its contents quantified. A comprehensive and systematic approach to analysis of pleural fluid in conjunction with the clinical presentation should allow the clinician to diagnose the cause of a pleural effusion in 75% of cases. A definitive diagnosis, such as the finding of malignant cells or specific organisms in pleural fluid, can be established in only one of four patients; however, a presumptive diagnosis, based on a clinical impression before thoracentesis, can be substantiated by pleural fluid analysis in an additional 50% of patients. Even with a nondiagnostic thoracentesis, pleural fluid analysis can be useful in excluding other possible causes of a pleural effusion, such as infection. Therefore, in three of four patients the cause of an effusion can be "diagnosed," and in >90% of patients information relevant to clinical decision making can be gained by pleural fluid analysis.

Indications and Contraindications

When a pleural effusion is suspected on physical examination and confirmed radiographically, a diagnostic thoracentesis should be performed in an attempt to establish the cause of the effusion. If the clinical diagnosis (e.g., uncomplicated congestive heart failure) is secure, it is reasonable to observe the patient's response to therapy and proceed with thoracentesis only when the clinical response is not appropriate. There are no absolute contraindications to diagnostic thoracentesis. Relative contraindications include a bleeding diathesis, anticoagulation, a small volume of pleural fluid, and mechanical ventilation. The needle should never be passed through an area of active skin infection. The patient on mechanical ventilation is not at increased risk for pneumothorax when undergoing thoracentesis, but tension pneumothorax is more likely to develop if the lung is punctured.

Technique

Diagnostic thoracentesis should be a simple and rapid procedure for the operator and impose minimal discomfort on the patient. Patient anxiety can be minimized greatly if the procedure is explained completely at the time informed consent is obtained. It is rarely necessary to administer atropine, narcotics, or sedative drugs for a diagnostic thoracentesis.

The selection of the site for thoracentesis is critical to a successful outcome. A chest radiograph should be available in the procedure room for review before site selection. The physical examination should dictate the precise placement of needle insertion. The site should be one to two interspaces below the level where the percussion note becomes flat and tactile fremitus decreases. With a free-flowing effusion, an area midway between the spine and the posterior axillary line should be selected, as the ribs are easily palpated in this location. When the interspace is selected, the needle should be passed over the superior surface of the rib to avoid possible laceration of the neurovascular bundle, which courses near the inferior rib margin. This is especially applicable in elderly patients, who tend to have tortuous intercostal arteries that may impinge on the intercostal space, so that the risk for laceration is increased. If the fluid is loculated or small, as demonstrated by decubitus radiographs, thoracentesis should be done under ultrasonic guidance. Thora-

centesis should be performed with the patient positioned exactly as during ultrasonography.

Good technique minimizes complications. The operator should maintain appropriate sterile technique and clean a wide area around the site selected for needle puncture. A 10% povidone-iodine solution decreases the usual cutaneous bacterial population by 85% for about 1 hour. The quaternary ammonium compounds, such as benzalkonium chloride, have a rapid onset of action, but their activity is antagonized by soaps and tissue constituents, and when these compounds are applied to the skin, they tend to form a film under which bacteria may remain viable. Furthermore, these compounds do not kill spores and require more than 5 minutes to decrease the bacterial population by 50%. The normal pleural space appears to have effective mechanisms for clearing bacteria; however, patients with severe pleural injury or immunosuppression probably are at increased risk for iatrogenic empyema if careful aseptic technique is not maintained.

If the skin, periosteum of the rib, and parietal pleura are properly injected with lidocaine, the patient should have minimal pain, similar to the discomfort associated with venipuncture. When pleural fluid is obtained by aspirating with the syringe containing lidocaine, the syringe and needle should be withdrawn and a 22-gauge needle, 1 1/2 inches long and attached to a 50-mL syringe, should be used along the same tract to obtain fluid for diagnostic evaluation. One milliliter of heparin (1:1000) should be added to prevent clotting of the fluid.

Occasionally the thoracentesis will be "dry." This may result from the absence of pleural fluid, incorrect needle placement, or a needle of inappropriate length. If air is obtained in the syringe, the lung has been punctured because the needle was placed superiorly to the effusion. If no air, or possibly blood, is obtained, the needle may have been inserted too inferiorly or been too short for an obese patient. If there are no adverse consequences of this misadventure, then appropriate adjustment of the technique usually results in a successful procedure. A longer needle should be used in a patient who is markedly obese.

Fifty milliliters of fluid is all that is necessary for complete pleural fluid analysis. The tests requested should be based on the clinical presentation. It is not clinically efficacious or cost-effective to request an entire battery of pleural fluid tests. It is probably cost-effective and clinically efficacious to order the following tests for all patients who undergo a diagnostic thoracentesis: total protein, lactate dehydrogenase (LDH), nucleated cell count and differential, and either a glucose or pH determination. Concomitant serum protein, LDH, and glucose levels should be measured; arterial pH should be measured if the pleural fluid pH is below 7.30 and acidemia is suspected. The aforementioned tests provide information that allows characterization of the fluid as a transudate or an exudate, narrows the differential diagnosis of an exudate, and indicates the degree of pleural inflammation and the acuteness of pleural injury. Gram, acid-fast bacilli (AFB), and potassium hydroxide (KOH) stains should be performed and pleural fluid cultured when infection is suspected. Pleural fluid cytology should be requested when malignancy is suspected or if an exudate is undiagnosed; lipid studies should be ordered when the fluid is milky, and immunologic studies should be performed if rheumatoid or lupus pleuritis is suspected. Amylase concentration should be measured when pancreatitis, pancreatic pseudocyst, esophageal rupture, or malignancy is considered.

Complications

Complications of diagnostic thoracentesis include pain at the needle insertion site, bleeding (local, intrapleural, or intra-abdominal), pneumothorax, empyema, and spleen or liver puncture. Pneumothorax is the most common clinically important complication of diagnostic thoracentesis and has been reported to occur in up to 10% of patients. The rate of pneumothorax correlates indirectly with operator experience. However, the pneumothorax usually is small and often can be treated expectantly. Liver or spleen puncture tends to occur when the patient is not sitting absolutely upright, because movement toward a recumbent position causes cephalad migration of the abdominal viscera. However, even if the liver or spleen is punctured with a small-bore needle, generally the outcome is favorable if the patient is not receiving anticoagulants and does not have a bleeding diathesis.

Pleural Fluid Analysis

Definitive Diagnosis

There are only a select number of diagnoses or causes of the effusion that can be established definitively by thoracentesis. These include malignancy, empyema, tuberculous pleurisy, fungal infection of the pleural space, lupus pleuritis, chylothorax, urinothorax, esophageal rupture, hemothorax, peritoneal dialysis, and extravascular migration of a central venous catheter (Table 1). Confirming the diagnosis of chylothorax does not establish the cause but provides evidence that the thoracic duct has been violated; lymphoma is the cause in >50% of cases. Esophageal rupture is the single entity associated with a pleural fluid having a high amylase concentration and a pH of <7.00. A pancreatic pleural effusion is associated with a high amylase concentration but the pH is virtually always >7.30. Some malignant pleural effusions have high amylase concentrations and the pH is >7.30 in two thirds of these patients; when the pH is low in malignant effusions, it rarely is <7.05. Empyema, tuberculous pleurisy, rheumatoid disease, and lupus pleuritis can all be associated with a low pleural fluid pH (<7.30), but the pleural fluid amylase concentration is less than the con-

TABLE 1. *Diagnoses or causes that can be established definitively by pleural fluid analysis*

Disease	Diagnostic pleural fluid tests
Empyema	Observation (pus, putrid odor); culture
Malignancy	Positive cytology
Lupus pleuritis	LE cells present
Tuberculous pleurisy	Positive AFB stain, culture
Esophageal rupture	High level of salivary amylase; pleural fluid acidosis (pH ≤ 7.00)
Fungal pleurisy	Positive KOH stain, culture
Chylothorax	Triglycerides (>110 mg/dL); lipoprotein electrophoresis positive for chylomicrons
Hemothorax	Hematocrit (pleural fluid/blood ratio >0.5)
Urinothorax	Creatinine (pleural fluid/serum ratio >1.0)
Peritoneal dialysis	Protein (<1 g/dL); glucose (300–400 mg/dL)
Extravascular migration of a central venous catheter	Observation (milky if lipids are infused); glucose pleural fluid/serum >1.0
Rheumatoid pleurisy	Characteristic cytology; pH 7.00; glucose <30 mg/dL; LDH > 1000 IU/L

comitant serum value. With extravascular migration of a central venous catheter, the resultant pleural effusion can be similar to the infusate and may be hemorrhagic and neutrophil-predominant because of trauma and inflammation. The pleural fluid-to-serum glucose ratio is >1.0; however, the pleural fluid glucose level is usually lower than that of the infusate, as glucose is transported rapidly from the pleural space.

Diagnostic Clues at the Bedside

Diagnostic clues can be obtained by gross inspection of the pleural fluid as it is being aspirated from the patient's chest (Table 2). A straw-colored fluid is typical of all transudates and minimally inflammatory exudative effusions, such as those seen in early malignancy, tuberculous pleurisy, and yellow nail syndrome. A bloody fluid in the absence of trauma suggests either malignancy, benign asbestos pleural effusion (BAPE), postcardiac injury syndrome (PCIS), or pulmonary infarction. A milky effusion suggests chylothorax but can be caused by a chyliform effusion (a lipid effusion that is not chyle with or without a high cholesterol level) or an empyema. Chylothorax signifies leakage of chyle from the thoracic duct, and the pleural fluid virtually always has a triglyceride concentration of >110 mg/dL; a triglyceride concentration of <50 mg/dL virtually excludes chylothorax. A chyliform effusion occurs in chronic pleural disease and is usually associated with a trapped lung, rheumatoid pleurisy, or tuberculous pleurisy, or is the result of pneu-

TABLE 2. *Diagnoses suggested by observations of pleural fluid*

Feature	Suggested diagnosis
Color	
Pale yellow (straw)	Transudate, some exudates
Red (bloody)	Malignancy, BAPE, PCIS, pulmonary infarction, trauma
White (milky)	Chylothorax or cholesterol effusion
Brown	Long-standing bloody effusion; rupture of amebic liver abscess
Black	*Aspergillus*
Yellow-green	Rheumatoid pleurisy
Color of enteral tube feeding	Feeding tube has entered pleural space
Color of central venous line infusate	Extravascular catheter migration
Character	
Pus	Empyema
Viscous	Mesothelioma
Debris	Rheumatoid pleurisy
Turbid	Inflammatory exudate or lipid effusion
"Anchovy paste"	Ruptured amebic liver abscess
Odor	
Putrid	Anaerobic empyema
Ammonia	Urinothorax

BAPE, benign asbestos pleural effusion; PCIS, post-cardiac injury syndrome.

mothorax therapy for tuberculosis. The diagnosis of a chyliform (cholesterol) effusion can be established by identifying cholesterol crystals on smears of the sediment; these rhomboid-shaped structures impart a lustrous sheen to the pleural fluid. Some chyliform effusions have high triglyceride levels; to differentiate between a chylothorax and a chyliform effusion that does not demonstrate cholesterol crystals, or if the triglyceride concentration is between 50 and 110 mg/dL, a lipoprotein electrophoresis should be performed to evaluate for the presence of chylomicrons, which are diagnostic for chylothorax.

When an amebic liver abscess ruptures into the pleural space, it produces an "anchovy paste"–like pleural aspirate that is a mixture of liver tissue that has undergone cytolysis, small pieces of liver parenchyma, and blood. The effusion is almost always right-sided. Amebae can be demonstrated in pleural fluid in <10% of patients. In patients with rheumatoid pleurisy, the fluid may have a yellowish-green tint or may appear to contain debris that results from exfoliation of necrotic visceral pleural rheumatoid nodules.

When fluid the color of the enteral feeding is aspirated from the pleural space, it confirms that a narrow-bore enteral feeding tube has passed through the tracheobronchial tree and into the pleural space. When the pleural fluid is similar to the infusate in a central venous line, extravascular catheter migration, which is most commonly associated with left-sided catheter placements through the jugular veins, has occurred. A viscous effu-sion suggests malignant mesothelioma because of the high levels of hyaluronic acid. A putrid odor is diagnostic of an anaerobic empyema, and the smell of ammonia suggests ipsilateral obstruction uropathy producing a urinothorax.

Transudates and Exudates

The characterization of pleural fluid as a transudate or an exudate is the next deductive step in pleural fluid analysis following observation of the aspirate. Transudates, largely because of imbalances in hydrostatic and oncotic pressures in the chest, can also result from movement of fluid from the peritoneal (cirrhosis) or retroperitoneal (urinothorax) spaces, or from iatrogenic causes, such as crystalloid infusion into a central line that has migrated extravascularly. Nevertheless, the diagnostic possibilities with a transudate are limited, and the diagnosis can usually be easily determined from the clinical presentation (Table 3).

In contrast, exudative effusions can be caused by a variety of diseases and present more of a diagnostic di-

TABLE 3. *Causes of transudative pleural effusions*

Cause	Comment
Effusion virtually always transudative	
Congestive heart failure	Acute diuresis can result in pseudoexudate
Cirrhosis	Rare without clinical ascites
Nephrotic syndrome	Usually subpulmonic and bilateral
Peritoneal dialysis	Massive effusion develops within 48 hours of initiating dialysis
Hypoalbuminemia	Edema fluid rarely isolated to pleural space
Urinothorax	Caused by ipsilateral obstructive uropathy
Atelectasis	Caused by increased intrapleural negative pressure; common in ICU setting
Constrictive pericarditis	Bilateral effusions
Trapped lung	Result of remote inflammation
Superior vena caval obstruction	Caused by acute systemic venous hypertension or acute blockage of thoracic lymph flow
"Classic exudates" that can be transudates	
Malignancy	Caused by early lymphatic obstruction, obstructive atelectasis, or concomitant disease
Pulmonary embolism	Incidence of 23%; caused by atelectasis
Sarcoidosis	Stage II and III disease
Hypothyroid pleural effusion	Transudates secondary to hypothyroid heart disease

lemma. Exudates result primarily from pleural and lung inflammation (pneumonia) or impaired lymphatic drainage of the pleural space (malignancy), and these in turn represent a capillary protein leak or decreased protein removal from the pleural space, respectively. Exudates can also result from the movement of fluid from the peritoneal space, as seen in acute or chronic pancreatis, chylous ascites, and peritoneal carcinomatosis. Disease in virtually any organ can cause exudative pleural effusions through a variety of mechanisms, including infection, malignancy, immunologic responses, lymphatic abnormalities, noninfectious inflammation, iatrogenic causes, and movement from below the diaphragm (Table 4).

The most practical method of distinguishing between transudates and exudates is measurement of serum and pleural fluid protein and LDH concentrations. If at least one of the following criteria is met, the fluid is virtually always an exudate, and if none is met, the fluid is virtually always a transudate: (1) pleural fluid protein-to-serum protein ratio of >0.5; (2) pleural fluid LDH-to-serum LDH ratio of >0.6; and (3) pleural fluid LDH >67% of the upper limits of normal for the serum LDH. Recent data using receiver operating characteristics (ROC) analysis suggest that an LDH concentration of 160 IU/L is the ideal cutoff point to separate transudates and exudates. Pleural fluid cholesterol appears to be a relatively good differentiating marker, with a level of 60 mg/dL as a cutoff; virtually all effusions with cholesterol levels of <60 mg/dL are transudative, and up to 10% of exudates have cholesterol levels of <60 mg/dL.

Transudates have characteristic, but not diagnostic, cellular and biochemical characteristics that support their noninflammatory pathogenesis. These effusions are usually straw-colored, nonviscous, and odorless. In approximately 80% of cases, the nucleated cell count is <1000/μL; it is rare to find a transudative effusion with a nucleated cell count of >10,000/μL. Eighty-five percent of transudative effusions have red blood cell counts of up to 10,000/μL, so the clinician cannot conclude that a serosanguinous effusion is not a transudate. Furthermore, serosanguinous transudative effusions do not become pseudoexudates by LDH criteria, possibly because extensive pleural space hemolysis would be required to affect pleural fluid LDH. Transudative effusions, because of their noninflammatory nature, are mononuclear-predominant and composed of lymphocytes, mesothelial cells, and monocytes-macrophages; it is extremely unusual for classic transudates to be neutrophil-predominant, and if found, this should suggest dual diagnoses. A low pleural fluid glucose level is not found in transudative effusions, and the pleural fluid pH is alkaline (with the exception of urinothorax) and exceeds the simultaneously obtained blood pH, usually in the range of 7.45 to 7.55.

In the acute stages of an exudate, the inflammatory response produces pleural fluid with high nucleated cell counts and a predominance of neutrophils. In the subacute or chronic stages, the exudative effusions may have low cell counts of <5000/μL with a predominance of mononuclear cells, usually lymphocytes.

Pleural Fluid Cells

The nucleated cell count in pleural fluid is virtually never diagnostic; however, counts of >50,000/μL usually are found only in parapneumonic effusions, usually empyema. Transudates generally are associated with nucleated cell counts of <1000/μL, and chronic exudates, as in malignancy and tuberculosis, with counts of <5000/μL. Patients with pleural fluid nucleated cell counts of >10,000/μL generally have substantial pleural inflammation, as can occur with pneumonia, pancreatitis, PCIS, and pulmonary infarction. When pleural fluid is grossly purulent, the nucleated cell count often is less than antici-

TABLE 4. *Causes of exudative pleural effusions*

Infectious	**Increased negative**
Bacterial pneumonia	**intrapleural pressure**
Tuberculous pleurisy	Atelectasis
Parasites	Trapped lung
Fungal disease	Cholesterol effusion
Atypical pneumonias	**Connective tissue disease**
Nocardia, Actinomyces	Lupus pleuritis
Subphrenic abscess	Rheumatoid pleurisy
Hepatic abscess	Mixed connective tissue
Splenic abscess	disease
Hepatitis	Churg-Strauss syndrome
Spontaneous	Wegener's granulomatosis
esophageal rupture	Familial Mediterranean fever
Iatrogenic	**Endocrine dysfunction**
Drug-induced	Hypothyroidism
Esophageal	Ovarian hyperstimulation
perforation	syndrome
Esophageal	**Lymphatic abnormalities**
sclerotherapy	Malignancy
Central venous	Yellow nail syndrome
catheter	Lymphangiomyomatosis
misplacement/	**Movement of fluid from**
migration	**abdomen to pleural**
Enteral feeding tube in	**space**
pleural space	Pancreatitis
Malignancy	Pancreatic pseudocyst
Carcinoma	Meigs' syndrome
Lymphoma	Carcinoma
Mesothelioma	Chylous ascites
Leukemia	Urinothorax
Chylothorax	
Other inflammatory	
Pancreatitis	
BAPE	
Pulmonary embolism	
Radiation therapy	
Uremic pleurisy	
Sarcoidosis	
PCIS	
Hemothorax	
ARDS	

pated, because lysis of neutrophils has occurred and the debris from these cells, in addition to fibrin and collagen, causes turbidity and purulence of the fluid.

The timing of thoracentesis in relation to the acute pleural injury determines the predominant cell in the exudate. Acute exudative pleural effusions are neutrophil-predominant. As the time from the acute insult to performance of thoracentesis lengthens, the effusion becomes mononuclear-predominant if pleural injury is not persistent. Diseases in which the patient is examined soon after the onset of symptoms, such as pneumonia, pulmonary embolism, and pancreatitis, usually are associated with neutrophil-predominant effusions.

Pleural fluid lymphocytosis, particularly lymphocyte counts of 85%–90%, suggests tuberculous pleurisy. However, lymphoma, sarcoidosis, and chronic rheumatoid pleurisy should be considered in the proper clinical setting. Carcinomatous pleural effusions have >50% lymphocytes in two thirds of cases. As the aforementioned diseases can be diagnosed by closed pleural biopsy, the presence of an unknown exudate and lymphocytosis is the prime indication for pleural biopsy. Approximately a third of patients with transudative pleural effusions have a predominance of lymphocytes; however, this finding is of no clinical relevance and does not indicate the need for pleural biopsy.

Pleural fluid eosinophilia (>10% of total nucleated cells are eosinophils) suggests a benign, self-limited pleural effusion associated with air or blood in the pleural space. Therefore, it is commonly seen following pleural space hemorrhage, pulmonary infarction, pneumothorax, or BAPE, or after thoracentesis. Pleural fluid eosinophilia is rare but not unknown in tuberculous pleurisy and is unusual with a malignant pleural effusion despite the high incidence of pleural space hemorrhage. When air or blood is not present with pleural fluid eosinophilia, parasitic disease (paragonimiasis, hydatid disease), fungal infection (histoplasmosis), and drugs (dantrolene, nitrofurantoin) should be considered. Approximately one third of eosinophilic pleural effusions are idiopathic; many of these effusions are probably caused by occult pulmonary embolism or BAPE, as these effusions are frequently bloody. Pleural fluid basophilia (>10% of total nucleated cells are basophils) is rare and suggests leukemic involvement of the pleura.

Mesothelial cells are predominant in transudative pleural effusions and are found to a variable degree in exudates. The presence of mesothelial cells in exudates is important, because if >5% of cells are mesothelial cells, tuberculous pleurisy is virtually excluded, and they may be confused with malignant cells. Mesothelial cells are scarce in the pleural space when there is diffuse pleural injury or fibrosis inhibiting exfoliation; this has been noted with empyema, rheumatoid pleurisy, after pleurodesis, and in chronic malignant effusions.

The pleural fluid macrophage has its origin in the circulating blood monocyte. The macrophage appears to modulate pleural injury and is called to the pleural space by pleural fluid neutrophil chemotaxins. The presence of macrophages is of no diagnostic value, but it is important not to confuse these cells with mesothelial cells, as the presence of macrophages does not exclude tuberculous pleurisy.

Finding a large number of plasma cells in pleural fluid suggests multiple myeloma with pleural involvement. A small number of plasma cells is nondiagnostic and has been observed in a spectrum of diseases ranging from congestive heart failure to malignancy.

The presence of blood-tinged pleural fluid is of minimal diagnostic value, as only a few drops of blood in 500 mL of fluid will result in hemorrhagic fluid. Up to 50% of exudates and 10%–15% of transudates may be sanguineous. The finding of more than 100,000 red blood cells per microliter suggests that the exudate is caused by trauma, malignancy, pulmonary embolism, PCIS, or BAPE. In the absence of trauma, malignancy is the most common cause of a frankly bloody pleural effusion. Determining whether the bloody effusion is real or caused by a traumatic thoracentesis frequently poses a dilemma. A traumatic thoracentesis is suggested by nonuniform color during aspiration, clotting of the fluid within several minutes, and the absence of hemosiderin-laden macrophages.

Pleural Fluid Chemistries

A low pleural fluid glucose concentration (<60 mg/dL, or pleural fluid-to-serum ratio of <0.5) narrows the differential diagnosis of the exudate to rheumatoid pleurisy, empyema, malignant effusions, tuberculous pleurisy, lupus pleuritis, and esophageal rupture. The mechanisms responsible for a low pleural fluid glucose concentration include decreased transport of glucose from blood to pleural fluid (malignancy, rheumatoid pleurisy) and increased glucose utilization by constituents of pleural fluid (empyema, malignancy). The lowest glucose concentrations are found in empyema and rheumatoid pleural effusions, with glucose being undetectable at times. In tuberculous pleurisy, lupus pleuritis, and malignancy, the glucose concentration when low is generally in the range of 30 to 55 mg/dL.

A pleural fluid pH of <7.30 with a normal blood pH is found in the same conditions associated with a low pleural fluid glucose concentration. Pleural fluid acidosis has been found with esophageal rupture (pH of 6.00), empyema (5.50–7.29), rheumatoid pleurisy (7.00), malignancy (7.05–7.29), and lupus pleuritis (7.05–7.29). The mechanisms responsible for pleural fluid acidosis are increased acid production by pleural fluid cells and bacteria (empyema), and decreased acid efflux from the pleural space because of pleuritis or pleural fibrosis (malignancy and rheumatoid pleurisy). A low pleural fluid pH has diagnostic, prognostic, and therapeutic implications in malignancy and parapneumonic effusions. In parapneumonic effusions, a pleural fluid pH of <7.10 suggests the need for chest tube drainage. In malignant pleural effusions, a pH value of <7.30 predicts a short survival time, an increased yield on pleural biopsy and cytology, and a poor response to pleurodesis.

An increased pleural fluid amylase concentration (above the upper limits of normal for serum, or a pleural fluid-to-serum ratio of >1.0) indicates one of four diagnostic possibilities: (1) acute pancreatitis, (2) pancreatic pseudocyst, (3) esophageal rupture, and (4) malignancy.

In addition to fulfilling one of the criteria defining an exudate, a high LDH level (>1000 IU/L) suggests empyema, rheumatoid pleurisy, or paragonimiasis involving the pleural space.

Immunologic Studies

A pleural fluid rheumatoid factor titer of 1:320 or higher is suggestive but not diagnostic of rheumatoid pleurisy. The finding of LE cells in pleural fluid is virtually diagnostic of lupus pleuritis. The likelihood of demonstrating LE cells in pleural fluid appears to be enhanced if the fluid is allowed to remain at room temperature for several hours before it is examined with Wright stain. An antinuclear antibody (ANA) titer of 1:160 or higher or a pleural fluid-to-serum ANA ratio of 1.0 or greater is suggestive but not diagnostic of lupus pleuritis. Pleural fluid complement levels are low in most patients with lupus pleuritis and rheumatoid pleurisy; this is true whether total hemolytic complement or complement components are measured.

Cytology

Cytology is a more sensitive test for the diagnosis of malignant pleural effusions than is percutaneous pleural biopsy, because pleural metastases tend to be focal and the latter is a blind sampling procedure. The yield of cytology increases as the disease becomes more advanced. With improved techniques, the yield from exfoliative cytology now approaches 90%–95%. If the clinician suspects a malignant effusion, several hundred milliliters of fluid should be removed at the initial diagnostic thoracentesis. This maneuver will not improve the yield on the initial study, but if the results are negative, a repeated procedure several days later may provide fluid with fewer degenerative cells and freshly exfoliated malignant cells. If the results of a second cytologic examination several days after the first are negative, a third examination soon after usually is nondiagnostic. Reasons for a true negative cytologic examination include improper handling of the specimen, variance of tumor type, and lack of interest and expertise of the cytopathologist.

Pleural Biopsy

Several techniques for percutaneous pleural biopsy have been available since the 1920s, but not until the 1950s, with the popularization of the Cope and Abrams needles, did routine bedside pleural biopsy become available to the clinician.

Percutaneous pleural biopsy is a simple bedside or outpatient procedure whose main indication is the evaluation of exudative effusions of unknown cause. The two diagnoses most commonly established by pleural biopsy are malignancy and tuberculosis. The diagnosis of rheumatoid pleurisy, fungal pleurisy (coccidioidomycosis, blastomycosis), sarcoidosis, and parasitic diseases, such as echinococcosis) also can be confirmed by pleural biopsy. Culturing *Coccidioides* from pleural tissue appears to be an excellent method of establishing the diagnosis of acute coccidioidal pleural effusion.

Demonstration of free-flowing fluid in the pleural space is imperative if complications are to be minimized. If doubt exists, confirmation before biopsy of fluid location by ultrasonography is recommended. The presence of pleural fluid is not a prerequisite for percutaneous pleural biopsy; if pleural symphysis does not exist, allowing air to enter the pleural space will separate the lung from the chest wall and allow the biopsy to be performed safely. If loculated pleural fluid is present, the biopsy should be done under ultrasonic guidance.

Contraindications to pleural biopsy include (1) pleural symphysis; (2) an uncooperative patient; (3) anticoagulation; (4) a bleeding diathesis, including moderate to severe azotemia, when a normal bleeding time cannot be ensured; (5) empyema; and (6) local cutaneous lesions (herpes zoster, pyoderma).

Technique

Proper positioning of the patient is important for any invasive procedure but particularly for pleural biopsy. The patient should be seated leaning backward in a chair with arms resting against the backrest or on a table to allow optimal patient comfort and ease of access of the operator to the posterior chest wall. Vasovagal episodes during pleural sampling are not uncommon in anxious patients; proper preparation of the patient, adequate local anesthesia, and preoperative administration of atropine virtually eliminate this complication.

A biopsy site should be chosen one to two intercostal spaces below the fluid level demonstrated on physical examination. Appropriate anesthesia of the parietal pleura and periosteum of the rib provides maximal patient comfort and cooperation. A skin incision parallel to the ribs with a No. 11 blade facilitates entrance to the pleural space of the 11-gauge outer cannula just above the superior border of the rib. When the outer cannula enters the pleural space, a characteristic pop is felt. After fluid is aspirated through the trocar, pressure is applied in the direction of the cutting needle, allowing the parietal pleura to be snagged. Several biopsy specimens should be obtained by rotating the trocar and cutting needle to different locations, with care taken to avoid the intercostal neurovascular bundle, which is more likely to be encountered with extreme cephalic or caudal angulation. The tissue is cut from the parietal pleura by advancing with a twisting motion (Cope needle) or rotating the inner cutting needle (Abrams needle). Three to five specimens should be taken from a single site. The pleural tissue should be placed in 10% formaldehyde for histologic examination and in sterile nonbacteriostatic saline solution for culture. If malignancy is the suspected diagnosis, only a single specimen needs to be cultured. If tuberculosis is likely, the specimen should be divided evenly between histology and culture.

Diagnostic Yield

The literature reports a wide range of diagnostic yields, from 30%–70% in patients with malignancy and 60%–95% in patients with tuberculous pleurisy. Patient population, biopsy technique, and the expertise of the operator, pathologist, and microbiology laboratory account for some of the variability. In a compilation of 14 series from the literature inclusive of 2893 pleural biopsies, 51% were nondiagnostic, 245 (75%) of 325 were positive for a confirmed diagnosis of tuberculous pleurisy, and 618 (57%) of 1080 were positive with a known diagnosis of carcinoma.

Sampling error has led to controversy as to the number, location, and sites for percutaneous pleural biopsy. A paucity of data exists regarding an adequate number of individual biopsy specimens to be taken at a single site, yet there is a suggestion that four or more improve the diagnostic yield. The sampling location usually is directed by the fluid level as determined on radiologic and physical examination. Thoracoscopy has demonstrated the nonuniform location of pleural metastasis. The highest yield would be expected from specimens obtained close to the diaphragm and midline, as pleural metastases tend to begin in the former location and spread toward the costal pleura and cephalad. Increasing the number of biopsy sites at one sitting does not appear to increase the diagnostic yield in either tuberculous pleurisy or malignancy. The stage of the malignancy at the time of pleural biopsy appears to be related to the diagnostic yield; more studies are positive in patients with far-advanced disease. The diagnostic yield is also high in patients with malignancy and a low pleural fluid pH (<7.30), as in advanced disease hydrogen ion efflux from the pleural space is impaired by increased tumor bulk and pleural fibrosis.

The primary indication for percutaneous pleural biopsy today is tuberculous pleurisy, as this test provides the highest diagnostic yield. With improvement in cytologic techniques, the yield of pleural fluid exfoliated cytology approaches 95% when the pleura is involved with malignancy; therefore, pleural biopsy rarely adds to the diagnosis. However, there are instances in which results of the cytologic examination are negative and the pleural biopsy findings are positive. Therefore, if findings of the first cytologic examination are negative and malignancy is suspected, a second procedure should include repeated cytologic examination with a single-site percutaneous pleural biopsy.

Complications

Potential complications of closed-chest pleural biopsy cover a spectrum ranging from pain at the needle insertion site to empyema; however, complications are unusual and generally of minimal clinical consequence. Pneumothorax, the most common and potentially important clinical complication, usually is small and is caused by the entrance of air through the needle into the pleural space, not by lung puncture. Small pneumothoraces have been reported in up to 15% of biopsies and usually can be treated expectantly. Site pain (reported incidence of 1%–15%) can be minimized with good technique and local anesthesia. Vasovagal reaction, reported in 1%–5% of patients, can virtually be eliminated with the use of atropine. The remaining complications, including hemothorax, transient fever, tumor seeding, site hematoma, subcutaneous emphysema, air embolism, biopsy of extrapleural tissue (liver and spleen), and empyema, occur in <1% of patients.

Thoracoscopy

Jacobaeus first described an endoscopic approach to serous cavities more than 80 years ago and published his experience in lysing pleural adhesions in the treatment of tuberculosis and the diagnosis of tumors based in pleura. The previously mentioned procedures were the major indications for thoracoscopy during the next two decades. Interest in thoracoscopy waned with the development of percutaneous needles for pleural biopsy. Recently, there has been a renewed interest in thoracoscopy because of better endoscopic optic systems, improved technology of the instrument itself, and interest in less invasive procedures. Today, thoracoscopy is used predominantly in the diagnostic evaluation of pleural effusions of unknown cause and for talc pleurodesis. Most procedures are performed using rigid thoracoscopes because of their superior optical systems, large working channels, and ease of maneuverability.

Usually, diagnostic thoracoscopy is performed under local anesthesia with small incremental doses of narcotics and a benzodiazepine. A chest tube is required after thoracoscopy. In diagnostic cases in which only the parietal pleura is sampled, a small chest tube can be used (16 to 20 French). With talc pleurodesis, a larger chest tube is placed and should remain in place until the pleural fluid drainage is <150 mL/d.

The diagnostic accuracy of thoracoscopy in pleural effusions of unknown cause varies depending on the duration of follow-up and the diagnostic methods employed, with the diagnostic accuracy in reported series ranging from 69%–96%. Although thoracoscopy is less invasive than formal thoracotomy and in certain circumstances is a better alternative than observation, it should not replace percutaneous needle biopsy. Although thoracoscopy is excellent for the diagnosis of metastatic cancer or mesothelioma, it should be unnecessary in the diagnosis of tuberculous pleurisy, as pleural biopsy culture and histology and pleural fluid culture will yield a diagnosis in the vast majority of patients. Furthermore, it is usually not helpful in the diagnosis of nonmalignant pleural disease, except to reveal the following: benign asbestos pleural plaques, which are large, white lesions that may resemble teeth; white patchy lesions of the visceral pleura with diffuse telangiectasia, seen in radiation pleuritis; a granular appearance on the pleural surface in rheumatoid pleurisy; and visceral and parietal pleural adhesions and gray-white plaques in tuberculous pleurisy.

Talc by poudrage is a highly effective method of pleurodesis for both malignant and nonmalignant pleural effusions. Talc slurry through a chest tube appears to have similar efficacy to talc poudrage and is less expensive, as the cost of thoracoscopy is avoided.

The mortality from diagnostic thoracoscopy in >4000 cases is <0.1%, comparable with the mortality of bronchoscopy with transbronchial biopsy. The potential complications, which are rare, include postoperative air leak, hemorrhage, hypotension, hypoxemia, subcutaneous emphysema, vagal syncope, and metastatic invasion of the access tract.

The only absolute contraindication is pleural symphysis. Cough, hypoxemia, severe cardiac disease, and coagulopathy are relative contraindications.

Open Pleural Biopsy

Although formal thoracotomy provides excellent visualization of the pleura and the opportunity to obtain the largest biopsy specimens, thoracoscopy has virtually replaced open pleural biopsy for the diagnosis of unknown pleural disease. However, in certain instances, as when attempting to establish definitively the diagnosis of malignant mesothelioma, which often requires a large amount of tissue, open pleural biopsy may be necessary. However, some clinicians have reported high diagnostic yields for malignant mesothelioma with thoracoscopy. Neither open pleural biopsy nor thoracoscopy always provides a diagnosis in unknown pleural disease, particularly with nonmalignant causes. At times, a malignancy is not discovered for months following open pleural biopsy; in these cases, the effusion was probably paramalignant at the time of the procedure.

BIBLIOGRAPHY

Adelman M, Albelda SM, Gottlieb J, Haponik EF. Diagnostic utility of pleural fluid eosinophilia. *Am J Med* 1984;77:915–920. *A review of 343 cases of pleural fluid eosinophilia showing that 28% were associated with air in the pleural space and that half of the cases of BAPE reported in the literature had pleural fluid eosinophilia.*

Albertine KH, Wiener-Kronish JP, Bastacky J, et al. No evidence for mesothelial cell contact across the costal pleural space of sheep. *J Appl Physiol* 1991;70:123–134. *Suggests that pleural liquid clearance is probably facilitated by liquid accumulation in dependent regions where lymphatic pathways exist.*

Albertine KH, Wiener-Kronish JP, Roos PJ, et al. Structure, blood supply, and lymphatic vessels of the sheep's visceral pleura. *Am J Anat* 1982;165:277–294. *A morphologic study of the visceral pleura of sheep. The blood supply of the entire visceral pleura was from the bronchial arteries.*

Albertine KH, Wiener-Kronish JP, Staub NC. The structure of the parietal pleura and its relationship to pleural liquid dynamics in sheep. *Anat Rec* 1984;208:401–409. *A morphologic study of the parietal pleura of sheep indicating that the parietal pleura plays a major role in pleural liquid and protein dynamics.*

Boutin C, Viallat JR, Cargnino P, Farisse P. Thoracoscopy in malignant pleural effusions. *Am Rev Respir Dis* 1991;124:588–592. *Documents the high diagnostic yield (87%) of properly performed thoracoscopy in 150 patients with malignant pleural effusions.*

Broaddus VC, Wiener-Kronish JP, Berthiaume Y, et al. Removal of liquid and protein by lymphatics in awake sheep. *J Appl Physiol* 1988;64:384–390. *Demonstrates in awake sheep with large hydrothoraces that pleural liquid and protein are removed at an hourly rate of 0.28 ± 0.01 mL/kg and that lymphatics are responsible for at least 98% of this removal.*

Collins TR, Sahn SA. Thoracentesis: complications, patient experience, and diagnostic value. *Chest* 1987;91:817–822. *A prospective study of the value and complications of pleural fluid analysis.*

Good JT Jr, King TE, Antony VB, Sahn SA. Lupus pleuritis: clinical features and pleural fluid characteristics with special reference to pleural fluid antinuclear antibodies. *Chest* 1983;84:714–718. *Details the clinical presentation, pleural findings, and diagnostic criteria in 14 patients with lupus pleuritis.*

Good JT Jr, Taryle DE, Maulitz RM, Kaplan RL, Sahn SA. The diagnostic value of pleural fluid pH. *Chest* 1980;78:55–59. *A pleural fluid pH of <7.30 was associated with empyema, malignancy, collagen vascular disease, tuberculosis, esophageal rupture, and hemothorax.*

Hsu C. Cytologic detection of malignancy in pleural effusion: a review of 5255 samples from 3811 patients. *Diagn Cytopathol* 1987;3:8–12. *The cytopathologic correlation with pleural biopsy was 96.5% accurate. The sensitivity of cytologic detections was 6.7% higher than that of pleural biopsy.*

Johnson WW. The malignant pleural effusion. A review of cytopathologic diagnoses of 584 specimens from 472 consecutive patients. *Cancer* 1985;56:905–909. *Of 5888 pleural fluid specimens, 584 contained malignant cells; 76% were carcinomas and 48% were adenocarcinomas. In 90.5% of patients, a cytopathologic diagnosis conclusive for malignancy was obtained from the first specimen of fluid.*

Kim KJ, Critz AM, Crandall ED. Transport of water and solutes across sheep visceral pleura. *Am Rev Respir Dis* 1979;120:883–892. *Studies of specimens of intact visceral pleura of sheep suggest that the transport properties of normal pleural tissue are unlikely to be responsible for differences in composition between interstitial and pleural fluid.*

Light RW, Erozan YS, Ball WC Jr. Cells in pleural fluid: their value in differential diagnosis. *Arch Intern Med* 1973;132:854–860. *An assessment of the value of pleural fluid cells in the assessment of pleural effusions with different causes.*

Light RW, MacGregor MI, Luchsinger PC, Ball WC Jr. Pleural effusions: the diagnostic separation of transudates from exudates. *Ann Intern Med* 1972;77:507–513. *Presents the criteria for separation of transudates from exudates.*

Menzies R, Charbonneau M. Thoracoscopy for the diagnosis of pleural disease. *Ann Intern Med* 1991;114:271–276. *In a prospective evaluation of patients referred for thoracoscopy, the authors show that thoracoscopy under local anesthesia is a safe procedure with an excellent diagnostic yield equivalent to that of thoracotomy.*

Negrini D, Ballard ST, Benoit JN. Contribution of lymphatic myogenic activity and respiratory movements to pleural lymph flow. *J Appl Physiol* 1994;76:2267–2274. *Demonstrates that intrinsic and extrinsic mechanisms account for a similar share of total pleural flow egress.*

Ryan CJ, Rogers RF, Unni KK, Hepper NC. The outcome of patients with pleural effusions of indeterminate causes at thoracotomy. *Mayo Clin Proc* 1981:56:145–149. *Reports on a 10-year experience at the Mayo Clinic of patients with undiagnosed pleural effusions who underwent open pleural biopsy.*

Sahn SA. Pleural fluid pH in the normal state and in diseases affecting the pleural space. In: Chretien J, Bignon J, Hirsch A, eds. *The Pleura in Health and Disease.* New York: Marcel Dekker; 1985:253–266. *Reviews the regulation of pleural fluid pH in the normal state and dysregulation in diseases of the pleura with clinical implications.*

Sahn SA. Pathogenesis and clinical features of diseases associated with a low pleural fluid glucose. In: Chretien J, Bignon J, Hirsch A, eds. *The Pleura in Health and Disease.* New York: Marcel Dekker; 1985:267–285. *Reviews the pathogenesis and clinical features of diseases associated with a low pleural fluid glucose.*

Sahn SA. The pleura. *Am Rev Respir Dis* 1988;138:184–234. *A comprehensive review of pleural anatomy, physiology, and diagnostic techniques, and of specific diseases of the pleura.*

Sahn SA. Thoracentesis and pleural biopsy. In: Shelhamer J, Pizzo PA, Parrilo JE, Masur H, eds. *Respiratory Disease in the Immunosuppressed Host.* Philadelphia: JB Lippincott; 1991:118–129. *Details the indications and contraindications, technique, and complications of thoracentesis and pleural biopsy.*

Sahn SA. The diagnostic value of pleural fluid analysis. *Semin Respir Crit Care Med* 1995;16:269–278. *A review of the cellular and biochemical findings of pleural fluid and their value in narrowing the differential diagnosis.*

Sahn SA, Good JT Jr. Pleural fluid pH in malignant effusions. Diagnostic, prognostic, and therapeutic implications. *Ann Intern Med* 1988;108:345–349. *Diagnostic yield on initial pleural fluid cytologic examination is greater in patients having malignant pleural effusions associated with a low pH (<7.30); additionally, such patients have a shorter mean survival and a poor response to chemical pleurodesis compared with patients having effusions with a normal pH (>7.30).*

Spriggs AI, Boddington NM. *The Cytology of Effusions.* 2nd ed. New York: Grune and Stratton; 1968. *A comprehensive work on the cytology of effusions.*

Staats BA, Ellefson RD, Boudahn LL, Dines DE, Prakash UB, Offord K. The lipoprotein profile of chylous and nonchylous pleural effusions. *Mayo Clin Proc* 1980;55:700–704. *Presents data on the usefulness of triglyceride concentrations in the diagnosis of chylothorax.*

Staub NC, Wiener-Kronish JP, Albertine KH. Transport through the pleura: physiology of normal liquid and solute exchange in the pleural space. In: Chretien J, Bignon J, Hirsch A, eds. *The Pleura in Health and Disease.* New York: Marcel Dekker; 1985:169–193. *A review of pleural liquid and protein exchange concluding that normal liquid and protein of the pleural space are primarily a function of the parietal pleura.*

Tomlinson JR, Sahn SA. Invasive procedures in the diagnosis of pleural disease. *Semin Respir Med* 1987;9:30–36. *Provides the yields from the literature on closed pleural biopsy, thoracoscopy, open pleural biopsy, and fiberoptic bronchoscopy in the diagnosis of pleural effusions.*

Wang N-S. The preformed stomas connecting the pleural cavity and the lymphatics in the parietal pleura. *Am Rev Respir Dis* 1975;111:12–20. *Demonstrates the stomata of the parietal pleura by scanning electron microscopy and shows that large particles and cells exit the pleural space by these structures.*

Yam LT. Diagnostic significance of lymphocytes in pleural effusion. *Ann Intern Med* 1967;66:972–982. *Discusses the diagnostic significance of pleural fluid lymphocytosis.*

Textbook of Pulmonary Diseases, 6th ed.
edited by G.L. Baum, J.D. Crapo, B.R. Celli, and J.B. Karlinsky,
Lippincott–Raven Publishers, Philadelphia, © 1998.

CHAPTER

13

Preoperative Evaluation and Relation to Postoperative Complications

James E. Hansen

INTRODUCTION

This chapter is designed to inform internists and surgeons, including pulmonologists and thoracic surgeons, of the pulmonary dysfunctions and complications that increase morbidity and mortality in patients undergoing surgical procedures, and to suggest a cost-effective method of assessing patients preoperatively. These pulmonary complications are especially likely to occur in patients who are older, obese, or smokers, who undergo thoracic or abdominal surgery, or who have lung or other organ system diseases or undergo lung resection.

PATHOPHYSIOLOGIC FEATURES OF MAJOR POSTOPERATIVE PULMONARY COMPLICATIONS

Atelectasis and Shunting with Hypoxemia

Lung volumes change quickly during anesthesia and surgery. In Fig. 1, the declines in both vital capacity (VC) and forced expiratory volume in 1 second (FEV_1) in the week after abdominal or thoracic surgery are striking and persistent, even though no lung was resected. Concurrently, alveolar-arterial differences in partial pressure of oxygen [$P(A-a)O_2$] increased. During surgery with general anesthesia, increases in $P(A-a)O_2$ and $P(A-a)CO_2$ (alveolar-arterial difference in partial pressure of carbon dioxide) could be attributed to decreases in lung compliance, increased shunting, increased pulmonary dead space, or decreased efficiency of ventilation secondary to

J. E. Hansen: Division of Respiratory and Critical Care Medicine, UCLA School of Medicine, Torrance, California 90509.

ventilation and perfusion mismatching—that is, mechanisms causing increases in venous admixture.

Altered mechanics of the chest wall and diaphragm, however, with a decrease in functional residual capacity (FRC), are the primary cause of the development of areas of atelectasis and secondary hypoxemia. Ventilation during anesthesia with gas mixtures low in nitrogen (N_2) may also accelerate air space collapse. Patients undergoing upper abdominal surgery who have the greatest reduction in FRC postoperatively also have the highest incidence of pulmonary complications. If patchy atelectasis is sought, it can nearly always be demonstrated roentgenographically during general anesthesia for upper abdominal surgery. The appearance of these areas of atelectasis during anesthesia in normal individuals correlates positively with the magnitude of shunting and can usually be cleared by application of positive end-expiratory pressure (PEEP) at 10 cm H_2O. Apparently, inhalation anesthetics inhibit hypoxic pulmonary vasoconstriction more than do intravenous anesthetics, thus tending to cause more overperfusion of poorly ventilated air spaces and greater hypoxemia.

Rarely in patients undergoing cardiac transplantation or in patients with severe lung disease who are undergoing resection, sufficient pulmonary hypertension develops to open a potentially patent foramen ovale and cause shunting from the right to left atrium, with very severe widening of the $P(A-a)O_2$. The diagnosis of a patent foramen ovale can be made by having the patient breath 100% O_2. Because of the resulting high alveolar and end-pulmonary capillary PO_2 and complete saturation of hemoglobin at these high pressures, the venous admixture resulting from the development of a right-to-left shunt reduces the measured PaO_2 in an almost linear fashion proportional to the size of the shunt.

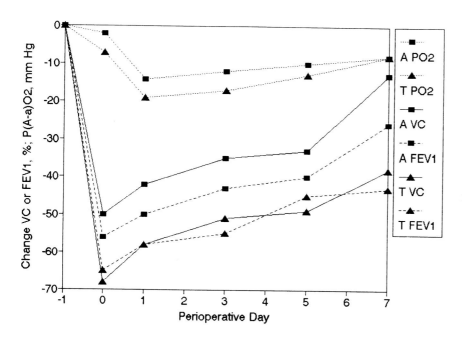

FIG. 1. Average change in spirometric values (%) and P(A-a)O₂ (mmHg) after thoracic (*T*) or abdominal (*A*) surgical procedures in 34 patients. (Modified with permission from Bryant LR, et al. Lung perfusion scanning for estimation of postoperative pulmonary function. *Arch Surg* 1972;104:52.)

Factors Predisposing to Postoperative Pneumonia

Impaired Transport of Mucus

Transport of mucus from the lower lobes and trachea is impaired for several days after upper abdominal surgery under general anesthesia, but only minimally after surgery of a lower extremity. It is well assessed by insufflation of the airways with tantalum. This transport deficiency, also associated with visible atelectasis, is probably related more to immobilization, diaphragmatic dysfunction, and ineffective coughing than to endotracheal intubation.

Aspiration

Aspiration of oral and gastric contents occurs occasionally in normal individuals during sleep. In the perioperative period, such aspiration of gastric or oropharyngeal contents into the tracheobronchial tree may cause pulmonary dysfunction resulting from acid burns, mechanical obstruction, or bacterial pathogens. Aspiration can easily occur during induction of anesthesia (if the stomach is not empty or emptied) whenever the endotracheal cuff is not properly inflated, or postoperatively if extubation is premature (before the gag reflex returns). Postoperatively, the use of a nasogastric tube may increase pulmonary aspiration.

Pre-existing Lung Infection

Both clinically evident and subclinical respiratory tract infection are associated with an increased risk for pneu-

monia. Carrel and colleagues found that pneumonia frequently developed in cardiac patients in whom immediate postsurgical tracheal aspirates were positive for microorganisms despite perioperative antibiotic therapy (8 of 26), but rarely in those with negative aspirates (1 of 72).

Impaired Coughing

Coughing to clear secretions in the postoperative period is especially difficult in the presence of postoperative chest and abdominal pain. Coughing is less effective in patients with obstructive lung disease and low expiratory flow rates.

Respiratory Failure

Postoperative respiratory failure commonly occurs in patients with severe obstructive lung disease undergoing thoracic or upper abdominal surgery. Preoperative CO₂ retention, obesity, sepsis, and shock all increase the probability of postoperative respiratory failure. Maede and colleagues showed that the ratio of abdominal to transdiaphragmatic pressure decreased postoperatively, indicating diaphragmatic weakness, and that the greatest reductions occurred in the 4 of their 20 patients who required mechanical ventilation for 2 to 6 days. The decrease in lung volumes and flow rates during the several days following chest or upper abdominal surgery, especially when combined with pain, weakness, and sedation, necessarily reduces the drive and ability of postoperative patients to ventilate and remove metabolically produced CO₂. The elimination of CO₂ rarely is a problem except in patients with significant lung disease. In these patients, the ability to ventilate may be not only seriously reduced but also inefficient, the latter attributable to an increase in the ratio of physiologic dead space to tidal volume (V_D/V_T). Postoperative infection with fever and increased metabolism (causing high CO_2 production) and the intraoperative insufflation of CO_2 during an abdominal endoscopic procedure are additional causes of acute respiratory acidosis and respiratory failure.

The degree of V_D/V_T abnormality can be calculated from the patient's estimated or measured CO_2 output and measurement of the arterial CO_2 and minute ventilation. In patients whose ability to ventilate is compromised, repeated assessments with changes in ventilator settings and body position may be necessary to reduce the V_D/V_T and optimize CO_2 removal. With anemia, heart failure, shock, or infection, ventilation with high O_2 or high ventilatory pressures can lead to further lung damage and failure.

Pulmonary Embolism

Pulmonary emboli are common sequelae of venous thrombosis in the deep veins of the leg. In one study, the incidence of deep venous thromboses in three groups of hospitalized patients was as follows: (1) 11% in those without any of the risk factors of advanced age, obesity, malignancy, recent surgery, or history of deep venous thromboses; (2) 50% in those with three risk factors; and (3) 100% in those with four or more risk factors. Another expert group estimates the incidence of deep venous thrombosis as follows: (1) approximately 10%–20% (high risk) in patients older than 40 years with a recent history of venous thrombosis, or those undergoing extensive abdominal or pelvic surgery for malignancy, or those undergoing major orthopedic surgery of a lower extremity; (2) approximately 2%–10% (moderate risk) in patients undergoing general surgery of >30 minutes' duration (risk increases progressively with advancing age, malignancy, congestive failure, obesity, varicose veins, prolonged immobilization, and paralysis); and (3) <1% (low risk) in patients having uncomplicated or minor surgery of <30 minutes' duration. In these three groups, the risk for fatal pulmonary embolism is approximately 1%–5%, 0.1%–1%, and <0.01%, respectively, with an overall risk for general surgery of approximately 1%. Despite this known high incidence, even now in a well-known academic medical center with a major interest in thromboembolic disease, a correct diagnosis was established before autopsy in only 30% of patients who had a fatal pulmonary embolism. Wheeler and Anderson further noted a low incidence of thromboembolic prophylaxis even in high-risk patients, ranging from 9%–56% in different New England hospitals.

RISK FACTORS

The following are some of the recognized risk factors contributing to an increase in pulmonary complications postoperatively.

Age

The maximal flow rates, FEV_1, VC, FEV_1/VC, and maximum voluntary ventilation (MVV) all decline with age, so that normal individuals have less ventilatory reserve and less ability to clear secretions by coughing as they age. Additionally, and probably related to the decrease in elastic recoil and resultant increase in residual volume (RV), the $P(A-a)O_2$ increases each year on average by approximately 0.4 mmHg. Thus, even without pulmonary, neuromuscular, or other organ disease processes, there is a gradual reduction in PaO_2 with aging and less reserve for the increased ventilatory requirements that may be needed postoperatively. Postoperative hypoxemia increases with advancing age. Of course, the more frequent occurrence of other systemic diseases with advancing age necessarily adds to the likelihood of postoperative problems.

Obesity

Obesity is a major cause of postoperative complications. At least two studies found that after upper abdominal surgery, obesity was the most important risk factor associated with clinically significant atelectasis. The incidence of both preoperative and postoperative hypoxemia increases strikingly with obesity and age and is worse in the supine position (Fig. 2). Such hypoxemia is primarily a consequence of the high proportion of regions with decreased ventilation without compensatory reduction in perfusion (low $\dot{V}_A/\dot{Q}$) at the lung bases, but it may be aggravated by reduced ventilatory drive associated with CO_2 retention or metabolic alkalosis. With moderate thoracic and abdominal obesity, the VC may remain within normal limits, but the expiratory reserve volume (ERV) inevitably declines, indicating that the resting position of the diaphragm is elevated. With extreme obesity, the VC and MVV may become significantly decreased below predicted values in the absence of intrinsic lung disease and despite normal general muscle strength. Thus, hypoxemia, hypercapnia, somnolence, sleep apnea, and pulmonary hypertension are common complications of even moderate obesity. As hypoxemia and atelectasis are common postoperative occurrences even in patients who are not obese, and ventilatory work is increased with truncal obesity, obese patients have multiple handicaps in the postoperative period. Additional disadvantages for obese patients are the requirements for larger doses of many anesthetics because of their high solubility in fatty tissue,

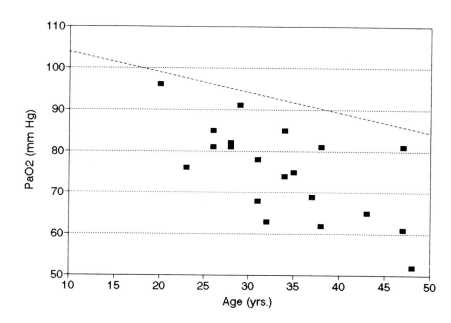

FIG. 2. Effect of age on PaO2 in morbidly obese, awake, supine patients. The *dotted line* is regressed from data of Sorbini and colleagues for normal adults, with a standard deviation of 4 mmHg. (Modified with permission from Vaughan RW, et al. Postoperative hypoxemia in obese patients. *Ann Surg* 1974;180:877.)

the longer time needed to eliminate anesthetics from the body, the longer time necessary to complete the surgical procedure, the increased acidity of gastric juice, and the increased frequency of aspiration of gastric contents. To this list can be added the higher incidence of diabetes mellitus and cardiovascular and thromboembolic diseases and the difficulties involved in postoperative ambulation and nursing care.

Surgical and Incisional Site

Evidence is overwhelming that the incidence of postoperative morbidity and mortality is closely linked to the site of surgical intervention. It should be recalled that with upper abdominal surgery or thoracic surgery without lung resection, the FEV_1 and VC are strikingly reduced as soon as they can be measured postoperatively and do not usually return to preoperative levels within 1 week. When possible, it is desirable to choose an incisional site in thoracic surgery associated with lesser postoperative discomfort. A higher rate of atelectasis and hypoxemia occurs with vertical than with horizontal laparotomies. The overall incidence of postoperative cardiopulmonary complications becomes progressively lower in patients undergoing lower abdominal, pelvic, and extremity surgery. However, the incidence of venous thromboses and pulmonary emboli is very high in patients undergoing hip and knee surgery.

Lung Disease

Although postoperative morbidity and mortality cannot be accurately predicted for every patient, patients with significant lung disease undergoing thoracic or abdominal surgery are at high risk. Both obstructive and restrictive lung

diseases are handicaps. However, the former carries a greater postoperative risk than the latter. In 1956, Miller and associates introduced a four-quadrant diagram based on the $FEV_{0.5}$ and VC, later modified by others, to categorize disturbed respiratory mechanics. This diagram graphically identifies relative postoperative risk in patients with obstructive, restrictive, and combined lung disorders (Fig. 3). All other things being equal, it can be noted in this diagram that the risk for postoperative ventilatory failure might be (1) slightly better than marginal in a patient with an FEV_1/VC of 50% and a VC or total lung capacity (TLC) that is 50% of predicted (i.e., moderate obstruction and moderate restriction); (2) prohibitive in a patient with an FEV_1/VC of 35% and VC or TLC that is 80% of predicted (i.e., severe obstruction and mild restriction); but (3) satisfactory in a patient with an FEV_1/VC of 70% and a VC or TLC that is 45% of predicted (mild obstruction and severe restriction). These differences in risk are logically related to the difficulty encountered by patients with obstructive disease in clearing airway secretions in the postoperative period.

Stein and colleagues noted that a reduced maximal expiratory flow rate ($FEF_{200-1200}$) was a potent predictor of postoperative pulmonary complications. Even patients with severe restrictive lung disease often have increased lung elastic recoil, can maintain satisfactory peak flow measurements, and can clear secretions adequately. On the other hand, patients with severe obstructive lung disease often have a very low $FEF_{200-1200}$ or peak flow readings and an ineffective cough. When either restrictive or obstructive lung disease has progressed to the stage at which CO_2 retention has occurred, the risk of surgery increases markedly. To oversimplify, the ''blue bloater'' chronic bronchitic patient is likely to be at greater risk than the ''pink puffer'' for the same severity of airways obstruction. The risk for complications in the asthmatic

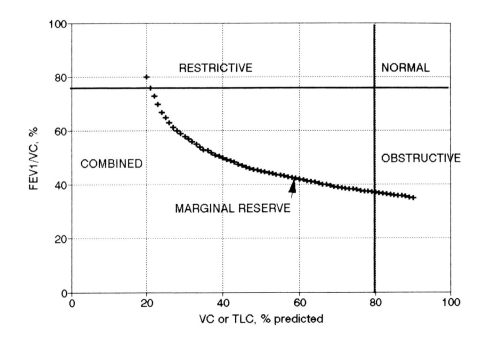

FIG. 3. Four-quadrant diagram for estimation of the relative risk of surgery in patients with lung disease. The *upper fourth* of the graph includes patients who are normal or have only restrictive lung disease; the *lower three fourths* includes patients with obstructive disease with or without restrictive lung disease. As a broad generalization, all patients below the marginal reserve line can be expected to require ventilatory support postoperatively. (Modified with permission from Hodgkin JE. Evaluation before thoracotomy. *West J Med* 1975; 122:104.)

patient is inversely related to the adequacy of control of the asthma before the time of surgery.

Resection of Lung Tissue

It is logical to expect that morbidity and mortality would be directly related to the amount of lung tissue resected. In many series, this expectation is obscured by patient selection, because those who are not expected to survive often do not have lung resected. More important than the amount of lung tissue removed is the ability of the remaining lung tissue to transfer O_2 and CO_2 between blood and environment through the processes of ventilation, diffusion, and perfusion. Thus, in those patients undergoing resection of a significant amount of lung tissue, it is wise to quantify the total lung function.

Smoking

It may be difficult to confirm statistically significant abnormalities in cardiovascular or pulmonary function in many smokers, even those who have smoked for long periods. Nevertheless, several studies do confirm that smokers, even those without demonstrable pulmonary or cardiovascular disease, are at increased risk for postoperative complications. For example, Wightman found a 15% incidence of postoperative complications (fever, productive cough, and abnormal chest findings) after abdominal surgery in smokers, compared with a 6% incidence in nonsmokers. Laszlo and colleagues found a 53% incidence of postoperative complications in smokers, versus a 22% incidence in nonsmokers. Carrel and coworkers prospectively evaluated 100 patients undergoing cardiac

surgery and found that the development of postoperative pneumonia was highly correlated with smoking, abnormal spirometry, and positive tracheal aspirates at the time of intubation. Poor oral hygiene, chronic cough, reduced ciliary function in the airways, likelihood of larger numbers of pulmonary bacterial pathogens, elevated carboxyhemoglobin levels, and the effects of nicotine on the cardiovascular system all contribute to the increased morbidity in smokers.

Cardiovascular, Neuromuscular, and Other Organ Disease

Patients with heart failure, recent myocardial infarction, or arrhythmia are at increased risk for postoperative cardiopulmonary complications, but moderate systemic hypertension is not a risk factor. Understandably, a recent stroke, psychosis or severe neurosis, degenerative neurologic processes, acute or chronic infections, damage to the upper airways or rib cage, compromised immunologic status, chronic drug or alcohol abuse, difficulty with mastication or swallowing, and chronic toxic or metabolic disorders all increase the likelihood of pulmonary morbidity.

Type and Duration of Anesthesia

Because of the many variables that influence selection of anesthetics and postoperative morbidity, it is difficult to compare different types or routes of anesthesia for the same operation. In two series of patients with severe obstructive lung disease, there was no difference in arterial oxygenation when general was compared with regional anesthesia for lower abdominal surgery. Clearly, the following are desirable: a smooth induction, adequate control of the airway and ventilation, adequate oxygenation without sudden shifts in acid-base status, reduction in atelectasis during and after surgery, adequate blood and fluid replacement, avoidance of other organ toxicity, and quick recovery from the anesthetic and muscle relaxant agents. There is consensus that the duration of the surgical procedure is much more significant than the type or route of administration of anesthesia.

PREOPERATIVE EVALUATION OF PATIENTS NOT UNDERGOING LUNG RESECTION

History and Physical Examination

It is trite but true that a good history and physical examination are extremely cost-effective and essential if unexpected morbidity and mortality are to be avoided. The history should include specific questions regarding duration and frequency of smoking; other drug history; dyspnea; activity level; cough frequency and characteristics; quantity and type of sputum production; intermittent wheezes or noisy breathing; chest pain, tightness, or distress; possible recent infections; toxic exposure; weight change; immobility; and venous insufficiency. Other major organ systems should not be ignored. For example, there is no significant cost associated with identifying patients with a high susceptibility to pulmonary embolism, who should receive appropriate prophylaxis. Likewise, Gracey and associates found that daily production of 2 oz or more of sputum was a valuable predictor of postoperative complications.

In the physical examination, poor oral hygiene, chest asymmetry, signs of airway disease, the duration (in seconds) of a complete forced expiration, body habitus, and evidence of clubbing, edema, or venous disease should be specifically noted. If the patient's subjective assessment seems inappropriate for objective physical findings, further evaluation is necessary. Wise physicians weigh their assessment of the patient's daily activity, exercise, and symptom status (or lack thereof) against the expected stress of surgery. We have all seen patients whose daily activity level is so low that they do not complain of dyspnea despite advanced heart or lung disease, and we regard highly those surgeons who walk or climb stairs with their patients before major surgery!

Roentgenography, Electrocardiography, and Other Laboratory Tests

A recent posteroanterior chest roentgenogram and electrocardiogram (ECG) should be obtained for anyone undergoing a significant surgical procedure. The necessity for other laboratory measures, including a hemogram, uri-

nalysis, blood chemistries, and smears or cultures of body fluids, depends on the surgery contemplated and the findings elicited or suspicions aroused during the history and physical examination.

Arterial Blood Gas Analysis

An arterial blood gas analysis is indicated for obese patients, patients with neuromuscular disease, and those with symptoms or signs suggestive of recent or current respiratory disease. An elevated $PaCO_2$, regardless of the cause, is a significant finding associated with high postoperative risk. A PaO_2 significantly below that predicted for the patient's age and body habitus indicates the need for further evaluation. Unexpected acid-base disturbances may also be detected from analysis of arterial blood gases and pH.

Spirometry

In general, we recommend simple spirometry for patients undergoing upper abdominal or thoracic surgery who are moderately to severely obese or who have a history of heavy smoking or symptoms or signs suggesting lung disease or heart failure. Spirometry is probably not cost-effective in asymptomatic patients or in mildly symptomatic patients undergoing surgery of an extremity. The important measures are FEV_1, VC, $FEF_{200-1200}$ or peak flow rate, and the directly measured MVV for 10 to 15 seconds. Except for body weight, visualization of the tracings, calculation of the FEV_1/VC, division of the VC into the inspiratory capacity and the ERV, and other measurements or calculations add little. It is especially important to measure the MVV directly in a patient who appears to be infirm or who is undergoing thoracic or upper abdominal surgery; inability to perform the MVV maneuver adequately gives warning that the patient may not be able to cooperate, coordinate, learn, or perform the necessary postoperative ventilatory maneuvers.

If airway obstruction is present, spirometry should be repeated after inhalation of a bronchodilator.

A review by Zibrak and associates criticized the methodology of earlier studies and concluded (in part) that "in upper abdominal surgery, spirometry and arterial blood gas analysis did *not* consistently have measurable benefit in identifying patients at increased risk for postoperative pneumonia, prolonged hospitalization, and death." This report went on to suggest that further critical investigation was required to reach a consensus regarding the role of preoperative pulmonary function tests in patients not undergoing lung resection.

We disagree. There is already significant evidence that preoperative spirometry is valuable in identifying patients at increased risk. Three decades ago, Stein and coworkers prospectively selected, at random, 100 ward patients admitted for surgical procedures. Of these, 32 did not have surgery because of lack of surgical indication and 5 were not operated on because of the severity of their cardiac or pulmonary disease. The 63 remaining patients were divided into two groups on the basis of their respiratory function. Group 1 patients had essentially normal lung function: $FEF_{200-1200}$ was >200 L/min (3.3 L/s) in 30 and was unmeasured in 3 patients; the single-breath O_2 test measured $\leq 2.5\%$ in 30 and was unmeasured in 3; and the estimated $PaCO_2$ was ≤ 41 mmHg in 28 and was unmeasured in 5. Group 2 patients had abnormal lung function: $FEF_{200-1200}$ was <200 L/min in 30 patients; the single-breath O_2 test measured $\geq 2.0\%$ in 18, $\leq 2.5\%$ in 8, and was unmeasured in 4; and the estimated $PaCO_2$ was ≥ 42 mmHg in 9, ≤ 41 mmHg in 18, and unmeasured in 3. Respiratory complications occurred in only one patient in group 1 and in 21 patients in group 2. In group 2, 7 of 9 patients undergoing thoracotomy and 11 of 12 undergoing abdominal surgery experienced complications.

The positive evidence from four more recent studies should be considered. First, Gracey and colleagues in a prospective study found that 6 of 35 patients with a midexpiratory flow rate (FEF_{25-75}) below 50% of predicted and forced vital capacity (FVC) below 75% of predicted (group A) required prolonged mechanical ventilation, whereas only 1 of 122 patients with values exceeding these (group B) required such ventilation after several types of surgery. Four of these 7 patients died. The total number of complications also differed significantly. Complications occurred in 12 of 35 patients (34%) in group A versus 15 of 122 patients (12%) in group B.

Poe and associates prospectively examined 209 patients undergoing elective cholecystectomy and postoperatively identified 21 with atelectasis, 8 with purulent bronchitis, and 2 with pneumonia. These 31 patients were hospitalized an average of 1.5 days longer than the others. Abnormal peak flow and the single-breath O_2 test were significant predictors of postoperative pulmonary complications, whereas reduced FVC was a significant predictor of prolonged hospitalization.

Vodinh and coworkers prospectively studied 153 patients undergoing nonurgent vascular surgery. In comparing 24 clinical and laboratory factors, they found postoperative respiratory complications were significantly higher only in those with a clinical chest abnormality, recent bronchitis, aortic surgery, longer duration of surgery, low FEV_1/VC, and low PaO_2. They concluded that spirometry and blood gas analysis were helpful in assessing risk.

Finally, Carrel and colleagues, in a prospective study of patients undergoing cardiac surgery, also demonstrated that incidence of postoperative pneumonia was correlated with abnormal results of preoperative lung function studies.

It is unlikely that any test can ever clearly distinguish between those who will or will not survive, or between those who will or will not have a specific complication. We suggest that spirometry and blood gas analyses should not be performed in everyone undergoing abdominal or thoracic surgery without lung resection, but that these tests are usually indicated for patients with asthma, chronic cough, sputum production, dyspnea, wheezing, poor exercise tolerance, congestive failure, weakness, or morbid obesity.

Gas Transfer and Lung Volume

Unless lung resection is contemplated or the patient has significant spirometric abnormalities, measurement of gas transfer (DLCO) and RV add cost and only infrequently provide additional information regarding operative risk.

Exercise Testing

If the patient has heart or lung disease or both, and the severity of the exercise limitation is uncertain, exercise testing with metabolic, ventilatory, gas exchange, blood pressure, and ECG measures may add information helpful in further assessing operative risk. Gerson and coworkers prospectively studied 177 geriatric patients undergoing abdominal and noncardiac thoracic surgery and included supine exercise testing in their multivariate analysis. They found that a patient's inability to perform 2 minutes of such exercise and raise the heart rate above 99 beats per minute (bpm) was the best single predictor of cardiac (14%), pulmonary (14%), or combined (22%) complications. There were 10 complications (9%) and 1 death (1%) in the group of 108 patients who could increase their heart rate to >99 bpm, and 29 complications (42%) and 5 deaths (7%) in the group of 69 patients who were unable to do so.

Because of the high perioperative mortality in elderly patients undergoing elective colorectal surgery or abdominal surgery for aortic aneurysm, Older and his colleagues successfully used noninvasive cardiopulmonary exercise testing with gas exchange measurements to screen 187 of 191 such patients over the age of 60. Forty-four had ECG tracings during exercise showing changes attributable to myocardial ischemia. Surgery was performed in the 187 screened patients, with an overall in-hospital mortality of 7.5%, 5.9% from cardiovascular causes. Mortality from cardiovascular causes was 18% in the 55 patients with an anaerobic threshold $\dot{V}O_2$ of <11 mL/min per kilogram, but was only 0.8% in the 132 patients with an anaerobic threshold that was ≥ 11 mL/min per kilogram. The association of an anaerobic threshold $\dot{V}O_2$ of <11 mL/min per kilogram and preoperative ischemia resulted in a mortality of 42%, whereas those with preoperative ischemia and a higher anaerobic threshold had a mortality of only 4%. In addition to recommending exercise testing with gas exchange measurements for major abdominal surgery in the elderly, they suggest that all patients with demonstrated preoperative myocardial ischemia or an anaerobic threshold of <11 mL/min per kilogram be admitted preoperatively for stabilization. The use of these policies has measurably reduced perioperative mortality.

Conclusions

Williams-Russo has commented that "preventing cardiac morbidity may be the best approach to reducing pulmonary morbidity." From the viewpoint of the patient, surgeon, and internist, we may unwisely evaluate the risks for morbidity and death by segregating the causes as "cardiovascular" or "pulmonary," as these systems are so clearly interrelated in real life.

In the individual patient, the risk of operative intervention needs to be weighed against the risk of other therapies or nontreatment of the patient's disorder. It is wise to delay surgery when the likely morbidity and mortality of thoracic or upper abdominal surgery can be reduced by active intervention (e.g., through weight loss, anticoagulation, antibiotic or corticosteroid therapy, or intensive bronchodilator therapy). If such delay significantly decreases the patient's chances for recovery or cure of the primary disorder, then only very brief interventions before a decision regarding surgery are warranted. Table 1 gives some broad guidelines suggestive of high morbidity and mortality in thoracic or upper abdominal surgery.

TABLE 1. *Some factors associated with high surgical mortality[a]*

Factor or test	Upper abdominal surgery	Lung resection[b]
Age >70 y	+	+
Abnormal ECG	+	+
FEV_1 <40% predicted	+	++
FEV_1/VC <40%	++	++
$FEF_{200-1200}$ <2 L/s	++	++
MVV <50% predicted	+	+++
D_LCO < 50% predicted	+	++
$PaCO_2$	++	+++
PaO_2 <60 mmHg	+	±
$\dot{V}O_2$max <15 mL/min/kg	++	+++

± indicates possible increase in mortality; +, some increase in mortality; ++, considerable increase in mortality; +++, very high increase in mortality.

[a] None of these factors or values should be used as absolute contraindications to surgery.

[b] Preoperative quantitative perfusion scans with preoperative FEV_1, MVV, D_LCO, and $\dot{V}O_2$max tests values are helpful in predicting same test values postoperatively after lung resection.

PREOPERATIVE EVALUATION OF PATIENTS UNDERGOING LUNG RESECTION

Initial Preoperative Assessment

All the evaluations considered for patients in whom lung resection is not planned, including D_LCO and lung volume measurements, are useful also in the patient being evaluated for lung resection. Commonly, lung resection is performed in malignant states, but similar evaluation is indicated for patients with decreased lung function resulting from inflammatory, traumatic, hereditary, or other disorders. Roentgenographic examinations will always be more complete, and endoscopy results may be available. Bronchodilator responsiveness becomes very important if ventilatory function is significantly reduced, and D_LCO should certainly be measured. If maximal inspiratory and expiratory pressures are low, preoperative pulmonary rehabilitation may reduce the incidence of postoperative complications.

In the earliest of several retrospective studies, Gaensler and coworkers found that the MVV was an important predictor of survival in patients undergoing lung resection for tuberculosis; if the preoperative MVV was <50% of predicted, 50% of the patients died, whereas if the MVV was >50% of predicted, only 1% of the patients died. Boushy and associates found that advanced age, severity of dyspnea, high RV, low gas transfer per lung volume (D_LCO/V_A), reduced FEV_1, and reduced MVV were all significant predictors of high morbidity and mortality. Confirming the value of the MVV, Didolkar and associates, in a retrospective study of resection for lung cancer, found that mortality from cardiopulmonary complications was much higher in those with an MVV that was <60% of predicted. There were no postoperative deaths in the nine patients older than 70 years who had a normal ECG and an MVV that was >60% of predicted.

Ferguson and coworkers retrospectively reviewed their results for lung resection in 237 patients (cancer in 203 and benign disease in 34). They took into account 38 different preoperative and operative risk factors and found, by logistic regression analysis, that the D_LCO was the most important predictor of postoperative survival and the sole predictor of pulmonary complications. For D_LCO values that were <60%, 61%–80%, 81%–100%, and >100% of predicted, postoperative mortality was 25%, 8%, 5%, and 0%, respectively, and pulmonary complications were 45%, 33%, 13%, and 11%, respectively.

Several investigators have utilized measures of pulmonary arterial pressure, pulmonary vascular resistance, and right ventricular injection fraction preoperatively and intraoperatively after pulmonary arterial clamping. These invasive measures are generally less useful than noninvasive exercise testing and quantitative scans in estimating postoperative morbidity and mortality.

Predicting Postoperative Function

When resting preoperative lung function, as measured by spirometry and DlCO, is significantly impaired, or when large portions of lung may be removed surgically, it is worthwhile to predict postoperative lung function to assess postoperative survival or quality of life. Bronchospirometry and the lateral position tests, introduced in the 1950s and 1960s, were of some assistance in predicting postoperative function, but they have now been supplanted by newer techniques.

Quantitative radioisotopic ventilation and perfusion scans are now commonly and effectively used to predict postoperative FEV_1, DlCO, and peak $\dot{V}O_2$ (Figs. 4 and 5). In each case, the expected postoperative FEV_1, DlCO, or peak $\dot{V}O_2$ is calculated by multiplying each preoperative value by the measured ratio of expected postoperative lung activity to preoperative total lung activity. For example, if 40% of the quantitatively measured perfusion scan activity occurs in the lung that is to be resected, the calculated postoperative DlCO or peak $\dot{V}O_2$ will be 60% of the preoperative DlCO or peak $\dot{V}O_2$. Ventilation scans or quantitative computed tomography (CT) can be similarly used to predict postoperative FEV_1 values. Using the ratio of the number of expected postoperative lung segments to the total number of preoperative segments tends to give an underestimate of postoperative function, because lung segments differ in size and because the removed segments are likely to be worse than those retained.

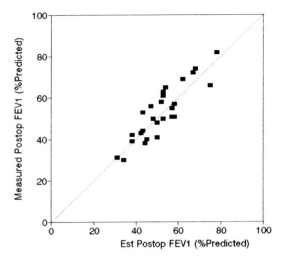

FIG. 5. Comparison of measured postoperative $\dot{V}O_{2max}$ and estimated postoperative $\dot{V}O_{2max}$ in 14 patients undergoing pneumonectomy. Estimated postoperative $\dot{V}O_{2max}$ was calculated from preoperative $\dot{V}O_{2max}$ and quantitative technetium Tc 99m perfusion scans. (Modified with permission from Corris PA, et al. Use of radionuclide scanning in the preoperative estimation of pulmonary function after pneumonectomy. *Thorax* 1987;42:285.)

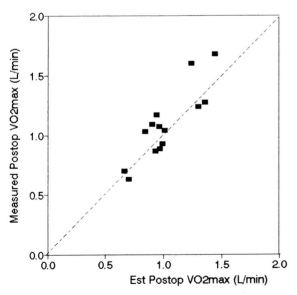

FIG. 4. Comparison of measured postoperative FEV_1 and estimated postoperative FEV_1 in 28 patients undergoing pneumonectomy. Estimated postoperative FEV_1 was calculated from preoperative FEV_1 and quantitative technetium Tc 99m perfusion scans. (Modified with permission from Corris PA, et al. Use of radionuclide scanning in the preoperative estimation of pulmonary function after pneumonectomy. *Thorax* 1987;42:285.)

Markos and coworkers prospectively studied by lung function tests and scintigraphy 55 consecutive candidates for lung cancer resection. Fifty-three underwent thoracotomy, with pneumonectomy in 18, lobectomy in 29, and no resection in 6. Postoperative FEV_1 and DlCO were well predicted from preoperative measures. There were only 3 deaths, all occurring in the 6 candidates who had a predicted postoperative FEV_1 of 40% or less. Wahi and associates reviewed 197 consecutive cancer patients undergoing pneumonectomy. Of the 14 perioperative deaths, 13 occurred in patients undergoing right pneumonectomy. Those with a predicted postoperative FEV_1 exceeding 1.65 L had lower mortality.

Pierce and colleagues found that the predicted postoperative product, which is the predicted postoperative FEV_1 times predicted postoperative DlCO, was the best predictor of surgical mortality in 54 consecutive patients with bronchogenic carcinoma. The mean values of their population were as follows: age, 67; FEV_1, 76% of predicted; DlCO, 85% of predicted; and peak $\dot{V}O_2$, 18.4 mL/min per kilogram. Pneumonectomy was performed in 11, lobectomy in 29, and lesser resection in 14. There were 48 survivors. Although peak $\dot{V}O_2$ values did not predict outcome, 2 of the 3 patients with peak $\dot{V}O_2$ values that were <14 mL/min per kilogram died in the perioperative period. In 331 candidates, Kearney and associates found that the primary predictor of resectional outcome was the absolute predicted postoperative FEV_1, but they did not analyze DlCO or peak $\dot{V}O_2$ values.

Exercise Testing

Two early studies showed the value of preoperative exercise testing in patients undergoing lung resection. Eugene and colleagues found that among 19 patients, death occurred in 3 of 4 patients with a peak $\dot{V}O_2$ of <1 L/min. In 22 patients, Smith and coworkers found no deaths and 10% morbidity if peak $\dot{V}O_2$ exceeded 20 mL/min per kilogram; 17% deaths and 67% morbidity with peak $\dot{V}O_2$ of 15 to 20 mL/min per kilogram; and 17% deaths and 100% morbidity if peak $\dot{V}O_2$ was <15 mL/min per kilogram.

Bechard and Wetstein prospectively evaluated 50 consecutive patients undergoing lung resection with the surgeon blinded to the preoperative peak $\dot{V}O_2$ values. Candidates for resection were required to have an FEV_1 of >1.7 L for pneumonectomy (10), 1.2 L for lobectomy (28), or 0.9 L for wedge resection (12). Mortality was 4% and other morbidity 12%. Both peak $\dot{V}O_2$ and anaerobic threshold measures predicted mortality and morbidity, but age, FVC, FEV_1, and MVV did not. Maurice and colleagues found 8 of 37 high-risk patients to have a peak $\dot{V}O_2$ of >15 mL/min per kilogram. All survived resectional surgery.

Walsh and colleagues prospectively evaluated 66 patients with potentially resectable non–small-cell lung cancer, considered to be high risks on the basis of preoperative FEV_1 that was $<40\%$ of predicted, predicted postoperative FEV_1 that was $<33\%$ of predicted, resting $PaCO_2$ exceeeding 45 mmHg, or at least two criteria indicating cardiac disease. In 20 patients with a peak $\dot{V}O_2$ of >15 mL/min per kilogram, there were no perioperative deaths and 40% complications. Among five patients with a peak $\dot{V}O_2$ of <15 mL/min per kilogram, there was one death. In this population, only surgical versus medical treatment and peak $\dot{V}O_2$ exceeding 15 mL/min per kilogram significantly predicted survival; age, FEV_1, $PaCO_2$, clinical stage, and T status did not. Bollinger and coworkers operated on 25 high-risk patients, with only three deaths. Lower preoperative or predicted postoperative peak $\dot{V}O_2$ values correlated with higher morbidity and mortality.

Conclusions

Physicians and surgeons are obligated to share information and expectations with patients before making final decisions on therapy. Assigning an exact risk to a major surgical procedure in the individual cancer patient is difficult, but multiple high-risk factors and common sense can dictate against surgical treatment. Debility and cardiovascular disease add to risk. Smoking cessation, vigorous bronchodilator therapy, and rehabilitating exercise therapy may help. Despite recent advances in therapy, I am not as optimistic as Olsen in believing that ''almost no one'' is inoperable. In a high-risk patient, measures of DL_{CO}, quantitative perfusion scan, and gas exchange exercise testing are all clearly useful in assessing risk. Because of differences in patient sex, size, and age,

both absolute and percent predicted values should be considered.

PREVENTION OF COMPLICATIONS

Preoperative Considerations

The more severe the risk of complications, the more important it is to take effective action preoperatively. Patients should stop smoking as soon as it is realized that surgery is likely, even if the patient has normal findings on pulmonary function tests. Cessation for even a few days is advantageous. Advantages of smoking cessation include an expected reduction in cough, improvement in ciliary function and mouth hygiene, reduction in lower airway pathogens, and reduction in carboxyhemoglobin levels. Warner and colleagues, in a blinded prospective study of patients undergoing coronary bypass surgery, found that postoperative pulmonary complications developed in approximately 1 of 3 of the current smokers, 5 of 9 of those who stopped smoking for less than 2 months, 1 of 7 of those who stopped smoking for more than 2 months, 1 of 9 of those who stopped smoking for 6 months or more, and 1 of 9 of those who had never smoked.

If the patient is obese and surgery can be delayed, weight reduction is advisable, especially if the surgery involves the thorax or upper abdomen. In those with hypoventilation and CO_2 retention, a weight loss of 10 to 20 kg may bring improvement. However, caloric and fluid intake should be adequate during the days immediately preceding major surgery.

We recommend intensive bronchodilator therapy for any patient with obstructive lung disease who shows evidence, either clinically or in the pulmonary physiology laboratory, of improvement with such treatment. Asthma should be cleared with steroids if necessary.

There is little evidence that routine antibiotic prophylaxis is beneficial, but recognized pulmonary infections should be aggressively diagnosed (smear and culture) and treated for several days preoperatively if feasible.

Several studies show that preoperative training in deep-breathing respiratory maneuvers reduces postoperative complications and is cost-effective in patients who undergo thoracic or upper abdominal surgery. Bartlett and coworkers emphasized that frequent inspiratory rather than expiratory maneuvers were essential. In a prospective study of 343 cholecystectomy patients, Thoren found roentgenographic atelectasis in 12% of those who performed preoperative and postoperative breathing exercise, 27% of those who performed postoperative breathing exercise only, and 42% of the control group. In patients undergoing abdominal surgery, Celli and associates found that clinical complications and duration of hospital stay were much diminished in patients who had respiratory treatment started 1 day before surgery and continued post-operatively than in a randomly selected control group. Roukema and colleagues prospectively randomized patients with noncompromised pulmonary status undergoing abdominal surgery into two groups. Group 1 consisted of 84 patients with no breathing exercises, whereas group 2 consisted of 69 patients treated with preoperative and postoperative exercises. Pulmonary complications occurred in 60% of group 1 versus 19% of group 2.

Stein and Cassara compared three groups of patients undergoing abdominal and thoracic surgery: (1) those considered to be of normal risk; (2) those considered, on the basis of pulmonary function tests, to be high-risk and who were not treated; and (3) those considered to be high-risk and who were treated intensively preoperatively with smoking cessation, bronchodilator drugs, inhalation of humidified gases, chest physiotherapy, and antibiotics when indicated. Postoperative pulmonary complications occurred in 1 of 17 patients in group 1, 14 of 20 patients in group 2, and 5 of 22 patients in group 3. We have often seen patients who were considered to be prohibitive risks for lung resection become acceptable risks after several weeks of intensive therapy.

Cardiovascular disease should be treated aggressively to minimize pulmonary edema, congestive failure, myocardial ischemia, arrhythmias, significant systemic or pulmonary hypertension, hypercoagulability, and the likelihood of postoperative thromboembolic disorders. Primary prophylaxis (i.e., the prevention of deep vein thromboses by drugs or physical methods) is cost-effective, may be life-saving, and should be used whenever possible in patients with high to moderate risk for thromboembolism. Primary prophylaxis consists of anticoagulation with low-dose heparin (5000 units subcutaneously 2 hours preoperatively, and then every 8 to 12 hours postoperatively without monitoring), adjusted-dose heparin (preoperative and postoperative dosage dependent on activated partial thromboplastin time), low-molecular-weight heparin, or oral anticoagulants. Alternatively, primary prophylaxis can consist of reduction in venous stasis with dihydroergotamine, intermittent pneumatic leg compression, or graduated compression stockings. The selection of specific primary prophylaxis depends on the site and type of surgery performed and the patient's other medical problems.

If aspiration occurs or is likely to occur, as in the obese patient, antacid therapy tends to minimize the expected pulmonary complications.

Intraoperative Considerations

To the best of our knowledge, there is no evidence that the route or type of anesthetic used affects the likelihood of postoperative pulmonary complications. Usually the anesthesiologist (on the basis of skill, training, and experi-ence) selects the most appropriate agents and route for the specific problem at hand. There is no clear evidence that spinal anesthesia is superior to general anesthesia in maintaining intraoperative and postoperative oxygenation, even in patients with severe obstructive lung disease, perhaps because of better control of the airways with general anesthesia. Among other things, the anesthesiologist attempts to maintain adequate cardiac output, oxygenation, CO_2 removal, and stable fluid and acid-base status; minimize arrhythmias, pooling of blood in extremities, and microatelectasis and macroatelectasis; and prevent aspiration of oral and gastric contents into the lung.

During laparoscopic cholecystectomy in which CO_2 is used for insufflation, a significant respiratory acidosis may develop in patients with cardiac or pulmonary disease. Because end-tidal CO_2 pressures may be misleading during such insufflation, arterial PCO_2 and pH should be monitored.

Postoperative Considerations

Ventilator support after recovery from anesthesia may be brief or prolonged. Continuous positive airway pressure (CPAP) or PEEP is usually helpful in improving oxygenation and CO_2 removal by decreasing atelectasis, improving $\dot{V}A/\dot{Q}$, and reducing barotrauma to the lung.

Hypoxemia can be reduced and ventilation of the lung bases improved by keeping the patient, especially if obese, in a sitting or semirecumbent position rather than in a supine position (Fig. 6).

Aggressive respiratory therapy to minimize atelectasis, increase FRC, improve oxygenation, and clear secretions is valuable and cost-effective. Previously, expiratory resistance and intermittent positive-pressure breathing were used frequently, but these have generally been discarded because of ineffectiveness, high cost, or barotrauma. Bronchodilator aerosol therapy alone is insufficient to improve lung volumes and oxygenation maximally after thoracic or upper abdominal surgery. There are many reports that compare the effectiveness of the following currently recommended modalities: (1) coughing and deep breathing (CDB) exercises; (2) sustained maximal inspiration or incentive spirometry (IS), using one of several available devices; (3) breathing with inspiratory resistance (IR); and (4) CPAP or PEEP by face mask. The major disadvantages of CDB, IS, and IR are the necessity for patient cooperation and the likely attendant increase in pain. PEEP or CPAP may be costlier and slightly increase the possibility of barotrauma or aspiration, but they hasten improvement in FRC and PaO_2 postoperatively in patients in whom atelectasis tends to develop. They may be detrimental to patients with severe emphysema, who are already hyperinflated because of highly compliant lung units.

Nearly all authors stress the necessity for frequent and

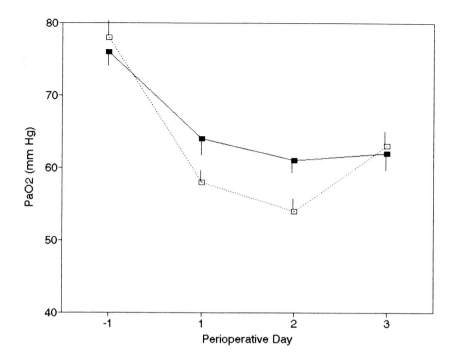

FIG. 6. Effect of body position on PaO$_2$ after abdominal surgery in 22 markedly obese patients. *Solid symbols* and *solid line* indicate semirecumbent position; *hollow symbols* and *dotted line* indicate supine position. (Modified with permission from Vaughan RW, Wise L. Postoperative arterial blood gas measurements in obese patients. Effects of position on gas exchange. *Ann Surg* 1975; 182:705.)

vigilant respiratory care in the high-risk population. Because of postoperative pain, analgesics may be necessary to improve coughing and deep breathing. With severe thoracic or abdominal pain, selective and repeated nerve blocks may help the patient's performance of ventilatory maneuvers.

It is important to reduce the likelihood of aspiration with good endotracheal tube and cuff care and good technique when giving nutritional support. If a nasogastric tube is used, it should be of small caliber. Overdistention of the stomach should be avoided.

Secondary prophylaxis for thromboembolism is more costly than primary prophylaxis but is still cost-effective and life-preserving. It consists of screening high-risk patients postoperatively with tests specific for venous thromboses (e.g., fibrinogen uptake, Doppler ultrasonography, impedance plethysmography, and venography), followed by full-dose anticoagulant therapy when test results are positive. Secondary prophylaxis should be used when prophylactic anticoagulation is desired but contraindicated (e.g., urgency of surgery, neurosurgery, spinal anesthesia) or when supplementation of primary prophylaxis is required in very high-risk patients.

BIBLIOGRAPHY

Bartlett RH, Gazzaniga AB, Geraghty TR. Respiratory maneuvers to prevent postoperative pulmonary complications. *JAMA* 1973;224: 1017–1021. *A review article stressing that maximal inspiratory efforts during the perioperative period are necessary to reduce the incidence of atelectasis, morbidity, and mortality.*

Bechard D, Wetstein L. Assessment of exercise oxygen consumption as preoperative criterion for lung resection. *Ann Thorac Surg* 1987;

44:344–349. *With surgeons blinded as to the results, 50 consecutive patients, with a mean age of 64 and selected on the basis of their FEV1, had resectional surgery. Low peak V̇O$_2$ values were significantly associated with high morbidity and mortality.*

Bollinger CT, et al. Lung scanning and exercise testing for the prediction of postoperative performance in lung resection candidates at increased risk for complications. *Chest* 1995;108:341–348. *Of 25 patients considered at high risk for resectional surgery (FEV$_1$ <2 L, DLCO <50% of predicted value, or FEV$_1$ and DLCO ≤80% of predicted value with a high dyspnea index), three died. Lower preoperative or predicted postoperative peak V̇O$_2$ values correlated with higher morbidity and mortality.*

Boushy SF, et al. Clinical course related to preoperative and postoperative pulmonary function in patients with bronchogenic carcinoma. *Chest* 1971;59:383–391. *One of a pair of analyses by this group of the relative importance of clinical, physiologic, and pathologic factors in the postoperative course of 124 patients with bronchogenic carcinoma.*

Bryant LR, et al. Lung perfusion scanning for estimation of postoperative pulmonary function. *Arch Surg* 1972;104:52–55. *Study quantitates the timing and extent of the declines in VC, FEV$_1$, and PaO$_2$ following thoracic and abdominal surgery.*

Carrel T, et al. Preoperative assessment of the likelihood of infection of the lower respiratory tract after cardiac surgery. *Thorac Cardiovasc Surg* 1991;39:85–88. *Tracheal aspirates were positive by Gram stain or culture in 26 of 100 patients undergoing cardiac surgery, and pneumonia often developed in these patients despite antibiotic prophylaxis. Cigarette smoking and abnormal spirometry findings were significantly more frequent in patients in whom pneumonia developed postoperatively.*

Celli BR, Rodriguez KS, Snider GL. A controlled trial of intermittent positive pressure breathing, incentive spirometry, and deep breathing exercises in preventing pulmonary complications after abdominal surgery. *Am Rev Respir Dis* 1984;130:12–15. *This study concludes that incentive spirometry may be the preferable method to reduce pulmonary complications.*

Consensus Conference. Prevention of venous thrombosis and pulmonary embolism. *JAMA* 1986;256:744–749. *The conclusions of experts in the United States are summarized.*

Corris PA, et al. Use of radionuclide scanning in the preoperative estimation of pulmonary function after pneumonectomy. *Thorax* 1987;42: 285–291. *In 28 pneumonectomy patients, preoperative perfusion and* ventilation scans, when combined with preoperative measures of FEV_1, VC, DLCO, and peak $\dot{V}O_2$, resulted in good estimates of the actual postoperative values for the latter four measures.

Didolkar MS, Moore RH, Takita H. Evaluation of the risk in pulmonary resection for bronchogenic carcinoma. Am J Surg 1974;127:700–703. A retrospective analysis of 258 patients undergoing pneumonectomy or lobectomy for bronchogenic carcinoma showing that a low value for MVV and abnormal ECG are important predictors of mortality from cardiopulmonary complications.

Eugene J, et al. Maximum oxygen consumption. A physiology guide to pulmonary resection. Surg Forum 1982;82:260–262. In this early study of 19 patients undergoing lung resection, preoperative spirometric values did not predict survival. Peak $\dot{V}O_2$ values of <1 L/min were associated with deaths in three of four patients; those with higher peak $\dot{V}O_2$ values survived.

Ferguson MK, et al. Diffusing capacity predicts morbidity and mortality after pulmonary resection. J Thorac Cardiovasc Surg 1988;96:894–900. This retrospective study of major pulmonary resection at the University of Chicago Medical Center analyzes a large number of preoperative and operative factors by regression and χ^2 methods. The authors conclude that the preoperative DLCO is the most important predictor of mortality and the sole predictor of postoperative pulmonary complications.

Gaensler EA, et al. The role of pulmonary insufficiency in mortality and invalidism following surgery for pulmonary tuberculosis. J Thorac Surg 1955;29:163–187. The first study showing the value of preoperative spirometry findings, especially the MVV, in predicting outcome of resectional lung surgery.

Gerson MC, et al. Prediction of cardiac and pulmonary complications related to elective abdominal and noncardiac thoracic surgery in geriatric patients. Am J Med 1990;88:101–107. The authors used supine cycle ergometry in 177 patients >65 years of age before thoracic or abdominal surgery. Of the multiple risk factors analyzed, cycle ergometry was of optimal value in risk stratification for both pulmonary and cardiac postoperative complications.

Gracey DR, Diverite MB, Didier EP. Preoperative pulmonary preparation of patients with chronic obstructive pulmonary disease. Chest 1979;76:123–129. An investigation of 157 patients with COPD undergoing surgery at Mayo Clinic after 2 to 3 days of preoperative pulmonary preparation. Respiratory complications and prolonged mechanical ventilation were more frequent in those undergoing extensive upper abdominal surgery and those with abnormal spirometry and $P(A-A)O_2$.

Hodgkin JE. Evaluation before thoracotomy. West J Med 1975;122:104–109. The author stresses the necessity of careful preoperative assessment in patients undergoing thoracotomy. He uses a four-quadrant diagram to show the importance of obstructive disease in reducing reserve.

Hull RD, Raskob GE, Hirsch J. Prophylaxis of venous thromboembolism. Chest 1986;89(Suppl):374S–383S. An excellent overview of this topic, including cost analysis.

Juhl B, Frost N. A comparison between measured and calculated changes in the lung function after operation for pulmonary cancer. Acta Anaesthesiol Scand Suppl 1975;57:39–45. The authors use both radioisotopic measures and segmental volumes to calculate postoperative lung function.

Kearney DJ, et al. Assessment of operative risk in patients undergoing lung resection. Importance of predicted pulmonary function. Chest 1994;105:753–759. Multiple preoperative measures and factors (not including DLCO or peak $\dot{V}O_2$) of 331 patients undergoing lung resection surgery were analyzed. A low predicted postoperative FEV_1 (expressed in liters, not as percent predicted) was the primary predictor of outcome.

Kristersson S, Lindell SE, Svanberg L. Prediction of pulmonary function loss due to pneumonectomy using ^{133}Xe-radiospirometry. Chest 1972;62:694–698. This is one of several studies from Sweden demonstrating the value of radioisotopic scans to predict postoperative lung function.

Laszlo G, et al. The diagnosis and prophylaxis of pulmonary complications of surgical operation. Br J Surg 1973;60:129–134. An early study showing a higher incidence of postoperative pulmonary complications in smokers.

Maede H, et al. Diaphragm function after pulmonary resection. Am

Rev Respir Dis 1988;137:678–681. A careful study of respiratory mechanics in 20 patients undergoing pulmonary resection.

Markos J, et al. Preoperative assessment as a predictor of mortality and morbidity after lung resection. Am Rev Respir Dis 1989;139:902–910. This prospective study of patients undergoing lung resection demonstrates that expressing postoperative predicted values for FEV_1 and DLCO as percent predicted is preferable to using absolute values. A predicted postoperative value of FEV_1 of >40% was associated with no mortality, whereas lower values were associated with 50% mortality.

Miller WF, Wu N, Johnson RL Jr. Convenient method of evaluating pulmonary function with a single-breath test. Anesthesiology 1956;17:480–493. Introduces the four-quadrant method of plotting the percentage of flow in a given time/total VC on the y-axis versus the total VC on the x-axis, allowing differentiation between normal function, and restrictive, obstructive, and combined ventilatory defects.

Morice RC, et al. Exercise testing in the evaluation of patients at high risk for complications from lung resection. Chest 1992;101:356–361. Thirty-seven patients with lung cancer were considered inoperable because the preoperative or predicted postoperative FEV_1 was <40% or <33% of predicted, respectively, or the $PaCO_2$ exceeded 45 mmHg. Eight of them had a peak $\dot{V}O_2$ of ≥15 mL/min per kilogram and were offered and survived resectional surgery.

Nakagawa K, et al. Oxygen transport during incremental exercise load as a predictor of operative risk in lung cancer patients. Chest 1992;101:1369–1375. A study of 31 patients using catheterization of the right side of the heart and exercise testing preoperatively. Because measures of O_2 delivery and anaerobic threshold (which can be measured noninvasively) were good discriminators, they recommend exercise testing "if the performance status of the patient looks poor or suspicious."

Nomori H, et al. Preoperative muscle training. Chest 1994;105:1782–1788. Patients with respiratory weakness have a higher risk for postoperative complications. Preoperative muscle training is of some benefit in patients undergoing thoracic surgery.

Older P, et al. Preoperative evaluation of cardiac failure and ischemia in elderly patients by cardiopulmonary exercise testing. Chest 1993;104:701–704. The authors found that an anaerobic threshold of <11 mL/min per kilogram associated with myocardial ischemia resulted in a mortality of 42% in their patients over age 60 undergoing abdominal surgery.

Olsen GN. Lung cancer resection. Who's inoperable? Chest 1995;108:298–299. An editorial suggesting that with modern techniques, the answer may be "almost no one."

Pierce RJ, et al. Preoperative risk evaluation for lung cancer resection: predicted postoperative product as a predictor of surgical mortality. Am J Respir Crit Care Med 1994;150:947–955. In 54 consecutive patients, the predicted postoperative product of FEV_1 and DLCO best identified surgical mortality. Age, PaO_2, $PaCO_2$, and other measures also predicted cardiac and respiratory complications.

Poe RH, et al. Can postoperative complications after elective cholecystectomy be predicted? Am J Med Sci 1988;295:29–34. In this prospective study at the University of Rochester, the sensitivity of abnormal spirometry was 42% and the specificity was 86% in predicting postoperative pulmonary complications in a general population of 209 patients undergoing cholecystectomy.

Putnam JB, et al. Predicted pulmonary function and survival after pneumonectomy for primary lung carcinoma. Ann Thorac Surg 1990;49:909–915. In a series of 139 patients, some individuals with stage III disease achieved substantial long-term survival, but survival was longer in those with left pneumonectomy and better preoperative spirometry.

Roukema JA, Carol EJ, Prins JG. The prevention of pulmonary complications after upper abdominal surgery in patients with noncompromised pulmonary status. Arch Surg 1988;123:30. Supervised breathing exercises in the perioperative period markedly reduced the incidence of postoperative pulmonary complications in 153 patients prospectively randomized before undergoing upper abdominal surgery.

Scuderi J, Olsen GN. Respiratory therapy in the management of postoperative complications. Respir Care 1989;34:281–291. This review summarizes the advantages and disadvantages of respiratory therapy modalities in the perioperative period.

Smith TP, et al. Exercise capacity as a predictor of post-thoracotomy morbidity. *Am Rev Respir Dis* 1984;129:730–734. *The authors evaluated 22 patients undergoing thoracotomy by routine spirometry, perfusion lung scanning, and gas exchange exercise testing. They found that only 1 of 10 patients with a peak $\dot{V}O_2$ of >20 mL/min per kilogram had a cardiopulmonary complication, whereas all 6 with a peak $\dot{V}O_2$ of <15 mL/min per kilogram had a complication. Predicted postoperative values of FEV_1 were similar in those with and without complications.*

Stein M, Cassara EL. Preoperative pulmonary evaluation and therapy for surgery patients. *JAMA* 1970;211:787–790. *An early report demonstrating that intensive perioperative pulmonary therapy reduces the incidence of morbidity and mortality in poor-risk patients identified by simple pulmonary function studies.*

Stein M, et al. Pulmonary evaluation of surgical patients. *JAMA* 1962; 181:765–770. *This early study demonstrated that simple pulmonary function tests in preoperative evaluation might helpfully influence patient selection, modify the approach of the surgeon or anesthetist, and indicate the need for prophylactic perioperative measures.*

Thoren L. Postoperative pulmonary complications: observations on their prevention by chest physiotherapy. *Acta Chir Scand* 1954;107:193–205. *This large and early study demonstrated the value of perioperative respiratory therapy in reducing complications following cholecystectomy.*

Vaughan RW, Wise L. Postoperative arterial blood gas measurements in obese patients: effect of position on gas exchange. *Ann Surg* 1975; 182:705–709. *Twenty severely obese patients undergoing abdominal surgery had low PaO_2 values, especially in the supine position. Hypoventilation resulting from metabolic alkalosis further accentuated the already-existing hypoxemia.*

Vodinh J, et al. Risk factors of postoperative pulmonary complications after vascular surgery. *Surgery* 1988;105:360–365. *This prospective study from France of 151 consecutive surgical patients, including 67 who underwent abdominal aortic surgery, found that risk factors for major postoperative respiratory complications were low FEV_1/VC, low PaO_2, recent bronchitis, chest deformation, and prolonged surgery. The authors conclude that preoperative spirometry and blood gas analysis provide valuable data for evaluating risk, superior to the classification of American Society of Anesthesiologists.*

Wahi R, et al. Determinants of perioperative morbidity and mortality after pneumonectomy. *Ann Thorac Surg* 1989;48:33–37. *A review of 197 patients undergoing pneumonectomy for lung cancer demonstrates that patients undergoing right pneumonectomy are at significantly higher risk.*

Walsh GL, et al. Resection of lung cancer is justified in high-risk patients selected by exercise oxygen consumption. *Ann Thorac Surg* 1994; 56:704–711. *Exercise testing proved very useful in helping decide operability in high-risk patients. All 20 patients in whom the peak $\dot{V}O_2$ was greater than 15 mL/min per kilogram survived.*

Warner MA, et al. Role of preoperative cessation of smoking and other factors in postoperative pulmonary complications: a blinded study of coronary artery bypass patients. *Mayo Clin Proc* 1989;64:609–616. *This prospective study of 200 patients undergoing coronary artery bypass surgery at the Mayo Clinic found postoperative pulmonary complications in one third of the current smokers but in only one ninth of those who had never smoked or who had stopped smoking for 2 or more months.*

Wasserman K, et al. *Principles of Exercise Testing and Interpretation.* 2nd ed. Philadelphia: Lea & Febiger; 1994. 479 p. *This text describes the physiology, method, interpretation, and utility of exercise testing using modern gas exchange techniques.*

Wheeler HB, Anderson FA. Prophylaxis against venous thromboembolism in surgical patients. *Am J Surg* 1991;161:507–540. *One of a series of publications in this journal issue illustrating the value of prophylaxis in preventing thromboembolism in the perioperative period.*

Wightman JAK. A prospective survey of the incidence of postoperative pulmonary complications. *Br J Surg* 1968;55:85. *After upper abdominal surgery, pulmonary complications are much higher in smokers than in nonsmokers.*

Williams-Russo P, et al. Predicting postoperative pulmonary complications. Is it a real problem? *Arch Intern Med* 1992;152:1209–1213. *A group of 278 patients undergoing elective general surgery were evaluated, but only 152 had spirometry and only 98 had arterial blood gas analyses. Pulmonary complications were more common in those with bronchitis, asthma, and heart disease.*

Wu MT, et al. Use of quantitative CT to predict postoperative lung function in patients with lung cancer. *Radiology* 1994;191:257–262. *In 38 patients, this technique reasonably accurately predicted postoperative FEV_1 and FVC values.*

Zeiher BG, et al. Predicting postoperative pulmonary function in patients undergoing lung resection. *Chest* 1995;108:68–72. *Sixty patients were studied by preoperative scans and preoperative and postoperative spirometry, with a calculation that each segment was exactly 1/19 of the lung. Predicted values tended to underestimate postoperative FEV_1 and FVC values.*

Zibrak JD, O'Donnell CR, Marton K. Indications for pulmonary function testing. *Ann Intern Med* 1990;112:763–771. *The report of a study group using a MEDLINE search in an attempt to assess critically other articles evaluating the role of preoperative pulmonary function testing in predicting postoperative outcomes.*

III DIFFERENTIAL DIAGNOSIS

Textbook of Pulmonary Diseases, 6th ed.
edited by G.L. Baum, J.D. Crapo, B.R. Celli, and J.B. Karlinsky,
Lippincott–Raven Publishers, Philadelphia, © 1998.

CHAPTER

14

Approach to the Clinical and Radiographic Evaluation of Patients with Common Pulmonary Syndromes

Gordon L. Snider · M. Elon Gale

INTRODUCTION

The invention of the stethoscope by Laennec early in the nineteenth century represented a quantum leap in the power of physicians to diagnose pulmonary diseases. The advent of radiographic imaging of the chest early in the twentieth century was an advance of equal importance; its full potential has not yet been realized, even with the invention of computed tomography (CT) about 25 years ago. The past four decades have seen the development and dissemination of other powerful tools: clinical pulmonary function testing, flexible fiberoptic bronchoscopy, ultrasonography, radionuclide scintiscanning, and improved laboratory evaluation of body fluids.

Despite the enormous advances these techniques have brought to our understanding of pulmonary diseases and the accuracy with which we can diagnose them, the physician's role in diagnosis remains undiminished. The medical history continues to be the single most powerful tool in the physician's armamentarium. It is the physician, using skills carefully honed during years of study, who separates the important from the unimportant data in the history, formulates a differential diagnosis, puts the laboratory studies into proper perspective with the history, and establishes the diagnosis. In this chapter, we present an approach to history taking and physical examination and briefly discuss the clinical and radiographic presentation of common pulmonary syndromes.

G. L Snider: Department of Medicine, Veterans Affairs Medical Center, Boston, Massachusetts 02130.

M. Elon Gale: Department of Radiology Veterans Affairs Medical Center, Boston Massachusetts 02130.

HISTORY

Patients with pulmonary disease most commonly seek medical attention because they are troubled by symptoms. Less often, they are referred to a physician because of an abnormal laboratory test result, such as a positive tuberculin test, or abnormal findings on a screening chest radiogram. Sometimes, patients are referred because of the presence of an extrapulmonary lesion known to be frequently associated with pulmonary disease, such as sarcoidosis involving the skin or eyes. The medical interview always begins with the patient's chief complaint.

Chief Complaint

The chief complaint should generally be recorded in the patient's own words; patient satisfaction is greater and the risk of the physician missing the patient's chief complaint is less if the patient is permitted to express major concerns fully and freely instead of simply responding to the physician's closed-ended questions. Each chief complaint is explored in detail. Questions should not be leading and should be expressed in words the patient can easily understand. The purpose is to permit the physician to evaluate the significance of the complaint; gathering of data and interpretation of the history proceed in parallel.

Patient's Assessment of Symptoms

It is important to involve patients in the diagnostic and therapeutic decisions that will affect their welfare. Is a symptom troubling the patient enough to justify ordering an expensive, perhaps invasive diagnostic test, or is the patient content with the physician's reassurance that a serious, potentially disabling or life-threatening condition is not present? What is the principle underlying the treatment plan? What is to be expected from the various drugs that have been prescribed, and are the expected effects immediate or delayed? What are the possible side effects of the drugs—immediate and delayed? If drugs are being used for symptom relief, as in the management of severe asthma, what options may the patient exercise as symptoms vary in severity? What changes of lifestyle are in order? Involving patients directly in their care (cooperative self-management) is an important ingredient in patient satisfaction and therapeutic success.

Pulmonary Symptoms

The number of pulmonary symptoms is limited: cough, expectoration of sputum, hemoptysis, chest pain, dyspnea, and wheezing. The precise manner of presentation of symptoms, the sequence in which they appear, the factors that worsen and alleviate them, and their response to treatment may be of value in suggesting the nature of the underlying disease process. For example, a cough with coryza and purulent sputum that abates with antibiotic treatment is compatible with an infectious bronchitis; a chronic cough with blood-streaked sputum in a cigarette smoker raises the suspicion of bronchogenic carcinoma.

Cough

Mechanisms

Cough may be defined as a forced expulsion of air associated with the generation of a harsh noise. Physiologically, cough is a reflex, forced expiratory event that comprises a rapid inspiration followed by an expiratory effort against a closed glottis, with rapid generation of a high intrapulmonary pressure. Sudden opening of the glottis is followed by an explosive expiration, which has the effect of moving excessive secretions or particulate material toward the mouth.

Cough may be initiated voluntarily or involuntarily. Irritant receptors located in the external auditory canal, larynx, trachea and large bronchi, pleurae, and stomach give rise to afferent stimuli that course centrally over the vagal nerves. The sensitivity of irritant receptors is greatest at the glottis and the main bronchial carina and diminishes rapidly after about the fourth-order bronchi. Thus, large amounts of secretion can pool in the distal airways without initiating a cough. Stimuli from the nose and paranasal sinuses travel centrally over the trigeminal nerve and from the pharynx over the glossopharyngeal nerve. Stimuli from the pericardium and the diaphragm

may initiate cough by afferent impulses coursing over the phrenic nerve. Efferent pathways include the vagus, phrenic, trigeminal, facial, hypoglossal, and accessory nerves as well as the intercostal and lumbar nerves innervating the intrinsic and accessory muscles of respiration.

Normally, secretions from the lungs and airways are removed by ciliary motion, which activates the mucociliary escalator and moves secretions toward the pharynx, where they are swallowed or expectorated. When this mechanism fails or is overwhelmed, cough takes over the critical role of maintaining the clearance function of the airways. The expiratory effort against a closed glottis, which is the first phase of a cough and lasts about 0.2 second, raises the intrapleural pressure to about 100 cm H_2O, although values as high as 300 cm H_2O may be reached. Opening of the glottis is followed by high-velocity, turbulent flow. As expiration proceeds, lung volume diminishes and dynamic compression of intrathoracic airways occurs. For a given flow, the linear velocity of gas is higher in an airway narrowed by dynamic compression than in one in which the normal geometry is maintained. If narrowing also occurs as a result of secretion in the airway, a pressure gradient is created that moves secretions toward the pharynx. These high linear velocities also set the secretions and bronchopulmonary tissues into vibration, creating the characteristic sound of a cough.

The effectiveness of cough may be impaired if any phase of the process is abnormal. The cough reflex may be suppressed by changes in irritant receptor function caused by narcotics, local or systemic anesthetics, or mucosal disease, as in bronchiectasis with severe destructive changes. Neurologic disease may affect any portion of the reflex pathways. Chest wall pain or asthenia resulting from age, illness, or neuromuscular disease may decrease the inspiratory effort preceding cough, thus decreasing the lengthening of expiratory muscle fibers required to develop a high intrapleural pressure against the closed glottis. Inspiratory as well as expiratory muscular dysfunction may result in a weak cough. Obstruction of air flow, as in asthma or emphysema, impairs the effectiveness of cough by decreasing the velocity of the flow of air available for moving secretions. Glottic closure is helpful but not essential for effective coughing; the pressure developed when the glottis is closed is 50%–100% greater than when a forced expiratory maneuver is carried out with the glottis open. Tracheotomized patients learn to carry out forced expiratory maneuvers that are effective in mobilizing their secretions, and persons with an intact glottis may elect to carry out forced, expiratory, coughlike maneuvers through a partially open glottis to minimize the pain induced by a forceful cough in the presence of acute tracheitis or chest wall pain.

The maximal expiratory pressure (MEP) is useful for assessing cough strength in patients with impaired muscle strength, and is likely a more accurate measure of cough strength than forced vital capacity. Patients with MEP values of 60 cm H_2O or more are able to generate sufficient peak flow to produce an effective cough.

Diagnostic Features

Cough of Recent Onset. Normal persons cough infrequently when they are well. The most common reason for the development of cough in a normal person is a viral respiratory infection. Such infections may be sporadic but more often occur in community epidemics or household or workplace clusters. One or more of coryza, sore throat, fever, chills, sweats, malaise, backache, retrobulbar pain, and postnasal discharge may accompany the cough. Cough may be nonproductive or productive, and an acute tracheitis may be accompanied by a tearing or burning substernal pain. The usual duration of cough resulting from an acute respiratory infection is 2 to 3 weeks, but occasionally the cough lingers much longer and is accompanied by wheezing that worsens after exercise or breathing cold air. Such patients show evidence of airways hyperreactivity on challenge with methacholine or cold air.

The history and physical findings of rhinopharyngitis, with or without middle ear disease, establish the diagnosis of cough resulting from an acute upper respiratory infection. A chest radiogram is not necessary to exclude pneumonia unless abnormalities are found on chest examination, or prostration is severe and persistent. Wheezing with cough of recent onset suggests air flow obstruction, possibly from asthma. Stridor indicates involvement of the upper airway.

Chronic cough. Cough that has persisted for more than 3 weeks may be considered to be chronic. However, it is not always easy to know whether chronic cough has been present; patients who have a mild repetitive cough (e.g., on arising) may either be unaware of it or misinterpret it as a natural phenomenon. The symptom will not be elicited unless the patient is asked whether cough occurs on arising, and sometimes it will come to light only after a family member has been questioned. It may also be helpful to determine whether cough described as of recent onset is really new or represents an exacerbation of a chronic condition. Finally, the recent cessation of a longstanding productive cough may indicate retention of bronchial secretions; this is observed occasionally in respiratory failure complicating chronic obstructive airways disease. Weakness, fatigability, fever, and night sweats suggest the presence of tuberculosis, other chronic infection, or malignancy. Physical examination, a chest radiogram, and simple laboratory studies are usually sufficient to establish these diagnoses.

The pioneering work of Irwin has established a diagnostic protocol, based on the locations of the afferent limb of the cough reflex, for investigating chronic cough that is not of obvious etiology. Some causes of chronic cough are listed in Table 1. Chronic bronchitis is the most common cause of chronic cough, occurring in up to 30% of cigarette smokers. The postnasal discharge syndrome is next most frequent. This syndrome is diagnosed when the patient describes a sensation of secretion dripping from the back of the nose into the throat, often with the need for frequent clearing of the throat. Physical examination reveals a cobblestone appearance of the oropharyngeal mucosa, sometimes with overlying mucoid or mucopurulent secretion.

Asthma is easy enough to diagnose when the patient describes episodic wheezing and shortness of breath. However, it must be remembered that asthma may present as only cough, with minimal expectoration and no wheezing. The cough is frequently precipitated by exposure to cold air or exercise and is often dry. An increase of >20% in FEV_1 (forced expiratory volume in 1 second) after administration of a sympathomimetic agonist aerosol, a positive result on a cold air or methacholine challenge test, or a therapeutic response to aerosol treatment with a β-adrenergic agonist support the diagnosis (Chapter 40).

Gastroesophageal reflux (GER) as a cause of chronic cough, with or without wheezing, is controversial. There is no question that some patients have chronic cough secondary to GER. Heartburn or regurgitation of acid material into the mouth may be caused by GER or a Zenker's diverticulum. These patients tend to cough more when lying down at night and respond promptly to treatment of the GER.

Troublesome cough may complicate the treatment of hypertension with angiotensin-converting enzyme inhibitors. Congestive heart failure is a common cause of chronic cough, and this is usually easily diagnosed from

---

TABLE 1. *Some causes of chronic cough*

Frequent
Chronic bronchitis (occurs in 30% of smokers)
Postnasal drip syndrome (caused by rhinitis ± sinusitis)
Asthma (may be variant, without wheezing)
Gastroesophageal reflux
Congestive heart failure
Cystic fibrosis
Chronic infections (tuberculosis, deep mycotic infections)

Infrequent
Occupational factors
Bronchiectasis
Psychogenic cough (may occur with stridor; is rarely nocturnal)
Interstitial lung disease
Bronchogenic carcinoma
Angiotensin-converting enzyme inhibitors
Pulmonary vascular disease
Tracheal compression (neck or mediastinal mass)
Recurrent aspiration (observed in the elderly and persons with swallowing disorders caused by neuromuscular disease; often accompanied by recurrent pneumonia)
Aspirated foreign body (rare in adults except with mental illness, mental retardation, or coma)

the history of heart disease, orthopnea, paroxysmal nocturnal dyspnea, exertional dyspnea, and the physical examination. The presence of chronic productive cough with purulent sputum, often in a nonsmoker, with or without evidence of patchy, persistent pneumonic disease on physical examination and chest radiography, should raise the possibility of cystic fibrosis, which is the most common genetic defect of Caucasians. The disease may present in adults with minimal or no gastrointestinal symptoms of pancreatic involvement (Chapter 73). Chronic cough is a frequent symptom in patients with bronchogenic carcinoma. Tracheal compression, sometimes in the neck, as by a goiter (Fig. 1), but more often in the region of the carina, may also give rise to a dry cough.

Occasionally, patients are observed with psychogenic cough. Such patients are usually young. The cough is frequent, sometimes with accompanying aphonia or stridor and a rather characteristic barking or brassy quality. The cough rarely disturbs sleep, although it may make work or attendance at school impossible. Psychologic abnormalities are not necessarily obvious, although they are usually detectable. The diagnosis is usually evident from the nature of the cough. An investigation to exclude organic disease is necessary, but clinical judgment must be exercised to keep the workup within reasonable bounds.

Complications of Cough. Cough syncope occurs mainly in middle-aged men who have chronic obstructive pulmonary disease (COPD). Fainting follows within 10 to 20 seconds of a paroxysmal cough that cannot be controlled by the patient. The mechanism is obscure; the fainting appears to be related to impairment of venous return and fall in cardiac output as a result of elevated intrathoracic pressure; at the same time, intracranial pressure is elevated by the transmitted intrathoracic pressure. The result is diminution of cerebral blood flow. Consciousness is usually promptly regained, and fatalities caused by this syndrome are rare.

Persistent cough may produce hoarseness. Large increases in muscular forces during severe cough may result in tearing of muscle fibers or rib fracture; the latter occurs most often in the posterior axillary line. Paroxysmal cough may cause headache and back pain. Chronic cough may contribute to recurrent inguinal hernia in men and to urinary incontinence in women. Persistent chronic cough seriously disrupts daily life and may be disabling.

Sputum

Mechanisms

A normal person produces between 10 and 40 mL of tracheobronchial secretion per day. The secretion, consisting primarily of an aqueous solution of mucous glycoprotein, is produced by the airways submucosal glands and goblet cells and is carried to the oropharynx by the mucociliary escalator. Increased amounts of secretion may be noted after eating, especially of highly seasoned food. The mechanism is most likely overflow vagal stimulation of the respiratory glands from intense gastric stimulation. Secretion may be stimulated in response to inhaled gaseous or particulate irritant substances. Inflammation of the respiratory tract also results in an increase in secretory activity, but the characteristics of the secretion are changed by the addition of pus cells, plasma proteins, and other inflammatory products, coming either from the bronchial walls or from the alveoli.

Differential Diagnostic Features

The quantity and quality of expectorated material are important features in bronchopulmonary diseases. The volume is usually best expressed by patients in some household unit of measurement, such as ounces, teaspoons, or tablespoons. Description of the secretions as clear and colorless (like egg white) indicates uninfected secretions; a yellow or green color indicates a purulent exudate. Purulence is most often the consequence of infection and the presence of neutrophilic leukocytes. However, large numbers of eosinophils can make sputum appear purulent. A fetid odor suggests anaerobic infection, as in aspiration lung abscess or necrotizing pneumonia. Rusty or brownish-red sputum is indicates the mixing of blood with the secretions, usually in an acute infectious process such as pneumococcal pneumonia.

In coal miners, the sputum may be black because of the presence of large amounts of anthracotic pigment; black sputum may sometimes occur long after work in the mines has ceased. Cigarette smokers may describe brownish sputum. A three-layered sputum with an uppermost frothy layer, a central mucous layer, and a thick bottom layer is said to be characteristic of bronchiectasis, but this nonspecific appearance may be seen in any bronchitic process with a large volume of secretions. Large amounts of mucoid sputum, up to a liter per day, are an

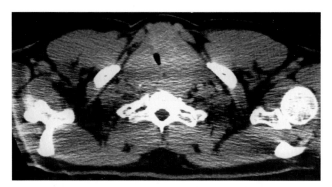

FIG. 1. Enlargement of the thyroid gland usually does not compress the trachea, which is supported by stiff cartilaginous rings. However, when a goiter becomes extremely large, as demonstrated here, the shape of the tracheal cross-section can be distorted and diminished.

unusual manifestation of alveolar cell carcinoma. Mucoid bronchorrhea may also be seen occasionally with chronic bronchitis. Fibrinous casts may be expectorated in the very rare plastic bronchitis syndrome, and ''pearls'' or wormlike structures comprised of bronchiolar casts are frequently expectorated in asthma. The latter are made up of eosinophils, desquamated bronchial epithelium, and Curschmann's spirals—spiral structures that consist of eosinophils and Charcot-Leyden crystals, which are eosinophil-derived. Brownish bronchiolar plugs may be observed in allergic bronchopulmonary aspergillosis.

The descriptions of sputum provided by patients are often inaccurate, and the physician should make every effort to look at secretions during the examination. Patients with chronic disease should be taught to differentiate between purulent and mucous secretions.

Hemoptysis

Mechanisms

Hemoptysis is defined as the expectoration of blood. The quantity of blood may vary from a few streaks mixed with bronchial secretions to an exsanguinating hemorrhage. The site of bleeding may be anywhere in the respiratory tract, including the nose or the mouth, and the mechanisms of bleeding are varied. The bronchial mucosa may bleed because of congestion from inflammation, often with accompanying superficial erosion of the overlying epithelium. Passively engorged blood vessels, as in mitral stenosis, may also bleed readily, either without evident cause or as a result of mucosal ulceration accompanying minor respiratory infections. Bleeding may result from ulceration of a tumor, such as a bronchial carcinoid or a bronchogenic carcinoma (Fig. 2). Indeed, hemoptysis

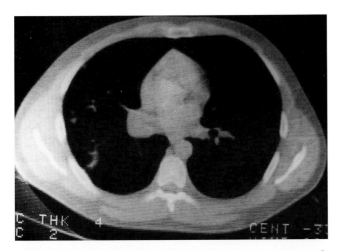

FIG. 2. This patient presented with dyspnea on severe effort; the findings on plain chest x-ray film were normal. On CT, the right hilum appeared to be enlarged. On bronchoscopy, this appearance was shown to be the result of complete occlusion of the bronchus intermedius by a bronchial carcinoid. Only minimal postobstructive parenchymal disease is present because of effective collateral air flow.

may occur as the bronchial wall is penetrated by an eroding structure, such as an infectious or noninfectious granuloma, a calcified lymph node, or an aortic aneurysm, which may be atherosclerotic, luetic, or dissecting. Rarely, in empyema, a ventricular-bronchial communication may cause massive hemoptysis. In bronchiectasis, the bronchial arteries undergo enlargement and extensive anastomosis with the pulmonary arteries; erosion into a bronchial artery with its systemic level of blood pressure may give rise to massive hemoptysis.

Blood may come from the pulmonary parenchyma, as from the vascular granulation tissue lining an anaerobic abscess (Fig. 3), a tuberculous abscess, an abscess of gram-negative bacillary or staphylococcal origin, or a mycetoma. If a blood vessel wall in an abscess is left unsupported by parenchyma, and especially if the blood vessel wall is eroded by the infectious process, hemorrhage may be massive and even exsanguinating. Hemorrhage commonly arises more simply from congested pulmonary parenchyma, as in pneumococcal pneumonia, or from engorged and necrotic parenchyma in pulmonary infarction (Fig. 4).

Differential Diagnostic Features

Patients describe hemoptysis in various ways. Pulmonary parenchymal or bronchial bleeding may be perceived as a bubbling sensation in the tracheobronchial tree, followed by the expectoration of blood. When underlying infection has been present, the patient may not be aware of any change in the quantity of secretion but may note blood mixed with mucus or replacing it. When bleeding is profuse, clots may be expectorated.

Bronchopulmonary bleeding may sometimes be manifested as vomiting of blood. Bleeding occurs during the night, and the blood reaches the oropharynx and is swallowed without the patient waking. The swallowed blood acts as an irritant and produces vomiting in the early morning hours. Roentgenographic and physical examination of the chest are therefore mandatory in the investigation of every patient with hematemesis. Hematemesis rarely masquerades as hemoptysis; the presence of gastrointestinal symptoms such as nausea and vomiting and a history of alcoholism or cirrhosis, sometimes with a past history of hematemesis, usually point to the correct diagnosis. The presence of food in a specimen of the bloody fluid and an acid pH suggest gastric origin. If the chest radiogram is negative, the presence of blood or ''coffee grounds'' material in the gastric aspirate settles the issue.

A history of epistaxis must be sought in patients with hemoptysis, because blood from the nasopharynx can be aspirated during the night and coughed up in the early morning. The nasopharynx should be examined in all patients with hemoptysis who have a negative chest radiogram.

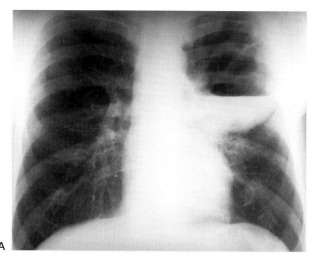

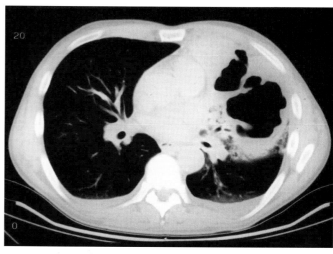

A

B

FIG. 3. A: Anaerobic lung abscess. On chest x-ray film, a large abscess cavity with an air-fluid level fills nearly the entire left upper lobe. Note that some streaky remnants of lung tissue remain visible, as do several smaller air-fluid levels. An area of pneumonia, seen here in the left infrahilar region, is commonly noted, reflecting infected but not yet necrotic lung adjacent to the abscess. B: On CT, the multilocular nature of the lung abscess is apparent. Small, air-containing structures in a region of perihilar pneumonia represent bronchiectasis and early foci of necrosis. Note the shaggy interior cavity wall, typical of lung abscess.

Small stones or gravel may be expectorated with blood in broncholithiasis, a condition in which calcium in granulomatous lymph nodes erodes through the bronchial wall, or a foreign body aspirated years earlier becomes calcified (Fig. 5). In the extremely rare catamenial hemoptysis, resulting from endometrial implants in the bronchial wall, the expectoration of blood occurs concomitantly with menstruation.

Table 2 provides a partial list of the more than 100 disease entities that can cause hemoptysis. Tuberculosis and bronchiectasis used to be the most common causes of hemoptysis. Erosive bronchitis in smokers with chronic bronchitis is now the most frequent cause of expectoration of blood, accounting for 40%–50% of all cases of hemoptysis. Bronchogenic carcinoma is the second most frequent cause of hemoptysis, underlying 20%–25% of all cases. Blood-streaked bronchitic sputum may be the only hint that a bronchogenic carcinoma has developed in a long-time smoker.

Massive hemoptysis, of which the most common causes

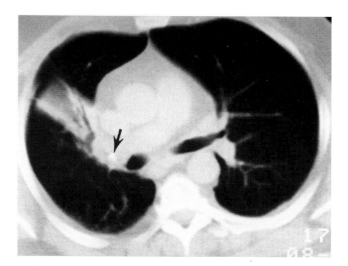

FIG. 4. This patient, with a cardiac valve replacement not clearly seen here, received excessive anticoagulant therapy with warfarin and presented with hemoptysis. In the right upper lobe, there is a dense opacification consisting of intraparenchymal hemorrhage. Unlike consolidations caused by infection, parenchymal hemorrhage tends to clear rapidly.

FIG. 5. CT demonstrates partial middle lobe collapse. Some patent bronchi are visible. A focus of calcification (arrow) is seen centrally near the origin of the middle lobe bronchus. At bronchoscopy, a broncholith composed of calcified and encrusted aspirated vegetable material was removed.

TABLE 2. *Some causes of hemoptysis*

Frequent
Chronic bronchitis
Bronchogenic carcinoma[a]

Infrequent
Bronchiectasis[a]
Tuberculosis
   Active[a]
   Inactive (post-tuberculous bronchiectasis)
Pulmonary contusion
Pulmonary abscess[a]
Bronchoarterial fistula[a]
Cardiogenic (mitral stenosis, pulmonary edema—
   pink sputum)
Aspergilloma[a]
Coagulopathy[a]
Pulmonary infarction
Idiopathic pulmonary hemosiderosis
Goodpasture's syndrome
Pulmonary telangiectasis[a]
Amyloidosis
Bronchiectasis[a]
Broncholithiasis
Sjögren's syndrome
Deep mycotic infection[a]
Bronchial adenoma
Metastatic carcinoma
Foreign body
Wegener's granulomatosis
Pseudohemoptysis (epistaxis, hematemesis, bleeding
   gums, malingering)

[a] Most frequent cause of massive hemoptysis.

are identified in Table 2, may be defined as expectoration of 600 mL or more of blood in 24 hrs. Hemoptysis of this magnitude is life-threatening and requires close monitoring and often urgent diagnostic and therapeutic intervention.

Chest Pain

Mechanisms

Pain in the chest may be derived from the chest wall (dermatomes T1-12), pleurae, trachea and main airways, mediastinum (including the heart and esophagus), and abdominal viscera. The parietal pleura is supplied with pain receptors; the visceral pleura is free of them. Pleuritic pain may be referred to the area of skin supplied by the same sensory roots that supply the area from which pain is arising. Thus, the pleurisy accompanying a right lower lobe pneumonia and involving dermatome T-11 may mimic the pain of acute appendicitis. The sensory fibers of the central tendon of the diaphragm run with the phrenic nerve (C3-4), and the pain of diaphragmatic pleurisy may be referred to the tip of the shoulder. Cardiac pain (T1-4) may radiate down the ulnar aspects of the arms, more often the left, and may radiate up into the jaws.

Visceral pain from the gallbladder, pancreas, or hepatic or splenic flexures of the colon may be referred to the epigastrium, substernal area, or lower thorax, as may the pain of upper abdominal peritonitis. A variety of other reactions may accompany severe chest pain. Autonomic reactions such as tachycardia and sweating may be observed; parasympathetic reactions include bradycardia, nausea, and vomiting. Skeletal muscle splinting may accompany severe pleuritic pain of any cause, and was present in the patient with malignant mesothelioma shown in Fig. 6.

Pain, like other sensory phenomena, is poorly understood, but it begins with a noxious stimulus generated mechanically or chemically as a result of tissue injury and inflammation. The chemical mediators released from inflamed tissues that initiate pain are beginning to be understood. Tissue receptors are activated and pain stimuli are transmitted via the peripheral afferent nervous system. Visceral pain is transmitted centrally via low-velocity, unmyelinated C-fibers; cutaneous and chest wall pain are transmitted by high-velocity, myelinated A-fibers.

The pain stimuli are processed in complex, incompletely understood ways by the central nervous system. This processing accounts for a variable dissociation of the central perception of pain from the magnitude of the peripheral stimulus. Many factors, such as emotion, depression, and competing stimuli, may influence the perception of pain. Visceral pain tends to be dull and poorly localized, whereas chest wall pain tends to be sharper and better localized.

Differential Diagnostic Features

History taking is the key to evaluating chest pain. There is only a weak relationship between the severity of chest pain and the importance of its underlying cause; accordingly, all chest pain must be taken seriously. The precise cause of chest pain cannot always be determined by taking a history and doing a physical examination, but it is generally possible to make a judgment as to whether the origin of the pain is the pleura, the chest wall, or the viscera, and to develop a diagnostic plan. Table 3 provides a partial list of causes of chest pain.

Pleural Pain. Chest pain that tends to be sharply localized, worsens during coughing, deep breathing, or motion of the trunk, and is relieved by maneuvers limiting the expansion of a particular part of the chest is very likely to be pleuritic in origin. The pain, which occurs more often at the lung bases than in the upper lung zones, may range in severity from mild and aching to excruciating. Worsening during respiratory motions is its hallmark. Pleuritic pain is caused by stretching of the inflamed parietal pleura. However, in chronic pleuritis, pain endings may no longer be stimulated despite roughening of the pleural surfaces, which continue to give rise to a loud rub.

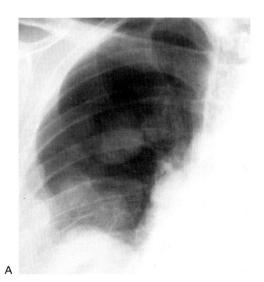
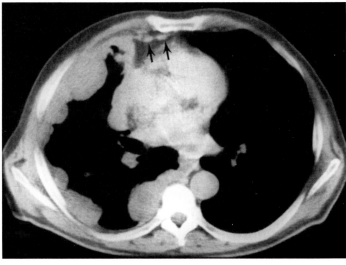

A   B

FIG. 6. A: Malignant mesothelioma presenting as multiple, large, rounded masses apparent in this right hemithorax. Some of the more centrally located lesions have the appearance of well-demarcated intraparenchymal lesions. However, others, which demonstrate broad, smooth margins merging with the chest wall, clearly have a pleural origin. **B:** It is evident on the corresponding CT image that there are no intraparenchymal lesions; rather, all the abnormalities are based in the pleura. Mesothelioma typically forms large, rounded lobules along the entire pleural surface. Microscopic invasion of the chest wall is poorly assessed on CT. Gross extension to other mesothelial surfaces, such as the contralateral pleura or peritoneum, can often be detected on CT. In this case, there is direct invasion (*arrow*) of pericardial fat immediately posterior to the sternum.

The rapidity of onset of the pain varies with its cause. Pleuritic pain accompanying a spontaneous pneumothorax or pulmonary infarct is usually sudden in onset. Pleurisy of viral origin or associated with pneumonia may be more gradual in onset and occurs in the context of an acute febrile, prostrating illness. Infection with coxsackievirus B produces a syndrome known as pleurodynia (Bornholm syndrome); this is characterized by fever, malaise, sore throat, debility, and anorexia and is followed by the sudden onset of muscular and pleuritic pain, with abdominal pain and muscle spasm in about half the cases. The disease runs its course in 3 to 7 days and may be complicated by a small pleural effusion. Tuberculous pleural effusion may be initially manifested by pleuritic pain and cough that subside rapidly. Parenchymal tuberculosis with overlying pleural disease, often occurring in the context of chronic systemic illness, may cause aching of the chest wall without a clear relation to respiration.

Pain Caused by Bronchopulmonary and Mediastinal Disorders. The lung parenchyma has no pain receptors. However, acute pulmonary diseases that involve the overlying pleura, such as pneumonia, lung abscess, and pulmonary infarction, cause pleuritic pain. Acute tracheobronchitis may give rise to substernal discomfort, with a tearing, rasping, sharp substernal pain on coughing. Mediastinitis causes a retrosternal, aching, oppressive sensation that can occasionally be severe. Chronic disorders of the large airways, such as tracheal or bronchial tumors, chondritis, or ulcers, do not cause pain. Mediastinal tumors are usually asymptomatic but can cause chest pain

if they compress or invade mediastinal structures or chest wall.

Pain Caused by Malignancy. The pain of a carcinoma invading the spine or ribs is generally well localized and of a severe, unremitting character (Fig. 7). With mesothelioma (Fig. 6) or metastatic carcinoma, as from a primary breast tumor, the pain may be more diffuse. Involvement of chest wall and nerve roots results in local, gnawing chest wall pain and radiation of the pain to the affected dermatomes. Thus, in Pancoast's syndrome, in which the brachial plexus is involved by an invasive primary lung tumor located peripherally in the extreme apex of the lung, there is pain in the shoulder, the scapular region, or the medial aspect of the arm and hand. The pain of this tumor sometimes masquerades as subacromial bursitis. The pain of vertebral metastases tends to be in the midline, often with girdle radiation, and may be associated with tenderness over the affected area. Intercostal neuropathy, which may result from irritation of an intercostal nerve by a costal metastasis or some other factor, may result in severe, lancinating, burning pain that is unilateral and segmental in distribution. There may be sensory loss or hyperesthesia over the affected dermatomes. Intercostal neuropathy is one cause of the postthoracotomy pain syndrome; traumatic neuroma in the thoracotomy scar and recurrent tumor are other causes.

Pain Originating in the Chest Wall. Fracture of a rib, either during trauma or spontaneously during cough, causes local pain in the affected area. The pain is severe, worsened by respiratory and trunk motion, and may be

TABLE 3. *Some causes of chest pain*

Pleural
Pleurisy (bacterial, viral, mycoplasmal)
Pneumothorax
Malignancy (primary and metastatic carcinoma, mesothelioma)
Hemothorax

Bronchopulmonary
Acute tracheobronchitis
Parenchymal disease involving pleura (pneumonia, abscess, infarct, carcinoma)
Pulmonary hypertension

Mediastinal
Mediastinitis
Mediastinal tumors

Chest wall
Rib fracture and costochondral dislocation
Neoplastic invasion
Nerve root, intercostal neuritis
Muscular pain
Chondritis
Xiphodynia
Precordial catch
Arthritic (spinal and costovertebral joints)
Herpes zoster
Mondor's disease

Cardiovascular
Cardiac ischemia
Aortic stenosis or regurgitation
Hypertrophic cardiomyopathy
Pericarditis
Mitral valve prolapse
Post-pericarditis and post-pericardiotomy syndrome
Dissecting aortic aneurysm
Aortic aneurysm

Gastrointestinal
Esophageal colic
Cholecystitis
Pancreatitis
Colonic distension syndromes

accompanied by a grating sensation during breathing. Local tenderness develops early, and a callus may be felt as the fracture heals. Costochondral dislocation, occurring from muscular effort or less frequently trauma, causes less severe, anterolateral chest pain.

The rare occurrence of subacute chondritis causes a dull, aching pain of the anterior chest wall that is not affected by breathing. The second, third, and fourth cartilages are most frequently involved, but the process can involve any costal cartilage or the xiphoid process. Disease of the thoracic spine may be associated with involvement of the costovertebral joints and cause discomfort or pain in the chest wall. Chest wall pain may be caused by damage to muscle fibers secondary to the severe muscular effort associated with coughing during an acute respiratory infection or with unusually severe exercise. Herpes zoster is often heralded by several days of neuritic pain

in the affected dermatomes; the pain persists during the cutaneous phase of the disease, and postherpetic neuralgia with its burning and paroxysmal lancinating pain may persist for long periods.

A rare cause of superficial chest wall pain is thrombosis of the superficial vein of the thoracic wall (Mondor's disease). The process is of unknown etiology but is self-limited. It may last several weeks; an initial acute phase is followed by an indolent phase, and a palpable subcutaneous cord over the lateral chest wall is its only sign.

Precordial catch is a pricking, precordial (left parasternal) pain, usually occurring at rest and often associated with emotional stress. The pain is variably worsened by deep inspiration, is not precipitated by effort, and tends to be transient and stabbing in character. It occurs more often in men than in women and is infrequently observed after the third decade. The pain is not caused by heart or lung disease and is probably of chest wall origin. The diagnosis is made by the characteristic history, negative physical findings, and appropriate laboratory tests performed to exclude visceral disease.

Cardiovascular Pain. The pain of cardiac ischemia results from an imbalance between the supply and demand of oxygen in the myocardium, and most often results from atherosclerotic coronary arteries. The pain of angina pectoris is induced by exercise, especially after a heavy meal or in cold or windy conditions. The chest pain is vague, diffuse, and ill-defined—that is, it is visceral in nature. Generally located substernally or in the anterior midline, it is described as constricting or squeezing, or as a weight on the chest. The pain may radiate down the medial aspect of the left arm (less often the right) or into the neck or mandible. Angina is relieved by rest or sublingual nitroglycerin. The pain of myocardial infarction is usually more persistent, lasting longer than 20 minutes, and is often accompanied by sweating, nausea, hypotension, dyspnea, and arrhythmias. Unstable angina occurs episodically at rest or with little provocation, and it may herald an impending myocardial infarction.

Cardiomyopathy may cause anginal chest pain, as may aortic stenosis and, to a lesser degree, aortic regurgitation. Mitral valve prolapse may be associated with sharp, stabbing chest pain not provoked by exertion; it is more frequent in female patients.

The pain of pericarditis is in the midline but not as distinctly substernal as the typical pain of myocardial ischemia. Because of the intimate association of the pericardium and the mediastinal pleura, pericardial pain often exhibits characteristics suggesting pleural involvement—it is worsened by inspiration and coughing. When the central tendon of the diaphragm is involved, the pain is referred to the trapezius ridge. Pericardial may be so severe that it mimics myocardial infarction, or be so mild and pleuritic in nature that acute pleurisy or pulmonary infarction become diagnostic considerations. The pain is often relieved by sitting up and leaning forward or by lying on the right side. Spontaneous pneu-

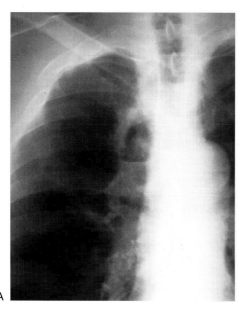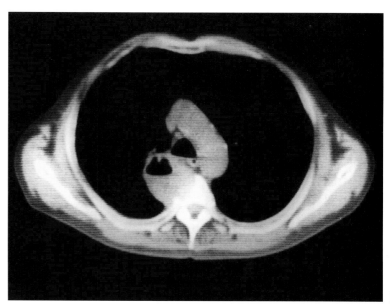

A   B

FIG. 7. A: A large mass is present in the right paramediastinal area. An air-fluid level is present within the central cavitary portion of the lesion, defining its approximate inner and outer margins. A small projection into the cavity from the lateral wall suggests the possibility of necrotizing tumor. The diagnosis of squamous cell carcinoma was confirmed by bronchoscopy. **B:** On CT, the entire anterolateral aspect of the adjacent vertebral body has been eroded. Chest wall invasion may be readily apparent or completely undetectable on CT.

momediastinum may also give rise to pain that has the characteristics of pericarditis.

Pain associated with acute pulmonary hypertension is similar to the pain of myocardial infarction, but the electrocardiographic and laboratory features of that disease are absent. The pain may be associated with multiple or massive pulmonary emboli or with an infectious process in a patient having a restricted pulmonary vascular bed or mitral stenosis. Its mechanism is unknown; it may be caused by the sudden distension of the main pulmonary artery and stimulation of mechanoreceptors.

Chest pain, usually excruciating and starting in an anterior substernal location, is the predominant presenting symptom in dissecting aneurysm of the aorta (Fig. 8). Unlike the pain of myocardial infarction, which waxes and wanes, this pain is usually maximal at onset. It is common for the pain to migrate posteriorly as the dissection propagates distally. Nondissecting aneurysm can produce continuous aching or lancinating pain in the chest, shoulder, and back by compressing the thoracic spinal nerves; bone erosion causes boring, intractable back pain.

Chest Pain Related to Gastrointestinal Disease. Recurrent noncardiac chest pain is a common clinical condition that is often frustrating to the physician. Such patients often have undergone angiography demonstrating normal or near-normal coronary arteries, but they continue to have angina-like chest pain that prompts repeated visits to the physician's office or emergency department. They have a low risk for myocardial infarction or cardiac death.

Spasm of the esophagus or esophageal colic is one important cause of such chest pain. The pain may mimic

cardiac pain perfectly. It ranges from mild to severe and may last from 5 or 10 minutes to many hours. The pain is usually substernal and may radiate down one or both arms, and into the neck, jaws, teeth, or epigastric area. Radiation through to the back suggests an esophageal origin, as does the association of heartburn and relief of pain by the ingestion of alkali or by changing from a recumbent to an upright position.

Proving that chest pain is of esophageal origin is often difficult. Different types of esophageal motility disorders have been described in association with chest pain: achalasia, diffuse esophageal spasm, "nutcracker" esophagus, and nonspecific motility disorder. However, the precise relation between these abnormal contractions and chest pain is far from clear; chest pain is frequently not present when motility disorders are being demonstrated in the laboratory, and motility disorders are often not associated with impaired esophageal function. Katz et al., reviewing the records of 910 patients studied manometrically for noncardiac chest pain, found abnormal motility in 28% during baseline manometry; diffuse spasm and achalasia were present in only 10% and 2% of subjects, respectively. Nutcracker esophagus and nonspecific motility disorders were most common, in 48% and 36%, respectively. Ambulatory pressure monitoring and monitoring of pH have also been widely studied to evaluate chest pain, as have provocative tests such as acid infusion and intravenous edrophonium.

Distension of the splenic flexure may cause left lower chest pain; the pain is usually relieved by passing flatus and is not related to breathing or trunk motion. Gallbladder disease may also give rise to epigastric and midline

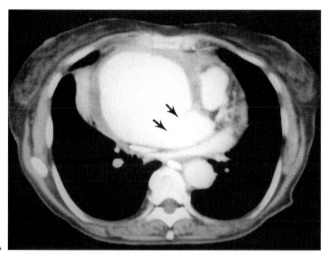 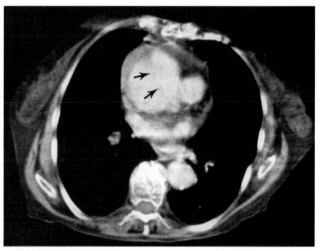

FIG. 8. A: In many cases, dissection of the aorta is easily seen on contrast-enhanced CT, as demonstrated in this example. Here, a large saccular component of the aneurysm at the root of the aorta bulges anteriorly and to the right into the sinus of Valsalva. The intimal flap is visible as a thin, dark, obliquely oriented line (*arrows*) at the posterior aspect of the large, contrast-enhanced aortic root. Note that the attenuation of the region immediately surrounding the aorta is higher than that of fat and normal soft tissue and is caused by leakage of blood into the pericardial sac, a portion of which encompasses the aortic root. **B:** In another patient with aortic dissection, the dilatation of the aorta is not as extensive. Some intrapericardial hemorrhage is seen anterior to the aortic root. The intimal flap (*arrows*) can again be seen, in this case oriented anteroposteriorly. Note in both cases the gentle curvature of the intimal flap toward one lumen or the other, a common appearance.

chest pain mimicking angina as well as to right upper quadrant abdominal pain. The history of gastrointestinal symptoms and the atypical nature of the chest pain are helpful in differential diagnosis.

Dyspnea

Dyspnea may be defined as discomfort associated with breathing and is a symptom of both pulmonary and cardiac disease. In taking the history, it is important to determine whether dyspnea occurs only on exercise or also at rest; if the symptom occurs only on exercise, what has been the time course of its development? If dyspnea occurs at rest, how is the symptom related to the time of day, eating, and body position? A partial listing of the causes of dyspnea is given in Table 4, and a simple categorization of the severity of dyspnea is given in Table 5. The flowing section briefly summarizes our knowledge of the mechanisms of dyspnea, including the contributions of the relatively new field of respiratory psychophysics.

Mechanisms

Dyspnea may be accounted for by a decrease in ventilatory capacity, an increase in ventilatory demand during exercise, or by the perception of increased breathing as being uncomfortable. Put somewhat differently, the symptom varies directly with the demand for ventilation and inversely with ventilatory capacity. The symptom is related to the

patient's perception of whether ventilation is appropriate to a particular level of activity. Thus, the expected increase in ventilation while climbing a flight of stairs quickly is not perceived as dyspnea; a similar level of ventilation while climbing three or four stairs would be perceived as dyspnea

TABLE 4. *Some causes of dyspnea*

Acute
Upper airway obstruction (laryngospasm, aspirated foreign body, neoplasm)
Asthma
Chest trauma (rib fracture, peumothorax, lung contusion, vascular rupture, bronchial rupture)
Pneumonia (pleural effusion may contribute)
Pulmonary embolism
Acute interstitial lung disease (hemorrhage, adult respiratory distress syndrome)
Cardiogenic pulmonary edema
Spontaneous pneumothorax

Chronic
Chronic obstructive pulmonary disease
Cystic fibrosis
Interstitial lung diseases
Pleural effusion
Fibrothorax
Chest wall abnormalities (kyphoscoliosis, neuromuscular disease, diaphragmatic paralysis)
Pulmonary vascular disease (primary pulmonary hypertension, organizing pulmonary emboli, veno-occlusive disease, vascular malformations)
Cardiovascular disease
Severe anemia
Psychogenic dyspnea

TABLE 5. *American Thoracic Society dyspnea scale*

Grade	Degree	Defining clinical characteristics
0	None	Not troubled with breathlessness except with strenuous exercise
1	Slight	Troubled by shortness of breath when hurrying on the level or walking up a slight hill
2	Moderate	Walks more slowly than people of the same age on the level because of breathlessness or has to stop for breath when walking at own pace on the level
3	Severe	Stops for breath after walking about 100 yards or after a few minutes on the level
4	Very severe	Too breathless to leave the house or breathless when dressing or undressing

by an observant patient. An increase in the effort required to produce a given level of ventilation, as in asthma, might also be perceived as dyspnea.

Decreased ability to move air in neuromuscular, obstructive airways, or cardiac diseases may cause dyspnea. Cardiopulmonary disease may increase ventilatory demand in many different ways, thereby causing dyspnea: hypoxemia, hypercapnia, increased hydrogen ion concentration, and increased reflex activity from the lungs, muscles, or central blood vessels. For example, ventilatory capacity is relatively well maintained in diffuse interstitial disease, but there is an increase in ventilatory demand and elastic work of breathing during exercise that gives rise to dyspnea. Dyspnea occurs in COPD primarily because of the decrease in ventilatory capacity and the increase in resistive work of breathing. However, none of these physiologic correlates of dyspnea provides an understanding of the sensory basis of dyspnea.

Differential Diagnostic Features

The duration of dyspnea, whether it is of gradual or rapid onset, whether it is episodic or continuous, and its relation to effort should all be determined. For example, gradual onset of dyspnea suggests slowly progressive disease of the heart, lungs, or musculoskeletal system. Rapid onset of dyspnea suggests an acute respiratory infection; sudden worsening of air flow obstruction, as in asthma; or a sudden event, such as a pulmonary embolus. Dyspnea produced by a level of exercise not previously causing discomfort suggests slowly progressive heart or lung disease or anemia. Dyspnea occurring only during exercise suggests slowly progressive disease; dyspnea occurring also at rest suggests heart failure of fluctuating severity or variable air flow obstruction. Breathlessness may be similar to that experienced during normal exercise, sug-

gesting that air flow obstruction is not present, or breathlessness may be associated with labored breathing (difficulty in moving air into or out of the chest), suggesting that airflow obstruction is present. The presence of airflow obstruction is confirmed if the dyspnea is associated with wheezing (whistling or musical noises in the chest). Sudden chest pain occurring with dyspnea suggests a pulmonary infarction, spontaneous pneumothorax, or myocardial infarction. An episode of aspiration may precede dyspnea associated with pneumonia. Hemoptysis occurring with the dyspnea may signal diffuse interstitial lung diseases, as in Goodpasture's syndrome or pulmonary hemosiderosis. Expectoration of frothy pink sputum and orthopnea suggest pulmonary edema. Coryza, malaise, cough, expectoration, and chest pain suggest an acute upper or lower respiratory infection.

Severe dyspnea in a patient without airflow obstruction or heart disease should suggest the possibility of a diffuse interstitial parenchymal process, pulmonary embolism, or primary pulmonary hypertension (Fig. 9). The presence of fine crackles on auscultation suggests interstitial lung disease; the signs of pulmonary hypertension should be carefully sought in the absence of crackles. Paroxysmal nocturnal dyspnea can occur with either left ventricular failure or obstructive airways disease. Obstructive airways disease is not usually accompanied by orthopnea, whereas left ventricular failure and bilateral diaphragmatic paralysis virtually always are.

Trepopnea, or dyspnea in one lateral position but not in the other, may be produced by unilateral lung disease, unilateral pleural effusion, or unilateral airway obstruction. Platypnea, or dyspnea in the upright position relieved by recumbency, may be produced by intracardiac shunts or vascular shunts in the lungs. Differentiation of dyspnea of cardiac origin from that of pulmonary origin usually depends on demonstrating whether cardiac or pulmonary disease is present. Sophisticated tests of cardiac and pulmonary function and exercise testing may at times be necessary to settle the question, or to determine the relative contributions of heart and lung disease when both are present.

Psychogenic dyspnea occurs in several forms. The syndrome usually presents as breathlessness unrelated to exertion, occurring in women more often than in men, usually in the third or fourth decades of life. If the patient is hyperventilating (i.e., breathing in excess of metabolic needs), the partial pressure of arterial carbon dioxide ($PaCO_2$) decreases, with a resultant decrease in cerebral blood flow. Lightheadedness, faintness, visual disturbances, numbness, and tingling of the fingers and perioral areas may be noted. Patients are often disproportionately anxious.

Another form of hyperventilation is sighing dyspnea. This occurs equally often in both sexes, may occur at any age, and is not usually accompanied by symptoms of hypocapnia or severe anxiety. The symptom may appear in patients with known heart or lung disease. The patient

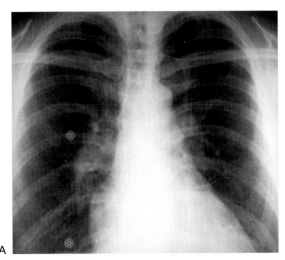

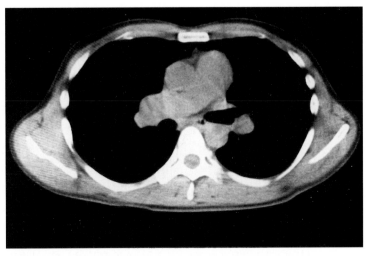

A   B

FIG. 9. A: On posteroanterior view of the chest in pulmonary hypertension, the central pulmonary arteries are enlarged and the peripheral arteries appear diminutive in size. On a lateral view, a hypertrophied right ventricle may be encroaching on the retrosternal air space. **B:** The diameters of the main and right pulmonary arteries are easily seen to be greater than the diameter of the adjacent aorta on CT of the mediastinum.

usually complains of not being able to get enough air at rest. Effort dyspnea is not present unless associated heart or lung disease is present, and then the effort dyspnea is different from the resting breathlessness. The patient usually describes how the expected deep visceral sensation of comfort or satisfaction in the epigastrium is not felt after a sighing inspiration. Consequently, the patient repeats a series of deep inspirations to attempt to produce this normal sensation. Because normally this sensation decreases and then disappears with successive sighs, the deep breaths do not have the desired effects, and the patient complains of being unable to ''fill the chest with air satisfactorily.'' A precipitating event can rarely be identified. A negative chest radiogram and electrocardiogram added to the negative findings on physical examination and a careful explanation of the nature of the symptoms are usually sufficient to produce relief.

Wheezing

Some patients with obstructive airflow disease may be aware of wheezing, but most are not and rather describe difficult breathing or a sense of tightness in the chest. Sounds generated by breathing may be heard only by family members. Wheezing may be audible only during recumbency. This symptom may suggest the possibility of asthma as the underlying cause in a patient with cough or dyspnea of obscure origin.

Stridor

Stridor is a harsh, blowing noise resulting from obstruction of the trachea or larynx by tumor (Fig. 10), bilateral

vocal cord paralysis, other forms of vocal cord dysfunction, tracheal compression, edema associated with inflammation, or the impaction of a foreign body. The airway must be narrowed to about 5 mm in an adult before stridor is produced. Stridor is mainly inspiratory, because air flow is more rapid during this respiratory phase. It has a characteristic crowing or musical sound. However, when upper respiratory tract obstruction is very severe and alveolar hypoventilation has occurred, stridor may be absent. Stridor may also be hysterical in origin.

Obstructive Sleep Apnea

Disorders of breathing associated with sleep have been reported with increasing frequency during the last four decades. Obstructive sleep apnea (OSA) is a condition in which 10 or more episodes of upper airway obstruction, each lasting 10 seconds or longer, are detected per hour of sleep. The resultant hypoxemia and impaired quality of sleep result in daytime hypersomnolence, a variety of cardiovascular abnormalities (arrhythmias, cor pulmonale), and neuropsychologic complications. The prevalence of OSA is not known, but it is estimated to affect 1%–2% of the population.

OSA should be suspected whenever excessive daytime sleepiness and snoring coexist. Obesity and alcohol abuse are well-known aggravating factors but need not be present. Nocturnal restlessness, choking spells, frequent urination at night, enuresis, and loss of libido are common. Morning headache and falling asleep during the day while working, engaging in conversation, or driving an automobile are all well-known features of this syndrome. An increased frequency of accidents at home, at work, or

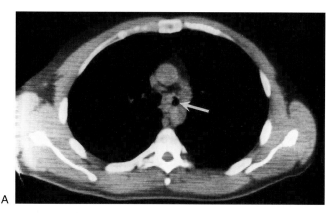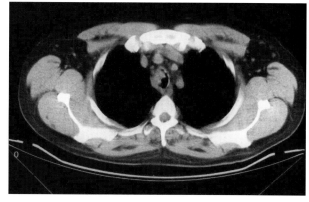

FIG. 10. A: This tracheal squamous papilloma originated near the carina. On inspiratory CT, it can be seen partially occluding the left main bronchus (*arrow*). On expiratory chest x-ray films and CT, there was significant air trapping in the left lung as the lesion created a ball valve effect. The partial obstruction also caused the patient to wheeze. **B:** This tracheal cylindroma demonstrates a lobular, intraluminal mass of soft-tissue density on CT. The affected portion of the tracheal wall is obscured by the neoplasm itself. Often, the bulk of a tracheal tumor is intraluminal rather than extraluminal.

while driving is common. It is essential to question the spouse or dwelling partner of the patient regarding these symptoms as well as snoring and apneic episodes during sleep, as the patient may be unable to give an account of them.

The presence of systemic hypertension, plethora associated with polycythemia, and evidence of pulmonary hypertension and cor pulmonale suggest OSA. Obesity, hypothyroidism, acromegaly, and maxillofacial or oropharyngeal abnormalities are predisposing factors, but none of these risk factors, including obesity, need be present. The diagnosis is established by polysomnography.

Systems Review and Social History

After the history of present illness has been completed, a careful review should be made of the function of other body systems. Joint pain with or without skin abnormalities may indicate the presence of a systemic disease, such as rheumatoid disease or sarcoidosis. Raynaud's phenomenon with thickening of the skin of the hands or face, possibly with dysphagia, suggests the possibility of progressive systemic sclerosis. A chronic skin ulcer may be evidence of systemic spread of a pulmonary fungal infection. Late afternoon fatigue, denoting a chronic inflammatory process in the body such as tuberculosis or a deep mycotic infection, may have been so insidious in onset as not to have reached the patient's awareness until the question is carefully put.

Tobacco-Smoking History

The tobacco-smoking history should be taken in a standard manner (Table 6). Patients should be asked if they currently smoke cigarettes. If the response is in the nega-

tive, the patient should be asked, "Did you ever smoke?" It is not rare for a patient with pulmonary disease, who has stopped smoking recently because of an alarming symptom such as hemoptysis, to answer negatively when asked, "Do you smoke tobacco?" The age when regular smoking began should be determined. The risk for lung cancer is inversely proportional to the age at which smoking was begun. The total number of years smoked should be calculated. If the patient has stopped smoking, the age at cessation of smoking should be recorded. For former smokers, the number of years of abstinence should be calculated; the risk for lung cancer drops with the duration of abstinence, approaching that of nonsmokers after 10 years, although some risk is nonreversible. The average amount of tobacco smoked per day (packs of cigarettes, number of cigars, ounces of pipe tobacco) during the patient's smoking lifetime should be noted, as it provides

TABLE 6. *The smoking history*

Age when started
- How old was the patient when regular smoking began?

Duration of smoking
- Were there periods when the patient stopped smoking?
- Is the patient currently smoking?
- At what age did the patient stop smoking?

Amount of tobacco smoked
- What is the average lifetime number of cigarettes smoked per day?
- What is the average lifetime number of cigars smoked per day?
- What is the average lifetime amount of pipe tobacco smoked per day?
- Pack-years of cigarettes smoked (average packs per day times number of years smoked) may be calculated, but as the only data recorded, this provides insufficient information.

a rough estimate of whether a patient is a light, medium, or heavy smoker.

Alcohol Use, Illicit Drugs, Sexual Preference

A detailed review of the use of alcoholic beverages should be routine because of the association of alcohol abuse and anaerobic, gram-negative, and other pulmonary infections (Fig. 11), as well as tuberculosis. Inquiry regarding the use of illicit drugs is essential; intravenous drug use is associated with septic pulmonary emboli, bacterial endocarditis, and human immunodeficiency virus (HIV) infection. A sexual history should be obtained. Male homosexuality, frequent use of prostitutes, anal intercourse by women, and heterosexual intercourse with intravenous drug users are risk factors for HIV infection and AIDS, with its panoply of unusual lung diseases (Fig. 12).

Medical Drug Use

A detailed record should be made of all drugs that have been taken for medical use, whether purchased over-the-

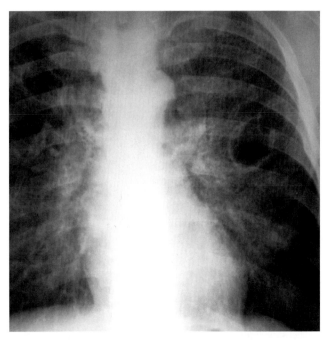

FIG. 12. The classic radiographic appearance of *Pneumocystis carinii* infection in an immunocompromised patient is that of hazy perihilar infiltrates, although the range is broad, from normal-appearing lungs to lobar consolidation. Parenchymal cystic and thin-walled cavitary changes have been associated with *Pneumocystis* infections, typically in the upper lobes. Two such cysts are evident in the left upper lobe of this AIDS patient with *P. carinii* infection.

counter or prescribed by a physician. The patient's history of allergic or toxic reactions to drugs should be noted. A large number of drug-induced lung diseases have been reported, and these have been summarized in recent reviews and are discussed in Chapter 22. Table 7 provides a list of the most common drug-induced pulmonary diseases.

Occupational History

The relationship of lung disease to occupation is not always clear. Current symptoms may be work-related. The patient may suggest the relationship or may answer affirmatively when asked the simple question of whether respiratory symptoms are worse at work. Support for the suspected relationship is provided if other workers at the same workplace have similar symptoms. Some disorders, like byssinosis (Chapter 35), are worse on the day of return to work after a weekend at home. Other disorders, such as air flow obstruction caused by diisocyanates, improve during weekends or vacations. The connection between occupational exposure and lung disease is much less evident when there is a long latent period between the onset of exposure and the appearance of symptoms (Figs. 13 and 14). The only way of knowing whether to consider seriously the diagnosis of an occupational

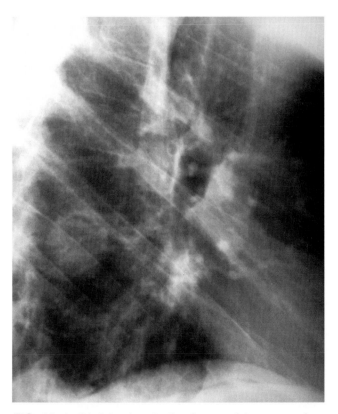

FIG. 11. In this lateral projection from an intravenous drug abuser, an abscess with a small air-fluid level is observed in the posterior segment of the lower lobe; additional parenchymal abscesses were seen elsewhere on other views. Lung abscesses associated with intravenous drug abuse or indwelling catheters tend to be smaller than those seen with underlying pneumonias; they also tend to be multiple and form cavities. In addition, abscesses in intravenous drugs abusers tend to demonstrate relatively rapid growth and cavitation.

TABLE 7. *Drug-induced pulmonary diseases*[a]

Parenchymal reactions
Pulmonary edema
  Aspirin, heroin, methadone, propoxyphen
Interstitial pneumonia
  Nitrofurantoin, gold salts, sulfasalazine
  Cytotoxic agents
    Alkylating agents: busulfan, cyclophosphamide,
      chlorambucil, melphalan
    Antibiotics: bleomycin, mitomycin
    Antimetabolites: methotrexate, azathioprine
    Nitrosoureas: BCNU (bischloroethylnitrosourea)
Pulmonary infiltrates with eosinophila
  Nitrofurantoin, methotrexate, penicillin, and many others
Diffuse interstitial lipidosis
  Amiodarone

Airways reactions
Chronic cough
  Angiotensin-converting enzyme inhibitors
Asthma
  Aspirin, nonsteroidal anti-inflammatory agents,
    β-adrenergic antagonists
Obliterative bronchiolitis
  D-penicillamine (treatment of rheumatoid disease and
    eosinophilic faciitis)

Pleural reactions
Drug-induced systemic lupus erythematosus
  Hydralazine, procainamide, isoniazid, phenytoin,
    D-penicillamine, and many others
Pleural effusion
  Dantrolene, and in association with parenchymal
    disease, busulfan, nitrofurantoin, amiodarone, and
    many others

Opportunistic infections
  Corticosteroids, cytotoxic agents

  [a] A partial listing.

pulmonary disease is to obtain an occupational history in systematic fashion.

All jobs (part-time and full-time) should be listed chronologically, with exact dates recorded if possible. Exactly what jobs were performed and what activity each entailed should be determined exactly—not just the name given to the job. Materials used should be identified, with the appropriate government agency called if necessary to determine the constituents of a substance with a brand name. The physician should obtain general estimates of the intensity of exposure and calculate a rough duration of exposure, should ask whether protective measures were used or recommended, and should inquire about ventilation in the plant. The interval between the start of the job and the beginning of symptoms should be determined. The physician should ask about examinations offered by the industry, such as chest radiograms. The environmental history should be completed with questions about exposures during hobbies or home activities, the presence of pets, use of humidifiers, and the geographic history.

PHYSICAL EXAMINATION

Inspection

Inspection is performed while the history is taken. It will be evident whether the patient is debilitated and chronically ill or presents the appearance of good health. It will also be evident whether the patient is dyspneic at rest, is cyanotic, or has a gross chest wall deformity. It is easy to see whether respirations are shallow or deep, slow or fast, but it is notoriously difficult to assess the

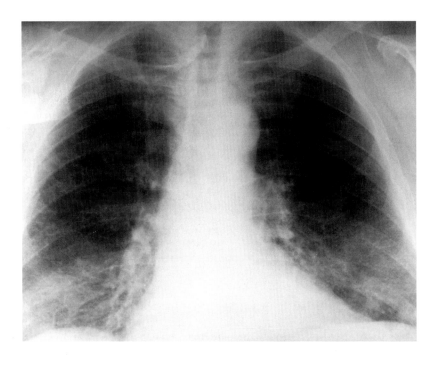

FIG. 13. The fine reticular pattern of asbestosis almost invariably tends to involve the lower lobes bilaterally. As the disease progresses, silhouetting of the diaphragm or cardiac borders by the interstitial lung disease may occur, and the appearance may be indistinguishable from that of idiopathic pulmonary fibrosis (Fig. 24). It is common to see either parenchymal asbestosis or asbestos-related pleural plaques; less commonly, both may be seen in the same patient.

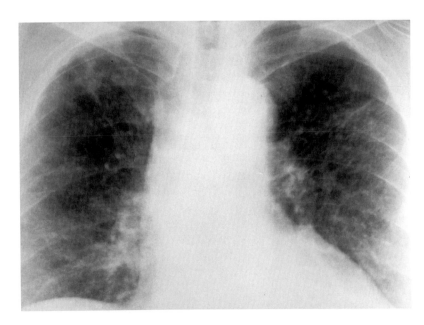

FIG. 14. Characteristic findings of silicosis are demonstrated throughout both lungs of this sandblaster: diffuse, small, scattered nodules, some calcified, with a slightly greater density in the upper lobes. In addition, a dense opacity has formed in the right upper lobe, representing a cicatrized conglomerate of multiple individual nodules. Secondary distortion and irregular contours of the hila are apparent.

effects of an altered breathing pattern on the adequacy of alveolar ventilation. The patient with rapid, shallow respirations may appear to be overbreathing when in fact dead space ventilation is excessive and alveolar ventilation is inadequate. Shallow respirations may be seen with myxedema or raised intracranial pressure; deep respirations are a characteristic feature of metabolic acidosis, as in diabetic ketoacidosis or renal failure.

Flaring of the alae nasi may accompany the rapid respiratory pattern in patients with severe pneumonia. Widespread and severe obstruction of the airways is signaled by noisy breathing and labored expiration, often with pursed-lip breathing and use of accessory muscles of respiration; retraction of the lower interspaces and supraclavicular fossae may be evident during inspiration. Supraclavicular retraction and use of accessory muscles is especially prominent with stridor. Periodic respiration, with intervals of regularly recurring apnea, occurs in cardiac failure, in narcotic and sedative drug overdose, and with increased intracranial pressure. The facial grimacing and sudden cessation of inspiration accompanying pleuritic pain may be dramatic.

Cyanosis

Cyanosis, or blueness of the skin and mucous membranes, is observed when more than 5 g of reduced hemoglobin is present per 100 mL of capillary blood in tissues. Thus, cyanosis may not occur during severe hypoxemia in the presence of anemia and is more evident with erythrocytosis than with a normal level of hemoglobin. Cyanosis may also be associated with methemoglobinemia or sulfhemoglobinemia. Interobserver variability in detecting cyanosis is high unless the arterial oxygen saturation is <85%; thus, cyanosis is an insensitive tool for

detecting hypoxemia. To avoid confusion with cyanosis resulting from venous stasis in cold fingers or toes, it is best to detect cyanosis by observing the tongue and oral mucous membranes. Sweating, coarse tremor, twitching, asterixis, drowsiness, and coma may accompany the hypercapnia that often complicates severe hypoxemia.

Digital Clubbing and Hypertrophic Osteoarthropathy

Digital clubbing may be defined as a focal enlargement of the subcutaneous tissue in the terminal phalanges of the digits, especially the dorsal surfaces; the mechanism is unknown. With rare exceptions, the process is bilateral; the toes as well as the fingers may be involved. Clubbing of the digits, although a most important finding in lung disease, is not specific for pulmonary disease and may be seen in inflammatory bowel disease, hepatic cirrhosis, congenital cyanotic heart disease, and bacterial endocarditis, and as a familial occurrence. Clubbing in pulmonary disease is most frequently found in association with neoplasms, particularly bronchogenic carcinoma, but may also be seen with mesothelioma and Hodgkin's disease. Clubbing can develop rapidly with suppurative lung disease, such as lung abscess; it is common with bronchiectasis and in cystic fibrosis of the pancreas. Clubbing is observed in about 15% of patients with interstitial lung disease and in patients with arteriovenous fistula of the lung. Among the pneumoconioses, clubbing is particularly prevalent in asbestosis.

Digital clubbing is almost never seen in tuberculosis unless the disease is complicated by suppurative bronchiectasis or is a complication of cyanotic congenital heart disease. Clubbing is not observed with chronic bronchitis and emphysema, and its occurrence with either condition should raise the possibility of complicating bronchogenic carcinoma.

In hypertrophic osteoarthropathy (HOA), periosteal new bone forms over the bones of the distal arms and legs, sometimes accompanied by symmetric arthritic changes involving the ankles, knees, wrists, and elbows. There may be thickening of the skin of the distal third of the arms and legs and, rarely, facial thickening. Digital clubbing is almost invariably also present, and there may be neurovascular changes of the hands and feet. The mechanism of HOA, like that of clubbing, is unknown. HOA is always associated with some underlying disease, most often an intrathoracic neoplasm, especially bronchogenic carcinoma; it may be seen with suppurative lung diseases. When joint involvement is prominent, a mistaken diagnosis of arthritis may be made.

The diagnosis of clubbing is made entirely from physical examination. The soft tissues at the base of the nail are spongier than normal. The hyponychial angle, the angle between the dorsum of the distal phalanx and a line connecting the cuticle and the hyponychium, is greater than the normal 195°. Mild clubbing may be difficult to recognize. As the process increases in severity, the shape of the distal digit is changed, with dorsal-palmar or side-to-side thickening. It is important not to confuse filbert nails (increased supero-inferior curvature of the nails) with clubbing. The absence of a spongy nail bed and a normal hyponychial angle are the clues to correct diagnosis. Radiographs of the distal bones of the leg and arm may reveal periosteal formation of new bone that is characteristic of HOA (Fig. 15).

Thorax

Inspection of the thorax is best carried out during the early part of the physical examination, with the patient sitting or standing, although the recumbent position is just as satisfactory for studying the patient's anterior aspect. Minor asymmetry of the thorax is common. In the defect known as *pectus excavatum,* the lower two thirds of the sternum is markedly depressed behind the frontal plane of the thorax. Other variants of this condition are horizontal grooves in the lower anterior thorax on one or both sides; similar horizontal grooves may remain after rickets in childhood. With pigeon breast (pectus carinatum), there is abnormal protrusion of the sternum anteriorly, especially in its upper part. This deformity may be idiopathic or may be acquired during childhood, most commonly as a result of chronic pulmonary overdistension in asthma or of severe cardiomegaly (Fig. 16).

The presence of thoracic kyphosis or kyphoscoliosis and swellings of the chest wall may be observed. These may denote the presence of an inflammatory process, such as a cold abscess, a tumor of the subcutaneous tissue or chest wall, or a necessitating empyema. Patients with an increase in anteroposterior diameter (e.g., with thoracic

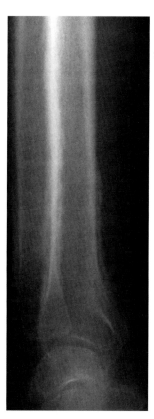

FIG. 15. Hypertrophic pulmonary osteoarthropathy typically involves the diaphyses and metaphyses of tubular bones of the extremities, often in a symmetric manner. In this patient with lung cancer, extensive periosteal new bone is evident along the cortical margins of the distal tibia and fibula.

kyphosis) need not have air flow obstruction. The increase in anteroposterior diameter often observed in emphysema is caused by an increase in functional residual capacity and total lung capacity.

As the chest is observed during respiration, a decrease or lag in motion on one side of the thorax may indicate the presence of underlying disease. Similarly, a flattening or drawing in of the chest, normally best observed in the supraclavicular fossae, may indicate the presence of an underlying fibrosing process. Differences in the two pectoral muscles (the right pectoral muscle may be larger in right-handed people) should be recognized and should not be confused with disease in the underlying lung. A completely immobile thorax is seen in ankylosing spondylitis with fusion of the costovertebral joints, or, rarely, in patients with severe bilateral pleural disease. The scars of an empyema drainage or thoracotomy should be noted. Engorged veins over the thorax and neck may be present in patients with superior vena caval obstruction. It should be remembered that expiratory filling of the neck veins is often seen in expiratory airways obstruction.

Palpation

Asymmetry or a decrease in movements that is suspected during inspiration may be confirmed by palpation

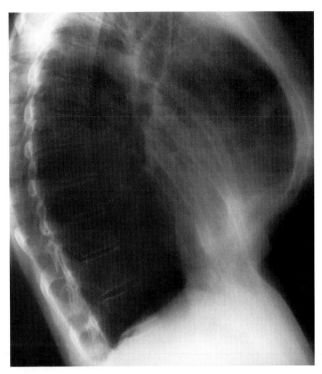

FIG. 16. In this lateral view of a patient with severe pectus excavatum, the heart is displaced posteriorly and superiorly by the lower sternum and xiphoid process. This deformity can cause silhouetting of the heart borders on the corresponding posteroanterior view, and it should not be mistaken for middle lobe or lingular disease. The normal downward slope of the ribs is accentuated as they bend toward their articulations with the sternum.

of the thorax. The location and nature of the apical cardiac impulse should be determined; lateral shifts of the apical impulse along with lateral displacement of the trachea are the main physical signs of a shift of the mediastinum from its usual midline position. The finding of a right ventricular lift at the end of systole, felt in the left parasternal area, denotes the presence of right ventricular hypertrophy. Palpable pulmonic valve closure should be looked for as an additional sign of pulmonary hypertension.

The transmission of the vibrations of the spoken voice to the chest wall (vocal fremitus) may be palpated. The intensity of vibration is increased with an increase in the loudness of the voice and a decrease in the pitch of the syllables used; hence, the common command to the patient to say ''99'' in a loud voice. As these vibrations are generally bilaterally asymmetric, being more intense over the right hemithorax than the left, it may be difficult to assess the significance of slight increases or decreases in vocal fremitus. However, it is usually easy to be certain of the complete absence of vibration. This denotes the presence of non-air-containing material in the thorax, such as fluid, that is totally absorbing the vibrations. Some degree of fremitus often persists with air in the pleural space, except when the pneumothorax is complete.

Percussion

The sound produced by percussion is determined by the combination of the sound made as the striking finger hits the pleximeter finger and the vibrations coming from the chest wall and the structures underlying it. Percussion over normally aerated lung produces vibrations that are maximal in the range of the natural frequency of the thorax (about 140 Hz in the average young adult man). When the lung is consolidated or the pleural space is filled with fluid, the percussion note is impaired. Relatively few added vibrations come from the underlying solid material, and the low-intensity, relatively high-pitched percussion note is predominantly caused by the sound of impact. A similar percussion note is generated by percussing over the liver. Percussion over an air-containing structure, such as a gas-filled stomach, tends to produce a louder note with a more musical quality (about 180 Hz with a harmonic at 360 Hz) than that produced by percussing over an aerated lung. Such a note is referred to as *tympanitic.*

Percussion is also useful for identifying the interface between the lung and solid structures. The interface between lung and liver, the outer margins of cardiac dullness, and the positions of the diaphragm may be readily determined. In identifying such an interface, a light, rapid percussion stroke should be used, and the pleximeter finger should be moved back and forth rapidly until the interface between normal and decreased percussion notes is accurately identified.

The exact characteristics of the percussion note vary over different parts of the thorax, depending on whether percussion is being carried out over chest wall covered only by subcutaneous tissue and skin, or whether muscles also cover the area. It should be recognized that even with the most vigorous percussion blow, vibrations do not come from a depth of more than 5 cm beneath the surface. It is not possible from percussion alone to differentiate between pleural fibrosis, pleural fluid, and pulmonary consolidation. When percussing over lung, it is generally sufficient to describe the percussion note as normal, dull, or absent. Hyperresonance may be found over a tension pneumothorax.

Auscultation

Careful clinical observations coupled with knowledge of lung physiology and the application of modern electronic technology have resulted in the development of new information regarding the genesis of the normal and adventitious sounds coming from the lungs. Recent reviews summarize much of this new information.

Sound Generation

The spectrum of normal hearing is 16 to 16,000 Hz, and most chest sounds are in the lower range of this spectrum (<1000 Hz), where the sensitivity of hearing is low. The intensity of a sound is determined by the amplitude of the vibrations, the distance the sound must travel, the medium through which the sound travels, and the amount of sound absorbed during the transit. The quality or timbre of a sound is determined by its harmonics or overtones and depends on the sound generator; we have no difficulty identifying whether the same note is played on an oboe, a violin, or a piano.

Sounds generated by the vibrations of gas bubbles in a liquid stream are termed *cavitation noise;* this mechanism may be involved in production of crackles. Sounds are also generated by complex turbulence when gas flows past a pole or a wire, through a tube into a cavity, or exits from a narrow nozzle. Flow visualization in models and casts of airways suggests that sounds are generated as gas develops turbulent flow just distal to the spurs or carinae of bifurcations in large and small airways.

The intensity of the sound generated in the airways, vibrations set up in airway walls, the direction of transmission of the sound, the nature of the material through which the sound is transmitted, the selective absorption of some sound frequencies but not others, and the reflection of sound from air-fluid interfaces all influence the characteristics of the sound detected through the stethoscope on the surface of the chest. The rate of sound transmission through lung tissue is 30 to 60 m/s, compared with 1530 m/s through soft tissue and 1600 to 1800 m/s through bone.

Breath Sounds

Auscultation over the normal lung (Fig. 17) reveals sounds having a murmuring quality; these vesicular or normal breath sounds contain a spectrum of frequencies between 100 and 500 Hz, with maximal intensity below 200 Hz. The sounds increase rapidly in intensity during inspiration, with no pause as expiratory sound begins. A rapid fall-off in intensity occurs during expiration, with little sound heard during the latter two thirds of expiration.

Auscultation over the trachea (Fig. 18) reveals a harsh, strident sound with almost equal intensity throughout inspiration and expiration, but with a distinct pause between the inspiratory and expiratory phase. Tracheal sounds contain frequencies up to about 1200 Hz, with loudest components below 900 Hz. Bronchovesicular breath sounds have features of tracheal and vesicular breath sounds; the sounds generated are harsher than vesicular sounds, are heard throughout expiration, and are similar in quality during the two phases of respiration. These sounds are normally heard only in the right infraclavicular region and posteriorly between the scapulae. There is much individual variation in the character of normal breath sounds, although they are constant in any one individual. The bronchial component is generally more evident in thin people.

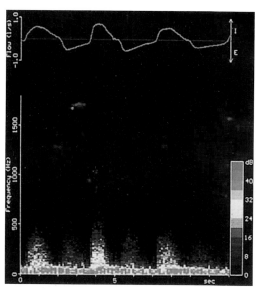

FIG. 17. Normal vesicular breath sounds. Sound spectrogram with simultaneous pneumotachogram (*top*); sound frequency in hertz (Hz) is represented on the ordinate, time (s) on the abscissa; colors designate sound intensity in decibels (dB) on the scale (*lower right*). Recorded over the left posterior lung base in a 13-year-old boy with cystic fibrosis. Note that inspiratory breath sounds are louder than expiratory sounds and that there is no pause between the respiratory phases. The frequencies are virtually all below 500 Hz and are most intense below 250 Hz. Contributions of low-frequency muscle and cardiovascular sound are visible. (Reproduced from Pasterkamp H. *R.A.L.E. Computer-Aided Instruction in Chest Auscultation with Digital Audio Presentation of Lung Sounds.* Winnipeg, Manitoba, Canada: PixSoft; 1990.) *See color plate 4.*

Calculations based on the size of the peripheral airways and the physics of gas flow in tubes show that air flow is laminar in the airways beyond the terminal bronchioles. Laminar air flow in small tubes does not produce sound. A widely accepted formulation is that the sounds heard over the periphery of the lungs are generated by turbulent air flow in the trachea and large bronchi. The sound travels at first through the gas contained in the large bronchi, but as the sound passes peripherally, airway caliber becomes too small for its transmission, and the sound energy is transmitted through lung tissue. The lung behaves as a band-pass filter, with a steep roll-off of frequencies above 200 Hz. Put differently, tracheal sounds are relatively rich in high frequencies. High-frequency absorption is characteristic of lung parenchyma; vesicular sounds that have passed through the most parenchyma have the smallest high-frequency component.

Consolidation of lung tissue (Fig. 19) with continued patency of the main bronchi results in the transmission of sounds from the large airways to the periphery with little change in their character. The sounds are similar to those heard over the cervical trachea and are termed *tubular* or *bronchial.*

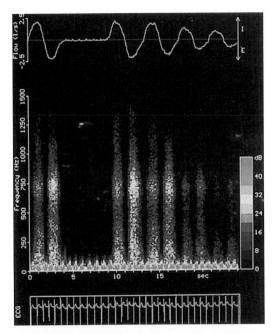

FIG. 18. Normal tracheal breath sounds. Sound spectrogram as described in Fig. 17, but with simultaneously recorded electrocardiogram (*bottom*). Recorded over the trachea at the suprasternal notch in a healthy, 26-year-old, male nonsmoker. The typical features of normal tracheal sounds are evident, with a broad frequency distribution, extending close to 1500 Hz during both inspiration and expiration, a slightly louder expiration, and a clear break (absence of respiratory sound) between the respiratory phases. During 5 seconds of breath holding and zero air flow, the contribution of low-frequency cardiovascular sounds becomes evident. The electrocardiogram helps to identify the high-intensity, low-frequency heart sounds. The dependence of sound intensity on air flow is obvious during the latter parts of this observation, when the subject was breathing more shallowly. (Reproduced from Pasterkamp H. *R.A.L.E. Computer-Aided Instruction in Chest Auscultation with Digital Audio Presentation of Lung Sounds.* Winnipeg, Manitoba, Canada: PixSoft; 1990.) *See color plate 6.*

Fluid, air, or scar tissue in the pleural space forms a sound barrier that diminishes the transmission of breath sounds, either because of altered absorption of sound, reflection at the lung pleural interface, or, in the case of pneumothorax, increasing acoustic mismatching of chest wall and underlying air. If the layer of fluid or scar tissue is thick enough, the sounds are absent. Some transmission of breath sounds through a pneumothorax persists except when the collection of air is large. Sounds of higher frequencies may pass through a thin layer of fluid, which gives the breath sounds at the upper borders of a large pleural effusion a bronchovesicular quality. Consolidation of lung tissue with accompanying occlusion of the segmental or lobar bronchi also results in a complete sound barrier, with obliteration of normal breath sounds. Similar principles govern the transmission of the whispered and spoken voice to the surface of the chest.

Spoken Voice

Recordings of the spoken vowels *E* and *A* over the periphery of the chest disclose that *E* results in lower-pitched vibrations reaching the periphery than is true for *A*. Sound recordings over consolidated lung tissue or over a thin layer of fluid reveal selective transmission of the vibrations from the *E*, with attenuation of the lower harmonics and increased transmission of the higher harmonics. The transmitted sound has both the recorded and spoken characteristics of an *A*, a phenomenon referred to as *E-to-A change* or *egophony.*

Whispered Voice

A similar phenomenon gives rise to increased transmission of the whispered voice, a finding termed *whispered pectoriloquy.* The whispered words ''one, two, three'' are normally heard over the periphery of the normal lung as three ill-defined murmuring or rushing sounds. However, the syllables are clearly identifiable when the transmitted whispered voice is heard over consolidated lung with pa-

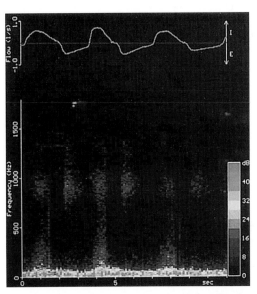

FIG. 19. Bronchial breath sounds. Sound spectrogram as described in Fig. 17, simultaneously recorded over the corresponding site on the right posterior lung base in the same patient as in Fig. 17. Pneumonia and consolidation of the right lower lobe were present, and bronchial breathing is evident. In comparison with the left side (Fig. 17), there is a decrease in intensity of breath sounds but an increase in high-frequency components extending above 1000 Hz. This is most evident during expiration; in contrast to the normal left side (Fig. 17), expiratory breath sounds are louder than inspiratory breath sounds. Contributions of low-frequency muscle and cardiovascular sound are visible. (Reproduced from Pasterkamp H. *R.A.L.E. Computer-Aided Instruction in Chest Auscultation with Digital Audio Presentation of Lung Sounds.* Winnipeg, Manitoba, Canada: PixSoft; 1990.) *See color plate 5.*

tent bronchi. Recordings show a marked increase in the intensity of sound transmitted between 200 and 600 Hz over consolidated lung, in contradistinction to the sharp cutoff of frequencies above 200 Hz in recordings made over a normal lung.

Adventitious Sounds

The adjective *adventitious* is reserved for sounds heard only in disease states. In recent years, a consensus has been reached that adventitious sounds arising from the lungs can be classified into continuous and discontinuous sounds. Continuous sounds are usually louder than the accompanying breath sounds, with a duration longer than 250 ms. Discontinuous sounds are explosive sounds, with a duration shorter than 20 ms. First described by Laennec, these sounds have been given a plethora of confusing names through the years by various authors. In the 1970s, the American Thoracic Society agreed on the terminology shown in Table 8.

Wheezes and Rhonchi

Wheezes and rhonchi are sounds whose duration is 250 ms or more. Wheezes have a hissing or less often a musical character. Their dominant frequency is 400 Hz; when wheezes are musical, harmonics of a relatively constant frequency of up to about 1000 Hz are generated. Rhonchi

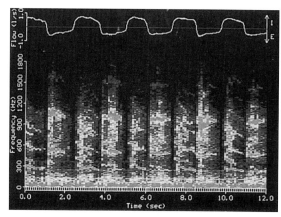

FIG. 20. Tracheal breath sounds in a patient with exercise-induced asthma. Sound spectrogram as described in Fig. 17. Polyphonic wheezing is present during both inspiration and expiration, seen as broad bands of intense sound with a narrow distribution of frequencies. Contributions of low-frequency muscle and cardiovascular sound are visible. (Reproduced from Pasterkamp H. *R.A.L.E. Computer-Aided Instruction in Chest Auscultation with Digital Audio Presentation of Lung Sounds.* Winnipeg, Manitoba, Canada: PixSoft; 1990.) *See color plate 7.*

are lower-pitched, with frequencies predominantly below 200 Hz (Figs. 20 and 21).

The best model for wheezes is thought to be sounds generated by uncoupled reeds, such as those of the oboe or clarinet. A disease process narrows the bronchus; as gas flows rapidly through the narrow region, the pressure falls because of the Venturi effect. Further narrowing occurs, almost to the point of closure, and opposite walls oscillate between the closed and nearly opened positions

TABLE 8. *Classification of common lung sounds*

Acoustic characteristics	American Thoracic Society nomenclature	Common synonyms
Discontinuous, interrupted sounds; loud, low in pitch	Coarse crackle	Coarse rale
Discontinuous, interrupted, explosive sounds; less loud, shorter in duration, and higher in pitch than coarse crackle	Fine crackle	Fine rale
Continuous sounds longer than 250 ms; high-pitched; dominant frequency 400 Hz or more; a hissing or musical sound	Wheeze	Sibilant rhonchus
Continuous sounds longer than 250 ms; low-pitched; dominant frequency about 200 Hz or less; a snoring sound	Rhonchus	Sonorous rhonchus

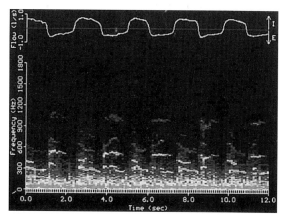

FIG. 21. Pulmonary breath sounds with wheezes. Sound spectrogram as described in Fig. 17. Sounds recorded over the right infraclavicular region in the same patient as in Fig. 20. Inspiratory and expiratory wheezes are seen as broad bands of intense sound with a narrow distribution of frequencies. The intensity of sound is less than in Fig. 20 and no sounds have frequencies higher than 900 Hz. (Reproduced from Pasterkamp H, et al. Digital respirosonography. *Chest* 1989;96:1405.) *See color plate 8.*

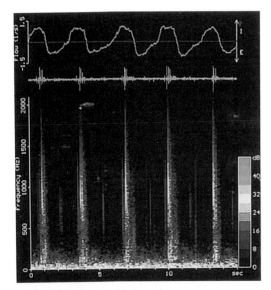

FIG. 22. Mid to late fine inspiratory crackles in a 60-year-old man with interstitial pulmonary fibrosis. These were recorded over the right posterior lung base. The broad frequency distribution is typical for fine crackles (coarse crackles would be contained largely below 1000 Hz). There are a few expiratory crackles as well. (Reproduced from Pasterkamp H. *R.A.L.E. Computer-Aided Instruction in Chest Auscultation with Digital Audio Presentation of Lung Sounds.* Winnipeg, Manitoba, Canada: PixSoft; 1990.) *See color plate 9.*

as air moves through, thus generating a sound. This mechanism of sound generation in collapsible tubes is known as *flutter*. The pitch of the note is determined by the tightness of the closure and by the mass and elastic properties of the solid structures set into vibration. The pitch of the sound is not affected by the length of the column of air in the airway. Thus, a high-pitched sound may be generated by marked narrowing of a main bronchus, as by tumor or fibrous stenosis, and a sound of similar pitch may also be generated from an orifice of comparable diameter in a small airway. Detailed reviews of the mechanism of wheeze generation have been published.

Wheezes vary widely in pitch, depending on the exact character of the narrowing in the bronchus. The bronchial obstruction that produces a wheeze may be caused by secretion, by an inflammatory or other structural change, or by dynamic compression of the airway. Because the airways narrow during expiration, wheezes are more frequent during expiration than inspiration.

Based on their time of appearance during forced respiration, wheezes may also be classified into one of two categories: random onset and simultaneous onset. Random-onset wheezes may be single or multiple, may be inspiratory or expiratory in timing, and may start and end at different times. The pitch of the sounds may vary considerably. The wheezes of asthma are an excellent example. Simultaneous-onset wheezes are expiratory sounds composed of several harmonically unrelated musical notes that tend to start and end simultaneously and

are generated during forced expiration in all types of chronic air flow obstruction. A large number of distant, high-pitched, piping wheezes become audible suddenly during a forced expiration, presumably as the equal pressure point migrates peripherally and sounds are simultaneously generated from dynamically compressed airways.

Simultaneous-onset wheezes can often be produced by normal persons performing a forced expiratory effort. The sound produced in normal persons occurs only during very severe effort, tends to be relatively low in intensity, and occurs only toward the end of expiration; with experience, the physician can learn from the amount of effort used whether the simultaneous-onset wheeze indicates disease or is a normal phenomenon. Random-onset wheezes may, of course, be heard in obstructive airways disease before the sudden onset of simultaneous-onset wheezing; they are never heard in normal persons. Simultaneous-onset wheezes may be the only wheezes heard in patients having severe obstructive air flow disease with scanty secretions.

Crackles

Crackles are short sequences of sound with a duration shorter than 20 ms and usually shorter than 10 ms. They range from one to 20 cycles; usually no more than five cycles exceed the noise level in the recording (Figs. 22 and 23). Crackles may be few in number or may occur as showers, so close together that the individual sounds

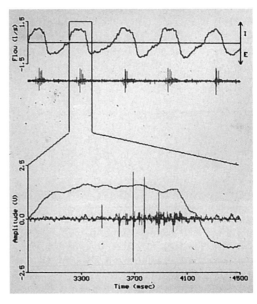

FIG. 23. The upper two records are the same as in Fig. 22. One expiration and a small part of the adjacent inspiration are shown on an expanded time-based display. The mid to late crackles are well shown. (Reproduced from Pasterkamp H. *R.A.L.E. Computer-Aided Instruction in Chest Auscultation with Digital Audio Presentation of Lung Sounds.* Winnipeg, Manitoba, Canada: PixSoft; 1990.) *See color plate 10.*

almost merge. Crackles occur during both inspiration and expiration, but they are more intense and more frequent during inspiration. The number of crackles heard tends to increase with increasing depth of respiration.

The words *fine, medium, coarse, wet,* and *dry* are often used by physicians to describe crackles but are not useful in distinguishing between disease categories. If the only information available is the character of the crackles, one cannot tell pulmonary edema from bronchopneumonia. There seems to be little purpose in dividing crackles into categories other than coarse and fine (Table 8). A recent study has confirmed the distinguishing characteristics of the fine crackles of interstitial lung disease in comparison with the coarse crackles of bronchiectasis, COPD, and congestive heart failure.

The mechanism of production of crackles is still unclear. They may be caused by air bubbling through secretions or by the sudden opening of a succession of small airways, with rapid equalization of pressures causing a series of implosive sound waves. In pneumonia and pulmonary edema, surfactant integrity is affected and respiratory air spaces readily collapse. In diffuse interstitial pulmonary fibrosis, thickening and distortion of the alveolar walls also result in instability of the air spaces, causing them to collapse during ordinary expiration, with the generation of crackles on the succeeding inspiration. Each collapsed respiratory air space opens suddenly at about the same lung volume in successive breaths as opening pressure is reached (Figs. 22 and 23).

In elderly patients without apparent lung disease, it is not uncommon to auscultate crackles at the lung bases that disappear as several deep breaths are taken. These are known as *atelectatic crackles.* Their likely mechanism is loss of surfactant with air space collapse. They disappear with successive deep breaths as surfactant is replenished and air space stability is restored. These crackles can be induced at the lung bases of normal young persons by having them breathe at low lung volume, especially if they breathe 100% oxygen, which washes out the nitrogen from the lungs and accentuates microatelectasis.

Crackles may be absent during ordinary respiration and become audible only during the deep inspiration that follows a cough or when the physician listens over the dependent lung with the patient in lateral recumbency. When the clinician must listen to a patient in lateral recumbency, it is important to remember that air motion is relatively smaller in the uppermost than in the lowermost lung. Thus, if the diseased lung is uppermost, the degree of expansion may not be sufficient to reach the critical opening pressure of the respiratory air spaces and thus generate crackles. On the other hand, when the same lung is listened to in the nether position, the increased proportion of ventilation going to that lung may generate crackles or wheezes. The same rationale applies in the evaluation of a patient who has symptoms of lung disease but negative findings on chest roentgenogram and no obvious findings when examined in the sitting position. The patient should be listened to in both lateral recumbent positions during ordinary and forced expiration, as well as in the upright position.

Showers of fine, mid to late inspiratory crackles are heard at the lung bases in interstitial lung diseases. These crackles ("velcro" crackles) sound like a velcro fastener being opened; they have a recurrent rhythm characterized by similar spacing and relative loudness. Fine crackles with these characteristics are heard in about 60% of patients with various forms of chronic interstitial pulmonary fibrosis but are heard in only about 20% of those with sarcoidosis and other granulomatous lung diseases. The fine crackles of interstitial lung disease appear to correlate with the pathologic severity of the disease, the evidence of radiographic honeycombing, and the severity of the physiologic abnormality (Fig. 24). Scanty expiratory crackles are also audible in interstitial lung disease.

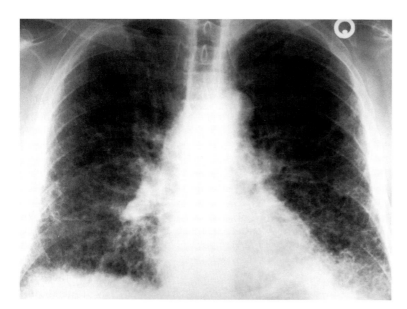

FIG. 24. Honeycombing is present, predominantly at the lung bases, in this case of severe interstitial pulmonary fibrosis. Note that fibrosis is so severe that the margins of the chest wall, diaphragm, and mediastinum are all rendered indistinct and shaggy. Early findings of interstitial pulmonary fibrosis may be seen on high-resolution chest CT before becoming visible on standard chest radiographs.

Crackles are heard in many lung disorders characterized by parenchymal disease: congestive heart failure, pneumonia, bronchiectasis, and cystic fibrosis. Crackles are also frequently heard early in inspiration in patients with chronic obstructive lung disease. These inspiratory crackles are coarse, loud, scanty, audible at the mouth as well as over the chest, and often associated with a few late-expiratory crackles. They are believed to be generated by air flowing through an airway intermittently occluded by mucus or a poorly supported bronchial wall.

Quiet breathing in normal persons is a virtually silent phenomenon, but in many patients with chronic bronchitis or an exacerbation of asthma, a noise is generated during inspiration that is audible with the naked ear at a distance from the mouth. A physician can often assess the presence of airways obstruction when noisy breathing is heard while speaking with the patient on the telephone.

Pleural Friction Rub

Pleural friction rubs are sounds heard over areas where roughened visceral and parietal pleurae rub over each other during respiration. The cause of the roughening is usually a fibrinous or organizing exudate. The characteristic grating or creaking sound is usually loudest at the end of inspiration, but a rub may be heard during both phases of respiration. Pleural friction rubs vary greatly from breath to breath and may be heard only during a deep respiration. They are usually most evident over the lower lateral and anterior thorax, because this is the location of greatest chest wall motion. Very loud rubs may produce palpable vibrations. Pleural friction rubs are usually readily identified, but it may sometimes be difficult to differentiate them from muscle sounds or from very coarse crackles.

Mediastinal Crunch

Mediastinal crunch is a series of crackles that are synchronous with the heartbeat and audible even when the breath is held. These crackles are produced by air in the areolar tissues of the mediastinum. The sound is often accentuated in left lateral recumbency. Mediastinal crunch is usually more sensitive than the chest roentgenogram in detecting mediastinal emphysema, but roentgenographic signs may precede mediastinal crunch when the air collects predominantly in the posterior mediastinum.

Adventitious Sounds Originating in the Chest Wall

Crackling sounds are produced when hair is trapped between the skin and stethoscope. Although these sounds may simulate crackles coming from the underlying lung, they tend to be closer to the ear and, with experience, are usually easily recognized. Firmer application of the stethoscope or wetting the skin stops them. Low-pitched rumbling, muffled, distant, sometimes roaring sounds may be heard during contraction of chest wall muscles. Muscle sounds may be varied by changing the patient's position. They often occur in a chilly or nervous patient who is shivering and are usually easily distinguished from crackles, which are higher-pitched and more discrete.

COMMON PULMONARY SYNDROMES

Pneumonia

The findings of parenchymal consolidation with patent bronchi vary depending on the completeness and extent of disease (Fig. 25). Chest wall motion, as determined by inspection and palpation, ranges from normal to impaired. Similarly, the percussion note ranges from normal to impaired. When consolidation is complete, the breath sounds heard over the periphery have a tubular quality, the spoken voice is increased in intensity, E-to-A change is present, and the syllables of the whispered voice can be clearly identified. Alterations in breath sounds and in spoken and whispered voice are less striking when the consolidation is patchy. Whispered pectoriloquy often gives a clear indication of the presence of consolidation, even when it is difficult to be certain of the significance of a slightly increased harshness and prolonged expiratory phase of the breath sounds. In general, increased transmission of the whispered voice is more easily identified than increased palpable vibration from the spoken voice or the E-to-A change.

In pneumonia, there may be no positive findings on physical examination if the process is interstitial, or if 1 to 2 cm of aerated lung separates the disease process from the chest wall surface. If the consolidated lung lies beneath the structures of the shoulder girdle, lung abnormalities may not be evident, even if the pneumonia extends to the visceral pleura.

When the consolidation is patchy and interspersed with aerated lung tissue, breath sounds and whispered voice sound changes may be minor, and crackles may be the major evidence of parenchymal lung disease. However, it must be stressed that in most instances crackles indicate the presence of parenchymal lung disease without establishing the nature of the process. The presence of crackles in a patient who has had tuberculosis or some other pulmonary problem but who is not acutely or severely ill may merely denote a residuum of the old disease. Conversely, crackles of recent origin or occurring in an acutely and severely ill patient make pneumonia a likely diagnosis.

When pulmonary consolidation is accompanied by an obstructed bronchus, the findings are very similar to those noted in pleural effusion—that is to say, motion of the thorax is decreased, vocal fremitus is absent, percussion

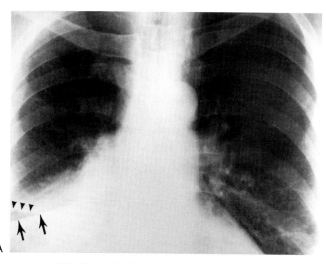

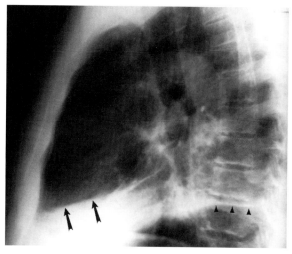

FIG. 25. A,B: Two regions of pneumonia are demonstrated in this patient, one lobar and one segmental. On the frontal view, the upper margin of a right middle lobe pneumonia is sharply demarcated by the minor fissure (*arrows*). More superiorly on the frontal view and posteriorly on the lateral view is a second segmental consolidation, also sharply demarcated inferiorly, in this case by a lower lobe superior accessory fissure (*arrowheads*). These consolidations are quite dense and do not demonstrate air bronchograms.

note is impaired, and breath and whispered voice sounds are absent. The findings are similar in patients with pleural fibrosis, except that there may be a decrease in the size of the ipsilateral hemithorax. With massive pleural effusion, the trachea and lower mediastinum may be shifted to the contralateral side; with pleural or pulmonary fibrosis, the mediastinal shift occurs to the ipsilateral side.

Obstruction of Air Flow

Moderate upper airway obstruction causes a sensation of difficult breathing but may produce few physical findings. As the obstruction becomes high-grade, wheezing and stridor become evident. The history and time course of onset are important. Slow progression in a smoker suggests the possibility of upper respiratory tumor. Sudden onset should raise the possibility of acute infection or aspiration of a foreign body. A history of endotracheal intubation suggests the possibility of tracheal stenosis.

There are few outward manifestations of abnormality in patients with mild air flow obstruction resulting from bronchial and bronchiolar disease or emphysema. In cases of moderate air flow obstruction, when the patient is asked to empty the lungs forcibly and completely, it is evident that expiration is prolonged and difficult, with incomplete pulmonary emptying. The degree of expiratory slowing may be estimated by measuring the forced expiratory time (normally 4 seconds or less) with a watch and a stethoscope. Auscultation over the larynx permits accurate determination of the end of expiration. Sounds are audible at this site at the low air flows occurring near residual volume (Fig. 18), when breath sounds are no longer audible over the lungs. As the process becomes severe, the

patient's distress is evidenced by labored breathing, use of the accessory muscles of respiration, inspiratory retraction of the supraclavicular fossae and lower interspaces, and positioning of the chest near total lung capacity.

Differentiation of air flow obstruction caused by asthma from that caused by chronic bronchitis or emphysema (COPD) depends on the history. Recent acute onset and a history of atopy or recurrent bouts of reversible air flow obstruction support the diagnosis of asthma. Slowly progressive worsening of symptoms, even with recent worsening, suggests COPD. It may not be possible to exclude emphysema with certainty in a chest radiogram taken during a severe asthmatic episode; loss of lung overdistension and attenuation of the vascular pattern in a film taken with the patient in remission establishes the diagnosis. Mild or moderate emphysema is not readily diagnosed in a plain chest radiogram unless bullae are present; CT of the chest is a much more sensitive diagnostic tool, although CT is not indicated for routine diagnostic evaluation.

The key finding of wheezes in chronic air flow obstruction was referred to earlier in the chapter, but it must be remembered that when airways obstruction is very severe, wheezes may completely disappear, along with a marked decrease in the intensity of breath sounds. The velocity of air flow is insufficient to generate sound. The reappearance of wheezes indicates diminished severity of airways obstruction, perhaps in response to treatment.

Pneumothorax

The findings in pneumothorax depend on the size of the pleural air space. Motion may be normal or diminished, fremitus may be decreased to absent, the percussion note is usually normal, and breath and whispered voice sounds are decreased to absent.

Pleural Effusion

The impaired percussion note in pleural effusion extends further paravertebrally and laterally than it does in the midscapular line. This is because no lung is present medially and laterally beneath the percussing fingers, whereas in the scapular line there is just a thin layer of fluid overlying the lung. Breath sounds with a bronchial character and an E-to-A change may frequently be heard over the thin layer of fluid at the upper end of an effusion. This physical finding may be helpful in determining the site for a thoracocentesis. Elevation of the diaphragm, as in ascites, hepatomegaly, or subphrenic abscess, may simulate the findings of a pleural effusion. The chest radiogram is of great help in diagnosing small pleural effusions when physical findings are normal or equivocal. The radiogram is the only way of diagnosing loculated pleural effusions that do not present on the chest wall.

Interstitial Pulmonary Fibrosis

Interstitial pulmonary fibrosis is defined as an inflammatory process of varying etiology involving the respiratory air space walls that is accompanied by varying amounts of fibrosis. Patients may be symptom-free and come to medical attention because of the findings in a chest radiogram. Others are seen with cough, which is usually nonproductive. Yet others seek attention because of effort dyspnea of recent onset. The history may give no hint of etiology. It may suggest the presence of a systemic disease; may reveal prior inhalation of a biologically active dust, such as asbestos or silica; or may reveal that the patient has lived in an area where an infection, such as one of the deep mycoses, is endemic. Alternatively, the patient's lifestyle may raise the possibility of HIV infection or may support a diagnosis of lung disease resulting from the intravenous injection of fibrogenic material, such as talc.

Physical examination usually discloses constant, fine, end-inspiratory crackles, which tend to be most evident at the lung bases. With advanced disease, the chest wall is diminished in volume at full inspiration, there may be right ventricular lift, and the pulmonic second sound may be accentuated, indicating the presence of pulmonary hypertension and right ventricular hypertrophy. The general examination may reveal the stigmata of a systemic disorder, such as rheumatoid disease.

The chest radiogram generally shows a diffuse parenchymal pulmonary infiltrate with a pattern that varies depending on the etiology of the process. When the plain chest radiographic findings are normal, the diagnosis may be supported by pulmonary function tests that show nor-

mal air flow, decreased vital and total lung capacity, deceased carbon monoxide diffusing capacity, and resting hypoxemia without hypercapnia that worsens with exercise. The presence of typical crackles also supports the diagnosis. The greater sensitivity of CT may reveal abnormalities not seen on the plain chest film. It is important when considering the differential diagnosis of the patient with dyspnea and normal parenchyma on CT to keep in mind the relatively rare occurrence of primary pulmonary hypertension. These patients often consult physicians for many months before the cause of their problems is established.

Deep Venous Thrombosis and Pulmonary Embolism

Each year in the United States, about 500,000 episodes of pulmonary embolism occur, which cause about 50,000 deaths. Hence, it is difficult for a practicing general physician or pulmonologist to long escape contact with this ubiquitous disease. Its underlying cause is predominantly deep venous thrombosis, risk factors for which include injury to the pelvis or lower extremities, surgery of the lower extremities, any surgical procedure requiring >30 minutes of general anesthesia, burns, pregnancy and the postpartum state, previous deep venous thrombosis, failure of the right side of the heart, prolonged bed rest, age >70 years, obesity, and use of estrogenic drugs. Deep venous thrombosis and pulmonary embolism should always be considered together. If a pulmonary embolus is suspected, a quest for the source of the embolus must follow immediately; the diagnosis of deep venous thrombosis must immediately raise the question of whether a pulmonary embolus is present.

Neither condition can be diagnosed on purely clinical grounds; deep venous thrombosis is confirmed only about half the time when clinical signs (pain, heat, redness, swelling) are present, and about half the proven incidents of recent-onset deep venous thrombosis are asymptomatic. Contrast venography, impedance plethysmography, and duplex ultrasonography are the three methods currently in use for diagnosing deep venous thrombosis (Chapter 66).

Prospective studies have shown that pulmonary embolism occurs in about 40% of patients with proven deep venous thrombosis. The most common symptoms of acute embolism are dyspnea and palpitations. Hemoptysis and pleuritic chest pain are consequences of infarction, which is an infrequent complication of embolism that occurs 12 to 36 hours after embolism. Angina, syncope, and recent onset of an arrhythmia may also accompany a pulmonary embolus. On examination, tachycardia and tachypnea may be observed. With severe embolism, signs of pulmonary hypertension may be present. The chest radiographic findings are usually normal. Large central emboli may produce enlargement of the hilar pulmonary artery shadow and give rise to peripheral oligemia. Atelectasis, which develops because of decreased surfactant production, may produce a shadow in the chest film. An infarct appears as a pleura-based shadow of any shape and is often accompanied by a pleural effusion.

A negative perfusion scintiscan excludes the diagnosis of pulmonary embolism. Perfusion defects when present are nonspecific. With larger defects, a ventilation scan in which defects match the perfusion is nondiagnostic. If the perfusion defects are well ventilated, the probability of embolus is high and the pulmonary angiogram can be bypassed. The pulmonary angiogram is the definitive test for pulmonary embolism (Chapter 66).

BIBLIOGRAPHY

Billings JA, Stoeckle JD. *The Clinical Encounter: a Guide to the Medical Interview and Case Presentation.* Chicago: Year Book; 1989. *A good review of interview techniques.*

Cahill BC, Ingbar DH. Massive hemoptysis. Assessment and management. *Clin Chest Med* 1994;15:147–167. *A useful review focusing on massive bleeding.*

Goldman L. Using prediction models and cost-effectiveness analysis to improve clinical decisions: emergency department patients with acute chest pain. *Proc Assoc Am Physicians* 1995;107:329–333. *A useful review.*

Irwin RS, Curley FJ. The treatment of cough; a comprehensive review. *Chest* 1991;99:1477. *A comprehensive article by experts in this field.*

Johnson D, Osborne LM. Cough variant asthma: a review of the clinical literature. *J Asthma* 1991;28:85. *A comprehensive review.*

Johnston H, Reisz G. Changing spectrum of hemoptysis; underlying causes in 148 patients undergoing diagnostic flexible fiberoptic bronchoscopy. *Arch Intern Med* 1989;149:1666. *A useful review of all types of hemoptysis.*

Light RW. *Pleural Diseases.* 2nd ed. Philadelphia: Lea & Febiger; 1990. *A helpful resource.*

Mahler DA, ed. *Dyspnea.* Mount Kisco, NY: Futura; 1990. *A comprehensive review.*

Mello CJ, Irwin RS, Curley FJ. Predictive values of the character, timing, and complications of chronic cough in diagnosing its cause. *Arch Intern Med* 1996;156:997–1003. *A comprehensive article by experts in this field.*

Meslier N, Charbonneau G, Racineux JL. Wheezes. *Eur Respir J* 1995; 8:1942–1948. *A useful review.*

Pasterkamp H, Carson C, Daien D, Oh Y. Digital respirosonography. *Chest* 1989;96:1405. *A useful review of digital respirosonography.*

Piirila P, Sovijarvi ARA, Kaisla T, Rajala HM, Katila T. Crackles in patients with fibrosing alveolitis, bronchiectasis, COPD, and heart failure. *Chest* 1991;99:1076. *A useful review.*

Richter JE. Gastroesophageal reflux as a cause of chest pain. *Med Clin North Am* 1991;75:1065. *A helpful review.*

Rosenow EC III, Limper AH. Drug-induced pulmonary disease. *Semin Respir Infect* 1995;10:86–95. *A masterful review.*

Smyrnios NA, Irwin RS, Curley FJ. Chronic cough with a history of excessive sputum production. The spectrum and frequency of causes, key components of the diagnostic evaluation, and outcome of specific therapy. *Chest* 1995;108:991–997. *A comprehensive article by experts in this field.*

Tatum JL, Jesse RL, Nicholson CS, Schmidt KL, Roberts CS, Ornato JP. Comprehensive strategy for the evaluation and triage of the chest pain patient. *Ann Emerg Med* 1997;29:116–125. *Two useful models.*

PULMONARY
PHARMACOLOGY

Textbook of Pulmonary Diseases, 6th ed.
edited by G.L. Baum, J.D. Crapo, B.R. Celli, and J.B. Karlinsky,
Lippincott–Raven Publishers, Philadelphia, © 1998.

CHAPTER

15 Aerosols

Lewis J. Smith

INTRODUCTION

Aerosols are defined as any mixture of solid or liquid particles or droplets that are stable as a suspension in air. They play an important role in respiratory medicine in several different ways. First, some aerosols (e.g., toluene diisocyanate, thermophilic actinomycetes) produce lung disease in susceptible individuals, whereas other aerosols worsen pre-existing disease (e.g., sulfur dioxide or ozone in asthma and chronic bronchitis). Second, aerosols are invaluable in diagnosing and assessing the severity of lung disease (e.g., radiolabeled aerosols to detect pulmonary embolism; aerosols containing methacholine, histamine, or distilled water to determine airway hyperreactivity). Third, they are used to treat an expanding list of lung diseases (e.g., asthma, cystic fibrosis) and to anesthetize the respiratory tract before diagnostic and therapeutic procedures, such as bronchoscopy. Finally, aerosols are used in research to define pathogenic mechanisms in several lung diseases (e.g., produce disease models in animals).

This chapter is designed to provide an overview of aerosols in respiratory medicine, including their physical characteristics and deposition patterns, the devices used to generate aerosols, the role of aerosols in the diagnosis and treatment of lung diseases, the unique features of aerosol delivery during mechanical ventilation, and the determinants of systemic bioavailability from aerosols. Several comprehensive reviews of aerosol generation, deposition, and therapy are available (see reference list) for those interested in more detailed information about this important area.

CHARACTERISTICS OF AEROSOLS

Aerosols are characterized as being of uniform (monodisperse) or varied (heterodisperse) size. Monodisperse aerosols have a geometric standard deviation less than 1.2 (see below). Environmental aerosols and aerosols used in clinical practice are heterodisperse. The range of particle size is wide: aerosols formed as condensation nuclei are usually between 0.001 and 0.1 μm in diameter, those created by cigarette smoke and automobile exhaust are between 0.1 and 1 μm, and aerosols formed by pollens and grinding or mining activity are most typically between 3 and 20 μm in diameter. Therapeutic aerosols tend to be in the 1- to 5-μm range. In general, very small particles are breathed in and out of the lung without being deposited. However, condensation nuclei can grow and coalesce to form particles in the 0.1- to 10-μm size range, which favors deposition in the lung. Large particles (10 μm) characteristically settle out of aerosols, especially if a holding chamber is used, and penetrate poorly into the lung.

Most aerosols generated are heterodisperse. They fit a log-normal distribution in which a plot of particle density (number of particles per given size) versus the logarithm of size yields a bell-shaped normal distribution curve (Fig. 1). The mass median aerodynamic diameter (MMAD) of an aerosol is the aerodynamic diameter around which the mass is centered. It takes into account aspects of particles that are difficult to measure (e.g., shape and density), and it is the key determinant of particle deposition in the lung.

L. J. Smith: Department of Medicine, Pulmonary Division, Northwestern University Medical School, Chicago, Illinois 60611.

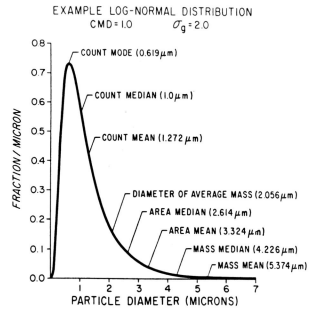

EXAMPLE LOG-NORMAL DISTRIBUTION
CMD = 1.0 σ_g = 2.0

FIG. 1. An example of the log-normal distribution in normalized linear form of aerosol particle sizes for a count median diameter (CMD) equal to 1 μM and a geometric standard deviation equal to 2. Particle density is on the y-axis and particle size is on the x-axis. (Reprinted with permission from *Aerosol Sci* 1971;2:289.)

The aerodynamic diameter (d_a) of a sphere is described as $d_a = d\sqrt{p}$, where d is the physical diameter of the particle and p is its density. The width of the size distribution is represented by the geometric standard deviation (σ_g), which is the ratio of the size below which 84.13% of the mass resides to that below which 50% of the mass resides. Values of σ_g of 1.2 indicate a narrow size distribution and define monodisperse aerosols. Although it is possible to generate aerosols with a narrow size distribution, most therapeutic aerosols have σ_g values of 1.6 to 2.0, indicating a broad size distribution, in which a proportion of the particles will likely not be deposited in the lung.

DEPOSITION OF AEROSOLS IN THE LUNG

The major mechanisms by which aerosols deposit in the lung are inertial impaction, sedimentation, and diffusion. Electrostatic precipitation and interception also play a role, but mostly under select circumstances. A particle deposits by impaction when its inertia is such that it is unable to continue to flow with the air stream as the air stream changes direction. This occurs in the upper airways when the air stream curves sharply in the nose, between the pharynx and the larynx, and in the lower airways at airway bifurcations. The degree of impaction is proportional to d^2Q, where d is the diameter of the particle and Q is the velocity of the air stream. As a result, the number of particles impacting increases with increasing flow rates, with larger particle size, with the acuteness of the angle through which the air stream turns, and with decreasing airway diameter.

Sedimentation is primarily responsible for the deposition of particles that do not impact a surface when entering the lung. Such particles, usually less than 5 μm in size, are subject to gravitational forces based on the square of their diameter. Sedimentation is enhanced by breath holding and slow, steady breathing.

Brownian diffusion is the major mechanism by which particles 0.5 μm in diameter deposit in the lung. These particles deposit in distal, nonairway lung units, and they comprise only a small fraction of the total pulmonary deposition of therapeutic aerosols. Deposition of condensation nuclei in the lung occurs mostly by diffusion.

Most aerosols are charged. As a result, electrostatic precipitation can contribute to the deposition of very small particles in the lung. Electrostatic precipitation may be most significant outside the lung, in that it increases the deposition of therapeutic aerosols in narrow plastic tubes and thereby decreases delivery to the lung, especially when dry powders are inhaled.

Interception occurs when the distance to a surface is less than the diameter of a particle. Its major role is in the deposition of fibers (e.g., fiberglass, asbestos) on airway walls. It is of little importance in the delivery of therapeutic aerosols.

The therapeutic relevance of particle size and its effects on deposition are apparent from reports indicating that for both ipratropium bromide and albuterol, particle sizes ≤2.8 μm provide optimal bronchodilation. Larger particles, which would be expected to exhibit greater upper airway impaction, are less effective.

FACTORS INFLUENCING AEROSOL DEPOSITION IN THE LUNG

For the purpose of describing particle deposition in the lung and the effects of various factors on deposition, the lung can be divided into three compartments: nasopharyngeal, tracheobronchial, and pulmonary. The major determinants of particle deposition are different for each. Inertial impaction is most important in the nasopharyngeal compartment, inertial impaction and sedimentation are both important in the tracheobronchial compartment, and sedimentation and diffusion are important in the pulmonary compartment (Fig. 2).

In addition to particle size, factors that can influence aerosol deposition in the lung include airway geometry, the breathing pattern, and the presence of airway disease. Normal subjects differ widely in airway geometry. In those with smaller conducting airways, central (i.e., tracheobronchial) deposition of aerosols is greater than in those with larger airways. Breathing pattern also can influence deposition. Rapid inspiration and inhalation of an

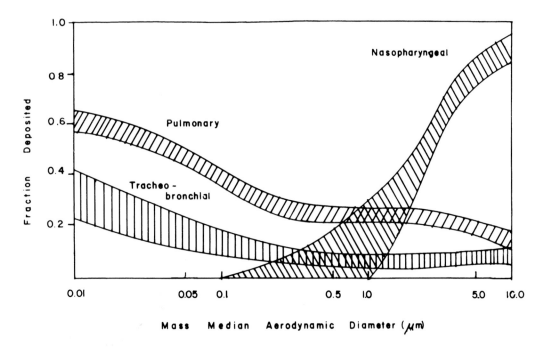

FIG. 2. Particle deposition in the respiratory tract, based on the three-compartment model of the International Committee on Radiation Protection. Each of the *shaded areas* indicates the variability of deposition for a given mass median (aerodynamic) diameter in each compartment when the geometric standard deviation varies from 1.2 to 4.5 and the tidal volume is 1450 mL. (Reprinted with permission from *Health Phys* 1966;12:173.)

aerosol that is injected into the air stream at the middle or end of an inspiration increase central deposition. In contrast, slow inspiration, aerosol inhalation at the beginning of a breath, and a breath hold at the end of inspiration increase peripheral (e.g., pulmonary) deposition. Increased minute ventilation, as occurs during exercise, increases particle deposition in the lung. However, the deposition pattern may be altered by changes associated with the increased minute ventilation, such as greater inspiratory flow rates and decreased ability to humidify the inspired particles fully (reduced hygroscopic growth).

Another factor influencing aerosol deposition is its tonicity. There may be growth or shrinkage of nonisotonic particles as they pass through humidified airways. Obviously, a change in particle size will alter the deposition pattern.

Airway narrowing resulting from any cause affects particle distribution in the lung. As explained above, this has been noted for normal subjects with airways of different sizes, but it is more pronounced in the presence of lung disease. Most diseases are associated with increased airway and decreased pulmonary deposition. For example, the reduced airway caliber of patients with cystic fibrosis enhances delivery to the tracheobronchial compartment by 200%–300%. A similar phenomenon is seen in patients with asthma and chronic obstructive lung disease from other causes.

The changes in deposition pattern produced by disease

and other factors have potential therapeutic and diagnostic implications that may differ depending on the specific drug or chemical administered. For example, the β-adrenergic agonist terbutaline produces an equivalent degree of bronchodilation and improvement in gas exchange regardless of whether it is deposited predominantly in the central airways or in the peripheral airways. In contrast, in patients with asthma, central deposition of methacholine produces a greater degree of bronchoconstriction than does peripheral distribution. Body position may also influence aerosol deposition. The importance of this phenomenon is obvious when aerosolized pentamidine is used to prevent *Pneumocystis carinii* pneumonia in immune-compromised patients. When a patient is in an upright position with a normal breathing pattern, less medication reaches the upper lung zones, and disease preferentially develops there.

Whether breathing is through the mouth or nose is another factor that can influence aerosol deposition. Because of the narrow nasal cross-sectional area (producing a high linear velocity), sharp bends, and hairs, most large particles (10 μm) and a high proportion of soluble gases are removed in the nose. Each of these features favors impaction. In addition, humidification causes growth of hygroscopic particles, further favoring impaction.

Finally, it is important to consider that deposition is different from retention. Retention reflects deposition plus clearance. Clearance mechanisms, including translocation of deposited particles, may have a major effect on the ability of aerosols to cause or treat disease. This concept is discussed in Chapter 2.

AEROSOL-GENERATING DEVICES

A number of inhalational devices are available to produce aerosols of respirable particles. They include pressurized metered-dose inhalers (MDI), nebulizers (jet and ultrasonic), and dry-powder inhalers. Each of these categories comprises several devices with differing characteristics. Production lots of the same device may vary such that particle distribution in the lung and the effects of the material being delivered are altered. When characterizing any aerosol-generating device, it is crucial to differentiate between the "metered" dose, the "delivered" dose, and the "respirable" dose. The metered dose is the dose filling and subsequently emptied from the metering device. The delivered dose is the dose exiting the device. The respirable dose is the dose exiting the device with an aerodynamic diameter of 6 μm or less.

Metered-Dose Inhalers

MDIs have achieved great popularity for the treatment of airways disease. Their advantages are that they are small and convenient to use, and they accurately deliver multiple doses of a drug. The drugs in MDIs are either dissolved or suspended as fine crystals in a liquid propellant mixture—usually chlorofluorocarbons (CFCs). Surfactants are added to increase the stability of the aerosolized suspensions. There are several disadvantages and problems associated with MDIs. One is the use of CFCs as a major component of the propellant. Their adverse impact on the atmosphere has resulted in a worldwide ban that will eventually make these chemicals unavailable for use in MDIs. It is anticipated that other chemicals will be adequate replacements. A second disadvantage is the sensitivity of the MDI to technique (e.g., inspiratory flow rate) and the difficulty some individuals have in coordinating triggering of the device and breathing pattern. If the MDI is triggered well after inspiration has begun, less drug reaches the lung and its distribution is not the same as when triggering occurs early during inspiration. A third problem is the initial rapid velocity imparted to the aerosol as it leaves the device. This can cause discomfort and coughing in some individuals, which may lead to discontinuation of the medication. In addition, a large number of particles deposit in the oropharynx, decreasing the dose available to the lung. It has been estimated that only about 10% of a drug dose is delivered to the lung from MDIs, while 80% or so is deposited in the oropharynx. A less commonly appreciated problem is the effect of environmental temperatures on particle size and therefore lung deposition. Lower temperatures result

in larger particles and decreased lung deposition. Keeping the device in an inside pocket rather than a purse and warming it in the hand before using it out of doors in cold weather should minimize this problem.

Several innovations have been devised to deal with some of the problems associated with MDIs. One is a breath-actuated device (Autohaler and others), which triggers the MDI valve at the start of inspiration. Also, initial velocity is lower, so that oropharyngeal deposition is decreased. However, individuals with arthritis or weakness involving the hand muscles may be unable to set the trigger. In addition, the device requires sealing the lips around the mouthpiece. This is at variance with recommendations by manufacturers of other devices that the MDI be placed a few inches outside the open mouth. A second innovation has been spacer devices. They come in a variety of sizes and shapes; costs and convenience also differ. All reduce the need to synchronize triggering of the inhaler with the onset of inspiration, and they decrease oropharyngeal and increase lung deposition. They are of greatest benefit in young children, the elderly, and in anyone inhaling corticosteroids or other medication with the potential for producing adverse events when deposited in the oropharynx.

Nebulizers

Nebulizers (jet, ultrasonic) are effective when high doses of drugs need to be administered. They are also appropriate for infants and young children, who cannot use hand-held devices. Their major advantages are that coordination with the respiratory cycle is not required, and they are effective even when patients have very low inspiratory flow rates. The major disadvantages are their large size and the need for an external power source. Both of these factors limit a patient's mobility.

Jet nebulizers produce an aerosol by moving a blast of air across a narrow nozzle into which liquid has been drawn according to the Bernoulli principle. When the air hits the liquid, small droplets are formed. Because the air stream is curved in the nebulizer before the aerosol exits, larger particles (10 μm) are removed. The distribution of particles generated by a nebulizer and subsequent deposition in the lung depend on the nebulizer (model, lot, and individual unit), the number and size of baffles, the diameter of the exhalation port tubing, the use of vents, gas flow rates, fill volume in the nebulizer reservoir, viscosity and surface tension of the solution, and ambient temperature and humidity. Because of these factors, it is important to know the specific characteristics of the unit being used and to follow the manufacturer's recommendations regarding proper operation carefully.

Ultrasonic nebulizers use a piezoelectric crystal, operating in the range of 1 to 3 MHz, that transforms high-frequency electric oscillations into mechanical oscillations, thereby providing energy for producing an aerosol. Output tends to be greater than from a jet nebulizer, but particle size is usually larger. With both types of nebulizers, much of the drug initially placed in the nebulizer remains there (on the walls) after the treatment is completed. Further, the concentration of the drug being administered may increase during the time the solution is being nebulized.

Dry-Powder Inhalers

Dry-powder inhalers have been available for years. They include the Spinhaler and Rotahaler, used to deliver a single dose of cromolyn sodium, albuterol, or beclomethasone from a capsule; the Diskhaler, which provides several doses of drug from a packet containing individual compartments; and the Turbohaler, which delivers as many doses of drug from a single container as a typical MDI.

The major advantages of dry-powder inhalers are breath actuation, which reduces difficulties with triggering the device at the start of inspiration, and the absence of CFCs. Disadvantages are those associated with any breath-actuated device—variable delivery at very low rates of flow (30 to 60 L/min) and the need to insert the device in the mouth and seal the lips. Nonetheless, these devices are very effective for delivering bronchodilators and corticosteroids to the lungs of patients with airway disease.

AEROSOLS FOR THE DIAGNOSIS AND TREATMENT OF LUNG DISEASE

Aerosols are used to diagnose and help control several lung diseases. The two most frequent and established diagnostic uses are for ventilation scans in suspected pulmonary embolism and for the identification and measurement of the severity of airway reactivity in patients suspected of having asthma. The principles and technical aspects of ventilation lung scanning are found in chapters on pulmonary embolism and ventilation-perfusion lung scan. Airway reactivity to a number of nonspecific (e.g, methacholine, histamine, distilled water) and specific (e.g., antigen) bronchoprovocation agents is determined by administering aerosols containing increasing concentrations of these substances while measuring the effect of each concentration on pulmonary function. The major advantage of performing bronchoprovocation testing with aerosols rather than administering these chemicals systemically is the elimination or reduction in systemic responses. Additional information on bronchoprovocation testing is found in chapters on asthma, airway reactivity, and bronchoprovocation testing.

Aerosols can also be used to measure peripheral airway size, epithelial permeability, regional ventilation, and gas mixing in the lung. For example, peripheral airway

size has been measured using a monodisperse di-2-ethylhexylsebacate aerosol with particles approximately 0.9 μm diameter. The results correlate well with mean lung density derived by chest computed tomography (CT) and with measurements of diffusing capacity and FEV_1. Alveolar epithelial permeability has been measured in numerous research studies using aerosols of technetium Tc99m DTPA (diethylenetriamine penta-acetic acid).

In addition to their value in diagnosing and managing lung disease, aerosols are invaluable for treatment. Saline aerosols are useful to add moisture to the airways to prevent and treat inspissated secretions. A more frequent use is for the delivery of drugs. The advantages of delivering drugs by this route are several. First, high therapeutic concentrations of some drugs can be achieved within the respiratory tract while systemic concentrations remain low and side effects are few. Some examples are aerosolized β_2-adrenergic agonists and corticosteroids for the treatment of asthma, antibiotics such as the aminoglycosides and amphotericin B, chemotherapeutic agents for the treatment of lung cancer, and cyclosporine for the prevention and treatment of lung allograft rejection. Second, aerosol delivery of some soluble and easily absorbed drugs provides a rapid and convenient route to the bloodstream. Atropine, lidocaine, and epinephrine fit into this category. Third, aerosols provide access for some enzymes, other proteins, and chemicals that ordinarily do not have access to the respiratory tract because of size or charge. Recombinant human deoxyribonuclease (DNase) for the treatment of cystic fibrosis, antioxidant enzymes such as catalase and superoxide dismutase, surfactant, and immune modifiers are just a few examples.

AEROSOL DELIVERY DURING MECHANICAL VENTILATION

Inhaled medications, especially bronchodilators such as β_2-adrenergic agonists and anticholinergic agents, are commonly administered to patients receiving mechanical ventilation. However, there is controversy as to the best method of delivery to such patients. For example, it has been reported that delivery of β_2-adrenergic agonists by MDI through a cylindrical chamber is superior to nebulizer delivery under *in vivo* and *in vitro* conditions. In contrast, others have suggested that even large doses of β_2-adrenergic aerosols administered by MDI to ventilated patients fail to have any appreciable physiologic effects, whereas nebulizers produce significant bronchodilation. Recently, studies using *in vitro* models of mechanical ventilation have examined the effect of different jet nebulizers and MDIs with actuator devices on the delivery of albuterol to the lung under various conditions. These studies suggest the following: (1) Adaptors play an important role in the ability of MDIs to deliver albuterol during mechanical ventilation; (2) important technical differences exist between these devices, which when not used properly can influence drug delivery; (3) spacer design is of prime importance for MDI effectiveness; (4) MDI delivery systems may be sensitive to humidification and synchronization with inspiration, such that delivery decreases with increased humidification and with lack of synchronization; and (5) jet nebulizers and MDI/actuator devices deliver comparable amounts of medication, but the latter require more direct therapist time.

It has also been shown that the delivery of an aerosol from an ultrasonic nebulizer during mechanical ventilation is inefficient and influenced by several factors, including the nebulizer used, the amount of solution placed in the nebulizer (more solution in some nebulizers results in a higher percentage of the total volume delivered to the lung), the addition of an aerosol storage chamber (increases delivery), the respiratory rate and minute ventilation (decreasing either one increases aerosol delivery), and inspiratory time (increasing this time increases delivery).

The important message is that under certain circumstances, aerosol drug delivery to patients receiving mechanical ventilation may be considerably less than anticipated. As a result, it may be necessary to give larger-than-usual doses of drug and titrate the dose according to effectiveness and toxicity.

DETERMINANTS OF SYSTEMIC BIOAVAILABILITY

It has been recognized for some time that the administration of certain medications via the airways can produce clinically significant systemic concentrations. Some examples are epinephrine, atropine, and lidocaine. The first two have been administered through endotracheal tubes during cardiopulmonary resuscitation. Systemic lidocaine toxicity with seizures is a serious complication during topical anesthesia for procedures such as bronchoscopy, especially when given to elderly individuals or those with liver disease.

The issue of systemic absorption and bioavailability is also important when drugs are delivered by aerosol to treat lung disease, especially as new inhaler delivery systems are designed to enhance lung deposition. An excellent review of this subject is provided by Lipworth. Systemic bioavailability is a consequence of absorption from the gastrointestinal tract and the lung. The amount of drug reaching the systemic circulation from the gastrointestinal tract depends on the amount deposited and the rate of first-pass metabolism in the liver. The systemic effects of inhaled corticosteroids absorbed from the gut appear to be limited by extensive first-pass metabolism. This has been reported to be 80% for beclomethasone, 89% for budesonide, and 99% for fluticasone. According to studies in which mouth rinsing, gargling, and the ingestion of

charcoal were used to reduce gut absorption, it appears that systemic bioavailability of these three corticosteroids is mainly determined by absorption across the lung vascular bed. A similar conclusion has been reached for the β_2-adrenergic agonist albuterol.

As a result, it should be anticipated that aerosol delivery systems that improve lung deposition will increase lung bioavailability and at the same time enhance systemic absorption. If so, it may be necessary, as more efficient drug delivery systems are developed, to re-examine the amount of medication administered by aerosol to patients with disease.

AEROSOLS IN RESEARCH

Studies have been performed in animals and humans using aerosols to define the role of environmental pollutants in human disease. Several investigators have explored the effects of oxidant and aerosol exposure on healthy subjects and patients with asthma. For example, by using sulfuric acid aerosols to sensitize the airways to ozone, it has been possible to quantify the effects of these pollutants on airway inflammation, physiology, and symptoms. Studies have also been performed with aerosols to test the validity of commonly used tests. One example is the commonly used technique of sputum induction to identify *Pneumocystis carinii* in the lung. Using an aerosol of technetium-labeled human serum albumin to measure lung clearance, it was found that sputum induction with 3% saline solution significantly increases tracheobronchial clearance rates.

In summary, aerosols play a major role in the diagnosis and treatment of lung disease. One can anticipate continued interest in this area, with increased use of aerosols to deliver new pharmacologic agents to treat lung diseases and also to deliver drugs that are rapidly inactivated in the gastrointestinal tract or liver to the systemic circulation, making it possible to bypass the intravenous and subcutaneous routes. However, caution must be exercised when this route of delivery is used, as the epithelium lining the lungs can be easily damaged. The potential local toxicity of agents delivered directly to the lung via aerosol must be considered and care taken to ensure this does not happen during the course of treatment.

BIBLIOGRAPHY

Beinert T, Brand P, Behr J, Vogelmeier C, Heyder J. Peripheral airspace dimensions in patients with COPD. *Chest* 1995;108:998–1003. *Monodisperse di-2-ethylhexylsebacate droplets in nitrogen were used to measure peripheral air space dimensions, and the results were compared with high-resolution CT-derived mean lung density, diffusion capacity, and FEV₁. The authors found good correlations with each of these measurements.*

Brain JD, Valberg PA. Deposition of aerosol in the respiratory tract. *Am Rev Respir Dis* 1979;120:1325–1373. *This concise, well-written overview of aerosols remains remarkably current.*

Collier JG, Dobbs RJ, Williams I. Salbutamol causes a tachycardia due to the inhaled rather than the swallowed fraction. *Br J Clin Pharmacol* 1980;9:273–274. *This brief report demonstrates that the systemic effects of β_2-adrenergic agonists are related to the amount of drug inhaled, not swallowed.*

Conneally E, Cafferkey MT, Daly PA, Keane CT, McCann SR. Nebulized amphotericin B as prophylaxis against invasive aspergillosis in granulocytopenic patients. *Bone Marrow Transplant* 1990;5:403–406. *Fifty milligrams of aerosolized amphotericin B twice daily may reduce the incidence of invasive aspergillosis in neutropenic patients, especially those cared for on open wards.*

Diot P, Morra L, Smaldone GC. Albuterol delivery in a model of mechanical ventilation. *Am J Respir Crit Care Med* 1995;152:1391–1394. *The authors used an in vitro model to compare the efficiency of jet nebulizers and MDIs with that of actuator devices to deliver albuterol in various conditions of mechanical ventilation. Both systems were effective if properly set up and used.*

Dubois J, Bartter T, Gryn J, Pratter MR. The physiological effects of inhaled amphotericin B. *Chest* 1995;108:750–753. *It is possible to give amphotericin B safely by the inhaled route for prophylaxis against fungal pneumonia. However, no information is provided about optimal dose and timing.*

Fuchs HS, Borowitz DS, Christiansen DH, et al. Effects of aerosolized recombinant human DNase on exacerbations of respiratory symptoms and on pulmonary function in patients with cystic fibrosis. *N Engl J Med* 1994;331:637–642. *Regular administration of aerosolized recombinant human DNase reduced respiratory symptoms, resulted in a slight improvement in pulmonary function, and was well tolerated.*

Fuller HD, Dolovich MB, Chambers C, Newhouse MT. Aerosol delivery during mechanical ventilation: a predictive in vitro lung model. *J Aerosol Med* 1992;5:251–259. *Using a lung model, the authors demonstrated that there are marked differences in aerosol delivery between nebulizers and an MDI plus a chamber, with the latter delivering more to the lung.*

Fuller HD, Dolovich MB, Posmituck G, Wong Pack W, Newhouse MT. Pressurized aerosol versus jet aerosol delivery to mechanically ventilated patients. *Am Rev Respir Dis* 1990;141:440–444. *The authors found a significantly greater efficiency of aerosol deposition to the lung in ventilator-dependent patients when an MDI plus aerosol-holding chamber was used than when a jet nebulizer was used.*

Harding SM. The human pharmacology of fluticasone propionate. *Respir Med* 1990;84 (Suppl A):25–29. *This study shows that fluticasone has virtually no oral bioavailability.*

Hickey AJ, Martonen TB. Behavior of hygroscopic pharmaceutical aerosols and the influence of hydrophobic additives. *Pharm Res* 1993;10:1–7. *A review of the important issue of hygroscopic growth of particles and how this can influence deposition.*

Hindle M, Chrystyn H. Relative bioavailability of salbutamol to the lung following inhalation using metered-dose inhalation methods and spacer devices. *Thorax* 1994;49:549–553. *Spacer devices improve pulmonary bioavailability of salbutamol and reduce the amount systemically available.*

Hultquist C, Wollmer PO, Eklundh G, Jonson B. Effect of inhaled terbutaline sulphate in relation to its deposition in the lungs. *Pulm Pharmacol* 1992;5:127–132. *The site of deposition may not be important for the bronchodilator effect of terbutaline.*

Kung M, Croley SW, Phillips BA. Systemic cardiovascular and metabolic effects associated with the inhalation of an increased dose of albuterol. *Chest* 1987;91:382–387. *Mouth rinsing and gargling reduce the total amount of albuterol delivered, but they do not reduce the magnitude of the systemic effects.*

Laube BL, Norman PS, Adams GK. The effect of aerosol distribution on airway responsiveness to inhaled methacholine in patients with asthma. *J Allergy Clin Immunol* 1992;89:510–518. *The bronchoconstrictor response to inhaled methacholine is greater after central rather than peripheral deposition, and increased heterogeneity in aerosol deposition increases airway reactivity to methacholine in patients with asthma.*

Leigh TR, Jones BE, Ryan P, Collins JV. The use of inhaled radioisotopes for measuring the effect of sputum induction on tracheobronchial clearance rates. *Nucl Med Commun* 1994;15:156–160. *The authors used a radiolabeled aerosol to test the effectiveness of a commonly used clinical procedure.*

Lipworth BJ. New perspectives on inhaled drug delivery and systemic bioactivity. *Thorax* 1995;50:105–110. *Well-referenced, clearly written review of the determinants of systemic bioavailability following aerosol delivery of medications. The emphasis is on β-adrenergic agonists and corticosteroids.*

Manthous CA, Hall JB, Schmidt GA, Wood LDH. Metered-dose inhaler versus nebulized albuterol in mechanically ventilated patients. *Am Rev Respir Dis* 1993;148:1567–1570. *Nebulized albuterol provides objective physiologic improvement, whereas albuterol administered by MDI through an adaptor does not. Furthermore, it is proposed that nebulizer treatments should be titrated to higher-than-conventional doses using toxic side effects and physiologic response to guide therapy.*

Martin FE, Harrison C, Tanner RJN. Metabolism of beclomethasone diproprionate by animals and man. *Postgrad Med J* 1975;51(Suppl 4):11–20. *Describes absorption and metabolism of inhaled beclomethasone diproprionate.*

Martonen TB. Mathematical model for the selective deposition of inhaled pharmaceuticals. *J Pharm Sci* 1993;82:1191–1199. *The author proposes a mathematical model to improve efficacy of aerosol therapy.*

Martonen T, Katz I, Cress W. Aerosol deposition as a function of airway disease: cystic fibrosis. *Pharm Res* 1995;12:96–102. *The reduced airway diameter in patients with cystic fibrosis increases the dose delivered to the tracheobronchial compartment by 200%–300%. Also, deposition is increased in more congested airways.*

Mercer TT. The deposition model of the task group on lung dynamic: a comparison with experimental data. *Health Phys* 1975;29:673–680. *The authors relate theoretical models of lung deposition and clearance to recent (at that time) experimental findings.*

Miller FJ, Martonen TB, Menosche MG, Graham RC, Spector DM, Lippmann M. Influence of breathing mode and activity level on the regional deposition of inhaled particles and implications for regulatory standards. In: Dodgson J, McCallum RI, Bailey MR, Fisher DR, eds. *Inhaled Particles.* Oxford: Pergamon Press; 1988:3–7. *Information is provided on how breathing pattern and physical activity affect particle deposition.*

Moren F, Newhouse MT, Dolovich MB. *Aerosols in Medicine: Principles, Diagnosis and Therapy.* New York: Elsevier; 1985. *Excellent monograph on key aspects of medical aerosols. The chapters are written by experts in the field.*

Oberdorster G. Lung clearance of inhaled insoluble and soluble particles. *J Aerosol Med* 1988;1:289–330. *This well-written article focuses on clearance mechanisms rather than deposition.*

O'Riordan TG, Greco MJ, Perry RJ, Smaldone GC. Nebulizer function during mechanical ventilation. *Am Rev Respir Dis* 1992;145:1117–1122. *Using an in vitro model, the authors found that nebulized aerosol delivery during mechanical ventilation is influenced by the type of nebulizer, treatment time, duty cycle, volume fill of the nebulizer, and presence of a humidification device. If these factors are defined, nebulizer systems can efficiently deliver medication to intubated, mechanically ventilated subjects.*

O'Riordan TG, Iacono A, Keenan RJ, Duncan SR, Burckart GJ, Griffith BP, Smaldone GC. Delivery and distribution of aerosolized cyclosporin in lung autograft recipients. *Am J Respir Crit Care Med* 1995;151:516–521. *The authors explored the factors determining the delivery and distribution of aerosolized cyclosporin A in the lungs of patients with severe allograft rejection. There was some relationship to regional ventilation, but a greater relationship to regional perfusion. They conclude that because of the great variability of deposition, direct measurement of regional deposition is necessary in the initial studies of the efficacy of aerosol therapy in these patients.*

Pedersen S, Steffensen G, Ohlsson SV. The influence of orally deposited budesonide after inhalation from a Turbuhaler. *Br J Clin Pharmacol* 1993;36:211–214. *Demonstrates that most of the systemically absorbed budesonide comes from that deposited in the airway.*

Phipps PR, Gonda I, Anderson SD, Bailey D, Bautovich G. Regional deposition of saline aerosols of different tonicity. *Eur Respir J* 1994;7:1392–1394. *The tonicity of aerosols appears to affect their distribution both through physical means (growth or shrinkage of the particles) and physiologic mechanisms (e.g., producing bronchoconstriction).*

Raabe OG. Deposition and clearance of inhaled aerosols. In: Witschi H, Nettesheim P, eds: *Mechanisms in Respiratory Toxicology.* Boca

Raton, FL: CRC Press; 1982:27–76 (vol 1). *Excellent, detailed description on aerosol behavior with extensive reference list.*

Ramsey BW, Dorkin HL, Eisenberg JD, et al. Efficacy of aerosolized tobramycin in patients with cystic fibrosis. *N Engl J Med* 1993;328:1740–1746. *Short-term, aerosolized, high-dose tobramycin is safe and effective in the treatment of patients with cystic fibrosis who have Pseudomonas aeruginosa endobronchial infection.*

Ryrfeldt A, Andersson P, Edsbacker S, Tonnesson M, Davies D, Pauwels R. Pharmacokinetics and metabolism of budesonide, a selective glucocorticoid. *Eur J Respir Dis* 1982;63(Suppl 122):86–95. *Demonstrates high topical potency and rapid metabolism of budesonide.*

Selroos O, Hulme M. Effect of a volumatic spacer and mouth rinsing on systemic absorption of inhaled corticosteroids from a metered-dose inhaler and dry-powder inhaler. *Thorax* 1991;46:891–894. *Illustrates that systemic absorption of corticosteroids inhaled from an MDI is reduced by using a spacer device, and that systemic absorption of corticosteroids inhaled from a dry-powder inhaler is reduced by mouth rinsing.*

Shek PN, Suntres ZE, Brook JO. Liposomes in pulmonary application: physicochemical considerations, pulmonary distribution and antioxidant delivery. *J Drug Target* 1994;2:431–432. *The authors discuss the benefits and problems associated with delivering drugs, in particular antioxidants, to the lung by means of liposome carriers.*

Tatsumura T, Koyama S, Tsujumoto M, Kitagawa M, Kagamimori S. Further study of nebulisation chemotherapy, a new chemotherapeutic method in the treatment of lung carcinomas: fundamental and clinical. *Br J Cancer* 1993;68:1146–1149. *5-Fluorouracil, along with its metabolites, accumulates in the trachea, bronchi, and regional lymph nodes of patients treated before surgery, suggesting that it is directly incorporated and metabolized in the respiratory tract. Also, an antitumor effect without significant adverse effects was found in a select group of patients with lung cancer.*

Thomas SH, O'Doherty MJ, Page CJ, Treacher DF, Nunan TO. Delivery of ultrasonic nebulized aerosols to a lung model during mechanical ventilation. *Am Rev Respir Dis* 1993;148:872–877. *This study, like that of O'Riordan et al., shows that delivery of an aerosol to the lung in mechanically ventilated patients depends on the nebulizer used, respiratory pattern, volume of fluid in the nebulizer, and the presence of a storage chamber.*

Thorsson L, Edsbacker S, Conradson TB. Lung deposition of budesonide from Turbuhaler is twice that from a pressurized metered-dose inhaler. *Eur Respir J* 1994;7:1839–1844. *Both systemic and pulmonary bioavailability of budesonide increases with the Turbuhaler. However, the increase in pulmonary bioavailability is greater than the systemic increase.*

Utell MJ, Frampton MW, Morrow PE, Cox C, Levy PC, Speers DM, Gibb FR. Oxidant and acid aerosol exposure in healthy subjects and subjects with asthma. Part II: Effects of sequential sulfuric acid and ozone exposures on the pulmonary function of healthy subjects and subjects with asthma. *Health Effects Institute* 1994;70:37–93. *This study illustrates how aerosols generated in the laboratory can be used to study the potential adverse health effects of environmental pollutants.*

Vidgren P, Vidgren M, Paronen P, Vainio P, Nuutinen J. Effects of Inspirease holding chamber on the deposition of metered-dose inhalation aerosols. *Eur J Drug Metab Pharmacokinet* 1991;3:419–425. *This spacer device increases deposition in the lung and decreases deposition in the mouth and upper airways.*

Wolff RK, Dorato MA. Toxicology testing of inhaled pharmaceutical aerosols. *Crit Rev Toxicol* 1993;23:343–369. *This review article examines the concept of how to determine if inhaled agents are safe. For example, people generally inhale through the mouth, whereas most laboratory animals inhale primarily through the nose.*

Zanen P, Go TL, Lammers J-WJ. The optimal particle size for parasympathetic aerosols in mild asthmatics. *Int J Pharm* 1995;114:111–115. *The optimal particle size to deliver ipratropium bromide to the lungs of patients with mild asthma was 2.8 μm. These authors previously demonstrated nearly identical findings for albuterol (Int J Pharm 1994;107:211–217).*

Textbook of Pulmonary Diseases, 6th ed.
edited by G.L. Baum, J.D. Crapo, B.R. Celli, and J.B. Karlinsky,
Lippincott–Raven Publishers, Philadelphia, © 1998.

CHAPTER

16

Theophylline and Glucocorticoids

Helen M. Hollingsworth

THEOPHYLLINE

Theophylline, or 1,3-dimethylxanthine, has been used as a bronchodilator in patients with asthma and chronic obstructive pulmonary disease (COPD) for more than 60 years. The specific mechanism of action of theophylline is not well understood, but it likely involves a constellation of effects, including phosphodiesterase inhibition and adenosine antagonism.

Mechanism of Action

Phosphodiesterase inhibitors reduce intracellular degradation of cyclic AMP, thus prolonging the intracellular effects of cyclic AMP: relaxation of bronchial smooth muscle and suppression of mast cell mediator secretion. Theophylline is a weak, nonselective phosphodiesterase inhibitor. In fact, at the usual therapeutic serum concentrations, it inhibits only 10%–20% of phosphodiesterase activity. For this reason, it remains controversial whether the bronchodilator activity of theophylline is predominantly a consequence of phosphodiesterase inhibition.

Another possible mechanism is adenosine inhibition. Adenosine is a naturally occurring purine nucleoside that has been shown to be a bronchoconstrictor in patients with asthma. Local adenosine concentrations increase with methacholine and allergen stimulation, presumably because of mast cell release. Theophylline selectively inhibits adenosine-induced bronchoconstriction at the usual therapeutic concentrations. Evidence against this mechanism is the observation that some methylxanthines that

are clearly active bronchodilators do not antagonize adenosine.

Other possible mechanisms of theophylline-induced bronchodilation include inhibition of the generation of contractile prostaglandins, modulation of intracellular calcium, and increased synergy between phosphodiesterase inhibitors and adenylate cyclase activators (e.g., β-adrenergic agonists).

Role of Theophylline as a Bronchodilator

Theophylline is less potent as a bronchodilator than are inhaled or subcutaneously injected β_2-adrenergic agents. It protects against exercise-induced bronchoconstriction, although it is not as effective as inhaled albuterol in terms of peak effect. On the other hand, sustained-release preparations of theophylline provide a longer duration of action than inhaled β_2-adrenergic agents, except salmeterol. This longer duration of action of 12- and 24-hr sustained-release preparations of theophylline can be helpful for patients with symptoms of nocturnal asthma or COPD.

When added to a regimen of inhaled corticosteroids and β_2-adrenergic agents, theophylline also reduces the frequency and severity of asthma symptoms in patients with moderately severe or severe chronic asthma. An additive, steroid-sparing benefit is seen when theophylline is added to a regimen of alternate-day prednisone or high-dose, daily inhaled beclomethasone.

In the setting of acute severe asthma, data are conflicting regarding the benefit of adding theophylline to the usual emergency regimen of nebulized adrenergic agents. On the other hand, theophylline may be beneficial in patients admitted to the hospital with status asthmaticus. In either situation, the drug should be continued and levels

H. M. Hollingsworth: Pulmonary Center, Boston University School of Medicine, Boston, Massachusetts 02118.

optimized in patients already on maintenance doses of theophylline.

In patients with COPD, even when spirometry findings are not improved, theophylline therapy is associated with a decrease in dyspnea. Theophylline also appears to benefit patients with COPD who are already taking ipratropium bromide and a β-adrenergic agent. Patients who have difficulty inhaling bronchodilator medication, despite education and the use of chamber or spacer devices, may derive greater benefit from orally administered theophylline.

Evidence for Anti-inflammatory Activity

Some patients with asthma experience significant deterioration when theophylline therapy is withdrawn. Because this deterioration appears greater than what would be expected based on the bronchodilating capacity of the drug, it has been hypothesized that theophylline has anti-inflammatory activity.

There is evidence that theophylline has weak anti-inflammatory activity. Although theophylline does not influence the immediate allergic response at moderate serum concentrations, it attenuates the bronchoconstriction associated with the late allergic response, possibly through an inhibitory effect on the cellular infiltration associated with the late-phase allergic response; theophylline reduces the levels of CD4 lymphocytes typically seen during this response. In patients with moderately severe asthma who are taking high-dose inhaled corticosteroids, withdrawal of theophylline results in an increase in CD4 and CD8 cells in the bronchial submucosa that correlates with a decrease in FEV_1 (forced expiratory volume in 1 second). Bronchial biopsy studies have shown a decrease in EG2-positive activated eosinophils immediately below the basement membrane in patients with mild asthma treated with theophylline. On the other hand, theophylline does not affect the increase in peripheral eosinophil counts associated with allergen challenge and does not inhibit allergen-induced increases in airway methacholine responsiveness, all evidence against significant anti-inflammatory activity.

Respiratory Muscle Effects: Force and Endurance

Theophylline has positive inotropic effects on normal diaphragm, but effects are hard to demonstrate if concentrations are in the normal therapeutic range. In patients with COPD, theophylline improves the strength of the fatigued diaphragm and makes the diaphragm more resistant to fatigue. These effects may help patients with asthma or COPD who are being weaned from mechanical ventilation, or are experiencing worsening of air flow obstruction.

Clinical Use

The specific indications for theophylline therapy may be found in Chapters 40 (Bronchial Asthma) and 43 (Clinical Aspects of COPD) of this book, and in recently published guidelines. Because of the narrow toxic-to-therapeutic window, use of this drug requires close attention to dosage, serum levels, and potential interactions with other drugs.

Once the decision has been made to initiate oral theophylline therapy in an adult, the drug should be started at a low dose (12 to 16 mg/kg daily, up to a maximum of 300 to 400 mg/d) and titrated slowly upward. The dose should be decreased if the patient experiences nausea, headache, tachycardia, or other side effects. The final daily regimen should be guided by the degree of symptom control, side effects, and measurement of serum levels; in general, one should aim for a therapeutic serum level of 5 to 20 μg/mL. Therapeutic serum levels should be lower in elderly patients with COPD, may be higher in younger patients with asthma, and should be between 8 and 12 μg/mL in pregnant women. The serum level should be measured about halfway into a dosing interval.

Shorter-acting theophyllines have been largely supplanted by 12- and 24-hr sustained-release preparations. Patients should be instructed to take medication at the same time each day with respect to meals. Theophylline has been used extensively in pregnancy without evidence of adverse effects for the neonatal, but serum levels need to be monitored closely and should not exceed 12 μg/mL.

The main indication for intravenous administration of theophylline is an inability to take oral medication or evidence of impaired gastrointestinal absorption. Otherwise, sustained-release oral preparations provide stable blood levels and are just as effective as systemically administered preparations.

Aminophylline, a salt of theophylline with 80% bioavailability, is frequently used for intravenous therapy. Patients with an adequate serum level on admission who are switched to intravenous therapy do not need a loading dose. If the theophylline level is subtherapeutic, a supplemental loading dose can be given: each milligram of aminophylline per kilogram of body weight will increase the serum concentration by 2 μg/mL. If the outpatient oral dose of theophylline is known, then the dose of aminophylline to be given over 24 hrs as a continuous infusion can be determined by multiplying the total daily dose of theophylline by 1.25. The loading dose for patients not previously on oral therapy is 2.5 to 5.6 mg/kg of lean body weight, given intravenously over 20 to 30 minutes. The usual maintenance dose of aminophylline is 3 to 9 mg/kg/hr.

Another alternative for intravenous use is anhydrous theophylline in 5% dextrose. The usual adult loading dose for this preparation is 5 mg per kilogram of lean body weight, and the usual maintenance dose is 2 to 8 mg/kg/hr.

The maintenance dose of both aminophylline and theophylline should be decreased in older patients, and in those who have liver disease, congestive heart failure, fever, or are taking interacting drugs. Higher initial infusion rates should be used for smokers and children. Daily determinations of serum concentration should guide further dose adjustments.

The theophylline dose should be adjusted during addition or withdrawal of medications that affect theophylline metabolism (Table 1). Because theophylline is metabolized in the liver by the P_{450} system, many medications that are similarly metabolized alter theophylline clearance or are themselves affected by theophylline. When in doubt about a potential drug interaction, it is important to educate patients regarding potential toxicity, to assess theophylline serum levels more frequently, and to consider empiric reductions in the theophylline dose. For instance, the theophylline dose should be reduced by half when patients are taking erythromycin, clarithromycin, quinolone antibiotics, zileuton, or oral contraceptives. Another macrolide antibiotic, azithromycin, is metabolized in the liver, but not by the cytochrome P_{450} enzymes, so adjustments in theophylline dose are not necessary. The theophylline dose should also be reduced by half when maintenance therapy with phenytoin, carbamazepine, or other P_{450} enzyme inducers is discontinued. Amoxicillin, cefaclor, co-trimoxazole, and doxycycline do not appear to interact with theophylline.

Adverse Effects

The most common adverse effects are nausea, abdominal discomfort, vomiting, diarrhea, diuresis, headache, and jitteriness. Side effects tend to increase as the serum level increases but may be seen with low therapeutic levels (5 to 10 μg/mL). Although excessively high serum levels are generally accompanied by nausea and abdominal discomfort, dangerous toxicity can develop in patients without these symptoms. Therefore, monitoring of serum levels is extremely important when therapy is initiated or changed, and then at 6- to 12-month intervals. Signs and symptoms associated with toxic levels include palpitations, premature ventricular contractions, atrial tachyarrhythmias, tremors, seizures, and gastrointestinal bleeding.

Treatment of Theophylline Intoxication

Theophylline poisoning may result from inadvertent iatrogenic overdose, patient error, or suicide attempt. Serious toxicity is associated with levels greater than 30 μg/mL, and serious adverse effects are more likely to be seen at any given blood level in patients with chronic intoxication than with acute overdose. Serum levels correlate poorly with occurrence of life-threatening events. Metabolic disturbances are more common with acute intoxication.

Electrocardiographic and hemodynamic monitoring are vital components of supportive care, because of the risk of cardiac arrhythmias. Sinus tachycardia and atrial and ventricular dysrhythmias are all manifestations of theophylline toxicity. Treatment is recommended only for serious arrhythmias causing unstable hemodynamics. Adenosine, verapamil, and digoxin have been used to treat supraventricular tachyarrhythmias, and lidocaine and phenytoin for ventricular arrhythmias.

Some patients require volume repletion, because of the diuretic effect of theophylline. Metabolic acidosis is common; conservative treatment is advisable. Hypokalemia, caused by hypercatecholemia and intracellular redistribution of potassium, is seen in 30% of patients with chronic intoxication and in 85% of patients with acute overdose. Frequently, potassium levels normalize spontaneously, and vigorous repletion is not necessary.

Seizures are usually treated with diazepam or phenobarbital; phenytoin is not recommended. Refractory status epilepticus may require general anesthesia with pentobarbital or thiopental and paralyzing agents. Prophylactic phenobarbital may be used for patients with serum levels $\geq$50 μg/mL, although this has not be studied in clinical trials.

Prevention of absorption is particularly important, because of the prevalent use of sustained-release theophylline preparations. Stomach emptying is recommended for patients who have ingested a large quantity of a slow-release preparation within 1 hour of seeking medical attention. Otherwise, it is better to inhibit absorption with 50 to 100 g of activated charcoal, given orally with 70%

TABLE 1. *Theophylline drug interactions*

Drugs that decrease theophylline clearance	
Allopurinol	Propofenone
Birth control pills	Propranolol
Calcium channel blockers	Quinolones
Cimetidine	Ranitidine
Clarithromycin	Tacrine
Erythromycin	Thiabendazole
Methotrexate	Troleandomycin
Mexiletine	Zileuton
Drugs that increase theophylline clearance	
Barbiturates	Rifampin
Phenytoin	
Other interactions with theophylline	
Increased lithium clearance	
Increased furosemide diuresis	
Enhanced β-adrenergic effects: "toxic synergism" (e.g., isoproterenol, ephedrine, albuterol)	
In combination with reserpine may result in tachycardia	
Decreased zafirlukast clearance	
In combination with ketamine may lower seizure threshold	
In combination with halothane may cause ventricular arrhythmias	

sorbitol (75 to 100 mL). This therapy enhances theophylline clearance in patients with moderate intoxication, but it should not be administered to patients who have depressed pharyngeal reflexes or are vomiting.

Charcoal hemoperfusion is indicated when the serum level is ≥ 80 μg/mL in acute intoxication; ≥ 60 μg/mL in chronic intoxication; or ≥ 40 μg/mL if the patient is 6 months of age greater than 60 years old, has significant liver or cardiac disease, or cannot tolerate activated charcoal. Hemodialysis doubles theophylline clearance and may be helpful when hemoperfusion is not available. It should be combined with oral activated charcoal therapy. Other modalities, such as peritoneal dialysis, plasmapheresis, and hemofiltration, are unlikely to be beneficial.

GLUCOCORTICOIDS

Glucocorticoids are effective in the treatment of a wide spectrum of pulmonary diseases because of their broad anti-inflammatory activity. Asthma, COPD, sarcoidosis, interstitial fibrosis, hypersensitivity pneumonitis, and bronchiolitis obliterans organizing pneumonia all respond significantly or partially to glucocorticoids. Unfortunately, glucocorticoids also have significant potential side effects that require careful monitoring and patient education. This section focuses on general concepts regarding the mechanisms of action, administration, and adverse effects of systemically administered glucocorticoids.

Mechanisms of Action

Recent research has increased our understanding of the cellular effects of glucocorticoids and provided insight into the reasons why glucocorticoids have such widespread anti-inflammatory effects. Glucocorticoids, when administered orally or intravenously, circulate in the blood either unbound or associated with cortisol-binding globulin. Free glucocorticoid (GC) diffuses into the cytoplasm of cells and binds to glucocorticoid receptors (GR) to form a GC-GR complex.

The GC-GR complex translocates into the cell nucleus and binds to DNA, resulting in either positive or negative modulation of gene transcription. Glucocorticoids also influence posttranscriptional events, such as RNA translation and protein synthesis and secretion (e.g., by altering the stability of certain cytokine messenger RNAs to change the intracellular steady state). Alternatively, the nuclear transcription factors NFκB and AP-1 may bind the GC-GR complex, preventing translocation into the nucleus.

Anti-inflammatory Effects

Glucocorticoids, through their effects on gene transcription and translation in many different cells, inhibit or suppress several steps in the inflammatory process. Glucocorticoids affect lymphocyte cytokine production, distribution, and activation in several ways. They inhibit transcription, directly or indirectly, of many cytokines, including interleukin-1 (IL-1), tumor necrosis factor-α (TNF-α), granulocyte-macrophage colony-stimulating factor (GM-CSF), IL-3, IL-4, IL-5, IL-6, and IL-8. Trafficking of leukocytes to sites of inflammation is diminished by glucocorticoids, because of a redistribution of lymphocytes out of the vascular compartment and a downregulation of adhesion molecules. Production of integrins and selectins is inhibited by glucocorticoids through their effect on IL-1 and TNF-α. Elaboration of vascular cell adhesion molecule-1 is indirectly reduced through the decrease in IL-4 and GM-CSF production. Suppression of IL-2 production is an important effect of glucocorticoids and results in decreased activation and proliferation of lymphocytes. Phospholipase A$_2$ release via the annexin family of proteins, which includes lipocortin-1, is inhibited, leading to decreased production of proinflammatory arachidonic acid metabolites. Fibroblast activity is downregulated, resulting in reduced synthesis and secretion of certain cytokines, collagen, and prostaglandins. Secretion of proinflammatory molecules by mast cells and basophils is suppressed, as is basophil activation and mediator release. Although mast cell mediator release is not directly inhibited, mucosal mast cell numbers are significantly reduced. Eosinophil accumulation at inflammatory sites is decreased, probably because of several glucocorticoid effects: decrease in circulating numbers of eosinophils, inhibition of synthesis of IL-4 and IL-5, inhibition of expression of adhesion molecules, and increased local apoptosis. Microvascular leakage of fluids is also decreased. IgE levels are decreased over time, possibly by immunoglobulin catabolism and inhibition of cytokines (e.g., IL-4) that promote IgE production.

Bronchial biopsy studies in patients with asthma who are taking inhaled budesonide or beclomethasone for 3 to 4 months have revealed a decrease in airway eosinophils, mast cells, and lymphocytes. This effect is not seen with inhaled terbutaline. A similar decrease in inflammatory cells is seen in bronchoalveolar lavage studies.

Clinical Pharmacology

Several different glucocorticoid analogues have been developed for clinical use. These compounds differ in their absorption and distribution characteristics, glucocorticoid receptor-binding affinities, elimination rates, topical versus systemic potencies, and mineralocorticoid activities. The choice of a specific analogue and dose depends on the disease being treated and its severity. These issues are reviewed in the chapters on individual diseases.

Certain general observations can be made about systemic glucocorticoid use. Smaller doses administered more frequently are more immunosuppressive than larger doses administered less frequently. A longer biologic half-life may be preferred to maintain the desired clinical effect through the day. However, when the duration of action extends through the night, the risk for hypothalamic-pituitary-adrenal (HPA) axis suppression and other glucocorticoid-related adverse effects increases. Topical or focal application of glucocorticoids results in less toxicity than systemic administration and is the preferred route of administration presuming the desired clinical affect can be achieved. Thus, airway diseases, such as asthma and COPD, can usually be managed with inhaled glucocorticoids, but pulmonary parenchymal diseases, such as interstitial pulmonary fibrosis, require systemic glucocorticoid therapy.

In balancing the need to suppress disease against the desire to protect the HPA axis, a compromise arrangement is to administer analogues with intermediate biologic half-lives (prednisone and methylprednisolone) in one to three doses during the day and early evening, but not at bedtime. As patients' symptoms improve, doses can be consolidated and reduced in frequency. When the prednisone equivalent dose is at or below 30 mg/d, attempts should be made to switch to an alternate-day dosing regimen to reduce further glucocorticoid-related morbidity and enhance recovery of the HPA axis. After patients have been on systemic glucocorticoid therapy for longer than 3 weeks, the glucocorticoid dose needs to be tapered gradually to allow recovery of the HPA axis; the longer the duration of therapy, the slower the taper.

Timing of the dose of oral glucocorticoids may affect the therapeutic result, especially if the disease exhibits diurnal variation. For instance, patients with asthma tend to have nocturnal symptoms when their disease flares. A late-afternoon dose of prednisone may provide better nocturnal symptom control than the usual morning dose.

Glucocorticoid Preparations

Several glucocorticoids are available in the United States for oral or parenteral use: hydrocortisone, prednisone, methylprednisolone, triamcinolone, dexamethasone, and Celestone. Hydrocortisone (half-life, 1.9 hours) is usually used for physiologic replacement or ''stress'' coverage, because of its rapid onset of action and long history of efficacy. It can be given orally or parenterally. Its mineralocorticoid effects are helpful in patients who need physiologic replacement, but they may be undesirable in patients requiring the medication for immunosuppression or anti-inflammatory activity.

Prednisone is a widely used oral glucocorticoid that is inactive until converted in the liver to prednisolone by reduction at the 11-keto position. Its relative potency is approximately four times that of hydrocortisone.

Methylprednisolone differs from prednisolone in having a methyl group in the 6α position; like prednisolone, it is active without hepatic conversion. The relative potency of methylprednisolone is five times that of hydrocortisone. Its mineralocorticoid effects are slightly less than those of prednisone, and it is available for both oral and intravenous use.

Triamcinolone is essentially devoid of mineralocorticoid activity. It is available as a suspension for intramuscular use. Its potency is about five times that of hydrocortisone. Response among patients is not uniform, but a single parenteral dose four to seven times the oral daily dose controls symptoms for about 4 days up to 4 weeks. Its major role is in treating patients who are noncompliant with oral medications.

Dexamethasone has very little salt-retaining effect, which is beneficial, but its biologic half-life is even longer than that of prednisone or methylprednisolone, increasing its potential to cause morbidity. Its relative potency is about 20 to 25 times that of hydrocortisone.

Celestone is a suspension of betamethasone sodium phosphate and betamethasone acetate available for intramuscular use. The onset of action of the betamethasone esters varies, so a single intramuscular injection may provide prompt as well as sustained glucocorticoid therapy, but this is variable. As with the use of intramuscular triamcinolone, the daily glucocorticoid effect in an individual patient is difficult to titrate. This drug is usually reserved for patients who are not able to take oral glucocorticoid preparations.

Glucocorticoid Resistance

Although glucocorticoids are the most effective anti-asthma medication currently available, some patients with chronic asthma do not experience the expected improvement in symptoms and pulmonary function following oral glucocorticoid administration. This phenomenon of glucocorticoid resistance has been explored most fully in patients with asthma, but it may also pertain in other diseases that can be treated with glucocorticoids.

One definition of glucocorticoid resistance is a lack of improvement of 15% in FEV_1 after 2 weeks of treatment with prednisone at a dose of 20 mg/d, or its equivalent. In addition to failing to show an improvement in respiratory function, some patients are resistant in that they do not exhibit the clinical features of hypercortisolism and their morning cortisol level is normal. These patients usually have familial glucocorticoid resistance, which is associated with normal glucocorticoid receptor binding but low numbers of receptors. Patients with acquired glucocorticoid resistance usually do experience glucocorticoid-induced side effects, including suppression of the morning cortisol level, with high-dose oral glucocorticoids. These patients have normal numbers of glucocorticoid receptors but exhibit decreased glucocorticoid receptor binding.

The first step in evaluating suspected glucocorticoid resistance is to determine whether the patient is adhering to the recommended dosing schedule and whether persistence of asthma triggers in the environment are responsible for the lack of response. Once these have been excluded, the most common cause for apparent glucocorticoid resistance is severe airway inflammation that ultimately requires higher corticosteroid doses over a more prolonged period. Other possible explanations would be decreased absorption or impaired metabolism of the active moiety.

In patients who have refractory asthma, the absorption and clearance of orally administered glucocorticoids should be assessed by measuring peak and trough blood levels of the specific glucocorticoid administered (available only in specialized laboratories), in addition to morning cortisol and total eosinophil levels. Enhanced plasma clearance of prednisolone or methylprednisolone has not been demonstrated to occur except in the presence of medications that enhance cytochrome P_{450} metabolism.

Another possible explanation for a lack of response to prednisone is a problem with the conversion of prednisone into biologically active prednisolone in the liver. This may be tested by administering methylprednisolone at a dose that is 80% of the usual prednisone dose and repeating spirometry after 2 weeks. If the problem is hepatic conversion of prednisone, the patient's symptoms will improve on methylprednisolone. Additionally, the total eosinophil count can be measured and compared during the two regimens.

Patients with familial glucocorticoid resistance, a rare autosomal dominant disorder with variable penetrance, have high circulating levels of cortisol and adrenocorticotropic hormone. These patients may also demonstrate signs and symptoms of excessive levels of nonglucocorticoid adrenal hormones (e.g., hypertension, hirsutism, menstrual irregularities, hyperkalemia). Measurement of endogenous cortisol levels helps to identify these rare patients. Referral to a specialized center for assessment of the cellular response to glucocorticoids may be necessary to complete the evaluation.

The treatment of glucocorticoid resistance depends on the exact mechanism (acquired or familial) and the degree of resistance. Conventional therapies, such as theophylline, salmeterol, terbutaline, ipratropium, nedocromil, or cromolyn, should be optimized in patients with asthma, while remembering that only the latter two medications have significant anti-inflammatory activity.

Steroid-sparing and other immunomodulatory therapies, such as methotrexate, cyclosporine A, intravenous immunoglobulin, and gold salts, may be considered, but studies have not shown dramatic responses in asthma. The 5-lipoxygenase inhibitor, zileuton, and the leukotriene receptor antagonist, zafirlukast, have recently been released and may be helpful in these patients. Another strategy is to try an alternate glucocorticoid analogue, such as oral methylprednisolone or triamcinolone, instead of prednisone. Ongoing, uncontrolled inflammation will likely require a course of high-dose, possibly intravenous, glucocorticoid therapy. Subsequently, the patient's glucocorticoid sensitivity is usually improved and the glucocorticoid dose can then be tapered.

Complications of Glucocorticoid Therapy

Oral glucocorticoid therapy is frequently associated with side effects that tend to become more serious and more prevalent as the dose and duration of therapy increase. Certain adverse effects, such as insomnia, emotional lability, increased appetite, and weight gain, are characteristically observed early in therapy. Insomnia can be decreased by consolidating most or all of the glucocorticoid dose to the early morning. Patient education and reassurance help with emotional instability, but serous problems in the face of an ongoing need for glucocorticoid therapy may require psychiatric assistance. Nutritional counseling helps to offset weight gain.

HPA axis suppression is to be expected when systemic therapy lasts longer than 3 weeks. After this time, steroid therapy needs to be tapered; the longer the duration of therapy, the slower the taper. The rate of tapering depends on the disease activity and the rate of adrenal recovery. When the dose of prednisone has been 30 mg/d for several weeks, a decrease in the daily dose of 10 mg every 1 to 3 weeks is usually acceptable. If the daily dose has been 20 mg, the decreases may be 5 mg every 1 to 3 weeks. With a daily dose of 10 mg, the incremental decreases may need to be 1 to 2 mg. When systemic glucocorticoid therapy is discontinued, a stimulation test with cosyntropin (Cortrosyn) can be used to determine whether the HPA axis has recovered.

Stress glucocorticoid coverage should be administered for 1 year after completion of systemic glucocorticoid therapy. Patients on high-dose inhaled glucocorticoids should also receive stress coverage during acute illnesses. Despite laboratory evidence of significant adrenal suppression with chronic glucocorticoid therapy, serious, clinically significant adverse events resulting from iatrogenic adrenal suppression are very rare.

Elevations in serum glucose are common during glucocorticoid therapy, but only in patients with underlying glucose intolerance. Patients need to be educated about signs and symptoms of hyperglycemia, and those who already require oral hypoglycemic agents or insulin should have frequent blood glucose determinations. Hypertension and acne usually occur in patients who have other underlying risk factors. Likewise, the risk for peptic ulcer disease appears to be more related to coexistent risk factors, such as nonsteroidal anti-inflammatory therapy.

The relative risk for infectious complications related to steroid therapy is about twice that of controls and varies according to the type of disease being treated, as well as the duration and intensity of therapy. The most common infectious side effect is oropharyngeal thrush, typically associated with inhaled steroids but also seen with oral steroid use, particularly when accompanied by antibiotic therapy. Patients who have never had varicella are at increased risk for generalized varicella and should receive hyperimmune immunoglobulin should they be exposed to someone with active varicella. Patients with a varicella skin rash should be treated with oral or intravenous acyclovir.

A controversial question has been whether all patients with a positive tuberculin skin test (purified protein derivative or PPD) who require glucocorticoid therapy should receive prophylaxis with isoniazid, assuming they have never previously received treatment. The current practice guideline is not to give isoniazid to patients who require intermittent steroid bursts for asthma. On the other hand, patients who require long-term glucocorticoid therapy should receive prophylactic isoniazid, barring other contraindications.

Steroids cause bone loss by decreasing the intestinal absorption and increasing the renal secretion of calcium. These changes in calcium metabolism result in lowering of serum calcium levels, which induces secretion of parathyroid hormone to facilitate resorption of calcium from bones. In a study of patients with asthma, long-term steroid treatment resulted in trabecular, but not cortical, bone loss, a pattern consistent with osteoporosis.

A reasonable strategy for patients receiving short, intermittent courses of oral glucocorticoid or high-dose inhaled glucocorticoid is to recommend that they ingest the recommended daily amounts of calcium (1500 mg in adults) and vitamin D for their age and follow a regimen of daily weight-bearing exercise for 30 to 60 min.

When patients begin long-term glucocorticoid therapy, it is important to assess the presence of other modifiable risk factors for osteoporosis, such as a sedentary lifestyle, menopause, overreplacement of thyroid hormone, and cigarette smoking. Sex hormones should be replaced if deficient. Bone density measurement of the hip and lumbar spine should be performed at baseline. If baseline bone density is adequate, primary prevention is accomplished by maintaining a daily calcium intake of 1500 mg/d through diet or supplements, and supplementing the dietary intake of vitamin D with 800 IU of vitamin D/day or 0.5 μg of calcitriol (1,25-dihydroxycholecalciferol) per day. Vitamin D supplementation maybe associated with hypercalcemia and hypercalciuria. It is recommended that serum and urinary calcium levels be measured 1 month into therapy. A low dose of a thiazide diuretic and sodium restriction can be initiated if the 24-hour urinary calcium excretion is 300 mg/d. Calcium and calcitriol supplementation may also need to be decreased. Six to 12 months after initiation of glucocorticoid therapy, a repeated bone density measurement will reveal whether this initial strategy has been successful, or whether further intervention is needed. If baseline bone density is low, consideration should be given to starting hormone replacement therapy, a bisphosphonate, or calcitonin. At this point, consultation with a rheumatologist or endocrinologist would be appropriate.

Osteonecrosis (avascular necrosis) of bone is a known complication of systemic glucocorticoid therapy, although the exact mechanism is not understood. Typically, it occurs in patients on long-term glucocorticoid therapy, but it has been described with short-term, high-dose therapy. The joints most commonly affected are the hips, knees, and shoulders. When the area involved is small, treatment can be conservative, with avoidance of weight-bearing activity and relief of pain using nonsteroidal anti-inflammatory agents or other analgesics. More severe cases require bone grafting or joint replacement.

Cataract development related to glucocorticoid administration is usually associated with higher doses and longer duration of therapy. Intraocular pressures should be monitored in patients on long-term systemic glucocorticoid therapy, because of the increased risk for glaucoma.

Steroid-induced myopathy is also associated with higher doses and longer duration of therapy. It may be a cause of diminishing exercise tolerance in the face of stable spirometry and usually improves as steroids are tapered.

Long-term systemic use of glucocorticoids in children may result in growth retardation. Studies are ongoing as to whether inhaled glucocorticoids alone have a significant effect on growth.

Relatively few adverse drug interactions have been described in association with glucocorticoid use. Phenobarbital, phenytoin, and carbamazepine increase cytochrome P_{450} activity, thereby reducing the effectiveness of prednisolone, methylprednisolone, and dexamethasone. Erythromycin and ketoconazole impair prednisolone and methylprednisolone elimination. Rifampin decreases the effectiveness of prednisolone and methylprednisolone. Cimetidine does not interact with prednisolone, methylprednisolone, or dexamethasone, but antacids decrease the bioavailability of prednisolone. Although there is no direct drug interaction, patients receiving insulin or oral hypoglycemic agents for glucose intolerance will likely need dose adjustments as glucocorticoid therapy is added or tapered.

BIBLIOGRAPHY

Allen DB, Mullen ML, Mullen B. A meta-analysis of the effect of oral and inhaled corticosteroids on growth. *J Allergy Clin Immunol* 1994; 93:967–976. *This meta-analysis of the effect of inhaled beclomethasone and prednisone on growth found no statistical evidence for growth impairment with even high daily doses of beclomethasone.*

Alvarez J, Surs W, Leung DYM, et al. Steroid-resistant asthma: immunologic and pharmacologic features. *J Allergy Clin Immunol* 1992; 89:714–721. *Mitogen-induced stimulation of peripheral blood mono-*

nuclear cells from steroid-sensitive asthmatic patients is inhibited in vitro by methylprednisolone, but not mitogen-induced stimulation of peripheral blood mononuclear cells from steroid-resistant asthmatic patients. Addition of troleandomycin appears to restore in vitro sensitivity to methylprednisolone.

American College of Rheumatology Task Force on Osteoporosis Guidelines. Recommendations for the prevention and treatment of glucocorticoid-induced osteoporosis. *Arthritis Rheum* 1996;39:1791–1801. *Recommendations for the prevention and treatment of glucocorticoid-induced osteoporosis in patients receiving glucocorticoid therapy for rheumatologic disease. The recommendations are probably also applicable to patients with pulmonary disease.*

ATS Statement. Standards for the diagnosis and care of patients with chronic obstructive pulmonary disease. *Am J Respir Crit Care Med* 1995;152:S77–S120. *Excellent overall reference on management of COPD, with special sections reviewing the role of theophylline in inpatient and outpatient management of COPD.*

Aubier M. Effect of theophylline on diaphragmatic and other skeletal function. *J Allergy Clin Immunol* 1986;78:787–792. *This study in normal subjects showed a 15% increase in diaphragmatic force (Pdi/Edi) after an infusion of 6 mg of aminophylline per kilogram of body weight.*

Barnes PJ, Greening AP, Crompton GK. Glucocorticoid resistance in asthma. *Am Rev Respir Dis* 1995;152:S125–S142. *Report of international workshop on familial and acquired forms of glucocorticoid resistance in asthma, with an excellent summary of molecular mechanisms of normal glucocorticoid response and possible mechanisms of glucocorticoid resistance.*

Beam WR, Weiner DE, Martin RJ. Timing of prednisone and alterations of airways inflammation in nocturnal asthma. *Am Rev Respir Dis* 1992;146:1524–1530. *A study of 10 asthmatic patients with nocturnal symptoms, comparing the effects of a single 50-mg dose of prednisone at 0800, 1500, and 2000 hours on morning FEV$_1$, morning levels of peripheral blood eosinophils, and bronchoalveolar lavage cell populations.*

Boumpas DT, Chrousos GP, Wilder RL, Cupps TR, Balow JE. Glucocorticoid therapy for immune-mediated diseases: basic and clinical correlates. *Ann Intern Med* 1993;119:1198–1208. *NIH conference report with excellent review of anti-inflammatory and immunosuppressive effects of glucocorticoids, in addition to a discussion of glucocorticoid adverse effects.*

Chrousos GP, Detera-Wadleigh SD, Karl M. Syndromes of glucocorticoid resistance. *Ann Intern Med* 1993;119:1113–1124. *NIH conference report on the pathophysiology, molecular mechanisms, evaluation, and management of familial glucocorticoid resistance.*

Cockcroft DW, Murdock KY, Gore BP, O'Byrne PM, Manning P. Theophylline does not inhibit allergen-induced increase in airway responsiveness to methacholine. *J Allergy Clin Immunol* 1989;83:913–920. *Sustained-release theophylline, given to six patients with atopic asthma, increased baseline PC20-methacholine and significantly reduced the early, but not the late, fall in FEV$_1$ following allergen challenge. The allergen-induced decrease in PC20-methacholine was not inhibited by theophylline but was inhibited by pretreatment with cromolyn. This raises doubt that theophylline has significant anti-inflammatory effect.*

Essayan DM, Lichtenstein LM. Phosphodiesterase inhibitors: yesterday, today and tomorrow. *Insights in Allergy* 1994;9:1–12. *Good discussion of the five classes of phosphodiesterase inhibitors, including theophylline, with regard to biochemistry and pharmacotherapy.*

Gaudreault P, Guay J. Theophylline poisoning: pharmacological considerations and clinical management. *Med Toxicol* 1986;1:169. *Discussion of theophylline elimination rates with recommended specific guidelines for charcoal hemoperfusion.*

Goldberg MJ, Park GD, Berlinger WG. Treatment of theophylline intoxication. *J Allergy Clin Immunol* 1986;78:811–817. *Strong recommendation for serial administration of activated charcoal for enhancement of theophylline elimination.*

Granneman GR, Braeckman RA, Locke CS, et al. Effect of zileuton on theophylline pharmacokinetics. *Clin Pharmakokinet* 1995;29:77–83. *Study showing that coadministration of zileuton and theophylline does raise theophylline serum levels.*

Huang D, O'Brien RG, Harman E, et al. Does aminophylline benefit adults admitted to the hospital for an acute exacerbation of asthma? *Ann Intern Med* 1993;119:1155–1160. *Examines benefit of intravenous aminophylline in 21 adult patients admitted to the hospital for asthma exacerbations. Patients in the aminophylline group required fewer albuterol nebulizer treatments and had a higher FEV$_1$ at 48 hours.*

Ip M, Lam K, Yam L, et al. Decreased bone mineral density in premenopausal asthma patients receiving long-term inhaled steroids. *Chest* 1994;105:1722–1727. *Study of the effect of inhaled glucocorticoids with or without intranasal glucocorticoids on bone mineral density in 30 asthmatic patients. The average daily dose of budesonide/beclomethasone was 1000 µg. Bone density of the femur and lumbar spine was decreased in female patients compared with healthy controls.*

Jenne JW. Two new roles for theophylline in the asthmatic? *J Asthma* 1995;32:89–95. *Raises possibility that theophylline still has a role in asthma, because of evidence for anti-inflammatory effects and role in preventing respiratory muscle fatigue.*

Jonasson S, Kjartansson G, Gislason D, et al. Comparison of the oral and intravenous routes for treating asthma with methylprednisolone and theophylline. *Chest* 1988;94:723–726. *Randomized but not blinded study of 28 patients admitted to the hospital with exacerbations of obstructive airways disease who received intravenous or oral methylprednisolone and aminophylline. Use of β-adrenergic agents was not controlled. No difference was found in terms of symptom improvement. If anything, the FEV$_1$ showed a greater increase in the oral medication group.*

Karpel JP, Kotch A, Zinny M, et al. A comparison of inhaled ipratropium, oral theophylline plus inhaled β-agonist, and the combination of all three in patients with COPD. *Chest* 1994;105:1089–1094. *Study showing an advantage to adding theophylline to a stable regimen of ipratropium bromide and albuterol.*

Larochelle GE, et al. Recovery of the hypothalamic-pituitary-adrenal (HPA) axis in patients with rheumatic diseases receiving low-dose prednisone. *Am J Med* 1993;95:258–264. *A study of rapid ACTH stimulation test responses in 44 rheumatology patients taking 5 mg of prednisone per day, showing spontaneous recovery of HPA axis function to normal or near normal levels. Recovery of HPA axis function did not depend on duration of steroid therapy.*

Lukert BP, Raisz LG. Glucocorticoid-induced osteoporosis: pathogenesis and management. *Ann Intern Med* 1990;112:352–364. *Editorial accompanying article by Ip and colleagues. A strong plea is made for preventive therapy of glucocorticosteroid-induced bone loss, even in patients on high-dose inhaled glucocorticoids.*

Mankin HJ. Nontraumatic necrosis of bone (osteonecrosis). *N Engl J Med* 1992;326:1473–1479. *Review of features and management of osteonecrosis (avascular necrosis).*

Murphy DG, McDermott MF, Rydman RJ, et al. Aminophylline in the treatment of acute asthma when β$_2$-adrenergics and steroids are provided. *Arch Intern Med* 1993;153:1784–1788. *Randomized, double-blinded, placebo-controlled emergency room study showing no advantage to adding aminophylline to inhaled β$_2$-adrenergics and glucocorticoids in terms of hourly peak flow.*

NHLBI/WHO Workshop Report. *Global Initiative for Asthma.* NIH/NHLBI Publication No. 95-3659. *Comprehensive and specific guidelines for asthma care, largely focusing on outpatient management and patient education. A new version is due for publication in 1997.*

Niki Y, Soejima R, Kawane H, et al. New synthetic quinolone antibacterial agents and serum concentration of theophylline. *Chest* 1987;92:663–669. *Six quinolone antibiotics were administered to healthy adults in combination with sustained-release theophylline. Variable effects on serum theophylline levels were found with the different preparations. Ciprofloxacin caused a more significant increase in serum theophylline level than norfloxacin, and norfloxacin more than ofloxacin.*

Pashko S, Simons WR, Sena MM, Stoddard ML. Rate of exposure to theophylline-drug interactions. *Clin Ther* 1994;16:1068–1077. *Computer analysis using Pennsylvania Medicaid Management System found 17,933 patients who filled at least one prescription for theophylline during the 15-month study period. Of these, 36.9% had prescriptions for at least one other medication known to affect theophylline metabolism.*

Rossing TH, Fanta CH, Goldstein DH, et al. Emergency therapy of asthma: comparison of the acute effects of parenteral and inhaled sympathomimetics and infused aminophylline. *Am Rev Respir Dis* 1980;122:365–371. *Study of 48 patients with acute asthma treated* *on an emergent basis. Both epinephrine and nebulized isoproterenol provided more rapid and greater improvement in FEV$_1$ at 1 hour than aminophylline.*

Sambrook P, Birmingham J, Kelly P, et al. Prevention of corticosteroid osteoporosis. *N Engl J Med* 1993;328:1747–1752. *Comparison of calcium, calcitriol, salmon calcitonin, and placebo in 103 patients on long-term corticosteroid therapy. Bone density of lumbar spine, femoral neck, and wrist were followed at 4-month intervals. Calcitriol and calcium prevented bone loss from the lumbar spine with or without calcitonin.*

Shannon M. Predictors of major toxicity after theophylline overdose. *Ann Intern Med* 1993;119:1161–1167. *Review of records of 249 patients referred to Massachusetts Poison Control System for theophylline overdose to determine predictors of toxicity. Chronic overmedication, peak serum level in patients with acute intoxication, and older age were risk factors for more serious toxicity.*

Shannon M, Lovejoy FH. Hypokalemia after theophylline intoxication: the effects of acute vs. chronic intoxication. *Arch Intern Med* 1989; 149:2725–2729. *Review of records of 88 patients with theophylline intoxication. Patients with acute intoxication were more likely to be hypokalemic and had lower levels than patients with chronic intoxication.*

Singer EP, Kolischenko A. Seizures due to theophylline overdose. *Chest* 1985;87:755–757. *Case report of two patients with prior neurologic injury in whom seizures developed at theophylline levels of 26 and 26.3 mg/dL, suggesting that special attention to serum levels is needed when theophylline is administered to patients with a history of neurologic injury.*

Sullivan P, Bekir S, Jaffar Z, et al. Anti-inflammatory effects of low-dose oral theophylline in atopic asthma. *Lancet* 1994;343:1006–1008. *Study looking at the effect of theophylline on migration of eosinophils into bronchial mucosa after allergen challenge.*

Szefler SJ. Glucocorticoid therapy for asthma: clinical pharmacology. *J Allergy Clin Immunol* 1991;88:147–165. *Review of pharmacology and drug interactions of oral and inhaled glucocorticoids used in the treatment of asthma.*

Szefler SJ, Bender BG, Jusko WJ, et al. Evolving role of theophylline for treatment of chronic childhood asthma. *J Pediatr* 1995;127:176–185. *Review article suggesting a role for theophylline in the treatment of asthmatic children who have poor inhaler technique, poor compliance with inhaled anti-inflammatory agents, or more severe disease.*

Urban RC Jr, Dreyer EB. Corticosteroid-induced glaucoma. *Int Ophthalmol Clin* 1993;33:135–139. *Report of glaucoma with oral and long-term topical glucocorticoid use.*

Ward AJM, McKenniff M, Evans, JM, Page CP, Costello JF. Theophylline—an immunomodulatory role in asthma? *Am Rev Respir Dis* 1993;147:518–523. *Twenty-one subjects with both early and late asthmatic responses to inhaled dust mite antigen were given slow-release theophylline or placebo in double-blinded fashion. Although methacholine responsiveness 24 hours after antigen challenge was not affected, the increase in peripheral blood CD4 and CD8 levels seen after antigen challenge was suppressed by theophylline.*

Wrenn K, Slovis CM, Murphy F, et al. Aminophylline therapy for acute bronchospastic disease in the emergency room. *Ann Intern Med* 1991; 115:241–247. *Randomized, placebo-controlled study of intravenous aminophylline in 133 adult patients with asthma or COPD, finding that aminophylline had no significant effect on patient satisfaction, physician assessment of response, spirometry, or peak flow, but was associated with a threefold decrease in hospital admission rate. Median serum theophylline concentration was 9.7 mg/L.*

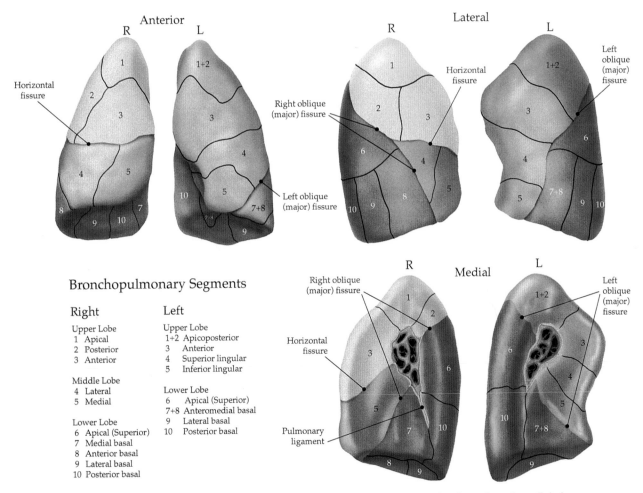

Anterior

R   L

Lateral

R   L

Horizontal
fissure

Right oblique
(major) fissure

Left oblique
(major) fissure

Horizontal
fissure

Left oblique
(major) fissure

Bronchopulmonary Segments

Right

Upper Lobe
1 Apical
2 Posterior
3 Anterior

Middle Lobe
4 Lateral
5 Medial

Lower Lobe
6 Apical (Superior)
7 Medial basal
8 Anterior basal
9 Lateral basal
10 Posterior basal

Left

Upper Lobe
1+2 Apicoposterior
3 Anterior
4 Superior lingular
5 Inferior lingular

Lower Lobe
6   Apical (Superior)
7+8 Anteromedial basal
9   Lateral basal
10   Posterior basal

Medial

R   L

Right oblique
(major) fissure

Left
oblique
(major)
fissure

Horizontal
fissure

Pulmonary
ligament

COLOR PLATE 1. Location of bronchopulmonary segments from anterior, lateral, and medial views.

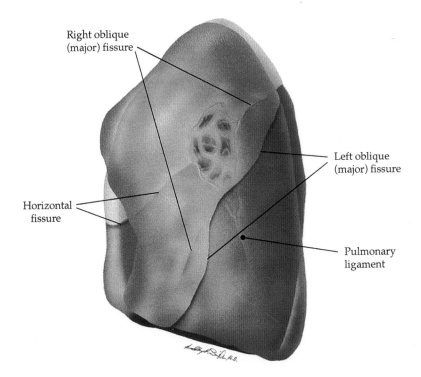

Right oblique
(major) fissure

Left oblique
(major) fissure

Horizontal
fissure

Pulmonary
ligament

COLOR PLATE 2. Left lateral view of the lungs. Partially translucent image of the left lung allows the right lung to be seen. The location of the major fissures and the horizontal fissure of the right lung are illustrated in the positions in which they would appear on a left lateral chest radiograph. Note that the major fissure on the right side lies slightly anterior and apical to the major fissure on the left side.

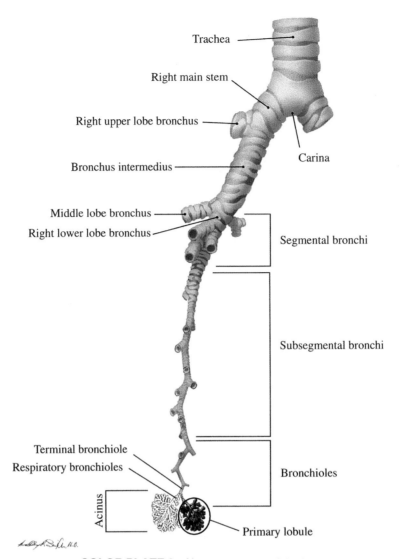

Trachea

Right main stem

Right upper lobe bronchus

Bronchus intermedius

Carina

Middle lobe bronchus

Right lower lobe bronchus

Segmental bronchi

Subsegmental bronchi

Terminal bronchiole

Respiratory bronchioles

Bronchioles

Acinus

Primary lobule

COLOR PLATE 3. Airway anatomy of the human tracheobronchial tree. This figure illustrates typical branching along one of the longer paths to a right lower lobe segment. In the normal human lung, there are approximately five to 15 branch points from a segmental bronchus to a terminal bronchiole. In a completely binary, symmetric branching system, 14 to 15 branch points from the trachea would be required to create the 43,000 terminal bronchioles in a human lung. Because many paths are shorter, there are also path lengths with >15 branch points from the trachea. Segmental bronchi are characterized by the presence of cartilaginous plates in their walls, whereas bronchioles contain smooth muscle in their walls but no cartilage.

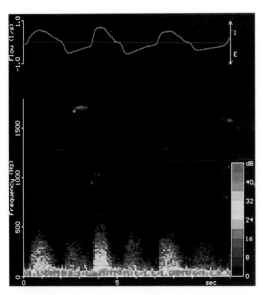

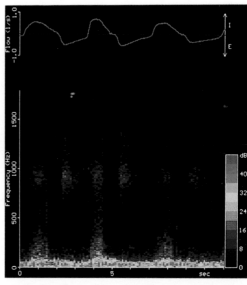

COLOR PLATE 4. Normal vesicular breath sounds. Sound spectrogram with simultaneous pneumotachogram (*top*); sound frequency in hertz (Hz) is represented on the ordinate, time (s) on the abscissa; colors designate sound intensity in decibels (dB) on the scale (*lower right*). Recorded over the left posterior lung base in a 13-year-old boy with cystic fibrosis. Note that inspiratory breath sounds are louder than expiratory sounds and that there is no pause between the respiratory phases. The frequencies are virtually all below 500 Hz and are most intense below 250 Hz. Contributions of low-frequency muscle and cardiovascular sound are visible. (Reproduced from Pasterkamp H. *R.A.L.E. Computer-Aided Instruction in Chest Auscultation with Digital Audio Presentation of Lung Sounds.* Winnipeg, Manitoba, Canada: PixSoft; 1990.)

COLOR PLATE 6. Normal tracheal breath sounds. Sound spectrogram as described in Color Plate 4, but with simultaneously recorded electrocardiogram (*bottom*). Recorded over the trachea at the suprasternal notch in a healthy, 26-year-old, male nonsmoker. The typical features of normal tracheal sounds are evident, with a broad frequency distribution, extending close to 1500 Hz during both inspiration and expiration, a slightly louder expiration, and a clear break (absence of respiratory sound) between the respiratory phases. During 5 seconds of breath holding and zero air flow, the contribution of low-frequency cardiovascular sounds becomes evident. The electrocardiogram helps to identify the high-intensity, low-frequency heart sounds. The dependence of sound intensity on air flow is obvious during the latter parts of this observation, when the subject was breathing more shallowly. (Reproduced from Pasterkamp H. *R.A.L.E. Computer-Aided Instruction in Chest Auscultation with Digital Audio Presentation of Lung Sounds.* Winnipeg, Manitoba, Canada: PixSoft; 1990.)

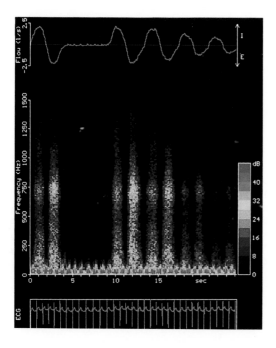

COLOR PLATE 5. Bronchial breath sounds. Sound spectrogram as described in Color Plate 4, simultaneously recorded over the corresponding site on the right posterior lung base in the same patient as in Color Plate 4. Pneumonia and consolidation of the right lower lobe were present, and bronchial breathing is evident. In comparison with the left side (Color Plate 4), there is a decrease in intensity of breath sounds but an increase in high-frequency components extending above 1000 Hz. This is most evident during expiration; in contrast to the normal left side (Color Plate 4), expiratory breath sounds are louder than inspiratory breath sounds. Contributions of low-frequency muscle and cardiovascular sound are visible. (Reproduced from Pasterkamp H. *R.A.L.E. Computer-Aided Instruction in Chest Auscultation with Digital Audio Presentation of Lung Sounds.* Winnipeg, Manitoba, Canada: PixSoft; 1990.)

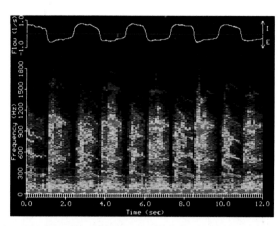

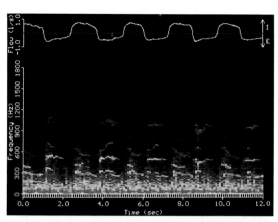

COLOR PLATE 7. Tracheal breath sounds in a patient with exercise-induced asthma. Sound spectrogram as described in Color Plate 4. Polyphonic wheezing is present during both inspiration and expiration, seen as broad bands of intense sound with a narrow distribution of frequencies. Contributions of low-frequency muscle and cardiovascular sound are visible. (Reproduced from Pasterkamp H. *R.A.L.E. Computer-Aided Instruction in Chest Auscultation with Digital Audio Presentation of Lung Sounds.* Winnipeg, Manitoba, Canada: PixSoft; 1990.)

COLOR PLATE 8. Pulmonary breath sounds with wheezes. Sound spectrogram as described in Color Plate 4. Sounds recorded over the right infraclavicular region in the same patient as in Color Plate 7. Inspiratory and expiratory wheezes are seen as broad bands of intense sound with a narrow distribution of frequencies. The intensity of sound is less than in Color Plate 7. No sounds have frequencies higher than 900 Hz. (Reproduced from Pasterkamp H, et al. Digital respirosonography. *Chest* 1989;96:1405.)

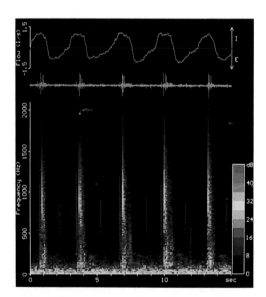

COLOR PLATE 9. Mid to late fine inspiratory crackles in a 60-year-old man with interstitial pulmonary fibrosis. These were recorded over the right posterior lung base. The broad frequency distribution is typical for fine crackles (coarse crackles would be contained largely below 1000 Hz). There are a few expiratory crackles as well. (Reproduced from Pasterkamp H. *R.A.L.E. Computer-Aided Instruction in Chest Auscultation with Digital Audio Presentation of Lung Sounds.* Winnipeg, Manitoba, Canada: PixSoft; 1990.)

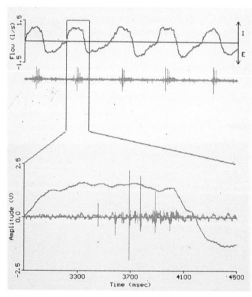

COLOR PLATE 10. The upper two records are the same as in Color Plate 9. One expiration and a small part of the adjacent inspiration are shown on an expanded time-based display. The mid to late crackles are well shown. (Reproduced from Pasterkamp H. *R.A.L.E. Computer-Aided Instruction in Chest Auscultation with Digital Audio Presentation of Lung Sounds.* Winnipeg, Manitoba, Canada: PixSoft; 1990.)

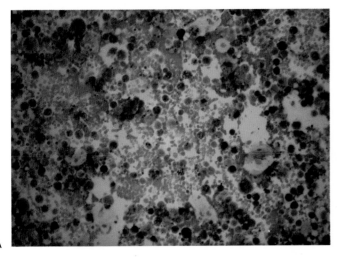
A

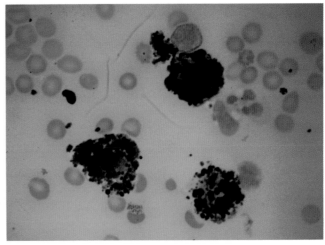
B

COLOR PLATE 11. A: Hemosiderin-laden macrophages. Photomicrograph of BAL fluid demonstrating numerous hemosiderin-laden macrophages with adjacent red blood cells indicating alveolar hemorrhage. Wright stain, low power. **B:** Photomicrograph of BAL fluid showing hemosiderin-laden alveolar macrophages stained blue by iron stain. Prussian blue stain, high power.

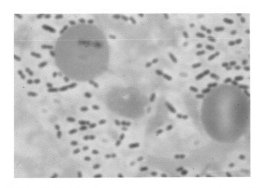

COLOR PLATE 12. *Streptococcus pneumoniae* in Gram's stain of sputum. x900.

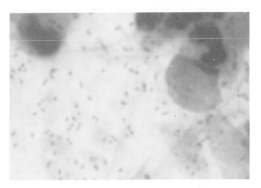

COLOR PLATE 13. *Haemophilus influenzae* in Gram's stain of sputum. X900.

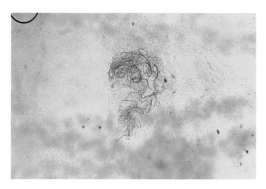

COLOR PLATE 14. Elastin fibers in a potassium hydroxide preparation of sputum.

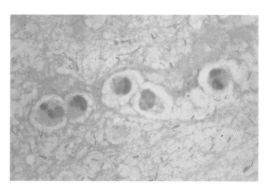

COLOR PLATE 15. *Pseudomonas* in sputum of a neutropenic patient. x900.

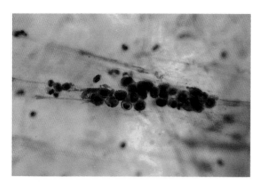

COLOR PLATE 16. Giemsa stain of endotracheal secretions showing intranuclear inclusions of HSV. Fever and diffuse interstitial pneumonia developed in this patient after coronary bypass surgery.

Textbook of Pulmonary Diseases, 6th ed.
edited by G.L. Baum, J.D. Crapo, B.R. Celli, and J.B. Karlinsky,
Lippincott–Raven Publishers, Philadelphia, © 1998.

CHAPTER

17 Surfactant

William W. Lunn · Jean E. Rinaldo

INTRODUCTION

In 1929, Von Neergard calculated that surface tensions in the alveoli and distal air spaces are large enough to cause collapse of the airways during normal lung functions. He postulated the existence of a substance capable of lowering airway surface tension. In 1955, two independent research laboratories isolated a material from the alveolar lining of lungs that was capable of dramatically lowering airway surface tension (surfactant). In 1959, Avery and Mead reported that alveolar washings from premature infants with infant respiratory distress syndrome (IRDS) lacked the normal amount of surface tension-lowering capacity. In 1961, it was shown that phospholipid isolated from the alveolar lining fluid of beef lungs possesses surface tension-lowering properties. These phospholipids contain hydrophilic and lipophilic moieties, which result in their forming a filmy monolayer over the aqueous alveolar luminal surface. Surfactant was found to be synthesized by type II pneumocytes and continually secreted into the air spaces, and to contain associated proteins with diverse biologic functions. Finally, in 1980, Fujiwara and associates reported the first successful use of exogenous surfactant therapy for infants with IRDS. Today, exogenous surfactant therapy for infants with IRDS is considered a clinical standard of care.

SYNTHESIS, METABOLISM, AND FUNCTIONS OF ENDOGENOUS SURFACTANT

Surfactant Lipids

Lipids constitute approximately 90% of surfactant isolated from human lungs. The lipid moiety comprises a

W. W. Lunn and J. E. Rinaldo: Pulmonary Division, Department of Medicine, Vanderbilt University, Nashville, Tennessee 37212.

mixture of phospholipids (90%) and other lipids (10%). The two principal phospholipids are phosphatidylcholine (PC), the most abundant phospholipid, and dipalmitoylphosphatidylcholine (DPPC), which may be the most important one. All phospholipids are structured so that they possess a polar head and a pair of hydrophobic tails, making them ideal molecules to form lipid-water interfaces, as they do in cell membranes. Most of the surface tension-lowering properties of surfactant reside in the DPPC molecule. It is the saturated palmitic acid residues that make the DPPC molecule unique, allowing them to be packed together tightly to form a monolayer with tensile strength at the air-fluid interface. The polar head of each DPPC molecule is charged, so that it has an affinity for molecules of water in the alveolar lining fluid. The long hydrophobic tails are directed away from water molecules and project into the air space. The repulsion of water molecules from the air-fluid interface results in a dramatic lowering of the surface tension in the air spaces (Fig. 1). The net effect is to retard the development of atelectasis and lung edema, to decrease lung compliance, and to diminish work of breathing. Some evidence suggests that the lipid component of surfactant may play a role in host defense, having been implicated in both bacterial killing and suppression of stimulated lymphocytes; most investigators believe that the surfactant-associated proteins play an important immunomodulatory role.

Surfactant-Associated Proteins

Proteins constitute approximately 10% of isolated surfactant. Most protein found in surfactant appears to have diffused in passively from serum. Only 20% is synthe-

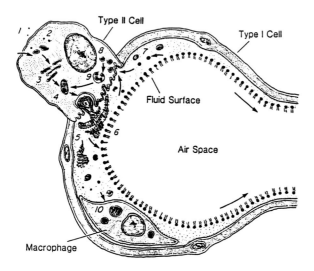

FIG. 1. Schematic diagram of a single alveolus emphasizing the movement of surfactant components through the type II cell and alveolar liquid. Components and compartments are not to scale. Key: *1,* surfactant precursors such as glucose, amino acids, and fatty acids; *2,* endoplasmic reticulum; *3,* Golgi apparatus; *4,* lamellar bodies; *5,* tubular myelin; *6,* surface film with adsorbed phospholipids; *7,* vesicular and myelin forms of surfactant possibly derived from material desorbed from the film; *8* and *9,* endocytotic compartments such as multivesicular bodies; *10,* alveolar macrophage. (From Hawgood S, Clements J. Pulmonary surfactant and its apoproteins. *J Clin Invest* 1990;86:1–6.)

sized locally. To date, three apolipoproteins (surfactant-associated proteins) have been well characterized: SP-A, SP-B, and SP-C. A fourth protein, SP-D, has been described, but there is debate in the literature regarding whether SP-D is a true apolipoprotein or simply a contaminating protein. Each surfactant-associated protein has a unique structure and function, summarized in Table 1.

SP-A is a large, collagen-like protein. It is the most ubiquitous surfactant-associated protein and appears to perform diverse functions critical to both surfactant homeostasis and immunoregulation. First, SP-A has been shown to assist in the conversion of newly secreted surfactant precursor into tubular myelin, believed to be the

intracellular source of the phospholipids and the surfactant film. SP-A also participates in the regulation of surfactant homeostasis by inhibiting surfactant synthesis and promoting surfactant uptake by type II pneumocytes. Second, SP-A has clearly been shown to regulate inflammation. It enhances the activity of pulmonary macrophages. Of interest, SP-A has structural similarities to C1q of the complement cascade, possibly accounting for its ability to activate macrophages. It appears that binding of SP-A to pulmonary pathogens such as *Mycobacterium tuberculosis* permits uptake of the organisms by a specific SP-A receptor on macrophages, suggesting that SP-A may function as a hapten as well as a nonspecific activator and suppressor of intra-alveolar inflammatory effector cells.

SP-B is a small, hydrophobic protein that appears to co-operate with SP-A in the formation of tubular myelin and possibly to play a role in the packing of surfactant precursor in lamellar bodies. Additionally, SP-B has been shown to enhance the spreading of surfactant lipids in a monolayer film. SP-C is another small, hydrophobic protein that is structurally similar to SP-B. The only known role of SP-C is that it functions like SP-B to enhance the spreading of surfactant lipids in the air spaces. SP-D is a recently described large glycoprotein that many investigators believe may function to enhance the clearance of microorganisms from the airways. Not much is known about SP-D at present. There is disagreement about whether SP-D is a surfactant apoprotein or a contaminating plasma protein.

Surfactant Synthesis, Secretion, and Uptake

The lipid and protein components of surfactant are synthesized in the type II pneumocyte. Surfactant lipid is made and stored in lamellar bodies within the cell. Stimulation of the type II pneumocyte may result in the secretion of surfactant material from lamellar bodies into the air space, where it is rapidly transformed into tubular myelin with the assistance of SP-A and SP-B. The precise pathways of surfactant-associated protein synthesis and incorporation into the lipid components of surfactant have

TABLE 1. *Surfactant-associated proteins*

	Protein structure	Functions
SP-A	Globular protein with a collagen-like domain and a short N-terminal; structural similarity to C1q	Assists in the formation of tubular myelin Enhances macrophage function Inhibits surfactant secretion Promotes reuptake of surfactant
SP-B	Small cationic protein with α-helix folding	Assists SP-A in tubular myelin formation Enhances spreading of lipid film in air-liquid interface
SP-C	Small cationic protein with α-helix folding	Enhances spreading of lipid film in air-liquid interface
SP-D	Large collagenous glycoprotein	Possible role in pulmonary host defense

TABLE 2. *Factors involved in regulating surfactant synthesis and secretion*

Promoters of synthesis	Promoters of secretion
Ambroxol	Ambroxol
cAMP	β-Agonists
β-Agonists	Estrogen
Estrogen	Mechanical ventilation
Glucocorticoids	Prostaglandins
Thyroxine	Thyroxine
Inhibitor of synthesis	Inhibitors of secretion
Testosterone	SP-A
	β-Blockers

eluded scientists to date. It is not clear whether the protein components become associated with the lipid components in the lamellar bodies, after secretion of tubular myelin into the air spaces, or both.

Several stimuli can induce surfactant synthesis and/or secretion in vitro (Table 2). These include glucocorticoids, β-adrenergic agonists, estrogen, and thyroxine, which share the ability to enhance both the synthesis and secretion of surfactant. Stretching of the lung via mechanical ventilation also results in surfactant secretion. Downregulators of surfactant secretion include SP-A and β-adrenergic blockers. Corticosteroids are an extremely important inducer of surfactant synthesis and is used for clinical purposes. Glucocorticoid levels rise dramatically in the normal fetus late in gestation just before the production of surfactant. Glucocorticoid treatment of pregnant women prior to giving birth to children at risk for IRDS increases the rate at which alveolar type II cells mature and the production of surfactant.

Studies of surfactant synthesis indicate that new surfactant is being generated continuously and is not degraded in the airways. Therefore, mechanisms for surfactant clearance must exist. Some of the excess surfactant is undergoes phagocytosis by alveolar macrophages or is removed from the airway by the mucociliary elevator. There appears to be a sophisticated system by which type II cells ''recycle'' DPPC by taking it up, packaging it back into lamellar bodies in the cytoplasm, and resecreting it. SP-A appears to mediate partly the reuptake of DPPC by type II pneumocytes. Impaired mechanisms for clearance and recycling may cause alveolar proteinosis, a disease characterized by excess surfactant accumulation in alveoli. Surfactant homeostasis is an area of vigorous ongoing research.

THERAPEUTIC USE OF EXOGENOUS SURFACTANT PREPARATIONS

As described above, surfactant is necessary to prevent atelectasis and lung edema, and to maintain normal lung compliance. As atelectasis, lung edema, and reduced lung compliance occur in IRDS and many acute lung disorders

in adults, it is not surprising that the effects of instilling exogenous surfactant into the lung have been the subject of considerable study. The therapeutic possibilities seem particularly attractive in critically ill patients undergoing mechanical ventilation, in whom there is ready access to a delivery conduit. Although the concept is superficially simple, practical issues have posed complex problems. Where will large quantities of human surfactant come from? Unlike many human bioactive substances, such as insulin, surfactant is predominantly lipid and thus cannot be cloned by recombinant DNA technology, so the molecular revolution has not solved the availability problem. Nor can human surfactant be isolated from human blood, like clotting factors or α_1-antiprotease; the human lung is presently the only source of human surfactant. Can animal surfactant be used? Can an artificial lipid surfactant be synthesized, and if so, what components of surfactant are most useful to instill? Must the human apoproteins be added? How can a large volume of liquid be delivered and spread evenly through the lung without causing respiratory compromise during delivery? These are some of the questions that must be answered prior to the use of surfactant as accepted practice.

Available Surfactant Preparations

The surfactant preparations may be divided into two groups: natural preparations and synthetic preparations. The natural surfactants are derived from animal sources, with bovine and porcine sources being the most common (Table 3). A natural surfactant can be prepared from human amniotic fluid, but this is not yet commercially available. Natural surfactants are either prepared by extraction from minced lung tissue or from lung lavage material. Lung lavage material has a theoretical advantage over minced lung material in that it contains less cellular and blood-derived contaminants, but obtaining it in large quantities is a laborious process. To date, there are no data from clinical studies to suggest that lung lavage preparations are more efficacious than lung mince preparations.

Several animal-derived surfactants are in clinical use. They differ considerably in composition, as both the extraction methods and addition of specific lipids may alter the final composition of the extract sold commercially. Surfacten was developed by the Fujiwara group in Japan and was the first surfactant preparation to be successfully employed to treat infants with IRDS. It is made from bovine lung mince and is supplied as a powder that must be reconstituted in sterile saline solution. Beractant is also prepared from bovine lung mince and is similar to Surfacten. It is supplied as a liquid and thus requires no mixing. Curosurf is prepared from porcine lung mince and is supplied as a liquid. It has the highest concentration of phospholipids (80 mg/mL) of all the natural surfac-

TABLE 3. *Natural surfactant preparations*

Name	Trade name	Source	Ingredients	Company
Surfactant TA	Surfacten	Bovine lung mince	Phospholipids, SP-B, SP-C, palmitic acid, tripalmitin	Tanabe (Tokyo, Japan)
Curosurf	Curosurf	Porcine lung mince	Phospholipids, SP-B, SP-C	Chiesi Farmaceutici (Parma, Italy)
Survanta	Beractant	Bovine lung mince	Phospholipids, neutral lipids, fatty acids, SP-B, SP-C, palmitic acid, tripalmitin	Abbott Laboratories (Chicago, IL)
Alveofact	Alveofact	Bovine lung lavage	Phospholipids, cholesterol, SP-B, SP-C	Thomas GmbH (Biberach, Germany)
Calf lung surfactant extract	CLSE	Calf lung lavage	Phospholipids, cholesterol, cholesterol esters, SP-B, SP-C	Privately produced in Canada
Infasurf	Infasurf	Calf lung lavage	Phospholipids, SP-B, SP-C	Forest Laboratories (St. Louis, MO)

tants. Alveofact is derived from bovine lung lavage material. In addition to phospholipids, it contains cholesterol and other lipids. Infasurf (CLSE) also contains cholesterol and cholesteryl esters in addition to phospholipids.

There are currently two synthetic surfactant preparations available, ALEC and Exosurf (Table 4). ALEC contains DPPC and other phospholipids but does not contain any surfactant-associated proteins. The phospholipid concentration is approximately 100 mg/mL, highest of all surfactant preparations. Exosurf contains DPPC, hexadecanol, and tyloxapol. Like ALEC, it does not contain any surfactant-associated proteins. The phospholipid concentration of Exosurf when diluted as directed is much lower than that of ALEC. It is not clear whether the lack of surfactant-associated proteins in these preparations is a disadvantage. A recent meta-analysis comparing Exosurf with natural surfactants suggested that improvements in lung compliance and oxygenation were delayed in infants treated with Exosurf in comparison with those treated with natural surfactants, but both natural surfactants and Exosurf were efficacious and resulted in a clear reduction in morbidity and mortality in treated infants, with no statistically significant difference in mortality rates. Large, prospective, controlled clinical trials would be helpful to determine if the natural surfactants are superior to synthetic preparations, but even if performed carefully, these studies would be extremely difficult to interpret because of the marked differences in the available natural and synthetic preparations and the likelihood that continu-

ous adjustments will be made in the composition of future preparations.

Methods for Delivery of Surfactant Therapy

The goal of administration of surfactant is to deliver the drug in a simple fashion that minimizes physiologic disturbances and spreads surfactant evenly through the lung. There are two obvious ways to attempt this: tracheal instillation or aerosolization. After Avery and Mead published their findings in 1959, scientists in the 1960s experimented with surfactant therapy for infants with IRDS. Aerosolized delivery of surfactant was employed by most investigators. No beneficial effect of treatment could be demonstrated. It was because of these difficulties that Fujiwara and colleagues chose direct tracheal instillation as the method of drug delivery in their landmark study. At present, all the manufacturers of commercially available surfactants recommend tracheal instillation as the method of choice for drug delivery, but there are considerable differences in the specifics of recommended delivery. Some companies advocate multiple dosing; others suggest directed positioning of patients after instillation to facilitate drug distribution.

Tracheal instillation has been proved effective in a large number of clinical trials involving thousands of patients. Tracheal instillation allows for drug to be delivered to airways that are not being ventilated, whereas aerosolized

TABLE 4. *Synthetic surfactant preparations*

Name	Trade name	Ingredients	Company
Artificial lung-expanding compound (ALEC)	Pumactant	DPPC, unsaturated phosphatidylglycerol	Britannia Pharmaceuticals (Redhill, England)
Exosurf	Exosurf	DPPC, hexadecanol, tyloxapol	Burroughs Wellcome (Research Triangle Park, NC)

DPPC, dipalmitoylphosphatidylcholine.

surfactant is delivered only to ventilated lung segments. Tracheal instillation techniques are relatively simple and do not require any specialized equipment. However, there are also disadvantages. First, patients must be intubated and on mechanical ventilation for the drug to be given. Repositioning and interruption of the ventilator circuit in hypoxemic patients may result in worsening hypoxemia. Also, as most of the surfactant preparations require large volumes of drug to be instilled, transient obstruction of the airways may occur and result in respiratory and hemodynamic instability.

Despite early disappointment with aerosol delivery, there is renewed interest in the use of this technique to circumvent the problems with tracheal instillation outlined above. Aerosolization is a noninvasive technique with which physicians, nurses, and respiratory therapists are familiar, making it readily acceptable. Significant problems remain. Aerosolization results in a smaller dose of surfactant delivered to the patient compared with tracheal instillation because of the inefficiency of the delivery devices currently available, especially in ventilated patients. When a jet nebulizer is used in the ventilator circuit at high flow rates, large particles impact in the inspiratory circuit and never reach the lung, whereas particles of 1 μ in diameter may be taken into the lung only to be exhaled. There may be foaming of the surfactant aerosol and subsequent malfunctioning of valves in the expiratory circuit. These technical difficulties remain to be overcome, and trials must be performed in humans to compare the clinical efficacy of aerosolized versus tracheally instilled surfactant.

A number of factors may influence the distribution of surfactant in the lungs, regardless of the mode of drug delivery employed. The type of surfactant preparation may be of importance. The natural surfactants containing SP-B and SP-C may spread more rapidly and evenly in the air-liquid interface of the alveoli. Some in vitro data suggest that the synthetic preparations, which lack surfactant-associated proteins, spread more slowly and have higher minimal surface tensions than the surfactants that contain proteins. The clinical significance of these findings is still uncertain. The volume of fluid instilled also influences the distribution of surfactant in the lung. A more homogeneous distribution of surfactant is achieved when it is given in larger volumes of vehicle. However, larger volumes are potentially hazardous, as they are associated with a greater frequency of respiratory and hemodynamic instability during and immediately after the instillation process. Finally, it is possible that the mode of ventilation may influence the distribution of surfactant after it is administered through the endotracheal tube. Standard practice has employed conventional, volume-cycled ventilatory modes after delivery of the drug. However, some investigators have studied the effect of high-frequency ventilation in animal models of lung injury. The results have been conflicting, so more research will

be required to determine whether ventilatory modes may significantly affect drug distribution.

CLINICAL APPLICATIONS OF SURFACTANT THERAPY

Infant Respiratory Distress Syndrome

IRDS is at present the only clinical condition for which surfactant instillation has been proved beneficial. The maturation of the fetal lung occurs late in the process of gestation. Type II pneumocytes begin to mature and develop lamellar bodies at approximately 24 weeks of gestation, but dramatic increases in the phospholipid concentration of amniotic fluid are not seen until approximately 28 weeks. Therefore, children born prematurely may not have a sufficient quantity of biologically active surfactant necessary to maintain normal lung function and are at risk for IRDS. More than 35 randomized, controlled trials of exogenous surfactant therapy for IRDS have been performed. The results, which have been dramatic, include a decreased incidence of pneumothorax, improved oxygenation, decreased dependence on mechanical ventilation, and a reduction of mortality. Clearly, the reduction in infant mortality rates observed in the 1980s in the United States was partially a consequence of the introduction of exogenous surfactant therapy.

Some now recommend surfactant therapy prophylactically in premature infants. Meta-analyses of data from clinical trials performed in the United States and abroad have answered important questions regarding surfactant therapy for IRDS. For example, it is clear that surfactant therapy given to infants in the delivery room who are at risk for IRDS is effective in lowering both the incidence and severity of the syndrome. However, trials comparing prophylactic therapy with rescue therapy have failed to demonstrate superiority of one style of treatment. Most investigators agree that prophylactic therapy should be given to infants at high risk for IRDS by someone with experience in neonatal resuscitation. Infants who are at low risk may be observed carefully for signs of respiratory insufficiency and treated if deterioration develops.

Some cases of IRDS do not respond to surfactant therapy. Approximately 10%–20% of infants treated with exogenous surfactant for IRDS fail to demonstrate any significant clinical response. These infants sometimes have been given an incorrect diagnosis and actually have other diseases, such as pneumonia or congenital heart disease. Meta-analyses suggest that other complications of prematurity, such as patent ductus atreriosis and interventricular hemorrhage, are unaffected by exogenous surfactant therapy.

Meconium Aspiration Syndrome

Meconium aspiration syndrome (MAS), which occurs secondary to fetal inhalation of meconium into the lungs, usually during labor, results in respiratory embarrassment shortly after birth. Infants with MAS may have hypoxemia, noncompliant lungs, and ventilator-associated barotrauma, just like infants with IRDS. Because MAS resembles IRDS clinically, many have postulated that meconium in the lungs of the neonate may interfere with the activity of surfactant. Experimental studies suggest reduced surface tension-lowering ability of surfactant after meconium contamination. In clinical and experimental studies, surfactant has resulted in improvements in lung compliance and oxygenation. The available data are promising, but randomized, controlled trials in a large number of patients need to be performed to establish a significant outcome benefit.

Congenital Diaphragmatic Hernia

Congenital diaphragmatic hernia (CDH) is a disorder in which the fetus develops with a defect in the diaphragm that allows abdominal contents to migrate into the thoracic cavity and compress the lung. This compression results in pulmonary hypoplasia, characterized by a reduced number of alveoli, and smooth-muscle hyperplasia in pulmonary arterioles. The hypoplastic lungs of these neonates are also deficient in surfactant. Infants with CDH are usually born at term and experience respiratory compromise early after birth. Surgery corrects the diaphragmatic defect, but the immature lung persists; the mortality rate for infants with CDH is approximately 30%–50%. Current data on exogenous surfactant therapy for infants with CDH are limited, but reports suggest that surfactant may improve oxygenation in these infants and facilitate support with mechanical ventilation. Further investigation of exogenous surfactant therapy for children with CDH is ongoing.

Adult Respiratory Distress Syndrome

Adult respiratory distress syndrome (ARDS) was named after IRDS because of the clinical similarities. Both syndromes are manifested by respiratory failure, poorly compliant lungs, alveolar flooding, and profound hypoxemia. Surfactant abnormalities and alveolar damage are present in each disorder. However, there are important differences. First, although alveolar damage is present in both syndromes, the alveolar injury occurs for different reasons. The primary abnormality in IRDS is immaturity of the lung and a primary deficiency of biologically active surfactant. This results in atelectasis in surfactant-poor areas and overdistention and hyperoxic exposure in alveoli in overventilated lung units. Overdistention and oxidant injury probably result in secondary alveolar disruption and injury. In contrast, an inflammatory alveolar injury is the primary pathophysiology of ARDS. The end result is alveolar disruption and pulmonary capillary leak-

age of serum proteins and water into the alveolar spaces. Surfactant processing and surface tension-lowering activity are impaired in this abnormal alveolar environment. Thus, the surfactant abnormalities in IRDS are fundamentally distinct from those of ARDS. Infants with IRDS cannot synthesize surfactant, whereas the surfactant in the lungs of patients with ARDS is inactivated by contaminating serum proteins, oxidants, and poorly characterized aberrations in surfactant homeostasis. This poses two questions in ARDS that are not relevant in IRDS: (1) Is the surfactant deficiency of ARDS an important factor in poor outcome or just an epiphenomenon? (2) Will exogenous administered surfactant function well in the ARDS inflammatory milieu? Neither question has been answered to date.

Available results of clinical trials are disappointing. As has often been the case with ARDS, small studies with encouraging results have been superseded by large, multicenter trials with negative findings, most recently a large, multicenter study of 498 patients with sepsis-induced ARDS, in which patients received treatment with either aerosolized Exosurf or placebo for 5 days. Preliminary summary data reported nationally suggested no differences in mortality, although final publication of the study is pending. There are a number of reasons that may explain the lack of efficacy. Exosurf lacks surfactant-associated proteins. The dose of surfactant employed was low, normalized to weight, and given in proportion to the usual dosage regimens for IRDS. On the other hand, employing large doses of surfactant in adults may be problematic because of the large volumes (70 to 300 mL, depending on the preparation) that are required. Also, as discussed above, a number of questions remain unanswered regarding the most efficient means of delivering the drug. Finally, there is the matter of timing. Unlike the onset of IRDS, the onset of ARDS is difficult to determine with precision, and the most severe respiratory failure may occur late as a result of nosocomial pneumonia or other complications. Should surfactant be administered as an adjunct to maximal ventilatory support, or should patients identified as being at risk for ARDS receive surfactant? Thus, the issue of surfactant therapy in ARDS perfectly illustrates the problems associated with translating this ''simple'' therapy into a practical regimen.

Future Applications

Surfactant, because of its beneficial effects of increasing lung compliance and oxygenation and preventing atelectasis, can be viewed as a nonspecific supportive therapy likely to provide physiologic benefit regardless of the nature of respiratory failure; it has therefore been postulated that exogenous surfactant therapy may be useful in a wide range of adult diseases, including pneumonia, pulmonary fibrosis, asthma, chronic bronchitis, and after lung transplantation. Surfactant abnormalities have been described in each of these disorders. However, all the problems associated with ARDS therapy might be expected to occur and even be exacerbated in this heterogeneous group of disorders, and no large, controlled trials in humans to date have demonstrated a benefit of exogenous surfactant therapy in any of them. However, speculation and optimism continue, and research is ongoing in each of these areas.

Despite the advances of the last 40 years of research, many questions regarding the function and metabolism of surfactant remain unanswered. As progress is made in understanding the mechanisms of surfactant function in health and disease, new treatment strategies may be designed. On the horizon, investigators are working to prepare more efficacious synthetic and natural surfactants, so-called ''designer surfactants'' containing higher concentrations of surfactant-associated proteins and a wider range of phospholipids. Others are working to improve dosing regimens and drug delivery. Finally, clinical studies are under way to study the effects of various surfactant preparations in a wide range of disorders, including ARDS, and as postoperative respiratory support after lung transplantation. Clearly, a vast potential market for effective surfactant therapy exists that will undoubtedly continue to drive research and product development in this area. It is hoped that patients with a variety of lung disorders will ultimately benefit.

BIBLIOGRAPHY

Anzueto A, Baughman R, Guntupalli K, DeMariaE, et al. An international, randomized, placebo-controlled trial evaluating the safety and efficacy of aerosolized surfactant in patients with sepsis-induced ARDS. *Am J Respir Crit Care Med* 1994;149:A567. *This abstract contains data for 498 patients enrolled in a trial to evaluate aerosolized Exosurf as treatment for sepsis-induced ARDS. The trial was negative, demonstrating no difference in mortality in the treated versus placebo group. A total of 725 patients were enrolled in this study, making it the largest of its kind, and final publication of all the data is pending at this time.*

Avery M, Mead J. Surface properties in relation to atelectasis and hyaline membrane disease. *Am J Dis Child* 1959;97:517–523. *This is the first report linking IRDS to an alteration of surfactant function. These investigators obtained saline extracts from the lungs of infants with IRDS and demonstrated that the surface tension-lowering ability of these extracts were impaired compared with those from lungs of normal infants.*

Boncuk-Dayanikli P, Taeusch H. Essential and nonessential constituents of exogenous surfactants. In: Robertson B, Taeusch H, eds. *Surfactant Therapy for Lung Disease.* New York: Marcel Dekker; 1995:217–238. *This article, which reviews the composition and functional properties of the available exogenous surfactants, is part of an excellent collection of review articles covering a range of topics in surfactant science and investigation.*

Comroe JH. Retrospectoscope: premature science and immature lungs. Part 1: Some premature discoveries. *Am Rev Respir Dis* 1977;116: 127–135. Part 2: Chemical warfare and the newly born. *Am Rev Respir Dis* 1977;116:311–323. Part 3: The attack on immature lungs. *Am Rev Respir Dis* 1977;116:497–518. *A truly wonderful review of the science leading up to the development of exogenous surfactant therapy.*

Fujiwara T, Chida S, Watabe Y, Maeta H, et al. Artificial surfactant therapy in hyaline membrane disease. *Lancet* 1980;1:55–59. *This is the first trial in which exogenous surfactant therapy was used successfully to treat children with IRDS.*

Hamm H, Fabel H, Bartsch W. The surfactant system of the adult lung: physiology and clinical perspectives. *Clin Investig* 1992;70:637–657. *A thorough review of the surfactant system of the adult lung and the potential role of exogenous surfactant therapy in a wide range of pulmonary diseases.*

Hawgood S, Poulain F. Functions of the surfactant proteins: a perspective. *Pediatr Pulmonol* 1995;19:99–104. *This review focuses on the functions of surfactant apolipoproteins and the implications for exogenous surfactant therapy.*

Jobe A. Techniques for administering surfactant. In: Robertson B, Taeusch H, eds. *Surfactant Therapy for Lung Disease.* New York: Marcel Dekker; 1995:309–324. *This eloquent discussion includes a review of various modes that may be employed to deliver surfactant to the lung. The author also reviews factors that may affect surfactant distribution.*

Lewis J, Jobe A. Surfactant and the adult respiratory distress syndrome. *Am Rev Respir Dis* 1993;147:218–233. *This ''state of the art'' discussion reviews the surfactant abnormalities accompanying ARDS, animal experiments suggesting exogenous surfactant therapy may be useful in laboratory models of acute lung injury, and the limited human data for surfactant therapy in ARDS.*

Lewis J, Veldhuizen R. Factors influencing efficacy of exogenous surfactant in acute lung injury. *Biol Neonate* 1995;67(Suppl 1):48–60. *This discussion reviews surfactant alterations in ARDS and factors that may influence the efficacy of exogenous surfactant therapy. Surfactant delivery method, timing of surfactant administration, dosing schedules, and types of surfactant preparations are covered in detail.*

Mercier C, Soll R. Clinical trials of natural surfactant extract in respiratory distress syndrome. *Clin Perinatol* 1993;4:711–735. *The authors discuss issues ranging from the development of natural surfactant extracts, to prophylactic versus rescue therapy for IRDS, to factors affecting response to therapy. Along the way, they provide the most extensive and careful review of randomized, controlled trials of exogenous surfactant therapy in IRDS.*

Tarnow-Mordi W, Soll R. Artificial versus natural surfactant—can we base clinical practice on a firm scientific footing? *Eur J Pediatr* 1994; 153 (Suppl 2):S17–S21. *These authors discuss the pros and cons of artificial and natural surfactants and review results from three trials comparing Exosurf and Survanta in infants with IRDS. They contend that because the difference in mortality rates in the two groups was not significant, it is unclear whether or not either preparation is truly superior.*

Walther F. Surfactant therapy for neonatal lung disorders other than respiratory distress syndrome. In: Robertson B, Taeusch H, eds. *Surfactant Therapy for Lung Disease.* New York: Marcel Dekker; 1995: 461–476. *This is the most extensive review covering the potential use of exogenous surfactant therapy for neonatal disease. The discussion includes meconium aspiration syndrome, congenital pneumonia, congenital diaphragmatic hernia, transient tachypnea of the newborn, and pulmonary oxygen toxicity.*

INFLAMMATORY AND INTERSTITIAL DISEASES

Textbook of Pulmonary Diseases, 6th ed.
edited by G.L. Baum, J.D. Crapo, B.R. Celli, and J.B. Karlinsky,
Lippincott–Raven Publishers, Philadelphia, © 1998.

CHAPTER

18 Interstitial Lung Diseases

Kenneth G. Saag · Joel N. Kline ·

Gary W. Hunninghake

GENERAL CONSIDERATIONS AND NOMENCLATURE

The interstitial lung diseases (ILD) are a group of disorders of both known and unknown etiology that are characterized by inflammation and fibrosis. Table 1 is a list of some of the pulmonary disorders commonly associated with ILD. This chapter covers two types of ILD of unknown cause: idiopathic pulmonary fibrosis (IPF) and ILD associated with the systemic rheumatologic disorders. The clinical presentation, physiology, pathology, and management of IPF are discussed first, and subsequently aspects of ILD associated with the systemic rheumatologic diseases.

IDIOPATHIC PULMONARY FIBROSIS

In the mid-1930s, Hamman and Rich first described a series of patients in whom developed what today is considered a variant of IPF. For a period of time, however, the term *Hamman-Rich syndrome* was used to denote most cases of pulmonary fibrosis. This term is now reserved for cases of acute interstitial pneumonitis (AIP) with a rapidly progressive and often fatal course. Several other names have been proposed for IPF, including *cryptogenic fibrosing alveolitis, diffuse interstitial lung disease,* and *interstitial pulmonary fibrosis.* Each of these names has merit; however, we refer to the disorder in this

K. G. Saag, J. N. Kline, and G. W. Hunninghake: Department of Internal Medicine, University of Iowa College of Medicine, Iowa City, Iowa 52246.

chapter as *IPF.* IPF has also been subdivided into usual interstitial pneumonitis (UIP) and desquamative interstitial pneumonitis (DIP). We recognize this classification and, when necessary, refer to differences between these two subdivisions of IPF. It should be noted, however, that many investigators do not use these terms and consider UIP and DIP as different manifestations of IPF.

Epidemiology

The prevalence of IPF has been estimated to be about 3 to 5/100,000. It is second only to sarcoidosis as a cause for ILD of unknown etiology. Prevalence estimates vary, however. For example, one study using a New Mexico lung disease registry estimated the prevalence of pulmonary fibrosis at 29/100,000 for male patients and 27/100,000 for female patients. This estimate may reflect the prevalence for the entire United States, or it may represent employment in local mining industries resulting in occult pneumoconiosis, migration of persons with chronic lung disease to New Mexico, or over-ascertainment of cases based on the use of administrative coding. In the New Mexico population, IPF accounted for 45% of all ILD. Based on autopsy studies, IPF may be 10 times more common than is clinically recognized. Few studies have examined ethnic or racial predilections for IPF; in one study of indigenous African patients, the clinical spectrum and frequency of illness were similar to those of other groups.

Although by definition ''idiopathic'' pulmonary fibrosis has no known cause, it is conceivable that inhaled particulate dust or other material could cause this disorder. Of interest, 70% of patients with presumed IPF had

TABLE 1. *Common cause of pulmonary fibrosis*

Idiopathic
  Idiopathic pulmonary fibrosis
  Familial pulmonary fibrosis
  Hamman-Rich syndrome
  Sarcoidosis
  Bronchiolitis obliterans organizing pneumonia
Systemic rheumatic disorders
  Rheumatoid arthritis
  Systemic lupus erythematosus
  Sjögren's syndrome
  Systemic sclerosis
  Dermatomyositis/polymyositis
  Mixed connective tissue disease
  Ankylosing spondylitis
Occupational
  Silicosis
  Asbestosis
  Berylliosis
  Coal worker's pneumoconiosis
  Hard metal pneumoconiosis
Infectious
  Fungal disease
  Postviral
Miscellaneous
  Sequelae to adult respiratory distress syndrome
  Hypersensitivity pneumonitis
  Drugs
  Oxygen toxicity
  Radiation toxicity

organic dust exposure in one study. Curiously, up to 40% of IPF patients may recall an antecedent viral-type illness accompanied by cough, fever, and malaise. However, despite intense investigation, there is no clear evidence implicating an infectious etiology for IPF.

The association between IPF and cigarette smoking has generated considerable interest. Of patients with IPF, 60%–80% are either current or former smokers. Cigarette smoking is a plausible IPF risk factor, as it may alter pulmonary immune function, reduce clearance of inhaled agents, and increase permeability of the respiratory epithelia. Cigarette smoking influences bronchoalveolar lavage fluid (BALF) cellularity and is the strongest independent predictor of increased BALF neutrophils and eosinophils (Table 2). Smoking may also cause respiratory bronchiolitis, an entity histologically similar to DIP; this may, in turn, lead to fibrosis.

Clinical Presentation

History

The typical patient with IPF is between 40 and 60 years of age. Symptoms of the disease frequently develop 1 to 2 years before the patient seeks attention. Men are affected slightly more commonly than women. Dyspnea at rest (and worsened by exertion) and a nonproductive cough are the most common symptoms. Constitutional symptoms of malaise and weight loss are seen in some cases. Even in the absence of a well-recognized rheumatologic disease, arthralgias without actual joint inflammation may be present.

The medical history, including a comprehensive symptoms review, occupational history, and family history, is invaluable in differentiating IPF from other types of ILD. A familial form of IPF, thought to be autosomal dominant with variable penetrance, has been described.

Sudden onset of respiratory symptoms with a clinical presentation suggestive of the adult respiratory distress syndrome (ARDS) (but for which no underlying cause is apparent) should raise suspicion of AIP or the Hamman-Rich syndrome. Individuals affected by AIP are often younger adults or even children. Although this disorder has a poor prognosis, patients who recover may have completely normal pulmonary function. Like AIP, bronchiolitis obliterans with organizing pneumonia (BOOP) may develop in an abrupt fashion, but it reflects a pattern

TABLE 2. *Comparison of BAL cellularity between patients with IPF and both nonsmoker and smoker volunteers[a]*

	Nonsmoker volunteers (n = 111)	Smoker volunteers (n = 19)	IPF study subjects (n = 83)
Cells/mL, $\times 10^4$	12.7±9.1[***]	48.9±40.2[*]	28.0±24.4
Macrophages/mL, $\times 10^4$	12.1±10.0[***]	47.4±39.6[**]	22.4±21.8
Lymphocytes/mL, $\times 10^4$	0.8±1.0	0.7±0.7	1.6±3.0
Neutrophils/mL, $\times 10^4$	0.1±0.2[***]	0.6±0.9[*]	2.8±7.3
Eosinophils/mL, $\times 10^4$	0.0±0.1[***]	0.1±0.2[***]	1.2±2.8
Percent lavage return	75.9±15.9	70.7±17.7	73.7±14.7

From Schwartz DA, Helmers RA, Dayton CS, Merchant RK, Hunninghake GW. Determinants of bronchoalveolar lavage cellularity in idiopathic pulmonary fibrosis. *J Appl Physiol* 1991;71:1688. Reproduced with permission.

[a] Values are means ± SD. Values for p were computed by comparing nonsmoker volunteers with patients having IPF and by comparing smoker volunteers with patients having IPF.

[*] $p < 0.01$; [**] $p < 0.001$; [***] $p < 0.0001$.

of injury in the small airways and the adjacent pulmonary parenchyma. It is often responsive to therapy and usually has a good prognosis.

Physical Examination

Physical examination findings generally include tachypnea, basilar crackles, and exercise-induced cyanosis. Chest crackles occur in 60%–75% of cases; typically they are fine and late in inspiration, and they are often described as "velcro rales." Crackles are more common in IPF than in other forms of ILD, such as sarcoidosis, and are thought to be associated with subpleural fibrosis. Mid- and late-expiratory crackles may be detected. These more subtle findings are believed to be caused by vibrations of the airway walls and may be a clinical indicator of disease severity. Clubbing is present in about 65% of cases of IPF. It occurs more commonly in men and may begin early in the disease course. Of note, full-blown hypertrophic osteoarthropathy is rare. In one study, clubbing correlated with the extent of smooth-muscle proliferation in fibrotic pulmonary lesions. With the onset of secondary pulmonary hypertension, signs of right-sided heart failure, such as jugular venous distension, an accentuated P_2 heart sound, and pedal edema, become apparent.

Evaluation for characteristic manifestations of systemic rheumatic disease, including physical examination findings and results of selected laboratory studies, complements the history in excluding ILD associated with specific illnesses.

Diagnostic Studies

Physiologic Evaluation

Results of pulmonary function studies are among the best indicators of the severity of IPF. Diminished single-breath diffusion capacity of carbon monoxide (D_LCO), in particular, is one of the earliest and most sensitive physiologic abnormalities of IPF. It has been recommended that D_LCO be corrected for alveolar volume (D_LCO/V_A, or KCO), because KCO is a more useful indicator of the severity of gas exchange impairment during exercise and the degree of pulmonary vascular involvement. It is not clear, however, whether D_LCO or KCO is the best index of impairment. Reduction in lung volumes typical of restrictive disease is also noted. The degree of reduction in lung volumes and increase in lung elastic recoil directly correlate with the extent of fibrosis. There is, however, a very poor correlation between lung volumes and inflammation. The reduction in lung volumes also causes a reduction in forced expiratory volume in 1 second (FEV_1) and forced vital capacity (FVC) as measured by spirometry. Because the reductions in FEV_1 and FVC are usually of equal magnitude, there is often

no evidence of airway obstruction. A widened alveolar-arterial gradient in partial pressure of oxygen [$P(A-a)O_2$], worsened by exertion, is also a useful parameter to monitor in patients with IPF.

Comorbid obstructive lung disease caused by cigarette smoking may complicate interpretation of pulmonary function data in patients with IPF, because of increased residual volume (RV) and functional residual capacity (FRC) resulting from trapping of air. The presence of both obstructive and restrictive lung diseases has opposite effects on measures of air flow and lung volumes, and smoking may appear to "normalize" these physiologic measures in IPF. The D_LCO is an accurate method of assessing lung function in patients with IPF who smoke and have obstructive lung disease. To confound matters further, small-airway obstruction is often present in early IPF, independently of smoking, and may influence physiologic parameters such as mid-expiratory flow rates. About two thirds of patients have morphometric and physiologic evidence of small-airway involvement, indicated by abnormalities of flow-volume curves and dynamic compliance.

Initially, it was thought that a fall in arterial PO_2 was most caused by diffusion abnormalities. More recent work suggests that arterial hypoxemia is explained best by ventilation-perfusion mismatch and to a lesser extent by a diffusion limitation. Patients with IPF have higher pulmonary arterial pressures both at rest and during exercise than patients who have other causes of ILD. Although pulmonary arterial hypertension may be mainly caused by destruction of blood vessel in fibrotic lung, pulmonary vasoconstriction caused by alveolar hypoxia is also important.

Physiologic changes in lung function during both exercise and sleep provide useful clues about the severity and functional consequences of IPF. Although exercise causes significant hypoxemia in most patients with long-standing IPF, there is generally little or no change in PCO_2. A small percentage of patients with early IPF may have normal or even improved levels of arterial blood gases during exercise. Pulmonary edema at maximal exercise, rather than inspiratory muscle fatigue, may account for exercise limitations observed in some patients with IPF. O_2 desaturation also develops in patients with IPF during REM sleep, similar to that seen in patients with chronic obstructive pulmonary disease (COPD). Insufficient ventilatory response to hypercapnia accounts for larger falls in O_2 saturation during sleep. Overall, O_2 desaturation during sleep is usually mild and less severe than that observed during exercise.

Like patients with COPD, patients with IPF expend about 120% of their predicted energy expenditure for body size. This is a principal component of the weight loss seen in IPF.

Quality-of-Life Evaluation

Quality-of-life considerations are of paramount importance in assessing disease severity and response to therapy. The sensation of dyspnea and limitations of physical activity are the most important considerations. Dyspnea may be quantitated (grades 1 through 4) in a simple and reliable manner, as outlined in the American Thoracic Society Shortness-of-Breath Scale. Various ordinal dyspnea scales, such as the Baseline Dyspnea Index (BDI), Medical Research Council (MRC) scale, and Oxygen-Cost Diagram (OCD), also provide semiquantitative information on disease-specific health-related quality of life (HRQL) and have good reliability. These measures of dyspnea are significantly associated with physiologic parameters of lung function. Severe breathlessness is correlated with lower resting DLCO and an accelerated ventilatory response to exercise. Dyspnea is related to reduced lung compliance and increased elastic work of breathing. In addition to dyspnea, other disease-associated factors clearly affect patients' quality of life. The Chronic Respiratory Questionnaire and the St. George's Respiratory Questionnaire evaluate a range of pulmonary symptoms. The short-form 36 (SF-36), a generic functional assessment instrument well validated for many chronic illnesses, has been used to measure HRQL in chronic obstructive pulmonary disease, and it correlates well with the BDI. For health outcomes research, a generic instrument such as the SF-36 may be preferred to disease-specific scales for comparing health states of patients having pulmonary disease with those of patients having other chronic conditions.

Both dyspnea and quantitative declines in pulmonary function are relevant to the determination of disability. Impairment rating may be defined by pulmonary function tests; 35.6% of patients with IPF are impaired, with an FVC of 50% or DLCO of 40%. This percentage is considerably higher than that for individuals with either sarcoidosis (12.1%), pneumoconiosis (13.6%), or asbestos exposure (1.1%).

Pulmonary Imaging

Plain Chest Radiography

Up to 10% of patients with IPF have normal chest x-ray findings despite significant functional impairment. When radiographic abnormalities are seen, the most characteristic finding is prominent bibasilar reticular or reticulonodular infiltrates (Fig. 1). These abnormalities progress to honeycombing late in the course of disease. Although the basilar findings are most easily appreciated on plain film radiograph, IPF is a diffuse process. Pleural findings on plain film are uncommon. To better quantitate and communicate plain radiographic findings, the International Labour Office (ILO) scoring system, developed for occupational lung disease, can be used. This scoring system is reliable and correlates to some degree with physiologic data. Table 3 describes demographic, clinical, and radiographic characteristics in a representative group of patients with IPF.

Computed Tomography

Computed tomography (CT) is superior to plain radiography in evaluating IPF. CT may also be more useful than chest radiography in assessing the location of disease and in suggesting sites for biopsy. CT has the advantage over plain radiographs of eliminating superimposition of structures, thereby allowing better definition of the type, severity, and distribution of abnormalities seen in IPF.

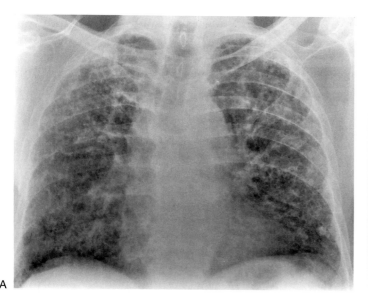
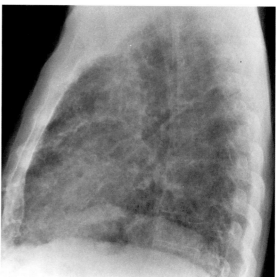

A   B

FIG. 1. Posteroanterior (**A**) and lateral (**B**) chest radiographs of a patient with IPF. A diffuse reticulonodular infiltrate is present throughout the lung with somewhat greater involvement peripherally. Cystic honeycombing is apparent in both lower lung fields.

TABLE 3. *Demographic, clinical, and radiographic characteristics of 24 patients with IPF*

Parameter	Value
Sex	
Male	15 (62.5%)
Female	9 (37.5%)
Age, y[a]	63.4 ± 12.5
Smoking history	
Never	8 (33.3%)
Formerly	14 (58.3%)
Currently	2 (8.3%)
Pack-years of cigarette smoking[a]	24.38 ± 21.79
Chest x-ray findings	
ILO category	
0	1 (4.2%)
1	10 (41.7%)
2	11 (45.8%)
3	2 (8.3%)
Pleural disease	
Present	5 (20.8%)
Absent	19 (79.2%)
Dyspnea class	
1	2 (8.3%)
2	8 (33.3%)
3	1 (4.2%)
4	6 (25%)
5	7 (29.2%)

From Hartley PG, Galvin JR, Hunninghake GW, et al. High-resolution CT-derived measures of lung density are valid indexes of interstitial lung disease. *J Appl Physiol* 1994;76:271. Reproduced with permission.

IPF, idiopathic pulmonary fibrosis; ILO, International Labour Office.

[a] Values are means ± SD.

Subpleural shadowing is well visualized on CT and predominates in the posterior lower lobes.

Fast scan times of 1 to 2 seconds allow high-resolution, thin-section scans (high-resolution CT). High-resolution CT is often performed with the patient both supine and prone to detect minimal pathologic changes. Cystic air spaces ("honeycomb" cysts) measuring 2 to 20 mm in diameter are detected in 90% of high-resolution CT scans, compared with 30% of plain radiographs. On high-resolution CT, IPF tends to have a patchy, peripheral distribution throughout the lung (Fig. 2). The presence of subpleural fibrosis seen in IPF by high-resolution CT may help differentiate it from sarcoidosis. High-resolution CT may be especially useful in the evaluation of patients with concomitant IPF and emphysema, who may have normal spirometric findings and lung volumes. Computer-aided diagnosis using clinical, plain radiographic, and high-resolution CT values is experimental but may prove useful in the future.

The utility of high-resolution CT for measuring disease severity and progression is controversial. A "ground-glass" appearance seen on high-resolution CT is thought to be indicative of active areas of inflammation, which may have potential therapeutic or prognostic importance.

Reticular patterns seen on high-resolution CT often correspond histologically with areas of fibrosis. Traction bronchiectasis and bronchiolectasis are often found in areas of fibrosis. Despite its many attributes and the increased sensitivity of high-resolution CT over plain radiographs, there are some significant limitations to this methodology. The overall sensitivity of high-resolution CT for biopsy-proven IPF is only 88%. Therefore, although sensitive, it may miss mild cases of IPF detected by biopsy or suggested by an abnormal DLCO. Parenchymal opacification ("ground-glass changes") detected by high-resolution CT may not be useful to guide therapy. For instance, it may be difficult with high-resolution CT to separate inflammation from fibrosis in all cases. In one study, ground-glass appearance correlated with inflammation in 65% and fibrosis in 54% of cases of diffuse lung disease. Ground-glass infiltrates have also correlated poorly with regions of inflammation in bleomycin-induced pulmonary fibrosis of rats. It is important to note that high-resolution CT provides only a limited sample of the chest and may miss a patchy process. On the other hand, IPF is diffuse and should therefore be an ideal disease to be studied using this technique. To minimize interobserver and intraobserver variability in interpretation of high-resolution CT and provide a quantitative measurement correlated with dyspnea and physiologic parameters, investigators have examined the utility of a computer-derived density analysis of lung parenchyma, with some success.

Gallium Scanning and Other Nuclear Imaging

Scanning with gallium citrate Ga 67 is a highly sensitive test for acute lung inflammation, but its very poor specificity limits its clinical usefulness. Further, the technique is poorly standardized, although computerized imaging methods may lessen the variability. Indium-labeled neutrophil scans have been successfully used in animal models to differentiate between normal animals and those having experimental alveolitis with increased neutrophils in the lung. Overall, ventilation-perfusion scans are not helpful in the routine assessment of IPF disease activity or in assessing response to therapy.

Magnetic Resonance Imaging and Positron Emission Tomography

The usefulness of magnetic resonance imaging (MRI) in detection and surveillance of IPF has been limited historically by long imaging times that require careful respiratory gating techniques to minimize artifact from respiratory movements. MRI provides qualitative rather than quantitative information about IPF. Positron emission tomography (PET) has been used in pilot studies to evaluate variations in pulmonary vascular permeability seen in IPF. The high cost and restricted availability of PET tech-

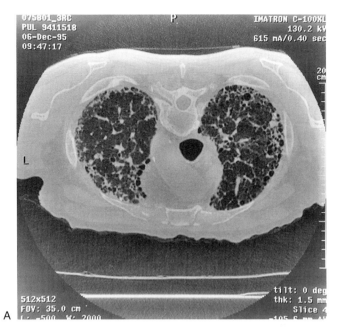

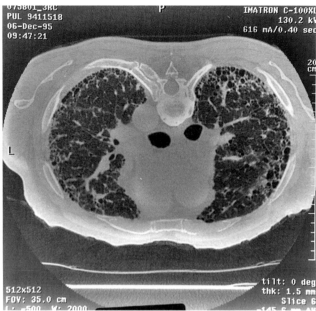

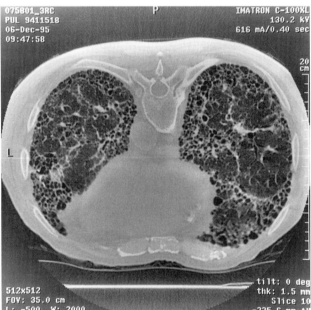

FIG. 2. High-resolution chest CT (1.5-mm slices) of a patient with IPF. Apical (**A**), midlung (**B**), and basilar (**C**) cuts are shown. These sections demonstrate marked peripheral fibrotic changes with cystic honeycombing most prominent at the bases of the lungs.

nology are likely to limit its common use. Neither modality has a role in the routine evaluation or management of IPF at this time.

Laboratory Studies

Although laboratory studies may be useful in excluding other causes of ILD, serum and urine biochemical and serologic studies are of limited value in the management of IPF. The erythrocyte sedimentation rate is elevated in approximately 50% of cases. Polyclonal gammopathy resulting from nonspecific B-cell activation is noted in about 75% of patients. Even in the absence of a clearly defined rheumatologic disorder, elevations are seen in

serum rheumatoid factor (30%) and antinuclear antibody (ANA) (15%). Measurement of serum levels of complement and immune complexes is nonspecific and not a reliable indicator of disease activity.

Bronchoalveolar Lavage

BAL is performed by instilling aliquots of saline solution through a flexible bronchoscope that has been "wedged" into a third- or fourth-order bronchus. With this technique, recovered fluid may be evaluated for cell number and differential analysis, cultures may be obtained, and secreted proteins can be identified and quantitated. BAL has been useful in the evaluation of lung cancer and infections. Its role in the management of IPF and other ILD has been controversial. Nevertheless, it can be extremely useful in the evaluation of alveolar inflammation, which can be used to establish a diagnosis, monitor response to therapy, and predict a patient's prognosis. Increased numbers of lymphocytes are seen in patients with more active inflammation and suggest an improved response to corticosteroid therapy. Neutrophils with or without eosinophils are increased in IPF BALF specimens, and neutrophilia portends a poor prognosis. BAL has been examined to assess its effectiveness as a surveillance and staging tool. BAL may be of limited value because technique is not standardized. Samples from different parts of the lung vary in cellularity, limiting reliability of BAL. It is important for both investigators and clinicians who plan to follow serial BAL in a particular patient to adopt standardized techniques to avoid high intrasubject variability. Correlation between BAL and high-resolution CT is essential to define better the role of BAL in assessment of inflammation. At the present time, BAL is still considered a research tool with no proven clinical utility in the management of IPF.

Lung Biopsy

The necessity to perform an open lung biopsy for the diagnosis of IPF is debated by many chest physicians. In the United Kingdom, the diagnosis is usually based on purely clinical grounds. Because IPF is a patchy disease, a negative or nonspecific transbronchial biopsy specimen may represent either an inadequate sample or a sample of an unaffected region of the lung. Several studies have also shown that the amount of tissue obtained by transbronchial lung biopsy is not sufficient to make a diagnosis of IPF. Transbronchial lung biopsy is often used, however, to exclude the presence of other disorders, such as hypersensitivity pneumonitis or BOOP. Many practitioners recommend an open lung biopsy for all patients with a negative transbronchial lung biopsy result if clinical suspicion of IPF is high. For many patients, open lung biopsy is required to establish a definitive diagnosis. Open lung biopsy is the "gold standard" for IPF diagnosis. With open lung biopsy, infectious and neoplastic processes can be excluded, and the specimen may provide some staging information useful for planning a treatment program. For diffuse pulmonary infiltrates of unknown etiology, open lung biopsy results in management changes in up to three quarters of all patients.

At the time of open lung biopsy, it is necessary to sample not only the most grossly affected areas, but also more central areas that are in earlier stages of the disease process. High-resolution CT before biopsy can be useful in localizing areas of particular interest. Although some disagree, it is recommended that the tip of the lingular segment and the right middle lobe be avoided, as these areas often have nonspecific changes. Open lung biopsy may result in serious complications 11%–23% of the time. This rate depends in part on the degree to which the patient is immunocompromised at the time of the procedure. The use of video-assisted thoracoscopic surgery, or thoracoscopy-guided lung biopsy, has significantly limited the need for open lung biopsy in selected centers. The diagnostic accuracy is essentially equal to that of open lung biopsy, and patients have less morbidity and shorter hospital stays.

Given the generally poor prognosis of IPF, coupled with the potential morbidity and mortality associated with open lung biopsy, many physicians decide to forego the surgical procedure when they strongly suspect the presence of IPF. Any decision to perform open lung biopsy must take into account the likelihood of the diagnosis without the test as well as the complications associated with its performance. Under certain circumstances, open lung biopsy may be omitted.

Pathology

On gross inspection, the lungs are small, with a nodular pleural surface. The subpleural areas of the lung parenchyma are most severely affected, with the development of honeycomb cystic changes in late-stage fibrosis. Fibrosis often occupies about 20% of the lung volume (Fig. 3).

From a histopathologic perspective, IPF can be divided into usual interstitial pneumonitis (UIP) and desquamative interstitial pneumonitis (DIP). DIP is characterized by mild inflammation of the alveolar interstitium, relative preservation of the alveolar architecture, and the presence of large numbers of macrophages in the alveolar air spaces. In UIP, the alveolar wall is thickened with inflammatory cells and connective tissue. There is often also a reorganization of the parenchyma. DIP and UIP may simply represent different stages of the same pathologic process. Of interest, different histopathologic patterns frequently are noted even in the same specimen.

Alveolitis is thought to be the initial abnormality in all cases of ILD. Infiltrates of lymphocytes and plasma cells are noted early in the disease, with interstitial edema and eventual loss of type I epithelial and capillary endothelial cells. Desquamation, indicative of an active inflammatory process, occurs when type II pneumocytes and alveolar macrophages fill the alveolar lumen. Type II pneumocytes proliferate in areas of less severe fibrosis, whereas cuboidal and metaplastic squamous epithelial cells renew epithelium in areas of very severe lung damage. Dense alveolar septal fibrosis occurs in later stages because of the accumulation of fibroblasts and collagen within the interstitium. The pleura is also abnormal in IPF; it thickens and becomes more vascular. It is lined by hypertrophied and hyperplastic mesothelial cells. The larger airways show increased amounts of muscle and glandular tissue.

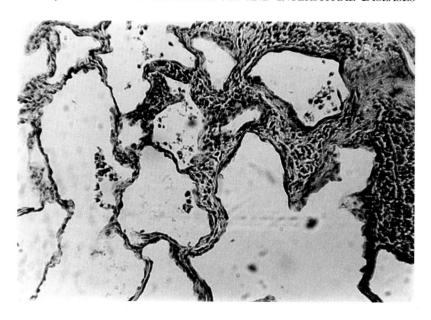

FIG. 3. Histology of open lung biopsy specimen from a patient with IPF. This reveals patchy dense fibrosis adjacent to normal alveoli. Original magnification × 200.

Histologic scoring systems have been developed by several groups to provide reproducible, standardized reporting techniques for clinical trials. Scoring systems use different pathologic parameters, such as the level of fibrosis and cellularity of specimens, which are uniformly interpreted by panels of pathologists. Semiquantitative systems are faster and may provide as much correlation with clinical parameters as more detailed morphometric analyses.

Ultrastructural features of IPF may be different from those observed in ILD associated with systemic rheumatologic disorders. Endothelial cell swelling and intracellular tubuloreticular structures are noted in patients with rheumatic disease-associated ILD, but not in IPF. These tubuloreticular structures are similar to those observed in viral pneumonia.

In AIP, in contrast to IPF, there are intra-alveolar hyaline membranes, interstitial septal widening, endothelial and epithelial damage, and fibroblast proliferation without extensive collagen deposition. These pathologic features are identical to findings in ARDS. However, ARDS often resolves without permanent damage, whereas fibrosis associated with hyperplastic type II pneumocytes often develops within a few weeks of onset of AIP. Pneumocytes proliferate, and the collapsed alveoli coalesce into a single thickened septum. Type I pneumocytes proliferate along the denuded basal lamina of the alveolar septa. As the disorder progresses, intra-alveolar exudates are incorporated into the alveolar wall, contributing to its thickness. Ultrastructural changes of AIP include folding of the alveolar septa with collapse of entire alveoli and apposition of their walls. Ultimately, honeycombing appears, occasionally within weeks, and the final histology of AIP is identical to that seen in IPF. In fact, it has been hypothesized that the sequence of lung injury in individual areas of the lung are similar in IPF and AIP.

Pathogenic Theories

IPF is most likely an immune-mediated illness, and it probably results from a host response to an as-yet-unknown respiratory antigen. Although many cells play important roles in perpetuating the immune response, tissue damage is predominantly mediated by alveolar macrophages and neutrophils. Macrophages directly damage the lung parenchyma and also attract and activate neutrophils and other inflammatory cells. Direct pulmonary damage is mediated by macrophage production of free oxygen radicals; alveolar macrophages are an important source of oxygen radicals in the lungs. Of interest, excessive production of free oxygen radicals in patients with IPF correlates with abnormal physiologic parameters. Macrophages release products chemotactic for neutrophils (leukotriene B_4), growth factors for fibroblasts (platelet-derived growth factors, fibronectin, and insulin-like growth factor), and proinflammatory cytokines (interleukin-1β and tumor necrosis factor-α). Macrophages release both IL-1β and its specific inhibitor, IL-1 receptor antagonist (IL-1RA); the IL-1β/IL-1RA ratio is increased in patients with IPF, resulting in a proinflammatory environment. Macrophages also recruit mesenchymal cells to the lung and activate them as part of the fibrotic process.

Neutrophils also appear to have a number of potential pathogenic roles in IPF. Neutrophils release oxidants and proteinases, like collagenase, that are locally destructive. In normal persons who do not smoke, very few neutrophils are seen in the lower respiratory tract, but in patients with active IPF, the neutrophil represents up to 20% of BALF cells. Eosinophils release similar compounds as well as other toxic products, such as eosinophil major basic protein.

As is true of all immunologic illnesses, lymphocytes

are central to the inflammatory cascade. B lymphocytes produce IgG, and IgG-containing immune complexes can be found in inflamed lung; although these complexes are associated with IPF, their pathogenic role is speculative. T lymphocytes may also play a prominent role, both in an autoimmune reaction against alveolar antigens and in enhancement of matrix production. Activated T cells produce cytokines that stimulate proliferation of fibroblasts and lead to increased collagen synthesis.

Mesenchymal cells of the interstitium synthesize type I collagen, type III collagen, fibronectin, and other matrix proteins prominent in fibrotic lungs. In IPF, these cells are numerous in the alveoli as well as in the interstitium. Both the amount of matrix proteins synthesized as well as their composition may be altered in IPF.

Treatment

As is true for many relatively rare, serious disorders of unknown cause, there is much dogma but few controlled studies evaluating IPF management. Because duration of disease is such a potent predictor of outcome, careful comparisons of therapeutic protocols are confounded by differing definitions and duration of disease. For most physicians, prednisone is the drug of first choice, and immunosuppressive agents are generally reserved for corticosteroid failures. Although early alveolitis is clearly more responsive to anti-inflammatory therapy than later, more fibrotic disease, improvements in survival with aggressive treatment are reported even in patients who have more advanced disease.

General Supportive Measures

As in the management of chronic obstructive lung disease, pulmonary rehabilitation and/or O_2 therapy are recommended for patients with limited exercise tolerance and severe arterial hypoxemia. O_2 therapy improved exercise tolerance in subjects with IPF in some but not in all studies. Continuous low-flow O_2 should be prescribed for all patients with demonstrated resting hypoxia, especially in the presence of cor pulmonale or polycythemia. Exercise- or sleep-induced desaturation should be treated with O_2 to maintain a saturation of 90%.

Vasodilators have been used in IPF as therapeutic agents for pulmonary hypertension. Isosorbide dinitrate, nitrendipine, nifedipine, and hydralazine have all been evaluated in small studies. Although nifedipine has been shown to blunt an exercise-induced increase in pulmonary vascular resistance in some studies, there is no clear evidence that any of the vasodilators have a role in the therapy of IPF. Use of these agents may be dangerous and lead to a worse outcome or even death.

Corticosteroids

Despite their significant short- and long-term toxic effects, corticosteroids remain the mainstay of therapy. Patients with highly cellular infiltrates have the best response to corticosteroids, but measurable improvements in pulmonary function are found in no more than 30% of cases. With corticosteroids, subjective improvement occurs in more than half of cases.

Early use of high-dose corticosteroid is recommended to provide the best chance for recovery. Improvement, if it is going to occur, is usually noted within several weeks. Corticosteroid therapy is begun with a daily dose of 0.5 to 1 mg of prednisone per kilogram of body weight, or the equivalent. Because of the toxicity of corticosteroids at this level, once improvement has been noted (or after 4 to 8 weeks), the dose is tapered to 20 mg/day or less.

Immunosuppressive Agents

Antimetabolites and cytotoxic drugs, broadly classified as immunosuppressive agents, have been used in numerous small clinical trials with variable results. The rationale for use of these drugs is based on both the need for steroid-sparing agents and the poor overall response of most patients to corticosteroids alone.

Azathioprine, typically administered at a dose of 2 to 3 mg/kg, has been used in conjunction with high-dose corticosteroids in several studies. As might be expected, the most favorable responses were noted in subjects with less fibrosis seen on biopsy. Favorable trends were noted in some of the studies, but there is still no clear evidence that this agent benefits patients with IPF. Azathioprine is generally well tolerated. In a few patients, evidence of significant hematologic abnormalities develops; therefore, careful monitoring of blood counts is imperative. A secondary malignancy is also a potential concern for patients.

Cyclophosphamide has also been used extensively in patients with IPF. Although several studies show benefits in isolated pulmonary parameters, others demonstrate no improvement or even a poorer outcome as a consequence of life-threatening infectious sequelae. A randomized, controlled trial of 43 patients with previously untreated IPF showed that the combination of prednisolone with cyclophosphamide was slightly superior to prednisolone alone in improving symptoms. Unfortunately, survival (although better in the cyclophosphamide group) was not significantly improved, and both groups demonstrated high overall mortality. Intermittent intravenous therapy, as biweekly pulses of between 500 and 1800 mg per dose) appears to be as effective as daily oral therapy. The benefits of cyclophosphamide may be attributable to the reduction of lung neutrophilia. With cyclophosphamide, improvement is slow, necessitating a prolonged course of up to 6 months with very careful hematologic monitoring for neutropenia. The risks for hemorrhagic cystitis and secondary malignancy, particularly uroepithelial and hematologic cancers, limit the long-term utility of this therapy. Intravenous administration may result in less bladder toxicity and allow easier monitoring of hematologic parameters. Of some concern is the development of interstitial pneumonitis secondary to cyclophosphamide therapy.

Chlorambucil, at doses between 2 and 6 mg daily, can be used as an alternate to cyclophosphamide in the treatment of IPF. It has the advantages of lower cost and an improved risk-benefit ratio, particularly because of less concern about urinary excretion of active metabolites. Close monitoring of blood counts is still very important. Preliminary studies suggest that the efficacy of chlorambucil is equivalent to that of cyclophosphamide.

Another agent with actions that may complement the effects of corticosteroids is cyclosporine A. This agent is a potent suppressor of T-lymphocyte function, and it could be useful in suppressing the cell-mediated immune responses in IPF. Because there is a high incidence of drug-induced hypertension and nephrologic toxicity associated with cyclosporine, and because there is no consensus regarding its usefulness in IPF, cyclosporine therapy is not standard at this time.

Miscellaneous Other Pharmacotherapeutic Agents

Low-dose oral colchicine is well tolerated, and it has been associated with an improvement in lung function in several small studies and case reports. Colchicine suppresses fibroblast function in vitro. The antimalarial agent chloroquine has also been successful in anecdotal use. D-penicillamine has been used to treat ILD associated with systemic sclerosis, and a small study reported better outcomes for patients with IPF who were taking this agent. Unfortunately, treatment-limiting hematologic toxicity, proteinuria, and dyspepsia are seen in a high percentage of penicillamine-treated patients.

Organ Transplantation

In selected patients with end-stage ILD, unilateral lung transplantation may provide a good functional result and can significantly improve quality of life. In terms of prolonging survival, 45% of IPF patients who receive a single lung are alive for 1 year or longer, and some have survived for up to 4 years after surgery. Unilateral transplant may be superior to total heart-lung transplant in terms of lowered surgical morbidity and mortality. In addition, single-lung transplantation potentially extends the opportunity for lung transplantation to twice the number of recipients. Physiologically, IPF and other restrictive lung diseases are most appropriate for single-lung transplantation. In these diseases, the native lung typically has very low compliance, so that ventilation and perfusion to the trans-

planted lung are better than in patients with emphysema who receive a single lung.

Monitoring Disease Activity

Because of the high mortality of IPF, survival is the most important marker of treatment success. Nevertheless, pulmonary function test results, bronchoscopic findings, and radiographic studies have a role in monitoring disease progression. In addition, Watters and colleagues have developed a clinical, radiographic, and physiologic (CRP) scoring system that correlates well with both pathologic changes and quality-of-life factors. In pulmonary function studies, a significant decline in D_LCO or FVC is indicative of a poor therapeutic response. The $P_{(A-a)}O_2$ gradient also can be followed, but this is somewhat variable and may not correlate well with disease progression.

Natural History and Prognosis

Despite optimal therapy, the 5-year survival for IPF remains no better than 50%. Although mean survival is estimated at 4 years, rare patients may persist with end-stage but stable fibrosis for periods of 20 years or more. A favorable response to treatment with corticosteroids is an excellent long-term prognostic factor. Symptoms of 1 year in duration also are associated with a better outcome. Younger age, female sex, less dyspnea, fewer radiographic abnormalities, absence of right-axis deviation on electrocardiogram, and higher arterial PO_2 are other demographic and clinical factors that predict longer survival. The survival of patients with advanced disease or progressive reductions in physiologic tests ($\geq 10\%$ in FVC or $\geq 20\%$ in D_LCO) is significantly worse. Cigarette smoking is the only potentially modifiable risk factor. It is associated with a poorer outcome in a dose-dependent manner. Despite the prompt response of some patients to therapy and apparent complete clinical remission, relapse can occur as many as 12 years later.

Respiratory failure from intractable hypoxemia accounts for many deaths in IPF (38.7%); this is frequently associated with the development of an acute pulmonary infection. The development of pulmonary hypertension and cor pulmonale is an indicator of imminent decline; this ultimately occurs in about 70% of patients with IPF. Other causes of death include heart failure, pulmonary embolism, and lung cancer.

Cancer

Bronchogenic cancer develops during the course of illness in approximately 5%–10% of patients with IPF. This represents an excess relative risk for lung cancer of almost

10 in comparison with a similar age- and sex-matched group. This risk ratio may be an underestimate, as many early lung carcinomas may be missed because of the shortened life expectancy of patients with IPF. It has been noted that the excess risk for cancer in male patients with IPF cannot be accounted for by cigarette smoking alone. Adenocarcinoma occurring in the periphery is the most common lesion, although all cell types have been described.

INTERSTITIAL LUNG DISEASE ASSOCIATED WITH SYSTEMIC RHEUMATIC DISORDERS

Many types of lung disease are associated with rheumatoid arthritis; the connective tissue disorders, including systemic lupus erythematosus (SLE), Sjögren's syndrome, systemic sclerosis (SSc), and dermatomyositis/polymyositis; mixed connective tissue disease (MCTD); and the seronegative spondyloarthropathies, principally ankylosing spondylitis. Of all the types of respiratory disorders associated with systemic rheumatic disorders, one of the most difficult to diagnose accurately and manage is ILD. Table 4 compares and contrasts IPF with two of the rheumatic diseases most commonly associated with ILD. The true prevalence of ILD in rheumatic disorders is unknown, and estimates vary depending on the diagnostic method used. Plain chest radiographs are least sensitive,

TABLE 4. *Comparison of common types of interstitial lung disease: clinical and pathologic manifestations*

	IPF	RA	SSc
Association with cigarette smoking	+++	++	−
Symptoms			
Pleurisy	+	++	+
Dyspnea	+++	++	+++
Signs			
Clubbing	+++	+	−
Nailfold capillary changes	−	−	+++
Arthritis	+	+++	+
Skin changes	−	+	+++
Serologic studies			
Rheumatoid factor	+	+++	−
Antinuclear antibodies	+	−	+++
Pulmonary function studies			
D$_{LCO}$ decline	+++	++	++
Lung volume reduction	+++	++	++
Pulmonary radiography			
Fibrosis	+++	++	++
Lung nodules	−	++	−
Pleural disease	−	+++	−
Response to therapy	poor	fair	poor
Association with pulmonary malignancy	++	+	++
Survival	poor	fair	poor

IPF, idiopathic pulmonary fibrosis; RA, rheumatoid arthritis; SSc, systemic sclerosis; D$_{LCO}$, diffusing capacity of lung for carbon monoxide; +, infrequent or mild; ++, occasional or intermediate; +++, very common or severe.

whereas pulmonary function tests detect lung disease at an earlier stage. High-resolution CT and BAL detect more subtle abnormalities not identified by other modalities. As in IPF, the gold standard of diagnosis remains histologic examination of an open lung biopsy specimen.

Rheumatoid Arthritis

Rheumatoid arthritis is the most common form of inflammatory arthritis, with a worldwide prevalence of 1%. It affects women more frequently than men, in a ratio of 3:1. Rheumatoid arthritis is a symmetric, inflammatory polyarthritis with a myriad of extra-articular features. Pulmonary manifestations range from common pleural effusions to rare bronchiolitis obliterans. The diagnosis of rheumatoid arthritis is based on the characteristic historical feature of morning stiffness, evidence on physical examination of swollen and tender joints, and supportive laboratory data, including a high titer of serum rheumatoid factors and characteristic bone erosion detected by radiograph. The American College of Rheumatology has developed rheumatoid arthritis classification criteria useful in clinical studies. Rheumatoid arthritis causes substantial morbidity, predominantly from progressive joint destruction, that results in a 50% work disability rate after 10 years of active disease. Rheumatoid arthritis also leads to premature mortality, shortening life expectancy by 8 to 13 years on average. Mortality is most often related to infectious illnesses. Rheumatoid arthritis is strongly associated with an increased frequency of the class II major histocompatibility complex (MHC) serotype HLA-DR4, and specific DR4 haplotypes (HLA-DRB1*0401 and *0404) predict more severe rheumatoid arthritis.

Epidemiology

Rheumatoid lung involvement may be manifested by many disease patterns. Although pleuropulmonary disease is seen quite often, ILD may be most common overall, based on series of patients undergoing lung biopsy.

Ellman and Ball were the first to link diffuse pulmonary fibrosis with rheumatoid arthritis. Since that time, numerous case series and several controlled studies have confirmed their observation. Many authors now refer to this entity as *rheumatoid arthritis-associated interstitial lung disease (RA-ILD)*. The reported prevalence of RA-ILD ranges from 2% to 40% of patients with rheumatoid arthritis. Variability in prevalence relates to different diagnostic modalities used to define this condition. Whereas only about 1%–5% of patients with suspected RA-ILD have abnormalities detected by plain chest radiography, the percentage of affected individuals increases dramatically if diagnosis is established by abnormal pulmonary function studies (about 40%) or abnormal tissue histology (up to 80% of patients).

Prior investigations into risk factors for RA-ILD have yielded disparate results. Although rheumatoid arthritis is three times more common in women than in men, RA-ILD has a stronger male predilection. Traditional measures of severity of rheumatoid arthritis, such as serum rheumatoid factor and subcutaneous nodules, Sjögren's syndrome, antirheumatic therapies, immunogenetic markers of disease severity (HLA-DR4 and HLA-B40), and cigarette smoking, all have been identified as potential predictors of RA-ILD, although other studies have failed to confirm these associations. The two risk factors that have generated the most interest have been cigarette smoking and serum rheumatoid factor. As in IPF, cigarette smoking has a consistently positive association with RA-ILD based on multiple epidemiologic analyses (Fig. 4). A positive correlation between rheumatoid factor titer and abnormal diffusion capacity has also been demonstrated. Cigarette smoking is also associated with elevated serum rheumatoid factor. It is uncertain whether rheumatoid factor plays an independent pathogenic role in RA-ILD or is only an epiphenomenon. In conjunction with rheumatoid factor, smoking may synergistically contribute to diminished DLCO. Whether cigarette smoking alone is responsible for many of the pulmonary features of rheumatoid arthritis is also a point of contention.

Many studies of RA-ILD have selected subjects with known pulmonary symptoms or have utilized control populations of patients without rheumatoid arthritis. Additionally, very few studies have been large enough to estimate with confidence the confounding risks of occupational exposures or infectious agents. Thus, knowledge about risk factors for the development of ILD in rheumatoid arthritis patients is limited.

Clinical Presentation

In all but a few studies, RA-ILD follows the development of joint disease, although the time interval from disease onset to lung involvement is often as short as 5 years. The medical history and physical examination are neither sensitive nor specific for the diagnosis of RA-ILD, but certain clinical features are common. In contrast to patients with IPF, many patients report symptoms of dyspnea or pleuritic chest pain. Clubbing has also been detected in some series, but less often than in IPF and

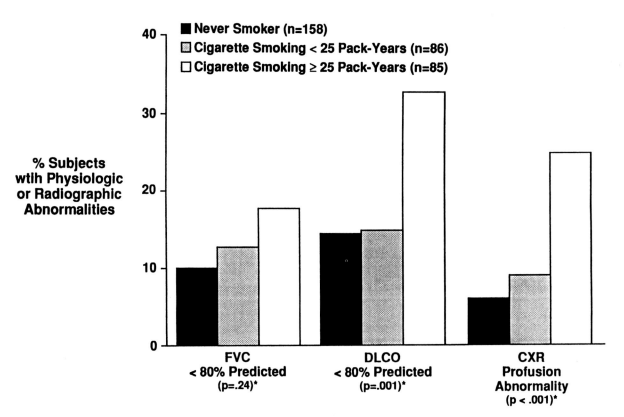

FIG. 4. Bar graph histogram demonstrating the association of cigarette smoking (expressed in pack-years) with abnormalities in pulmonary function studies (diffusion capacity of carbon monoxide [*DLCO*], forced vital capacity [*FVC*]) and chest radiograph (*CXR*) profusion abnormalities (interstitial infiltrates). Values for *p* are for the χ^2 trend test. (Reproduced with permission from Saag KG, Kolluri S, Koehnke RK, Georgou TA, Rachow JR, Hunninghake GW, Schwartz DA. Rheumatoid arthritis lung disease; determinants of physiologic and radiologic abnormalities. *Arthritis Rheum* (1996;39:1714. Reproduced with permission.)

usually later in the course of the disease. Chest crackles are strongly correlated with radiographic changes. Recurrent bronchitis with sputum production may occur in well-established RA-ILD. A surprisingly low percentage of patients with RA-ILD have pulmonary disease-related disability. This may be because physical disability resulting from rheumatoid arthritis limits patients' functional status and precludes exertional activities strenuous enough to produce pulmonary symptoms.

Diagnostic Studies

Physiologic Evaluation

Pulmonary function tests suggest a diagnosis of RA-ILD in a high percentage of clinically significant cases. Abnormality in diffusion capacity is the best predictor of fibrosis on biopsy. Indeed, reductions in diffusion capacity may precede other extra-articular manifestations of rheumatoid arthritis in many patients. Frequently, the coexistence of both restrictive and obstructive airway disease in cigarette smokers with rheumatoid arthritis confounds the interpretation of pulmonary function test abnormalities. In these patients, although both lung volumes and flows may be normalized, DLCO can be markedly reduced. Obstructive changes may also result from coexisting bronchiectasis or bronchiolitis obliterans. Because of the high concurrence of chronic disease-associated anemia, in rheumatoid arthritis it is necessary to adjust the DLCO reading for the hemoglobin level.

Pulmonary Imaging

Characteristic ILD findings are present on chest radiographs in about 12% of patients with rheumatoid arthritis. The plain radiographic appearance is identical to that of IPF except for an increased prevalence of nodules and pleural thickening. High-resolution CT can be used to identify very early evidence of RA-ILD, which may not be visible on plain radiographs. High-resolution CT often reveals fibrotic changes in the periphery, similar to those of IPF, as well as subpleural nodules and cavitations that are unique to RA-ILD. Some patients with rheumatoid arthritis who have abnormalities visible on high-resolution CT but not on plain x-ray films also have physiologic abnormalities. The clinician must be aware that the significance of high-resolution CT abnormalities in asymptomatic patients without other diagnostic abnormalities is unclear from both a therapeutic and prognostic perspective.

Laboratory Studies

No serologic study is sufficiently accurate to assist in the diagnosis of RA-ILD. As noted, serum rheumatoid factor is a strong predictor of RA-ILD, but it is not a good screening test. A study of 600 patients with rheumatoid arthritis and controls identified the ANA as a potential marker of disease.

Bronchoalveolar Lavage and Lung Biopsy

Although BAL is of greater value in excluding infectious and neoplastic causes of ILD, it may provide usefully prognostic information in RA-ILD. Both neutrophilic and lymphocytic alveolitis have been described in the BALF of patients with RA-ILD. As in IPF, elevated lymphocyte counts in BALF occur early in RA-ILD, whereas a neutrophilic predominance is found later in the disease process. Despite the value of BAL, the gold standard in the diagnosis of interstitial fibrosis is histopathologic examination of open lung biopsy specimens. In the absence of nodules that raise the index of suspicion, and because results are unlikely to alter clinical therapy, open lung biopsy is less often performed in RA-ILD than in IPF.

Pathology

The histologic features of RA-ILD are nearly indistinguishable from those of IPF. Biopsies show thickened alveolar septae and in some cases alveolar cell hyperplasia. Lymphocytic infiltration of the alveolar wall and cuboidalization of the type I pneumocytes are also present. Features that help differentiate RA-ILD from IPF include the prominent lymphocytic infiltrates, hyperplasia of lymphoid follicles, and characteristic rheumatoid pulmonary nodules. Rheumatoid nodules in the lung, the only pulmonary lesion specific to rheumatoid arthritis, impart a better prognosis. Disease based in the pleurae is more common in RA-ILD than in IPF and may help further separate the two entities.

Treatment and Prognosis

The treatment of RA-ILD is confounded by the fact that many of the traditional therapies used to manage both the articular and extra-articular manifestations of rheumatoid arthritis may also cause pulmonary toxicity. Intramuscular gold, cyclophosphamide, and methotrexate have all been linked to pneumonitis that may mimic early pulmonary fibrosis. Because methotrexate is currently the most commonly used second-line agent for the treatment of rheumatoid arthritis, pulmonary toxicity attributable to this therapy is of special concern. Unfortunately, there are no pathognomonic findings of methotrexate pneumonitis, and like RA-ILD, it may present with nonspecific bilateral reticulonodular or interstitial infiltrates. In one study, methotrexate did not cause restrictive disease or abnormalities with gas exchange, but instead it was associated with air trapping. Although some studies have suggested that methotrexate, gold, or D-penicillamine may be independent risk factors for RA-ILD, most investigations have failed to substantiate these associations.

Careful monitoring of RA-ILD progression is crucial in guiding therapy, as many potential therapeutic agents may cause significant iatrogenic morbidity. Therapy of early, symptomatic RA-ILD consists of high-dose corticosteroids, usually given as 1 mg of prednisone per kilogram of body weight, or the equivalent. It is important to start corticosteroids early in the inflammatory phase, as more advanced fibrotic disease is steroid-resistant. For RA-ILD that is refractory to corticosteroids or necessitates protracted high-dose therapy, cyclophosphamide, methotrexate, and more recently cyclosporine have been used with anecdotal success.

Survival statistics for RA-ILD are limited. For many individuals with mild disease, the prognosis is better than for IPF. However, among patients with extensive manifestations, the 5-year survival rate for RA-ILD is reported to be as low as 39%. Prognosis is significantly improved if a component of the fibrosis appears to be drug-related. As in IPF, histologic findings of UIP portend a particularly bad prognosis. Likewise, very rare upper lobe fibrosis, akin to ankylosing spondylitis, is also a poor prognostic factor. Lastly, bronchogenic carcinoma can complicate rheumatoid arthritis. Controversy surrounds the potential independent roles of cigarette smoking, commonly used immunosuppressive agents, and the underlying rheumatoid arthritis disease process in carcinogenesis.

Systemic Lupus Erythematosus

SLE is a heterogeneous multisystem disorder of unknown cause with a predilection for young black and Asian women. SLE is diagnosed on the basis of a constellation of characteristic symptoms, signs, and laboratory abnormalities. Because SLE is a clinical diagnosis and there are no pathognomonic features, SLE is both underdiagnosed and overdiagnosed by many physicians. It is estimated that the average patient with lupus waits for 2 years from the time of symptom onset until a correct diagnosis is achieved. Although some individuals, particularly those with discoid skin lesions, have a milder disease course, organ involvement affecting the kidneys, central nervous system, or respiratory tract is associated with significant morbidity and premature mortality.

Epidemiology

The most common form of lupus lung disease is pleurisy with or without pleural effusions; pleuropulmonary disease has an overall prevalence in SLE of about 70%. In addition, both acute and chronic ILD frequently develops in SLE. In most cases, ILD occurs in patients who have had other serious SLE-associated organ disease, although it may rarely precede the development of frank SLE. Studies that assess the frequency of lupus lung disease are predominantly small, uncontrolled investigations that suffer from referral and selection biases. Clinically significant ILD occurs in 3% of adult patients with SLE. However, physiologic abnormalities are noted in up to 88% of cases.

Several independent reviews have shown that parenchymal lung disease coincides directly with other manifestations of SLE in 20% of cases. In autopsy series of SLE, infection, congestive heart failure, coagulopathy, and O_2 toxicity account for the majority of the pulmonary abnormalities. These studies, however, are potentially limited by the selection of specific subsets of SLE patients likely to undergo autopsy and of those seen in referral centers.

Clinical Presentation

Numerous pulmonary SLE syndromes have been defined that present with clinical parameters suggestive of ILD.

Acute Lupus Pneumonitis

This fulminant process almost always develops in patients with established SLE. Patients are acutely ill, with the rapid development of tachypnea, dyspnea, fever, cough, and occasionally blood-tinged sputum. Physical examination and laboratory studies demonstrate cyanosis and hypoxemia, and chest examination with radiography reveals prominent alveolar consolidation findings. The most important differential diagnostic considerations are elimination of both conventional and atypical infectious etiologies. Of concern, up to 75% of patients with acute lupus pneumonitis have persistent lung dysfunction after resolution of the acute process.

Chronic Interstitial Disease

Chronic ILD may develop independently of acute pneumonitis or as its sequela. Dyspnea both at rest and with mild exertion is the predominant symptom. Cough and pleuritic chest pain each are reported in about two thirds of cases. Unlike IPF, chronic ILD is associated with pleuritis in about 40% of cases. Clubbing of the digits is also considerably less common than in IPF and is perhaps secondary to decreased digital perfusion resulting from Raynaud's phenomenon. Chronic ILD is more common in the subset of SLE patients who display overlapping features of scleroderma, such as edema of the hands and abnormalities of the nailfold capillaries.

Acute Reversible Hypoxemia

A syndrome of reversible hypoxemia has been observed in hospitalized SLE patients that is independent of pulmonary parenchymal infiltrates. This presentation has been attributed to pulmonary leukoaggregation in SLE patients who are acutely ill. These white cell clumps lead to substantial ventilation-perfusion mismatching.

Acute Pulmonary Hemorrhage

The sudden development of severe pulmonary insufficiency coupled with hemoptysis and rapidly progressive infiltrates should raise strong concerns about pulmonary hemorrhage. Pulmonary hemorrhage may complicate acute lupus pneumonitis or can occur independently. Unexpected elevation in DLCO, blood visualized by bronchoscopy, and hemosiderin-laden macrophages visible on biopsy all support this very serious complication.

Shrinking Lung Syndrome

Shrinking lung syndrome is another type of lupus-associated lung disease that may mimic ILD. Basilar atelectasis is a frequent radiographic finding that can be at least partially attributed to this pathologic process. Shrinking lung syndrome is not an intrinsic pulmonary disorder, but rather is caused by diaphragmatic dysfunction and respiratory muscle weakness that result in restrictive physiologic parameters and an elevated diaphragm. Some lupus patients may also demonstrate decreased respiratory muscle strength in the absence of chest radiographic abnormalities.

Diagnostic Studies

Physiologic Evaluation

Pulmonary function tests are the most sensitive indicators of chronic ILD in SLE. Diminished lung volumes, low diffusion capacity, and abnormal compliance occur in both acute and chronic lupus ILD. In one study, DLCO was reduced in 72% and lung volumes in 49% of all patients with SLE. Of younger patients with SLE (mean age, 15.5 years), restrictive pulmonary function test defects were found in 35% and diminished DLCO in 25%. Decreased ability to generate inspiratory and expiratory pressures is observed in patients with diaphragmatic dysfunction. Curiously, in SLE patients without known lung disease, a significant and progressive longitudinal decline occurs in small-airway physiologic parameters but not in lung volumes or DLCO. These changes are independent of smoking history.

Pulmonary Imaging

Plain radiographic findings are often normal early in the course of chronic lupus ILD. In contrast, in both later stages of chronic lupus ILD and acute lupus pneumonitis, prominent lower lobe infiltrates are present. Chest radiographs show abnormalities in about 30% of chronic ILD cases. As in other forms of ILD, high-resolution CT may noninvasively suggest the diagnosis of lupus ILD. A ground-glass appearance suggestive of more active inflammation has been correlated with a better response to therapy.

Laboratory Studies

ANA is detectable in the sera of 95% of patients with SLE. The most common ANA pattern is diffuse (also called *homogeneous*), but the peripheral (or rim) pattern is more specific. Although higher levels of antibodies to native (double-stranded) DNA and lower serum complement fractions are associated with more aggressive SLE in some patients, similar associations with lung disease have not been substantiated. Based on small series, the presence of antibodies to U1-RNP as well as SSA (Sjögren's syndrome antigen A) appears to be predictive of chronic restrictive lung disease and a decreased DLCO. Because of very poor specificity, assays for immune complexes are not recommended for either the diagnosis or surveillance of SLE pneumonitis.

Bronchoalveolar Lavage and Lung Biopsy

Particularly with acute infiltrates, BAL is often necessary to exclude infectious causes. Some authors advocate repeated BAL as a measure of response to therapy, but this approach cannot be strongly advocated in SLE, as there is no evidence of improved management or outcome based on BAL findings.

Pathology

Many of the pathologic lesions of SLE lung disease are at least partially attributable to immune complex deposition. In acute pneumonitis, interstitial edema, hyaline membranes, acute alveolitis, arteriolar thrombosis, intra-alveolar hemorrhage, and alveolar cell hyperplasia are all seen on histology. Immune complexes are identified in alveolar walls, interstitium, and near small vessels.

The pathology of chronic ILD is nearly identical to that of IPF. Chronic inflammatory cell infiltrates and deposition of immunoglobulins and complement are seen in the interstitium. In a large autopsy series, interstitial inflammatory infiltrates and thickening were ubiquitous, but significant fibrotic changes were not found. In this same series, the pattern of alveolar septal loss and panacinar emphysema was similar to the fibrosis of mild SSc. Rarely, lymphocytic interstitial pneumonitis has been seen in SLE. Thorough searches for chronic infectious agents have been consistently unrevealing in both acute and chronic lupus lung disease.

Treatment and Prognosis

After all types of both typical and opportunistic infections have been excluded, treatment of acute lupus pneumonitis begins with O_2 therapy, to correct hypoxemia, and moderate doses of corticosteroids (typically started at 1 mg of methylprednisolone per kilogram per day in divided doses). If pulmonary disease is refractory to this regimen, pulse methylprednisolone at 1 g/d, often for 3 days, has been advocated along with the concomitant use of immunosuppressive agents, such as intravenous cyclophosphamide. Plasmapheresis also has been used in rapidly deteriorating patients with anecdotal success.

The management of chronic ILD is more controversial. Treatment decisions should be geared toward alleviating symptoms, as few data exist to suggest that therapy alters disease progression. Chronic fibrosis indicated by irreversible honeycombing and the absence of inflammatory alveolitis is poorly, if at all, responsive to therapy. Pharmacotherapy should be reserved for patients with some evidence of an active inflammatory disease process, which is more likely to respond to the traditional agents. When treatment is indicated, corticosteroids remain the mainstay of the therapeutic armamentarium. They are usually administered as 40 to 60 mg of prednisone per day, or the equivalent. Steroid-sparing therapy with azathioprine or oral cyclophosphamide should be considered in refractory cases, or when treatment is necessary for a protracted period. Careful monitoring of physiologic studies and chest radiographs provides guidance on response to treatment.

Acute lupus pneumonitis carries a 50% mortality rate. Because improved chemotherapeutic regimens have increased the survival of patients with nonpulmonary manifestations of SLE, the final outcome of patients who have SLE associated with chronic lung disease often depends on the development of pulmonary hypertension and cor pulmonale. Reports of successful heart-lung transplantation in patients who have lupus-associated pulmonary hypertension without pulmonary fibrosis raise the hope that this therapy may be successful in patients with end-stage lupus lung diseases.

Sjögren's Syndrome

Sjögren's syndrome is an autoimmune exocrinopathy defined by the constellation of keratoconjunctivitis sicca and xerostomia. Sjögren's syndrome occurs as both a primary disorder and as a secondary condition in other rheumatologic disorders—most commonly, rheumatoid arthritis, SSc, and SLE. Although most patients with Sjögren's syndrome have symptoms limited to the exocrine glands, a myriad of well-described extraglandular features range from renal tubular acidosis to central nervous system lesions. Although Sjögren's syndrome is typically a benign lymphoproliferative disorder, progression to pseudolymphoma and frank B-cell lymphoma are uncommon but well-described disease transformations.

Epidemiology

The most common pulmonary manifestation of Sjögren's syndrome is desiccation of the airway (xerotrachea), leading to chronic cough and recurrent tracheobronchitis. Other types of pulmonary abnormalities that have been described include obstructive airway disease, lymphocytic interstitial pneumonitis (LIP), chronic interstitial fibrosis, pseudolymphoma, and pulmonary lymphoma. Pulmonary disease of all types occurs in up to 75% of patients with primary Sjögren's syndrome. In one study, significant pulmonary involvement was noted in 9% of 343 patients with Sjögren's syndrome. ILD detected in Sjögren's syndrome may begin as an LIP but can progress to frank pulmonary fibrosis. LIP is seen in about 1% of cases of Sjögren's syndrome, whereas nonlymphocytic ILD is observed in approximately 4% of patients with Sjögren's syndrome. More than half of all patients with Sjögren's syndrome and LIP also have rheumatoid arthritis; therefore, it is hard to know which pathologic process is directly responsible for this pulmonary condition. Not surprisingly, pulmonary involvement is both more common and more severe in secondary rather than in primary Sjögren's syndrome. Smoking is not a proven risk factor for the development of pulmonary disease in Sjogren's syndrome, as it is in RA-ILD and IPF.

Clinical Presentation

Characteristic clinical features of Sjögren's syndrome include sicca symptoms and, less commonly, salivary gland enlargement. Extraglandular tissues that can be involved include those of the central nervous system, gastrointestinal tract (primary biliary cirrhosis), and kidney (type II renal tubular acidosis). In one cross-sectional study, >40% of patients with recently diagnosed Sjögren's syndrome had respiratory symptoms in the absence of physical signs or radiographic evidence of lung disease. Dyspnea on exertion is a common complaint in these patients. Cough and pleuritic chest pain are also reported frequently and correlate with lymphocytosis on BAL. Wheezing is infrequently reported and clubbing is uncommonly seen except in patients in whom end-stage pulmonary fibrosis develops. The initial presentation of pulmonary Sjögren's syndrome may be misdiagnosed as an infectious pneumonia, because of the fevers and pulmonary symptoms and signs noted above. Pneumothorax also has been reported as a complication of LIP.

Diagnostic Studies

Physiologic Evaluation

D$_L$CO is diminished in about 19%–25% of patients with primary Sjögren's syndrome, often in the absence of radiographic abnormalities. The abnormality of diffusion capacity is more severe if Raynaud's phenomenon is present. Positive findings in biopsy specimens of minor salivary glands are correlated with a reduction in lung function. Although restrictive pulmonary disease patterns are most commonly reported, tests indicative of abnormalities in small-airway function also can be seen in the same patient.

Pulmonary Imaging

Bibasilar interstitial infiltrates are the most common plain radiographic finding of LIP. Nodular chest lesions secondary to atypical lymphoid hyperplasia are seen in the setting of pseudolymphoma. Most nodules are small, peripheral areas of consolidations, frequently containing air bronchograms. Multiple isolated nodules with better-defined margins, a more central location, and mediastinal adenopathy should raise concern of a transformation to a malignant pulmonary lymphoma.

Laboratory Studies

Although a variety of autoantibodies are frequently present in the serum of patients with Sjögren's syndrome, including rheumatoid factor (found in the majority of cases of both primary and secondary), ANA (70% of primary), SSA/Ro (70% of primary), and SSB/La (50% of primary), these serologic markers are generally indicative of nonpulmonary extraglandular disease and have very little bearing on pulmonary manifestations. Elevated levels of β_2-microglobulin are found in patients with lymphoproliferative complications and in subjects with obstructive airway disease.

Bronchoalveolar Lavage and Lung Biopsy

Patients with primary Sjögren's syndrome have a higher percentage of lymphocytes in their BALF than do normal controls, a finding potentially consistent with their underlying disease process.

Pathology

LIP consists mostly of large and small mature B lymphocytes and plasma cells. LIP is analogous to other aspects of Sjögren's syndrome; however, instead of infiltration of exocrine glands, the lungs are invaded by lymphocytes. Prolonged LIP may be complicated by amyloidosis. Pulmonary fibrosis can occur late in LIP, although a lymphocytic predominance may persist.

Lymphoproliferation in Sjögren's syndrome can progress to a pseudolymphoma. Pseudolymphoma is often heralded by a rising IgM level and the presence of germinal centers on lung biopsy. If malignant transformation follows, there is a notable decline in the IgM level, generalized hypogammaglobulinemia, and disappearance of rheumatoid factor. Patients usually have Sjögren's syndrome for 15 years or longer before malignant lymphoproliferation develops. If lymphoma occurs, the lungs are involved in at least 20% of cases.

An additional lymphoproliferative disorder that is included in the differential diagnosis of pulmonary Sjögren's syndrome is lymphomatoid granulomatosis. In this disorder, there is a proliferation of T lymphocytes (rather than the B lymphocytes of Sjögren's syndrome) and lesions exhibit angiodestructive infiltration, with frequent involvement of the upper airways in addition to the lungs. There are rare reports of concurrent lymphomatoid granulomatosis in patients with pre-established Sjögren's syndrome.

Although the cause of Sjögren's syndrome and its pulmonary syndromes are unknown, interesting work has focused on the potential role of viruses, such as the Epstein-Barr virus and retroviruses, as possible etiologic agents. Deposition of circulating immune complexes followed by complement activation appears to account partially for the pulmonary manifestations.

Treatment and Prognosis

Standard treatment of ILD associated with Sjögren's syndrome is not well established. In addition to general supportive measures, corticosteroids are often recommended for treatment of LIP despite an absence of good data to provide clear support for their beneficial use. Chloroquine has also been used successfully in case reports.

Pseudolymphomatous transformation is believed to merit aggressive chemotherapy with combined corticosteroid and alkylating agent regimens (chlorambucil or cyclophosphamide). When feasible, resection of lymphomatous mass lesions affords another therapeutic option.

Systemic Sclerosis

SSc, also called *scleroderma,* is a rare autoimmune disorder characterized by progressive fibrosis of the skin, vasculature, and internal organs. Estimates of the prevalence of SSc range from as few as 2 to as many as 265/100,000 people, and the predominance of women in their 50s is significant. Hidebound skin of the digits and distal extremities is the most characteristic finding of this disorder. Systemic sclerosis is subdivided into diffuse (dSSc) and limited (lSSc) variants. Limited SSc, or CREST (an acronym for *c*alcinosis, *R*aynaud's phenomenon, *e*sophageal dysmotility, *s*clerodactyly, and *t*elangiectasia), has a significantly better short-term prognosis, with a paucity of proximal skin, renal, and intestinal involvement. However, over the long term, the life span of patients with CREST is also reduced, often because of the development of pulmonary hypertension. In the recent past, survival from dSSc was decreased most significantly by hypertensive renal crisis and end-stage renal disease. The advent of angiotensin-converting enzyme inhibitors has revolutionized the modern approach to dSSc and has significantly improved the short-term prognosis. Although pulmonary disease in dSSc is third in frequency, behind skin and gastrointestinal manifestations, it is now the most lethal feature of SSc. Interstitial pulmonary fibrosis remains one of the most difficult-to-manage aspects of this disabling and life-shortening disorder.

Epidemiology

Pulmonary disease is estimated to occur in 70%–85% of patients with SSc. The exact prevalence of lung disease is difficult to determine because of the rarity of SSc, difficulties with characterization of SSc subtypes, and the inaccurate diagnosis of the variable pulmonary pathologies. Although the percentage of ILD in dSSc is much higher, and although most serious end-stage fibrosis occurs in dSSc, ILD is also described in patients with lSSc. Severe restrictive lung disease appears more likely to develop in African-American men with cardiac involvement than in other demographic groups.

Intense interest has focused on potential environmental factors that may predispose to SSc, and such interest has been further increased by the development of scleroderma-like disorders, such as the 1981 toxic oil syndrome and the eosinophilia-myalgia syndrome caused by adulterated L-tryptophan. Of particular interest with respect to lung disease, exposure to silica may increase a person's risk for development of SSc 25- to 100-fold. More recently, attention has focused on the putative role of augmentation mammoplasty and the implantation of silicone elastomers in the development of SSc. Despite numerous associations noted in case reports and series of patients, large epidemiologic studies as yet have failed to confirm a significant association between exposure and disease.

Clinical Presentation

Sclerodermatous skin changes and Raynaud's phenomenon are frequent and striking physical findings that greatly aid in the differential diagnosis. Symptoms of pulmonary disease in SSc include dyspnea on exertion and an occasional dry cough. The presence of abnormal nailfold capillary loops with vessel dropouts, dilations, and severe ectasia help establish the diagnosis of an underlying connective tissue disorder and predict more severe pulmonary disease as manifested by a diminished DLCO. Pulmonary symptoms rarely antedate the skin manifestations of SSc, although cases of scleroderma *sine* scleroderma have been described. Hemoptysis, in some cases secondary to bleeding telangiectases, occurs uncommonly. SSc is associated with the development of significant impairment; the overall work capacity of patients with SSc is only 50% of the predicted normal. Although pulmonary disease contributes to this functional impairment, myocardial ischemia, ventricular arrhythmias, and limitations in locomotor function are also significant cofactors.

Diagnostic Studies

Physiologic Evaluation

Abnormalities in pulmonary function testing are detected in up to 70% of patients with CREST, often in the absence of symptoms or chest radiographic evidence of parenchymal disease. Decline in DLCO is more strongly correlated with abnormalities in nailfold capillaries than are decrements in lung volumes. Although 20% of patients with SSc who are nonsmokers have an isolated reduction in DLCO, they have a good prognosis overall in regard to pulmonary morbidity and mortality. A decline in DLCO in lSSc may be caused by Raynaud's phenomenon of the pulmonary vasculature. An increase in dead space ventilation in various connective tissue diseases associated with Raynaud's phenomenon lends credence to the theory of redistribution of blood flow resulting from pulmonary Raynaud's phenomenon. Whether pulmonary Raynaud's phenomenon coincides with digital Raynaud's phenomenon and how commonly pulmonary Raynaud's phenomenon occurs in SSc are matters of current controversy.

Pulmonary Imaging

In dSSc, diffuse or bibasilar infiltrates are the typical findings. A bibasilar reticulonodular pattern is also seen in cases of lSSc with pathologic evidence of UIP. As in ILD of other causes, the chest radiograph, albeit more specific, is considerably less sensitive for early ILD than are pulmonary function tests.

High-resolution CT has been evaluated as a diagnostic and surveillance tool for ILD in SSc. It is better than plain radiography in detecting interstitial pulmonary abnormalities that may indicate early disease, such as ground-glass opacities, and reticular abnormalities consistent with fibrosis. High-resolution CT showed changes consistent with ILD in 19 of 21 patients with SSc; in comparison, unequivocal ILD abnormalities were revealed by plain chest x-ray films in only 8 subjects. Areas of inflammatory ground-glass appearance on high-resolution CT correlate well with BAL findings of elevated percentages of eosinophils.

Laboratory Studies

ANA is present in the majority of patients with SSc, most commonly in a speckled pattern on immunofluorescence. Two serologic markers are of particular clinical interest in SSc: antibodies to centromere (ACA), detected in about 50%–80% of patients with limited disease, and anti-Scl-70 (an antibody to DNA topisomerase I), seen in one third of patients with diffuse SSc. Although ACA is generally protective for lung involvement, anti-Scl-70 predicts restrictive lung involvement and other ominous visceral disease in many studies. In one study, antihistone antibodies, seen commonly in drug-induced lupus, were predictive of more severe pulmonary fibrosis in SSc.

Bronchoalveolar Lavage and Lung Biopsy

BAL is touted by many as a useful tool for accurately identifying patients with SSc and active alveolitis who may respond to aggressive anti-inflammatory therapy. Neutrophil influx associated with increased collagen production may be an early pathologic finding in SSc-associated pulmonary fibrosis. Collagenase activity is significantly elevated in patients with BAL neutrophilia, suggesting an increased level of matrix turnover. However, a lymphocyte predominance is more frequently seen in many patients, particularly if they have secondary Sjögren's syndrome. Increased ratios of lymphocytes to granulocytes are associated with milder impairment in physiologic parameters.

Pathology

Interstitial fibrosis, bronchiolectasis with cyst formation, and intimal proliferation with medial hypertrophy of small pulmonary vessels are the classic histologic findings of ILD associated with dSSc. Based on open lung biopsy specimens in which IPF was compared with SSc, endothelial or epithelial injury and focal lymphoid hyperplasia may differentiate SSc from IPF. Raynaud's phenomenon of the lungs may account for some of the changes noted on pulmonary function studies and may play a role in the development of secondary pulmonary hypertension. Both lung fibrosis and vascular hyperplastic changes are common in SSc and may independently contribute to right-sided heart failure. Patients with lSSc can have pathologic features of UIP, particularly those who present with bilateral lower lobe infiltrates.

Treatment and Prognosis

No pharmacologic agent has been identified that is of unequivocal value in modifying the natural course of lung disease in SSc. Notwithstanding, therapeutic interventions may be indicated for severe pulmonary disease if diagnostic evidence of an active inflammatory process is found. For instance, in patients with rapidly declining lung function and an increased proportion of lymphocytes on BAL, high doses of corticosteroids and immunosuppressive therapy are reasonable. This regimen may lead to a decrease in pulmonary inflammation, as assessed by BAL. Based on retrospective data analysis and open-label trials, cyclophosphamide appears to improve FVC over time and should likely be added to corticosteroids in patients with refractory, inflammation-related pulmonary decline. Because of its ability to interrupt molecular cross-linking of collagen, D-penicillamine has been of considerable interest to many investigators as a potential disease-modifying agent in SSc. Despite negative findings in several studies, three small studies support a small but statistically significant benefit for D-penicillamine in treating lung disease. However, the true clinical benefits may be very limited. Further, poor patient tolerance and the hematologic and renal toxicity (of concern in a patient population at already at high risk for kidney disease) associated with D-penicillamine have substantially dampened enthusiasm for its use. A long-term study of high versus low-dose D-penicillamine is currently under way and, it is hoped, may resolve still unanswered questions about its clinical role in SSc-associated lung disease.

Several experimental therapies loom on the horizon. Small, open-label studies of interferon-γ (IFN-γ) have shown no serious adverse effects from this agent, and in one study patients treated with IFN-γ showed mild improvement in some pulmonary parameters. IFN-γ cannot be advocated as an effective conventional therapy at this time. In open-label trials and retrospective reviews, potassium p-aminobenzoate has been demonstrated to produce modest softening effects in sclerodermatous skin, and in one investigation it resulted in a slower decrease in vital capacity and DLCO.

Based on data from an inception cohort, the estimated 5-year survival rate for all patients with SSc is about 70%. However, the natural history of SSc is highly variable, and a large percentage of patients have a protracted disease course with survival in excess of 20 years. Worsening of ILD in SSc is less rapid than in IPF, and patients with fibrosis secondary to SSc may have a better long-term prognosis than those with other fibrotic lung diseases. Isolated impairment in DLCO (≤55% predicted) does not indicate a poor prognosis. Although abnormalities in static lung compliance and diffusing capacity may worsen over time, the lung volumes did not appreciably deteriorate in one large series of untreated patients followed on average for 3 years. Abnormal cardiopulmonary signs and, in particular, severely impaired gas exchange (DLCO 40% of predicted) are associated with significantly worse survival in several series. Patients with long-term SSc tend to have a rate of decline in pulmonary function tests not substantially different from that of the general population, but this could be partially because of a survival bias. Anti SSA/Ro, the autoantibody seen most often in Sjögren's syndrome and potentially predictive of lung disease in SLE, is also a poor pulmonary prognostic marker in SSc based on results from small studies.

Death was caused by pulmonary hypertension in 60% of cases in one of the largest prospective series of patients with both dSSc and lSSc. Although pulmonary hypertension is a more common outcome in lSSc, secondary pulmonary hypertension may develop in patients with dSSc after years of pulmonary fibrosis. For patients with advanced interstitial disease in whom secondary pulmonary hypertension and cor pulmonale develop, long-term O₂ therapy at home may significantly lower pulmonary vascular resistance and improve quality of life and survival. Once cor pulmonale with peripheral edema has developed, the 5-year mortality rate for patients with SSc is 70%. In a subset of patients with severe pulmonary vascular changes, rapidly progressive respiratory failure and severe pulmonary hypertension often develop, and these patients die quickly.

Independently of cigarette smoking but in relation to pulmonary fibrosis, SSc confers an increased risk for lung cancer, with increased risks estimated at 4- to 17-fold. Alveolar cell carcinoma in particular, as well as lymphoma and leukemia, has been reported most commonly. Small-cell carcinoma of the lung in the absence of a history of smoking has also been noted.

Idiopathic Inflammatory Myopathy

The idiopathic inflammatory myopathies (IIM) comprise a group of illnesses including polymyositis (PM), dermatomyositis (DM), and inclusion body myositis. The IIM are rare, with 5 to 10 new cases per million per year in the United States. These related yet distinct disorders all produce nonsuppurative muscle inflammation that leads to weakness and disability. Inclusion body myositis, a disorder of older Caucasian men characterized by both distal and proximal weakness, is the least prevalent of the three condition and seldom has associated respiratory

features; it is not discussed further here. Despite differing histopathologic findings and putative immunologic mechanisms, PM and DM have many characteristics in common, including a predilection for the proximal musculature and a spectrum of pulmonary disorders.

Epidemiology

Lung disease of all types occurs in up to 50% of cases of DM/PM. Pulmonary disease in IIM commonly occurs through four processes: (1) aspiration from bulbar weakness, (2) ventilatory insufficiency resulting from myositis of the chest wall and diaphragm, (3) secondary infection, and (4) ILD. The first three entities are discussed in Chapter xx; the remainder of this section focuses on IIM-associated ILD. Either radiographic or physiologic evidence of ILD is estimated to occur in from 5%–30% of large series of IIM. Ethnic and racial variation in prevalence of IIM-associated ILD is uncertain, but in one Japanese series radiographic evidence of ILD was reported in 81% of cases.

Clinical Presentation

Patients with IIM note prominent bilateral proximal weakness that inhibits simple activities of daily living. In patients with DM, a prominent, scaly erythroderma erupts in a v-shaped distribution on the chest and back. Over the knuckles of the proximal interphalangeal and metacarpophalangeal joints of the hands, a scaly rash known as *Gottron's papules* is nearly pathognomonic for DM. A heliotrope rash, a purplish edematous discoloration over the eyelids, is also often noted. Constitutional symptoms of fatigue, fevers, and weight loss are additional harbingers of IIM, and it is difficult to determine whether these are caused by myopathy or pulmonary pathology.

In as many as one third of cases, lung disease antedates muscle involvement or occurs in patients with only minimal myopathy. The antisynthetase syndrome, named for the response to autoantibodies to aminoacyl transfer RNA synthetase (discussed below), is an IIM variant in which seronegative, nonerosive arthritis, fevers, "mechanic's hands," Raynaud's phenomenon, and ILD can strongly overshadow a mild or even clinically insignificant myopathy. Clubbing is uncommon in IIM-associated ILD but has been reported.

Diagnostic Studies

Physiologic Evaluation

Although ILD associated with IIM frequently causes physiologic abnormalities similar to those of IPF, additional physiologic parameters, such as maximal ventilatory volume (MVV) and inspiratory effort, should be measured. If results of these studies are abnormal, they point toward respiratory muscle weakness as an explanation for at least a component of the pulmonary findings.

Laboratory Studies

At a minimum, minor but usually striking elevations of muscle enzymes such as creatinine kinase and aldolase are almost always present at some point in the disease course of all patients with IIM. Diagnosis of PM/DM is ultimately confirmed based on characteristic abnormalities present on electromyographic recordings and muscle biopsy specimens. Elevations in erythrocyte sedimentation rate nonspecifically mirror changes in disease activity or herald the development of opportunistic infections. The ANA is elevated in a small percentage of cases, often indicative of antisynthetase antibodies. One of the most exciting serologic associations is the established relationship between antisynthetase antibodies and IIM-associated ILD.

Antibodies to histidyl tRNA synthetase, known as *anti-Jo-1*, occur in 25% of patients with DM/PM. Of special interest, this antibody is found in 50% of patients with IIM and concomitant ILD. The presence of this antibody in patients with IIM, therefore, should raise concern for concomitant ILD. Additionally, a small percentage of patients have antibodies to signal recognition protein (SRP), and they are less likely to have ILD. Autoantibodies to other amino tRNA synthetases have also been identified but are less strikingly associated with lung disease.

Bronchoalveolar Lavage and Lung Biopsy

The need for BAL and/or lung biopsy is uncertain. Histopathologic and BAL data may predict therapeutic response, but this has not been shown to significantly alter management or outcome.

Pathology

A mononuclear cell infiltration of the muscle and surrounding tissue with fiber degradation, regeneration, and fibrosis are the major systemic features of PM and DM. Of note, DM is not simply PM with a rash; it is a humorally mediated disease with immune complex deposition in the perimysium and a perivascular vasculitis that is presumed to be responsible for the pathology. PM results from lymphocytic infiltration of the true muscle fibers and is the manifestation of a cell-mediated immune process.

In the lungs, histologic features are typical for interstitial pneumonitis resembling IPF. Investigators have identified three major histopathologic groups for IIM-associated ILD that have prognostic significance: BOOP,

UIP, and diffuse alveolar damage (DAD). Patients with BOOP had the best prognosis, while those with DAD fared the worst. A histologic finding seen more commonly in hypersensitivity pneumonitis than in ILD, Masson bodies and intra-alveolar buds are prominent in many cases of IIM-associated ILD. Immune complex deposition in the lungs has not been frequently detected in IIM-associated ILD. Several cases of pulmonary cryoglobulin deposition have been documented.

From a pathogenic perspective, antibodies to Jo-1 have been observed only in patients with myositis. An interesting line of investigation has detected amino acid homology between the Jo-1 antigen and the genomic RNA of certain picornaviruses. The authors speculate that as in pathogenic mechanisms proposed for other autoimmune disorders, such as reactive arthritis, molecular mimicry could lead to tissue damage. Curiously, patients with antisynthetase syndrome (antibodies to Jo-1) typically have an abrupt onset of symptoms in the spring of the year.

Treatment and Prognosis

High-dose corticosteroids, initiated with at least 1 mg of prednisone per kilogram of body weight, or the equivalent, in divided doses, forms the starting point for regimens directed at both the muscle disease and newly diagnosed pulmonary involvement. Methotrexate is a commonly used second-line agent for general manifestations of IIM, and despite its own association with pneumonitis, it is safe to use in IIM-associated ILD. Although some authors question the efficacy of cyclophosphamide in IIM, given its potential value in other types of ILD and anecdotal reports of its success in IIM, it is prudent to consider this agent if the patient is failing with other options. Cyclosporine has also led to improvement in patients with steroid resistant IIM-associated ILD. The effective use of intravenous immunoglobulin for refractory myositis has been reported in several case series and at least one controlled trial. Although study end points included only measures of motor function and no mention was made of lung involvement, given the reasonable safety of this therapy, it should be strongly considered as an early second-line agent.

For many patients, adequate control of muscle inflammation is achieved with anti-inflammatory agents. Notwithstanding, a significant percentage of individuals continue to require a maintenance dose of corticosteroid to avoid relapse. In these patients, sustained morbidity and even mortality may ultimately ensue from the treatment. With respect to IIM-associated ILD, response to corticosteroids and other immunosuppressive agents is variable. Some studies report very disappointing results, with up to 60% mortality despite aggressive therapy. In another series, the 5-year mortality rate for IIM with ILD was 40%. ILD with minimal myopathy is a poor prognostic sign.

An association between IIM and malignancy has been suspected for many years, and well-conducted population-based studies now fully support both a higher incidence of cancer and a higher rate of mortality from cancer. Adenocarcinoma (particularly ovarian cancer) is reported most commonly. Some authorities advocate aggressive cancer screening for all patients with newly diagnosed IIM. Based on the need to consider patient comfort and safety, avoid false-positive results that can occur with excessive testing, and constrain health care costs, we recommend a thorough physical examination (including breast, genital, and rectal examinations) and prudent use of age-appropriate and clinically directed cancer-screening modalities (i.e., Pap test, mammogram, flexible sigmoidoscopy) for all patients with newly diagnosed IIM.

Mixed Connective Tissue Disease

The term *mixed connective tissue disease* (MCTD) was coined in 1972 by Sharp to describe a subset of patients with connective tissue disease who have overlapping features of SLE, SSc, and idiopathic inflammatory myopathy. The initial cases described had a set of common clinical and laboratory features that, in addition to pulmonary disease, frequently included erosive inflammatory arthritis with diffuse hand swelling, esophageal dysmotility, myopathy, Raynaud's phenomenon, high-titer speckled ANA, antibodies to U1-RNP, and an absence of antibodies to Smith (Sm) and double-stranded DNA (dsDNA).

Not all experts agree that MCTD merits a separate diagnostic label. Physicians experienced in caring for patients with connective tissue diseases recognize that many patients with the idiopathic inflammatory disorders have variable presentations and often do not present with "classic" features of any one particular diagnostic entity. As such, it has been suggested that the MCTD paradigm is conceptually flawed, as it may not identify a unique patient population, provide direction on specific treatment options, or offer guidance on prognosis.

Epidemiology

Most of the pulmonary reports on MCTD have focused on pulmonary hypertension. However, ILD may be more frequent and severe in MCTD even than in SSc. In one series, 80% of all patients with MCTD had pulmonary disease, and 69% of the asymptomatic patients had pulmonary dysfunction on physiologic tests, chest radiographs, or both.

Clinical Presentation

The most common and worrisome pulmonary feature of MCTD, significant pulmonary hypertension, cannot be accurately predicted based on symptoms, signs, or laboratory data. Pleural effusions, not commonly seen in SSc, may aid in the differential diagnosis. When ILD occurs in MCTD, it mimics that seen in SSc.

As in the other connective tissue disorders, reduction in diffusion capacity is the single most sensitive test to show physiologic dysfunction in MCTD. Despite abnormal physiology, chest radiographs demonstrated identifiable abnormalities in only 21% of cases. A lower lobe predominance has been described most commonly. The features of patients who have SLE with U1-RNP and those of patients with scleroderma overlap; they include edematous hands and nailfold capillary loop abnormalities.

Treatment and Prognosis

Authors report pulmonary improvements in 38%–86% of patients with MCTD who are treated with corticosteroids and/or cyclophosphamide. Patients may have fatal outcomes related to respiratory disease, in part because the disease may not be diagnosed until it is far advanced. Pulmonary outcome is worse if features are more characteristic of SSc.

Seronegative Spondyloarthropathies

This group of heterogeneous disorders includes ankylosing spondylitis, psoriatic arthritis, reactive arthritis (Reiter's syndrome), and arthritis associated with bowel inflammation. Although these conditions are in many ways heterogeneous, they share common features, including inflammatory arthritis of the spine and sacroiliac joints, enthesopathy (inflammation at the insertion of ligaments and tendons into bones), an association with HLA-B27, and a spectrum of similar mucocutaneous lesions. The occurrence of ILD in ankylosing spondylitis is the best described, although similar changes have been reported in psoriatic arthritis with a lower frequency.

Clinical Presentation

Noninfectious fibrobullous disease of the lung upper lobes is nearly pathognomonic for ankylosing spondylitis. The abnormality usually appears late in the disease course and does not correlate with severity of extrapulmonary disease. In a series of 2080 patients with ankylosing spondylitis seen at the Mayo Clinic, the prevalence was 1.3%.

The pulmonary process often begins unilaterally, with linear opacities on radiographs. As it advances, these changes can be seen in both apices, and bullae gradually develop. In advanced cases, pleural thickening and cavitary disease can occur and are not uncommonly confused with tuberculosis.

Pathology

Specimens show intra-alveolar fibrosis, hyalinized connective tissue, and degeneration of elastic fibrils. Despite extensive investigations, no infectious organism has been identified as an etiologic agent for these lesions.

Treatment and Prognosis

In one large study of 836 patients with ankylosing spondylitis, the number of cases of respiratory disease was 1.5 times higher than expected. Although many of the problems are caused directly by the fibrobullous disease, secondary infection of bullae with bacteria, mycobacteria, or fungi (particularly *Aspergillus*) may lead to considerable morbidity and mortality.

BIBLIOGRAPHY

Baughman RP, Shipley RT, London RG, Lower EF. Crackles in ILD: comparison of sarcoidosis and fibrosing alveolitis. *Chest* 1991;100: 96–101. *This study compared auscultory to high-resolution CT findings and suggests that subpleural fibrosis is necessary but not sufficient for rales. Honeycomb changes were not correlated with crackles.*

Bitterman PB, Rennard WI, Keogh BA, Wewers MD, Adelberg S, Crystal RG. Familial IPF: evidence of lung inflammation in unaffected family members. *N Engl J Med* 1986;314:1343–1347. *Gallium scans and BAL in 17 clinically unaffected members of three families with strong IPF pedigrees showed increased BALF macrophages or increased neutrophils in eight subjects, four of whom had positive gallium scans.*

Cervantes-Perez P, Toro-Perez AH, Rodriguez-Jurado P. Pulmonary involvement in rheumatoid arthritis. *JAMA* 1980;243:1715–1719. *This is one of the largest series of open lung biopsies in rheumatoid arthritis. Interstitial lung disease was the most notable feature. Of further interest, more than half the patients were asymptomatic despite histologic abnormalities.*

Constantopoulos SH, Papadimitriou CS, Moutsopoulos HM. Respiratory manifestations in primary Sjögren's syndrome: a clinical, functional, and histologic study. *Chest* 1985;88:226–229. *Of 36 patients with primary Sjögren's syndrome, 75% had evidence of respiratory involvement. Diffuse interstitial lung disease was most common and present in 25% of cases.*

Davies D. Ankylosing spondylitis and lung fibrosis. *Q J Med* 1972;164: 395–417. *This is one of the first reports to describe an association of apical pulmonary fibrosis with ankylosing spondylitis. The authors emphasize that apical lesions may cavitate and become colonized by Aspergillus.*

Dayton CS, Schwartz DA, Helmers RA, et al. Outcome of subjects with idiopathic pulmonary fibrosis who fail corticosteroid therapy. Implications for further studies. *Chest* 1993;103:69–73. *About half of patients failing treatment with prednisone stabilized with cyclophosphamide treatment. Clinical data, including pulmonary function tests, did not predict which patients would die after beginning this therapy.*

Eisenberg H, Dubois EL, Sherwin RP, Balchum OJ. Diffuse interstitial lung disease in systemic lupus erythematosus. *Ann Intern Med* 1973; 79:37–45. *Eighteen patients with SLE had restrictive lung disease well characterized by clinical and physiologic parameters.*

Greenwald GI, Tashkin DP, Gong H, Simmons M, Duann S, Furst DE, Clements P. *Am J Med* 1987;83:83–90. *During an average of 3 years, pulmonary physiologic studies did not show significant deterioration, suggesting a reasonably slow progression of systemic sclerotic lung disease.*

Groen H, Wichers G, ten Borg EJ, vander Mark TW, Wouda AA, Kallenberg CGM. Pulmonary diffusing capacity disturbances are related to nailfold capillary changes in patients with Raynaud's phenomenon with and without an underlying connective tissue disease. *Am J Med* 1990;89:34–41. *This report illustrates the importance of nailfold capillary loop abnormalities in predicting intrinsic pulmonary dysfunction, particularly as defined by a low diffusion capacity of carbon monoxide.*

Hakala M. Poor prognosis in patients with rheumatoid arthritis hospitalized for interstitial lung fibrosis. *Chest* 1988;93:114–118. *Forty-nine patients with interstitial lung disease associated with rheumatoid arthritis had a median survival of only 3.5 years, with a 5-year survival rate of 39%.*

Hamman L, Rich AR. Acute diffuse interstitial fibrosis of the lungs. *Bull Johns Hopkins Hosp* 1944;74:177–206. *The original description of Hamman-Rich syndrome.*

Hartley PG, Galvin JR, Hunninghake GW, et al. High-resolution CT-derived measures of lung density are valid indexes of interstitial lung disease. *J Appl Physiol* 1994;76:271–277. *This study examines the validity of computer-assisted analysis of high-resolution CT images in interstitial lung disease. The investigators determined that computer-assisted analysis can provide clinically meaningful assessment of parenchymal lung involvement.*

Haupt HM, Moore GW, Hutchins GM. The lung in systemic lupus erythematosus: analysis of the pathologic changes in 120 patients. *Am J Med* 1981;71:791–798. *Parenchymal abnormalities attributable to lupus were found in 18% of 120 patients; five had interstitial fibrosis and 11 had interstitial pneumonitis.*

Hunninghake GW, Gadek JE, Kawanami O, Ferrans VJ, Crystal RG. Inflammatory and immune processes in the human lung in health and disease: evaluation by bronchoalveolar lavage. *Am J Pathol* 1979;97: 149–206. *This early study showed that BAL is a useful tool for the evaluation of inflammation in the lung.*

Hunninghake GW, Kalica AR. Approaches to the treatment of pulmonary fibrosis. *Am J Respir Crit Care Med* 1995; 151(3 Pt 1):915–918. *This workshop summary reports that current therapies for pulmonary fibrosis have little impact on disease progression or outcome, and suggests that future research be directed toward therapies based on new understandings of pathogenesis.*

Hyde DM, King TE Jr, McDermott T, Waldron JA Jr, Colby TV, Thurlbeck AF, Ackerson L, Cherniack RM. Idiopathic pulmonary fibrosis: quantitative assessment of lung pathology. *Am Rev Respir Dis* 1992;146:1042–1047. *A panel of pathologists developed a semiquantitative pathology scoring system to overcome the limits of qualitatively assessing inflammatory (exudative) and fibrotic (reparative) components in IPF. They found that a semiquantitative method reliably assessed the relative degree of inflammation and fibrosis compared with a more detailed morphometric analysis of specific histopathologic features.*

Hyland RM, Gordon DA, Broder I, Davies GM, Russell ML, Hutcheon MA, Reid GD, Cox DW, Corey PN, Mintz S. A systematic controlled study of pulmonary abnormalities in rheumatoid arthritis. *J Rheumatol* 1983;10:395–405. *This large, prospective evaluation identified cigarette smoking, extra-articular rheumatoid arthritis features, level of rheumatoid arthritis disease activity, and treatment with either oral corticosteroids or gold as the most important risk factors for pulmonary abnormalities in rheumatoid arthritis.*

Johnson MA, Kwan S, Snell NJC, Nunn AJ, Darbyshire JH, Turner-Warwick M. Randomized controlled trial comparing prednisolone alone with cyclophosphamide and low-dose prednisone in combination in cryptogenic fibrosing alveolitis. *Thorax* 1989;44:280–288. *Patients were randomized to moderate-dose prednisone versus cyclophosphamide plus alternate-day prednisone. The findings of this study suggest that cyclophosphamide in combination with low-dose prednisone is at least as effective as a course of high-dose steroids followed by an alternate-day low-dose regimen. Cyclophosphamide in the dose used in this study was associated with limited toxicity, which was rapidly reversible when the drug was discontinued. Many patients, however, failed to respond to either therapy.*

Kelly C, Gardiner P, Pal B, Griffiths I. Lung function in primary Sjögren's syndrome: a cross-sectional and longitudinal study. *Thorax* 1991;46:180–183. *A comprehensive study of 100 patients with primary Sjögren's syndrome demonstrating a strong relationship between reduction in lung function and histologic evidence of Sjögren's syndrome. The authors conclude that lung disease is sometimes an early feature of primary Sjögren's syndrome and may progress over a relatively short period.*

Kline JN, Schwartz DA, Monick MM, Floerchinger CS, Hunninghake GW. Relative release of interleukin-1β and interleukin-1 receptor antagonist by alveolar macrophages. A study in asbestos-induced lung disease, sarcoidosis, and idiopathic pulmonary fibrosis. *Chest* 1993; 104:47–53. *This study examined the relative release of the pro-inflammatory cytokine IL-1β and its specific inhibitor IL-1RA by cultured alveolar macrophages in IPF, sarcoidosis, and asbestos-induced lung disease. Each of these disorders causes an increase in the ratio of IL-1β to IL-1RA, but this altered ratio may be caused by an increase in IL-1β, a decrease in IL-1RA, or both.*

Lee P, Langevitz P, Alderdice CA, Aubrey M, Baer PA, Baron M, Buskila D, Dutz JP, Khostanteen I, Piper S, Ramsden M, Rosenbach TO, Sukenik S, Wilkinson S, Keystone EC. Mortality in systemic sclerosis (scleroderma). *Q J Med* 1992;82:139–148. *This prospective analysis of >230 scleroderma patients demonstrates that pulmonary manifestations, particularly pulmonary hypertension, are the most frequent cause of death.*

Matthay RA, Schwarz JI, Petty TL, Stanford RE, Gupta RC, Sahn SA, Steigerwald JC. Pulmonary manifestations of systemic lupus erythematosus: review of 12 cases of acute lupus pneumonitis. *Medicine* 1974;54:397–409. *This early report of acute lupus pneumonitis also reviews other pulmonary manifestations of SLE.*

Miller FW. Myositis-specific autoantibodies: touchstones for understanding the inflammatory myopathies. *JAMA* 1993;270:1846–1849. *This is a comprehensive review of autoantibodies associated with inflammatory myopathies. The authors discuss the association of anti-Jo-1 antibody with interstitial lung disease.*

Muller NL, Staples CA, Miller RR, Vedal S, Thurlsbeck WM, Ostrow DN. Disease activity in IPF: CT and pathologic correlation. *Radiology* 1987;165:731–734. *This retrospective study suggests that high-resolution CT findings (patchy areas of parenchymal air space consolidation in the periphery) correlate well with disease activity and histologic cellularity. All four patients with little disease activity on CT progressed despite steroids. These observations suggest a role for high-resolution CT in predicting steroid responsiveness.*

Nugent KM, Peterson MW, Jolles H, Monick MM, Hunninghake GW. Correlation of chest roentgenograms with pulmonary function and bronchoalveolar lavage in interstitial lung disease [see comments]. *Chest* 1989;96:1224–1227. *Classification of interstitial lung disease by size and profusion of abnormal lung markings was used to evaluate patients with nonoccupational interstitial lung disease. No correlation was found between this classification system and either severity of illness (determined by pulmonary function tests) or BAL cellularity.*

Panos RJ, Mortenson RL, Niccoli SA, King TE Jr. Clinical deterioration in patients with IPF: causes and assessment. *Am J Med* 1990;88:394–404. *A review of previous studies showing that cardiovascular and lung cancer deaths are common in IPF. Disease-associated complications and adverse drug effects need to be distinguished from IPF progression when therapeutic response or outcome is assessed.*

Patterson CD, Harville WE, Pierce JA. Rheumatoid lung disease. *Ann Intern Med* 1965;62:685–697. *This very large hospital-based analysis shows a low prevalence of radiographically evident interstitial lung disease in > 700 patients with rheumatoid arthritis.*

Peterson MW, Monick M, Hunninghake GW. Prognostic role of eosinophils in pulmonary fibrosis. *Chest* 1987;92:51–56. *BALF eosinophilia may be a prognostic indicator of progressive lung disease in patients with IPF.*

Raghu G, Depaso WJ, Cain K, Hammar SP, Wetzel CE, Dreis DF, Hutchinson J, Pardee NE, Winterbauer RH. Azathioprine combined with prednisone in the treatment of IPF: a prospective double-blind, randomized, placebo-controlled clinical trial. *Am Rev Respir Dis* 1991;144:291–296. *This study randomized 27 IPF patients to prednisone or prednisone plus azathioprine. Results favored the prednisone-plus-azathioprine combination, but survival benefit (after adjustment for age) was not apparent until after 3 to 4 years of treatment.*

Roschmann RA, Rothenberg RJ. Pulmonary fibrosis in rheumatoid arthritis: a review of clinical features and therapy. *Semin Arthritis Rheum* 1987;16:174–185. *This is the most comprehensive up-to-date review of pulmonary fibrosis in rheumatoid arthritis.*

Saag KG, Kolluri S, Koehnke RK, Georgou TA, Rachow JR, Hunninghake GW, Schwartz DA. Rheumatoid arthritis lung disease: determinants of physiologic and radiologic abnormalities. *Arthritis Rheum* 1996;39:1711–1719. *One of the largest analyses to show a dose-responsive significant association between cigarette smoking and rheumatoid arthritis interstitial lung disease.*

Schwartz DA, Helmers RA, Dayton CS, Merchant RK, Hunninghake GW. Determinants of bronchoalveolar lavage cellularity in idiopathic pulmonary fibrosis. *J Appl Physiol* 1991;71:1688–1693. *BALF from patients with IPF contained greater numbers of neutrophils and eosinophils than that from normal volunteers, regardless of smoking status. The numbers of macrophages, neutrophils, and eosinophils was strongly associated with smoking history among the IPF patients.*

Schwartz DA, Helmers RA, Galvin JR, et al. Determinants of survival in idiopathic pulmonary fibrosis. *Am J Respir Crit Care Med* 1994; 149(2 Pt 1):450–454. *The authors performed a survival analysis on 74 patients with IPF over a 4-year mean observational period. Decreased survival was associated with male sex, initial pulmonary function abnormalities, radiographic findings, and cultured alveolar macrophage release of prostaglandin E².*

Schwartz MI, Matthay RA, Sahn SA, Stanford RE, Marmorstein BL, Scheinhorn DJ. Interstitial lung disease in polymyositis and dermatomyositis: analysis of six cases and review of the literature. *Medicine* 1976;55:89–104. *This is the first review of interstitial lung manifestations of inflammatory muscle disease. The authors compare and contrast their 13-year experience with previous reports.*

Schwartz DA, Merchant RK, Helmers RA, Gilbert SR, Dayton CS, Hunninghake GW. The influence of cigarette smoking on lung function in patients with idiopathic pulmonary fibrosis. *Am Rev Respir Dis* 1991;144(3 Pt 1):504–506. *Cigarette smoking was significantly associated with decreased DLCO and increased TLC, FRC, and RV in IPF. The FEV₁/FVC ratio was not related to smoking status in IPF patients.*

Schwartz DA, Van Fossen DS, Davis CS, et al. Determinants of progression in idiopathic pulmonary fibrosis. *Am J Respir Crit Care Med* 1994; 149(2 Pt 1):444–449. *This study examined progression of IPF and determined correlates of decline in pulmonary function. Although there was an overall improvement during the study period in TLC and DLCO, cigarette smoking, severe dyspnea, and treatment with cyclophosphamide were each associated with declining lung function.*

Silberstein SL, Barland P, Grayzel AI, Koerner SK. Pulmonary dysfunction in systemic lupus erythematosus: prevalence classification and correlation with other organ involvement. *J Rheumatol* 1980;7:187–195. *Abnormal diffusion capacity was the most common finding in this series of 43 SLE patients undergoing pulmonary function studies. Of note, DLCO did not fully correlate with other clinical or diagnostic measures of pulmonary disease.*

Stack HBR, Choo-Kang, Heard BE. The prognosis of cryptogenic fibrosing alveolitis. *Thorax* 1972;27:535–542. *This classic, descriptive study of 96 IPF patients followed for 17 years revealed excess cardiovascular and lung cancer deaths. The mean survival from the time of diagnosis was 4 to 5 years, although some patients survived more than 10 years. Younger age, female sex, increased cellularity, and steroid responsiveness predicted a better survival, whereas worse dyspnea, FVC, and lower PO₂ at presentation predicted a worse outcome.*

Staples CA, Muller NL, Vedal S, Abboud R, Ostrow D, Miller RR. UIP: Correlation of CT with clinical, functional, and radiologic findings. *Radiology* 1987;162:377–381. *Twenty-three patients with IPF were studied retrospectively. CT better estimated disease extent and showed more honeycombing than chest radiograph. CT correlated fairly well with dyspnea score (r = .62) and diffusing capacity (r = .64), but not with other pulmonary function tests.*

Steen VD, Conte C, Owens GR, Medsger Jr TA. Severe restrictive lung disease in systemic sclerosis. *Arthritis Rheum* 1994;37:1283–1289. *This large review of >800 patients from a scleroderma data bank demonstrated moderate or severe restrictive disease in 40% of systemic sclerosis patients. African-American men with pulmonary and cardiac disease had the worst prognosis.*

Strimlan CV, Rosenow III EC, Weiland LH, Brown LR. Lymphocytic interstitial pneumonitis: review of 13 cases. *Ann Intern Med* 1978; 88:616–621. *This review of 13 cases of lymphocytic interstitial pneumonitis included three patients with coexistent Sjögren's syndrome.*

Sullivan WD, Hurst DJ, Harmon CE, Esther JH, Agia GA, Maltby JD, Lillard SB, Held CN, Wolfe JF, Sunderrajan EV, Maricq HR, Sharp GC. A prospective evaluation emphasizing pulmonary involvement in patients with mixed connective tissue disease. *Medicine* 1984;

63:92–97. *This longitudinal evaluation of 34 patients with mixed connective tissue disease identified pulmonary disease in 80% of patients.*

Tazelaar HD, Viggiano RW, Pickersgill J, Colby TV. Interstitial lung disease in polymyositis and dermatomyositis; clinical features and prognosis as correlated with histologic findings. *Am Rev Respir Dis* 1990;141:727–733. *Three major types of interstitial lung disease in inflammatory myopathy were identified: bronchiolitis obliterans organizing pneumonia, usual interstitial pneumonia, and diffuse alveolar damage. Histologic subclassification was a better predictor of survival than radiography or clinical presentation.*

Tukianen P, Taskinen E, Holsti P, Korhola O, Valle M. Prognosis of cryptogenic fibrosing alveolitis. *Thorax* 1983;38:349–355. Retrospective analysis of 100 patients with IPF and ILD-CTD (33%) treated with prednisone for at least 3 years. *Early objective functional improvement was present in 30% of IPF patients. Longer survival was noted in younger patients, especially with shorter duration of symptoms, less radiographic abnormality, or less abnormal difference. The most favorable prognosis was early response to steroids.*

Vergnon J-M, Barthélémy J-C, Riffat J, Boissier C, Claudy A, Emonot A. Raynaud's phenomenon of the lung: a reality both in primary and secondary Raynaud syndrome. Chest 1992;101:1312–17. *This report lends strong support to the concept of pulmonary Raynaud's phenomenon.*

Watters LC, King TE, Cherniack RM, Waldron JA, Standord RE, Willcox ML, Christopher KL, Schwarz MI. BAL neutrophils increase after corticosteroid therapy in smokers with IPF. *Am Rev Respir Dis* 1986;133:104–109. *Ten IPF smokers had no difference in histologic findings compared with nonsmokers, but five of six smokers treated with steroids had a subsequent increase in BALF neutrophils, even as their clinical condition improved.*

Watters LC, King TE, Schwarz MI, Waldron JA, Stanford RE, Cherniack RM. A clinical, radiographic and physiologic scoring system for the longitudinal assessment of patients with IPF. *Am Rev Respir Dis* 1986;133:97–103. *A composite clinical-radiographic-physiologic IPF scoring system demonstrated a good correlation with cellularity and severity assessed by histology.*

Weese WC, Levine BW, Kazemi H. Interstitial lung disease resistant to corticosteroid therapy. *Chest* 1975;67:57–60. *An example of early IPF treatment literature. This case series describes three patients with ILD refractory to steroids who responded to azathioprine or cyclophosphamide.*

Weiss W. Smoking and pulmonary fibrosis. *J Occup Med* 1988;30:339. *This literature review describes experimental animal, human histologic, and radiographic evidence that cigarette smoking leads to pulmonary fibrosis.*

Wells AU, Cullinan P, Hansell DM, Rubens MB, Black CM, Newman-Taylor AJ, Du Bois RM. Fibrosing alveolitis associated with systemic sclerosis has a better prognosis than lone cryptogenic fibrosing alveolitis. *Am J Respir Crit Care Med* 1994;149:1583–1590. *Despite histologic and radiologic similarities, IPF had an increased risk for mortality three times greater than that of interstitial lung disease associated with systemic sclerosis.*

Textbook of Pulmonary Diseases, 6th ed.
edited by G.L. Baum, J.D. Crapo, B.R. Celli, and J.B. Karlinsky,
Lippincott–Raven Publishers, Philadelphia, © 1998.

CHAPTER

Immunologically Mediated Lung Diseases

19

Jeffrey L. Curtis · Mark Schuyler

PULMONARY IMMUNE DEFENSE MECHANISMS

The lungs are defended by a successive series of mechanisms that for the most part prevent deposition of pathogens in the alveoli and eliminate those that do arrive there. The first line of pulmonary defense against infections consists of mechanical impediments to aspiration, such as cough and glottic closure. These mechanisms are largely defeated by tracheal intubation and anesthetics, which in part accounts for the increased risk for pneumonia in critically ill patients.

Deposition of airborne particles depends on aerodynamic size (See Chapter 1). Inhaled particles with an aerodynamic diameter than 2 to 5 μm seldom reach the distal air spaces, because they become trapped in the nose or conducting airways. Repeated branching of the airways is another physical facet of lung defense; it induces local turbulence, which causes particles to impinge at branch points. In these sites, particles are trapped in airway mucus and are carried away by normal ciliary motility and the mucociliary escalator. Particles in the 2- to 5-μm size range can remain in inspired air and be deposited in the alveoli. Of course, larger particles may also reach the alveoli when aspirated. Mucociliary clearance does not extend beyond the respiratory bronchioles. Thus, particles that reach the alveoli must be handled by cellular defenses.

Small numbers of pathogens reaching the alveoli can be contained by resident phagocytes without recruitment of bloodborne inflammatory cells. Alveolar lining fluid is also bacteriostatic, in part because of its high concentration of free fatty acids and in part because of the opsonic activity of specific proteins, notably surfactant protein A (SP-A) and immunoglobulins (Ig). Pathogens can at times survive these mechanisms, either because they arrive in large numbers, or because they are intrinsically resistant to elimination by them. In this case, recruitment of bloodborne phagocytes and specific immune responses must be mounted to aid in elimination. Because parenchymal inflammatory and immune responses have considerable potential to interfere with gas exchange, their development is under tight regulation.

Although this chapter focuses largely on the destructive aspects of immune mechanisms, it is important to recall that these potent processes have evolved precisely because they normally prevent pulmonary infection efficiently with minimal impact on the gas exchange function of the lungs. The introductory sections of this chapter detail the cellular and soluble components of pulmonary immune defense, describe the regulation of pulmonary immune response generation, and detail the mechanisms that control the recruitment of activated inflammatory cells to sites of pulmonary inflammation.

Cellular Effectors

The molecules on the surface of human leukocytes are named by a unique cluster of designation (CD) numbers. CD numbers are assigned by an international workshop; as of the Fifth International Workshop on Leukocyte Differentiation Antigens, held in November 1993, 130 CD numbers have been assigned. The characteristics of several important CD molecules are listed in Table 1.

The predominant phagocyte in the normal alveolar space is the alveolar macrophage (AM). These cells com-

J. L. Curtis: Department of Internal Medicine, The University of Michigan Medical Center, Ann Arbor, Michigan 48109-0360.

M. Schuyler: Department of Medicine, University of New Mexico School of Medicine, Albuquerque, New Mexico 87108.

TABLE 1. *CD number of important molecules*

Molecule	Alternate name	Distribution	Characteristics
CD1		Thymocytes, DC, B cells	Class I-like MHC molecules
CD2		T	Adhesion and costimulatory T-cell molecule
CD3		T	Multichain structure that constitutes invariant portion of T-cell receptor
CD4		T subset	T-cell receptor for class II MHC
CD8		T subset	T-cell receptor for class I MHC
CD14		Mø, G	LPS receptor; a GPI-linked protein
CD16		NK, Mø, G	FcγR III, found in GPI-linked form on NK and transmembrane form on Mø and G
CD25		Activated T, B, Mø	Inducible component of high-affinity IL-2 receptor
CD28		Activated T	Homodimeric T-cell costimulatory molecule, receptor for CD80
CD31		P, leukocytes, EC	Adhesion molecule that forms homotypic interactions during leukocyte transmigration of EC
CD40		B, Mø, DC, EC	Costimulatory molecule that for germinal center B cells prevents apoptosis
CD44		T, B, G	Hyaluronate receptor
CD45	Leukocyte common antigen	Leukocytes	Tyrosine phosphatase with multiple isoforms, used to identify a cell as being bone marrow-derived
CD56		NK	
CD62L	L-selectin	T, B, G	Adhesion molecule
CD62E	E-selectin, ELAM	EC, P	Inducible adhesion molecule
CD62P	P-selectin	P, EC	Inducible adhesion molecule
CD80	B7-1	DC, B, Mø	Essential costimulatory molecule for T-cell activation
CD90	Thy-1	T, thymocytes, brain	GPI-linked protein of uncertain function, used to identify T cells

B, B cells; DC, dendritic cells; EC, endothelial cells; G, granulocytes; Mø, macrophages; NK, natural killer cells; P, platelets; T, T cells; IL, interleukin; MHC, major histocompatibility complex; LPS, lipopolysaccharide.

prise 2%–5% of parenchymal cells in the normal human lung. Most AM are derived from bloodborne monocytes, although local macrophage proliferation may contribute to maintenance of AM numbers in the normal state. The primary function of AM is to ingest and eliminate foreign materials entering the alveoli. States in which AM are overwhelmed by substances that have undergone phagocytosis, as in silicosis or alveolar cell proteinosis, are characterized by increased susceptibility to opportunistic infections. AM avidly bind particles opsonized by IgG or complement because of their high-density surface expression of three classes of Fc receptors (FcR) and of two classes of complement receptors (CR1 and CR3). However, to combat certain intracellular pathogens successfully, notably *Mycobacterium tuberculosis*, AM must be activated by lymphocyte-derived cytokines, such as interferon-γ (IFN-γ) or granulocyte-monocyte colony-stimulating factor (GM-CSF). Absence of these activating signals appears to be the principal cause of the increased susceptibility to opportunistic infections in AIDS. Activated AM secrete a wide variety of important enzymes, cytokines, and other mediators (e.g., complement components C1q, C2, C3, and C5) that are essential for clearance of opsonized organisms and immune complexes. Alternatively, AM can be induced (by signals that are currently

uncertain) to differentiate along an alternative pathway with chiefly secretory activity. Secretory AM produce platelet-derived growth factor (PDGF), fibronectin, and insulin-like growth factor-1 (IGF-1). These factors probably are important in repair of lung injury as in wound repair elsewhere in the body, but they also may contribute to lung fibrosis by stimulating fibroblast recruitment and survival and collagen secretion. In addition to AM, the normal lungs contain interstitial macrophages. It is uncertain whether these cells, far less well characterized than AM, are an independent cell type or an intermediary stage between monocytes and AM.

Dendritic cells are the primary antigen-presenting cell in the airways and lung parenchyma. Dendritic cells are a type of bone marrow-derived cell unrelated to monocytes and macrophages. Antigen exposure induces large numbers of dendritic cells to be recruited to the airway epithelium. Dendritic cells carry antigens back to regional lymph nodes, where the dendritic cells bind to and potently activate naïve T cells. Hence, there is considerable experimental interest in manipulating dendritic cell numbers and function to control asthma and to facilitate protective immunization. Two types of dendritic cell are found in the lungs and in T-cell zones of lymph nodes: Langerhans cells (which express CD1 and contain Birbeck granules) and interdigitating or lymphoid dendritic cells (which do not express CD1 or contain Birbeck granules). Whether Langerhans cells and interdigitating dendritic cells are distinct cell types or different stages of the same lineage is unclear. Langerhans cells are increased in the bronchoalveolar lavage fluid (BALF) of smokers and are prominent in the lesions of eosinophilic granuloma. Demonstration of increased numbers of cells that are CD1$^+$ (by immunofluorescence) or that contain Birbeck granules (by electron microscopy) in BALF supports a diagnosis of eosinophilic granuloma. A third type of dendritic cells, follicular dendritic cells, is found within the lungs only in the B-cell zones of organized lymphoid tissue. The origin of follicular dendritic cells and their relationship to other dendritic cells are uncertain. Follicular dendritic cells retain immune complexes on their surfaces for prolonged periods, and therefore provide one explanation for the remarkable persistence of immune memory at sites of previous antigenic stimulation within the lungs.

Lymphocytes are crucial for the generation and regulation of all specific immune responses. Lymphocytes are divided into three major lineages: T cells, B cells, and natural killer (NK) cells. They are found in the normal lung in the following ratios: T cells, 70%–80%; B cells, 10%; NK cells, 10%.

T cells are central to the generation of protective and destructive immune response by their secretion of immunoregulatory cytokines; additionally, some are cytotoxic T lymphocytes (CTL). T cells are identified by surface expression of CD2, CD3, or Thy-1 (CD90). Almost all human T cells express either CD4 or CD8 surface receptors, which determine the class of major histocompatibility complex (MHC) molecules to which the T cell responds. CD4$^+$ T cells primarily induce (''help'') both antibody production by B cells and maturation of CD8$^+$ CTL. A small group of CD4$^+$ function as class II-restricted CTL. CD8$^+$ T cells either mediate cytotoxicity or suppress other immune effector cells. Both CD4$^+$ T cells and CD8$^+$ T cells secrete cytokines, as discussed below.

Regardless of whether they express CD4 or CD8, mature T cells express a heterodimeric T-cell antigen receptor (TCR). In the vast majority, this TCR is composed of $\alpha\beta$ chains; these cells mediate virtually all the functions conventionally associated with T lymphocytes. The minority of T cells, which have $\gamma\delta$ variable chains, have been suggested to provide immune surveillance of mucosal surfaces. In some anatomic sites (e.g., skin and female urogenital tract), $\gamma\delta$ T cells exhibit very limited junctional diversity, suggesting that they should recognize a very restricted antigen repertoire. However, restricted diversity is not the case for lung $\gamma\delta$ T cells in the lungs. Despite the fact that $\gamma\delta$ TCR$^+$ cells have been isolated from the lungs or pleural spaces of humans and experimental animals, especially during the primary response to mycobac-

teria, most T cells in normal lung, in pulmonary granulomas, or adjacent to pulmonary tumors bear $\alpha\beta$ TCR.

B cells produce antibody when activated, secrete some cytokines, and serve as antigen-presenting cells for memory T cells. Initial B-cell activation leads to IgM secretion, whereas secretion of other Ig isotypes requires T cell-derived cytokines, which induce class switching of B cell Ig genes. B cells are identified by expression of surface Ig or B220 (a subspecies of CD45).

Most immunologists recognize NK cells as a separate lineage of lymphocytes, although the relationship of natural killer cells (NK) to lymphokine-activated killer (LAK) cells induced by high dose treatment with interleukin-2 (IL-2) remains controversial. NK cells require no prior activation or immunization to mediate their functions, which include cytotoxicity and cytokine production. Thus, NK cells are an important component of the innate immune system discussed below (see Innate Versus Specific Immunity). Human NK cells can be identified by surface expression of CD16 and CD56. How NK cells recognize their targets, tumors, and possibly other dividing cells, as well as some pathogens, is not understood. Within the lungs, NK cells are found primarily in the interstitium and are poorly represented in BALF. Some investigators have detected very little functional activity of human pulmonary NK cells, possibly because of the suppressive effects of AM and surfactant. NK cell deficiency is an extremely rare condition manifested by life-threatening relapsing herpesvirus and polymicrobial infections.

Neutrophils are rarely found in the alveoli or interstitium of normal subjects. However, the normal pulmonary vasculature contains a large population of neutrophils, which, because of their size, pass through alveolar capillaries much more slowly than do erythrocytes. In response to chemoattractants such as C5a, bacterial products such as lipopolysaccharide or formylmethionine-containing peptides, platelet-activating factor (PAF), leukotriene B$_4$ (LTB$_4$), or IL-8, these intravascular neutrophils are readily activated and recruited into the lung parenchyma. During transmigration, activated neutrophils can release three types of products destructive to lung parenchyma: reactive oxygen products, proteolytic enzymes, and products of lipid peroxidation. The reactive oxygen products of the respiratory burst (superoxide, hydrogen peroxide, hydroxyl radicals, and hypochlorous acid) react with essentially all cellular components, causing denaturation and cross-linkage of proteins, changes in the permeability of plasma membranes and cellular organelles, and base modifications or strand breakage in nucleic acids. Proteolytic enzymes such as elastase and metalloproteinases released from neutrophil granules can digest all components of the lung interstitium. Neutrophil oxidants act synergistically with these enzymes to cause local tissue damage; hypochlorous acid inactivates the proteolytic inhibitors (including α_1-antitryptase) that would otherwise check the action of neutrophil elastase. Oxidants are also essential for activation of neutrophil collagenase. Finally, lipid peroxidation products, especially LTB_4 and PAF, cause changes in vascular permeability and are chemotactic for neutrophils, eosinophils, and lymphocytes. For these reasons, it should not be surprising that the presence of increased numbers of neutrophils in BALF correlates with a poor prognosis in pulmonary fibrosis. Nevertheless, neutrophils are clearly important in clearance of certain pathogens from the alveoli (to a larger degree than previously recognized) and can also carry particles to regional lymph nodes for initiation of specific immune responses.

Eosinophils are a second type of granulocyte possessing considerable potential for tissue destruction via release of their granular proteins: major basic protein (MBP), eosinophil peroxidase, eosinophil cationic protein, and eosinophil-derived neurotoxin. MPB can damage epithelial cells directly; it also activates basophils, mast cells, neutrophils, and platelets. Major basic protein (MBP) may also increase airways hyperresponsiveness by blocking inhibitory M2 cholinergic receptors. Eosinophil degranulation is not inhibited by glucocorticoids.

Mast cells are increasingly recognized as integral components in the pulmonary immune response to various stimuli in addition to IgE. For instance, degranulation of mast cells can be triggered by complement fragments (C3a or C5a), eosinophil MBP, or substance P. On degranulation, mast cells liberate large quantities of LTB_4 and LTC_4, as well as prostaglandin D_2 (PGD_2) and PAF. These substances are potently chemotactic for inflammatory cells, and may increase the accessibility to the lung parenchyma of serum proteins such as immunoglobulins and complement components. Mast cells produce a spectrum of cytokines (IL-3, IL-4, IL-5, GM-CSF) similar to that of Th2 T cells (described below). Mast cell proteases, which constitute 20% of the cellular weight, can activate the Hageman factor-dependent pathways linking the complement, fibrinolytic, and kinin pathways. Additionally, cultured murine mast cells induce fibroblast proliferation in vitro through secretion of an uncharacterized soluble factor. Together with the observation of large numbers of mast cells in the lungs in idiopathic pulmonary fibrosis and chronic hypersensitivity pneumonitis, these findings suggest that mast cells may be important in the generation of pulmonary fibrosis.

Type II alveolar epithelial cells are known chiefly for their capacity to secrete surfactant and to serve as a regenerative source for epithelium in the damaged lungs. However, based on recent studies showing their capacity to express class II MHC molecules and to elaborate IFN-γ and GM-CSF, type II cells should also be considered as important components in pulmonary host defense.

Humoral Aspects of Pulmonary Host Defense

The humoral elements, including Ig and complement cascade components, are the early warning system of the respiratory tract against inhaled and aspirated pathogens. Ig and complement components opsonize pathogens, identifying them as foreign and facilitating their ingestion. Both of these humoral elements can directly lyse some pathogens (certain viruses by immunoglobulins, many bacteria by complement components). Products of complement activation are also chemotactic for phagocytic cells.

All the major Ig isotypes have been identified in bronchial secretions, although IgM and IgE are present in only minute quantities. IgA predominates in the upper and proximal airways. Most IgA appear to be secreted locally; at least 90% is dimeric (secretory) IgA linked by the J components. IgA is not an opsonin and does not activate complement. Instead, it blocks attachment of potentially pathogenic bacteria.

The concentration of IgG rises progressively in the lower respiratory tract until it predominates over IgA in BALF. IgG probably enters the lungs largely by transudation from the serum in normal hosts, whereas the increased relative amounts of IgG in the lower respiratory tracts of smokers may come from local secretion. The major known role of IgG is complement-independent neutralization of viruses. IgG, especially of subclasses IgG_1 and IgG_3, efficiently opsonizes a variety of pathogens. AM have subclass-specific Fc receptors for IgG_1 and IgG_3. IgG_4, which does not fix complement and for which macrophages do not have Fc receptors, functions largely as a reaginic or cytophilic antibody that counteracts IgE by sterically hindering its binding to its cell-surface receptors.

Experimentally, antibody-secreting cells have been observed to persist within lung parenchyma for years after local antigenic stimulation. Deficiencies of IgG and especially of subgroups IgG_2 and IgG_4 are associated with chronic sinopulmonary infections. Although panhypogammaglobulinemia usually causes devastating immunodeficiency, the infections associated with IgG subclass deficiencies may be subtle and largely limited to the lungs. In cystic fibrosis, hydrolysis of alveolar IgG with removal of the Fc fragment by pseudomonal metalloproteinase may lead to impaired opsonization.

The complement system is analogous to the clotting or kinin pathways in its sequential activation of proteolytic factors that in turn activate the next downstream component. The central factor in the complement system is C3, which can be activated by either of two major pathways (Fig. 1). The classic pathway is usually activated by antigen-antibody complexes (immune complexes). Binding of the Fab portion of an antibody molecule activates the Fc portion, which is then capable of binding and activating the first three components of the classic pathway: C1q, C1s, and C1r. The proteolytic portion of this interaction, activated C1s, cleaves its targets C2 and C4 into an active complex (C4b,2a), called *classic C3 convertase*. By contrast, the more phylogenetically ancient

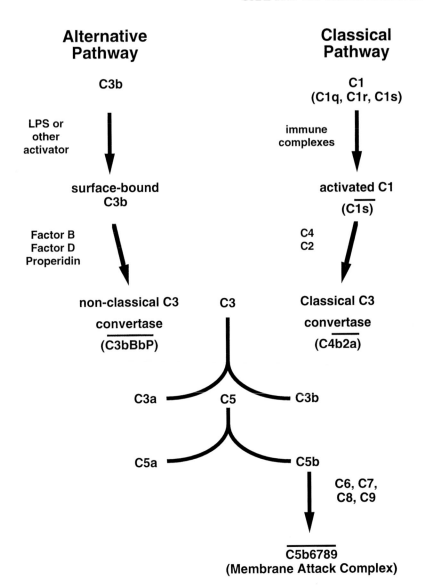

FIG. 1. Complement pathways. See text for explanation.

alternative complement pathway is activated directly by complex polysaccharides such as fungal zymosan and bacterial lipopolysaccharide, leading to production of alternative C3 convertase (C3b,Bb). Both pathways converge to cleave C3 into C3b, which in turn activates the alternative pathway in a positive feedback loop to produce more C3 convertase. Consequently, the complement system can rapidly deposit large amounts of C3 on targets. Both of these convertases can also activate C5 to produce a cytotoxic terminal attack complex consisting of C5b,6,7,8,9. This sequential family of enzymes, each activating the next, provides for powerful amplification of inflammatory signals.

Proteolytic cleavage of C4, C3, and C5 produces high-molecular-weight fragments (C4b, C3b, and C5b), which attach to the target, and diffusible low-molecular-weight fragments or anaphylatoxins (C4a, C3a, and C5a), which mediate inflammation. Anaphylatoxins increase vascular permeability, induce contraction of smooth muscles, including those of the bronchi, and induce noncytotoxic release of histamine from mast cells and basophils.

Complement contributes to host defense against some pulmonary infections. Experimentally, mice depleted of complement by cobra venom factor have impaired clearance of *Streptococcus pneumoniae* or *Pseudomonas aeruginosa*, but not of *Klebsiella pneumoniae* or *Staphylococcus aureus*. Normal function of the classic complement pathway appears essential for clearance of immune complexes from the bloodstream, and patients with inherited deficiencies of C2 or C4 are at markedly increased risk for development of systemic lupus erythematosus. Massive activation of the complement system in gram-negative and gram-positive bacteremias may be one factor that mediates lung injury in the sepsis syndrome.

Because of its immense potential to destroy host tissues, the complement system is tightly regulated by a series of related plasma and membrane glycoproteins, called the *regulators of complement activation (RCA) cluster*. The RCA cluster comprises six proteins: decay accelerating factor (DAF, CD55), complement receptors type 1 (CR1, CD35) and type 2 (CR2, CD21), C4-binding protein (C4-bp), factor H, and membrane cofactor protein (CD46). The genes for all six are tightly clustered on the long arm of chromosome 1. RCA proteins regulate complement activation by interacting with C3b and C4b bound to targets or as part of C3 convertases via either of two mechanisms. The first mechanism is decay accelerating activity, by which the protease component of the C3 convertase (C2a or Bb) is cleaved from C4b or C3b, respectively. The second regulatory mechanism is cofactor activity, by which a cofactor protein binds to the C3b or C4b, rendering it susceptible to degradation by a plasma serine protease, factor I. There are additionally complement regulatory proteins outside the RCA. The serum protein C1 inhibitor antagonizes complement activation by releasing C1r and C1s from C1q, thereby blocking the classic pathway. Deficiency of C1 inhibitor causes angioedema. Mammalian membranes also possess an inhibitor of C8 binding, CD59, which prevents insertion of the membrane attack complex.

Cytokines in Immune Lung Defense and Disease

Cytokines are low-molecular-weight peptides (usually 20 kDa) that mediate intracellular communication and regulate cellular homeostasis, inflammation, and repair. Because they were originally identified through their production by and action on leukocytes, several cytokines have been termed *interleukins* (*IL*). However, it is now recognized that many cytokines can be produced by pulmonary interstitial and parenchymal cells, indicating that these cells can participate actively in both defense and immune injury of the lungs.

As of 1996, there are 17 commonly accepted interleukins (IL-1 through IL-17). For a peptide mediator to be recognized as an interleukin, it must have been molecularly cloned. This requirement prevents the previous confusion in which the same substance was referred to by multiple names based on bioassays (e.g., T-cell growth factor for IL-2). For purely historical reasons, such important, well-characterized cytokines as tumor necrosis factor-α (TNF-α), transforming growth factor-β (TGF-β), and IFN-γ have not been assigned numbers as interleukins.

Most cytokines may have both stimulatory or inhibitory actions, depending on the cellular target and the concurrent actions of other cytokines. Attempting to explain the complexity of these interactions, Kunkel and associates have advanced the concept of cytokine networking, which highlights the dependence of cytokine secretion by certain cell types on more proximal cytokines (e.g., dependence of secretion of IL-8 by pulmonary fibroblasts on macrophage-derived IL-1 or TNF). Sporn and Roberts have likened the complex interplay of cytokines to a cellular signaling language, suggesting that the ultimate response of a target cell is determined by a number of different messages received concurrently at the cell surface. It is likely that individual immunologic lung diseases are not caused by deficiencies or excessive activities of single cytokines, but rather by the net effect of inflammatory and anti-inflammatory cytokines and other mediators.

Although most cytokines are produced by and affect a broad range of cell types, it is conceptually useful to divide these cytokines into three broad groups: inflammatory cytokines, lymphokines, and chemokines. The biochemical attributes of several important cytokines are summarized in Table 2.

Inflammatory cytokines, which have both paracrine and endocrine effects, are secreted principally by monocytes/macrophages and by parenchymal cells. This group of cytokines consists of IL-1, TNF, IL-6, and IL-12, all of which have broad ranges of cellular targets. There are two varieties of IL-1, products of distinct genes: IL-1α, produced primarily as a cell-associated protein by endothelial cells, and IL-1-β, primarily a secreted protein. Although sharing only 26% homology at the amino acid level, these peptides interact with the same receptor with identical activities. IL-1 is secreted by macrophages in response to bacterial products and to phagocytosis of other particles. In response to macrophage-derived IL-1, endothelial cells and fibroblasts elaborate additional IL-1, thereby amplifying the inflammatory response. IL-1 induces endothelial cell expression of adhesion molecules and is chemotactic for lymphocytes. Prolonged local secretion of IL-1 is central to granuloma formation, especially in sarcoidosis. IL-1 is important as a competence factor for lymphocytes and as an inducer of angiogenesis and fibrosis. Distant effects of IL-1 include fever, anorexia, somnolence, leukocytosis, and decreased pain perception. A very important recent observation is the dynamic interplay between IL-1 and IL-1 receptor antagonist protein (IRAP), a pure receptor antagonist that blocks all effects of IL-1.

TNF-α (also called *cachectin*), also secreted in response to lipopolysaccharide and probably other pathogenic products, mediates most of the toxic effects of the sepsis syndrome. Of course, TNF also has a protective role, as it is chemotactic for inflammatory cells and activates neutrophils and endothelial cells. TNF-α appears to play a crucial role in the chronic interstitial pneumonitis associated with graft-versus-host disease and in experimental immune complex disease. TNF-β (also called *lymphotoxin*), a related protein, is secreted by cytotoxic lymphocytes. Although only 30% homologous to TNF-α, lymphotoxin binds to the same receptor and causes a similar range of effects.

IL-6 is a multifunctional mediator produced by a wide

TABLE 2. *Biochemical attributes of cytokines*

Cytokine	M_r^a	Structure	Source[b]	Target
Monokines				
IL-1	17.5	Monomer	Mø/M (E, F)	B, E, F, H, N, T
TNF-α	17	Homotrimer	Mø/M (F, T)	E, F, H, Mø/M, N
IL-6	23–30	Monomer (multiple isoforms)	Mø/M (E, F, T)	B, E, F, H, T
IL-12	35, 40	Heterodimer	Mø/M	T, NK
Lymphokines				
IL-2	15–17	Monomer	T	B, T, Mø/M
IL-3	20–26	Monomer	T	MC, N (other hematopoietic)
IL-4	20	Monomer	T, MC	B, T
IL-5	22	Homodimer	T, MC	B, Eo
IL-10	18	Homodimer	B, Mø/M, T	
IFN-γ	20–24	Heterodimer	T	B, Eo
GM-CSF	14–35	Monomer	T (E, F, M)	Eo, MC, Mø/M, N
Chemokines				
IL-8	6.5	Monomer	Mø/M, N (E, F, H)	N, T

IL, interleukin; TNF-α, tumor necrosis factor-α; GM-CSF, granulocyte-macrophage colony-stimulating factor; IFN-γ, interferon-γ; B, B lymphocyte; E, endothelial cell; Eo, eosinophil; F, fibroblast; H, hepatocyte; M, monocyte; Mø, macrophage; MC, mast cell; N, neutrophil; NK, natural killer cell; P, platelet; SM, smooth muscle cell; T, T lymphocyte.
[a] Relative molecular weight of subunits (kilodaltons).
[b] Major source of cytokine (minor sources in parentheses).

variety of cell types (including T cells, AM, mast cells, endothelial cells, and fibroblasts) in response to IL-1 and TNF-α. IL-6 has both local and systemic actions, with many of its effects overlapping or synergizing with those of IL-1 and tumor necrosis factor (TNF). For example, IL-6 is the major inducer of hepatic acute-phase reactants and is itself an endogenous pyrogen. It also induces terminal differentiation of B cells and T cells. IL-6 stimulates hematopoiesis by synergizing with IL-3 to induce stem cells to enter the cell cycle. IL-6 was originally described as IFN-β_2, but is now known to be unrelated to the other interferons.

IL-12 is a heterodimeric protein produced primarily by phagocytes in response to bacterial products and to a lesser degree by B cells and connective tissue mast cells. IL-12 acts as a growth factor for activated NK cells and T cells. It importantly pushes the balance of immune responses toward cell-mediated immunity by upregulation of IFN-γ.

Lymphokines, secreted primarily by lymphocytes, have complex regulatory actions that account for many of the differences between nonspecific inflammation and specific immune responses. This group consists of IL-2, IL-3, the various colony-stimulating factors (of which only GM-CSF is considered here), IFN-γ, IL-4, and IL-5. Lymphocytes are also potent secretors of IL-6 and have the capacity to elaborate TNF-α and TNF-β.

IL-2 is an essential growth factor for most T cells and some B cells. IL-2 also increases the cytotoxic activity of monocytes and macrophages, and, at least in pharmacologic dosages, results in endothelial cell damage. Local secretion of IL-2 within the lungs is especially prominent in active pulmonary sarcoidosis.

IL-3 is a growth factor for precursors of multiple hemato-

poietic lineages and for mast cells. It also may regulate the function of mature monocytes and eosinophils. Granulocyte-monocyte colony-stimulating factor (GM-CSF), in addition to stimulating the growth of granulocyte and monocyte precursors, potentiates microbial killing and production of IL-1 and TNF-α by mature macrophages, neutrophils, and eosinophils. GM-CSF potently inhibits neutrophil migration, immobilizing neutrophils at sites of inflammation. GM-CSF also increases phagocyte longevity at sites of inflammation by blocking apoptotic cell death.

IL-4 and IL-5, typically secreted together by both CD4$^+$ T cells and mast cells, regulate allergic responses by affecting multiple cell types. IL-4 is required for the generation of both primary and secondary IgE responses. Many actions of IL-4 antagonize those of IFN-γ, although both IL-4 and IFN-γ induce class II major histocompatibility complex (MHC) expression. Both IL-4 and IL-5 are growth and differentiation factors for B cells and T cells. IL-5 is chemotactic for eosinophils. IL-5 also supports the growth and differentiation of eosinophils and lengthens their survival in tissues by preventing their elimination by apoptosis. IL-5 further acts on basophils to increase their release of histamine and leukotrienes.

IFN-γ is perhaps best known as the major macrophage-activating factor; it increases AM expression of Fc receptors and phagocytic capacity. IFN-γ also increases the adhesiveness of endothelial cells for lymphocytes and induces expression of class II MHC molecules on macrophages and endothelial cells, permitting them to become antigen-presenting cells. IFN-γ antagonizes the isotype-regulating actions of IL-4 and IL-5 on B cells. Additionally, IFN-γ is a growth factor for fibroblasts, suggesting that it may be important in both normal wound repair and in fibrosis. Because steroids inhibit the release of IFN-γ

in vitro, one of their important therapeutic actions infibrotic lung diseases may be to inhibit fibroblast proliferation.

IL-10 is a 178-amino acid glycoprotein (expressed as noncovalently linked homodimers) that appears to be a natural brake on immune responses. IL-10 was initially identified as a T-cell product that suppressed production of other T-cell cytokines, especially IFN-γ and IL-3. Subsequently, other cell types, including AM, have been shown to produce IL-10. IL-10 decreases production of TNF-α, IL-12, and the chemokines MIP-1α and MIP-2 (discussed below). IL-10 also decreases expression of class II MHC, of the adhesion molecules ICAM and VCAM, and of the co-stimulatory molecule B7-1 (CD80) on several types of antigen-presenting cells. IL-10 inhibits T-cell proliferation in vitro both by these effects and by directly inhibiting IL-2 mRNA elaboration.

A major conceptual breakthrough in understanding immunoregulation is the observation that CD4$^+$ T cells can be divided into at least two mutually exclusive subsets, Th1 and Th2, based on the range of lymphokines they secrete. Th1 cells produce IL-2 and IFN-γ, whereas Th2 cells produce IL-4, IL-5, and IL-10; both subsets can produce IL-3, GM-CSF, and TNF. These two subsets differ in function: Th1 cells mediate delayed-type hypersensitivity reactions, activate macrophages for microbicidal functions, and induce IgG$_1$ and IgG$_{22}$, whereas Th2 cells provide superior help for antibody responses and induce IgG$_4$ and IgE. The two subsets are also mutually inhibitory. IFN-γ (produced by Th1 cells) inhibits growth of Th2 cells, whereas IL-10 (produced by Th2 cells) inhibits cytokine secretion by Th1 cells. CD8$^+$ T cells principally secrete a Th1-like spectrum of cytokines, although examples of Th2-producing CD8 clones exist.

In some cases, the cytokine profile and hence the nature of the host response appears to be directed into one of two mutually exclusive patterns, namely, Th1-predominant delayed-type hypersensitivity responses or Th2-predominant antibody-forming responses. The classification of CD4$^+$ T cell clones into Th1 and Th2 subsets is well established in mice, in which strain differences in the balance between these two subsets lead to either fatal infection or protective immunity for several different pathogens. The classification also appears to pertain to humans. Whether dysregulation of the balance between these cross-regulatory T-cell subsets underlies any immunologic lung diseases, especially asthma, is a matter of active study. Th2 cells may play an important regulatory role in normal immune responses by limiting the tissue-damaging effects inherent in responses of Th1 cells and activated macrophages.

Chemokines form a large supergene family of small cytokines that possess important chemotactic, activating, and angiogenesis-influencing properties. Cross-linkage of internal cysteine residues is believed to render chemokines highly resistant to proteolytic degradation. Based on the position of the terminal four cysteine (C) residues, two major subfamilies of chemokines are distinguished: C-X-C (α) chemokines have an amino acid between the two cysteine residues, whereas C-C (β) chemokines do not. Distinction of these two subfamilies is important, as they differ in target specificity. C-X-C chemokines are predominantly chemotactic for granulocytes, whereas C-C chemokines are chemotactic for mononuclear cells. Both C-X-C and C-C chemokines can be elaborated by a wide variety of cell types, although there is a degree of stimulus specificity for their production. Recent evidence indicates that chemokines play a variety of roles other than leukocyte chemotaxis. For example, individual chemokines can promote or inhibit the proliferation of blood vessels during wound repair or tumor growth. One receptor for C-C chemokines, CC-CKR-5, was very recently identified as a cofactor in entry of wild-type HIV into cells.

IL-8 is the prototypic C-X-C chemokine. IL-8 is very potently chemotactic for neutrophils; some investigators have also suggested it is chemotactic for lymphocytes. IL-8 is a major cause of neutrophil recruitment in cystic fibrosis, bronchiectasis, chronic bronchitis, and empyema. Interestingly, elaboration of IL-8 is induced in pulmonary epithelial cells by neutrophil elastase and in mesothelial cells by asbestos. Signal transduction of IL-8, like that of other chemotactic stimuli such as f-MLP and C5a, occurs via GTP-binding proteins and activation of phosphatidyl-inositol-specific phospholipase C. Other C-X-C chemokines include ENA-78, *gro*-α, IP-10, MIP-2, and PF4.

Monocyte chemotactic peptide-1 (MCP-1) is the prototypic C-C chemokine. MCP-1 is a 13-kDa glycosylated, heparin-binding protein produced by AM, fibroblasts, and pulmonary epithelial and endothelial cells. It is chemotactic in vitro for T cells and monocytes. MCP-1 is induced by lipopolysaccharide (LPS), IL-1, TNF-α, IL-4, IFN-γ, TGF-β, and PDGF. MCP-1 plays a crucial role in host defense against gram-negative organisms. Other C-C chemokines include MCP-2, MCP-3, RANTES, MIP-1α, and MIP-1β.

Innate Versus Specific Immunity

Recognition of infectious agents, especially bacteria, elicits a rapid and vigorous response of neutrophils and monocytes. This initial response does not depend on prior immunization, as does the specific immune response. Instead, this innate or natural immune response relies on a phylogenetically more primitive system that recognizes danger signals found on pathogens but not on mammalian cells. Examples of such danger signals are repeated polysaccharides, mannan, LPS, or formylated peptides. Recognition of such signals mobilizes a vigorous but nonspecific response characterized by complement activation and recruitment of phagocytic cells. The alternative complement pathway is always activated in an antibody-independent fashion, via recognition of repeated polysaccharides (especially those lacking sialic acid) or LPS. However, even in the absence of specific antibody, complement activation can occur via the classic pathway following recognition of C-reactive protein, mitochondrial membranes, or naked DNA.

The best-understood danger signal to which the innate immune system responds is LPS of gram-negative bacteria. LPS is recognized by phagocytic cells owing to two proteins, CD14 and LPS-binding protein (LBP). CD14 is a 55-kDa glycoprotein expressed both as a membrane receptor linked to GPI (glycerol phosphatidylinositol) and as an abundant (3 g/mL) soluble serum protein (sCD14). Each CD14 molecule directly binds 1 to 2 LPS molecules. Recent evidence suggests that CD14 can bind other microbial products, including those of gram-positive organisms and possibly fungi. Binding of LPS to CD14 is markedly accelerated by the transfer protein LBP. LBP also catalyzes the transfer of LPS from CD14 to serum lipoproteins, which renders LPS biologically inactive. This process provides a means for temporally limiting responses to only newly formed LPS.

LPS is an extremely potent stimulant for phagocytic cells to produce IL-1, TNF-α, and IL-12. Sepsis is a failure to contain locally the response to LPS or other microbial products, resulting in dangerously high quantities of these inflammatory cytokines circulating throughout the body. Phagocytic cell production of IL-12 early in immune responses appears to be a crucial bridge between innate and specific immunity. IL-12 production biases responses towards cell-mediated Th1 responses and away from IgE secretion. LPS also nonspecifically activates components of specific immunity (e.g., by polyclonally activating B cells to secrete IgM). LPS inhaled in large amounts causes cotton worker's pneumoconiosis.

Recent evidence suggests that CD4$^+$,NK1.1$^+$ cells, another apparent component of innate immunity, constitute an antigen-independent pathway that provides IL-4 necessary to initiate Th2 immune responses. These natural T (NT) cells express a relatively invariant TCR and are activated by the nonclassic MHC class I-like CD1 molecules on macrophages. This capacity explains the otherwise puzzling dilemma of how Th2 responses can be initiated without pre-existing Th2 T cells.

RECRUITMENT OF INFLAMMATORY AND IMMUNE CELLS TO SITES OF INFLAMMATION

Enormous strides have been made in the last decade toward understanding the molecular basis of leukocyte recruitment. Considerable effort has been expended in this investigation, because it is widely anticipated that it will lead to the development of novel immunomodulatory therapies. This process involves an interaction in which both the leukocyte and the endothelial cell are active participants. Recruitment is a complex phenomenon facilitated by activation of either the leukocyte or the endothelial cell. For example, neutrophil activation leads to cytoplasmic stiffening, which increases retention within the pulmonary microvasculature. Endothelial cell activation rapidly leads to upregulation of a variety of adhesion receptors, detailed below. An additional means of arresting groups of activated leukocytes, even within the lumina of larger vessels, is adhesion of individual leukocytes to each other. These interactions (mediated by a host of receptor/ligand interactions, including LFA-1/ICAM, CD2/LFA-3, and CD44/hyaluronate) can contribute to tissue injury by leukostasis, as in cerebral lupus and possibly in sepsis.

The process of leukocyte recruitment can be divided into seven steps, each of which is controlled by multiple cell surface receptors and cytokines: (1) leukocyte rolling along endothelium; (2) leukocyte triggering; (3) firm adhesion to endothelial cells; (4) transmigration of the endothelial layer; (5) penetration of the vascular basement membrane; (6) migration through extracellular matrix into parenchyma; and (7) selective tissue retention.

Videomicroscopy studies indicate that neutrophils roll along vascular endothelia, making transient interactions that probably facilitate leukocyte arrest at sites of inflammation. Together with considerations of physical size, rolling probably accounts for the large pool of marginated neutrophils and lymphocytes within the pulmonary vasculature. In the case of neutrophils, rolling is mediated by the interaction of L-selectin with endothelial cell ligands bearing the sialylated carbohydrate sLEX. Initial adhesion of neutrophils to activated endothelia appears to be mediated in a similar fashion when carbohydrate determinants on the neutrophil are recognized by the inducible endothelial ligands E-selectin (CD62E) and P-selectin (CD62P). A subgroup of human memory T lymphocytes also binds to E-selectin, whereas other lymphocytes bind to the lymphocyte-specific endothelial ligand, VCAM, via the action of VLA-4 (CD29/CD49d). Expression of these endothelial ligands is regulated by inflammatory cytokines: IL-1 and TNF-α induce ICAM-1 and E-selectin, and together with IL-4 induce VCAM.

Triggering appears to be mediated by chemokine receptors that recognize chemokines presented by an endothelial cell surface protein such as CD44. Triggering increases the stability of the initial adhesion through rapid changes in the avidity of binding of leukocyte β_2-integrin receptors such as LFA-1 (CD11a/CD18) and MAC-1 (CD11b/CD18). Both of these β_2-integrins interact with ICAM-1 on the surface of endothelial cells. Changes in avidity are followed by changes in receptor density that result in firm adhesion and the transformation of the leukocyte from a spherical cell to an ameboid, motile cell. Transmigration of endothelial cells depends on leukocyte β_2-integrins such as LFA-1 and on the homotypic interaction of CD31 on both leukocytes and endothelial cells. Interdigitation of CD31 is believed to act like a zipper, allowing reversible disruption of the endothelial cell tight junctions, permitting leukocyte transmigration without fluid leakage. LFA-1 is increased on human memory T cells, and has been suggested to be increased by IL-1.

Penetration of vascular basement membrane requires enzymatic digestion, which is mediated by leukocyte metalloproteinases, especially plasminogen activator bound to its receptor, and collagenases. It is likely that secretion of these potent enzymes, as well as of high concentrations of cytokines such as TNF, account in part for immune-mediated damage to vessel walls. The reparative phase of this immune angiitis can involve vessel wall fibrosis, resulting in some cases of pulmonary hypertension seen in association with a variety of interstitial lung diseases. Directed migration is necessary for inflammatory cells to arrive at sites of inflammation; migration is clearly increased by some cytokines *in vitro*. IL-1, IL-2, IL-4, IL-8, and IFN-γ are all chemotactic for lymphocytes in vitro. RANTES, a C-C chemokine, is selectively chemoattractant for memory T cells.

Finally, selective retention is probably an important component of immune response generation. Lymphocytes are recruited to sites of inflammation nonspecifically (i.e., without regard to antigen specificity), but they are retained if activated by recognition of antigen, as described below. Selective retention could be mediated by the matrix-binding domains of the β_1-integrins VLA-4, VLA-5, and VLA-6, which are upregulated on human memory T cells. Chemokines and inflammatory cytokines could increase selective retention both by increasing surface expression and binding avidity of these adhesion receptors, and by acting at high doses as migration inhibition factors.

Generation of Pulmonary Immune Responses

To generate protective immune responses, nonself antigens must be recognized by lymphocytes. Each lymphocyte clone bears an antigen receptor that generally recognizes only a single antigen. B cells can be activated directly by binding of antigen to surface immunoglobulin molecules. However, in most biologically relevant cases, B-cell maturation to an immunoglobulin-secreting cell requires specific interactions with CD4$^+$ T cells through both receptor-mediated and cytokine-mediated interactions. Both of these interactions generally require recognition of the same antigen by the T cell and the B cell. This requirement is called a *cognate interaction*. Thus, T-cell help is mediated primarily by direct cell-to-cell contact, permitting considerable control over which individual B cells produce antibody.

T-cell activation is required to initiate and maintain immune responses to virtually all antigens of clinical relevance. T cells have heterodimeric antigen receptors composed of $\alpha\beta$ or $\tau\delta$ chains, which recognize antigen only as fragments in the context of appropriate MHC molecules on specialized antigen-presenting cells (Fig. 2). T cells are activated when they receive two types of signals. The first signal consists of recognition of polypeptide fragments displayed by MHC molecules of antigen-presenting cells. Antigen is recognized by a macromolecular complex consisting of (1) antigen-specific variable chains of the T-cell antigen receptor (TCR), (2) an MHC restriction element (CD4 or CD8), and (3) a signal-transduction complex collectively called *CD3*.

CD8$^+$ T cells respond to antigen presented by class I MHC molecules, whereas CD4$^+$ T cells respond to antigen presented by class II MHC molecules. Class I MHC molecules present intracellular antigens, especially viral products. Class I MHC molecules are constitutively expressed by virtually all cell types. In contrast, class II molecules are constitutively expressed only by a few cell types, notably B cells and dendritic cells; however, class II MHC expression can be induced on many cell types by IFN-γ. Because of this requirement for antigen presentation in conjunction with MHC molecules, regulation by lymphokines of the MHC expression of parenchymal cells such as fibroblasts and endothelial cells is central to the control of immune responses. Class II MHC molecules present extrinsic antigens, which enter the antigen-presenting cell by phagocytosis or pinocytosis.

A second type of signal, which is antigen-nonspecific and termed *co-stimulatory*, is required for complete activation leading to cell division. True co-stimulatory molecules fulfill two criteria. First, these molecules provide signals necessary (together with TCR or CD3 ligation) for activation of naïve T cells. Second, in their absence, stimulation via TCR or CD3 not only fails to activate the T cell but in certain settings induces it to become refractory to further stimulation or even die by apoptosis. Hence, the fate of an activated T cell can be determined by co-stimulatory signals during activation.

The best-understood of these necessary co-stimulatory receptors is CD28. Signaling through CD28 leads to IL-2 mRNA stabilization. CD28 recognizes two ligands displayed by antigen-presenting cells, B7-1 (CD80) and B7-2 (CD86). Human AM are deficient in expression of B7-1 and B7-2, even when stimulated with IFN-γ. Proliferation of human CD4$^+$ T cells to recall antigen or anti-CD3 in the presence of AM improves if CD28 is cross-linked. These findings indicate that deficient co-stimulation through CD28 is a major reason for poor function of antigen-presenting cells, and suggest that AM may induce T-cell unresponsiveness or apoptosis. A second true co-stimulatory T-cell molecule is gp39, the ligand for CD40. CD40 is highly expressed by B cells and DC. Co-stimulatory activity that does not meet these two criteria has also been ascribed to adhesion molecules, includ-

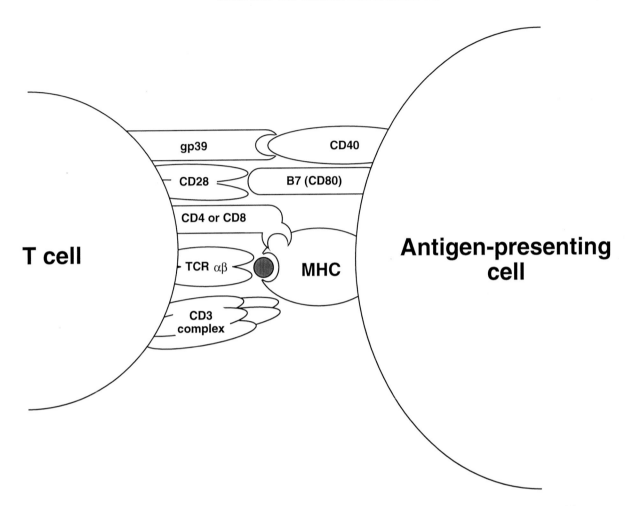

FIG. 2. Schematic representation of receptors involved in T-cell activation. Antigen is recognized in the context of the MHC molecule on the antigen-presenting cell by a complex including the TCR, the CD3 complex, and CD4 or CD8. T-cell co-stimulatory molecules, including CD28 and gp39, provide necessary second signals to permit completion of the cell cycle.

ing CD44, and β_1-integrins such as VLA-4 or β_2-integrins such as LFA-1. Proliferation of mitogen-activated lymphocytes is increased when these molecules are ligated. The conventional interpretation is that improved adhesion to the antigen-presenting cells increases proliferation because of enhanced signaling through TCR or CD3.

Lymphocyte Distribution and Recirculation

Thus, generation of immune responses is constrained both by the relative paucity of antigen-specific lymphocytes for any given determinant and by the necessity that antigenic determinants be presented by immunocompetent cells. The solution that has evolved to solve both of these constraints is drainage of antigens to lymph nodes, between which virgin lymphocytes continuously recirculate. In this way, the few lymphocytes specific for any given antigen have a greatly increased likelihood of being activated efficiently.

Lymphocytes enter organized lymphoid tissue principally by adhering to and crossing specialized postcapillary venules, known for their hypertrophied ("heightened") endothelial cells as *high endothelial venules* (*HEV*). HEV endothelial cells express unique ligands, called *vascular addressins,* to which lymphocytes adhere. Lymphocyte recirculation is not random, but instead appears to be organized into several anatomic recirculatory circuits. One circuit involves the skin and extremities draining into the peripheral nodes. This circuit is controlled by the lymphocyte receptor L-selectin (CD62L), which binds an endothelial addressin called *glyCAM*. The other well-characterized circuit involves migration of IgA-secreting B cells from Peyer's patches to intestinal lamina propria. This circuit is controlled by the $\alpha_4\beta_7$-integrin on lymphocytes, which binds an endothelial addressin called *Mad-CAM,* an immunoglobulin supergene family member.

Lymphocytes are found within the lung in four distinct anatomic compartments: (1) a marginated intravascular pool that differs in composition from peripheral blood, (2) the interstitium, (3) the alveolar spaces, and (4) organized lymphoid tissue. Organized lymphoid tissue includes lymphoid aggregates, both encapsulated and unencapsulated. Traditionally, bronchus-associated lymphoid tissue (BALT) is considered a part of the lymphoid compartment of the lung. BALT consists of nodules of unencapsulated lymphoid tissue lacking germinal centers, initially described in a variety of animal species. BALT nodules lie in immediate apposition to airways; their lymphocytic areas are separated from the airway lumina by a single layer of specialized epithelium (lymphoepithelium), through which lymphocytes and possibly antigens are believed to pass. However, the importance of organized intrapulmonary lymphoid tissue, especially BALT, in the generation of pulmonary immune responses has been questioned by some recent investigators. In fact, compared with that of experimental animals, the lung parenchyma of healthy humans contains relatively little organized lymphoid tissue and few parenchymal lymphocytes. Therefore, pulmonary immune responses are likely initiated in regional lymph nodes and mediated largely by recruitment of lymphocytes and other leukocytes from extrapulmonary sources, as discussed above.

Nevertheless, large numbers of lymphocytes can be released from enzyme-digested fragments of human lung tissue (probably reflecting recovery of cells from all four anatomic compartments, especially the marginated intravascular compartment), suggesting that overall the lung contains a large number of lymphocytes. Results of studies that have compared the phenotype and function of lymphocytes recovered from the lungs of patients with interstitial lung diseases indicate that alveolar lymphocytes closely resemble lymphocytes recovered from minced lung tissue (interstitial plus some organized lymphoid tissue). Thus, analysis of BALF is generally believed to reflect accurately processes occurring in the lung interstitium.

It has been suggested that the lungs and upper airways are part of the gastrointestinal circuit, comprising along with the gut, breast, and urogenital tract what has been called a *common mucosal immune system*. Supporting this hypothesis, BALT morphologically resembles gut-associated lymphoid tissue (GALT), such as Peyer's patches. Moreover, in adoptive transfer experiments, lymphocytes derived either from bronchus-associated lymphoid tissue (BALT) or from Peyer's patches repopulated both the lungs and the gut with IgA-bearing cells, whereas lymphocytes derived from peripheral lymph nodes did not. However, a number of findings are difficult to reconcile with the hypothesis that the lung parenchyma is part of a common mucosal immune system. Studies in several species have shown that lymphoblasts isolated either from bronchial nodes or from efferent pulmonary lymph localize to the lungs significantly better than to the gut or peripheral nodes. Moreover, two groups of investigators have found that antigen priming of the tra-

chea does not result in significant dissemination of memory cells to the gut. These data argue that the lungs and their draining lymph nodes are not part of a common mucosal immune system, but instead constitute a separate recirculatory circuit. Also consistent with a separate pulmonary circuit of lymphocyte recirculation, experimental studies show that the initial immune response to intratracheal antigens occurs in the bronchial lymph nodes. This observation has led to the proposal that primary immune responses in lung parenchyma develop by recruitment of lymphocytes activated in these nodes back to the lungs. To date, however, no mechanism has been proposed to explain this postulated recruitment of lymphocytes back to lung parenchyma. In summary, despite compelling evidence from in vivo studies, it is uncertain whether there is a distinct recirculatory circuit involving the lung and bronchial lymph nodes, and if so, how important such a circuit is in the maintenance of immunologic lung diseases.

Analysis of surface markers shows that lung T cells are predominantly primed cells, that is, they are the progeny of cells that have been activated previously by encounter with an antigen. At present, it seems likely that accumulation of primed T cells in the normal lung results from their increased expression of adhesion receptors; however, in immunologic lung diseases like sarcoidosis, local lymphocyte proliferation may contribute as well.

In vitro studies have shown multiple factors that could limit lymphocyte activation and proliferation within the lungs. AM are poor antigen-presenting cells compared with other mononuclear phagocytes. Their poor antigen-presenting cellular function is explained by limited expression of class II MHC molecules in some species and by secretion of inhibitory factors, including prostaglandin E_2 (PGE_2), IL-1 receptor antagonist, TGF-β, and reactive nitrogen intermediates. In vitro, rodent and human AM block proliferation of mitogen-activated lymphocytes *in vitro* without interfering with CD3 downmodulation, CD25 expression, or IL-2 elaboration. AM also inhibit the antigen-presenting cellular function of pulmonary dendritic cells. Although AM can transport particles to mediastinal nodes to initiate immune responses, eliminating AM *in vivo* increases the pulmonary immune response, suggesting that their net effect is inhibitory. Alveolar lining fluid inhibits lymphocyte proliferation in vitro, in part because of its lipid components. BALF of sensitized guinea pigs before challenge with inhaled mycobacterial antigens increases pulmonary inflammation, supporting an immunosuppressive effect of normal alveolar lining fluid *in vivo*. Alveolar epithelial cells may also directly suppress lymphocyte proliferation via PGE_2 and by a mechanism not involving surfactant phospholipid or prostaglandins. Hence, factors secreted by both AM and alveolar epithelial cells appear able to block proliferation (but not necessarily cytokine secretion) of activated lymphocytes recruited to the lungs during pulmonary immune responses.

The factors that regulate physiologic immune responses to prevent prolonged interference with gas exchange are incompletely understood. Antigen elimination, through macrophage ingestion, is probably very important. Some lymphocytes migrate out of the lungs, probably to contribute to specific immune memory against pathogens. Recent evidence suggests that many activated lymphocytes die in the lungs by apoptosis, as do the majority of neutrophils and eosinophils. There are excellent teleologic reasons why lymphocyte apoptosis should contribute to immune response termination. By eliminating obsolete clones, apoptosis prevents competition with clones expanding in subsequent responses. Apoptosis also eliminates potentially autoreactive cells, especially activated B cells, which can produce novel autoantibodies during Ig gene hypermutation. The role of immunosuppressive cytokines, especially IL-10 and TGF-β, is just beginning to be explored, and it may lead to novel immunomodulatory therapies.

ALLERGIC PULMONARY TISSUE INJURY

There is evidence that four standard types of allergic tissue injury are operative in the lungs and play important roles in the pathogenesis of many of the interstitial and immunologically mediated diseases discussed later in this chapter. One should remember that such classifications are by no means absolute, because in an actual disease process several types of hypersensitivity are likely to be operative, either simultaneously or at different stages of the disease.

Type I (Anaphylactic) Tissue Injury

Antigen characteristically reacts with specific antibody of the IgE class, which is attached to a basophil or mast cell by means of its Fc fragment. Both tissue mast cells and circulating basophils concentrate IgE on their surfaces; the surface of one cell contain 500,000 IgE molecules. IgE fixes to a glycoprotein receptor site on the cell membrane, resulting in an arrangement permitting exposure of the antibody-combining sites (Fab) to the surrounding milieu. Cross-linking of two IgE antibody molecules by specific antigen aggregates the corresponding IgE and receptor sites and results in the initiation of a series of cellular biochemical events culminating in the expulsion of secretory granule contents. The biochemical events involved in the secretory process have been well described, and they include an extracellular Ca^{++}-dependent conversion of a membrane-associated serine esterase from its precursor to an activated form. Among the many preformed granule-associated and newly synthesized mediators released during type I (IgE-mediated) reactions are histamine; the leukotrienes C, D, and E; eosinophil chemotactic factor of anaphylaxis (ECFA);

heparin; superoxide dismutase (SOD); peroxidase; prostaglandins; thromboxanes; PAF; neutrophil chemotactic factor of anaphylaxis (NCFA); bradykinin; major basic protein; and a wide variety of inflammatory factors of anaphylaxis that may be important in so-called late-phase reactions. Once these mediators are discharged or synthesized, they are active for finite periods. For example, histamine is destroyed by several enzymes found in all tissues. Other enzymes, proteases, or peptidases specifically destroy mediators such as leukotrienes and ECFA, and the prostaglandins are metabolized by dehydrogenases and reductases. Many of these mediators, before their deactivation, promote vasodilation and smooth muscle contraction, which are the pathophysiologic hallmarks of IgE-mediated allergic tissue injury. Activation of the complement cascade is not involved in this type of reaction, although effects identical to those noted in IgE-mediated reactions can be produced after nonimmunologic activation of the alternative pathway of complement. For example, the C5a component of complement can trigger release of all the above-mentioned mediators through a non-IgE-dependent mechanism. In the respiratory tract, it is well recognized that type I allergic tissue injury is operative in the production of uncomplicated seasonal allergic rhinitis and true allergic bronchial asthma.

Type II (Cytotoxic) Tissue Injury

Type II allergic tissue injury involves the reaction of specific complement-fixing antibody of the IgG or IgM class with an antigenic component of the cell or with an antigen or hapten firmly bound to a cell surface, which in turn causes activation of the complement cascade and resulting cell damage or death. An example of type II, cytotoxic allergic tissue injury at the pulmonary level might be that of Goodpasture's syndrome. The finding of complement receptors on the surface of AM and the detection of C3 bound to AM in lung biopsy specimens from patients with farmer's lung disease also suggests that type II reactions may be involved, to a minor extent, in the pathogenesis of certain forms of hypersensitivity pneumonitis.

Type III Allergic Tissue Injury

Type III allergic tissue injury (Arthus or serum sickness reactions) is produced by soluble circulating immune complexes, generally under conditions of slight antigen excess, that theoretically become trapped under endothelial cell linings along capillary membranes. There is mounting evidence that increased small-vessel permeability as a result of an antecedent type I allergic reaction plays an important role in allowing localization and entrapment of immune complexes in vessel walls and along basement membranes. Immune complexes then interact with serum complement and activate the complement sequence. The resulting complement-induced neutrophil chemotaxis ultimately leads to tissue destruction (basement membrane or endothelial cell damage plus necrosis and vasculitis) caused by lysosomal enzyme release. In tissue spaces such as the lung under conditions of relative antigen excess, complexes may tend to be insoluble and be removed by the reticuloendothelial system. In general, the organ or area of deposition of soluble immune complexes will determine the clinical picture. Serum sickness, the classic example of this type of reaction, was commonly seen in humans after administration of antitoxins or antibacterial sera prepared in nonhuman species (e.g., it may be seen after repeated administration of horse antitoxins). Currently, it is more commonly noted after administration of some drugs, including antibiotics, particularly penicillin and sulfonamides. The presence of serum precipitins, the time course of development of lung lesions, and the demonstration of dual type I and type III skin test reactions in some patients with hypersensitivity pneumonitis suggest that this mechanism may be partly involved in pathogenesis. However, other more recent evidence strongly indicates that AM activation and cell-mediated (delayed) hypersensitivity (type IV) play a more prominent role in production of these lesions. The histologic findings in lung biopsy specimens from patients with hypersensitivity pneumonitis also usually do not reveal the hemorrhagic necrosis, vasculitis, and polymorphonuclear cell infiltration characteristic of type III allergic reactions.

Type IV Allergic Tissue Injury

Type IV allergic tissue injury (delayed or cell-mediated hypersensitivity) is mediated through sensitized T cells plus other recruited effector lymphocytes and macrophages rather than through circulating or fixed antibodies, as in the previous three types. After antigen contact with sensitized cells, there is generally a latent period of 24 to 72 hrs before clinical expression of a type IV reaction. Complement is not involved in the reaction. The characteristic histologic lesions seen in type IV allergic tissue injury involves infiltration of tissues with the two effector cells of these reactions, lymphocytes and macrophages, often in a perivenular distribution. On contact with antigen, specifically sensitized T cells release lymphokines, which either directly lead to or augment the characteristic reactions of type IV allergic tissue injury.

Type IV allergic reactions can be passively transferred by specifically sensitized lymphocytes or by an enzyme-resistant dialyzable crude extract of lymphocytes called *transfer factor*. This factor may play an important role in converting nonsensitized lymphocytes to specific antigen-responsive cells, although more recent evidence suggests that it acts in a nonspecific manner. The production of certain lymphokines, such as interferon-γ, on exposure of sensitized lymphocytes to antigen forms the basis for in vitro assays of the type IV reaction, as are employed in the diagnosis of certain forms of hypersensitivity pneumonitis.

Expression of cell-mediated immunity and of specific antibody reflect the activity of different types of CD4$^+$ T cells. T cells include CD4$^+$ (helper) and CD8$^+$ (suppressor/cytotoxic) subsets. CD4$^+$ cells can be divided into Th1, Th2, or Th0 subsets according to their patterns of cytokine secretion. Th1 cells preferentially secrete IL-2, IFN-γ, and TNF-β; activate macrophages; and are responsible for cell-mediated immunity reactions and T-cell toxicity. Th2 CD4$^+$ cells secrete IL-4, IL-5, IL-9, IL-10, and IL-13; provide help for immunoglobulin (particularly IgE and IgG$_4$) secretion; enhance eosinophil production, survival, and activity; and promote mast cell maturation and proliferation. Development of either a predominant Th1 or Th2 response in mice depends on many factors, including attributes of the antigen, site of delivery, adjuvant used, and type of antigen-presenting cell encountered. Cytokines secreted by one CD4$^+$ subset inhibit the development of the reciprocal subset, leading to a predominance of one of the subsets and polarization of the immune response. Th0 cells secrete a mix of cytokines characteristic of both Th1 and Th2 cells and may represent progenitors of both Th1 and Th2 cells. The above models developed in mice have not been entirely confirmed in humans in the sense that Th1 and Th2 cells may not exist as exact counterparts in humans. However, the concept that the cytokine milieu (derived from many possible sources, such as CD4$^+$, CD8$^+$, NK, mast cells, and γδ T cells) at the time of CD4$^+$ cell differentiation determines the later pattern of cytokine secretion and function is valid. More recently, CD8$^+$ cells have been found to differentiate into Tc1 and Tc2 subtypes, with cytokine secretion profiles apparently similar to those of Th1 and Th2 CD4$^+$ cells.

EOSINOPHILIC PULMONARY SYNDROMES

In adult animals, most eosinophils are produced in the bone marrow and released into the blood; emergence time is generally 60 to 80 hrs and the half-life in the circulation is 8 to 12 hrs, but tissue half-life is approximately 24 hrs. T lymphocytes are necessary participants in the production of soluble eosinophilopoietic factors such as IL-3, IL-5, and GM-CSF by immunologic mechanisms in vitro and *in vivo*. Immunologically elicited eosinophilia is independent of B lymphocytes and antibody formation.

Eosinophils are positioned predominantly in tissues, but full expression of their unique functional capabilities requires directed influx, accumulation, and activation at sites of specific tissue reactions. Many distinct factors from several sources are known to be selectively chemotactic for eosinophils, including certain complement components, ECFA, certain leukotrienes, lymphokines, and chemokines. IL-4 selectively induces the appearance of specific adhesins (VCAM-1) on endothelial cells that interact specifically with eosinophils and basophils. This might explain the intermediate steps by which certain stimuli lead to the accumulation of eosinophils in tissue. As in the case of other leukocytes, eosinophils can respond to a variety of fluid phase and particulate stimuli with increased adherence, expression of membrane receptors, phagocytosis, cytotoxicity, enhancement of certain synthetic activities, lysosomal degranulation, and oxidative metabolism.

Eosinophilic granules contain a wide array of enzymes comparable with those in neutrophil lysosomes; however, the eosinophil lacks lysozyme, and there are many other major differences in enzyme content between eosinophils and neutrophils. Some eosinophilic granule enzymes and several cationic polypeptides that are present predominantly in eosinophils are of special importance in pulmonary eosinophilias and hypersensitivity reactions. At least three different cationic polypeptides are major constituents of eosinophilic granules. These are MBP and two eosinophilic cationic proteins (ECP). Eosinophils are capable of generating superoxide and hydroxyl radicals at rates higher than those observed in neutrophils, and the production of superoxide by eosinophils remains at maximal levels for several hours. The specificity and intensity of the microbicidal activity of eosinophils differs substantially from those of other leukocytes in that eosinophils have less bactericidal capacity. Other specialized functions of eosinophils, however, are operative in the destruction of metazoan nematodes, trematodes, and cestodes known to be characteristically associated with eosinophilia. The most striking degrees of eosinophilia are found during the tissue-invasive or tissue-migratory phases of helminthic infections. At least two different populations of eosinophils can be distinguished by density. Hypodense eosinophils are activated according to the criteria of partial degranulation, increased oxygen consumption and deoxyglucose uptake, cytotoxicity against schistosomes, LTC_4 production, and expression of certain receptors for IgG, IgE, and complement. An increased number of hypodense eosinophils are found in some patients with asthma and may be the mediators of tissue damage in some of the syndromes described below.

Eosinophilic infiltrates around invading helminths and ticks have been documented for some time. Eosinophils adhere to helminths by C3b- and IgG-dependent mechanisms. They then degranulate and deposit granule-associated proteins on the surface of the helminth, leading to the appearance of microscopic defects in the organism's cuticle. ECPs are 10-fold more active in this regard than MBP. The efficiency of helminthicidal activity of eosinophils is enhanced markedly by ECFA and LTB_4.

Several monokines and lymphokines also enhance eosinophilic helminthicidal activity.

Downregulatory eosinophilic activities are attributable to certain factors, including PGE_2, which suppresses the release of mediators by mast cells; MBP, which binds heparin; and a set of specific enzymes capable of degrading mediators. In addition, mast cell granules are ingested by intact eosinophils. Pertinent to the discussions in this text are the fact that at concentrations attained in the airways, MBP is capable of injuring bronchial epithelial cells and increasing airways permeability to luminal factors. It is clear that eosinophils are tissue cells with the capacity to augment and prolong or inhibit and terminate immediate and late-phase reactions evoked by mast cells and basophils. The net outcome of eosinophil-mast cell interactions at any time during the hypersensitivity response is likely a function of the relative number of each type of cell and their degree of activation. Eosinophils alone and in concert with mast cells and macrophages thus have the potential to participate in host defense or to promote processes that injure host tissues. The finding of elevated concentrations of specific eosinophilic constituents in sputum and lung tissues of patients with asthma and other inflammatory lung diseases of suspected allergic origin emphasizes the importance of further analysis of the eosinophil in normal lung function and lung diseases. Although eosinophilia can occur in association with many illnesses, it is generally most prominent in diseases affecting organ systems in contact with the external environment—namely, the skin, gastrointestinal tract, and respiratory tract. The eosinophilic involvement of the lung in many of these syndromes is well defined and of considerable clinical importance. The clinical features of eosinophilic syndromes are reviewed in the following sections.

The group of miscellaneous pulmonary eosinophilias generally characterized by eosinophilic radiodensities with or without peripheral blood eosinophilia is poorly understood and ill-defined. These eosinophilias are assumed to represent some type of altered immunologic response to exogenous allergens or infectious agents, but the etiologic agents and immunopathogenic mechanism involved usually are not known.

In 1952, Crofton and co-workers described these disorders as *pulmonary eosinophilias* and divided them into five general categories, with some degree of overlap, as follows:

Group 1: Pulmonary eosinophilia (Loeffler's syndrome); pulmonary infiltrates with eosinophilia (PIE syndrome)
Group 2: Prolonged pulmonary eosinophilia
Group 3: Tropical eosinophilia
Group 4: Pulmonary eosinophilia with asthma
Group 5: Pulmonary lesions of polyarthritis nodosa

Crofton clearly recognized the inadequacy of this classification and, in an attempt to create order out of this heterogeneous group of diseases, decided that the generic term *pulmonary eosinophilia* could be used for the entire group. Despite many other useful classifications of this type, there are still few new data available concerning the immunopathogenesis and etiology of these diseases, with the exception of allergic bronchopulmonary aspergillosis (ABPA).

Loeffler's Syndrome

Loeffler's syndrome was described in 1932 as a benign and often symptomless association of transient migratory or successive pulmonary infiltrates and peripheral blood eosinophilia, generally lasting for 20 days. Because of the benign nature of this syndrome, few if any of the clinically documented cases were studied morphologically. Pulmonary eosinophilia that is more prolonged (group 2 of Crofton, lasting 6 months or longer) and frequently has a more severe clinical course has also been characterized. Overall, the primary features of Loeffler's syndrome are a high degree of peripheral eosinophilia together with rapidly fluctuating, varied, and fleeting chest roentgenographic shadows and a benign course. This syndrome has often been associated with infestation of parasites, including *Ascaris, Strongyloides, Necator americanus, Fasciola hepatica,* and *Entamoeba histolytica* among others.

Other, more severe types of pulmonary eosinophilia with features unlike those described by Loeffler and characterized by weight loss, high fever, and night sweats have also been described. These cases (chronic eosinophilic pneumonia) have usually been associated with massive pulmonary radiodensities in a pattern of a "negative image" of pulmonary edema, with peripheral but not central radiodensities. Despite the often life-threatening nature of these disorders, corticosteroid therapy usually induces complete clinical recovery and clearing of roentgenographic abnormalities within a few days, although symptoms may promptly recur on cessation of therapy. Patients tend to be middle-aged, Caucasian women with a history of asthma.

In all cases of suspected Loeffler's syndrome or chronic eosinophilic pneumonia, appropriate skin tests and serologic tests should be performed with various *Aspergillus* species in view of the emergence of ABPA and its increasing recognition in the United States.

Drug-Induced Eosinophilia

Pulmonary eosinophilia may occur after the administration of a variety of drugs, including para-aminosalicylic acid, penicillin, nitrofurantoin, chlorpropamide, sulfonamides, aspirin, acetaminophen, beclomethasone, carbamazepine, chlorpromazine, imipramine, mephenesin, methotrexate, naproxen, diclofenac, certain phenylephrine-containing nose drops, penicillamine, tetracycline, cromolyn sodium, inhaled pentamidine isethionate, inhaled heroin, and crack cocaine. An extensive list of drugs reported to be directly or indirectly associated with adverse pulmonary actions was compiled by Rosenow, and the subject of drug-induced pulmonary disease is discussed in more detail in Chapter 22 in this text. In many cases, the relationship between eosinophilia or other lung lesions and drug administration is primarily anecdotal, but in others peripheral or pulmonary eosinophilia is clearly associated with drug administration.

A specific cause of eosinophilia with pulmonary infiltrates caused by ingestion of a drug was identified in subjects who used L-tryptophan as a sleeping aid. It is likely that a contaminant (designated as *peak E*) found in some lots of L-tryptophan is responsible for the syndrome. Although pulmonary involvement is not uniform in the eosinophilia-myalgia syndrome, dyspnea and cough occur in 60%–70% of reported cases and pulmonary radiodensities occur in approximately 20%–50% of such cases. The radiodensities tend to be basilar and resemble those seen in interstitial fibrosis. Histologically, there is pulmonary vasculitis and perivasculitis associated with a mild chronic interstitial pneumonitis. Pleural effusions, arterial hypoxemia, and pulmonary hypertension are common. BAL during acute illness demonstrates an increased number of eosinophils. Lavage several months after onset of symptoms may indicate lymphocytosis with a predominance of CD8[+] cells. Respiratory failure may result from muscle weakness.

Tropical Eosinophilia

Peripheral blood eosinophilia and asthma with or without eosinophilic infiltrates have been commonly associated with various parasitic infestations. The term *tropical eosinophilia,* a symptom complex of dyspnea, fever, intense eosinophilia, pulmonary infiltrates with or without wheezing, and weight loss, as defined by Weingarten, has been used to refer to many of these conditions. Unfortunately, the term has gradually come to be applied to virtually any case of pulmonary or blood eosinophilia occurring in a person who resides in a tropical area.

Intriguingly, in some cases of tropical eosinophilia, the pulmonary radiodensities can be minimal, whereas generalized lymphadenopathy and eosinophilia are far more prominent. It is not known why primarily pulmonary eosinophilic manifestations develop in some patients and more pronounced lymphadenopathy develops in others. Characteristics of tropical eosinophilia include extreme peripheral blood eosinophilia (generally 3000 eosinophils per cubic millimeter), often high titers of anti-filarial antibody, and extreme elevation of serum IgE, typically to 1000 ng/mL. In classic cases of tropical filarial eosinophilia caused by *Wuchereria bancrofti,* there is an absence of circulating microfilariae in the presence of high anti-filarial antibody titers. Lung biopsies, when performed in these cases, show varying degrees of parenchymal changes and, in more acute phases of the illness, patchy pulmonary lesions consisting of histiocytic and eosinophilic infiltrates in the alveolar, interstitial, and peribronchial spaces. With longer duration of disease (up to several months), massive eosinophilic pneumonias with occasional abscesses develop. In even more chronic cases, of several years' duration, marked fibrosis is often apparent.

Diethylcarbamazine is the drug of choice in patients with tropical eosinophilia. Most patients show considerable improvement after 2 weeks on this drug in a dose of 6 to 8 mg/kg/day, although relapses may be noted.

Many roundworm larvae and other parasites have also been reported to be associated with pulmonary eosinophilic infiltrates and wheezing. Among these are *Necator* (hookworm), *Toxocara, Ascaris, Strongyloides,* microfilariae (*Wuchereria bancrofti*), *Ancylostoma braziliense* (creeping eruption), *Trichuris trichiura, Fasciola hepatica,* and others. Some of these diseases may be associated with type I (IgE-mediated) hypersensitivity in view of positive wheal and flare skin reactions to antigens derived from certain roundworms. Precipitating and complement-fixing antibody to parasites has also been detected in the sera of patients with some of these conditions.

Pulmonary Eosinophilias Induced by Fungi, Bacteria, and Related Agents

Certain fungal, bacterial, insect, and related antigens can produce eosinophilia and pulmonary radiodensities with asthma and, at times, alveolitis. Among these are inhaled mites, grain dusts, coffee dusts, grain weevils (*Sitophilus granarus*), and proteolytic enzymes derived from *Bacillus subtilis,* the latter being used in the preparation of washing powders. These agents commonly produce asthma, and only occasional cases of eosinophilic or related pneumonia have been reported. Only one of such induced conditions—ABPA, which is associated with fungal antigens, namely *Aspergillus fumigatus* and a few other fungal species—has been well described.

Allergic Bronchopulmonary Aspergillosis

The previously described ill-defined diseases characterized as PIE syndrome, Loeffler's syndrome, or chronic pulmonary eosinophilia stand in sharp contrast to the well-described entity of ABPA, which also presents a pattern of wheezing, peripheral blood and sputum eosinophilia, and fluctuating pulmonary infiltrates. With the original general description of ABPA by Hinson and colleagues in 1952 and the development of diagnostic tests for the disease, many of the ill-defined eosinophilic pneumonias continue to fall into this better-defined category.

ABPA has long been known to be common in the United Kingdom, where it is the cause of 50%–80% of the cases of pulmonary eosinophilia. Originally, it was not recognized with great frequency in the United States and was considered a rarity. However, an increasing number of cases are being recognized, and some patients with asthma without evident ABPA have evidence of central bronchiectasis, the hallmark of ABPA. This raises the possibility that unrecognized ABPA may be common in the asthmatic population. It is likely that the syndrome is being missed in this country because of lack of availability or inadequate use of diagnostic tests and lack of familiarity with the syndrome.

There are no absolute criteria for the diagnosis of ABPA, but the disease is to be clearly distinguished from the two other forms of aspergillosis originally described by Hinson and co-workers—namely, the saprophytic form (aspergilloma, mycetoma) and the septicemic or pyemic form characterized by generalized mycotic abscesses and granuloma. McCarthy and Pepys, in an extensive review of 143 cases of ABPA, noted the following features: (1) intense blood and sputum eosinophilia; (2) wheezing and transitory pulmonary radiodensities (Fig. 3); (3) evidence of type I and type III skin reactions to *A. fumigatus;* (4) positive sputum cultures for *A. fumigatus* in 50% of cases; (5) the expectoration of brownish, tough sputum plugs containing fungal mycelia (Fig. 4); (6) the presence of serum precipitating antibody to *A. fumigatus* or related *Aspergillus* antigens by conventional double gel diffusion analysis (Fig. 5); and (7) the presence of central bronchiectasis (Fig. 6). Other strongly supportive features of the disease are dual (immediate and late) bronchial responses on bronchoprovocation challenge testing with *A. fumigatus* antigen, and dramatically elevated levels of serum total IgE, particularly after episodes of eosinophilic pneumonitis, with gradual return of serum IgE to normal during quiescent periods.

There are no population-based studies of the incidence or prevalence of ABPA in unselected asthmatic patients. However, Schwartz and associates found that 28% of asthmatic patients seen in private allergy practice in Cleveland, Ohio, had positive immediate-type *Aspergillus* skin test reactivity. In a later study, these authors reported that 10%–28% of 100 asthmatic patients with positive *Aspergillus* skin test reactivity had ABPA according to sets of criteria that either included central bronchiectasis (10%) or did not include demonstrable central bronchiectasis (28%), as well as the presence of serum IgE and IgG anti-*Aspergillus* antibody or serum precipitins. Therefore, an estimate of the prevalence of ABPA in asthmatic patients is 2.5%–7%. Clearly, more community-based studies of the incidence and prevalence of ABPA are indicated.

Clinical Features and Sequelae

ABPA is almost always a complication of asthma, in that almost all patients with ABPA have had a previous

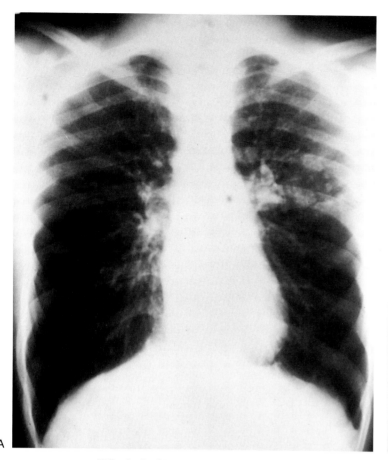

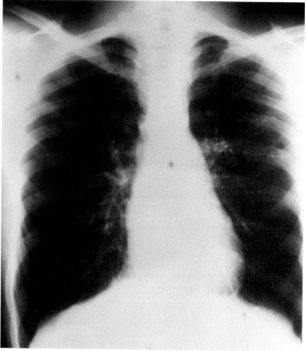

A

B

FIG. 3. A: Chest roentgenogram of a patient with ABPA at the time of hospital admission. Note the radiodensities in the left upper lobe. **B:** Chest roentgenogram of the same patient as in A after 1 week of corticosteroid therapy. Note almost complete resolution of the radiodensity in the left upper lobe.

diagnosis of asthma. Acute symptoms are wheezing, localized transitory pulmonary infiltrates, chest pain, cough, and production of mucoid or mucopurulent sputum, often containing brownish flecks or plugs (Fig. 4). These symptoms usually occur in atopic individuals with a previous history of asthma and may occur in familial aggregates. This is not surprising, considering the familial nature of atopy and exposure to common sources of *Aspergillus* species. The disease often is incorrectly diagnosed as tuberculosis, bronchiectasis, or bacterial pneumonia. Although many patients in whom the disease initially is detected demonstrate isolated skin reactivity to *Aspergillus* antigens later in life, younger patients with the disease appear to have a high incidence of atopic respiratory disease and broad patterns of positive wheal and flare skin reactivity to common inhaled allergens. Wheezing, roentgenographic shadows, intensity of eosinophilia, and serum IgE response appear to be worse during the autumn and winter months, when *Aspergillus* spores are usually more prevalent in the atmosphere. At times, a source of *Aspergillus* can be identified, such as moldy marijuana, a municipal leaf-compost site, garden mulch, or a soy sauce and bean brewery.

Patients with an early onset of asthma often demonstrate a lengthy interval (mean, 24 years) between the onset of wheezing and initial detection of pulmonary radiodensities. This does not hold for the late-onset group, suggesting that intense and prolonged antigen stimulation is necessary for induction of ABPA in atopic subjects. During initial episodes, reversible airways obstruction is the rule, but obstruction tends to become more fixed later during the course of the disease, although cor pulmonale and pulmonary hypertension rarely are noted. Progressive central bronchiectasis commonly associated with upper lobe fibrosis is frequently present in chronic cases and often is a hallmark of the disease. A protracted course extended over many years with multiple episodic flares is the rule.

Patterson and colleagues reported their experience with 84 patients with ABPA followed for a mean of 5 years. They found that ABPA could be divided into five stages: acute (I), remission (II), exacerbation (III), corticosteroid-dependent asthma (IV), and fibrosis (V). Only 16 of the patients remained in remission, with most being in the corticosteroid-dependent asthma stage (38 patients) or the fibrotic stage. Most of the eligible patients (not in

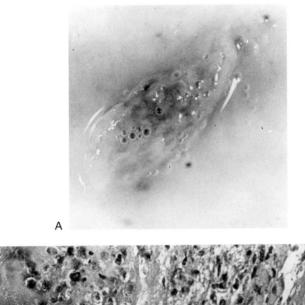

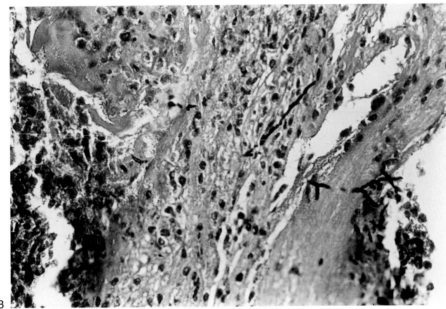

FIG. 4. A: Bronchial plug expectorated by a patient with ABPA. The plug is a cast of a medium-sized bronchus, is golden brown, and is composed of *Aspergillus* mycelial elements. **B:** An expectorated bronchial plug, composed of degenerating cells, mucus, amorphous debris, and *Aspergillus* organisms (branching, septate, methenamine silver-positive structures). Gomori's methenamine silver stain, ×400.

the fibrotic stage) experienced an exacerbation of ABPA despite alternate-day glucocorticoid therapy. This confirms the findings of earlier studies that ABPA tends to recur. It further implies that most patients with ABPA require long-term corticosteroid therapy and that doses sufficient to control asthma may not prevent flares of ABPA.

When patients with stage V disease (fibrosis) are considered separately, two subgroups are evident. The first includes those with low FEV_1 (forced expiratory volume in 1 second) 6 months after initiation of therapy (mean, 0.8 L). These patients have a very poor prognosis, all dying within 7 years (most of respiratory failure). Patients in the second group have less severe obstruction of air flow (mean FEV_1, 1.3 L) and survive 3 to 8 years taking

moderate doses of glucocorticosteroids. These data are consistent with a beneficial effect of glucocorticosteroid therapy.

Roentgenographic Changes

Radiologic features of ABPA can be classified as acute or chronic changes. Chronic changes occur as a result of repeated episodes of acute disease and are often associated with physiologic impairment.

Acute Changes. Parenchymal abnormalities are the most common, manifested in 80%–90% of patients by the presence of ill-defined homogeneous radiologic shadows, without evidence of volume loss, that may be either lim-

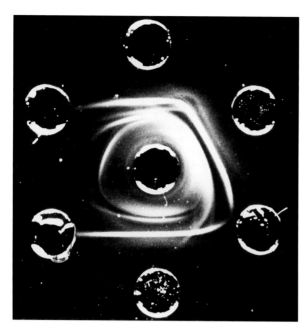

FIG. 5. Precipitin lines to *M. faeni* ("Ouchterlony" or double diffusion in agar technique). Central well contains serum from a patient with farmer's lung disease. Outer wells contain different preparations of *M. faeni* antigen. Note the multiple lines and lines of identity between the antigen preparations.

ited (5 to 15 mm) or massive (lobar) in extent. These shadows can appear in any part of the lung but predominate in the upper lobes. They often resolve (e.g., are fleeting) after expectoration of a bronchial plug but tend to recur in the same location. Half of the episodes of homogeneous shadows (consolidation) leave permanent residue, mainly ring shadows. Corticosteroid therapy hastens resolution. Homogeneous shadows presumably are caused by bronchial obstruction with plugs, localized eosinophilic pneumonia, or both. Fig. 3 depicts the chest x-ray films of a patient with ABPA on admission to the hospital and 1 week later after glucocorticosteroid therapy.

Bronchial abnormalities occur in 50%–70% of episodes of acute ABPA and are manifested as tramline, parallel line, and ring shadows (which represent normal or abnormal bronchial walls) and "toothpaste" and "gloved-finger" shadows (which represent intrabronchial exudate). Tramline shadows are the thickened walls of undilated bronchi, so the distance between the walls is that of a normal bronchus. Parallel line shadows represent walls of bronchiectatic bronchi; the distance between the walls is greater than normal. Ring shadows are either bronchiectatic bronchi seen *en face* or small abscesses. When a normal or bronchiectatic bronchial segment becomes filled with exudate, tramline or parallel line shadows change to toothpaste shadows. Removal of the intrabronchial exudate may cause the tramline or parallel line shadows to reappear. Tramline, parallel line, and toothpaste shadows not only are present in patients with ABPA

but also may occur in patients with asthma but no ABPA and those with cystic fibrosis and other pulmonary diseases.

Mucoid impaction of bronchi occurs in 15%–30% of patients with ABPA. A proximal impaction of large bronchi (toothpaste shadow) may extend into second-, third-, and fourth-order bronchi. Involvement of several second-order bronchi results in gloved-finger radiodensities, which are tubular radiodensities, 2 to 3 cm long and 5 to 8 mm wide, that branch distally from the hilus and represent dilated branching bronchi filled with inflammatory exudate (Fig. 7). These occur in 10%–20% of episodes of acute ABPA. Thirty percent of episodes of mucoid impaction of bronchi in ABPA cause permanent changes to bronchial walls.

Atelectasis of a lobe or a lung with evidence of shrinkage from occlusion of a bronchus by a plug is present in 10%–20% of patients with acute ABPA. Perihilar radiodensities simulating hilar adenopathy occur in 40% of episodes of ABPA. These represent central dilated bronchi filled with fluid and debris, associated with perihilar

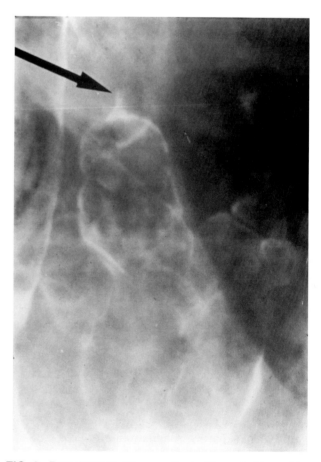

FIG. 6. Bronchogram from a patient with central bronchiectasis and ABPA. Note the greatly dilated proximal bronchi with normal distal bronchi (*arrow*). This is characteristic of central bronchiectasis. Note also the branching of the dilated bronchi, so that a gloved-finger radiodensity would result if the bronchiectatic cavity was filled with exudate.

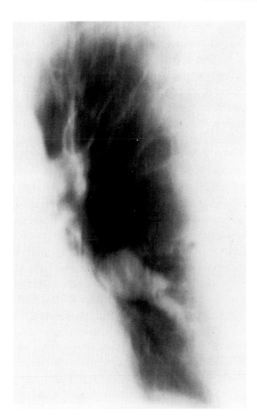

FIG. 7. Gloved-finger radiodensity in a patient with ABPA. This represents thick exudate in dilated third- and fourth-order bronchi, including branches.

parenchymal infiltrates. Other acute changes include abscesses with air-fluid levels (10%–20%), diffuse nodulation (10%–20%), avascular areas (10%), and signs of hyperinflation (10%–30%). Pleural effusion occurs in 5% of episodes.

Chronic Changes. Chronic changes reflect permanent histologic abnormalities resulting from repeated acute episodes of ABPA. Bronchial wall changes (tramline, parallel line, and ring shadows) may persist. In addition, because pulmonary fibrosis generally occurs at these sites, the upper lobe usually is involved in chronic ABPA. Physiologic impairment in patients with fibrosis is often significant. The incidence of pulmonary fibrosis in patients with ABPA varies from none of 20 patients followed for 44 months to 18 of 50 patients (36%) followed for 11 years and is directly related to the frequency of acute episodes of ABPA. The association between ABPA and interstitial fibrosis with upper lobe predominance is so strong in Great Britain that a patient with this radiologic finding, a negative tuberculin skin test, and a positive immediate *Aspergillus* skin test reaction is considered to have ABPA.

Central bronchiectasis is apparently a unique feature of ABPA (Fig. 6). In contrast to saccular bronchiectasis, in which small bronchi and bronchioles are dilated, central bronchiectasis is associated with normal small bronchi

and bronchioles. This probably is the result of growth of *Aspergillus* only in relatively large (second-, third-, and fourth-order) bronchi, with localized damage to bronchial walls and no injury to smaller bronchi. This peculiar pattern of bronchiectasis can occur even when chest radiographic findings are normal, presumably as a result of relatively few episodes of ABPA insufficient to cause tubular or ring shadows. In instances of severe bronchiectasis, the characteristic changes can be visible on plain films or tomograms without bronchographic dye. It should be noted that bronchography is associated with more complications in asthmatic patients than in normal subjects and that 4 of 16 patients with ABPA who underwent bronchography in the early experience of the Northwestern group had adverse reactions to dye.

High-resolution computed tomography (CT) of the chest detects central bronchiectasis in 35%–40% of the bronchi of patients with ABPA. Interestingly, 5%–15% of the bronchi of control subjects (asthmatic patients with skin test reactivity to *Aspergillus* but without a diagnosis of ABPA) also demonstrate central bronchiectasis. Thus, it is possible that central bronchiectasis is more common than previously appreciated in asthma and may not be unique to ABPA. Alternatively, some of the *Aspergillus*-sensitive asthmatic patients may have ABPA. The resolution of this question awaits further development of specific and sensitive diagnostic tests. In a direct comparison, using bronchography as the gold standard, high-resolution CT was 100% sensitive in detecting central bronchiectasis in patients with ABPA. When individual bronchial segments were compared, CT was 83% sensitive and 92% specific. In view of these findings, the safety and noninvasive nature of CT negates the need for bronchography in patients with suspected ABPA. Table 3 lists the radiologic features of ABPA.

Diagnostic Considerations

Positive sputum cultures for *A. fumigatus* are found in 50% of the patients, often associated with brownish flecks

TABLE 3. *Radiologic features of allergic bronchopulmonary aspergillosis*

Abnormality	Approximate frequency, %
Central bronchiectasis	100
Homogeneous shadows ("fleeting infiltrates")	80–90
Parallel line shadows	70
Ring shadows	45
Lobar shrinkage	35
Toothpaste shadows	35
Honeycomb shadows (pulmonary fibrosis)	25
Tramline shadows	20
Atelectasis	20
Cavitation	15
Gloved-finger shadows	10

or sputum plugs containing *Aspergillus* mycelia. Such positive cultures may have little clinical meaning, however, because *A. fumigatus* is ubiquitous and many patients with chronic lung disease have positive *Aspergillus* sputum cultures.

Most patients with ABPA also demonstrate serum precipitating antibody against *A. fumigatus*. However, anti-*Aspergillus* and related antifungal antibody is detectable in the population at large when more sensitive procedures are employed, strongly suggesting that antifungal antibody *per se* only reflects environmental exposure to ubiquitous antigens. Also, precipitins diminish remarkably after treatment with corticosteroids and may be undetectable after 2 years, only to reappear following another episode of pneumonitis.

There are significant problems with antigen preparations used to test for the presence of sensitization to *Aspergillus*. Crude *Aspergillus* antigen from either culture supernatant or mycelia are used clinically. Because these materials include a variety of proteins (including proteolytic enzymes), lipids, lipoproteins, and other substances, and because the method of preparation is not standardized, there are substantial differences between different preparations. The precipitin test with crude *A. fumigatus* is adequately sensitive for practical diagnostic purposes but is inadequate for specificity. Serum IgE and IgG anti-*Aspergillus* antibodies are higher in patients with ABPA than in comparable *Aspergillus*-sensitive asthmatic patients without ABPA. There is some evidence that serum IgA (particularly IgA_1) antibody against *Aspergillus* increases before and during flares of ABPA. It is possible that selected serologic and immunologic findings (skin test reactivity, elevated serum IgE, elevated levels of serum IgE and IgG anti-*Aspergillus* antibody) in patients without demonstrable central bronchiectasis represent a stage of ABPA (ABPA-serologic or ABPA-S). It remains to be seen how frequently ABPA-S precedes ABPA-central bronchiectasis (ABPA-CB) and whether therapy can influence this progression.

There is substantial overlap of antibody levels of asthmatic patients with ABPA and those without ABPA but with positive skin test reactivity to *Aspergillus*. This has led to efforts to purify various *Aspergillus* components to increase specificity. The level of IgE antibodies that react with a concanavalin A nonbinding fraction has been reported to distinguish between *Aspergillus*-sensitized asthmatic patients with and without ABPA. A major 18-kD allergenic *Aspergillus* protein cloned and expressed in bacteria has been useful in distinguishing asthmatic patients or patients with cystic fibrosis with ABPA from those with sensitization to *Aspergillus* but without ABPA, in that sera from patients with ABPA exhibit more IgE and IgG_4 anti-*Aspergillus* antibody. However, some patients with ABPA who had positive skin test reactivity to commercial *Aspergillus* preparations had negative skin tests to the recombinant protein. This illustrates the issue

of proper antigen selection. It is likely that different patients respond to slightly different antigenic *Aspergillus* epitopes, so that it is unlikely that any purified antigen will detect all patients with ABPA.

In addition to serologic assays, stronger diagnostic evidence for the role of hypersensitivity to *A. fumigatus* in ABPA comes from the demonstration of dual immediate type I and late or type III skin reactions to this agent. In most patients with ABPA, positive skin tests have been more reliable than precipitins as diagnostic aids. Dual skin reactions also correlate with the elicitation of similar dual early and late bronchial and nasal responses to *Aspergillus* antigen on provocative challenge. There is, however, considerable controversy over the type of reagent best suited to elicit the dual skin test response. There is also controversy over whether the late skin test response represents a local type III immune complex-mediated reaction or a late-phase IgE-dependent reaction. The controversy over the optimal reagent might be expected in view of the lack of precise information on characterization and purification of appropriate antigens. Pepys and McCarthy originally used a saturated ammonium sulfate precipitated protein extract of *A. fumigatus* prepared according to the method of Longbottom, but most preparations marketed today for skin testing consist of crude extracts of the mat and spores. All these agents seem satisfactory, provided that sufficiently high concentrations of the crude antigen are employed. Skin test reactive materials are also present in culture filtrates of the organisms, but there are no adequate studies comparing culture filtrates with mycelial extracts, nor are there any standards of potency for these extracts. In addition, there is a problem with specificity of the skin test in ABPA. In a group of asthmatic patients without aspergillosis and a group of normal subjects, skin tests were positive in 12% and 4%, respectively. There is also evidence to indicate the antigens that react in the skin are not among those detected with a precipitin test and that the *Aspergillus* antigens that elicit IgE antibodies in patients with ABPA do not elicit IgG antibodies.

In addition to skin tests, precipitins, and other immunoassays, lymphocyte stimulation studies with *Aspergillus* antigens have been employed as diagnostic aids in allergic aspergillosis. Lymphocyte proliferation in response to *Aspergillus* antigens may be a feature of ABPA. In one study comparing antigen-induced lymphocyte transformation, precipitins, and skin reactivity, it was noted that patients with aspergilloma had a low incidence of wheal and flare skin reactivity and low lymphocyte responses to *Aspergillus* antigens *in vitro* but extremely high levels of precipitins. On the other hand, patients with ABPA all have immediate positive wheal and flare reactivity but low levels of precipitins. The invasive cases of *Aspergillus* were too heterogeneous to characterize completely.

A limited number of BAL specimens from patients with ABPA have demonstrated increased numbers of neutrophils and eosinophils and increased concentrations of IgG,

IgA, and IgM antibodies directed against *Aspergillus* antigens, suggesting local production of these antibodies.

ABPA can occur in patients with cystic fibrosis with an incidence of up to 1% annually and a prevalence of 10%–15%. Because patients with cystic fibrosis without ABPA are subject to episodes of fleeting radiodensities (infectious pneumonia and atelectasis) and have bronchiectasis, an increased prevalence of atopy, and a higher prevalence of *Aspergillus* colonization of the respiratory tract and sensitization to *Aspergillus* compared with age-matched controls, the diagnosis of ABPA can be difficult to establish. There is some evidence that cystic fibrosis patients with ABPA exhibit increased levels of serum IgE and IgG (especially IgG$_1$ and IgG$_4$) antibodies to *Aspergillus* and evidence of lymphocyte sensitization when compared with cystic fibrosis patients without ABPA. In addition, peripheral blood B cells from patients with cystic fibrosis and ABPA secrete increased amounts of IgE, and T cells secrete factors that increase B-cell IgE production (perhaps IL-4). Many of the indicators of sensitization to *Aspergillus* in such patients wane spontaneously, so that it can be difficult to determine the importance of these indicators in a patient with cystic fibrosis. In any case, new pulmonary densities in conjunction with deterioration of pulmonary function tests, evidence of sensitization to *Aspergillus,* and elevation of serum IgE in some patients with cystic fibrosis respond to the addition of corticosteroids to antibiotic therapy.

Immunopathogenesis

Currently, there is some evidence to support the contention that a combination of IgE-mediated type I hypersensitivity and immune complex-mediated type III hypersensitivity plays an important role in inducing ABPA. In ABPA in humans, inhibition of type I pulmonary reactions with cromolyn sodium has also prevented the occurrence of subsequent late bronchial pulmonary provocation challenge reactions, whereas the administration of corticosteroids inhibits the late, but rarely the early, responses. In addition, human serum that contains high levels of IgE antibody, when injected intradermally into primates, leads to increased translocation of specific IgG-containing human hyperimmune serum into the skin sites. These findings suggest that deposition of immune complexes is facilitated by IgE antibody acting as a ''gatekeeper.'' Other evidence for a possible role of type I and type III hypersensitivity in ABPA is obtained from the appearance of dual skin reactivity and pulmonary lesions in a primate challenged by aerosol with *Aspergillus* antigen following passive infusion of serum from a patient with the disease who had both precipitins and reaginic activity against *A. fumigatus.* In contrast, similar challenge after passive transfer of serum containing anti-*Aspergillus* reaginic activity with no precipitins failed to produce such lesions on challenge. There are many alternative explanations for

the pathogenesis of ABPA. In view of the high levels of IgE (as high as 90,000 ng/mL of serum) and the fact that most of this IgE is not specific for *A. fumigatus,* Patterson has suggested that *A. fumigatus* growing in the respiratory tract may result either in stimulation of helper T cells for IgE production (i.e., Th2 cells) or of B lymphocytes capable of producing IgE. The Th2 characteristics of *Aspergillus*-specific CD4$^+$ cell lines derived from peripheral blood of patients with ABPA supports this hypothesis. There is also mounting evidence that pharmacologic intermediates such as ECFA and leukotrienes (i.e., LTB$_4$) released by basophils during type I reactions can attract eosinophils to the site of the initial allergic reaction, resulting in late-phase IgE-dependent eosinophilic reactions. Eosinophil-derived cationic proteins, MBP, and peroxidase are all capable of further stimulating mast cells and basophils to release mediators, and they can damage pulmonary tissues directly as well. Finally, mediators released from eosinophils, such as LTC$_4$, can act as further late-phase bronchoconstrictors and secretagogues for bronchial glands and epithelial cells. These late reactions are not precipitin-dependent and are not associated with deposition of complement or immunoglobulin. Furthermore, they can be inhibited by agents that inhibit the type I reaction. It is likely that such a mechanism involving attraction of eosinophils to the site of intense type I allergic reactions by chemotactic agents released during the reaction will be shown to be important in the production of many types of eosinophilic pneumonia.

Although attractive, the preceding formulation does not explain the distinction between those asthmatic patients with positive skin tests to *Aspergillus* and circulating IgG anti-*Aspergillus* antibody but without ABPA (25%–30% of unselected asthmatics) and those asthmatic patients in whom ABPA develops (probably 5% of unselected asthmatics). A possible explanation is the observation that circulating basophils from patients with ABPA release more histamine when exposed to both *Aspergillus* antigen and anti-human IgE. This suggests that asthmatic patients in whom ABPA is destined to develop have abnormal basophils that release more mediators on contact with *Aspergillus.* The basis for this abnormality (intrinsic to the cell or a result of exposure to serum factors) has not been elucidated.

Pathologic Features

Lung biopsy of confluent patchy infiltrates demonstrates an interstitial granulomatous infiltrate with a predominance of eosinophils. MBP (derived from eosinophils) is present in the interstitium and in macrophages as well as in activated lymphocytes (increased expression of IL-2R). Mucous plugs containing eosinophils and Charcot-Leyden crystals may be visible in large bronchi, and their presence correlates with shadows seen on chest roentgenograms. Bronchial biopsy generally demonstrates basement membrane thickening, mucosal edema, hypertrophy of mucous glands and smooth muscle, infiltrates of neutrophils and eosinophils, atrophic cilia, some mucous plugs firmly attached to the bronchial wall with profuse intraluminal mucopurulent secretions, and areas of bronchial wall squamous metaplasia.

It should be noted that the tissue reaction in ABPA overlaps with those of other clinical, radiologic, and pathologic entities. Mucoid impaction of the bronchus is often present in ABPA, although it can occur without evidence of sensitization to *Aspergillus*. Eosinophilic pneumonia can be present in ABPA and is believed to be the cause of many of the fleeting radiologic shadows. Finally, the pathologic entity of bronchocentric granulomatosis (BCG) as described by Katzenstein and associates is often found in ABPA. Katzenstein's series of 23 patients with BCG included 10 with asthma. Nine had eosinophilic pneumonia, nine had fungi present in resected specimens, and four had positive serum precipitins to *Aspergillus*. Skin testing was not reported in this series. It is probable that some of these patients had ABPA. Therefore, one of the common causes of BCG may be ABPA. In this regard, Bosken and associates reported that 18 of 18 excised lungs from patients with ABPA demonstrated mucoid impaction of the bronchus, BCG, or both.

Prognosis

There is a lack of prospective population-based studies of the outcome of patients with ABPA. It is clear that some patients progress to end-stage pulmonary fibrosis with cor pulmonale and that some maintain stable pulmonary function tests for many years. Because reports of ABPA originate from referral centers (and thus may not be representative of all patients with ABPA), it is difficult to determine the fate of unselected ABPA patients. In a retrospective study, Malo and coworkers found that after 5 years asthmatic patients with ABPA had more compromised pulmonary physiologic tests than did asthmatic patients without ABPA. Both groups (asthmatics with and without ABPA) had features of asthma (decreased flow rates, increased lung volumes), but asthmatic patients with ABPA tended to exhibit decreased diffusing capacity and total lung capacity. This is compatible with the superimposition of a restrictive defect (pulmonary fibrosis associated with bronchiectasis) on a pre-existing obstructive defect (asthma).

Therapy

Treatment of ABPA is directed toward three goals: treatment of the symptoms of asthma, resolution of acute symptoms of ABPA, and prevention of permanent lung damage. Therapy consists of 40 to 60 mg prednisone daily in divided doses for 2 weeks. The prednisone is rapidly tapered to a maintenance dosage, 0.5 mg/kg on alternate days, and is maintained at that level for 3 months. It should be noted that this schedule is empiric, as there have been no formal studies of different glucocorticoid schedules. Flares can occur while a patient is taking low-dose corticosteroids. Follow-up consists of monthly, and then bimonthly, serum analyses of IgE levels and chest radiographs for 2 to 3 years. If there are no flares, monitoring can be at semiannual intervals, as most patients destined to have recurrent episodes have their first flare within 3 years after the first episode. However, it should be noted that an occasional patient may have a flare after an extended remission.

Systemic glucocorticoid treatment (20 to 40 mg of prednisolone per day) significantly hastens clearing of pulmonary radiodensities, so that 4 weeks after the onset of infiltrates, 58% of the new radiodensities cleared in treated patients, in contrast to 23% in untreated patients. In addition, clinical symptoms of asthma, expectoration of bronchial plugs, and sputum production remitted more quickly in treated patients. Permanent lung damage, as manifested by new persistent pulmonary radiodensities, is less frequent if patients are treated. Safirstein and associates, in a retrospective review of patients followed for 5 years, found that therapy with as little as 7.5 mg of prednisone daily prevented the appearance of new radiologic shadows, whereas new persistent shadows appeared in 7 of 19 patients who were not treated with steroids. Capewell and associates, in another retrospective study, found that treatment with 20 mg or more of prednisolone per day was associated with more frequent resolution of radiodensities and peripheral blood eosinophilia, in comparison with treatment with no drug or 20 mg/d.

Twenty percent to 35% of ABPA flares are asymptomatic and can be detected only radiologically. In addition, some patients with ABPA experience only one episode during their lifetimes, and others exhibit flares only at long intervals. This has led to attempts to identify those patients with ABPA most likely to benefit from glucocorticoid therapy. Such patients would be those with frequent flares of acute ABPA resulting in chronic radiologic changes and physiologic impairment.

The striking increase in total IgE in patients with acute ABPA has been used to monitor patients. Most of the IgE is not directed against *Aspergillus* antigens but rather is nonspecific. Total serum IgE increases during flares of ABPA and in some instances before flares. This has led to the recommendation that serial IgE determinations be obtained and patients be treated on the basis of rising concentrations of IgE. Although *Aspergillus* is a potent stimulus for IgE production, it is not the only cause of rising IgE levels. Reed's group demonstrated that most (9 of 13), but not all, increases in serum IgE levels in ABPA were associated with flares. Therefore, it is somewhat precarious to initiate corticosteroid therapy solely on the basis of increasing serum IgE.

The following treatment regimens cannot be recommended and have not been demonstrated to be effective in controlled studies, although there have been anecdotal reports of effectiveness: (1) hyposensitization therapy with *Aspergillus* species (which may cause immediate bronchospasm, would also raise IgG levels to *Aspergillus,* and could theoretically worsen the disorder); (2) inhaled corticosteroids; (3) systemic or inhaled antifungal agents, such as ketoconazole, natamycin, or itraconazole.

Allergic Bronchopulmonary Mycosis

Recently, a series of cases that clinically resemble ABPA, without evidence of sensitivity to *Aspergillus* but with evidence of sensitization to dematiaceous hyphomycetes *Curvularia* and *Drechslera, Candida, Helminthosporium, Fusarium, Rhizopus, Penicillium, Torulopsis, Bipolaris,* or *Pseudallescheria boydii,* have been reported. The course of this illness (allergic bronchopulmonary mycosis) is currently unknown but presumably resembles that of ABPA. However, it appears that most instances of allergic bronchopulmonary fungal disease are caused by exposure to *Aspergillus,* although other fungi rarely can cause a similar clinical and radiologic syndrome.

Other Forms of Pulmonary Eosinophilia

In addition to ABPA and the forms of eosinophilia described in this chapter, one must consider several other types of pulmonary eosinophilia in the differential diagnosis. Among these are allergic granulomatous angiitis, a probable variant of polyarteritis, characterized by severe asthma and intense peripheral blood eosinophilia plus prominent granulomatous infiltrates and Churg-Strauss vasculitis.

Hypereosinophilic syndrome, a separate form of pulmonary eosinophilia, is defined by peripheral and bone marrow eosinophilia and infiltration of multiple organs by mature eosinophils. Any organ system may be involved, but characteristically the lung, heart, skin, muscle, and central nervous system are more prominently affected. The heart is almost uniformly affected, and the lungs are involved in 50% of cases. This disease take several forms. A more benign form consisting of hypereosinophilia with lung involvement and angioedema is often responsive to steroids. In other patients, severe cardiac or central nervous system impairment develops that is unresponsive to either steroids or cytotoxic agents, and in a few cases overt eosinophilic leukemia with documented cytogenic abnormalities develops. Because this disease is of unknown etiology, one must rule out parasitic, allergic, or other autoimmune or related etiologies. The most common pulmonary defect in hypereosinophilic

syndrome appears to be a paroxysmal nocturnal cough without airways obstruction. A few patients have underlying asthma. Treatment depends on proving the existence of progressive organ system involvement. In this event, corticosteroid therapy is initiated, and if a response does not occur, treatment with hydroxyurea and occasionally vincristine may result in improvement. When patients are unresponsive to steroids, hydroxyurea often has altered survival rates significantly.

Finally, in the United Kingdom, where ABPA constitutes 50%–80% of all pulmonary eosinophilic pneumonias, those pulmonary eosinophilias that do not fulfill the diagnostic criteria for ABPA are considered merely as a single category of cryptogenic pulmonary eosinophilia. In describing 27 cases of this syndrome, McCarthy and Pepys noted that the cryptogenic form was associated with a lesser degree of blood and sputum eosinophilia when compared with ABPA and that it more frequently involved younger women. There was also no seasonal predilection in the cryptogenic variety. Cough and sputum production were not prominent, and the brownish mucous plugs noted in ABPA rarely were seen. These patients did not have a type I or type III skin test reaction to *Aspergillus,* high levels of circulating total IgE, or cytophilic antibody directed to *Aspergillus,* and did not progress to the bronchiectasis, fibrosis, and atelectasis that are often noted in ABPA. The fact that systemic polyarteritis was ultimately diagnosed in several patients of this series with cryptogenic eosinophilia suggests that many of these cases were perhaps variants of allergic granulomatous angiitis.

Acute Eosinophilic Pneumonia

Recently, a small number of patients with acute onset of fever, diffuse radiodensities, and hypoxemia, at times progressing to adult respiratory distress syndrome (ARDS), with a high proportion of eosinophils in bronchoalveolar lavage (BAL) specimens and sputum and many eosinophils in the pulmonary parenchyma, have been described. Peripheral blood eosinophilia is usually present during the course of the illness, but often not at presentation. The chest radiographic densities are diffusely distributed and not peripheral and therefore are different from those described in chronic eosinophilic pneumonia. CT demonstrates diffuse bilateral ground-glass densities, micronodules, or both. These patients do not have evidence of parasitic infection or atopic disease. Mild cases of acute eosinophilic pneumonia improve rapidly without specific therapy, whereas more severe cases respond promptly to corticosteroid therapy with no permanent sequelae. In some patients, acute eosinophilic pneumonia is related to exposure to environmental fungi or ascarids, with some evidence of sensitization to these antigens. The relationship of this syndrome to other forms of PIE and ARDS is unknown.

HYPERSENSITIVITY PNEUMONITIS

The term *hypersensitivity pneumonitis* (or *extrinsic allergic alveolitis,* the British term) denotes a group of lung diseases caused by inhalation of a wide variety of different materials that are usually organic and always antigenic. The stereotypic clinical events are transient fever, hypoxemia, myalgias, arthralgias, dyspnea, and cough that occur 2 to 9 hrs after exposure and resolve in 12 to 72 hrs without specific treatment.

Hypersensitivity pneumonitis was first clearly described in Dr. Jon Finsen's doctoral thesis in 1874, when he described *heykatarr* in Iceland.

"This is a chronic chest disease. I do not know its incidence, as my observations thereupon are incomplete. The disease occurs only in winter, or rather during the time when the animals are kept inside, and is found only in the man whose job it is to loosen the hay in the barn and handle it before it is fed to cattle. The hay is always more or less dusty and has to be shaken to eliminate the dust before it is used as fodder. When this dust is inhaled, especially when the harvesting has been difficult and the hay has moulded in the barn, the man who works with the hay becomes ill with this disease, which lasts as long as he continues the same occupation, but usually disappears in summer. The disease expresses itself by cough, rather scant expectoration, and chest heaviness, especially in the evening (the hay is usually loosened in the afternoon, i.e., when it is intended to be given in the evening and the next morning). When examining the chest of those men, I have on a few occasions found signs of bronchitis, but in most cases I have never found anything abnormal. I have never had the occasion to examine a patient during an acute episode."

This syndrome was described again in British farmers in the 1930s and called *farmer's lung disease.* Dr. Finsen's description is notable for the association of the illness with a particular environmental exposure, its relationship to the season of the year, its occurrence several hours after exposure, the nature of the symptoms, and even the association with bronchitis. Many other diseases have since been described that exhibit the same clinical features and are denoted as hypersensitivity pneumonitis. Despite the terms *hypersensitivity* and *allergic,* hypersensitivity pneumonitis is not an atopic disease and is not associated with increases in IgE or eosinophils. Drug reactions are sometimes described as representing hypersensitivity pneumonitis, usually because certain BALF findings resemble those in hypersensitivity pneumonitis. However these reactions are not hypersensitivity pneumonitis, as the inciting agent is administered systemically and the pathogenic mechanisms are likely different from those of hypersensitivity pneumonitis.

Table 4 is a listing of currently described examples of hypersensitivity pneumonitis.

Some of these diseases have apparently disappeared from the originally described clinical settings (e.g., bagassosis in Louisiana) but presumably exist in areas with similar agricultural or industrial settings, and other diseases are being newly recognized (e.g., potato riddler's lung and machine operator's lung). Both the disappearance of previously described examples of hypersensitivity pneumonitis and the appearance of new examples are the consequence of changing agricultural and/or industrial practices that result in changes of exposure of subjects to antigenic material that can cause hypersensitivity pneumonitis. At the present time, farmer's lung disease, bird fancier's disease, ventilator lung, and Japanese summer-type hypersensitivity pneumonitis (in Japan) are the most commonly recognized forms of hypersensitivity pneumonitis.

Recognition of new examples of hypersensitivity pneumonitis usually requires a cluster of new cases with a unifying exposure history. Because complete occupational and vocational histories are at times not obtained from patients with pneumonia, it is likely that substantially more examples of hypersensitivity pneumonitis exist that have not yet been recognized and described. For example, introduction of a new metal-working fluid led to recognition of machine operator's lung in an auto parts manufacturing facility because of the clustering of cases and a common, unusual exposure (pseudomonads in cooling fluid).

Clinical Presentation

There are two different clinical presentations of hypersensitivity pneumonitis.

Acute hypersensitivity pneumonitis (dyspnea, nonproductive cough, myalgias, chills, diaphoresis, lassitude, headache, and malaise) occurs 2 to 9 hrs after a particular exposure, peaks typically between 6 and 24 hrs, and resolves without specific treatment in 1 to 3 days (sometimes longer after a particularly intense exposure). Patients exhibit fever, tachypnea, bibasilar rales, and occasionally cyanosis. Fig. 8 diagrams the course of acute hypersensitivity pneumonitis. There is peripheral blood leukocytosis with neutrophilia and lymphopenia, but not eosinophilia, and BAL neutrophilia.

Chronic hypersensitivity pneumonitis is characterized by progressively more severe dyspnea, nonproductive cough, weight loss, and often anorexia in a patient exposed to a recognized cause of hypersensitivity pneumonitis. Symptoms are usually present for months to years. There is typically no fever, but tachypnea and bibasilar dry rales are usually present. Symptoms and signs of cor pulmonale are not uncommon at presentation. In general, clubbing occurs infrequently, although Selman, using retrospective chart review, reported clubbing in up to 50% of subjects with pigeon breeder's disease in Mexico City.

A proportion (20%–40%) of patients with chronic hypersensitivity pneumonitis first have symptoms of chronic bronchitis (e.g., chronic productive cough), some even

TABLE 4. *Currently described examples of hypersensitivity pneumonitis*

Disease	Antigen source	Probable antigen	References
Plant products			
Farmer's lung disease	Moldy hay	Thermophilic actinomycetes *M. faeni* (*S. rectivirgula*) *T. vulgaris* *Aspergillus* sp.	Pepys J, et al. *Lancet* 2: 607–611, 1963.
Bagassosis	Moldy pressed sugarcane (bagasse)	Thermophilic actinomycetes *T. sacchari* *T. vulgaris*	Salvaggio J, et al. *Am J Med* 46: 538–544, 1969.
Mushroom worker's disease	Moldy compost and mushrooms	Thermophilic actinomycetes *M. faeni* *T. vulgaris* *Aspergillus* sp. Mushroom spores	Cox A, et al. *Eur Respir J* 1: 466–468, 1988.
Suberosis	Moldy cork	*Penicillium* sp.	Avila R, et al. *Lancet* 1: 620–621, 1968.
Malt worker's lung	Contaminated barley	*Aspergillus clavatus*	Riddle H, et al. *Thorax* 23: 271, 1968.
Maple bark disease	Contaminated maple logs	*Cryptostroma corticale*	Emanuel D, et al. *NEJM* 274: 1413–1418, 1966.
Sequoiosis	Contaminated redwood dust	*Graphium* sp. *Pullularia* sp.	Cohen H, et al. *Am J Med* 43: 785, 1967.
Soybean lung	Soybeans in animal feed	Soybean hull antigens	Zubeldia JM, et al. *J Allergy Clin Immunol* 95: 622–626, 1995.
Wood pulp worker's disease	Contaminated wood pulp	*Alternaria* sp.	Schleuter D, et al. *Ann Intern Med* 77: 907–914, 1972.
Wood dust HP	Contaminated wood dust	Bacillus subtilis *Alternaria* sp.	Sosman AJ, et al. *NEJM* 281: 977–980, 1969.
Compost lung	Compost	*Aspergillus* sp. *T. vulgaris*	Vincken W, et al. *Thorax* 39: 74–75, 1984.
Cheeseworker's disease	Cheese or cheese casings	*Penicillium* sp.	Campbell J, et al. *Am Rev Respir Dis* 127: 495–496, 1983.
Wood trimmer's disease	Contaminated wood trimmings, at times in sawmills	*Rhizopus* sp. *Mucor* sp.	Belin L, *Int Arch Allergy Appl Immunol* 82: 440–443, 1987.
Thatched roof disease	Dried grasses and leaves	*Saccharomonospora viridis*	Blackburn C, et al. *Lancet* 2: 1396, 1966.
Greenhouse lung	Greenhouse soil	*Aspergillus* sp. *Penicillium* sp. *Cryptostroma corticale*	Yoshida K, et al. *Arch Environ Health* 48: 260–262, 1993.
Coffee worker's lung	Green coffee dust	Unknown	Van Toorn D. *Thorax* 25: 399–405, 1970.
Potato riddler's lung	Moldy hay around potatoes	Thermophilic actinomycetes *M. faeni* *T. vulgaris* *Aspergillus* sp.	Greene JJ, et al. *Ir Med J* 78: 282–284, 1985.
Tobacco worker's disease	Mold on tobacco	*Aspergillus* sp.	Huuskonen MS, et al. *Br J Indust Med* 41: 77–83, 1984.
Wine grower's lung	Mold on grapes	*Botrytis cinerea*	Popp W, et al. *Prax Klin Pneumol* 41: 165–169, 1987.
Woodman's disease	Mold on bark and fuel chips	*Penicillium* sp.	Dykewicz MS, et al. *J Allergy Clin Immunol* 81: 455–460, 1988.
Soy sauce brewer's lung	Fermentation starter for soy sauce	*Aspergillus oryzae*	Tsuchiya Y, et al. *J Allergy Clin Immunol* 91: 688–689, 1993.
Domestic allergic alveolitis	Decayed wood	Fungi *Serpula lacrymans* *Leucogyrophana pinastri* *Paecilomyces variottii* *Aspergillus fumigatus*	Bryant DH, et al. *Allergy Proc* 12: 89–94, 1991.

TABLE 4. *Continued*

Disease	Antigen source	Probable antigen	References
Plant products			
Riding school lung	Hay in horse stall	Thermophilic actinomycetes *M. faeni* (*S. rectivirgula*) *T. vulgaris*	Kristiansen JD, et al. *Acta Paediatr Scand* 80: 386–388, 1991.
Stipatosis	Esparto grass (*Stipa tenacissima*) used to make plaster	Esparto grass antigens	Gamboa PM, et al. *Allergol Immunopathol* 18: 331–334, 1990.
Animal products			
Pigeon breeder's disease	Pigeon droppings	Altered pigeon serum (probably IgA) Pigeon bloom (derived from feathers)	Reed C, et al. *JAMA* 193: 261–265, 1965.
Turkey handler's disease	Turkey products	Turkey proteins	Boyer RS, et al. *Am Rev Respir Dis* 109: 630–635, 1974.
Chicken breeder's lung	Chicken feathers	Chicken feather proteins	Warren CP, et al. *Am Rev Respir Dis* 109: 672–677, 1974.
Bird fancier's lung	Domestic and wild bird products	Bird proteins	Burdon JG, et al. *Am Rev Respir Dis* 134: 1319–1320, 1986.
Duvet lung	Duvet and pillow	Goose proteins	Haitjema T, et al. *Thorax* 47: 990–991, 1992.
Laboratory worker's HP	Rat fur	Rat urine protein	Carroll K, et al. *Clin Allergy* 5: 443–456, 1975.
Pituitary snuff taker's disease	Pituitary powder	Vasopressin	Harper L, et al. *Ann Intern Med* 73: 581–584, 1970.
Shell lung	Oyster or mollusk shell	Shell proteins	Orriols R, et al. *Ann Intern Med* 113: 80–81, 1990.
Miller's lung	Grain weevils in wheat flour	*Sitophilius granarius* proteins	Lunn J, et al. *Br J Indust Med* 24: 158–162, 1967.
Sericulturist's lung	Silk worm larvae	Silk worm larvae proteins	Nakazawa T, et al. *Thorax* 45: 233–234, 1990.
Reactive chemicals			
TDI HP	Toluene di-isocyanate	Altered proteins (albumin + others)	Yoshizawa Y, et al. *Ann Intern Med* 110: 31–34, 1989.
MDI HP	Diphenylmethane di-isocyanate	Altered proteins	Vandenplas O, et al. *Am Rev Respir Dis* 147: 338–346, 1993.
HDI HP	Hexamethylene di-isocyanate	Altered proteins	Selden AI, et al. *Scand J Work Environ Health* 15: 234–237, 1989.
TMA HP	Trimetallic anhydride	Altered proteins	Baur X. *J Allergy Clin Immunol* 95: 1004–1010, 1995.
Other			
Ventilator lung	Contaminated humidifiers, dehumidifiers, air conditioners, heating systems	Thermophilic actinomycetes *T. candidus* *T. vulgaris* *Penicillium* sp. *Cephalosporium* sp. Amebae *Klebsiella* sp. *Candida* sp.	Banaszak E, et al. *NEJM* 283: 271–276, 1970.
Basement lung	Contaminated basement (sewage or mold)	*Cephalosporium* sp. *Penicillium* sp.	Patterson R, et al. *J Allergy Clin Immunol* 68: 128–132, 1981.
Sauna taker's disease	Sauna water	*Aureobasidium* sp.	Metzger WJ, et al. *JAMA* 236: 2209–2211, 1976.
Detergent worker's disease	Detergent enzymes	*Bacillus subtilis*	Berson SA, et al. *NEJM* 284: 688—690, 1971.

TABLE 4. *Continued*

Disease	Antigen source	Probable antigen	References
Other			
Japanese summer house HP	House dust ?Bird droppings	*Trichosporon cutaneum*	Shimazu K, et al. *Am Rev Respir Dis* 130: 407–411, 1984.
Hot tub lung	Mold on ceiling	*Cladosporium* sp.	Jacobs RL, et al. *Ann Intern Med* 105: 204–206, 1986.
Tractor lung	Contaminated tractor cab air conditioner	*Rhizopus* sp.	O'Connell M, et al. *J Allergy Clin Immunol* 95: 779–780, 1995.
Machine operator's lung	Contaminated metal-working fluid	*Pseudomonas* sp.	Bernstein DI, et al. *Chest* 108: 636–641, 1995.
Fertilizer lung	Contaminated fertilizer	*Streptomyces albus*	Kagen S, et al. *J Allergy Clin Immunol* 68: 295–299, 1981.
Sax lung	Saxophone mouthpiece	*Candida albicans*	Lodha S, et al. *Chest* 93: 1322, 1988.

without radiologic parenchymal densities on standard chest radiographs. There is substantial morphologic evidence of bronchitis in the large airways of patients with farmer's lung disease. As most patients with hypersensitivity pneumonitis are nonsmokers without any other cause for the development of chronic bronchitis, these symptoms are likely to be a result of hypersensitivity pneumonitis and may correlate with evidence of airway hyperreactivity in patients with chronic hypersensitivity pneumonitis.

The reasons for the different clinical presentations (acute and chronic) of hypersensitivity pneumonitis are not clear, but they could include differences of intensity and duration of exposure (i.e., low intensity and long duration tending to cause chronic hypersensitivity pneumonitis, and high intensity and short duration tending to cause acute hypersensitivity pneumonitis). This is most clearly demonstrated in hypersensitivity pneumonitis caused by exposure to birds. Bird fancier's disease (chronic exposure to low amounts of bird antigens) is associated with chronic hypersensitivity pneumonitis. Pigeon breeder's disease presents differently in different geographic areas. Intermittent exposure of pigeon breeders to large amounts of pigeon antigens in the United States and Europe is associated with acute disease and a good prognosis, whereas chronic exposure to a few

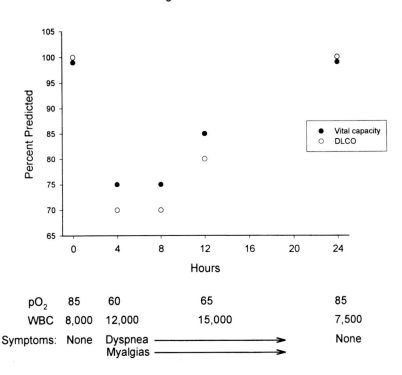

FIG. 8. Diagram of a typical episode of acute pigeon breeder's disease induced by exposure to pigeon serum at 0 h.

household pigeons in Mexico is associated with chronic disease and a much poorer prognosis. In the United States and Europe, pigeon breeders keep their animals in an enclosure separate from their living areas and visit it periodically, so that exposure is intermittent. In Mexico, birds are kept in living quarters, so that exposure is continuous. It is of interest that bird antigens can persist in a room for a substantial length of time (18 months) after removal of the birds, so that Mexicans with pigeon breeder's disease would be expected to be exposed to pigeon antigens for prolonged periods of time even after removal of the pigeons. Therefore, pigeon breeder's disease in Mexico resembles bird fancier's disease in the United States and Europe in type of exposure, clinical presentation, and prognosis, and differs from pigeon breeder's disease in the United States and Europe. Because the relevant antigens are similar in these two examples of bird-associated hypersensitivity pneumonitis, it is likely that type of exposure, not antigen characteristics, determines clinical presentation and prognosis.

Although the recognition of a new example of hypersensitivity pneumonitis is usually associated with the acute presentation of hypersensitivity pneumonitis, most patients with well-recognized types of hypersensitivity pneumonitis have chronic disease. This might be related to the difficulties in establishing a link between chronic disease and chronic exposure, as opposed to the relative ease in making the association of acute disease and acute exposure.

The above discussion indicates that hypersensitivity pneumonitis, and particularly chronic hypersensitivity pneumonitis, may be more prevalent than is readily apparent and may be a cause of some cases of idiopathic pulmonary fibrosis. Detailed histories are not always obtained from patients with idiopathic pulmonary fibrosis, serum antibody to the agent responsible for hypersensitivity pneumonitis tends to wane after cessation of exposure, and high-resolution CT scans of the chest in chronic hypersensitivity pneumonitis can resemble those of idiopathic pulmonary fibrosis, so it is possible that some patients with idiopathic pulmonary fibrosis have chronic hypersensitivity pneumonitis.

Radiology

In acute hypersensitivity pneumonitis, chest radiographs demonstrate diffuse, poorly defined nodular radiodensities, at times with areas of ground-glass radiodensities or even consolidation. These radiodensities tend to occur in the lower lobes and spare the apices. Linear radiodensities (presumably representing areas of fibrosis from previous episodes of acute hypersensitivity pneumonitis) may also be present. The nodular and ground-glass densities tend to disappear after cessation of exposure, so that the chest radiograph findings may be normal after resolution of an acute episode of hypersensitivity pneu-

monitis. Figure 9 demonstrates radiologic resolution of acute hypersensitivity pneumonitis. High-resolution CT often demonstrates ground-glass densities better than chest radiographs and at times reveals a diffuse increase of pulmonary radiodensity, but findings may also be normal after resolution of an acute episode. Pleural effusions or thickening, calcification, cavitation, atelectasis, localized radiodensities (coin lesions or masses), and intrathoracic lymphadenopathy are rare.

In chronic hypersensitivity pneumonitis, diffuse linear and nodular radiodensities with upper lobe predominance, sparing of the bases, and volume loss (Fig. 10) are apparent on chest radiographs. Pleural effusions and thickening are very unusual, although subcutaneous emphysema (presumably as a consequence of pleural rupture caused by bronchiolitis and lobular overinflation) has been reported.

High-resolution CT of patients with chronic hypersensitivity pneumonitis demonstrates several patterns. Most commonly, there are multiple centrilobular nodules, 2 to 4 mm in diameter, throughout the lung fields, with some areas of ground-glass radiodensities, especially in the lower lobes (Fig. 11). The nodules are seldom attached to the pleura or bronchovascular bundles, as they are in sarcoidosis, and the border between the nodules and the surrounding lung is well demarcated. There are also well-delineated areas of increased radiolucency; these are presumably overinflated pulmonary lobules subserved by partially occluded bronchioles. The ground-glass densities and micronodules tend to resolve after cessation of exposure. Although these findings are suggestive of hypersensitivity pneumonitis, they are found in only a subset (50%–75%) of patients with hypersensitivity pneumonitis, and high-resolution CT findings in hypersensitivity pneumonitis can resemble those of idiopathic pulmonary fibrosis. Cormier reported a substantial prevalence of mild to moderate emphysema detectable by high-resolution CT in nonsmoker patients with farmer's lung disease. It is not clear if this represents lobular overinflation or emphysema. Magnetic resonance imaging (MRI) is inferior to high-resolution CT in demonstrating anatomic detail, but it is equal to CT in demonstrating ground-glass areas and may be useful in determining the course of ground-glass densities without necessitating radiation exposure.

Epidemiology

The prevalence of hypersensitivity pneumonitis is quite variable in different populations, presumably related to differing intensity, frequency, and duration of inhalation exposure. Among pigeon breeders, 8%–30% of those who are members of pigeon-breeding clubs and participated in surveys exhibited pigeon breeder's disease. Among farmers, 0.5%–5% have symptoms compatible with farmer's lung disease. The prevalence of symptoms is decreased in farms that use hay-drying methods that

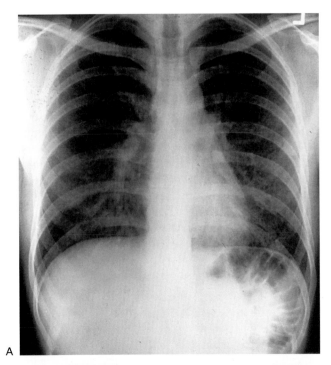

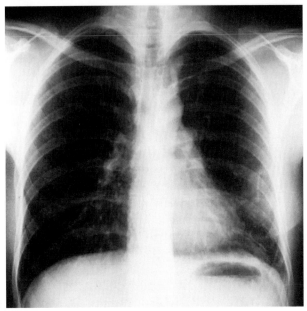

FIG. 9. A: Chest radiograph of a patient with pigeon breeder's disease having symptoms of fever, dyspnea, and bibasilar rales. The patient had kept pigeons for 5 years and was seen with fever, dyspnea, and myalgias approximately 8 hours after cleaning the pigeon coop. He had serum antibody to pigeon dropping extract. Note 2- to 3-mm nodules bilaterally in lower lobes. **B:** Chest radiograph of the same patient 2 weeks later. No specific treatment was given. Note clearing of the lower lobe nodules and the staples in the left chest from the open lung biopsy.

reduce exposure to the responsible antigens and is increased following a wet summer season.

The population at risk and the season of the year of occupance vary with the type of hypersensitivity pneumonitis. For example, most cases of farmer's lung disease occur in cold, damp climates in late winter and early spring, when farmers (usually men) use stored hay to feed their livestock. Pigeon breeder's disease occurs chiefly in men in Europe and the United States; it occurs predominantly in women in Mexico because of differing patterns of exposure, but there is no seasonal preference in either population. Bird fancier's disease in Europe and the

United States occurs in subjects who keep domestic birds and does not exhibit a predilection for either sex. Japanese summer-type hypersensitivity pneumonitis occurs mostly in women not employed outside the home from June to September in warm, moist areas of Japan.

Unlike what occurs in other pulmonary diseases, there is a remarkable predominance of nonsmokers (80%–95%) among patients with all types of hypersensitivity pneumonitis, substantially greater than the proportion of nonsmokers in similarly exposed subjects who are not ill. The mechanisms of this striking phenomenon are unknown, but they could include smoking-induced alter-

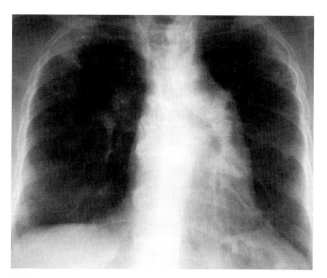

FIG. 10. Chest radiograph of a patient with bird fancier's disease who was first seen with progressive dyspnea and weight loss. She had kept two or three parakeets in her home for the past 15 years and did not notice episodic fever or acute dyspnea. Her serum was positive for precipitins to parakeet serum, and she had severe restrictive disease and resting hypoxemia. Note the diffuse radiodensities, loss of volume of the upper lobes, and pulmonary hypertension.

ations of lung defense mechanisms or immunologic reactivity. This clinical finding indicates that active smoking weighs substantially against a diagnosis of hypersensitivity pneumonitis.

An important feature of hypersensitivity pneumonitis is the great variability in susceptibility among exposed populations and the apparent resistance to illness of most exposed individuals. Possible reasons include differences of exposure or differences among hosts, either inborn or acquired. There are no differences in the prevalence of atopy or of HLA-A, -B, -C, or -DR haplotypes in exposed subjects with and without hypersensitivity pneumonitis.

There is an increased prevalence of HLA-DPβ1 glutamate 69 in berylliosis, a disease with many similarities to hypersensitivity pneumonitis, but HLA-DP haplotypes have not been reported in hypersensitivity pneumonitis. The prevalence of hypersensitivity pneumonitis, unlike that of most other lung diseases, is not increased but rather is substantially decreased in cigarette smokers. This protection against development of hypersensitivity pneumonitis in smokers extends to serum antibody, so that smokers have a lower prevalence of serum antibody than apparently equally exposed nonsmokers. The reasons for these phenomena are unknown but could include depression of immune responses to antigen delivered to the lung, which is well documented in smokers.

Pathology

Lung biopsy specimens (almost always from patients with chronic hypersensitivity pneumonitis) show chronic interstitial inflammation with infiltration of plasma cells, mast cells, histiocytes, and lymphocytes, usually with poorly formed nonnecrotizing granulomas. There is often bronchiolitis and sometimes (25%–50%) bronchiolitis obliterans (Fig. 12). Organizing pneumonia is often also present, so that 15%–25% of patients with hypersensitivity pneumonitis have bronchiolitis obliterans with organizing pneumonia (BOOP). Conversely, in patients with recognized BOOP, hypersensitivity pneumonitis may be the cause. Interstitial fibrosis is often present to a varying extent. Unlike what is seen in sarcoidosis, the interstitial inflammatory cell infiltrate is distal as well as proximal to the granulomas. The granulomas do not occur in groups and do not tend to occur near bronchi or in subpleural locations; they are often adjacent to bronchioles and usually occur singly. These characteristics help to differentiate hypersensitivity pneumonitis from sar-

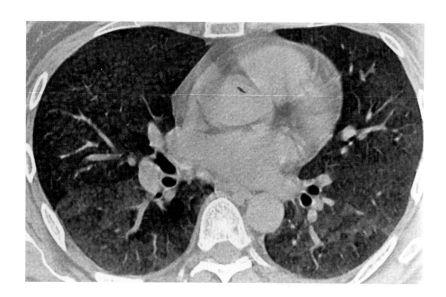

FIG. 11. High-resolution CT of a non-smoker with exposure to both birds and shells who had progressive dyspnea, weight loss, hypoxemia, and a restrictive ventilatory defect. Note the diffuse nodular radiodensities in the lower lobes with areas of ground-glass densities posteriorly.

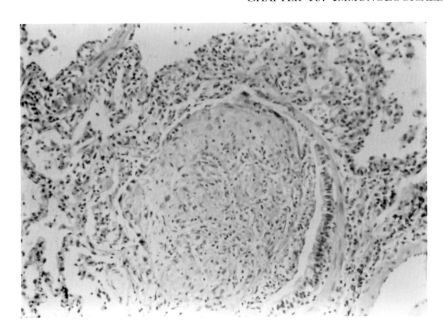

FIG. 12. Bronchiolitis obliterans in the same patient with pigeon breeder's disease as in Fig. 9.

coidosis. Giant cells, at times with Schaumann or asteroid bodies or cholesterol clefts, are present both within and outside the granulomas. Foamy AM are often observed in patients with hypersensitivity pneumonitis caused by bird exposure (Fig. 13). Vasculitis and eosinophilia are not evident.

The specific histologic changes of hypersensitivity pneumonitis, when present, can be diagnostic. However, the granulomas and respiratory bronchiolitis may not be present years after cessation of exposure, so that only interstitial inflammation and fibrosis remain. Therefore, these changes are quite specific, but their sensitivity is unknown.

Differential Diagnosis

The symptoms, signs, and laboratory findings of acute hypersensitivity pneumonitis can resemble those of many other lung diseases, including pulmonary edema, bronchoalveolar cell carcinoma, organic dust toxic syndrome (ODTS), and some forms of pneumoconiosis. Acute hypersensitivity pneumonitis is most often confused with infectious pneumonia (usually thought to be of viral or mycoplasmal origin) and at times with psittacosis in subjects exposed to birds.

ODTS has been described in some of the same populations exposed to materials that cause hypersensitivity

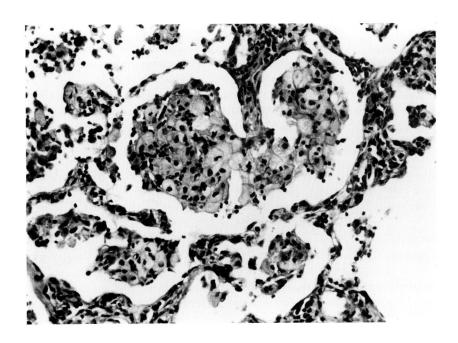

FIG. 13. Foamy alveolar macrophages in the same patient as in Fig. 10.

pneumonitis. ODTS, which occur in a larger proportion of the exposed population than hypersensitivity pneumonitis, is characterized by transient fever, dyspnea, nonproductive cough, peripheral blood leukocytosis, and BALF neutrophilia; unlike hypersensitivity pneumonitis, however, it is not associated with chest radiographic changes, permanent lung damage, or prior sensitization (as indicated by the absence of serum antibodies). Endotoxin, activated complement, and cytokine released from AM have been implicated as mediators of ODTS. Patients who present with ODTS tend to have had a more intense exposure of shorter duration than those who present with farmer's lung disease.

Exposure to the same agents that cause ventilator lung may result in humidifier fever. This is characterized by fever, chills, myalgias, arthralgias, headache, malaise, cough, dyspnea, peripheral blood leukocytosis, and arterial hypoxemia that begins 4 to 12 hrs after exposure. Some investigators report decreased lung volumes with normal flow rates (''restrictive pattern'') and decreased diffusing capacity, whereas others report normal lung volumes and diffusing capacity. The clinical syndrome remits after 12 to 24 hrs without specific therapy. Symptoms and signs are exaggerated after exposure that follows a period of no exposure (such as vacation or a weekend), but then they become blunted despite continued exposure (''Monday illness''). Monday illness with tolerance to apparently the same exposure later in the work week also occurs in byssinosis and metal fume fever. All signs and symptoms of humidifier fever remit after cessation of exposure, and no permanent physiologic or roentgenologic changes occur. Serum antibodies to thermophilic organisms are rarely present, but antibodies are often present to extracts of humidifier water or slime, gram-negative and gram-positive bacteria (*Bacillus, Flavobacterium, Pseudomonas, Streptomyces*), fungi (*Cephalosporium, Penicillium, Sporotrichum, Aspergillus, Fusarium, Mucor, Phoma, Rhizopus*), or amebae.

There is evidence that some cases of humidifier fever may be caused by endotoxin. Many of the symptoms of humidifier fever can be reproduced by exposure to endotoxin. Rylander described a printing factory in which symptoms of humidifier fever developed in 20 of 50 workers. The humidifier water was heavily contaminated with pseudomonads and endotoxin, and airborne endotoxin was detected in the factory atmosphere when the humidifier was operating. However, other investigators have not detected endotoxin in humidifier water using a pyrogen assay, so that the role of endotoxin in humidifier fever is uncertain.

Treatment consists of removing subjects from exposure to contaminated humidifier water by frequent cleaning of the humidifiers or by changing their job location. It is frequently difficult to clean humidifiers permanently, as any agent used to cleanse water must be removed before humidifiers can be put back in use, so that workers are not exposed to the cleansing agent. Prognosis in humidifier fever after removal from exposure seems to be excellent, as no permanent physiologic or roentgenologic changes occur.

Chronic hypersensitivity pneumonitis resembles idiopathic pulmonary fibrosis, and in some instances the two are indistinguishable. The differential diagnoses includes pulmonary fibrosis of other causes (chemotherapeutic agents, radiation, inhaled toxins, sarcoidosis, idiopathic pulmonary fibrosis, pneumoconiosis) and heart failure.

A thorough and complete occupational and vocational history is essential to diagnose both forms of hypersensitivity pneumonitis. The history should seek to establish a link between a particular exposure (at work, home, or elsewhere) and previous episodes of pneumonia. Information about other exposed individuals with similar symptoms should be sought.

If the history suggests a relationship between exposure and pulmonary symptoms, evidence of sensitization and the nature of the pulmonary inflammatory response should be determined. Sensitization is indicated by the presence of serum antibody to an agent known to cause hypersensitivity pneumonitis. A large proportion of lymphocytes in BALF (usually >40%) is suggestive of hypersensitivity pneumonitis, although many other pulmonary processes can cause BALF lymphocytosis.

Evidence of repetitive appropriate symptoms and laboratory and radiologic abnormalities associated with exposure to a particular environment is sufficient to diagnose hypersensitivity pneumonitis. In questionable instances, a natural exposure (i.e., documentation of appropriate symptoms and laboratory abnormalities after exposure to an environment suspected of causing hypersensitivity pneumonitis) can be used to diagnose hypersensitivity pneumonitis. A natural exposure challenge should not be considered positive unless there is objective evidence of a change in temperature, total peripheral white blood cell number, chest radiograph or high-resolution CT, or increased alveolar-arterial gradient as reflected by the development or worsening of decreased arterial oxygen tension. In some patients, lung biopsy may be required to differentiate hypersensitivity pneumonitis from other causes of diffuse pulmonary inflammation and/or fibrosis. Transbronchial lung biopsy specimens often do not provide sufficient material to establish fully the presence and interrelationships of granulomas, bronchiolitis, and interstitial inflammation, so that either open or thoracoscopic lung biopsy is often required.

Deliberate aerosol inhalation exposure to the suspected antigens should not be performed outside research settings because of the lack of standardized antigens, the possibility of severe adverse effects from the inhaled material in a sensitized person, and the need to demonstrate the lack of a reaction in normal subjects without prior exposure to the same material, thereby possibly inducing sensitization in previously unsensitized individuals.

Terho and colleagues have established major and minor criteria for the diagnosis of farmer's lung disease. An adaptation of their criteria follows.

Major criteria for hypersensitivity pneumonitis:

1. Evidence of exposure to appropriate antigen by history or detection of serum antibody
2. Symptoms compatible with hypersensitivity pneumonitis
3. Findings compatible with hypersensitivity pneumonitis on chest radiographs or high-resolution CT

Minor criteria:

1. Bibasilar rales
2. Decreased diffusing capacity
3. Arterial hypoxemia, either at rest or during exercise
4. Pulmonary histologic changes compatible with hypersensitivity pneumonitis
5. Positive natural challenge
6. BALF lymphocytosis

The diagnosis is confirmed if the patient fulfills all the major criteria and at least four of the minor criteria, and if all other diseases with similar symptoms can be ruled out (e.g., sarcoidosis). Normal chest radiographic findings are acceptable if pulmonary histology is compatible with hypersensitivity pneumonitis. A normal result of high-resolution CT eliminates the possibility of active or chronic hypersensitivity pneumonitis but is possible between acute episodes, so that a normal CT result is acceptable if compatible pulmonary histologic changes are present.

Laboratory Findings

In addition to peripheral blood leukocytosis with neutrophilia, usually BALF lymphocytosis is present (typically 40%–80% of BALF cell number increased two- to fourfold) when BAL is performed 5 days or more after the last exposure. Earlier lavage (especially <48 hours after exposure) is characterized by BALF neutrophilia. BALF lymphocytosis, at least in dairy farmers, is related to continued antigenic exposure and not to the presence of disease, and it does not predict outcome. In most instances of hypersensitivity pneumonitis, the BALF lymphocytes are virtually all $CD3^+$ with a relative increase of $CD8^+$, cells so that the CD4/CD8 ratio is <1. Many of the $CD8^+$ cells express CD57, a marker of cytotoxic cells, and also express CD25 (the IL-2 receptor) and other activation markers. However, the BALF CD4/CD8 ratio is 1 in ventilator lung, some cases of bird fancier's disease, and some cases of farmer's lung disease in Japan, although the BALF CD4/CD8 ratio is <1 in Japanese summer-type hypersensitivity pneumonitis. These differences between Japanese and non-Japanese patients with some types of hypersensitivity pneumonitis might be re-

lated to different types of exposure, differing periods of time between last important exposure and BAL, or genetic differences. In support of the importance of timing between last exposure and lavage, Soler demonstrated that cessation of exposure is associated with an increase of BALF $CD8^+$ cells. There is some suggestion that an increase of BALF $CD8^+$ cells is associated with protection against pulmonary fibrosis. BALF NK cell activity is increased in patients with hypersensitivity pneumonitis who continue to be exposed to the responsible antigen. The killer cell activity is found in cell populations with characteristics of both NK cells and non-NK cells, including LAK cells. Most of the $CD3^+$ cells are TCR $\alpha\beta^+$, but there is an increase of TCR $\gamma\delta^+$ cells and some tendency towards T-cell oligoclonality as demonstrated by increased $V_{\beta}8$, $V_{\beta}6$ and $V_{\beta}5$ TCR usage in some patients with hypersensitivity pneumonitis. BALF macrophages display many aspects of activation, including spontaneous secretion of TNF-α and IL-1 and expression of CD25. Monokines that can activate macrophages and cause chemotaxis of $CD8^+$ cells (i.e., MIP-1α, MCP-1, and IL-8) are present in BALF and AM from patients with acute hypersensitivity pneumonitis. Mast cells, often with ultrastructural markers of degranulation, are increased in both the lung parenchyma and BALF of patients with hypersensitivity pneumonitis. The concentration of IgG, IgM, IgG, and albumin are increased in BALF, presumably as a result of pulmonary inflammation. BALF histamine and tryptase is increased in some patients with acute hypersensitivity pneumonitis.

Virtually all patients with hypersensitivity pneumonitis have easily demonstrable antibody (typically IgG, IgM, and IgA) to the offending material in serum and often also in BALF. A multitude of methods have been used to demonstrate antibody (ELISA and variants, indirect immunofluorescence, complement fixation, latex agglutination, counterimmunoelectrophoresis, radioimmunoassay, Western blot). As most clinical studies have used simple agar diffusion ("Ouchterlony") methods to detect antibody, this is considered the standard method, but other methods are also acceptable (Fig. 5). The key issue is the ability of the antigen to detect antibody in the serum of patients with hypersensitivity pneumonitis. This varies with the methods of bacterial growth (for bacterial antigens) and of extraction of soluble antigens from either cultured material or material that causes hypersensitivity pneumonitis (e.g., hay in farmer's lung disease, bird droppings in bird fancier's disease). Because antigen preparations are not standardized, it is difficult to be confident of the meaning of a negative result unless the antigens have been tested against panels of sera from patients with and without hypersensitivity pneumonitis, so that reports of a negative hypersensitivity pneumonitis panel do not exclude the diagnosis of hypersensitivity pneumonitis. At times, it is useful to use antigens prepared from the environment suspected of causing hypersensitivity pneumonitis. This is especially important in patients with ventilator lung.

Serum antibody is also present in many subjects who are exposed but not ill, in virtually the same amounts as in patients with hypersensitivity pneumonitis. Therefore, the presence of antibody indicates exposure and sensitization and not necessarily disease. There is some suggestion that the presence of IgG and IgA antibody to *Trichosporon cutaneum* correlates with symptoms in subjects with Japanese-type hypersensitivity pneumonitis, whereas IgG antibody alone correlates with exposure but no symptoms. This correlation of exposure and symptoms with IgA antibody is not found in pigeon breeders or farmers. In asymptomatic pigeon breeders, the prevalence of antibody to pigeon antigens is 30%–60%. In farmers, the prevalence of anti-*Micropolyspora faeni* serum antibody is 2%–27%. The occurrence of serum antibody is not consistently related to apparent exposure (i.e., hours or intensity of exposure) in most instances of hypersensitivity pneumonitis. This may be related to a threshold effect, in that most exposures are above the minimum required to induce antibody and increases above that threshold are not associated with increases of the prevalence of antibody. In addition, serum antibody tends to wane after cessation of exposure, so that patients with chronic hypersensitivity pneumonitis who have not been exposed for some time may not have demonstrable antibody. In farmer's lung disease, approximately 50% of patients with initially positive serum antibody to *M. faeni* (*Saccharopolyspora rectivirgula*) lose demonstrable antibody 6 years after cessation of exposure. Farmers who continue to farm also lose detectable antibody (35%–50% in 5 years), and in some asymptomatic farmers initially without serum antibody, antibody later develops without farmer's lung disease. In pigeon breeder's disease and bird fancier's disease, approximately 50% of patients with initially positive serum antibody to avian antigens lose demonstrable antibody 2 to 3 years after cessation of exposure. Therefore, it is possible no serum antibody will be detectable in patients with hypersensitivity pneumonitis, either because an inappropriate antigen is used or because antibody has waned since the last exposure.

Nonspecific markers of inflammation, such as sedimentation rate and C-reactive protein, are often elevated during an acute episode of hypersensitivity pneumonitis. There are a few reports of increased prevalence of rheumatoid factor in patients with hypersensitivity pneumonitis. Antinuclear antibody or other autoantibodies are not present. There is increased uptake of gallium 67 in the lungs of patients with active hypersensitivity pneumonitis, which declines with improvement of the disease. Serum angiotensin-converting enzyme is not elevated, as it is in sarcoidosis.

Skin tests (of either immediate or delayed type) to detect sensitization to the suspected antigens are not useful, as extracts of agents that cause hypersensitivity pneumo-

nitis produce nonspecific reactions that do not indicate sensitization and do not discriminate between sensitized and unsensitized subjects. In addition, preparations of antigens that cause hypersensitivity pneumonitis are not readily commercially available. Early reports indicated that some patients with hypersensitivity pneumonitis demonstrate 4- to 8-hour skin test reactivity ("Arthus type"), which correlates with the presence of serum antibody. However, the presence of this reaction does not add information important in the diagnosis of hypersensitivity pneumonitis, as antibody can be readily detected in serum.

Tests designed to detect cell sensitization (most commonly antigen-induced lymphocyte proliferation or lymphokine secretion) are not useful in the clinical diagnosis of hypersensitivity pneumonitis, although they have been performed in specialized research settings. Patients with hypersensitivity pneumonitis have depressed delayed-type skin reactivity to recall antigens, similar to that observed in patients with sarcoidosis.

Pulmonary function tests typically demonstrate a restrictive ventilatory defect with small lung volumes, normal or increased flow rates, increased lung elastic recoil, and usually decreased diffusing capacity. There is frequent occurrence of a mild obstructive defect and increased upstream airway, resistance probably related to either bronchiolitis or emphysema. Arterial hypoxemia with hypocapnia, reflecting an increased alveolar-arterial oxygen gradient, is common either at rest or after exercise.

Many (20%–40%) patients with hypersensitivity pneumonitis exhibit increased nonspecific airway reactivity, which may be related to increased numbers of mast cells in the lung and BALF or to bronchial epithelial damage, and in some (5%–10%) clinical asthma develops. The increased airway reactivity and asthma tend to diminish after cessation of exposure.

Pathogenesis

Multiple immunologic markers present in subjects with hypersensitivity pneumonitis suggest that immune mediation is important in the pathogenesis of this syndrome. In addition, the necessity for previous sensitization (indicated by the presence of serum antibody in virtually all patients with hypersensitivity pneumonitis) suggests immunologic mediation.

The presence of serum antibody in patients with hypersensitivity pneumonitis and the timing of symptoms after exposure (2 to 9 hrs) led to the hypothesis that hypersensitivity pneumonitis represents an example of immune complex-mediated lung disease. However, the presence of antibody in subjects who are exposed but not ill, the lack of correlation between the presence of serum antibody and abnormalities on pulmonary function tests, the lack of evidence of complement consumption during acute exposure, the pathologic features that include granulomatous changes, and findings from animal models strongly suggest that cell-mediated immune processes are very important in hypersensitivity pneumonitis.

Many of the agents responsible for hypersensitivity pneumonitis can act as adjuvants and are particulate (promoting retention of antigen within the lung for prolonged periods of time), persistent, and nondegradable. They can interact with humoral mediators (complement and antibody) and cells in the lung to produce inflammation. The agents can induce injury by causing polymorphonuclear leukocytes and macrophages to release phlogistic substances such as reactive oxygen compounds, proteolytic enzymes, and products of arachidonic acid metabolism (prostaglandins and leukotrienes). The agents can also cause the production and release of IL-1, TNF-α and IL-6 from macrophages and lymphokines (IL-2, interferon-γ, and B-cell growth and differentiation factors) from lymphocytes. Injury to the lung caused by the above factors could enhance pulmonary exposure to inhaled antigen, which might promote immunologic sensitization and subsequent further pulmonary damage. The result of all these processes is pulmonary inflammation.

In animal models of hypersensitivity pneumonitis, T cells and macrophages are central in the induction and expression of hypersensitivity pneumonitis. Macrophage-derived cytokines, such as IL-1α, IL-6, TGF, and TNF-α, seem to play a central role in models involving intrapulmonary administration of materials that cause hypersensitivity pneumonitis.

Administration of cyclosporine A ameliorated pulmonary lesions in animals subjected to airway challenges with *Thermoactinomyces vulgaris,* another agent causing hypersensitivity pneumonitis, and nude mice did not exhibit pulmonary lesions of hypersensitivity pneumonitis after exposure that produced lesions in thymus-intact littermates. Ability to express pulmonary lesions can be transferred with T cells from sensitized mice. Pulmonary fibrosis induced by repeated challenges with *M. faeni,* but not an increase of BALF inflammatory cells, can be reduced by administration of anti-CD11a, implicating integrins in the processes that lead to fibrosis in this model.

Adoptive transfer models of hypersensitivity pneumonitis allow differentiation between direct lung damage (toxicity), sensitization (the development of antibody and cellular reactivity), and the results of immunologic reactions (the interaction of antigen with antibody and/or cells). We have developed such a model in inbred guinea pigs and mice that allows transfer of susceptibility to *M. faeni* by cultured cells from sensitized animals.

Culture of peritoneal exudate, spleen, or peripheral or lung-associated lymph node cells with a soluble extract of *M. faeni,* the agent that causes farmer's lung disease, confers the ability to induce susceptibility to pulmonary injury in recipients of transferred cells 4 days after an intratracheal injection of *M. faeni.* The pulmonary injury

is characterized by increased number of mononuclear cells in the lungs in both perivascular and peribronchiolar locations. This phenomenon depends on sensitization of the donor with *M. faeni,* culture with soluble *M. faeni,* and the number of transferred cells, and it persists for at least 8 weeks after cell transfer. Serum from sensitized animals cannot transfer experimental hypersensitivity pneumonitis. Three different mouse strains (C3H/HeJ, SJL/J, and C57Bl/6) do not differ in response. The post-culture cells responsible for transfer are CD3$^+$, CD4$^+$, CD8$^+$, and SIGM$^-$ T cells. Development of cells able to transfer depends on the presence of CD3$^+$ and CD4$^+$ but not CD8$^+$ cells at the onset of culture. The transferring cells are a mixture of naïve and memory (as defined by CD44, CD45RB, and L-selectin, markers) CD4$^+$ cells. The presence of recipient CD3$^+$ and CD4$^+$ but not CD8$^+$ cells is required for expression of adoptive experimental hypersensitivity pneumonitis. IFN-γ and IL-2 are present in substantial quantities in culture supernatants, suggesting a predominance of Th1 CD4$^+$ cells. The presence of serum IgG$_4$ antibody to pigeon antigens correlates with lack of symptoms in pigeon breeders. As IgG$_4$ is an immunoglobulin isotype that is induced by IL-4 and suppressed by IFN-γ, this suggests that hypersensitivity pneumonitis may be characterized by predominance of Th1 type immunologic reactivity.

Prognosis and Treatment

Prognosis varies considerably with the type of hypersensitivity pneumonitis or even the geographic location. For example, farmer's lung disease has a good prognosis in Quebec, even in farmers who continue to farm. However, in Finland it often results in significant physiologic impairment and even death. Pigeon breeder's disease in the United States and Europe has an good prognosis, whereas the same disease in Mexico has a 30% 5-year mortality. The reasons for these differences are not clear, but they likely include differences in the antigen, differences in the nature of the exposure, or both.

Removal from exposure to the offending antigens is usually sufficient to effect a resolution of symptoms and physiologic abnormalities within a few days for acute hypersensitivity pneumonitis and within a month for chronic hypersensitivity pneumonitis. In some patients, symptoms and signs of pulmonary fibrosis persist more than 6 months, which suggests a poor outcome. Removal from exposure completely is most effective, but cleaning of the environment in situations in which removal is impractical (e.g., Japanese summer-type hypersensitivity pneumonitis) can prevent further episodes of hypersensitivity pneumonitis. There is one report of resolution of symptoms of hypersensitivity pneumonitis after installation of filters in an air-conditioning system, which greatly lowered mold colony counts. Pigeon lofts in which litter materials designed to absorb pigeon excreta are not used have significantly lower levels of airborne pigeon antigens than lofts in which litter material is used. It is not known whether avoidance of litter materials is associated with a decrease in pigeon breeder's disease.

Systemic glucocorticosteroids are sometimes required to treat severe disease, although there is no formal evidence that such treatment is associated with long-term improvement in symptoms or radiologic or pulmonary function test abnormalities. The usual treatment is 40 to 60 mg of prednisone or prednisolone per day for 2 weeks, followed by a gradual decrease to no medication within 1 to 2 months. Patients with farmer's lung disease treated with prednisolone demonstrated slightly more rapid resolution of some radiologic abnormalities (ground-glass opacities) and physiologic abnormalities (slight improvement of diffusing capacity, no difference in lung volumes or arterial oxygen tension) than did untreated patients. However, there were no differences between the groups 6 months after the diagnosis of hypersensitivity pneumonitis. The above evidence suggests that systemic steroids may slightly increase the rate of resolution of acute pulmonary inflammation but have little or no effects on chronic residue of hypersensitivity pneumonitis. Inhaled glucocorticosteroids, nonsteroidal anti-inflammatory agents (cromolyn or nedocromil), and systemic immune modulators are not indicated in the treatment of hypersensitivity pneumonitis.

If patients are removed from exposure before permanent radiologic or physiologic abnormalities develop, the prognosis is excellent, with little evidence of long-term ill effects. If removal from exposure is impossible, the use of efficient masks during exposure can result in the prevention of acute hypersensitivity pneumonitis and is associated with an excellent prognosis. If exposure persists, some patients (proportion unclear, but probably 10%–30%) will progress to diffuse pulmonary fibrosis with resultant cor pulmonale and premature death. Mortality from farmer's lung disease is reported to be between 0% and 20% and usually occurs after 5 years of recurrent symptoms, although there are a few case reports of death after acute massive exposure to antigen. The prognosis varies considerably with different types of hypersensitivity pneumonitis. In general, long-term, relatively low-level exposure seems to be associated with a poorer prognosis, whereas short-term, intermittent exposure is associated with a better prognosis. This is well illustrated by pigeon breeder's disease, which in the United States and Europe has an excellent prognosis; most patients were asymptomatic and no deaths had occurred 10 years after diagnosis in a group of 24 patients with pigeon breeder's disease. In contrast, for patients in Mexico City who have pigeon breeder's disease, the mortality is 30% after 5 years. Unfortunately, many patients who present with chronic hypersensitivity pneumonitis also have pulmonary fibrosis and physiologic abnormalities that are only partially reversible after cessation of exposure.

Markers of pulmonary inflammation at the time of presentation, such as a high proportion of BALF lymphocytes, neutrophils, or mast cells, or the presence of procollagen III, hyaluronic acid, fibronectin, and fibroblast growth factors in BALF, do not predict outcome.

In conclusion, hypersensitivity pneumonitis is an immunologically mediated lung disease in which T cells and macrophages play important roles. It is diagnosed by a careful history and appropriate laboratory tests. Avoidance of exposure is usually associated with a good prognosis. Because of constantly changing environmental exposures, new examples of hypersensitivity pneumonitis are constantly being described and represent a continuing challenge to astute clinicians.

BIBLIOGRAPHY

Allen JN, Pacht ER, Gadek JE, Davis WB. Acute eosinophilic pneumonia as a reversible cause of noninfectious respiratory failure. *N Engl J Med* 1989;321:569–574. *First description of acute eosinophilic pneumonia.*

Ando M, Arima K, Yoneda R, Tamura M. Japanese summer-type hypersensitivity pneumonitis. Geographic distribution, home environment, and clinical characteristics of 621 cases. *Am Rev Respir Dis* 1991; 144:765–769. *Description of summer-type hypersensitivity pneumonitis, the most common form of hypersensitivity pneumonitis in Japan.*

Banham SW, McSharry C, Lynch PP, Boyd G. Relationships between avian exposure, humoral immune response, and pigeon breeder's disease among Scottish pigeon fanciers. *Thorax* 1986;41:274–278. *Survey of 277 Scottish pigeon breeders found 30% with serum antibody, a 10% prevalence of pigeon breeder's disease, and a striking increase of nonsmokers in patients with pigeon breeder's disease.*

Barbee RA, Callies Q, Dickie HA, Rankin J. The long-term prognosis in farmer's lung. *Am Rev Respir Dis* 1968;97:223–231. *Description of prognosis of the first group of patients with farmer's lung disease described in North America.*

Berman J. Lymphocytes in the lung: should we continue to exalt only BALT? *Am J Respir Cell Mol Biol* 1990;3:101–102. *This editorial describes the evidence that BALT is relatively unimportant in humans.*

Berman JS, Beer DJ, Theodore AC, Kornfeld H, Bernardo J, Center DM. Lymphocyte recruitment to the lung. *Am Rev Respir Dis* 1990; 142:238–257. *The classic review of the mechanisms of lung lymphocyte recruitment.*

Butcher EC. Leukocyte-endothelial cell recognition: three (or more) steps to specificity and diversity. *Cell* 1991;67:1033–1036. *This review succinctly describes the popular model for the sequential steps regulating leukocyte recruitment to sites of inflammation.*

Chelen CJ, Fang Y, Freeman GJ, Secrist H, Marshall JD, Hwang PT, Frankel LR, DeKruyff RH, Umetsu DT. Human alveolar macrophages present antigen ineffectively due to defective expression of B7 costimulatory cell surface molecules. *J Clin Invest* 1995;95:1415–1421. *As the title indicates, absence of essential co-stimulation is a crucial reason why alveolar macrophages are poor antigen-presenting cells.*

Coleman A, Colby TV. Histologic diagnosis of extrinsic allergic alveolitis. *Am J Surg Pathol* 1988;12:514–518. *Excellent description of the histologic criteria for hypersensitivity pneumonitis.*

Cox G, Crossley J, Xing Z. Macrophage engulfment of apoptotic neutrophils contributes to the resolution of acute pulmonary inflammation in vivo. *Am J Respir Cell Mol Biol* 1995;12:232–237. *Ingestion of effete and dying neutrophils by macrophages prevents release of many toxic compounds and limits lung toxicity during resolving inflammation.*

Doerschuk CM, Downey GP, Doherty DE, English D, Gie RP, Ohgami M, Worthen GS, Henson PM, Hogg JC. Leukocyte and platelet margination within microvasculature of rabbit lungs. *J Appl Physiol* 1990;

68:1956–1961. *Studies from these investigators have highlighted the role of physical constraints, such as cell size and cytoskeleton-dependent cell stiffness, in leukocyte passage through the pulmonary vasculature.*

doPico GA. Health effects of organic dusts in the farm environment. Report on diseases. *Am J Ind Med* 1986;10:261–265. *Description of organic dust toxic syndrome.*

Dranoff G, Crawford AD, Sadelain M, Ream B, Rashid A, Bronson RT, Dickersin GR, Bachurski CJ, Mark EL, Whitsett JA, et al. Involvement of granulocyte-macrophage colony-stimulating factor in pulmonary homeostasis. *Science* 1994;264:713–716. *Transgenic mice unable to produce GM-CSF develop a syndrome identical to human alveolar proteinosis, suggesting that normal macrophage function is essential to prevent this idiopathic condition.*

Drent M, van Velzen-Blad H, Diamant M, Wagenaar SS, Hoogsteden HC, van den Bosch JM. Bronchoalveolar lavage in extrinsic allergic alveolitis: effect of time elapsed since antigen exposure. *Eur Respir J* 1993;6:1276–1281. *BALF neutrophilia soon after antigen exposure and lymphocytosis later.*

Fearon DT, Locksley RM. The instructive role of innate immunity in the acquired immune response. *Science* 1996;272:50–53. *This review, part of an entire journal issue dedicated to elements of immunity, advances the notion that innate immunity not only provides a hard-wired rapid response system for responding to pathogens, but also determines to which antigens the acquired immune system will respond.*

Freedman PM, Ault B. Bronchial hyperreactivity to methacholine in farmer's lung disease. *J Allergy Clin Immunol* 1981;67:59–63. *Patients with hypersensitivity pneumonitis express bronchial hyperreactivity.*

Gariepy L, Cormier Y, Laviolette M, Tardi A. Predictive value of BAL cells and serum precipitins in asymptomatic dairy farmers. *Am Rev Respir Dis* 1989;140:1386–1389. *BALF findings and serum antibody do not predict outcome in exposed farmers in Quebec.*

Gleich G, Adolphson C, Leiferman K. The biology of the eosinophilic leukocyte. *Annu Rev Med* 1993;44:85–101. *Eosinophils are characterized by specific cytoplasmic granules and include cationic toxins targeted to helminths, protozoa, bacteria, and other cells.*

Harmsen AG, Muggenburg B, Snipes M, Bice D. The role of macrophages in particle translocation from lungs to lymph nodes. *Science* 1985;230:1277–1280. *This article elegantly demonstrates that particle-containing macrophages migrate from the alveoli to the mediastinal lymph nodes.*

Hinson K, Moon A, Plummer N. Bronchopulmonary aspergillosis. A review and a report of eight new cases. *Thorax* 1952;7:317–333. *First modern description of ABPA.*

Janeway CA, Bottomly K. Signals and signs for lymphocyte responses. *Cell* 1994;76:275–285. *Brief review of the state-of-the-art understanding on the signals regulating lymphocyte activation.*

Janis EM, Kaufmann SH, Schwartz RH, Pardoll DM. Activation of $\tau\delta$ T cells in the primary immune response to *Mycobacterium tuberculosis*. *Science* 1989;244:713–716. *Study illustrates the role of this alternate T-cell population in mucosal defense.*

Katzenstein A, Liebow A, Friedman P. Bronchocentric granulomatous, mucoid impaction, and hypersensitivity to fungi. *Am Rev Respir Dis* 1975;111:497–537. *Classic paper describing the interrelationships among bronchocentric granulomas, mucoid impaction, and ABPA.*

Knutsen AP, Mueller KR, Levine AD, Chouhan B, Hutcheson PS, Slavin RG. Asp fI CD4+ Th2-like T-cell lines in allergic bronchopulmonary aspergillosis. *J Allergy Clin Immunol* 1994;94:215–221. *Important support for the concept that ABPA is a reflection of Th2 cell overactivity.*

Kokkarinen JI, Tukiainen HO, Terho EO. Effect of corticosteroid treatment on the recovery of pulmonary function in farmer's lung. *Am Rev Respir Dis* 1992;145:3–5. *Glucocorticosteroid treatment causes slightly more rapid improvement of pulmonary function tests after 1 month, but there is no difference from no treatment after 6 months.*

Lenschow D, Walunas T, Bluestone J. CD28/B7 system of T-cell co-stimulation. *Annu Rev Immunol* 1996;14:233–258. *Detailed review of the signaling pathways whereby the CD28/B7 receptor/ligand system mediates T-cell and B-cell regulation.*

Lynch DA, Rose CS, Way D, King TE Jr. Hypersensitivity pneumonitis: sensitivity of high-resolution CT in a population-based study. *AJR*

Am J Roentgenol 1992;159:469–472. *Description of high resolution CT findings in hypersensitivity pneumonitis.*

Marathias KP, Preffer FI, Pinto C, Kradin RL. Most human pulmonary infiltrating lymphocytes display the surface immune phenotype and functional responses of sensitized T cells. *Am J Respir Cell Mol Biol* 1991;5:470–476. *This study provided groundbreaking data on the expression of adhesion molecules on human lung lymphocytes.*

McWilliam AS, Nelson D, Thomas JA, Holt PG. Rapid dendritic cell recruitment is a hallmark of the acute inflammatory response at mucosal surfaces. *J Exp Med* 1994;179:1331–1336. *Data suggest that influx of dendritic cells during acute inflammation acts as surveillance for opportunistic viruses and that this system is operative at a limited number of mucosal tissue sites.*

Moore VL, Fink JN. Immunologic studies in hypersensitivity pneumonitis—quantitative precipitins and complement-fixing antibodies in symptomatic and asymptomatic pigeon breeders. *J Lab Clin Med* 1975;85:540–545. *Quantities of serum antibodies overlap between asymptomatic exposed persons and patients with pigeon breeder's disease.*

Orriols R, Morell F, Curull V, Roman A, Sampol G. Impaired nonspecific delayed cutaneous hypersensitivity in bird fancier's lung. *Thorax* 1989;44:132–135. *Patients with hypersensitivity pneumonitis have impaired delayed-type skin test reactivity.*

Pabst R, Binns RM. Lymphocytes migrate from the bronchoalveolar space to regional bronchial lymph nodes. *Am J Respir Crit Care Med* 1995;151:495–499. *These immunofluorescence staining experiments demonstrate that lymphocytes may leave the lung to migrate widely throughout the body. It is likely that these cells contribute to specific immune memory against pathogens.*

Pabst R, Binns RM, Licence ST, Peter M. Evidence of a selective major vascular marginal pool of lymphocytes in the lung. *Am Rev Respir Dis* 1987;136:1213–1218. *Using an elegant perfusion system in the pig, this study demonstrates the existence of a sizeable population of lymphocytes associated with the pulmonary vasculature, and thus available for rapid recruitment into lung parenchyma. Intra-arterial injection shows that trapping of intravenously injected cells in the lungs is a specific process, not simply embolization.*

Panchal N, Pant C, Bhagat R, Shah A. Central bronchiectasis in allergic bronchopulmonary aspergillosis: comparative evaluation of computed tomography of the thorax with bronchography. *Eur Respir J* 1994;7:1290–1293. *Direct comparison of bronchoscopy and CT in ABPA.*

Patterson R, Greenberger PA, Castile RG, Yee WF, Roberts M. Diagnostic problems in hypersensitivity lung disease. *Allergy Proc* 1989;10:141–147. *Example of a hypersensitivity pneumonitis screen giving false-negative results and delaying the diagnosis of hypersensitivity pneumonitis.*

Patterson R, Greenberger PA, Halwig JM, Liotta JL, Roberts M. Allergic bronchopulmonary aspergillosis. Natural history and classification of early disease by serologic and roentgenographic studies. *Arch Intern Med* 1986;146:916–918. *Description of staging system for ABPA.*

Perez-Padilla R, Salas J, Chapela R, Sanchez M, Carrillo G, Perez R, Sansores R, Gaxiola M, Selman M. Mortality in Mexican patients with chronic pigeon breeder's lung compared with those with usual interstitial pneumonia. *Am Rev Respir Dis* 1993;148:49–53. *Mortality from pigeon breeder's disease in Mexico is 30% in 5 years (i.e., much higher than that in the United States and Europe).*

Reed C. Variability of antigenicity of *Aspergillus fumigatus*. *J Allergy Clin Immunol* 1978;61:227–229. *Description of variability of different preparations of clinically used antigens.*

Reeder W, Goodrich B. Pulmonary infiltration with eosinophilia (PIE syndrome). *Ann Intern Med* 1952;36:1217–1240. *Introduction of the term PIE syndrome.*

Schlossman S. *Leucocyte Typing V: White Cell Differentiation Antigens. Proceedings of the Fifth International Workshop and Conference in Boston, 3–7 November, 1993.* Oxford: Oxford University Press; 1995.

Schlossman SF, Boumsell L, Gilks W, Harlan JM, Kishimoto T, Morimoto C, Ritz J, Shaw S, Silverstein RL, Springer TA, Tedder TF, Todd RF. CD antigens 1993. *J Immunol* 1994;152:1. *These two publications describe the long and the brief views of the most recent workshop to define human leukocyte surface antigens.*

Schuyler M, Gott K, Shopp G, Crooks L. CD3+ and CD4+ cells adoptively transfer experimental hypersensitivity pneumonitis. *Am Rev Respir Dis* 1992;146:1582–1588. *CD4+ cells adoptively transfer experimental hypersensitivity pneumonitis.*

Shelhamer JH, Levine SJ, Wu T, Jacoby DB, Kaliner MA, Rennard SI. NIH conference. Airway inflammation. *Ann Intern Med* 1995;123: 288–304. *Summary of the wide variety of pathways, mediators, and cells that mediate and regulate both acute and chronic inflammation of the airways.*

Sporn MB, Roberts AB. Peptide growth factors are multifunctional. *Nature* 1988;332:217–219. *This influential review advances the concept that cytokines may be understood not as substances with invariant properties, but as terms in an intercellular language.*

Strieter RM, Kunkel SL. The immunopathology of chemotactic cytokines. *Adv Exp Med Biol* 1993;351:19–28. *Location and function of the chemotactic cytokines that play critical roles in regulating airway inflammation.*

Thepen T, Van Rooijen N, Kraal G. Alveolar macrophage elimination in vivo is associated with an increase in pulmonary immune response in mice. *J Exp Med* 1989;170:499–509. *This group pioneered the use of liposomes that selectively deplete alveolar macrophages.*

Warren C, Tse K, Cherniack R. Mechanical properties of the lung in extrinsic allergic alveolitis. *Thorax* 1978;33:315–321. *Description of increased upstream resistance in hypersensitivity pneumonitis.*

Weiss SJ. Tissue destruction by neutrophils. *N Engl J Med* 1989;320: 365–376. *Summary of neutrophil function and the multiple pathways whereby they are activated and mediate tissue injury.*

Yoshida K, Ando M, Sakata T, Araki S. Prevention of summer-type hypersensitivity pneumonitis: effect of elimination of *Trichosporon cutaneum* from the patients' homes. *Arch Environ Health* 1989;44: 317–322. *Cleaning the environment of molds can prevent further episodes of hypersensitivity pneumonitis.*

Yoshimoto T, Bendelac A, Watson C, Hu-Li J, Paul WE. Role of NK1.1[+] T cells in a Th2 response and in immunoglobulin E production. *Science* 1995;270:1845–1847. *This report describes an unusual cell type that provides an explanation for source of IL-4 needed to induce Th2 differentiation of naïve T cells, especially for help in IgE production. Because these cells recognize antigen presented by CD1[+] antigen-presenting cells, dysregulation of CD1 expression may be one cause of atopy.*

Textbook of Pulmonary Diseases, 6th ed.
edited by G.L. Baum, J.D. Crapo, B.R. Celli, and J.B. Karlinsky,
Lippincott–Raven Publishers, Philadelphia, © 1998.

CHAPTER

20 ► Systemic Sarcoidosis

Lynn T. Tanoue · Jack A. Elias

INTRODUCTION

Between 1865 and 1875, Sir Jonathan Hutchinson is believed to have encountered the first case of what we now recognize as sarcoidosis. In 1889, Besnier described a patient with raised violaceous facial lesions that he called *lupus pernio*. His report was followed by one by Tenneson describing the presence of granulomas and the absence of tubercle bacilli in similar skin lesions. In 1899, Boeck described a patient with pronounced lymphadenopathy and multiple nodules of the skin, face, and back. When these lesions were examined histologically, Boeck was struck by their close resemblance to a sarcoma and gave them the name *benign sarcoid*. Schauman in 1914 and Kuznitsky and Bittorf in 1915 recognized that sarcoid skin lesions, lupus pernio, and visceral lesions were all part of the same multisystem disorder. This important observation set the stage for the recognition of sarcoidosis as a distinct entity. In the years since its recognition, sarcoidosis has been the topic of intense investigation. These studies have shed light on some of the clinical manifestations, epidemiologic characteristics, and pathogenic mechanisms of the disease. However, although commonly encountered and frequently diagnosed, sarcoidosis is still poorly understood. Its etiology is unknown, our knowledge of its pathogenesis is incomplete, and its diagnosis, staging, and treatment are steeped in controversy. In this chapter, we have attempted to outline the areas of certainty and uncertainty regarding this disor-

der. We also hope to provide a rational approach that can be used for evaluating and treating affected patients.

DEFINITION

A number of attempts have been made to formulate a definition of sarcoidosis. In 1948, the National Academy of Sciences proposed a definition that was essentially an extensive clinical definition of the manifestations of the disease. In 1976, the Subcommittee on Classification of the Seventh International Conference on Sarcoidosis proposed the following definition:

> Sarcoidosis is a multisystem granulomatous disorder of unknown etiology most commonly affecting young adults and presenting with bilateral hilar adenopathy, pulmonary infiltration, and skin or eye lesions. The diagnosis is established most securely when clinical or radiographic findings are supported by histologic evidence of widespread noncaseating epithelioid granulomas in more than one organ or by a positive Kveim-Siltzbach skin test. Immunologic features are depression of delayed-type hypersensitivity, suggesting impaired cell-mediated immunity and increased or abnormal immunoglobulins. There may also be hypercalciuria with or without hypercalcemia. The course and prognosis may correlate with mode of onset. An acute onset with erythema nodosum heralds a self-limited course and spontaneous resolution, whereas an insidious onset may be followed by relentless progressive fibrosis. Corticosteroids relieve symptoms and suppress inflammation and granuloma formation.

This definition is dated, overly descriptive, and its sheer bulk limits its utility. It is more useful to define sarcoidosis as a systemic granulomatous disorder of unknown etiology. In this definition there are three points that need

L. T. Tanoue and J. A. Elias: Department of Internal Medicine, Yale University School of Medicine, New Haven, Connecticut 06510.

emphasis: that sarcoidosis is a systemic disorder, that it is a granulomatous disorder, and that, despite many attempts, its etiologic agent or agents are unknown.

EPIDEMIOLOGY

The majority of patients with sarcoidosis are either asymptomatic or have such trivial symptoms that they do not bother to consult a physician. This makes an accurate assessment of the incidence of sarcoidosis in the United States difficult. Best estimates are that sarcoidosis in the United States occurs in 1 in 10,000 people per year, making for some 22,500 cases annually. Within the United States, sarcoidosis is 10 times more frequent in black than in white persons. It was thought to be particularly prevalent in the southeastern states. However, more recent epidemiologic studies have cast some doubt on this latter contention, as corrections of previous studies for differences in black and white population densities and new case-matched studies have shown that the incidence of sarcoidosis in the south and southeast is similar to that in other parts of the United States.

In parts of the world where mass radiographic screening is performed, more accurate estimates of the prevalence of sarcoidosis can be obtained. These studies have shown a prevalence rate of 64/100,000 in Sweden and 20/100,000 in the United Kingdom. Interestingly, rates as high as 200/100,000 are noted among Irish women of childbearing age, whereas the disease is quite rare in China and southeast Asia.

ETIOLOGY

The granulomatous lesions in sarcoidosis are similar to those caused by infectious agents, such as mycobacteria and fungi, or inorganic agents, such as zirconium and beryllium, and to those seen in hypersensitivity reactions to organic agents, such as thermophilic actinomycetes. These similarities have caused many to speculate that infectious agents or organic or inorganic dusts may be etiologic in sarcoidosis. Particular interest has been directed at the possibility that sarcoidosis is the result of an unusual host response to a common agent, or the result of an infection by, or inhalation of, a poorly characterized agent. Efforts to test these speculations have been ongoing for many years. These studies have failed to observe consistent associations between the occurrence of sarcoidosis and a person's place of birth, place of residence, or personal history of allergies, drug ingestion, exposure to pets, or occupational exposure. In addition, contentions that common and exotic agents such as viruses (including human immunodeficiency virus, or HIV-2), corynebacteria, fungi, and pine pollen play an etiologic role have not stood up under close scrutiny. The polymerase chain reaction (PCR) has recently been used to reinvestigate the

role mycobacteria play in this disorder. Using this technique, some investigators have reported enhanced detection of mycobacterial DNA in patients with sarcoidosis. These studies overall had a high rate of false-positive PCR reactions. In contrast, others have found mycobacterial DNA in only a small minority of patients with sarcoidosis. As a result, it cannot be concluded that *Mycobacterium tuberculosis* is etiologic in the majority of cases of sarcoidosis. Additional studies will be required to clarify this issue.

Epidemiologic studies have demonstrated that sarcoidosis is commonly encountered in people from northern Europe, is more common in American blacks than American whites, and can cluster in families. These observations suggest that genetic predisposition may be an important variable in disease acquisition. However, to date, no consistent mode of inheritance has been found. In addition, most studies have shown no consistent association between human leukocyte antigen (HLA) type and disease. The report that sarcoidosis is five and a half times as frequent in American blacks that are HLA-Bw15-positive than in those lacking this antigen is interesting, but it will require additional confirmation.

PATHOLOGY

The histologic features of sarcoidosis consist of varying degrees of granulomatous inflammation, interstitial pneumonitis, and tissue fibrosis. Which of these lesions predominates depends on the stage of the patient's disease.

Granulomatous Inflammation

The epithelioid granuloma is the characteristic lesion of sarcoidosis. These granulomas are usually not necrotic. When necrosis occurs, it is usually minimal and confined to the central portions of the lesion. The granulomas are usually distinct, even when densely clustered. Epithelioid cells and multinucleated giant cells are found in the center of the granulomas. They are intermingled with and surrounded by macrophages, monocytes, and lymphocytes (Fig. 1). In some cases, the granulomas are surrounded by fibroblasts and fibroblast-derived connective tissue products. The epithelioid cells are felt to be derived from tissue macrophages and are approximately 20 μm in diameter and 25 to 45 μm in length. They have ample, pale-staining cytoplasm, well-defined boundaries, and a central or eccentrically placed oval nucleus. Ultrastructural studies reveal abundant mitochondria, abundant rough and smooth endoplasmic reticulum, large numbers of vesicles, and a well-developed Golgi apparatus, suggesting that these cells have an enhanced secretory capacity. The multinucleated giant cells are believed to form from fused epithelioid cells. They are 150 to 300 μm in diameter and resemble the epithelioid cells ultrastructurally.

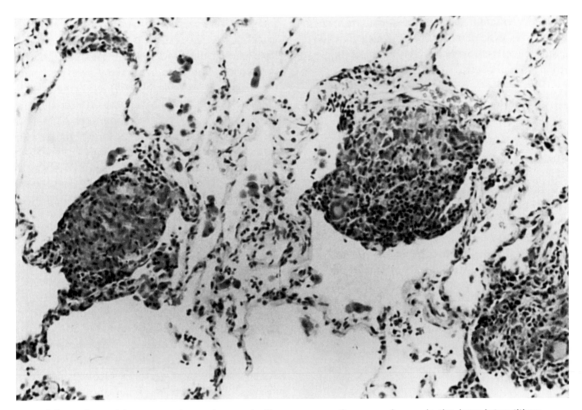

FIG. 1. Lung biopsy specimen demonstrating noncaseating granulomas in the lung interstitium.

The lymphocytes in and around these granulomas are often larger and contain more organelles than their circulating relatives. Characterization using monoclonal antibodies has shown that most of the T cells express the CD4 (OKT4) antigen, which is usually associated with a helper/inducer phenotype, and a minority express the CD8 (OKT8) antigen, which is usually associated with a cytotoxic/suppressor phenotype. As a result, the ratio of helper/inducer lymphocytes to cytotoxic/suppressor lymphocytes (CD4/CD8 ratio) in sarcoid granulomas is increased and parallels that noted in the cells obtained by bronchoalveolar lavage (BAL).

Noncaseating granulomas may be found in any organ in the body. In the lung they tend to be peribronchial, interstitial, and subpleural in location. Perivascular granulomas are also commonly noted. These lesions rarely extend past the vascular adventitia, and luminal distortion and endothelial cell disruption are rare. True vasculitis can be found in 42%–67% of lung biopsy specimens in sarcoidosis. However, in the vast majority of cases, the vasculitis is a minor aspect of the lesion. When vasculitis is prominent, alternative diagnostic possibilities should be considered, such as necrotizing sarcoidal vasculitis or Wegener's granulomatosis.

Interstitial Pneumonitis

Although the epithelioid granuloma is the characteristic lesion of sarcoidosis, it is probably not the first lesion to be present. The granulomas are preceded by, and then noted in conjunction with, an interstitial pneumonitis characterized by macrophages and lymphocytes, the majority of which are T cells. The macrophages and lymphocytes in these infiltrates appear to be activated, as they are larger and contain more organelles than corresponding cells in the circulating pool. The exact relationship between the intensity of the interstitial pneumonitis and the density of granuloma formation is not understood. The possibility that the granulomas are a consequence of the interstitial pneumonitis may explain why most studies find that the granulomas are most prominent when the interstitial pneumonitis is least intense, and vice versa.

Tissue Fibrosis

The interstitial pneumonitis and granulomatous inflammation seen in sarcoidosis are dynamic processes. Some lesions remain cellular for an extended period of time. In contrast, the majority resolve, either spontaneously or in response to steroid therapy. Approximately 75%–80% of these resolving lesions heal with preservation of the normal parenchymal architecture. In the rest, the fibroblasts at the periphery of the granulomas proliferate and increase their production of collagens and other matrix molecules. As a result, the granuloma is replaced in a centripetal fashion with scar tissue. In the process, normal alveolar and bronchial architecture are distorted and the pulmonary vascular surface area is compromised. Bronchiectasis and cystic parenchymal lesions can result, and in the most severe cases, honeycombing and pulmonary hypertension can occur.

IMMUNOPATHOGENESIS

Sarcoidosis is the prototypic example of a compartmentalized immune response. Heightened cell-mediated immunity is seen within the lung and at other sites of disease involvement. In contrast, depressed cell-mediated immunity, often with cutaneous anergy, is seen in the peripheral circulation. Studies during the last few decades have added significantly to our understanding of the cellular events involved in the inflammatory and fibrotic phases of this disease. As a result, we have an improved understanding of the state of activation and effector function of the cells in sarcoidal infiltrates, a picture of how these alterations mediate pulmonary inflammation, and a preliminary understanding of the role that cytokines may play in granuloma formation.

T Cells

In sarcoidosis, helper T lymphocytes accumulate at sites of disease activity. The ratio of helper (CD4$^+$) to suppressor (CD8$^+$) cells is increased in bronchoalveolar lavage fluid (BALF). The T cells that accumulate in the lungs of patients with sarcoidosis and are found in BALF are activated, as they express markers of cell-surface activation, such as the major histocompatibility complex (MHC) DR antigen, the VLA-1 late activation antigen, and the interleukin-2 (IL-2) receptor (Tac antigen). Unlike unstimulated T lymphocytes, they also spontaneously produce a variety of cytokines, including IL-2, interferon-γ (IFN-γ), monocyte chemotactic factor (MCF), and a factor (possibly IL-6) that induces the differentiation of B cells to immunoglobulin-secreting cells. The IL-2 that is produced by sarcoid T cells appears to bind to the IL-2 receptor and stimulates T-cell proliferation in an autocrine and/or paracrine fashion. Interestingly, although BALF T cells are spontaneously activated, like peripheral lymphocytes, their response to "recall" antigens such as purified protein derivative (PPD) and *Candida* is decreased. The reason for this is not clear. This decreased memory function may explain in part the cutaneous anergy observed clinically in some patients with sarcoidosis.

T cells recognize foreign antigens via their T-cell receptors (TCR). Each T cell expresses a receptor for a unique antigen. The diversity of receptors necessary to encode an appropriately diverse immune repertoire is generated by creating TCR that differ in the constant (C), joining (J), and variable (V) regions of the two proteins that make up the heterodimeric TCR complex. In an attempt to identify the agent(s) causing the lymphocytosis in sarcoidosis,

the TCR on the surface of BALF and peripheral blood lymphocytes have been extensively studied. These studies have shown that BALF T lymphocytes are not a clonal population. Some studies have, however, detected a distinct bias for the use of TCR with the V$_\beta$8 and V$_\alpha$2.3 variable region subtypes and the C$_\beta$1 constant region subtype. Others have reported subgroups of individuals who have sarcoidosis with expression in blood or lung of one or more of five V$_\beta$ gene families (V$_\beta$5, V$_\beta$8, V$_\beta$15, V$_\beta$16, V$_\beta$18). These findings suggest that T-cell activation in sarcoidosis is not a nonspecific process. Instead, the lymphocytosis appears to be a specific response to a limited number of antigens.

The majority of T cells in sarcoidosis lesions express α and β TCR proteins (e.g., they are $\alpha\beta$ T lymphocytes). However, a subgroup of individuals with sarcoidosis has been reported in which the BALF T lymphocytes contain $\gamma\delta$ TCR. This observation is quite interesting, as $\gamma\delta$ T cells may play an important role in the cellular immune response to mycobacterial antigens and mucosal immunity. Immunohistochemical studies, however, have failed to detect $\gamma\delta$ T cells within sarcoid lymph nodes. This discrepancy has not yet been resolved. However, it may reflect differences in the kinetics of T-cell accumulation, as $\gamma\delta$ T cells may be found only at sites of active early alveolitis.

T-Lymphocyte Subsets

Recent studies of murine, and to a lesser extent human, lymphocytes have demonstrated the existence of subpopulations of cells based on the patterns of cytokines that they produce. Two major subpopulations of CD4 (and other) lymphocytes have been noted, Th1 (T helper) and Th2 cells. Th1 cells produce IFN-γ and IL-2, cytokines that are important in macrophage activation. These cells are felt to be mediators of delayed-type hypersensitivity responses. In contrast, Th2 cells express IL-4 and IL-5, cytokines that are important in antibody-mediated responses, IgE class switching, and eosinophilia. Th2 cells are therefore felt to be mediators of humoral and eosinophil-mediated disorders, such as atopy and allergy. These lymphocyte subsets also cross-regulate each other, with Th1 cell-derived IFN-γ downregulating the cytokine production and proliferation of Th2 cells, and Th2-derived Il-4 and Il-10 having similar inhibitory effects on Th1 cells. In addition, the macrophage-derived cytokines IL-10 and IL-12 play an important role in the regulation of these processes, with IL-12 augmenting Th1 responses and IL-10 augmenting Th2 responses.

The Th1-Th2 paradigm provides a theoretical explanation for why cell-mediated immunity dominates in some circumstances, whereas antibody-based responses predominate in others. A variety of lines of evidence suggest that Th1-mediated processes play an important role in sarcoidosis. A variety of experimental granulomatous models have been shown to be Th1-mediated. In addition, BALF studies of patients with sarcoidosis have demonstrated increased levels of IFN-γ, IL-2, and IL-12 and low or undetectable levels of IL-4, IL-5, and IL-10. Similarly, T cells from the lungs of patients with sarcoidosis produce exaggerated amounts of IL-1 and IFN-γ. Additional experimentation will be required to confirm the impression that sarcoidosis is a Th1-predominant disorder.

Monocytes/Macrophages

Monocytes, macrophages, epithelioid cells, and giant cells are important participants in the alveolitis of patients with sarcoidosis. The macrophages appear to be activated in vivo, because, in contrast to the alveolar macrophages of normal persons, they spontaneously release proinflammatory cytokines, such as IL-1, IL-6, tumor necrosis factor (TNF), granulocyte colony-stimulating factor (G-CSF), and granulocyte-macrophage colony-stimulating factor (GM-CSF), and secrete increased quantities of 1,25-dihydroxyvitamin D, angiotensin-converting enzyme, and reactive oxygen metabolites, such as hydrogen peroxide. Sarcoid alveolar macrophages also have an increased capacity to present antigen compared with normal macrophages. This may reflect the increased adhesiveness of sarcoid macrophages and lymphocytes. In accord with this concept, sarcoid alveolar macrophages express increased amounts of the cellular surface adhesion molecules leukocyte function-associated antigen-1 (LFA-1) and intercellular adhesion molecule-1 (ICAM-1). In addition to secreting cytokines, these macrophages express cell surface IL-2 receptors and can thus be activated by the IL-2-secreting T cells at sites of inflammation.

Fibroblasts

Fibroblasts have been traditionally thought of as effector cells that, under the influence of T cells and macrophages, produce matrix components, such as collagen. The demonstration that IL-1 and TNF regulate fibroblast production of types I and III collagen has provided additional support for the concept that dysregulated cytokine production by activated mononuclear cells can lead to fibroblast activation and tissue fibrosis in sarcoidosis. It is now being increasingly appreciated, however, that fibroblasts are also important immune effector cells at sites of inflammation. IL-1 and TNF can induce fibroblast production of a wide variety of cytokines, including IL-6, monocyte chemotactic peptide-1 (MCP-1), IL-8, IL-11, leukemia inhibitory factor, G-CSF, and GM-CSF. IL-6, MCP-1, and the CSFs may be particularly important in sarcoidosis. IL-6 activates the acute-phase response, B-cell immunoglobulin production, and T-cell proliferation;

MCP-1 recruits fresh peripheral blood monocytes to sites of inflammation; and the CSFs activate local macrophages. IL-1 and TNF can also increase the adherence of T lymphocytes to lung fibroblasts, a mechanism by which fibroblasts may contribute to the compartmentalized activation of T cells seen in this granulomatous disorder.

Mechanisms of Tissue Inflammation in Sarcoidosis

Inflammatory responses in the sarcoid lung are therefore regulated, at least in part, by a complex network of interacting cytokines. The majority of the alveolar macrophages in the lung are derived from circulating blood monocytes. They enter the lung along chemotactic gradients and have a limited but definite capacity to proliferate locally. Infectious agents and/or noxious stimuli that reach the lung via the airways can activate resident macrophages to produce TNF, IL-6, IL-8, transforming growth factor-β (TGF-β), platelet-derived growth factor (PDGF), modest amounts of soluble IL-1β, and insulin-like growth factor (IGF). IL-8, in conjunction with IL-1, TNF, activated complement fragments, and other chemotactic agents, activates and recruits leukocytes to the lung. This recruitment is at least partially a consequence of cytokine-enhanced endothelial cell adhesion molecule expression. The cytokines also interact with antigen-presenting cells (such as alveolar macrophages and/or dendritic cells) to activate T lymphocytes. Activated T lymphocytes express high-affinity IL-2 receptors and produce a variety of cytokines, most notably IL-2, IFN-γ, and IL-6. IL-2, as noted above, acts in an autocrine and/or paracrine fashion to stimulate lymphocyte proliferation. IFN-γ and IL-2 activate local macrophages, and IL-6 contributes to the proliferation and terminal differentiation of B lymphocytes into antibody-producing plasma cells. IL-1, TNF, and other moieties also stimulate local stromal cells, such as fibroblasts, to produce cytokines such as IL-6, MCP-1, IL-1α, and colony-stimulating factors. These proinflammatory molecules further augment local T-cell and B-cell responses and activate local macrophages. The IL-1, TNF and IL-6 that are produced also enter the systemic circulation, where they stimulate the production of acute-phase proteins and induce fever. In addition, TGF-β, IL-1, PDGF, and IGF may also stimulate the fibrotic response, as under appropriate circumstances each can stimulate fibroblast proliferation and/or collagen production.

As noted above, the alveolar macrophages and T cells in the lungs of patients with sarcoidosis appear to be activated in vivo. These cells express cytokine receptors and produce, in an exaggerated fashion, many of the cytokines responsible for the interactions noted above. Specifically, alveolar macrophages express IL-2 receptors and produce IL-1, TNF, GM-CSF, PDGF, and TGF-β. T-cell IL-2 receptor expression and IL-2, IFN-γ, and MCF production are also augmented. The IFN-γ that is produced may be a key mediator in the pathogenesis of this disorder, as IFN-γ activates macrophage IL-1 production, 1,25-dihydroxyvitamin D production, hydrogen peroxide production, IL-2 receptor expression, and macrophage fusion into multinucleated giant cells. MCF encourages monocyte entry into sites of inflammation, and the IL-1 and TNF that are produced activate stromal cell IL-6 production. IL-1, TNF, and IL-6 induce fever and stimulate the heightened acute-phase response characteristically seen in patients with sarcoidosis. The elevated levels of IL-6 may also contribute to the polyclonal hypergammaglobulinemia seen in this disorder.

The Kveim Reaction

It has been known since 1941 that in patients with sarcoidosis a localized cutaneous nodule often develops 2 to 6 weeks after intradermal injection of an extract of spleen or lymph node from another patient with sarcoidosis. Biopsy specimens of these Kveim-Siltzbach test lesions exhibit histopathologic similarities to sarcoid granulomas. Moreover, Kveim-Siltzbach lesions and sarcoid granulomas have a similar distribution of OKT4$^+$ and OKT8$^+$ lymphocytes and a similar distribution of specific Vβ and T-cell subsets. Despite these similarities, there are several reasons why the Kveim reaction cannot be classified as a true immunologic response. First, a delayed-type hypersensitivity reaction becomes positive within 48 to 72 hours and resolves within a week. In contrast, Kveim nodules develop after 4 to 6 weeks and persist for several months. Second, despite an intensive search, a specific antigen has not been identified in this material. Attempts to induce patient lymphocytes to proliferate or secrete cytokines after in vitro exposure to Kveim material have been largely unrewarding.

CLINICAL MANIFESTATIONS

The manifestations of sarcoidosis in persons who come to medical attention vary with their ethnic and racial background and the degree to which the local medical community utilizes chest radiographic screening that would detect milder or asymptomatic forms of the disease. Sarcoidosis can involve and cause symptoms in virtually any organ in the body. A detailed description of every manifestation is beyond the scope of this chapter. Instead, attention is focused on the major modes of presentation and patterns of organ involvement.

Presentation

As many as 50% of patients with sarcoidosis are asymptomatic at the time of diagnosis. Physicians become aware of these patients as a result of abnormalities noted incidentally on chest x-ray films that have been performed for other reasons. Patients who are symptomatic at the time of presentation generally have pulmonary, ocular, dermatologic, or systemic complaints (Table 1). Overall, pulmonary symptoms are noted in 15%–40% of patients presenting with sarcoidosis. Shortness of breath, dyspnea on exertion, cough, and substernal chest pain are common. Between 10% and 32% percent of patients with sarcoidosis present with skin lesions. Erythema nodosum is seen approximately twice as often as the other, more specific skin manifestations, and is frequently found in association with fever, malaise, and polyarthralgias. Maculopapular lesions, nodules, and ulcers also can be presenting manifestations. Granulomatous infiltration of old scars resulting in swelling, purple discoloration, and occasionally tenderness also may cause the patient to seek medical attention. Approximately 10%–25% of patients present with ocular symptoms, most commonly caused by acute uveitis and consisting of redness of the eye, tearing, cloudy vision, and photophobia. This type of acute ocular involvement is often seen in association with erythema nodosum and bilateral hilar adenopathy. Systemic symptoms are reported by approximately 40% of patients and are more common in blacks and Asians from the Indian subcontinent. The fever is usually mild, and weight loss is usually limited to 5 to 15 lb within the preceding 3 months. However, temperatures as high as 104°F, more severe weight loss, and night sweats, anorexia, fatigue, and myalgias are well described.

Intrathoracic Involvement

Respiratory tract involvement is the most common manifestation of sarcoidosis. In 90% of patients, signs

TABLE 1. *Presenting complaints of patients with sarcoidosis*

Complaint	Percentage of patients
Asymptomatic	12–35
Systemic	15–40
Fatigue	20–30
Malaise	15
Weight loss	20–30
Fever	15–22
Night sweats	15
Weakness	10
Chills	10–15
Respiratory	15–40
Cough	30–40
Dyspnea	20–30
Sputum production	10–12
Hemoptysis	1–3
Chest pain	15–25
Skin lesions	10–28
Ocular symptoms	10–20
Joint complaints	5–17
Neurologic symptoms	2–5
Cardiac symptoms	1–5

and symptoms of respiratory sarcoidosis are present at some time during the disease. The true incidence of respiratory involvement may actually be higher, as biopsy specimens of patients with sarcoidosis whose lungs are radiographically and physiologically normal often reveal granulomas. Parenchymal lung involvement and lymph node enlargement are the most common thoracic manifestations. Airway, pleural, and blood vessel involvement are also well documented.

Lymph Node and Parenchymal Involvement

By international convention, a staging system for sarcoidosis has been devised based on the appearance of a patient's chest x-ray film (Table 2). Up to 8% of patients present with stage 0 disease. They have evidence of extrathoracic disease and normal chest x-ray findings. As mentioned, a high percentage of these patients have granulomas on lung biopsy, indicating subclinical involvement of the pulmonary parenchyma. Approximately 40%–60% of patients present with stage I disease. The chest x-ray films of these patients demonstrate bilateral hilar lymphadenopathy, with or without paratracheal adenopathy, but without radiographically apparent lung infiltrates. Stage II radiographs are noted in 15%–30% of patients at the time of diagnosis. These radiographs demonstrate bilateral hilar adenopathy (with or without paratracheal adenopathy) with associated lung field involvement. The remaining 10%–15% of patients with sarcoidosis present with stage III radiographs, which show lung field involvement only. Patients without adenopathy whose lung field involvement is notable for severe pulmonary fibrosis, volume loss, cysts, bullae, and honeycombing are defined as having stage IV disease by some (but not all) investigators (Fig. 2).

Radiographically, bilateral hilar adenopathy is the most common pattern of lymph node involvement in sarcoidosis. This enlargement can be striking, causing some to refer to the lymph nodes as ''potato'' nodes. Paratracheal adenopathy has been reported in up to 71% of cases. This adenopathy is less common on the left, because the left paratracheal lymph nodes are located more posteriorly, are smaller in size, and are fewer in number than their counterparts on the right. Aortopulmonary window and

subcarinal adenopathy are noted in 33%–75% and approximately 21% of patients, respectively. By virtue of their location, these lymph nodes can, on rare occasion, cause symptoms by compressing the esophagus and nearby bronchi and vessels. When sarcoidosis causes anterior mediastinal lymph node enlargement, hilar adenopathy is almost always present. Lymphomas, metastatic malignancies, and other pathologic conditions must be strongly considered when isolated anterior mediastinal adenopathy is present. Similarly, posterior mediastinal adenopathy and unilateral hilar adenopathy are rare in sarcoidosis and should cause the physician to pursue other diagnostic possibilities. Parenchymal involvement in sarcoidosis can take on a variety of radiographic appearances. It is most commonly symmetric, diffuse and reticular, reticulonodular, or finely nodular in appearance. Symmetric bilateral lesions of the upper lobe or lesions predominant in the mid-lung field are also well documented, as are diffuse alveolar infiltrates. Unilateral disease, multiple large nodules, and even solitary nodules have been reported. However, alternative diagnostic possibilities must always be looked for when these patterns are noted. When sarcoidosis progresses, the parenchymal infiltrates become coarser and coalesce, and pulmonary architecture becomes distorted. This can cause the development of bronchiectasis, cysts, bullae, and, at worst, a honeycombed lung with volume loss, signs of pulmonary hypertension, and cor pulmonale.

Computerized tomography (CT) and magnetic resonance imaging (MRI) of the chest are more sensitive than plain chest radiographs, as they can reveal focal pulmonary parenchymal abnormalities in patients with stage O or stage I disease by chest radiograph. It has been suggested that the presence of ground-glass densities on CT in sarcoidosis and other infiltrative lung diseases may correlate with an inflammatory state likely to be responsive to treatment. The practical value of this information in terms of prognosis or correlation with functional status remains to be determined.

The architectural distortion that takes place in patients with advanced sarcoidosis predisposes them to a number of complications. Areas of cavitation and bronchiectasis are susceptible to repeated infections. In addition, mycetoma caused by *Aspergillus* (and rarely other fungi) can form in these cavities and have been reported in as many as 40% of patients with cavitary disease. Progressive pleural thickening in the area around a cavity may be the earliest indication that an aspergilloma is forming. CT may be useful in demonstrating these structural abnormalities. Diagnosis requires the presence of IgG-precipitating antibodies to the fungus and demonstration of a mycetoma in the cavity by conventional chest radiography or CT. These aspergillomas can cause hemoptysis that, on occasion, may be life-threatening. Treatment of patients with mycetoma and massive hemoptysis is often problematic, as their underlying respiratory insufficiency precludes

TABLE 2. *Staging of sarcoidosis by chest radiograph*

Stage	Radiographic abnormality
0	None
I	Hilar, mediastinal, or paratracheal adenopathy
II	Hilar, mediastinal, or paratracheal adenopathy with pulmonary parenchymal abnormalities
III	Pulmonary parenchymal abnormalities without adenopathy
IV	Fibrobullous pulmonary paraenchymal disease without adenopathy

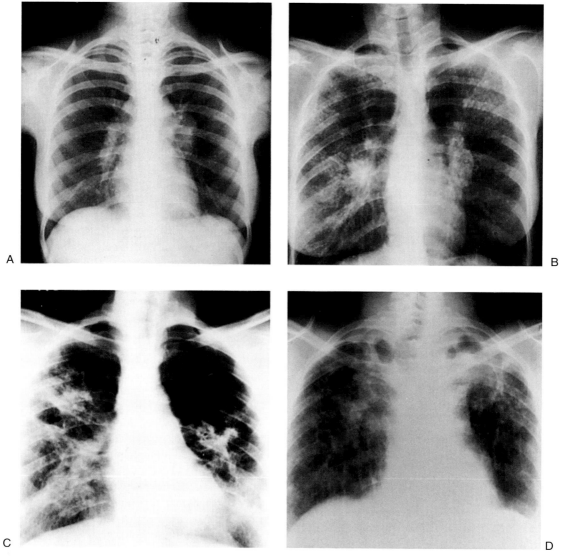

FIG. 2. Radiographs illustrating the different stages of sarcoidosis. **A:** Stage I. Bilateral hilar adenopathy and paratracheal adenopathy with normal lung fields. **B:** Stage II. Bilateral hilar adenopathy with interstitial lung field involvement. **C:** Stage III. Lung field involvement only. **D:** Stage IV. Severely fibrotic lungs with volume loss and cyst formation.

surgery for some and increases the risk of surgery for the others. In patients who cannot be treated surgically, anecdotal evidence suggests that bronchial arterial embolization and intracavitary instillation of amphotericin B may be useful. Less commonly, in patients with mycetoma a hypersensitivity reaction develops to the colonized fungus. This can be manifested as a bronchospastic lung disorder with many of the clinical and immunologic characteristics of allergic bronchopulmonary aspergillosis.

Airways Involvement

Endobronchial biopsy specimens reveal a granulomatous infiltration of the mucosa and submucosa in 30%–70% of patients with sarcoidosis. At its mildest,

this involvement does not alter the appearance of the bronchial mucosa. When more severe, nodules are seen, and a cobblestone pattern has been described. As in the interstitium of the lung, this granulomatous infiltration can lead to a fibrotic reaction causing fixed lesions and, in its most severe form, diffuse bronchial stenosis with bronchial occlusion (Fig. 3). Endobronchial involvement can be seen in all radiographic stages of the disease. The lesions may cause airway narrowing, atelectasis, and ventilation-perfusion mismatching. The clinical manifestations of patients with severe endobronchial involvement are often different from those of the usual patient with sarcoidosis. Like patients with asthma, chronic obstructive pulmonary disease (COPD), or upper airway obstruction, they can have repeated pneumo-

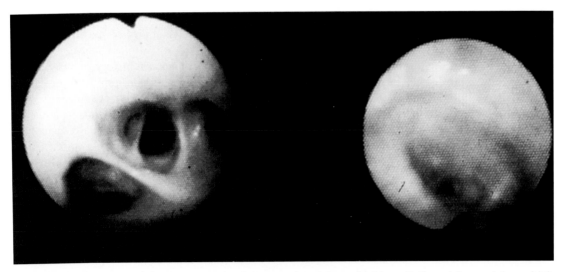

FIG. 3. Comparison of the appearance of a normal endobronchial tree (*left*) and the endobronchial tree of a patient with bronchial stenosis caused by sarcoidosis (*right*).

nias and bronchitis and experience dyspnea, stridor, chronic cough, and recurrent episodes of bronchospasm. Bronchiectasis may also result.

Pleural Involvement

Pleural involvement in sarcoidosis is relatively uncommon, occurring in 1%–12% of patients. This involvement can be manifested as pleural thickening, pleural effusion, or spontaneous pneumothorax. Effusions occur with equal frequency on the right and left and are bilateral 33% of the time. They are usually small or moderate in size. Massive effusions are rare. Pleural biopsy may show non-caseating granulomas, and presumably this granulomatous infiltration is the cause of the effusion. Vascular compression from mediastinal adenopathy is rarely a cause of pleural effusion in patients with sarcoidosis. The pleural fluid is usually exudative, occasionally hemorrhagic, and usually shows a predominance of lymphocytes. An increase in eosinophils may also be seen. Effusions have been described in patients with all radiographic stages of sarcoidosis. However, they are more common in patients with widespread parenchymal lung disease and have not been reported as the sole manifestation of the disease. The presence of a pleural effusion in a patient with sarcoidosis must always be interpreted with caution, and other causes of pleural disease, including tuberculosis, mycotic or bacterial infections, congestive heart failure, and malignancies, must always be considered. The natural history of pleural effusions in sarcoidosis is not totally known. Most appear to resolve without gross residua, either spontaneously or in association with steroid therapy. Progression to chronic pleural thickening has been reported.

Spontaneous pneumothorax in sarcoidosis is usually caused by the rupture of subpleural blebs or the necrosis of subpleural granulomas. This occurs most commonly in patients with advanced fibrotic lung disease with upper lobe bullae, but it can also occur in patients with stage O or stage I disease.

Pulmonary Vasculature

Granulomatous vasculitis involving both arteries and veins has been described in patients with sarcoidosis but is generally asymptomatic. On rare occasions, it can cause pulmonary hypertension.

Pulmonary Physiology

In 1940, Bruce and Wassen demonstrated a reduction in vital capacity and total lung capacity in the first study of the lung function of patients with sarcoidosis. Subsequent studies have confirmed these observations and have demonstrated that although the pulmonary physiologic parameters of some patients with sarcoidosis are normal, in most cases they are not. Like most other interstitial lung diseases, sarcoidosis commonly causes restrictive physiology and a gas transfer abnormality. The restrictive defect is manifested by reduced lung volumes and decreased lung compliance in the presence of normal large-airway function. The gas transfer abnormality is characterized by a reduced diffusing capacity for carbon monoxide.

Dysfunction of large and small airways resulting from the peribronchial distribution of granulomas is also an important component of the pathophysiology of sarcoidosis. Large-airways obstruction with a decreased FEV_1/FVC ratio is noted in a minority of patients. It has been described in all radiographic stages of sarcoidosis but is more common in patients with stage III or stage IV disease. It is usually caused by bronchial distortion and/or bronchiectasis from granulomas, edema, and scarring. It is rarely reversible and may cause symptoms of wheezing and dyspnea. If appropriately tested for, small-airways dysfunction can be seen in the majority of patients with sarcoidosis. These alterations are the result of peribronchial and endobronchial involvement or airways hyperreactivity and can be seen in all radiographic stages of the disease.

Patients with normal or mildly abnormal pulmonary function tests usually have normal alveolar-arterial oxygen gradients, normal arterial blood gases, and normal exercise tests. Occasionally, exercise testing unmasks modest abnormalities in the alveolar-arterial oxygen gradient, even in patients with stage O or stage I sarcoidosis. As the disease worsens, the alveolar-arterial oxygen gradient at rest increases. This is followed by exercise-induced desaturation and then hypoxia at rest. When carbon dioxide retention is noted, it is almost always the result of advanced disease, often with incipient respiratory failure.

The fact that a significant percentage of patients with stage O or stage I disease on chest x-ray films have restrictive pulmonary function demonstrates that pulmonary function tests are more sensitive in detecting parenchymal lung disease than are chest radiographs. Increases in alveolar-arterial oxygen gradient with exercise may be the most sensitive physiologic parameter, followed by the carbon monoxide diffusing capacity and then the vital capacity. Overall, the degree of physiologic impairment in sarcoidosis correlates with the radiographic stage of disease. Patients with stage O or stage I disease usually have mild physiologic derangements, and patients with stage III or stage IV disease tend to be the most severely restricted (and/or obstructed). The overlap between these categories is large enough, however, to make it difficult and not clinically useful to predict a given patient's pulmonary function from the radiographic stage.

Studies of structure-function relationships in sarcoidosis have shown that pulmonary function tests generally correlate with the overall severity of morphologic changes on lung biopsy. Patients with normal or minimally abnormal pulmonary function tend to have mild inflammatory changes with minimal fibrosis on biopsy. Patients with severely abnormal pulmonary function tend to have more extensive inflammatory changes and/or severe fibrotic changes on biopsy. However, these studies have also shown that the correlation between physiologic abnormalities and pulmonary histology has limitations. Pulmonary function tests may differentiate extremes of histology but do not accurately differentiate moderate from severe disease. In addition, pulmonary function tests do not distinguish the degree to which a defect is caused by interstitial pneumonitis, granulomas, or fibrosis. Thus, in a given individual at a single point in time, pulmonary function tests cannot predict with absolute certainty the severity, character, or reversibility of the histologic lesion that is present.

Studies of the natural history of sarcoidosis have demonstrated that pulmonary physiologic alterations over time tend to correlate with changes in the severity and activity of disease. Patients whose parenchymal lesions are improving roentgenographically usually have an improvement in their vital capacity and diffusing capacity. Similarly, patients whose parenchymal sarcoidosis is radiographically stable or worsening usually exhibit declines in their vital capacity and/or diffusing capacity. The correlations between histologic severity, disease progression, and pulmonary function provide the rationale for the use of pulmonary function tests in the ongoing evaluation of patients with sarcoidosis. It is important to point out, however, that at the present time there are no pulmonary function criteria that allow the clinician to predict accurately the natural history or response to therapy of a given patient.

Extrathoracic Manifestations

Ophthalmic

In 1936, Heerfordt's syndrome of uveitis, salivary gland involvement, seventh cranial nerve palsy, and fever was recognized to be a form of sarcoidosis. Subsequent studies have shown that the eye and adnexa are involved in 11%–60% of patients with sarcoidosis and that ocular involvement is an important cause of morbidity in this disorder. The types of ocular disease noted in patients with sarcoidosis can be conveniently classified according to whether they involve the anterior eye, the posterior eye, or the orbit and other structures.

The anterior structures of the eye are involved in 80%–90% of patients with ophthalmic sarcoidosis. Granulomatous uveitis and granulomatous conjunctivitis are the two most common lesions. Iris nodules, band keratopathy, and interstitial keratitis occur far less frequently. The granulomatous uveitis can be acute or chronic. Patients with acute uveitis can experience the sudden onset of unilateral optic injection with tearing, blurred vision, and photophobia. Physical examination often reveals circumcorneal ciliary injection, aqueous cells and flares, and "mutton fat" keratitic precipitates. In contrast, chronic uveitis develops more slowly and insidiously. It may be unilateral or bilateral, and when symptomatic, it usually causes pain and blurring of vision. Although keratitic precipitates are often noted, ciliary injection can be absent. Chronic uveitis can lead to adhesions between the iris and lens, glaucoma, cataract formation, and blindness. Chronic uveitis is often seen in association with other manifestations of chronic sarcoidosis, such as lupus pernio, cutaneous plaques, bone lesions, and pulmonary fibrosis. Granulomatous involvement of the conjunctivae occurs in 10%–60% of patients. These conjunctival lesions can appear as tiny, translucent, pale yellow conjunctival follicles. Biopsy specimens of normal-appearing conjunctivae also can show granulomatous inflammation. This involvement can be asymptomatic or cause irritation, resulting in a gritty feeling in the eye.

The posterior structures of the eye are involved in approximately 25% of patients with ocular sarcoidosis. The retina, vitreous, and optic nerve can all be affected. Chorioretinitis, periphlebitis, and chorioretinal nodules are the most frequent lesions. Periphlebitis may be associated with visible evidence of lymphocytic infiltration of venous walls, termed "candle wax drippings." Cellular aggregates (particularly CD4$^+$ T lymphocytes), hemorrhage and opacities in the vitreous, and local neovascularization are less common. Optic nerve involvement in sarcoidosis can take a number of forms. Papilledema resulting from increased intracranial pressure, optic atrophy, papillitis, optic neuritis, and optic disk granulomas are all well documented. Ninety-five percent of patients with posterior eye involvement also have anterior eye involvement. In addition, the presence of posterior eye involvement should alert the clinician to possible concomitant central nervous system disease, as the incidence of central nervous system involvement is increased in these patients.

Granulomatous infiltration of the lacrimal gland is the most common form of orbital involvement, occurring in 5%–15% of patients with ocular sarcoidosis. It is usually bilateral, often associated with parotid swelling, and can be the sole ocular manifestation. Chronic mass effect from extralacrimal soft-tissue involvement may also be seen. Hyposecretion of tears may occur with any of these and can cause a severe sicca syndrome mimicking that of Sjögren's syndrome. Retro-orbital granulomas are a less common orbital manifestation of sarcoidosis that have been reported to cause unilateral proptosis and hamper extraocular muscle function.

Lymphadenopathy

Granulomatous infiltration of lymph nodes is found in up to 95% of patients with sarcoidosis and may be solely microscopic. Granulomatous involvement may cause visible and palpable adenopathy that is usually symmetric and rarely massive. The nodes tend to be firm, rubbery, discrete, mobile, and painless and are rarely associated with changes in the overlying skin, ulceration, or sinus formation. All major lymph node groups can be involved. Cervical, axillary, epitrochlear, and inguinal lymphadenopathies are found in the order noted. The cervical lymph nodes are enlarged on the right more often than on the left and in the posterior triangle more often than in the anterior triangle. Preauricular, postauricular, submaxillary, submental, mesenteric, and retroperitoneal nodes

also can be enlarged. Occipital lymphadenopathy is rare. Massive involvement of retroperitoneal or abdominal lymph nodes may rarely cause abdominal discomfort sufficient to warrant systemic therapy.

Cutaneous Involvement

Cutaneous involvement is seen in 20%–50% of patients with sarcoidosis and can be conveniently divided into two categories: nonspecific, nongranulomatous lesions and specific, granulomatous lesions. Erythema nodosum is the principal nongranulomatous skin lesion, occurring in 9%–17% of patients. Most commonly it is manifested as subcutaneous, erythematous, tender nodules that involve the anterior tibial and other extensor surfaces. Its onset is usually sudden, and its appearance may herald the beginning of the disease. It may be accompanied by a flulike syndrome with fever, fatigue, and polyarthralgia. In addition, it often exists in association with acute uveitis, an elevated sedimentation rate, and bilateral hilar adenopathy. As the lesions of erythema nodosum resolve, they become ecchymotic (erythema contusiformis) and can leave localized areas of hyperpigmentation. Biopsy specimens of erythema nodosum reveal a septal panniculitis. Erythema nodosum is not specific for sarcoidosis. The clinical picture and histology of erythema nodosum associated with sarcoidosis are indistinguishable from those of erythema nodosum associated with other diseases. However, the presence of erythema nodosum in sarcoidosis appears to have prognostic import. Patients presenting with erythema nodosum, polyarthralgias, and bilateral hilar adenopathy (Löfgren's syndrome) have a particularly favorable outcome, with at least 90% experiencing a spontaneous resolution of their disease within 6 to 12 months. In addition, in white patients, erythema nodosum alone may correlate with an improved prognosis.

Granulomatous skin lesions occur in 10%–35% of patients with sarcoidosis. In general, their presence confers an unfavorable prognosis, suggests a higher likelihood of extensive disease, and may warrant local or systemic treatment. Lupus pernio is a granulomatous lesion that is specific for sarcoidosis. It is a chronic, violaceous, nodular or plaquelike eruption on the nose, cheeks, and ears (Fig. 4) and can be associated with fusiform swelling and mutilation of the fingers. Its onset is usually insidious, its course is usually chronic, and it commonly results in significant scarring and deformity. It is most common in women between 40 and 60 years of age and is often associated with other manifestations of chronic sarcoidosis, such as pulmonary fibrosis, bone lesions, uveitis, and upper respiratory tract involvement. Granulomatous infiltration also may cause papules, plaques, nodules, ulcers, ichthyosiform lesions, psoriasis-like lesions, and scarring alopecia. Scarring is not a frequent outcome of these lesions, as it is in lupus pernio.

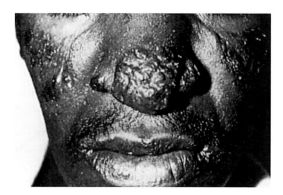

FIG. 4. Raised lesions of lupus pernio.

Neuroendocrine Involvement

Sarcoidosis causes clinically detectable nervous system disease in 10% of patients. Pathologic studies have shown that subclinical nervous system infiltration occurs in up to 15% of patients. Among patients with clinical neurosarcoidosis, 50%–75% have neurologic manifestations as their presenting feature. Multiple neurologic lesions are present in one third of such patients. Any structure in the central or peripheral nervous system may be involved, resulting in a wide spectrum of clinical disease. Neurosarcoidosis may cause significant morbidity. It is also associated with a 10% mortality rate, which is approximately twice that of sarcoidosis in general.

A basal granulomatous meningitis is the most common pathologic lesion in the central nervous system of patients with sarcoidosis. It is clinically apparent in approximately two thirds and pathologically present in virtually all patients with central nervous system involvement. The basal predilection of these lesions explains the frequent involvement of the optic nerve, optic chiasm, pituitary, hypothalamus, and periventricular areas. This granulomatous meningitis also can extend along the perivascular space and disrupt the local parenchyma and vascular structures.

Cranial nerve involvement has been reported in 24%–73% of patients with neurosarcoidosis. Seventh (facial) nerve involvement is the most common neurologic manifestation of sarcoidosis. It usually presents as a unilateral peripheral lesion but may also occur bilaterally or in association with other cranial nerve abnormalities. The resulting palsy generally resolves spontaneously, but relapses can occur and result in sequelae such as spasms and contractions. The optic nerve is the next most frequently involved cranial nerve; symptoms and signs include decreased or blurred vision, papilledema, optic atrophy, visual field defects, and pupillary abnormalities. Visual evoked potentials may be abnormal in an asymptomatic patient with optic nerve involvement. Cranial nerves IX and X are the third most commonly involved cranial nerve complex in sarcoidosis; their involvement results in dys-

phagia, hoarseness, an absent gag reflex, an immobile soft palate, and vocal cord dysfunction. The eighth cranial nerve is the fourth most commonly affected; involvement results in deafness, vertigo, and a sensory-neural hearing loss.

Peripheral nerve involvement has been noted in 15%–18% of patients with sarcoidosis presenting as a mononeuropathy or polyneuropathy with sensory and/or motor abnormalities. As a result, pain, paresthesias, muscle weakness, and depression of tendon reflexes may be found. In one series, ulnar and peroneal nerves were the most frequently involved. A Guillain-Barré–like syndrome has also been described.

Meningeal involvement, with aseptic meningitis, has been reported to be present in 64% of patients with neurosarcoidosis, although most are asymptomatic. In these patients, examination of the cerebrospinal fluid generally shows hyperproteinorrhachia, hypoglycorrhachia, and a lymphocytic pleocytosis. Cerebrospinal fluid levels of angiotensin-converting enzyme are elevated in 55% of patients. Cerebrospinal fluid levels of angiotensin-converting enzyme must be interpreted with caution, however, as similar elevations may be found in the setting of bacterial meningitis and tumors of the central nervous system. In patients with known systemic sarcoidosis and suspected neurosarcoidosis, an elevated level of angiotensin-converting enzyme in the cerebrospinal fluid may be helpful in following disease progression or response to therapy.

Hypothalamic-pituitary abnormalities have been noted in approximately 25% of patients with neurosarcoidosis. These patients manifest signs and symptoms caused by (1) anterior pituitary insufficiency, (2) abnormalities of water metabolism, and (3) compression or infiltration of the nearby optic chiasm. The pituitary and hypothalamus can be separately involved. Most studies show extensive infiltration and/or mass lesions in the hypothalamus, with a lesser degree of pituitary involvement. Central diabetes insipidus is the most common manifestation of hypothalamic sarcoidosis. Hypothalamic hyperphagia has also been described. Anterior pituitary insufficiency most commonly presents as gonadal dysfunction with decreased libido, impotence, or amenorrhea, and less commonly as hypothyroidism or adrenal insufficiency. A significant percentage of these patients have elevated prolactin levels and normal pituitary responses to hypothalamic releasing hormones, suggesting that the hypothalamus and hypothalamic stalk are the major sites of involvement.

The abnormal water metabolism that is found in most patients with hypothalamic-pituitary sarcoidosis appears to be of multifactorial origin. In some patients it is the result of partial or complete diabetes insipidus. Other patients appear to have primary abnormalities of thirst. Either or both these abnormalities may result in chronic hypernatremia.

Granulomatous masses may involve any part of the central nervous system. Whereas most of these are diffuse or infiltrating, some are manifested as space-occupying lesions. The clinical presentation of these lesions is not significantly different from that of mass lesions caused by other processes and can include headaches, seizures, localized neurologic dysfunction, papilledema, and uncal or cerebellar tonsillar herniation.

Intracranial hypertension can occur in sarcoidosis as a result of a number of mechanisms. Involvement of the ependyma and choroid plexus can alter cerebrospinal fluid dynamics. Chronic meningitis can cause obliteration of the subarachnoid space and aqueductal stenosis, and intraventricular granulomas can cause outlet obstruction of the fourth ventricle.

The symptoms that result from central nervous system lesions in sarcoidosis can vary depending on the anatomic site of the infiltrative process and the degree to which intracranial pressure is increased. Increased intracranial pressure can cause headache, nausea, vomiting, lethargy, and cranial nerve palsies. Cortical infiltration can mimic cerebrovascular accidents, and basal ganglion involvement can lead to a wide range of extrapyramidal manifestations, including choreiform movements, hemiballismus, and parkinsonism. Seizures occur in 5%–22% of patients with neurologic sarcoidosis. *Grand mal* seizures are most common, but partial, jacksonian, psychomotor, and myoclonic seizures can occur. The presence of seizures is generally associated with a poor prognosis. Patients may respond to corticosteroid therapy. Low-dose wholebrain radiation therapy has also been described as potentially beneficial.

Vascular compromise, manifested as strokes or transient ischemic attacks, rarely occurs in sarcoidosis. This is surprising, as perivascular and vascular infiltration of the meningeal and cerebral vessels, often with local infarction, is well described pathologically. Spinal cord involvement is also extremely rare in sarcoidosis; when present, it is caused by local meningeal involvement with extramedullary compression or intramedullary mass formation.

The diagnosis of neurosarcoidosis is generally facilitated by evidence of sarcoidosis in other organs. Compatible neurologic findings supported by CT, MRI, or cerebrospinal fluid data in the setting of histologic confirmation from other tissues may be adequate for diagnostic purposes. However, this may not obviate the need to examine neurologic tissue in situations in which other etiologies cannot adequately be ruled out.

The diagnosis of nervous system sarcoidosis in the absence of other manifestations of sarcoidosis may be extremely difficult. Biopsy of neurologic tissue or tissue from other, seemingly less involved organs (such as the lung or conjunctivae) may be necessary. Guidance for these biopsies may be provided by CT, MRI, pulmonary function tests, slit-lamp examination, or gallium scanning.

The abnormalities noted with these studies are, however, often not specific for sarcoidosis.

Muscle

Skeletal muscle involvement in sarcoidosis can be documented in up to 80% of patients. In the vast majority, this involvement is asymptomatic. Symptomatic muscle disease may be manifested as nodules, myalgias, and frank myopathy. Acute myopathy, although rare, is more common in women. It presents as a polymyositis-like syndrome with muscle pain, weakness, and tenderness. Chronic myopathy is somewhat more common and generally poorly responsive to corticosteroids. It presents with the gradual onset of weakness and wasting and is associated with elevated levels of muscle enzymes and a myopathic electromyogram.

Liver

Although the liver is involved pathologically in 60%–90% of patients with sarcoidosis, clinically significant hepatic disease is infrequent. Small periportal granulomas are noted most commonly. A nonspecific mononuclear cell infiltrate with varying degrees of fibrosis can also be seen. The majority of patients are asymptomatic and have only low-grade increases in serum alkaline phosphatase, transaminases, or bilirubin levels. In some cases, modest hepatomegaly may be found. In a minority of patients, more serious involvement may take the form of chronic hepatocellular injury with secondary cirrhosis, hepatic encephalopathy, portal hypertension, or bleeding esophageal varices. Cases of Budd-Chiari syndrome have been reported. Sarcoidosis may also be associated with chronic intrahepatic cholestasis, which can be difficult to differentiate from primary biliary cirrhosis, and with extrahepatic biliary tract obstruction resulting from granulomatous involvement of the hepatic duct and surrounding lymph nodes.

Hepatic sarcoidosis may also be manifested as a fever of unknown origin (FUO). Patients with hepatic sarcoidosis presenting with FUO often also have abdominal organ, spleen, and lymph node involvement.

Spleen

Granulomatous infiltration of the spleen occurs in up to 60%–90% of patients with sarcoidosis; disease is usually clinically silent. Splenomegaly develops in 5%–15% of patients; in a minority of these, complications such as hypersplenism, splenic rupture, portal hypertension, and abdominal pain develop. Sarcoidosis is only one of many disorders that cause splenic granulomas. Thus, it is important to interpret splenic granulomas in the clinical context in which they are noted.

Heart

The most common cardiac abnormality in sarcoidosis is cor pulmonale, resulting from severe pulmonary disease. Primary cardiac involvement also occurs and is clinically recognizable in 3%–5% of patients. Granulomas, however, are found in up to 30% of patients with sarcoidosis at autopsy. No portion of the heart is immune to granulomatous infiltration. The myocardium is most frequently involved, with the left ventricular free wall being affected most commonly. Involvement of the ventricular septum, the right ventricular free wall, and the atrial wall follow in order of decreasing frequency. When the left ventricle is involved, the granulomas are most commonly located in the papillary muscles and the free wall below the papillary muscles. The extent of infiltration and scarring and its proximity to vital structures such as the atrioventricular node and conduction pathways appear to be crucial determinants of the clinical import of cardiac involvement. The abnormalities that result from these lesions are quite varied, including arrhythmias, bundle branch blocks, congestive heart failure, mitral regurgitation, ventricular aneurysms, pericardial effusions, and sudden death.

Ventricular tachycardia is the most frequent major arrhythmia occurring in patients with cardiac sarcoidosis. Its appearance usually indicates extensive inflammatory scarring of the heart. Ventricular fibrillation and atrial arrhythmias are less commonly noted. When atrial arrhythmias exist, they are usually the result of atrial dilatation arising from left ventricular dysfunction and not the result of direct granulomatous infiltration. Complete heart block and bundle branch blocks also occur. They are usually caused by involvement of the cephalad portion of the intraventricular septum near the atrioventricular node and conduction bundles, respectively.

Valvular disease occurs in 3% of patients. Mitral regurgitation is well described and may be the result of papillary muscle dysfunction caused by infiltration of the papillary muscle or the left ventricular free wall below the papillary muscle. More often, the lesion is the result of altered papillary muscle dynamics resulting from left ventricular dilatation or dysfunction.

Extensive ventricular involvement can cause congestive heart failure. Ventricular aneurysms that exacerbate congestive failure and arrhythmias can also form. An association between long-term corticosteroid therapy and the development of aneurysms has been reported. However, definitive documentation that steroid therapy predisposes to aneurysm development is still lacking.

There are a number of reasons why establishing a clinical diagnosis of cardiac sarcoidosis may be problematic. First, the clinical manifestations of the disease—chest pain, palpitations, congestive heart failure, electrocardiographic changes, syncope, and light-headedness—are also manifestations of other, more common cardiac disorders. Second, when sarcoidosis causes cardiac dysfunction, it often does not cause dysfunction in other organ systems. Thus, the majority of patients with cardiac sarcoidosis do not have overt lung, eye, or skin involvement that might cause a physician to suspect this disorder.

As many as half of all patients with cardiac sarcoidosis may have electrocardiographic abnormalities. Ventricular arrhythmias are evident in up to 22% of patients. Because of this, Holter monitoring has been suggested as part of the routine evaluation of patients with sarcoid. Subclinical cardiac dysfunction can occasionally be detected by cardiopulmonary exercise testing. Endomyocardial biopsies are useful when they yield myocardial granulomas, but a nonspecific lymphocytic myocarditis is commonly encountered. In addition, the diagnostic sensitivity of endomyocardial biopsies is likely quite variable, given the patchy distribution of granulomatous changes in the heart and the inability of the procedure to obtain samples from the area of the heart that is likely involved. Lastly, a number of investigators have described a pattern of inhomogeneity of thallium uptake in the myocardium of patients with cardiac sarcoidosis. Involved areas are visualized as thallium defects at rest, which then disappear with exercise. This "reverse distribution" pattern is the opposite of that seen during thallium imaging in patients with ischemic coronary disease. The sensitivity and specificity of the "reverse distribution pattern" has not been defined. It is clear that the criteria for patient selection for exercise testing, endomyocardial biopsy, and thallium scanning are poorly defined, and the prognostic significance of cardiac abnormalities found are still unknown.

Electrolyte Abnormalities

Approximately 11% of patients with sarcoidosis are hypercalcemic. The hypercalcemia tends to be episodic in patients with acute sarcoidosis and persistent in patients with chronic disease. It can be mild or severe and life-threatening, and in some patients it is the sole reason for treatment with systemic steroids. Hypercalciuria occurs in 15%–60% of patients with sarcoidosis. When severe, it can cause nephrolithiasis, nephrocalcinosis, and renal insufficiency.

The hypercalcemia and hypercalciuria of sarcoidosis are at least partially a consequence of increased intestinal calcium absorption. This increased absorption is the result of elevated levels of 1,25-dihydroxyvitamin D caused by the accelerated conversion of 25-hydroxyvitamin D to 1,25-dihydroxyvitamin D. The increased 1-hydroxylation occurs in a parathyroid hormone-independent fashion in the macrophages of sarcoidal granulomas. Thus, sunlight exposure worsens the hypercalcemia seen in these patients.

Increased osteolysis also appears to play a role in the calcium disorder seen in some patients with sarcoidosis. This heightened resorption may may be a direct effect of osseous granulomas, or of bone-resorbing soluble factor(s) such as osteoclast-activating factor.

Kidney

Renal insufficiency in sarcoidosis is generally the result of hypercalcemia and/or hypercalciuria. Granulomatous changes are noted in the kidneys of 4%–40% of patients but rarely cause clinically significant renal dysfunction.

Granulomatous renal arteritis, glomerulonephritis, and altered renal tubular function have been rarely reported. Some investigators feel that sarcoid nephritis is a steroid-responsive disorder. Others believe that although steroid responses can be seen, relapses are common, and renal failure often occurs within 5 years of the clinical onset of the disease.

Joints

Joint signs and symptoms occur in approximately 10%–35% of patients with sarcoidosis. The major manifestations are an acute and chronic polyarthritis.

The acute polyarthritis is seen early in the course of the disease. It is usually a symmetric peripheral arthritis and periarthritis that most commonly involves the ankles and knees, and less commonly the elbows, wrists, and the small joints of hands and feet. Histologically, there is a nonspecific inflammatory synovitis. The clinical presentation includes pain, tenderness, restricted motion, soft-tissue swelling, and joint effusions that can be transient and occasionally precede other signs of the disease. This form of joint involvement is frequently seen in association with bilateral hilar adenopathy, fever, and erythema nodosum (Löfgren's syndrome), and is generally associated with a high rate of spontaneous remission. Erythrocyte sedimentation rates may be elevated. In the absence of bone involvement, radiographic studies are usually normal or reveal soft-tissue swelling. Rarely, periarticular osteoporosis is noted. Acute polyarthritis occurs more commonly in women than in men. It also is more likely to develop and be associated with uveitis, erythema nodosum, and spontaneous remission in individuals who are HLA-B8-positive.

A relapsing chronic polyarthritis develops in 3%–6% of patients with chronic sarcoidosis. Some of these patients have had a previous episode of acute sarcoid polyarthritis, but the majority have not. The shoulders, knees, wrists, ankles, and small articulations of the hands are most commonly involved. Erythema nodosum and fever are uncommon. This involvement can be asymmetric and is rarely monarticular. Radiographic studies reveal soft-tissue swelling, periarticular osteoporosis, mild narrowing of the joint space, and well-defined eccentric erosions. In addition, articular destruction and collapse may result from inflammatory extension into subchondral bone. Histologically, the process is characterized by a granulomatous inflammation of the synovium, articulations, and tendon sheaths. Synovial fluid analysis reveals increased protein, increased leukocytes, and occasionally a lymphocytosis of the joint fluid.

Bone

Osseous involvement occurs radiographically in 1%–13% of patients and is generally associated with chronic sarcoidosis. It is more common in blacks than in whites and is rarely seen without chronic cutaneous lesions (such as lupus pernio), ocular sarcoidosis, and overt lung involvement. Radiographically, sarcoidosis can affect the skeleton in a focal or generalized and usually asymmetric fashion and can cause osteolytic and, less commonly, osteosclerotic lesions. In all cases, these lesions are not specific for sarcoidosis, radiographically resembling the lesions of other diseases. Osteoporosis, cortical thinning, well-defined cysts, and rarefactions are the usual types of lytic lesions. They are encountered most frequently in the hands, with the wrists and feet being less commonly involved. When diffuse, they can cause a latticework or honeycomb pattern. In general, they are not associated with periosteal reactions or sinus tracts, and the joints are not involved except when bone adjacent to the joint is destroyed. Osseous sarcoidosis is generally asymptomatic except in cases in which soft-tissue swelling or bony deformity causes local symptoms. The prognosis for the small number of patients with progressive destructive bony changes is poor, as these lesions tend to be unresponsive to treatment.

Upper Respiratory Tract

Sarcoidosis involves the upper respiratory tract in approximately 2%–6% of patients. Although occasionally seen as an isolated lesion, it is most common in symptomatic patients with manifestations of chronic sarcoidosis, including lupus pernio. The nasal mucosa, pharynx, larynx, nasal bones, and palate can all be involved. Sarcoidosis causes the nasal mucosa to appear erythematous and granular. Epistaxis, stuffiness, crusting, and nasal discharge are common symptoms. In addition, adhesions, polypoid lesions, submucosal nodules, ulcerations, septal perforations, paranasal sinus extension, osteolytic destruction of the nasal bone, and saddle-nose deformities have all been described. Biopsies of the nasal turbinate may need to be performed to differentiate sarcoidosis from other nasal disorders.

Hematologic Manifestations

Hematologic manifestations of sarcoidosis include anemia, lymphopenia, eosinophilia, and thrombocytopenia. Of these, lymphopenia is the most common, occurring in more than half of patients with active disease. A low CD4 count is seen in the peripheral blood, although BAL often reveals an increased number of CD4 cells. Examination of the bone marrow may reveal granulomatous changes.

ESTABLISHING THE DIAGNOSIS

To establish the diagnosis of sarcoidosis, three criteria must be met: (1) The patient's clinical and radiographic presentation must be compatible with sarcoidosis, (2) a biopsy must demonstrate noncaseating epithelioid cell granulomas, and (3) other causes of granulomatous infiltration must be carefully excluded.

The first criterion for diagnosis is usually not difficult to meet, even though the clinical presentation of sarcoidosis varies widely depending on the type and extent of organ involvement. Tissue biopsy specimens can be obtained from a number of sites in the body. The sensitivity of some biopsy techniques for making the diagnosis of sarcoid are detailed in Table 3. The optimal site from which to take a specimen depends on the clinical manifestations, personal preferences, and the procedures that are performed proficiently at a given institution. The gold standard procedure is thoracotomy with open lung biopsy and lymph node sampling, which yields noncaseating granulomas in 90%–100% of patients with sarcoid. Muscle biopsy, scalene node biopsy, and mediastinoscopy also have high sensitivity. However, because of the invasive nature of these procedures and their small but definite incidence of serious complications, they are not the initial diagnostic procedure of choice. Thoracoscopic biopsy may also have a high yield. However, experience with this approach is still quite limited. At our institution, bronchoscopy with transbronchial biopsies is often the procedure of first choice. Because granulomas tend to congregate in the peribronchial area, the diagnostic yield of transbronchial biopsy is high. The procedure can be performed with topical anesthesia in an awake patient with minimal discomfort, and the risk for major complications (pneumothorax, bleeding, respiratory distress) is low. With bronchoscopy, granulomas are obtained in 70%–90% of patients with Stage I disease, 85%–95% of patients with Stage II disease, and 80%–90% of patients with Stage III disease. To achieve this level of sensitivity, it is recommended that at least 4–10 biopsies be obtained. 85%–95% of patients with stage II disease, and 80%–90% of patients with stage III disease. An added advantage of bronchoscopy is that it allows other specimens to be collected for cytologic and microbiologic examination to help rule out other conditions.

Biopsy of the skin, conjunctivae, salivary glands, and lacrimal glands may also reveal the diagnosis. Skin biopsies are useful only when the skin is clinically involved by lesions other than erythema nodosum. Biopsies of normal skin and erythema nodosum lesions provide little help in establishing the diagnosis. For conjunctival biopsy to be optimally sensitive, biopsy of clinically involved conjunctivae is necessary, and the fixed tissue must be carefully sectioned and intensively examined. The utility of

TABLE 3. *Selected biopsy sites in sarcoidosis*

Site	Percentage of patients with sarcoidosis having a positive biopsy result	Comments
Skin	30–90	Biopsy of normal skin or erythema nodosum of little value
Liver	75	Large number of diseases cause hepatic granulomas; must be interpreted with caution
Muscle	50–85	Optimal sensitivity requires large biopsy specimen with intensive sectioning and pathologic examination
Conjunctiva	10–60	
Minor salivary gland	58	
Lacrimal gland	21	Higher sensitivity if only enlarged gland or glands that take up gallium 67 are sampled
Scalene lymph node	47–82	
Mediastinoscopy		
Stage I	90–95	
Stage II	90–95	
Stage III	50–60	
Bronchoscopy with transbronchial biopsy		Optimal sensitivity requires up to 4–10 biopsy specimens
Stage I	70–90	
Stage II	85–95	
Stage III	90–100	
Open lung biopsy	90–100	

blind biopsies of normal conjunctivae is still controversial. Similarly, lacrimal biopsies are positive most frequently when the gland is enlarged or positive on gallium scan.

The third criterion for diagnosing sarcoidosis is the exclusion of other causes of tissue granulomatosis (Table 4). Mycobacterial infection, fungal infection, berylliosis, hypersensitivity pneumonitis, granulomatous vasculitis, foreign-body granulomas, and granulomatous reactions in lymph nodes draining malignancies all need to be considered. Mycobacterial and fungal infections can usually be excluded by appropriate staining and culturing of tissue and secretions. However, the proper use and utility of PCR are still being evaluated. In addition, although up to 50% of patients with sarcoidosis are anergic, they usually demonstrate cutaneous sensitivity to tuberculin when actively infected with *M. tuberculosis*. A thorough history may be all that is required to rule out berylliosis and hypersensitivity pneumonitis. When hypersensitivity pneumonitis needs to be considered in greater depth, IgG-precipitating antibodies to the suspected causal antigen should be sought. The beryllium-induced blast transformation assay may be used to make a diagnosis of berylliosis. Histologic examination alone may be adequate to rule out the granulomatous vasculitides, foreign-body granulomas, and concomitant malignancies. If uncertainty remains, a biopsy specimen from a second site may be required.

Clinical findings and liver biopsy may not allow the physician to differentiate with confidence chronic intrahepatic cholestasis caused by sarcoidosis from primary biliary cirrhosis. Assays for serum antimitochondrial antibodies can be helpful in these cases, because they are positive in 99% of patients with primary biliary cirrhosis and are usually negative in sarcoidosis. In addition, the demon-

stration of extrahepatic granulomas can be used to support a diagnosis of sarcoidosis.

Crohn's disease also can be difficult to differentiate from sarcoidosis. Both are characterized by the presence of noncaseating granulomas and may be associated with similar dermatologic, hepatic, and ocular lesions. In addition, patients with Crohn's disease may have abnormalities on pulmonary function tests and increased numbers of OKT4$^+$ lymphocytes on BAL. At present, these two diseases are probably best distinguished on the basis of clinical differences. Crohn's disease is usually localized to the digestive tract. In contrast, sarcoidosis is a systemic disease with prominent respiratory, ophthalmic, and cutaneous lesions.

Asymptomatic patients with normal physical examination findings and bilateral hilar adenopathy and patients with bilateral hilar adenopathy and erythema nodosum or uveitis have sarcoidosis with such a high frequency that biopsy confirmation of the diagnosis may not be necessary. This view, however, remains somewhat controversial. Many still feel that histologic confirmation of the diagnosis is essential, as infections, particularly tuberculosis and fungal infections, and neoplasms, particularly lymphomas and primary lung cancers, can cause asymptomatic hilar adenopathy.

Gallium 67 scanning, measurement of serum angiotensin-converting enzyme levels, and BAL with analysis of the recovered cell populations were felt to provide highly specific information allowing a diagnosis of sarcoidosis. However, all these tests are not sufficiently sensitive or specific to be used alone to establish the diagnosis. Gallium scans are positive in only two thirds of patients with sarcoidosis, and increased gallium uptake is seen in many other inflammatory lung disorders. Whereas gallium uptake in cranial, mediastinal, and hilar areas has been postulated to be helpful in diagnosing sarcoidosis, the specificity of these patterns is problematic. Serum levels of angiotensin-converting enzyme are elevated in only 50%–80% of patients with sarcoidosis. Although rare, angiotensin-converting enzyme levels can also be elevated in a wide spectrum of granulomatous and nongranulomatous disorders (Table 5). A predominantly lymphocytic BALF is also not specific for sarcoidosis, being present in hypersensitivity pneumonitis, berylliosis, lymphomas, and tuberculosis.

A positive Kveim-Siltzbach test result has also been proposed as specific for sarcoidosis. The test is performed by injecting a sterile suspension of sarcoidal tissue intradermally. In patients who have a positive Kveim test result, a nodule will form at the site of the injection in 2 to 6 weeks. The test is then completed by taking a biopsy sample of the nodule and demonstrating that it contains noncaseating granulomas. Many investigators have reported that with properly standardized extract, the test is sensitive and specific for sarcoidosis. However, it is positive most often in patients with typical sarcoidosis. It is

TABLE 4. *Differential diagnosis of noncaseating granulomas*

Infectious diseases
    Mycobacteria
    Fungi
    Leprosy
    Syphilis
    Cat scratch disease
    Parasitic infection
Inflammatory diseases
    Sarcoidosis
    Berylliosis
    Hypersensitivity pneumonitis
    Granulomatous vasculitides
    Eosinophilic granuloma
    Foreign body reactions
    Biliary cirrhosis
    Crohn's disease
Neoplastic diseases
    Lymphoma
    Carcinoma
Other
    Hypogammaglobulinemia

TABLE 5. *Selected diseases in which elevated serum levels of angiotensin-converting enzyme have been reported*

Sarcoidosis
Gaucher's disease
Leprosy
Amyloidosis
Multiple myeloma
Lymphoma
Berylliosis
Farmer's lung
M. avium-intracellulare infection
Hyperthyroidism
Alcoholic hepatitis
Diabetes with retinopathy
Histoplasmosis
Silicosis

far less sensitive in patients with atypical presentations, in whom additional diagnostic studies must be performed. In addition, the test delays a diagnosis by 2 to 6 weeks. Kveim biopsy findings can be difficult to interpret, and patients cannot receive corticosteroid therapy until the test is completed. At present, the lack of readily available standardized antigen extract and the availability of other reliable diagnostic procedures has markedly reduced the use of the Kveim-Siltzbach test in the United States.

EVALUATING THE EXTENT AND SEVERITY OF ORGAN INVOLVEMENT

The extent and severity of organ involvement in sarcoidosis must be assessed when the disease is first diagnosed and periodically thereafter. Assessment must be tailored to the individual patient. There are, however, a number of tests that should be considered for all patients. A complete blood cell count and platelet count provide information about the patient's hematologic profile. Periodic chest x-ray studies and pulmonary function testing help to assess a patient's lung involvement. Initial pulmonary function testing should include spirometry, lung volumes, and diffusing capacity. Patients without obstructive physiology can then be followed with serial measurements of vital capacity and diffusing capacity. An electrocardiogram is adequate initial screening for cardiac involvement in patients without cardiac symptoms. Periodic slit-lamp examinations should be obtained regardless of whether ocular signs or symptoms are present. Liver function tests, including alkaline phosphatase levels, provide an indication of hepatic involvement. Serum calcium, blood urea nitrogen, and creatinine levels should be checked, and a 24-hour urine calcium collection should be performed. These tests may be repeated as necessary to assess therapeutic response.

PROGNOSIS

The majority of patients with sarcoidosis have a good prognosis. In approximately two thirds of patients, the disease resolves spontaneously with minor or no residua. In the other third of patients, the disease smolders or worsens. Overall, 15%–20% of patients suffer a permanent loss of lung function, and approximately 5% die of the disorder. These deaths are most commonly caused by respiratory failure with cor pulmonale and right-sided heart failure. Hemoptysis secondary to bronchiectasis or aspergillomas, arrhythmias resulting from cardiac involvement, nervous system involvement, and uremia are less common causes of death. A number of variables appear to have prognostic import. Those that correlate with a good prognosis include an acute disease presentation plus the presence of erythema nodosum (in whites), acute iritis, a stage I radiograph, and few manifestations of extrathoracic disease. Poor prognostic variables include an insidious disease presentation plus a stage III or IV chest radiograph, bone involvement, lupus pernio, chronic uveitis, upper respiratory tract involvement, bronchial involvement, cor pulmonale, nephrocalcinosis, and hepatomegaly. Genetic background also may have prognostic import. American blacks have a worse prognosis than American whites. In addition, HLA-B8 has been associated with spontaneous disease resolution, and HLA-B13 has been associated with a chronic, persistent form of the disorder.

A rough correlation exists between radiographic stage and the course of intrathoracic disease. Patients with stage I disease have the best prognosis, with approximately 50%–80% experiencing spontaneous radiographic resolution within 1 to 5 years. Approximately 10% of these patients maintain stage I radiographs for long periods of time, and 15%–30% progress to stage II to stage IV disease. Patients presenting with stage II radiographs have a somewhat less favorable prognosis. Approximately 40%–60% of these patients experience a spontaneous radiographic resolution or remission. The remainder have a chronic stage II radiograph or progress to stage III or stage IV disease. Patients with stage III radiographs have the worst prognosis, with spontaneous radiographic resolution occurring only 12%–35% of the time. The remaining patients usually maintain their stage III radiographs, with only 5%–10% progressing to stage IV disease.

ASSESSMENT OF DISEASE ACTIVITY

The signs and symptoms of sarcoidosis can be the result of inflammation or fibrosis. Inflammatory lesions are felt to be potentially reversible, whereas fibrotic lesions are not. Chronic inflammation in sarcoidosis has also been postulated to lead to tissue fibrosis. As a result, it has been assumed that treatment decisions might be made on a more rational basis and a patient's response to anti-inflammatory agents predicted more accurately if patients with active inflammation could be differentiated from those with largely fibrotic disease. This would allow the physician to identify and aggressively treat the patients who are at the greatest risk for development of tissue fibrosis and most likely to benefit from the therapeutic intervention. It would also allow the physician to avoid steroid-induced side effects in patients who are likely to improve spontaneously or not respond to steroid therapy. Clinical signs and symptoms and physiologic abnormalities provide some prognostic data. However, their utility in an individual patient is limited. As a result, a number of other assessment techniques have been employed. Gallium 67 radioisotope scanning, determination of serum angiotensin-converting enzyme activity, and evaluation of BALF have received the most attention.

Angiotensin-Converting Enzyme

Angiotensin-converting enzyme, a normal constituent of the endothelium, converts angiotensin I to angiotensin II. Leiberman et al. reported that in contrast to normal controls, 15 of 17 patients with clinically active sarcoidosis had increased levels of serum angiotensin-converting enzyme. Subsequent studies showed that angiotensin-converting enzyme was aberrantly produced in these patients by granulomatous tissue. Initial reports suggested that angiotensin-converting enzyme levels could be used for diagnosis and assessment of disease activity. Unfortunately, elevated serum levels of angiotensin-converting enzyme are found in only 50%–75% of patients with clinically active sarcoidosis, and the enzyme may be elevated in a number of other conditions, such as hepatic cirrhosis, hyperthyroidism, and diabetes mellitus (Table 5). When elevated, enzyme levels do seem to correlate with the clinical activity in some patients. However, subsequent studies have found angiotensin-converting enzyme determinations to be no more sensitive than chest radiographs in determining the need for treatment. In addition, it has been reported that steroid therapy may lower serum angiotensin-converting enzyme levels independently of changes in disease activity. Thus, the clinical utility of serum angiotensin-converting enzyme levels in staging sarcoidosis remains unsettled.

Gallium 67 Scanning

Another staging procedure, often used in conjunction with BAL, is radioisotope scanning with gallium 67. After intravenous injection, this isotope is actively taken up by inflammatory tissue and accumulates in the lungs and other involved organs of patients with clinically active sarcoidosis. Gallium 67 scanning may provide an index of macrophage activation in patients with sarcoidosis, because it appears that alveolar macrophages are the primary pulmonary inflammatory cells that incorporate gallium 67. As with BAL, the value of this technique in staging has been called into question. However, it may be useful in separating fibrotic from inflammatory disease, and in localizing extrapulmonary sites of disease activity. Gallium 67 scanning is relatively noninvasive and is easily performed serially. The disadvantages of this technique are that it is nonspecific, expensive, and difficult to quantitate, and it exposes the patient to radiation.

Bronchoalveolar Lavage

In the early 1980s, investigators defined two groups of patients with sarcoidosis based on the proportion of T lymphocytes in their BALF. Patients with 28% T lymphocytes in their BALF were said to have "high-intensity alveolitis," and those with 28% BALF T lymphocytes had "low-intensity alveolitis." It was proposed that patients with high BALF lymphocyte counts, particularly in association with positive gallium scans, are likely to deteriorate clinically. However, several studies have raised questions about the usefulness of BALF lymphocyte counts alone as a measure of disease activity, response to therapy, or prognosis. Two prospective studies in patients with newly diagnosed, untreated sarcoidosis followed for long periods of time showed no correlation between BALF lymphocyte counts and initial radiographic findings, pulmonary function abnormalities, need for steroid treatment, and, importantly, long-term outcome. Foley and co-workers found that an increase in the BALF lymphocyte count and CD4/CD2 ratios were actually associated with an improved prognosis. The lack of correlation between BALF lymphocyte counts and disease activity and prognosis has also been noted by Ceuppens and co-workers. They did find, however, that a decrease in or return to normal of the T-cell helper-suppressor ratio accompanied or preceded clinical and radiologic improvement and response to corticosteroid therapy. Thus, quantification of lung T cells does not provide usable prognostic information. In addition, the utility of BALF histamine, angiotensin-converting enzyme, procollagen III aminopeptide, fibrinogen, and vitronectin levels in predicting disease chronicity or the development of fibrosis remains to be proved. Other soluble BALF components, including immunoglobulins, surfactant proteins, reactive oxygen species, and antiproteases, have also been evaluated. Correlation of their presence in lavage fluid with prognosis or disease progression remains an area of ongoing investigation.

BALF cytokine levels might provide prognostic information. Alveolar macrophages from patients with sarcoidosis have been demonstrated to express increased levels of mRNA for TNF-γ, IL-6, IFN-γ, GM-CSF, and IL-1.

It has been suggested that increased levels of each of these cytokines as well as of interleukin-8 in BALF may parallel disease activity. Whether measurements of these and other cytokines in BALF will prove clinically useful in predicting the prognosis of sarcoidosis is unknown.

Measurement of potential serum markers of disease activity may also be useful in this regard. A soluble form of the IL-2 receptor (sIL-2R) is released by activated T cells in many granulomatous disorders. As sIL-2R is easily detectable in serum, several investigators have attempted to use sIL-2R levels to stage disease activity. These studies have found that the levels of sIL-2R are markedly increased in the serum of patients with active sarcoidosis, are significantly lower in patients with inactive disease, and fall with clinical improvement. Although the levels of serum sIL-2R correlate well with clinical parameters, their correlation with BALF T-cell counts, CD4/CD8 ratios, and BALF T-cell HLA-DR expression is poor. If these promising early reports are substantiated, the measurement of serum sIL-2R or BALF levels of sIL-2R may prove to be useful in predicting activity of sarcoidosis.

In summary, measurement of BAL cell profiles, soluble protein levels and cytokine levels, gallium scanning, and serum ACE levels have not been consistently shown to be good predictors of disease progression or response to therapy in patients with sarcoidosis. It is clear, however, that at some centers and in some patients, these assays, particularly if used in serial fashion, have been useful in prognosis and prediction of therapeutic response. At present, it is not clear if the conflicting reports in the literature reflect the true lack of utility of these assays or differences in the patient populations being studied. At present, these tests cannot be relied upon to the exclusion of clinical judgement in making decisions regarding patient management. Thus, until more information is available and newer assays are tested further, it seems most prudent to use traditional criteria, including clinical symptoms, pulmonary function tests, and chest radiographs, as well as indices of inflammation in assessing patients with sarcoidosis.

TREATMENT

It is not necessary to treat all patients with sarcoidosis. Decisions regarding treatment must be individualized, and are best based on individual manifestations of the disease and the clinical course of a given patient.

Extrapulmonary Disease

There is general agreement that systemic therapy with corticosteroids is indicated for any patient with life- or organ-threatening disease and for patients with refractory or progressive organ involvement (or symptoms) that have not responded to topical or symptomatic therapy. Some of the indications for systemic steroids in patients with extrapulmonary sarcoidosis are shown in Table 6. When systemic therapy is required for life-threatening disease, it is recommended that treatment be initiated with 40 to 60 mg of prednisone, given orally, once each day. After a clinical response has been achieved, the daily dose may be tapered by 5 to 10 mg/month. When the daily dose has been reduced to the equivalent of 20 mg of prednisone per day, a schedule of 40 mg on alternate days may be instituted. In patients without life-threatening complications, treatment may be initiated with 40 to 60 mg of prednisone on an alternate-day regimen. This dose is slowly tapered during the next 12 to 18 months, with the rate of taper and ultimate duration of therapy tailored to the clinical status of the patient. If disease reactivation occurs during dose reduction, the daily or alternate-day dose of prednisone should be increased by 10 mg and this dose administered for 2 to 3 months before tapering is attempted again. Some patients may require prolonged or even lifelong therapy.

It is important to realize that parenteral corticosteroid is not required for all extrapulmonary manifestations of sarcoidosis. Topical steroids are often effective in the treatment of anterior uveitis. Intradermal steroids, chloroquine, methotrexate, and retinoids may cause regression of sarcoid skin lesions, and nonsteroidal anti-inflammatory agents are useful in controlling joint pain and systemic manifestations of sarcoidosis. Colchicine is considered to be particularly effective in the treatment of the arthralgias and periarthritis of sarcoidosis, and mild hypercalcemia can occasionally be managed with hydration, a low-calcium diet, and avoidance of sunlight and vitamin D. Ketoconazole may also be useful in the treatment of hypercalcemia and hypercalcuria, as it decreases the synthesis of 1,25-dihydroxyvitamin D.

Pulmonary Disease

The present treatment of patients with pulmonary sarcoidosis remains a subject of considerable controversy. Given the variability in clinical course, the high rate of spontaneous remission, and the lack of reliable indicators of prognosis, the criteria for initiating and altering systemic treatment with corticosteroids remain ill-defined. This controversy is augmented by the realization that although steroids cause radiographic and functional improvement, their ability to alter the natural history of sarcoidosis is difficult to document.

Some authors advocate treatment of all patients with pulmonary sarcoidosis regardless of symptoms or physiologic abnormalities. Most, however, feel that only patients who are symptomatic or whose condition is deteriorating should be treated. An approach in accordance with this view is summarized below.

TABLE 6. *Extrapulmonary sarcoidosis: indications for systemic treatment*

Affected organ/disorder	Clinical findings	Remarks
Heart	Arrhythmia, conduction blocks, heart failure, sudden death	Antiarrhythmics, inotropic agents, diuretics, and pacemaker should be used when indicated.
Eye	Anterior uveitis, posterior uveitis, papilledema	Topical steroids alone may be adequate for anterior disease.
Hypercalcemia, hypercalciuria		Treatment is indicated if condition unresponsive to hydration, reduction in calcium and vitamin D intake, and avoidance of sunlight.
Central nervous system peripheral neuropathy	Variable	Treatment is indicated in most cases. Surgical treatment may be necessary in some situations (e.g., hydrocephalus). One third of patients will relapse as treatment is withdrawn.
Kidney	Nephrotic syndrome, renal compromise	Rare.
Spleen	Cytopenia, massive splenomegaly	
Pituitary, hypothalamus	Diabetes insipidus, pituitary insufficiency (rare)	
Liver	Cholestatic hepatitis, severe involvement	Patients with asymptomatic elevations in liver function tests do not require treatment.
Skin	Lupus pernio, skin infiltration	Systemic treatment is indicated if condition unresponsive to topical or intralesional treatment. Chloroquine, methotrexate and retinoids may be useful.
Bone	Symptomatic or disfiguring lesions	Colchicine may be beneficial.
Arthritis	Acute polyarthritis	Treatment with anti-inflammatory agents is usually adequate.
	Chronic polyarthritis	Anti-inflammatory agents deserve trial before use of steroids.

1. Patients with stage I disease are often asymptomatic and usually have normal or near normal pulmonary function. They should be carefully observed with serial chest radiographs and pulmonary function tests initially every 3 months. If disease progresses radiographically or if pulmonary function significantly declines (15% decrease in lung volumes or diffusing capacity), treatment with steroids should be initiated.

2. Patients with stage II or stage III disease with normal or near normal pulmonary function and minimal symptoms should be followed serially and treated if they progress as described for stage I patients. Patients presenting with significantly abnormal pulmonary function (lung volumes and/or diffusing capacity 65% of predicted) warrant an empiric trial of steroids. The indices of inflammation noted above are often helpful in defining parameters of disease activity that can be followed in these patients. Clinical status and pulmonary function should also be monitored and chest radiographs taken periodically.

3. Patients presenting with fibrobullous disease (advanced stage III or stage IV) also warrant an empiric trial of steroids. Although the likelihood of reversing fibrotic changes is small, patients with concomitant pulmonary inflammation may improve significantly with therapy.

4. Patients with severe, end-stage lung disease despite treatment may be candidates for single lung or heart-lung transplantation. Referral to an appropriate transplantation center should be made, preferably before the onset of cor pulmonale.

These recommendations parallel those recently made by Sharma in a commentary for the American Thoracic Society.

There is little agreement as to the amount of steroid necessary to adequately treat pulmonary sarcoidosis. Initial dosages, daily versus alternate day regimens, and schedules for tapering vary institutionally and among practitioners. The response (or lack thereof) of the individual patient will largely dictate his or her regimen. In severe cases of pulmonary sarcoidosis, up to 60 mg of prednisone daily may be used as an initial dose. In most other cases, a lower prednisone dose of 40–60 mg every other day can be used from the outset. The patient is then observed on therapy for up to several months.

In patients who appear to respond, the initial prednisone dose (40–60 mg/day) is maintained for 3 to 6 months and then reduced by 5 to 10 mg every 1 to 3 months. This usually results in a total duration of therapy of between 12 and 15 months. In patients who do not respond, steroids are tapered and discontinued more rapidly.

Relapses can occur during the treatment period. When a relapse occurs, the most recent effective dose should be reinstituted for 2 to 3 months and then tapering should be attempted. A few patients require lifelong steroid therapy, although usually at relatively low doses. Others have remissions, only to have reactivation of disease years later. For these reasons, most patients with sarcoidosis should remain under observation indefinitely and have their disease activity periodically reassessed.

Agents Other Than Steroids

The use of cytotoxic agents in the treatment of refractory sarcoidosis is based on uncontrolled studies that claim or refute therapeutic success with a variety of agents. Methotrexate has been used in uncontrolled trials in low doses (e.g., 10 mg/week) with some success, particularly in patients with severe skin involvement. Long-term therapy with methotrexate carries the risk for hepatotoxicity. Serial liver biopsies may be required to monitor this potential problem. Cyclophosphamide, azathioprine, and chlorambucil have also been used and appear to be of limited value. Cyclosporine has been reported in case studies to be of benefit in pulmonary sarcoidosis refractory to corticosteroids. Thalidomide has also been reported to be of benefit in one case of cutaneous and pulmonary sarcoidosis. There are no known advantages of any of these agents. The choice between these drugs is best dictated by the clinician's familiarity with each and the patient's clinical presentation. In cases in which active sarcoidosis is not adequately treated with high-dose steroids or in which the patient cannot tolerate steroids because of side effects, a trial of one of these agents may be warranted.

Transplantation

End-stage organ failure may develop in patients with severe sarcoidosis. In such situations, transplantation of solid organs, including lung, heart, liver, and kidney, has been successfully performed. It has been well documented that noncaseating granulomas can be seen in lung and heart allografts after transplantation. This finding appears to be specific for patients with sarcoidosis and is not observed in allografts of patients who have undergone transplantation for other diseases. Fortunately, clinical disease caused by recurrent sarcoidosis in the transplanted organ is uncommon. This may be in part a consequence of the uniform use of immunosuppressive agents to prevent transplant rejection. As sarcoid recurrence in allografts appears to be associated with little in the way of clinical symptoms or organ dysfunction, transplantation remains a viable option for patients with sarcoidosis-induced end-stage organ failure.

Interestingly, there have been case reports in which sarcoidosis appears to have been transmitted via organ donation. Experience is not yet broad enough to determine if subsequent clinical manifestations related to sarcoidosis will be severe enough to exclude persons with sarcoidosis from organ donation.

BIBLIOGRAPHY

Athos L, Mohler JG, Sharma OP. Exercise testing in the physiologic assessment of sarcoidosis. *Ann N Y Acad Sci* 1986;465:491 (Johns CJ, ed. *Tenth International Conference on Sarcoidosis and Other Granulomatous Disorders*). *Study of cardiopulmonary exercise testing in 39 patients with sarcoidosis. Maximal exercise was associated with significant abnormalities in gas exchange, which correlated with radiographic staging.*

Balbi B, Moller DR, Kirby M, Holroyd K, Crystal RG. Increased numbers of T lymphocytes with gamma/delta positive antigen receptors in a subgroup of individuals with pulmonary sarcoidosis. *J Clin Invest* 1990;85:1353. *This study is reflective of a growing appreciation of the importance of T-lymphocyte subpopulations in sarcoidosis.*

Besnier E. Lupus pernio de la face: synovites fomagueuses symétriques des extrémités supérieures. *Ann Dermatol Syphilol* 1989;10:333. *One of the original descriptions of lupus pernio.*

Boeck C. Multiple benign sarcoid of the skin. *J Cutan Genitourinary Dis* 1899;17:543. *Boeck's classic article on sarcoidosis of the skin.*

Bost TW, Riches DWH, Schumacher B, Carre PC, Rhan TZ, Martinez JAB, Newman LS. Alveolar macrophages from patients with beryllium disease and sarcoidosis express increased levels of mRNA for tumor necrosis factor-α and interleukin-6 but not interleukin-1β. *Am J Respir Cell Mol Biol* 1994;10:506–513. *One of a number of recent articles reporting cytokine profiles in BALF from patients with sarcoidosis. In this study, evaluation of alveolar macrophage cytokine gene expression was notable for elevation of macrophage mRNA for the proinflammatory cytokines TNF-α and IL-6.*

Ceuppens JL, Lacquet LM, Marien G, Demedts M, van den Eeckhout A, and Stevens E. Alveolar T-cell subsets in pulmonary sarcoidosis: Correlation with disease activity and effect of steroid treatment. *Am Rev Respir Dis* 1984;129:563–568.

Churg A, Carrington CB, Gupta R. Necrotizing sarcoid granulomatosis. *Chest* 1979;76:406–413. *Clinicopathologic review of 12 patients with necrotizing sarcoid granulomatosis. The follow-up of these patients suggests that this entity does not behave like other forms of angiocentric granulomatosis, but rather follows a course that parallels more typical forms of sarcoidosis.*

Clarke D, Mitchell AW, Dick R, James GD. The radiology of sarcoidosis. *Sarcoidosis* 1994;11:90–99. *Comprehensive overview of the radiographic evaluation of sarcoidosis.*

Consensus Conference. Activity of sarcoidosis. *Eur Respir J* 1994;7:624–627. *Concise and practical overview of the utility of available parameters to assess disease activity in sarcoidosis.*

Daniele RB, Rossman MD, Kern JA, Elias JA. Pathogenesis of sarcoidosis. *Chest* 1996;89:174. *Helpful overview of cellular mechanisms involved in the pathogenesis of sarcoidosis. This summary provides a good framework for subsequent studies detailing individual aspects of inflammatory and fibrotic processes in the lung.*

du Bois RM. Corticosteroids in sarcoidosis: friend or foe? *Eur Respir J* 1994;7:1203–1209. *Commentary on corticosteroids for the treatment of sarcoidosis.*

Elias JA, Freundlich B, Kern JA, Rosenbaum T. Cytokine networks in the regulation of inflammation and fibrosis in the lung. *Chest* 1990;97:1439. *Overview of the networking of cytokines and their role(s) in the regulation of inflammation and fibrosis. This article extensively outlines the complex interplay that occurs among cells involved in inflammatory processes in the lung.*

Foley NM, Coral AD, Tung K, Hudspith BN, James DG, and Johnson NM. Bronchoalveolar lavage cell counts as a predictor of short term outcome in pulmonary sarcoidosis. *Thorax* 1989;44:732–738.

Forman JD, Klein JT, Silver RF, Liu MC, Greenlee BM, Moller DR. Selective activation and accumulation of oligoclonal V_β-specific T cells in active pulmonary sarcoidosis. *J Clin Invest* 1994;94:1533–1542. *Using molecular analysis of T-cell receptor gene expression, this study provides evidence that the granulomatous response in sar-*

coidosis preferentially involves αβ⁺ T cells expressing a limited number of V_β genes.

Girgis RE, Basha MA, Maliarik M, Popovich J Jr, Iannuzzi MC. Cytokines in the bronchoalveolar lavage fluid of patients with active pulmonary sarcoidosis. *Am J Respir Crit Care Med* 1995;152:71–75. *One of a number of recent reports detailing cytokine profiles in BALF in patients with sarcoidosis. In this study, levels of the proinflammatory cytokines IL-6 and IL-8 were elevated.*

Groen H, Hamstra M, Aalberst R, Van Der Mark TW, Koeter GH, Postma DS. Clinical evaluation of lymphocyte subpopulations and oxygen radical production in sarcoidosis and idiopathic pulmonary fibrosis. *Respir Med* 1994;88:55–64. *Lymphocyte populations in BALF differed among patients with pulmonary and extrapulmonary sarcoidosis and idiopathic pulmonary fibrosis.*

Harrison BDW, Shaylor JM, Stokes TC, Wilkes AR. Air flow limitation in sarcoidosis—a study of pulmonary function in 107 patients with newly diagnosed disease. *Respir Med* 1991;85:59. *Study of 107 patients with newly diagnosed sarcoidosis demonstrating that air flow limitation is the most common physiologic abnormality seen on pulmonary function testing.*

Hunninghake GW, Crystal RG. Pulmonary sarcoidosis: a disorder mediated by excess helper T-lymphocyte activity at sites of disease activity. *N Engl J Med* 1981;305:429. *Original description of the presence of large numbers of helper T cells and increased helper-suppressor T-cell ratios in the lungs of patients with sarcoidosis and high-intensity alveolitis.*

Hutchinson J. Recurring ophthalmitis with opacities in the vitreous: Mabey's malady. *Arch Surg* 1892;4:361. *Original description of sarcoidosis.*

Israel HL, Albertine KH, Park CH, Patrick H. Whole-body gallium 67 scans. Role in diagnosis of sarcoidosis. *Am Rev Respir Dis* 1991;144:1182. *Commentary on patterns of gallium scanning seen with sarcoidosis, and on the utility of this technique in the diagnosis of sarcoidosis.*

Israel HL, Karlin P, Menduke H. Factors affecting outcome of sarcoidosis. Influence of race, extrathoracic involvement, and initial radiologic lung lesions. *Ann N Y Acad Sci* 1986;465:609. *Subjects in this study were monitored for a mean length of 9.3 years. Factors influencing clinical progression/recovery included race and extrathoracic involvement, but not the initial radiographic stage.*

James DG, Sherlock S. Sarcoidosis of the liver. *Sarcoidosis* 1994;11:2–6. *Review of hepatic sarcoidosis, including an extensive differential of causes of granulomatous inflammation in the liver.*

Janis EM, Kaufmann SHE, Schwartz RH, Pardoll DM. Activation of γδ T cells in the primary immune response to *Mycobacterium tuberculosis. Science* 1989;244:713–716. *One of the original descriptions of the role of γδ T cells in granulomatous inflammation.*

Keicho N, Kitamura K, Takaku F, Yotsumoto H. Serum concentration of soluble interleukin-2 receptor as a sensitive parameter of disease activity in sarcoidosis. *Chest* 1990;98:1125. *In the search for reliable clinical parameters of disease activity, a number of serum markers have been examined, although none has proved definitively useful. Serum soluble IL-2R is one such potential parameter. The clinical utility of such markers remains to be proved.*

Koerner SK, Sakowitz AJ, Applemen RI, Becker NH, Schoenbaum SW. Transbronchial lung biopsy for the diagnosis of sarcoidosis. *N Engl J Med* 1975;293:268. *Sentinel description of the high diagnostic yield of transbronchial biopsy for histologic confirmation of sarcoidosis.*

Kuznitsky E, Bittorf A. Boecksches sarkoid mit detiligung innes organe. *Munch Med Wochenschr* 1915;62:1349. *One of the original descriptions of sarcoidosis as a multiorgan disease.*

Le Guludec D, Menad F, Faraggi M, Weinmann P, Battesti JP, Valeyre D. Myocardial sarcoidosis. Clinical value of technetium 99m sestamibi tomoscintigraphy. *Chest* 1994;106:1675–1682. *Comparison of the diagnostic sensitivity of thallium 201 scintigraphy and technetium 99m sestamibi tomoscintigraphy for myocardial sarcoidosis.*

Lieberman J, Schleissner LA, Nosal A, Sastre A, and Mishkin FS. Clinical correlations of serum angiotensin-converting enzyme (ACE) in sarcoidosis: A longitudinal study of serum ACE, 67-gallium scans, chest roentgenograms, and pulmonary function. *Chest* 1983;84:522–528.

Liebow AA, The J. Burns Amberson Lecture—pulmonary angiitis and granulomatosis. *Am Rev Respir Dis* 1973;108:11–18. *Extensive classic clinicopathologic discussion of pulmonary angiitis and granulomatosis, including Liebow's original description of necrotizing sarcoid granulomatosis.*

Lohmann-Matthes M-L, Steinmuller C, Franke-Ullmann G. Pulmonary macrophages. *Eur Respir J* 1994;7:1678–1689. *Comprehensive review of pulmonary macrophages, covering cellular origin and localization, metabolic functions, surface markers, and cytokine production.*

Lower EE, Baughman RP. Prolonged use of methotrexate for sarcoidosis. *Arch Intern Med* 1995;155:846–851. *Nonrandomized trial evaluating the safety and efficacy of methotrexate in patients with sarcoidosis. Fifty patients who completed at least 2 years of methotrexate therapy were monitored.*

Mangiapan G, Hance AJ. Mycobacteria and sarcoidosis: an overview and summary of recent molecular biological data. *Sarcoidosis* 1995;12:20–37. *Extensive review taking a new look at the proposed relationship between sarcoidosis and mycobacterial infection using molecular techniques (polymerase chain reaction).*

Martinez EJ, Orens JB, Deeb M, Brunsting LA, Flint A, Lynch JP. Recurrence of sarcoidosis following bilateral allogeneic lung transplantation. *Chest* 1994;106:1597–1599. *One of several reports documenting recurrence of sarcoidosis after lung transplantation.*

Meyrier A, Valeyre D, Bouillon R, Paillard F, Battesti JP, Georges R. Different mechanisms of hypercalciuria in sarcoidosis. Correlations with disease extension and activity. *Ann N Y Acad Sci* 1986;465:575 (Johns C, ed. *Tenth International Conference on Sarcoidosis and Other Granulomatous Disorders*). *Good review of mechanisms of hypercalciuria in sarcoidosis.*

Muller-Quernheim J, Pfeifer S, Mannel D, Strausz J, Ferlinz R. Lung-restricted activation of the alveolar macrophage/monocyte system in pulmonary sarcoidosis. *Am Rev Respir Dis* 1992;145:187. *In this study, alveolar macrophages isolated from the lungs of patients with active sarcoidosis spontaneously released TNF-α and IL-1, whereas peripheral blood monocytes from these same patients did not. This observation supports the concept of compartmentalized activation of cells involved in the inflammatory process in sarcoidosis.*

Roberts WC, McAllister HA, Ferrans VJ. Sarcoidosis of the heart: a clinicopathologic study of 35 necropsy patients (group I) and review of 78 previously described necropsy patients (group II). *Am J Med* 1977;63:86. *Extensive study of the histopathology of cardiac sarcoidosis.*

Rochester CL, Elias JA. Cytokines and cytokine networking in the pathogenesis of interstitial and fibrotic lung disorders. *Semin Respir Med* 1993;14:389–415 (Rhagu G, ed. *Interstitial Pulmonary Disorders*). *Comprehensive review of cytokines and cytokine networking in interstitial lung diseases, including sarcoidosis.*

Satorre J, Antle CM, O'Sullivan R, White VA, Nugent RA, Rootman J. Orbital lesions with granulomatous inflammation. *Can J Ophthalmol* 1991;26:174. *Extensive review of causes of granulomatous inflammation of the orbit.*

Schauman J. *Sur le Lupus Pernio. Memoire Présenté en Novembre 1914 à la Société Française de Dermatologie et Syphilégraphic pour le Prix Zambaco.* Stockholm: PA Norsledt och Soness Furlag; 1934. *One of the original descriptions of lupus pernio.*

Scott TF. Neurosarcoidosis. *Neurology* 1993;43:8–12. *Review of neurosarcoidosis, including a brief summary of cerebrospinal fluid findings.*

Selroos O. Sarcoidosis and pregnancy: a review with results of a retrospective survey. *J Intern Med* 1990;227:221–224. *Interesting retrospective analysis of 38 pregnant women with sarcoidosis, including a literature review of the topic.*

Shammas RL, Movahed A. Sarcoidosis of the heart. *Clin Cardiol* 1993;16:462–472. *Review of cardiac sarcoidosis, including clinical manifestations, diagnostic techniques, treatment, and management.*

Sharma OP. Pulmonary sarcoidosis and corticosteroids. *Am Rev Respir Dis* 1993;147:1598–1600. *Commentary on the role of corticosteroids in the treatment of sarcoidosis, including recommendations for dosage and duration of therapy.*

Sharma OP. Myocardial sarcoidosis. A wolf in sheep's clothing. *Chest* 1994;106:988–990. *Commentary on diagnosis, evaluation, and treatment of cardiac sarcoidosis.*

Sharma OP, Sharma AM. Sarcoidosis of the nervous system. A clinical approach. *Arch Intern Med* 1991;151:1317. *Good review of neurosarcoidosis, with extensive bibliography.*

Shijubo N, Imai K, Shigehara K, Honda Y, Koba H, Tsujisaki M, Hinoda Y, Yachi A, Ohmichi M, Hiraga Y, Abe S. Soluble intercellular adhesion molecule-1 (ICAM-1) in sera and bronchoalveolar lavage fluid of patients with idiopathic pulmonary fibrosis and pulmonary sarcoidosis. *Clin Exp Immunol* 1994;95:156–161. *One of a number of studies demonstrating the compartmentalized immune response in sarcoidosis. In this study, patients with sarcoidosis were found to have normal levels of circulating ICAM-1 but had increased levels of ICAM-1 in BALF.*

Takemura T, Matsui Y, Oritsu M, Akiyama O, Hiraga Y, Omichi M, Hirasawa M, Saiki S, Tamura S, Mochizuki I, Mikami R. Pulmonary vascular involvement in sarcoidosis: granulomatous angiitis and microangiopathy in transbronchial lung biopsies. *Virchows Archiv A Pathol Anat* 1991;418:361. *Pathologic study of 174 cases of sarcoidosis showing a significant (53%) prevalence of granulomatous angiitis and microangiopathy.*

Tanoue LT, Elias JA. Cytokines and interstitial lung disease. In: Leff A, ed. *Pulmonary and Critical Care Pharmacology and Therapeutics.* New York: McGraw-Hill; 1996:275–284. *Overview of cytokines and cytokine interactions in interstitial lung disease, including sarcoidosis, with extensive bibliography.*

Teirstein AS, Lesser M. Worldwide distribution and epidemiology of sarcoidosis. In: Fanburg BL, ed. *Sarcoidosis and Other Granulomatous Diseases of the Lung.* New York: Marcel Dekker; 1983:101–134 (vol 20; chapter 4). *Description of the worldwide epidemiology of sarcoidosis, broken down by continent and country.*

Tenneson M. Lupus pernio. *Bull Soc Fr Dermatol Syphilol* 1892;3:417. *One of the original descriptions of sarcoidosis of the skin.*

Thomas PD, Hunninghake GW. Current concepts of the pathogenesis of sarcoidosis. *Am Rev Respir Dis* 1987;135:747–760. *Extensive, well-written review of sarcoidosis, including clinical manifestations, pathology, etiology, and immune pathogenesis.*

Vandenplas O, Depelchin S, Delaunois L, Delwiche JP, Sibille Y. Bron-choalveolar lavage immunoglobulin A and G and antiproteases correlate with changes in diffusion indices during the natural course of pulmonary sarcoidosis. *Eur Respir J* 1994;7:1856–1864. *An evaluation of BALF immunoglobulin and antiprotease levels and T4/T8 lymphocyte ratios as potential predictive markers for changes in diffusion indices in patients with sarcoidosis. The authors point out that duration of disease is important in the evaluation of potential parameters of disease activity.*

Verstraeten A, Demedts M, Verwilghen J, van den Eeckhout A, Marien G, Lacquet LM, Ceuppens JL. Predictive value of bronchoalveolar lavage in pulmonary sarcoidosis. *Chest* 1990;95:560. *One of multiple studies examining lymphocyte populations in BALF. As in other reports, a high ratio of T4 cells to T8 cells and a high lymphocyte count are consistent with an alveolitis, but do not predict course or prognosis of disease.*

Weissler JC. Southwestern Internal Medicine Conference. Sarcoidosis: immunology and clinical management. *Am J Med Sci* 1994;307:233–245. *Overview of immunopathogenesis of sarcoidosis with commentary on clinical management.*

Wilson JD, Castillo M. Magnetic resonance imaging of granulomatous inflammations: sarcoidosis and tuberculosis. *Top Magn Reson Imaging* 1994;6:32–40. *Discussion of the role of magnetic resonance imaging in the diagnosis of neurosarcoidosis.*

Winterbauer RH, Moores KD. A clinical interpretation of bilateral hilar adenopathy. *Ann Intern Med* 1973;78:65. *Sentinel article examining 100 patients with bilateral hilar adenopathy. Bilateral hilar adenopathy in patients without symptoms and with negative physical examination was felt always to be associated with sarcoidosis. The authors propose that biopsy confirmation in these cases is not necessary.*

Wollschlager C, Khan F. Aspergillomas complicating sarcoidosis. A prospective study in 100 patients. *Chest* 1984;86:585. *A comprehensive examination of aspergilloma complicating sarcoidosis.*

Textbook of Pulmonary Diseases, 6th ed.
edited by G.L. Baum, J.D. Crapo, B.R. Celli, and J.B. Karlinsky,
Lippincott–Raven Publishers, Philadelphia, © 1998.

CHAPTER

21

Major Pulmonary Disease Syndromes of Unknown Etiology

Joseph P. Lynch, III · Ganesh Raghu

INTRODUCTION

Pulmonary inflammation and fibrosis may concur in the context of myriad acute and chronic disorders affecting the lung parenchyma or small airways (e.g., bronchioles). The etiologies of these various disorders have not been clarified, but clinical, radiographic, and physiologic features are often distinctive and overlap between the various disorders. These heterogeneous chronic interstitial lung diseases (CILD) share many of the following clinical features: exertional dyspnea; bilateral infiltrates on chest radiographs; physiologic abnormalities of restrictive lung defect, decreased diffusing capacity (DLCO), and increased alveolar-arterial oxygen gradient [$P(A - a)O_2$] at rest or with exertion; absence of pulmonary infection and neoplasm; and histopathologic features of inflammation and fibrosis, with or without granulomatous or vascular lesions in the pulmonary parenchyma. Some of the CILD primarily involve alveolar walls and interstitium, but proximal airways may be involved incidentally. In addition, a group of disorders preferentially involve the small airways (terminal and respiratory bronchioles); the distal alveolar spaces may be involved incidentally or may be spared. Disorders affecting the small airways alone are usually characterized by exertional dyspnea; clear chest radiographs with preserved or increased lung volumes; physiologic defects of airways obstruction, air trapping, impaired DLCO, and widened $P(A - a)O_2$; absence of infection and neoplasm; histopathologic features of con-

stricted small-airway lumina (i.e., constrictive or obstructive bronchiolitis). The spectrum of clinical, radiographic, physiologic, and histopathologic manifestations is wide, and significant overlap between these diverse disorders exists.

Many of these CILD are discussed in detail elsewhere in this text, and their features are not reiterated here; they include idiopathic, collagen vascular-associated, and radiation- or drug-induced pneumonitis/fibrosis; pneumoconiosis and pneumonitis of occupational or environmental origin; sarcoidosis; eosinophilic pneumonias; hypersensitivity pneumonitis; and rare inherited diseases (e.g., neurofibromatosis, tuberous sclerosis, Hermansky-Pudlak syndrome, metabolic storage disorders, and hypocalciuric hypercalcemia). This chapter discusses in detail selected major disease syndromes of unknown etiology exhibiting distinctive clinical, radiographic, or histopathologic features. The clinical course and treatment of these diverse disorders are variable and are discussed in detail in the following sections.

DISEASES OF THE BRONCHIOLES AND SMALL AIRWAYS

Bronchiolitis Obliterans with Organizing Pneumonia

A wide spectrum of inflammatory disorders may involve terminal and respiratory bronchioles, resulting in diverse clinical syndromes. The literature is confusing, as the terms *bronchiolitis obliterans* (with or without organizing pneumonia), *cryptogenic organizing pneumonia, obliterative (mural) bronchiolitis,* and *organizing pneumonia* have often been used interchangeably to refer to a heterogeneous group of bronchiolar inflammatory disorders with diverse clinical expression. We first review bronchiolitis obliterans organizing pneumonia (BOOP),

J. P. Lynch III: Division of Pulmonary and Critical Care Medicine, Department of Internal Medicine, University of Michigan Medical Center, Ann Arbor, Michigan 48109-0360.

G. Raghu: Division of Pulmonary and Critical Care Medicine, Department of Internal Medicine, University of Washington Medical Center, Seattle, Washington 98195.

also called *cryptogenic organizing pneumonia.* BOOP may complicate collagen vascular disease, exposures to toxic fumes or pharmacologic agents, organ transplantation (e.g., bone marrow or lung), or specific pulmonary infections (e.g., *Legionella,* viruses, *Mycoplasma* species). When no cause can be elicited, the term *idiopathic BOOP* or *idiopathic cryptogenic organizing pneumonia* has been applied. BOOP is characterized by a subacute process, focal alveolar infiltrates (mimicking pneumonia), and granulation tissue obstructing small bronchioles and extending into the lung parenchyma. The prognosis and clinical expression of BOOP differ markedly from those of other disorders involving small bronchioles, to be discussed later (e.g., obliterative bronchiolitis, diffuse panbronchiolitis, respiratory bronchiolitis).

Epidemiology

The precise incidence of BOOP is not clear, as many cases have likely erroneously been ascribed to other disorders (e.g., desquamative interstitial pneumonitis, eosinophilic pneumonia, pulmonary fibrosis). BOOP probably has been underrepresented in the literature, as cases lacking histologic confirmation have not been reported. In 1985, Epler and colleagues identified 67 patients with BOOP (17 of whom had collagen vascular disease) gleaned from a review of 2500 open lung biopsies performed from 1950 to 1980. Investigators at Ohio State University detected 16 cases of BOOP within a 4-year period, accounting for 4% of referrals for obstructive lung disorders. Cordier et al. detected 16 cases of BOOP in 6 years at a leading referral center in France. Katzenstein

and colleagues identified 24 cases by retrospective review of pathologic files at the University of Alabama from 1972 to 1984. These and other studies suggest that even large referral centers diagnose only two to four cases of BOOP annually. BOOP usually presents in the fifth through sixth decades of life, but persons of any age may be affected. There is no sex predominance.

Clinical Features

Nonproductive cough, dyspnea, fever, weight loss, and malaise are typical presenting features. Despite pronounced constitutional symptoms in some patients, extrapulmonary involvement does not occur. The course is usually subacute, with symptoms developing within 2 weeks to 6 months. An antecedent upper or lower respiratory tract infection or flulike illness is noted in 40%–60% of patients within 1 to 3 months of onset of symptoms. Crackles are present on physical examination in 60% of patients; 40% manifest a mid-inspiratory squeak. Despite the presence of airways obstruction, overt wheezing is rare. Clubbing is not a feature of BOOP, as in is in several other CILD. No characteristic laboratory aberrations are noted. The eythrocyte sedimentation rate is elevated in 80% of cases; one third exhibit leukocytosis.

Chest Radiographic Findings

Chest radiographs reveal single or multiple segmental or lobar alveolar infiltrates in more than two thirds of patients (Fig. 1). A basilar predominance is more com-

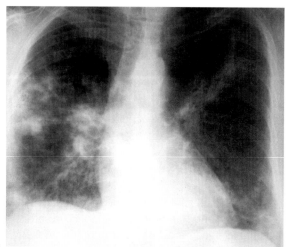

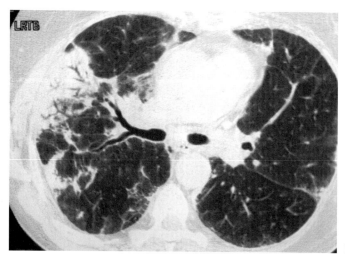

A

B

FIG. 1. A: Bronchiolitis obliterans organizing pneumonia. PA chest radiograph from a 67-year-old woman demonstrates patchy bilateral infiltrates. She had been given three prior courses of antibiotics by her personal physician during the preceding 7 weeks because of persistent cough, fever, and dyspnea, with no improvement. Changes revealed by transbronchial lung biopsy were consistent with BOOP, and corticosteroids (1 mg of prednisone per kilogram of body weight per day) were initiated. **B:** CT demonstrates dense alveolar infiltrates with striking air bronchograms in the periphery of the right lung.

mon, but any lobe can be affected. Patchy, unilateral or bilateral air space consolidation, often with air bronchograms, has been noted in 62%–79% of patients. In some patients, the infiltrates migrate or wax and wane, either spontaneously or in apparent response to antibiotics. The fleeting nature of these infiltrates may cause them to be mistaken for pneumonia, particularly when patients have been treated with antibiotics. Dense lobar infiltrates with consolidation contrast sharply with the interstitial nature of infiltrates seen in idiopathic pulmonary fibrosis (IPF) and many other CILD. However, diffuse reticulonodular infiltrates, indistinguishable from those of IPF or other CILD, are noted in 20%–40% of cases of BOOP (Fig. 2). In 4%–10% of cases, chest radiographic findings are normal or exhibit only hyperinflation. Pleural effusions, cavitary lesions, and intrathoracic lymphadenopathy are not features of BOOP. The pattern on chest radiographs influences prognosis. Dense alveolar infiltrates are associated with a pronounced component of organizing pneumonia, a more acute course, and greater responsiveness to corticosteroids (Fig. 3). By contrast, a diffuse reticulonodular or interstitial pattern has been associated with a more chronic course and lower rate of response to therapy.

High-Resolution Thin-Section Computed Tomography

High-resolution thin section computed tomography (CT) typically reveal single or multiple focal alveolar nodular infiltrates or areas of consolidation (with air bronchograms) (Figs. 1B and 3B). In some cases, a feeding vessel or bronchus leading into the area of consolidation or nodular opacity may be seen. Reticulonodular interstitial infiltrates are noted in one quarter of patients. Other findings include ground-glass opacities and peribronchiolar nodules extending into the lung parenchyma in a centrifugal fashion from involved airways. Honeycombing is not seen in BOOP. Pleural effusions are observed in <10% of patients and are rarely prominent. Mediastinal lymphadenopathy has been noted, but is usually minor (lymph nodes <1.5 cm in size).

Pulmonary Function Tests

A restrictive defect, with reductions in lung volumes (e.g., vital capacity, total lung volume) is characteristic of BOOP. Other physiologic aberrations include reduced D_LCO, hypoxemia, and a widened $P(A - a)O_2$. Despite the involvement of small airways, a purely obstructive defect is rare (except in smokers). The lack of obstruction has been attributed to the patchy nature of airway involvement. Some regions are completely obstructed (resulting in loss of entire units and reduced lung volumes), whereas other areas are spared. Bronchodilators are generally ineffective. Functional deficits may markedly improve or normalize following corticosteroid therapy.

Histopathologic Features

The histologic hallmark of BOOP is polypoid masses of granulation tissue filling (and obstructing) terminal and respiratory bronchioles and alveolar ducts (Fig. 4). The plugs of loose granulation tissue are composed of aggregates of inflammatory cells, edematous fluid, debris, fibrin, and fibrous connective tissue. The inflammatory infiltrate is composed of lymphocytes, plasma cells, foamy macrophages, and scattered polymorphonuclear leukocytes, eosinophils, and multinucleated giant cells. Extension of the inflammatory process to contiguous alveolar ducts and alveolar spaces results in the "organizing pneumonia" component. Fibrous connective tissue (e.g., fibroblasts, myofibroblasts, collagen) may extend from the small-airway lumina into the alveolar spaces, but extensive fibrosis or honeycombing is lacking. Even when extensive consolidation is present, the alveolar architecture is preserved. These histologic features have variably been ascribed to organizing pneumonia, lipoid pneumonia, cholesterol pneumonia, and resolving pneumonia. Other distinctive features of BOOP include bronchocentricity and patchy involvement; these features can readily be appreciated on low-power magnification of lung biopsy specimens. This "organizing pneumonia" component has been associated with an excellent prognosis and high rate of response to corticosteroid therapy. Histologic features

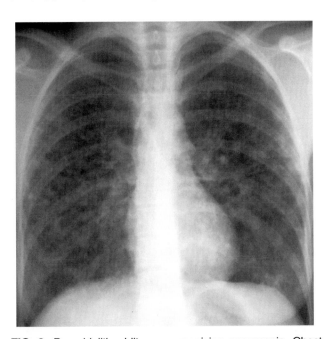

FIG. 2. Bronchiolitis obliterans organizing pneumonia. Chest radiograph demonstrates diffuse reticulonodular infiltrates in a 27-year-old woman who presented with a 6-week history of cough and progressive dyspnea. Transbronchial lung biopsies demonstrated features consistent with BOOP. Corticosteroid therapy (60 mg of prednisone daily for 1 month, with a subsequent taper) was initiated, with complete resolution of symptoms and normalization of chest radiograph. (Reproduced with permission from Neagos GR, Lynch JP III. Making sense out of bronchiolitis obliterans. *J Respir Dis* 1991:12;807.)

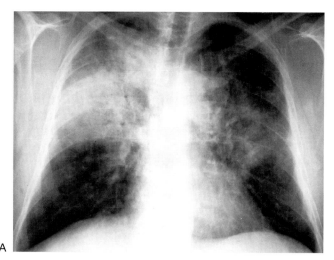

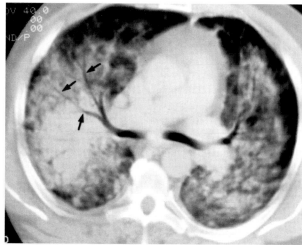

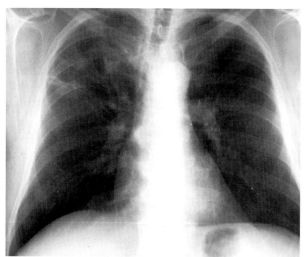

FIG. 3. A: Bronchiolitis obliterans organizing pneumonia. PA chest radiograph from a 62-year-old man demonstrates confluent alveolar infiltrates in both upper lobes with extensive air bronchograms. He had been treated with broad-spectrum parenteral antibiotics for 2 weeks without improvement and with worsening findings on chest radiographs. **B:** High-resolution CT from the same patient demonstrates confluent alveolar infiltrates and striking air bronchograms (*arrows*). Transbronchial lung biopsies demonstrated typical features of BOOP. Corticosteroids were initiated, and the process resolved during the next few weeks. **C:** PA chest radiograph from the same patient 3 weeks after institution of corticosteroid therapy demonstrates nearly complete resolution of alveolar infiltrates.

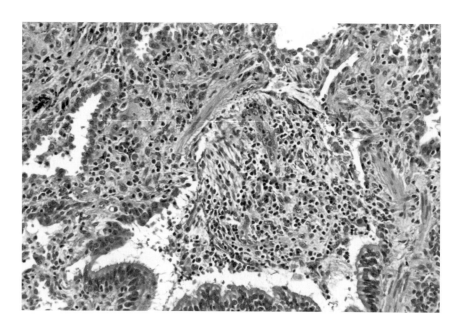

FIG. 4. Bronchiolitis obliterating pneumonia. Photomicrograph of open lung biopsy specimen demonstrates a plug of organizing granulation tissue within a respiratory bronchiole. A peribronchiolar mononuclear inflammatory cell infiltrate is also evident. H&E stain, oil immersion. (Reproduced with permission from Neagos GR, Lynch JP III. Making sense out of bronchiolitis obliterans. *J Respir Dis* 1991:12;801.)

of BOOP overlap with those of other inflammatory lung disorders (especially hypersensitivity pneumonitis, desquamative interstitial pneumonitis, chronic eosinophilic pneumonia, and pulmonary infections). Foamy macrophages in alveolar spaces may erroneously suggest the diagnosis of desquamative interstitial pneumonitis (DIP). BOOP differs from constrictive or mural bronchiolitis obliterans (to be discussed later), which is characterized by fibrous connective tissue obliterating bronchioles and alveolar ducts but lacks an intense inflammatory component. Fiberoptic bronchoscopy with bronchoalveolar lavage (BAL) and transbronchial lung biopsies (TBB) can substantiate the diagnosis of BOOP in some cases, provided the salient histologic features are present and alternative causes have been reliably excluded. BAL in BOOP reveals increases in polymorphonuclear leukocytes (often exceeding 40%), with less striking increases in eosinophils or lymphocytes. These findings are nonspecific. Patients who have marked increases in BAL fluid lymphocytes generally have a more acute course, more prominent component of organizing pneumonia, and higher rate of corticosteroid responsiveness compared with patients who have low or normal BAL lymphocyte counts. Increases in BAL neutrophils or eosinophils have limited prognostic value. Given the patchy nature of BOOP and the small sample size of TBB, video-assisted thoracoscopic lung biopsy should be performed in equivocal or nondiagnostic cases.

Pathogenesis

Although the pathogenesis has not been elucidated, BOOP likely represents a distinctive and stereotypic host response to diverse injurious or inflammatory stimuli. The frequent association of antecedent viral or respiratory tract infection in idiopathic BOOP suggests that inhaled antigens may induce bronchiolar or alveolar injury. The histologic features of BOOP are usually of uniform age, suggesting that BOOP is an inflammatory reaction to one injurious stimulus, not to recurrent injury. Immune complex deposition in response to inhaled antigens may elicit a brisk inflammatory response. The prominence of neutrophils and neutrophil products in BAL fluid suggests a role for neutrophils in the pathogenesis. However, lymphocytes and macrophages undoubtedly are also important. The evolution of the lesions depends on the balance between the inflammatory process and reparative mechanisms (e.g., fibrosis, remodeling).

Therapy

Corticosteroids are the cornerstone of therapy for BOOP. Studies assessing optimal dose or duration of corticosteroid therapy for BOOP have not been performed. Most investigators advocate initial treatment with prednisone (1 mg/kg/day), but lower doses may be adequate in mild cases. Favorable responses are achieved with corticosteroids in 60%–80% of cases. Symptomatic improvement may be evident within 2 to 3 days; radiographic resolution usually ensues within 1 to 4 weeks. Corticosteroid therapy has been associated with marked reduction in BAL fluid neutrophils, collagenase activity, and myeloperoxidase activity in responding patients. The dose and rate of taper of corticosteroid need to be individualized according to clinical symptoms and results of chest radiographs and pulmonary function tests. In patients showing prompt and dramatic responses to corticosteroids, the dose may be tapered to 40 mg/day within 2 to 6 weeks. A more gradual taper may be appropriate for patients with persistent disease. The dose of prednisone may be tapered to 20 to 30 mg on alternate days within 4 to 6 months, provided patients remain in continuous remission. Because of the potential for relapse with premature discontinuation of therapy, low-dose corticosteroids should be continued for a minimum of 12 to 18 months unless serious adverse effects develop. Prolonged therapy may be required for selected patients exhibiting a propensity to relapse. Serious sequelae associated with BOOP are rare. Pulmonary fibrosis occurs in <20% of patients and fatalities in 3%–10%. Immunosuppressive or cytotoxic agents should be considered in patients failing to respond or experiencing adverse effects of corticosteroids. Data evaluating these agents are limited to anecdotal cases and small series.

Rapidly Progressive BOOP

A subset of patients with BOOP exhibit a more fulminant course, leading to death or severe fibrosis and honeycombing. Cohen et al. articulated the clinical features of 10 such patients seen at three medical centers from 1979 to 1992. The onset of symptoms was rapid (ranging from 3 days to 2 months). Bilateral basilar crackles were noted in 9 of 10; all had dyspnea and hypoxemia. Nine required mechanical ventilatory support. All but one patient were current or former smokers. Possible etiologic factors included connective tissue disease, nitrofurantoin, gold, and exposure to birds. BAL (performed in five patients) demonstrated increases in eosinophils and/or neutrophils. Histopathologic features were consistent with BOOP, but features of diffuse alveolar damage, alveolar septal inflammation, end-stage fibrosis, and honeycombing were also present. Despite aggressive therapy with corticosteroids in all patients (five of whom also received immunosuppressive agents), seven died. Although data regarding therapy are limited, we advise treating with ''pulse'' methylprednisolone (1000 mg daily for 3 days), followed by high-dose prednisone (1 mg/kg per day for 2 weeks, with a gradual taper). Cyclophosphamide or azathioprine should be added for steroid-recalcitrant cases.

Obliterative Bronchiolitis (Constrictive Bronchiolitis)

Obliterative bronchiolitis (OB) is a rare disorder characterized by progressive fibrosis and obliteration of bronchiolar lumina, resulting in progressive dyspnea and air flow obstruction. The terms *constrictive bronchiolitis, mural bronchiolitis,* and *pure bronchiolitis obliterans* are synonymous. Most cases of OB have occurred in the context of specific underlying disorders or risk factors, including collagen vascular disease (particularly rheumatoid arthritis), inhaled toxins, drugs (e.g., penicillamine), lung or bone marrow transplantation, infection, and diverse autoimmune, inflammatory, and vasculitic disorders. When no associated disorder can be identified, the term *idiopathic* is used. The prevalence is not known, but idiopathic OB is much less common than BOOP. Turton and colleagues detected 10 patients with OB among 2094 patients with airways obstruction. Five had rheumatoid arthritis; two had an antecedent chest infection; three cases were idiopathic. Many cases of OB diagnosed before 1985 likely represented BOOP.

Clinically, OB differs markedly from BOOP in clinical features, prognosis, and responsiveness to therapy. Patients with OB present with dyspnea and severe air flow obstruction, which progresses relentlessly during weeks to months. Severe reductions in FEV_1 and FEV_1/FVC ratio are characteristic. Air trapping (increased residual volume, or RV) or hyperinflation (increased total lung capacity, or TLC) are common associated features. Chest radiographic findings are usually normal or demonstrate only hyperinflation. However, diffuse reticular or finely nodular shadows, reflecting peribronchiolar inflammation and fibrosis, may be observed. High-resolution CT may reveal peribronchiolar nodular infiltrates and patchy increases in attenuation, accentuated by expiration, which reflect localized air trapping.

Histopathology

Obliterative (constrictive) bronchiolitis is centered on membranous and respiratory bronchioles and is characterized by fibrosis in submucosal and peribronchiolar regions, encircling and encroaching bronchiolar lumina. Necrotic bronchiolar epithelial cells and a mixed polymorphous inflammatory infiltrate may be seen. As the lesion progresses, peribronchiolar fibrosis dominates, resulting in concentric narrowing (and cicatrization) of bronchiolar lumina. Intrabronchial tufts of granulation tissue and extension to the alveolar interstitium are not seen, as they are in BOOP. The lesions are patchy and may be missed, even on open lung biopsy, unless several sections are reviewed. Remnants of destroyed bronchioles may occupy only a few millimeters; the surrounding lung parenchyma may be normal. Serial sections and trichrome stains may be required to identify the progressive narrowing of the caliber of bronchiolar lumina and the peribronchiolar scars. Late findings including bronchiolectasia with mucostasis, distortion of airway walls, bronchial metaplasia, and smooth-muscle hyperplasia.

Therapy

OB typically progresses relentlessly to severe air flow obstruction and ultimately death. In contrast to BOOP, OB rarely responds to therapy. Because of the devastating course, high-dose corticosteroids or immunosuppressive or cytotoxic agents are generally tried, but results have been disappointing.

Bronchiolitis Obliterans Complicating Bone Marrow Transplantation

Bronchiolitis obliterans is a well-recognized complication of bone marrow transplantation, principally in allogeneic recipients manifesting chronic graft-versus-host disease in skin, mucous membranes, liver, or extrapulmonary sites. Bronchiolitis obliterans complicates allogeneic bone marrow transplantation in 10%–12% of long-term survivors with graft-versus-host disease. The prevalence in allogeneic recipients without graft-versus-host disease or autologous recipients is rare (<1%). Bronchiolitis, occasionally with fibrinous obliteration of lumina, is the cardinal feature on lung biopsy or necropsy. The clinical course is indolent, developing 1.5 to 10 months after transplantation. Pulmonary symptoms include cough (60%), dyspnea (50%), wheezing (25%), or coldlike or flulike symptoms (25%). Declines in FEV_1 and VC and increases in RV are characteristic. Chest radiographic findings are normal or reveal mild hyperinflation in 80% of affected patients. In the remaining patients, reticular or finely nodular infiltrates may be noted. The diagnosis of OB can be presumed in bone marrow transplant recipients with a chronic course, progressive air flow obstruction, and lack of evidence for infection. BAL may be adequate in this context to exclude infection. TBB is more specific, but the risk may not be justified, particularly when thrombocytopenia or severe air flow obstruction is present. Prognosis is poor. Augmented immunosuppression is usually administered, but improvement occurs in <20% of patients.

Bronchiolitis Obliterans Complicating Lung Transplantation

Bronchiolitis obliterans, believed to represent a form of chronic lung allograft rejection, complicates lung or heart-lung transplantation in 30%–60% of recipients. Clinically, OB is characterized by progressive airways obstruction, cough, dyspnea, and recurrent lower respiratory tract infections. OB develops 9 to 18 months following lung or heart-lung transplantation. The lesion is never seen in the first 60 days after transplantation. Prevalence approximates 30% by 2 years after transplantation. By 5 years, OB syndrome develops in >50%. Histologically, bronchiolitis obliterans in affected lung allografts is similar to constrictive bronchiolitis or pure bronchiolitis obliterans, described earlier. Dense fibrous plaques narrow or obliterate the small airways. Submucosal and epithelial mononuclear cell infiltrates may be present, but the dense perivascular lymphocytic infiltrates characteristic of acute allograft rejection are lacking. Concomitant features include mucostasis, foam cells in distal airways, and epithelial metaplasia. Lymphocytic bronchitis or bronchiolitis, characterized by peribronchiolar and peribronchial lymphocytic infiltrates, but without fibrosis, may be a precursor of OB in some recipients. Risk factors for development of OB include recurrent episodes of acute allograft rejection, cytomegalovirus (CMV) pneumonitis, large-airway ischemic injury in the initial period after transplantation, heightened immunologic activity against the donor (as assessed by the primed lymphocyte test), and enhanced cell-mediated cytotoxicity. CMV infection may upregulate class I and II histocompatibility (HLA) antigens on epithelial and endothelial cells, thereby amplifying the process. Lung or heart-lung transplant recipients with OB demonstrate submucosal and intraepithelial mononuclear cell infiltrates, enhanced expression of class II HLA antigens on bronchiolar epithelial and lung endothelial cells, and increased number of dendritic cells (e.g., antigen-presenting cells) in the airways. These features support the premise that OB is a form of chronic lung allograft rejection. In other organ allografts, chronic rejection is associated with disappearance or dissolution of structures within the allograft [e.g., vanishing bile duct syndrome (liver), disappearance of renal tubules (kidney), accelerated coronary artery disease (heart)].

The course of OB is indolent. Asymptomatic reductions in expiratory flow rates (e.g., $FEF_{25\%-75\%}$, FEV_1) usually precede the onset of clinical symptoms. Initial symptoms are nonproductive cough, "bronchitis," or "chest cold." Physical examination findings are usually unimpressive, but rales or rhonchi develop later. Chest radiographic findings are usually normal, but hyperinflation or bronchiectatic changes develop in the late phases. Once airways obstruction occurs on pulmonary function tests, a downhill course is nearly inevitable. A rapid course (with fall in FEV_1 below 40% of predicted) can occur as early as 3 to 4 months in some patients. In others, pulmonary function stabilizes after an initial decline. Gas exchange is preserved until late in the course. Airways become colonized with *Pseudomonas aeruginosa*, *Staphylococcus aureus*, or *Aspergillus* species. Progressive dyspnea ensues, which may culminate in respiratory failure. The diagnosis of OB can be established by TBB in more than 75% of affected patients. Because the lesion is patchy, a negative biopsy result does not exclude OB. In this context, a clinical diagnosis of OB syndrome can be made if a sustained and progressive loss in FEV_1 (>15% decline) or $FEF_{25\%-75\%}$ (>25% decline) has been documented and alternative causes of airways obstruction have been excluded.

Once developed, OB typically worsens, but the rate of progression is highly variable. Augmented immunosuppression with pulse methylprednisolone, antilymphocytic agents (e.g., antilymphocyte sera or globulin, OKT3 antibody), FK506, and aerosolized cyclosporine have been tried for OB or OB syndrome, with anecdotal successes. However, sustained remissions are unusual, and most patients experience continued or persistent decline in pulmonary function. Because the prognosis in untreated patients is dismal, most investigators treat OB aggressively with two to four cycles of augmented immunosuppression. The risk-to-benefit ratio of this approach is uncertain, as the rate of complications and short-term and long-term efficacy have not been well defined. In our experience, response to therapy is rarely dramatic. The lesions stabilize (often for 6 to 24 months) in some patients, but one third or more of affected recipients die of respiratory failure within 2 to 3 years of onset of symptoms. Secondary bacterial or fungal pneumonias may accelerate the course. Aggressive treatment and prophylaxis of airway infections may reduce the risk for secondary infections and prolong survival. It is hoped that prophylactic regimens against CMV and improved operative techniques to reduce large-airway ischemia may lower the incidence of OB. Repeated transplantation has been performed in patients with progressive OB refractory to augmented immunosuppressive therapy. Success with repeated transplantation has been less than with initial transplant procedures. Given the scarcity of donor organs, repeated transplantation for OB is controversial.

Follicular Bronchiolitis

Follicular bronchiolitis, a rare disorder most commonly seen in association with rheumatoid arthritis or other connective tissue disorders, exhibits features that overlap with those of OB and BOOP. The relationship of follicular bronchiolitis to these other bronchiolar disorders is not clear. Pulmonary function tests may reveal restriction or airways obstruction. In contrast to OB, which results in intramural or intraluminal compression and distortion of bronchioles, follicular bronchiolitis typically compresses bronchioles externally from lymphoid follicles. A pronounced lymphocytic infiltration within bronchiolar walls may also be evident. Chest radiographs demonstrate reticular or reticulonodular opacities, corresponding to these peribronchiolar cellular infiltrates. The prognosis is more favorable than in OB, as approximately 50% respond to corticosteroid therapy.

Respiratory Bronchiolitis

Respiratory bronchiolitis is a rare disorder of cigarette smokers with features overlapping with those of BOOP. Lung biopsy reveals clusters of pigmented, golden-brown macrophages in respiratory and membranous (terminal) bronchioles and adjacent alveolar spaces. Chronic inflammation and fibrosis may be present but are invariably mild. Most patients are asymptomatic or note mild cough or dyspnea. Chest radiographic findings may be normal or demonstrate accentuated bronchopulmonary markings ("dirty lungs") resembling those of chronic interstitial pneumonitis. Constitutional symptoms, fever, or dense alveolar infiltrates do not occur in respiratory bronchiolitis, as they do in BOOP. Prognosis has been favorable, but data have been derived from a few small series.

The histologic lesion termed *respiratory bronchiolitis* was initially described by Niewoehner and associates in 1974 as an incidental necropsy finding in young asymptomatic smokers who died of nonpulmonary causes. The cardinal feature was clusters of pigmented macrophages in respiratory and terminal bronchioles. The macrophages had abundant cytoplasm with finely, granular, golden-brown pigment. The coarse granules typical of hemosiderin were absent. Peribronchiolar inflammation or fibrosis was noted but was never severe. This lesion was referred to as *small-airways disease* and was believed to represent a reaction to cigarette smoke with minimal clinical significance. In 1987, Myers and colleagues described a similar lesion in six smokers in whom open lung biopsies had been performed for suspected CILD. Four of the cases were identified during a review of all open lung biopsies at the University of Alabama from 1972 to 1984; two additional cases had been referred for pathologic consultation. All were heavy smokers, usually in the third or fourth decade of life. Five had mild symptoms of cough or dyspnea. Chest radiographs demonstrated bilateral interstitial or reticulonodular infiltrates in five. The dominant histologic feature was aggregates of pigmented macrophages within respiratory and terminal bronchioles and adjacent alveolar ducts and spaces. Electron microscopy demonstrated numerous phagolysosomes and "smoker's inclusions" within alveolar macophages. Severe fibrosis or honeycombing was uniformly absent. The prognosis was excellent. In 1989, Yousem et al. extracted 18 cases of respiratory bronchiolitis from the open lung biopsy files of Boston University and an extensive pulmonary pathology consultation collection. All 18 patients were smokers; mean age was 36 years. Symptoms were mild and were limited to cough, dyspnea, or sputum production. Chest radiographs revealed bilateral reticulonodular infiltrates, with a basilar predominance, in 13 patients (72%). Chest radiographic findings were normal in five patients (28%). Pulmonary function tests revealed consistent reductions in diffusing capacity; mild degrees of airway obstruction, with preserved lung volumes, were also

noted. Open lung biopsies demonstrated pigmented macrophages in bronchioles and alveolar spaces, with bronchiolar and peribronchiolar inflammation or fibrosis. Severe fibrosis or honeycombing was never evident. The clinical course was benign. Symptoms resolved in 13 patients (81%); five (19%) remained stable; none worsened. Symptoms improved in 12 of 15 following cessation of smoking. Of three patients who continued to smoke, symptoms persisted in two. Only two patients were treated with corticosteroids; symptoms improved in both. Since these sentinel reports, the clinicopathologic syndrome of respiratory bronchiolitis-associated ILD has been further characterized. Cough, dyspnea, and sputum production are the predominant symptoms. Bilateral basilar rales are noted in 40% of patients; clubbing does not occur. Chest radiographs may show fine reticulonodular interstitial infiltrates, bronchial wall thickening, and ring shadows with normal lung volumes. High-resolution CT has been performed in only a few patients. Fine irregular nodules (2 to 3 mm) are most characteristic. Additional features include foci of patchy ground-glass opacities, atelectasis, emphysema, and peripheral blebs. BAL profiles in respiratory bronchiolitis are similar to those of smokers and do not manifest the striking neutrophilia observed in BOOP. Histologically, the strictly peribronchiolar distribution of respiratory bronchiolitis contrasts with the patchy, subpleural involvement noted in usual interstitial pneumonitis (UIP). Honeycombing, a cardinal feature of UIP, is absent in respiratory bronchiolitis. Intraalveolar accumulation of macrophages may be observed in DIP. The process is uniform and diffuse with DIP and lacks the peribronchiolar distribution seen in respiratory bronchiolitis. The prognosis in respiratory bronchiolitis is excellent, even in the absence of therapy. No deaths have been attributed to respiratory bronchiolitis, and serious pulmonary fibrosis is rare. However, data are limited, and long-term observational studies involving large numbers of patients with respiratory bronchiolitis are lacking. Smoking cessation is the cornerstone of therapy. Corticosteroids should be reserved for patients with persistent or progressive symptoms despite smoking cessation.

Diffuse Panbronchiolitis

Diffuse panbronchiolitis (DPB) is a chronic, progressive bronchiolar inflammatory disorder characterized by pansinusitis, cough, sputum production, diffuse micronodular shadows on chest radiographs, progressive bronchiectasis, and increases in cold-agglutinating antibodies. Panbronchiolitis shares many features with cystic fibrosis, but these disorders are unrelated. The etiology of DPB is not known, but a strong genetic basis is evident. Virtually all cases have been described in Japan and Korea. Fewer than 10 patients with DPB have been described in the United States. More than 60% of patients with DPB express HLA-B54, an antigen restricted to Oriental populations. The incidence of HLA-B54 is 10%–11% in Japanese and Chinese populations and 3% in Koreans. By contrast, HLA-B54 is invariably lacking in Caucasians, blacks, Hispanics, and American Indians.

Clinical Features

Characteristically, chronic sinusitis begins in the second or third decade of life. Chronic cough, sputum production, and bronchiectasis follow 10 or more years after the onset of sinusitis. In time, colonization of the lower respiratory tract with *Hemophilus influenzae* and eventually *P. aeruginosa* develops. Once colonization with *P. aeruginosa* occurs, the course accelerates. Repetitive suppurative infections lead to progressive respiratory failure. Pulmonary function tests in DPB demonstrate airways obstruction, hypoxemia, and air trapping (increased RV). Chest radiographs demonstrate widely disseminated, small (1 to 4 mm), ill-defined nodules, with a predilection for the lung bases. Lung volumes may be normal or increased during the early phases, but destruction of bronchioles and lung parenchyma eventually results in volume loss. Ring shadows, tramlines, and dilated, ectatic bronchioles reflect cystic bronchiectasis. High-resolution CT reveals diffuse nodular and rounded opacities (representing fluid-filled or inflamed bronchioles), dilated bronchi and bronchioles, bronchiolectasis, and cystic bronchiectasis. In contrast to BOOP, DPB is not characterized by dense focal alveolar infiltrates. BAL reveals intense neutrophilia (typically exceeding 40%); lymphocytes are usually normal or slightly increased. Erythrocyte sedimentation rate and levels of C-reactive protein are usually elevated. Serum immunoglobulins are normal or increased. Persistent elevation of polyclonal cold-agglutinating antibodies is a distinctive feature. Although circulating antibodies against *Mycoplasma pneumoniae* are absent, many patients respond clinically to long-term therapy with erythromycin, suggesting an infectious etiology.

Histologic Features

The distinctive early lesion of DPB are small, poorly circumscribed nodules centered on respiratory bronchioles (bronchiolocentric). These nodules correspond to dense peribronchiolar and intraluminal infiltrates of acute and chronic inflammatory cells. An alveolar component is lacking or minimal. The walls of respiratory bronchioles are thickened; airway lumina may be filled with mucus or intraluminal neutrophils. Foamy macrophages and proliferating lymphoid follicles are common associated features. As the disease advances, destruction of bronchiolar walls results in bronchiolectasis and proximal bronchiectasis. Narrowing and obliteration of bronchiolar lumina, ectatic

bronchioles, hypersecretion of mucus, and cystic destruction of proximal bronchioles and bronchi may ensue. Histologic features of DPB overlap with those of obliterative (constrictive) bronchiolitis, but the high frequency of sinus and lower respiratory tract infections and bronchiectasis characteristic of DPB are lacking in OB.

Therapy

The prognosis of DPB is poor, with a 5-year survival from the time of diagnosis of 40%; 10-year survival is 25%. Corticosteroids or immunosuppressive agents are not efficacious and may exacerbate infections. Long-term low-dose erythromycin (600 mg/d) ameliorates symptoms and chest radiographic and physiologic findings in some cases, and is recommended. Its impact on long-term prognosis has not been defined. The mechanism of action of erythromycin is not clear, as the dose is below the minimal inhibitory concentration (MIC) for most pathogenic organisms cultured from sputum.

Bronchocentric Granulomatosis

Bronchocentric granulomatosis (BCG), a granulomatous inflammatory disorder involving and destroying bronchi and bronchioles, was initially described in 1973 by Averill Liebow, a renowned pulmonary pathologist. Bronchial walls were infiltrated and replaced by inflammatory cells (predominantly eosinophils, lymphocytes, and mononuclear cells), with extensive necrosis. Bronchial lumina were filled with necrotic exudate, inflammatory cells (particularly eosinophils), epithelioid cells, and multinucleated giant cells. Foci of organizing pneumonia were observed in the distal alveolar spaces and interstitium. Pulmonary vessels contiguous to involved bronchi were often surrounded by inflammatory cells, but true vasculitis was lacking. Predominant clinical manifestations included fever, cough, malaise, dyspnea, and wheezing. Chest radiographs demonstrated patchy infiltrates, consolidation, mucoid impaction, or atelectasis. We are reluctant to make the diagnosis of BCG, as virtually all cases are associated with a specific underlying disease. Asthma or allergic bronchopulmonary aspergillosis (ABPA) has been noted in 30%–50% of cases of BCG. In this context, blood or tissue eosinophilia, increased serum IgE levels, or intrabronchial *Aspergillus* hyphae may be found. Findings of BCG have been described in Wegener's granulomatosis, rheumatoid arthritis, BOOP, and diverse infectious etiologies. It is likely that BCG represents a hypersensitivity response to a variety of intrabronchial antigens rather than a specific disease entity. Therapy should be directed to the underlying disease. Corticosteroids are highly efficacious for ABPA or asthma. When BCG is caused by an infectious granulomatous process (e.g., tuberculosis, fungal infection, nocardiosis, echinoccosis), antimicrobial therapy directed against the responsible organism may be curative.

PULMONARY VASCULITIS

Systemic necrotizing vasculitis involving the lung occurs primarily in the context of the granulomatous vasculitis syndromes (e.g., Wegener's granulomatosis, Churg-Strauss angiitis, lymphomatoid granulomatosis) or pulmonary-renal syndromes (e.g., microscopic polyangiitis, pauci-immune glomerulonephritis). Classic polyarteritis nodosa rarely involves the lung. Pulmonary arterial aneurysms are well-recognized complications of Takayasu's disease. Pulmonary hemorrhage (usually caused by capillaritis) rarely complicates Behçet's disease or Henoch-Schönlein purpura.

Antineutrophil Cytoplasmic Antibodies

Circulating autoantibodies directed against cytoplasmic components of neutrophils and monocytes (e.g., ANCA) are frequently found in patients with necrotizing small-vessel vasculitis, associated with pulmonary capillaritis or glomerulonephritis. ANCA with differing antigenic specificities have been noted and have differing prognostic and clinical significance. Antibodies with antigenic specificity for proteinase 3 exhibit a cytoplasmic pattern on immunofluorescence (c-ANCA); antibodies with antigenic specificity for myeloperoxidase (MPO) exhibit a perinuclear pattern (p-ANCA). Antibodies with distinct antigenic determinants are observed in different types of vasculitis. c-ANCA (PR3-ANCA) are detected in 70%–93% of patients with untreated Wegener's granulomatosis and may be found in patients with microscopic polyangiitis (MPA) or Churg-Strauss syndrome (CSS). More than 50% of patients with MPA, CSS, or pauci-immune glomerulonephritis demonstrate circulating p-ANCA (MPO-ANCA), whereas p-ANCA is rarely found in Wegener's granulomatosis. Detectable ANCA (typically p-ANCA) are present in <20% of patients with macroscopic polyarteritis nodosa (PAN). c-ANCA is relatively specific for small-vessel vasculitis (>90% specificity), but p-ANCA may be observed in a myriad of inflammatory disorders in which vasculitis is lacking (e.g., collagen vascular disease, inflammatory bowel disease).

Wegener's Granulomatosis

Wegener's granulomatosis, the most common of the pulmonary granulomatous vasculitides, typically involves the upper respiratory tract (e.g., sinuses, ears, nasopharynx, oropharynx, trachea), lower respiratory tract (bronchi and lungs), and kidneys, with varying degrees of disseminated vasculitis. Major histologic features include a necrotizing vasculitis involving small vessels (i.e., arterioles, venules, and capillaries), extensive necrosis, and granulomatous inflammation. The estimated prevalence of Wegener's granulomatosis is between 1.3 to 3 cases per 100,000 persons per 5-year period. The peak incidence is in the fourth through sixth decades of life; children or adolescents are rarely affected. There is no sex predominance.

Clinical Features

Clinical manifestations are protean, and virtually any organ can be involved. Upper airway symptoms often dominate. Pulmonary involvement occurs in more than two thirds of patients; glomerulonephritis, in 55%–85%. Although Wegener's granulomatosis usually involves multiple organs, limited variants exist involving only one or two organs. This subset of patients has a more favorable prognosis. DeRemee proposed a staging classification based on involvement of ear, nose, throat (E), lung (L), and kidney (K), to stratify patients with single or multiorgan involvement. Other diagnostic criteria proposed by the American College of Rheumatology in 1990 include nasal or oral inflammation, abnormalities on chest radiographs, abnormal urine sediment, and granulomatous inflammation on biopsy. Many classic features lacking in the early phases of the disease may evolve months or even years after the initial presentation. High titers of circulating c-ANCA may support the diagnosis in the appropriate clinical context, even when histologic features are not definitive. However, the specificity of c-ANCA has been challenged.

Upper Airway Involvement

The upper respiratory tract (e.g., sinuses, ears, nasopharynx, oropharynx, trachea) is involved in >90% of patients. Chronic persistent sinusitis, epistaxis, and otitis media are often the presenting and dominant clinical features of Wegener's granulomatosis, but they are often mistakenly thought to represent allergic or infectious etiologies. Sinus radiographic or thin-section CT findings are abnormal in >85% of patients with Wegener's granulomatosis. Thickening or clouding of the sinuses is characteristic; erosion or destruction of sinus bones may occur. Secondary pyogenic sinus infections are common and may be difficult to distinguish from exacerbations of Wegener's granulomatosis. Otologic involvement occurs in 30%–50% of patients. Otalgia and refractory otitis media are common early symptoms of Wegener's granulomatosis. Chronic otitis media, chronic mastoiditis, or hearing loss develops in 15%–25% of patients. The nasopharynx is involved in 60%–80% of patients. Clinical manifestations include epistaxis, nasal septal perforation, persistent nasal congestion or pain, and mucosal ulcers.

Saddle nose deformity, resulting from destruction of the nasal cartilage, occurs in 10%–25% of patients. Sore throat or hoarseness may reflect ulcerations or granulomatous involvement of the pharynx or vocal cords. Despite the propensity for Wegener's granulomatosis to affect the upper respiratory tract, histologic confirmation may be difficult. Biopsy specimens of upper airway lesions often demonstrate nonspecific findings of necrosis and chronic inflammation. The cardinal histologic features of vasculitis and granulomatous inflammation may be lacking. A review of 126 biopsy specimens from upper airway or nasopharyngeal lesions in patients with Wegener's granulomatosis seen at the National Institutes of Health revealed the triad of granulomas, vasculitis, and necrosis in only 16% of specimens. Dual features of vasculitis plus granulomas or vasculitis plus necrosis were each noted in 21% of patients. Generous samples of involved sites or samples from additional sites are critical to substantiate the diagnosis. Ocular involvement occurs in 20%–50% of patients with Wegener's granulomatosis. Manifestations may be superficial (e.g., conjunctivitis, scleritis), but uveitis, vasculitis, or compression of the optic nerve may lead to blindness in 2%–9% of patients. Proptosis from a retro-orbital granulomatous inflammatory process has been described in 10%–22% of patients and may compromise the blood supply to the optic nerve. In this context, surgical decompression may be required in patients failing to respond to aggressive medical therapy.

Involvement of Trachea and Bronchi

Stenosis or narrowing of the trachea or major bronchi from granulomatous involvement develops in 10%–30% of patients with Wegener's granulomatosis. The rate of asymptomatic involvement of major airways is even higher. Tracheal or bronchial involvement is nine times more common in female patients and is usually associated with severe sinusitis. Tracheal stenosis is usually circumferential and localized, extending only 3 to 5 cm below the glottis. However, more extensive involvement of the distal trachea or main bronchi may occur. A recent study from the Mayo Clinic cited endobronchial abnormalities in 30 of 51 patients (59%) with Wegener's granulomatosis undergoing bronchoscopy. Four (13%) had tracheal or bronchial stenosis. Extensive endobronchial abnormalities were noted in 11 patients with normal chest radiographic findings. Ulcerating tracheobronchitis was the most common lesion and eventually resulted in progressive stenosis in seven patients followed on a long-term basis. Persistent dyspnea or wheezing may reflect scarring at the site of previous endobronchial inflammation. Stridor or wheezing is a clinical clue to the development of large-airway (trachea or main bronchi) stenosis. Truncation (flow rate limitation) of the inspiratory portion of the flow-volume loop is a sensitive indicator of physiologi-

cally significant upper airway obstruction. When the site of obstruction is fixed, both inspiratory and expiratory portions are affected (Fig. 5). Bronchoscopy or spiral CT more objectively quantitates the degree of airway stenosis. Histologic confirmation of the diagnosis is difficult, as endobronchial biopsies usually demonstrate nonspecific changes (e.g., necrosis or inflammation). In the Mayo Clinic study, endobronchial biopsy specimens fulfilled specific histologic criteria for Wegener's granulomatosis in only 3 of 17 patients. Serum titers of c-ANCA did not correlate with endobronchial inflammation. Severe stenosis of large airways may necessitate treatment with YAG (yttrium-argon-garnet) laser, dilation, or placement of Silastic airway stents. Severe upper airway obstruction may mandate tracheostomy. Tracheal reconstruction has been successfully performed in patients with severe tracheal stenosis refractory to medical therapy but is a formidable undertaking.

Lung Involvement

Pulmonary symptoms (e.g., cough, dyspnea, hemoptysis) are noted in approximately one third of patients with Wegener's granulomatosis, caused by parenchymal ne-

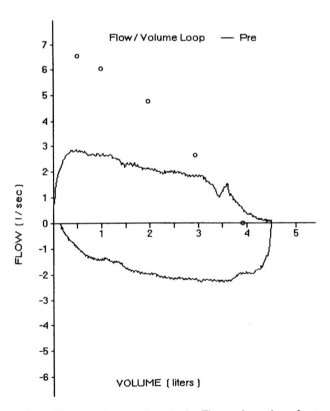

FIG. 5. Wegener's granulomatosis. Flow-volume loop from a 34-year-old woman with tracheal (subglottic) stenosis caused by Wegener's granulomatosis. Note the truncation of both inspiratory and expiratory limbs, consistent with fixed upper airway obstruction.

crosis, endobronchial inflammation and cicatrix formation, or alveolar hemorrhage. Pulmonary function tests may demonstrate airways obstruction (particularly when endobronchial involvement is prominent), restriction, or mixed patterns. Despite a relatively low prevalence of clinical symptoms, abnormalities on chest radiographs are noted in more than 80% of patients at some point during the course of the disease. Single or multiple nodules or nodular infiltrates are characteristic; cavitation is noted in one quarter (Fig. 6). Other features include focal pneumonic infiltrates (Fig. 7), large mass lesions (Fig. 8), pleural effusions, stenosis of trachea or bronchi, or atelectasis. Hilar or mediastinal lymphadenopathy has only rarely been described. Extensive alveolar or mixed interstitial alveolar infiltrates may be seen in patients with pulmonary capillaritis and alveolar hemorrhage (Fig. 9). Open (or thoracoscopic) lung biopsy is usually required to substantiate the diagnosis of pulmonary Wegener's granulomatosis. When focal pulmonary infiltrates or nodules are present, the triad of vasculitis, granulomas, and necrosis can be found in >90% of patients by surgical biopsy. By contrast, the yield of endobronchial or transbronchial lung biopsies is only 3%–18%. Massive alveolar hemorrhage is a rare but potentially fatal complication of Wegener's granulomatosis, reflecting diffuse injury to the pulmonary microvasculature. In this setting, rapidly progressive glomerulonephritis is present in >90% of patients. By contrast, 40% manifest upper airway symptoms. The role of surgical lung biopsy in the setting of diffuse alveolar hemorrhage is controversial. Histopathologic features are usually nonspecific. Alveolar hemorrhage dominates. Inflammation and necrosis of the alveolar capillaries

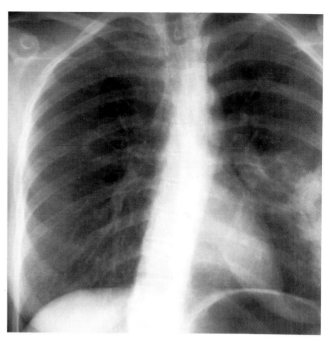

FIG. 7. Wegener's granulomatosis. PA chest radiograph demonstrates dense focal alveolar infiltrates in an 18-year-old female patient with sinusitis, cough, fever, and cutaneous nodules. Serum antineutrophil cytoplasmic antibody was positive (c-ANCA titer of 1:1200). Skin biopsies demonstrated a leukocytoclastic vasculitis. Sinus biopsies revealed a granulomatous necrotizing vasculitis consistent with Wegener's granulomatosis. Chest radiographs normalized within 2 weeks of initiation of cyclophosphamide and prednisone therapy.

(termed *capillaritis*) may be noted, but the granulomatous vasculitis or extensive parenchymal necrosis characteristic of Wegener's granulomatosis at other sites is lacking. For severe pulmonary hemorrhage, we believe the risk of surgical lung biopsy outweighs the benefit. A presumptive diagnosis of diffuse alveolar hemorrhage (DAH) can often be established on the basis of clinical and radiographic features, circulating c-ANCA, and bronchoscopy with BAL. Large numbers of hemosiderin-laden macrophages, bloody or serosanguinous BAL fluid, and absence of infectious etiologies support the diagnosis of DAH (Fig. 10). Biopsy of extrapulmonary sites of involvement may substantiate the diagnosis. However, DAH is a medical emergency requiring aggressive therapy with intravenous pulse methylprednisolone (1 g daily for 3 days) pending the results of a diagnostic workup with biopsies and ancillary laboratory studies. Conventional therapy with oral cyclophosphamide and a tapering regimen of corticosteroids are appropriate once the diagnosis of Wegener's granulomatosis has been confirmed.

Renal Involvement

Glomerulonephritis (pauci-immune) occurs in 70%–85% of patients at some point in the course of the disease,

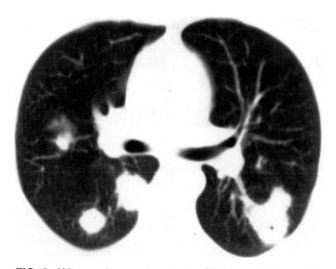

FIG. 6. Wegener's granulomatosis. CT demonstrates multiple focal nodules in a 40-year-old man. Open lung biopsy demonstrated a necrotizing granulomatous vasculitis consistent with Wegener's granulomatosis. (Reproduced with permission from Orens JB, Sitrin RC, Lynch JP III. The approach to nonresolving pneumonia. *Med Clin North Am* 1994: 78;1160, Fig. 8B.)

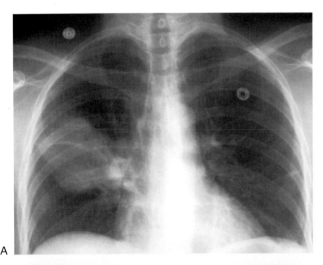

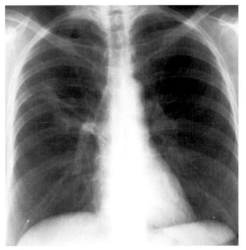

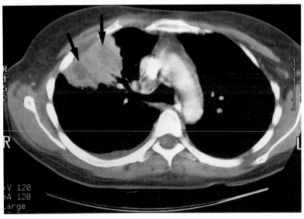

FIG. 8. A: Wegener's granulomatosis. PA chest radiograph demonstrates right upper lobe mass in a 36-year-old woman with leukocytoclastic vasculitis, fever, sinusitis, and cough. **B:** CT in the same patient reveals a mass lesion in the anterior segment of the right upper lobe with areas of focal necrosis (*arrows*). Transbronchial lung biopsies demonstrated granulomatosis vasculitis with extensive necrosis and a polymorphous inflammatory cell infiltrate consistent with Wegener's granulomatosis. **C:** PA chest radiograph from same patient 5 weeks after initiation of therapy with cyclophosphamide and prednisone, showing nearly complete resolution of right upper lobe mass.

but only 11%–17% of patients exhibit severe renal insufficiency at presentation. Granulomatous vasculitis is observed in <8% of renal biopsy specimens from patients with Wegener's granulomatosis. The characteristic renal lesion of Wegener's granulomatosis is a segmental focal glomerulonephritis. With more fulminant forms, a necrotizing, crescentic glomerulonephritis is observed. Immune complexes have been noted in a minority of cases. These histologic findings are nonspecific and can be found in diverse immune-mediated or infectious disorders. Clinically evident renal insufficiency may be subtle and progress indolently. Microscopic hematuria or proteinuria precedes detectable abnormalities of renal function. Once renal failure is present, rapid progression may ensue within days or weeks. Aggressive and prompt institution of therapy is mandatory to avert irreversible renal damage. Even in oliguric renal failure, substantial recovery of renal function can be achieved in most patients. Chronic renal failure remains a major cause of death, and 10%–30% of patients with Wegener's granulomatosis eventually require long-term dialysis. Renal transplantation has been successfully accomplished in patients with end-stage renal disease in whom Wegener's granulomatosis is in complete remission. Recurrence of Wegener's granulomatosis has been rare following transplantation.

Other rare urologic complications of Wegener's granulomatosis include necrotizing vasculitis involving the ureters, penis, or prostate (anecdotal reports).

Central or Peripheral Nervous System Involvement

Central or peripheral nervous system involvement occurs in <4% of patients at initial presentation, but eventually it develops in 10%–34%. Mononeuritis multiplex or polyneuritis accounts for >50% of neurologic complications. Other manifestations include cerebral infarction or hemorrhage, cranial nerve palsies, focal deficits or seizures from cerebral mass lesions, diabetes insipidus (secondary to granulomatous involvement of the hypothalamus), quadriparesis or paraparesis (reflecting involvement of the spinal cord microvasculature), generalized seizures (reflecting meningeal involvement), and visual loss (from compression of the optic nerve or vasculitis of the vasculature). Vasculitis of the central nervous system has only rarely been confirmed histologically, because of inaccessibility or risks associated with biopsies. The diagnosis is usually supported by histologic confirmation at extraneural sites or by noninvasive studies (e.g., electromyelogram, magnetic resonance imaging, or CT of the brain)

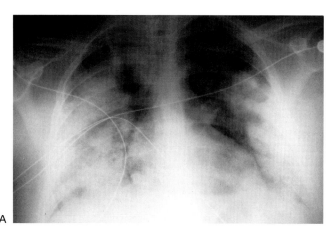

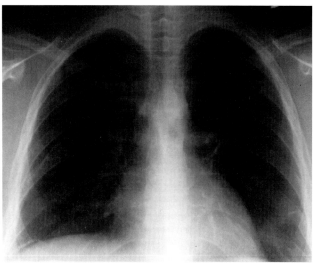

FIG. 9. A: Alveolar hemorrhage caused by Wegener's granulomatosis. PA chest radiograph from a 13-year-old girl demonstrates extensive, confluent alveolar infiltrates. She presented with severe dyspnea, fever, and hemoptysis. Urinalysis demonstrated microscopic hematuria and proteinuria. Open lung biopsy demonstrated massive pulmonary hemorrhage and capillaritis but no granulomas. Review of a prior sinus biopsy demonstrated extensive necrosis and inflammatory exudate with occasional multinucleated giant cells but no definite vasculitis. Pulse methylprednisolone, followed by oral prednisone and cyclophosphamide, was instituted. **B:** PA chest radiographs from the same patient 3 weeks later demonstrate complete clearing of the alveolar infiltrates. After institution of therapy, she remained asymptomatic. Cyclophosphamide was discontinued after 15 months, and prednisone was discontinued after 18 months.

in patients with neurologic symptoms and previous documentation of Wegener's granulomatosis. Cerebral angiography is ill advised, because the small vessels affected in Wegener's granulomatosis are below the sensitivity of angiography. In some patients, biopsy of the sural nerve or other affected nerves may substantiate the diagnosis.

Other Organ Involvement

Constitutional features (e.g., malaise, fatigue, fever, weight loss) occur in one third or more of patients with Wegener's granulomatosis. Nondeforming polyarthritis involving medium and large joints occurs in two thirds of patients and parallels activity of the systemic disease. Articular symptoms usually remit with cytotoxic or corticosteroid therapy. Cutaneous lesions are present in 40%–50% of patients during the course of the disease. Manifestations are protean and include palpable purpura, subcutaneous nodules, papules, petechiae, ulcers, and nonspecific erythematous or maculopapular rashes. Skin biopsy may demonstrate granulomatous vasculitis with necrosis but most often reveals nonspecific changes of leukocytoclastic vasculitis. Cardiac involvement is rarely documented

ante mortem, but prevalence rates of 10%–15% have been estimated. Coronary arteritis and pericarditis are the most common clinical features. Cardiomyopathies, conduction defects, and fatal arrhythmias may reflect necrotizing vasculitis or granulomatous inflammation involving the myocardium or coronary arteries. Gastrointestinal manifestations (e.g., abdominal pain, diarrhea, hemorrhage, and perforation) have been cited in <5% of patients with Wegener's granulomatosis. This may in part reflect inaccessibility of lesions or lack of an aggressive diagnostic approach. In a review of the literature, granulomatous or vascular lesions within the gastrointestinal tract were found in 23 of 59 necropsies performed in patients with Wegener's granulomatosis.

Histopathology

The cardinal histopathologic features of Wegener's granulomatosis include a necrotizing vasculitis affecting arterioles, venules, and capillaries; granulomatous inflammation; geographic parenchymal necrosis; hemorrhagic infarcts; and areas of fibrosis. Well-formed sarcoidlike granulomas are uncommon, but multinucleated

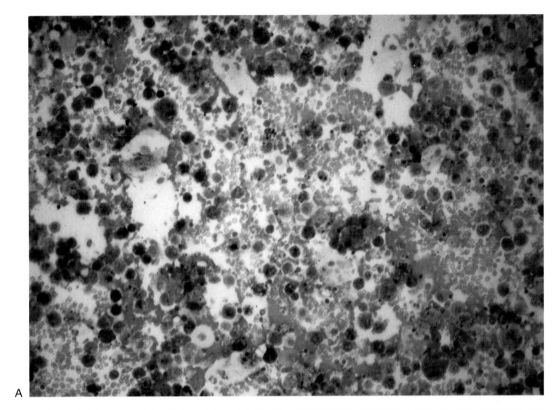

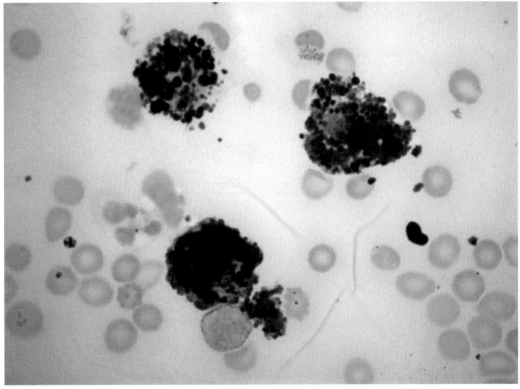

FIG. 10. A: Hemosiderin-laden macrophages. Photomicrograph of BAL fluid demonstrating numerous hemosiderin-laden macrophages with adjacent red blood cells indicating alveolar hemorrhage. Wright stain, low power. **B:** Photomicrograph of BAL fluid showing hemosiderin-laden alveolar macrophages stained blue by iron stain. Prussian blue stain, high power. *See color plate 11.*

giant cells, epithelioid cells, and collections of histiocytes are usually evident in involved organs. Vascular walls are infiltrated by mononuclear cells and neutrophils, with occasional multinucleated giant cells and eosinophils (Fig. 11). Fibrinoid necrosis and thrombosis within vascular lumina are early findings. Later, fibrosis of vascular walls may result in stenosis or obliteration of the lumina. A pronounced fibroblastic component, with concentric rings of collagen and connective tissue matrix, may be present. These histologic features may not be found if small or nonrepresentative biopsy specimens are obtained. Granulomas and vasculitis of small vessels may be observed with infections (particularly with mycobacterial and fungal etiologies). Thus, special stains should be performed in any granulomatous or necrotic lesion to exclude infectious causes.

Laboratory Features

Anemia, thrombocytosis, or leukocytosis has been noted in 30%–40% of patients with Wegener's granulomatosis. Leukopenia or thrombocytopenia is rare in the absence of cytotoxic therapy. Peripheral blood eosinophilia is not a feature of Wegener's granulomatosis. Polyclonal hypergammaglobulinemia occurs in up to 50% of patients. Serum complement levels are normal or elevated. Circulating immune complexes have been found but are of no clinical value in either the diagnosis or follow-up. Renal function tests (serum creatinine, blood urea nitrogen) and urinalysis should be obtained in all patients initially. Striking increases in erythrocyte sedimentation rate and levels of C-reactive protein are characteristic of active, generalized disease. However, erythrocyte sedimentation rate or levels of C-reactive protein can be normal with active disease, particularly when only a single site is involved. Serial determinations of the erythrocyte sedimentation rate or levels of C-reactive protein are useful in monitoring the disease but are nonspecific, as elevations may occur in the presence of coexisting infections. c-ANCA are helpful in the initial diagnosis of Wegener's granulomatosis and in monitoring response to therapy. Increases in c-ANCA have been noted in >90% of patients with active generalized Wegener's granulomatosis, and in 40%–70% of patients with active regional Wegener's granulomatosis. Changes in c-ANCA usually correlate with disease activity and are unaffected by intercurrent infections. However, c-ANCA titers may persist in 30%–40% of patients even after complete clinical remission has been achieved. Serial determinations of c-ANCA provide a useful adjunct to the clinical data, but treatment decisions should not rely exclusively on c-ANCA titers.

Pathogenesis

The cause of Wegener's granulomatosis is unknown. The preponderance of disease in the upper and lower respiratory tracts, the intensity of mononuclear infiltrates, and the granulomatous character are consistent with an exaggerated cellular immune response to inhaled antigen(s). Increases in serum immunoglobulins, B-cell activity, circulating autoantibodies (c-ANCA), and immune

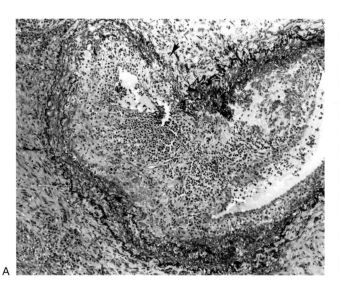

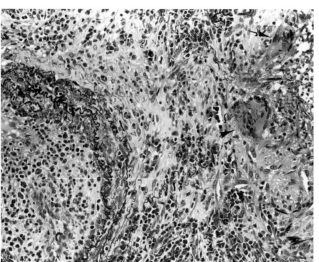

A

B

FIG. 11. A: Wegener's granulomatosis. Photomicrograph of lung biopsy specimen demonstrates transmural inflammation of a small vessel with partial destruction of elastin framework (*arrow*). Note the inflammation of the intima and marked narrowing of the vascular lumen. Pentachrome stain. (Courtesy of Andrew Flint, M.D., Department of Pathology, University of Michigan Medical Center.) **B:** Photomicrograph of lung biopsy specimen demonstrating multinucleated giant cells surrounding necrotic debris (*arrows*). A markedly inflamed blood vessel is present in the left portion of the field. Pentachrome stain. (Courtesy of Andrew Flint, M.D.)

complexes suggest that humoral mechanisms are also operative. The presence of polymorphonuclear leukocytes in the inflammatory vasculitic process, and of circulating autoantibodies directed against neutrophil cytoplasmic components, suggest a role for neutrophils and c-ANCA in the pathogenesis and evolution of the disorder. Exacerbations of Wegener's granulomatosis during intercurrent infections, and the frequent relapses observed in patients with Wegener's granulomatosis who are chronic nasal carriers of *S. aureus*, suggest that infections may amplify the inflammatory process, possibly by eliciting an antibody and acute-phase response.

Therapy

Before therapy became available, >80% of patients with Wegener's granulomatosis died within 3 years of onset of symptoms, usually of progressive renal insufficiency. Corticosteroids improved survival modestly. In the 1970s, the introduction of cyclophosphamide led to dramatic improvement in prognosis and survival. Oral cyclophosphamide (1 to 2 mg/day) combined with corticosteroids (1 mg/kg/day, with taper) is the treatment of choice for Wegener's granulomatosis. Remissions are achieved in 70%–93% of patients with this regimen; early mortality has been <15%. Late sequelae of vasculitis (e.g., cerebrovascular accidents, myocardial infarction, renal failure, hypertension) or complications of cyclophosphamide therapy (e.g., opportunistic infections, neoplasms) contribute to long-term mortality and morbidity. The dose of cyclophosphamide may need to be adjusted to maintain acceptable blood counts (particularly a leukocyte count of >3000/mm3). Corticosteroids ameliorate many of the inflammatory manifestations of Wegener's granulomatosis and are important as adjunctive therapy. The dose of corticosteroid needs to be individualized according to the clinical response and presence or absence of adverse effects. We attempt to taper to alternate-day prednisone (e.g., 60 mg every other day) within the first 2 to 3 months. Thereafter, we taper the prednisone gradually by 10-mg decrements every 1 to 3 months, until a maintenance dose of 15 to 20 mg every other day is achieved. Thereafter, the rate of taper may be slowed. Cyclophosphamide should be continued for a minimum of 12 months after complete clinical and laboratory remission has been achieved. Shorter duration of therapy has been associated with unacceptably high rates of relapses and late sequelae. Relapses occur in 20%–50% of patients as the regimen is tapered or discontinued, but reinstitution of therapy is usually efficacious. Prolonged therapy may be required in patients exhibiting a propensity to relapse. Unfortunately, cyclophosphamide is associated with a myriad of complications. Opportunistic infections (particularly herpes zoster) occur in 20%–30% of patients receiving cyclophosphamide. Other complications include bone marrow toxicity, pulmonary toxicity, alopecia, gastrointestinal symptoms (e.g., nausea, vomiting, diarrhea, hepatotoxicity), stomatitis, infertility, and oligospermia. Cyclophosphamide may induce both solid and hematologic neoplasms. Malignant lymphomas or hematologic malignancies have been noted in 1%–3% of patients with Wegener's granulomatosis who are receiving cyclophosphamide. Hemorrhagic cystitis occurs in 30%–50% of patients but is severe in <6% of patients. A recent, long-term study of 146 patients with Wegener's granulomatosis treated with cyclophosphamide cited seven cases of transitional cell carcinoma of the bladder. Antecedent hematuria had been noted in all patients. The risk for bladder carcinoma correlated with duration and total dose of cyclophosphamide therapy; cigarette smoking may amplify the risk. The incidence of bladder cancer following first exposure to cyclophosphamide is 5% at 10 years and 16% at 15 years. The risk persists for many years after discontinuation of cyclophosphamide. Serial urinalyses at 3- to 6-month intervals are advised in patients receiving cyclophosphamide and are sensitive in detecting bladder carcinomas. The presence of hematuria (macroscopic or microscopic) warrants cystoscopy. Intermittent intravenous high-dose (pulse) cyclophosphamide has been used to treat Wegener's granulomatosis, but results have been unimpressive. Early responses were noted in 13 of 14 patients treated with pulse cyclophosphamide in a nonrandomized trial at the National Institutes of Health. However, sustained remissions were achieved in only three patients (21%). Pulse cyclophosphamide is less toxic than daily oral cyclophosphamide but is less effective and is not recommended.

Other Therapeutic Options

In view of the rarity of Wegener's granulomatosis, prospective, randomized trials assessing therapy have not been performed. Anecdotal successes have been noted with other immunosuppressive or cytotoxic agents (e.g., azathioprine, methotrexate, and chlorambucil), but we consider these agents as second-line. Chlorambucil (Leukeran) may be oncogenic, and data are limited evaluating its efficacy as therapy for Wegener's granulomatosis. We do not employ chlorambucil in the treatment of Wegener's granulomatosis. Azathioprine (Imuran) is clearly less effective than cyclophosphamide, but it may be effective in maintaining remissions in patients experiencing adverse effects from cyclophosphamide. In an early report from the National Institutes of Health, cyclophosphamide successfully induced remissions in all 10 patients whose disease had been refractory to therapy with azathioprine. Azathioprine cannot be considered a first-line agent. Oral methotrexate, administered once weekly, may be used for patients with Wegener's granulomatosis in whom serious adverse effects develop from cyclophosphamide. A recent prospective (but nonrandomized) study at the National Institutes of Health treated 42 patients who had non–life-threatening Wegener's granulomatosis with oral methotrexate (mean dose, 20 mg/week) combined with corticosteroids. Treatment regimens before entry into the study included no prior therapy (16); corticosteroids alone (14); corticosteroids plus trimethoprim/sulfamethoxazole (6); cyclophosphamide plus corticosteroids (4); azathioprine (2). The four patients receiving cyclophosphamide were switched to methotrexate because of toxicity (hemorrhagic cystitis or leukopenia). All other patients had failed to achieve remissions with prior treatment regimens. Exclusion criteria included acute renal failure, pulmonary hemorrhage, serum creatinine levels of >2.5 mg%, and chronic liver disease. However, all patients had active disease at entry into the study, including glomerulonephritis in 21 (50%) and lung involvement in 22 (52%). Methotrexate was initiated at a dose of 0.3 mg/kg once weekly and was increased to tolerance up to a maximal dose of 20 to 25 mg once weekly. Prednisone was initiated at a dose of 1 mg/kg daily and gradually tapered as improvement occurred. Remissions were achieved in 30 of 42 patients (71%). Median time to remission was 4.2 months. Of the 30 patients achieving remission, 11 (36%) relapsed at a mean of 29 months. A second remission was induced in six of eight patients following a second course of methotrexate and prednisone. Toxicity was generally mild, but *Pneumocystis carinii* pneumonia developed in four patients (two of whom died). Methotrexate pneumonitis developed in three, which resolved with cessation of therapy. Asymptomatic elevation in transaminases was noted in 24% and always resolved with reduction of dose. Titers of c-ANCA did not correlate with disease activity. These data are encouraging and support the use of methotrexate plus prednisone in patients experiencing adverse effects from cyclophosphamide and as initial therapy in patients with mild Wegener's granulomatosis. Additional data are required to evaluate the role of methotrexate as therapy for Wegener's granulomatosis more fully.

Trimethoprim/Sulfamethoxazole

Anecdotal responses have been observed with trimethoprim/sulfamethoxazole (T/S), but firm data affirming the efficacy of T/S are lacking. In a nonrandomized clinical trial, DeRemee and colleagues at the Mayo Clinic cited favorable responses with T/S in a subset of patients with Wegener's granulomatosis. DeRemee added T/S to a previously failing regimen of cyclophosphamide/prednisone in 31 patients with indolent but progressive Wegener's granulomatosis. Favorable responses were noted in 26 patients; late relapses were observed in four patients in this group. In addition, T/S was given as initial therapy in 15 patients with limited Wegener's granulomatosis. In

this context, 14 responded; only three experienced late relapses. On the basis of these favorable results, DeRemee advocated T/S (one double-strength tablet twice daily) as initial therapy for patients with limited disease (lacking renal disease or generalized vasculitis) or for patients with progressive disease despite cyclophosphamide and corticosteroids. If no improvement was evident after 8 weeks, prednisone and/or cyclophosphamide were introduced. Although other investigators have cited favorable responses with T/S, data are limited. A prospective study at the National Institutes of Health found that T/S (alone or combined with corticosteroids) as initial therapy for Wegener's granulomatosis was ineffective in all nine patients. Nonetheless, a role for T/S in attenuating the course of the disease is plausible. Stegeman and colleagues evaluated the efficacy of T/S in preventing relapses in patients with Wegener's granulomatosis who were in remission during or after treatment with cyclophosphamide and prednisone. Patients were randomized to either T/S (160 mg trimethoprim/800 mg sulfamethoxazole) twice daily or placebo in addition to conventional treatment with cyclophosphamide and prednisone. At 24 months of follow-up, 82% of patients assigned to T/S were in remission, compared with only 60% in the placebo group. The annual rate of respiratory and nonrespiratory infections was also lower in the T/S group. Titers of ACNA did not differ between groups. Although this study did not address T/S as primary (initial) therapy for Wegener's granulomatosis, T/S did reduce the rate of relapses in patients with Wegener's granulomatosis following conventional treatment with cyclophosphamide/prednisone. Its mechanism of action is not known, but T/S may suppress autoantibody formation by direct antimicrobial effects or by indirect immunosuppressive or anti-inflammatory effects. Relapses of Wegener's granulomatosis are more frequent coincident with respiratory infections or in patients with chronic nasal carriage of *S. aureus*. Low-grade bacterial infection may prime neutrophils to express target antigens (e.g., c-ANCA) on the cell surface and may trigger local immune responses. The antimicrobial effect of T/S may abrogate these effects, thus limiting neutrophil activation and further tissue damage. Although these data are intriguing, the role of T/S has not been defined. In view of its low toxicity, T/S may be considered as adjunctive therapy in patients with persistent, indolent disease despite cyclophosphamide and corticosteroids. We do not believe T/S should supplant conventional therapy with cyclophosphamide/corticosteroids.

Polyarteritis Nodosa

Classic (macroscopic) polyarteritis nodosa (PAN) is a necrotizing vasculitis involving small and medium-sized muscular arteries. PAN differs from Wegener's granulomatosis in that microscopic vessels (e.g., small arterioles, venules, capillaries) are spared, and a granulomatous component is lacking in PAN. Macroscopic aneurysms involving the renal, mesenteric, or hepatic arteries can be demonstrated by angiography in more than two thirds of patients. Clinical manifestations predominantly affect the kidneys, gastrointestinal tract, central nervous system, skin, heart, and viscera. Clinical lung involvement complicates PAN in <2% of cases. Most previous reports of PAN with lung involvement probably represented either Churg-Strauss Syndrome (CSS) or microscopic polyangiitis (MPA). These entities are discussed in detail later in this chapter. Circulating ANCA (typically p-ANCA) have been detected in <20% of patients with PAN. By contrast, circulating ANCA (typically c-ANCA) are found in most patients with Wegener's granulomatosis, MPA, or CSS. Most cases of PAN are primary or idiopathic, but secondary forms (e.g., caused by hepatitis B virus or tumor antigens) are well recognized. Patients with PAN and hepatitis B antigenemia are usually treated with antiviral therapies in combination with plasmapheresis or immunosuppressive agents. For PAN without hepatitis B antigenemia, corticosteroids (alone or in combination with cyclophosphamide) are the mainstay of therapy. Five-year survival exceeds 75% but may be worse in the presence of adverse prognostic factors (e.g., gastrointestinal tract or central nervous system involvement, renal failure, loss of >10% of body weight, age of >50 years). The optimal doses of corticosteroid have not been delineated in randomized trials. For mild to moderate cases, initial therapy with prednisone (1 mg/kg per day for 1 month), followed by a gradual taper, is reasonable. For more severe or fulminant cases, we initiate therapy with high-dose intravenous methylprednisolone (500 to 1000 mg daily for 3 days), followed by oral prednisone (1 mg/kg/day or the equivalent) for 4 to 6 weeks. The dose of corticosteroid and rate of taper need to be individualized according to the response and clinical course. Cyclophosphamide is a highly effective drug for PAN, even in steroid-refractory cases. We routinely add oral cyclophosphamide (2 mg/kg/day) to corticosteroids, but some investigators reserve this agent for more severe or steroid-recalcitrant cases. Randomized European multicenter trials cited higher response rates (and fewer relapses) in regimens employing oral cyclophosphamide plus corticosteroids compared with corticosteroids alone. Survival did not differ between groups. Intravenous pulse cyclophosphamide (administered once monthly) may be less toxic than oral cyclophosphamide and appears to be equally efficacious. Patients responding to therapy with cyclophosphamide should be continued on this agent for at least 1 year after induction of remission. Relapses warrant reinstitution of therapy with corticosteroids plus cyclophosphamide. Plasmapheresis can be considered as adjunctive therapy in patients with fulminant PAN refractory to conventional therapy but should not be used routinely. In two randomized trials (that included patients with PAN or CSS), the addition of plasma exchange to prednisone or prednisone and cyclophosphamide did not improve prognosis or mortality.

Microscopic Polyangiitis

Microscopic polyangiitis (previously termed *overlap polyangiitis syndrome*) has clinical and histopathologic features overlapping with those of classic PAN and CSS. Predominant clinical manifestations are glomerulonephritis and pulmonary capillaritis (manifested as alveolar hemorrhage), but other organs may be involved. Microscopic polyangiitis is rare, with an estimated prevalence of 2.4 cases per million (range, 0.9 to 5.3). Mean age at onset is approximately 50, but all ages may be affected. There is a slight male predominance. As its name implies, microscopic polyangiitis (MPA) involves small vessels (arterioles, venules, and capillaries). MPA appears to be identical to what Zeek termed ''hypersensitivity angiitis'' in 1952. In the mid-1980s, the term *microscopic polyarteritis* was adopted to distinguish this disorder from macroscopic (classic) PAN. Capillaries are invariably involved in MPA, but arterioles may be spared. Thus, the term *microscopic polyangiitis* has replaced *microscopic polyarteritis*. Circulating ANCA (usually c-ANCA) have been demonstrated in a majority of patients with MPA, suggesting a possible relationship with other ANCA-associated pulmonary vasculitides (e.g., Wegener's granulomatosis and CSS). The defining criteria for MPA are less crisp than those for either Wegener's granulomatosis or CSS. In 1994, a panel of experts convened at the Chapel Hill Consensus Conference to provide defining criteria for vasculitis. MPA and PAN were distinguished primarily by histologic features. Small vessels (capillaries, venules, arterioles) were invariably involved in MPA but were always spared in classic PAN. Medium-sized or small arteries could be affected in either MPA or PAN. Granulomas were absent in both disorders.

Clinical Features

The predominant manifestations of MPA are alveolar hemorrhage and rapidly progressive glomerulonephritis, features rarely seen in classic PAN. The clinical features of MPA were articulated by Savage and colleagues in 1985. A necrotizing, crescentic glomerulonephritis with few or no immune deposits (termed *pauci-immune*) is characteristic of MPA. Alveolar hemorrhage occurs in 30%–50% of patients and is often the dominant (and most life-threatening) manifestation (Fig. 12). A prodromal respiratory illness precedes the onset of vasculitis in one third of patients. Arthralgias and myalgias may be prominent. Sinus or upper airway involvement may occur but is rarely a prominent or presenting feature. Oral ulcers have been noted in up to 21% of patients with MPA and may mimic Wegener's granulomato-

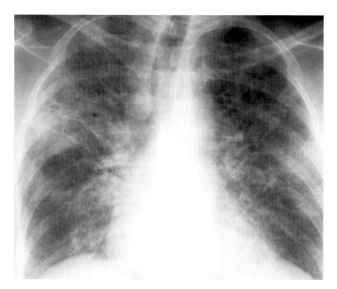

FIG. 12. Alveolar hemorrhage caused by microscopic polyangiitis. PA chest radiograph demonstrates diffuse alveolar infiltrates involving all lobes. Within 24 hours, the infiltrates worsened and severe respiratory failure developed; mechanical ventilatory support with positive end-expiratory pressure (PEEP) at 16 cm H$_2$O was required to achieve acceptable oxygenation. Because of the severity of respiratory failure, no lung biopsy was performed. Urinalysis demonstrated numerous red cells and occasional red cell casts. Serum creatinine level was 1.4 mg%. One gram of pulse methylprednisolone (Solu-Medrol) was administered daily for 3 days. Renal biopsy demonstrated glomerulonephritis and a necrotizing vasculitis involving renal arterioles; no granulomas were present. Cyclophosphamide was instituted (2 mg/kg daily) and corticosteroids were continued. Within 5 days, the infiltrates had cleared completely and serum creatinine level was 0.6 mg%.

sis. Cutaneous involvement (leukocytoclastic vasculitis) is common. Renal infarcts, renal vasculitis, and visceral aneurysms, cardinal features of PAN, are rarely observed in MPA. Peripheral neuropathy occurs in 50%–80% of patients with PAN, but in only 10%–20% of patients with MPA. Circulating immune complexes and rheumatoid factor have been noted in 40% of patients with MPA and antinuclear antibodies in 21%. These nonspecific tests have been supplanted by ANCA, which have been detected in 50%–90% of patients with MPA. By contrast, ANCA are present in <20% of patients with PAN. Several features of MPA (e.g., circulating ANCA, small-vessel vasculitis, glomerulonephritis, and pulmonary capillaritis) may be observed in patients with Wegener's granulomatosis or CSS. Both of these latter vasculitic disorders exhibit a granulomatous component, which is lacking in MPA. Asthma or eosinophilia (in blood or tissue), characteristic features of CSS, are not found in MPA. A firm diagnosis of MPA requires that these alternative diagnoses be definitely excluded.

Histopathology

Like other ANCA-associated vasculitides, MPA principally affects small arterioles, venules, and capillaries. A granulomatous component is lacking and eosinophils are rare or absent, in contrast to what is observed in CSS and Wegener's granulomatosis. Immune complexes are nondetectable or present in only small amounts in involved tissue (*pauci-immune*).

Treatment

Diverse regimens employing prednisone, azathioprine, cyclophosphamide, and plasmapheresis, alone or in combination, have been used to treat MPA. Because of the rarity of MPA, data regarding therapy are limited. Treatment regimens have been extrapolated from studies that have incorporated patients with MPA, CSS, and PAN. In this context, overall survival appeared to be similar with various regimens, including corticosteroids alone, corticosteroids plus oral cyclophosphamide, corticosteroids plus intravenous cyclophosphamide, corticosteroids plus plasma exchange, and corticosteroids plus cyclophosphamide plus plasma exchange. Plasmapheresis adds another level of complexity and should be reserved for fulminant or refractory cases. Most investigators use oral cyclophosphamide (2 mg/kg/day) and corticosteroids (1 mg/kg/day, with gradual taper), similar to the regimen used in Wegener's granulomatosis. Favorable responses are achieved in >80% of cases; 10-year survival exceeds 70%. As with Wegener's granulomatosis, treatment should be continued for a minimum of 1 year after complete clinical and laboratory remission has been achieved.

Churg-Strauss Angiitis (Allergic Angiitis and Granulomatosis)

CSS, also termed *allergic angiitis and granulomatosis,* was originally reported in 1951 by Churg and Strauss, who described 13 patients with asthma, peripheral eosinophilia, constitutional symptoms, and systemic necrotizing vasculitis. These investigators noted that CSS shares histologic features with PAN, but is distinct from classic PAN. In 1957, Rose and Spencer identified 32 patients with asthma and features consistent with CSS from a necropsy series of 111 patients with PAN. Only sporadic reports of CSS were described during the next two decades. In 1977, Chumbley and co-workers reviewed 30 patients with CSS seen at the Mayo Clinic during a 24-year period. A review of the files of the Armed Forces Institute of Pathology in 1981 revealed only four cases of CSS. As of 1982, only 138 cases of CSS had been published. The annual incidence of CSS has been estimated at 2.4 cases per million. In 1984, Lanham and colleagues reported 16 additional patients with CSS (only eight of whom had histologic confirmation of vasculitis) seen at a large referral hospital in England during a 6-year period, and suggested that the rarity of CSS in part reflected the stringent criteria required for the diagnosis.

They suggested that the diagnosis of CSS could be made even when not all classic criteria (e.g., necrotizing vasculitis, extravascular granulomas, tissue eosinophilia) were present. A concept of ''limited forms'' of CSS, analogous to limited Wegener's granulomatosis, has been suggested. Cardinal features required for the diagnosis include an allergic diathesis and eosinophilic component (either in blood or tissue).

Clinical Features

Pulmonary involvement (characteristically manifested as asthma) is present in virtually all patients. Focal alveolar infiltrates are present on chest radiograph in 30%–70% of cases. Diffuse alveolar hemorrhage is a rare complication. Pulmonary nodules or cavitary lesions are rarely observed in CSS, as they are in Wegener's granulomatosis. Typically, a history of atopy and asthma precedes the development of vasculitis by months or even years. Hay fever, nasal polyposis, allergic rhinitis, and sinusitis are noted in more than two thirds of patients. Otolaryngeal manifestations include nasal crusting or nasal polyposis in up to 75% of patients with CSS and nasal perforation in 5%. Peripheral blood eosinophilia is usually prominent during the asthmatic and vasculitic phases. Increasingly severe and more frequent exacerbations of asthma precede the development of necrotizing vasculitis. Constitutional symptoms are usually prominent. Fever, weight loss, or malaise are noted in >90% of patients. Arthralgias or myalgias occur in one third of patients. Central or peripheral neurologic involvement occurs in 40%–63% of patients with CSS. Peripheral neuropathy or mononeuritis multiplex predominates; cerebral infarction has rarely been described. Cutaneous manifestations (e.g., subcutaneous nodules, purpura, or petechiae) occur in two thirds of patients. Skin biopsy may demonstrate nonspecific findings of leukocytoclastic vasculitis; when dense eosinophilic infiltrates are noted, the diagnosis of CSS is strongly suggested. Cardiac involvement occurs in 30%–50%. Cardiac failure and pericarditis are the most common clinical manifestations. Cardiac involvement may reflect primary coronary vasculitis or eosinophilic endocarditis with associated fibrosis. Abdominal viscera are involved in 20%–40%. Abdominal pain or perforation of a viscus resulting from ischemia are well-recognized complications. Renal failure is rare with CSS, but hypertension develops in nearly 50% of patients. The mean age of onset is in the middle to late 40s, but the range is wide (14 to 75 years). Laboratory studies demonstrate elevations in the erythrocyte sedimentation rate and blood eosinophil counts in >80% of patients during acute exacerbations. Both erythrocyte sedimentation rate and blood eosinophil counts usually correlate with activity of disease. Circulating ANCA (both p-ANCA and c-ANCA) have been noted in a majority of patients with CSS.

Histopathology

The salient histologic features of CSS include a necrotizing vasculitis involving small arteries and veins, with eosinophilic and granulomatous components. The pronounced eosinophilic and granulomatous character distinguishes CSS from other pulmonary vasculitides. Eosinophilic infiltration of vascular walls is usually striking; mononuclear cells, neutrophils, and occasional multinucleated giant cells are also present. Granulomas and eosinophils in extravascular tissues are hallmarks of the disorder. Palisades of histiocytes and giant cells surround a central eosinophilic core. The diagnosis can be supported even when histologic features are not definitive, provided the clinical and laboratory features are characteristic. The lesions in diffuse alveolar hemorrhage demonstrate nonspecific findings of capillaritis.

Therapy

Corticosteroids have been the mainstay of therapy, with remissions in >80% of patients. Immunosuppressive and cytotoxic agents have also been tried. Prospective, randomized trials (that enrolled patients with PAN or CSS) have evaluated various medical regimens, including corticosteroids alone; corticosteroids plus oral cyclophosphamide; corticosteroids plus pulse cyclophosphamide; corticosteroids plus plasma exchange; and the combination of corticosteroids, cyclophosphamide, and plasma exchange. Long-term (10-year) survival is similar with the various regimens (3-year survival, 80%–90%; 10-year survival, 72%–78%). Pulse (once-monthly intravenous high-dose) cyclophosphamide was comparable with oral cyclophosphamide and steroids for PAN or CSS. Given the high remission rate with corticosteroids and the potential late sequelae associated with cytotoxic agents, we consider prednisone as first-line therapy for mild to moderate cases of CSS (1 mg/kg/day for 4 weeks, followed by a gradual taper). Oral cyclophosphamide (2 mg/kg/day) is added for more fulminant cases or when unfavorable prognostic features are present [e.g., proteinuria >1 g/day, severe gastrointestinal involvement, cardiomyopathy, renal insufficiency (serum creatinine levels of >1.6 mg%), or central nervous system involvement]. Asthma, polyarthritis, myalgias, ophthalmologic signs, weight loss, or cutaneous involvement do not influence prognosis. For fulminant or refractory cases, more rapid control of the disease can be accomplished with aggressive combination therapies. In this context, pulse methylprednisolone (1 g daily for 3 days) followed by oral prednisone (1 mg/kg/day) combined with cyclophosphamide (2 mg/kg/day) is advised. Plasma exchange may be added in patients failing or experiencing adverse effects from therapy, but it has been associated with an increased risk for infectious complications. Plasmapheresis may be given three times per week for the first 2 to 3 weeks, and at decreasing frequency during the next 2 to 4 months.

Lymphomatoid Granulomatosis

Lymphomatoid granulomatosis (LYG) was initially described in 1972 as a necrotizing vasculitic disorder having several features in common with Wegener's granulomatosis and atypical lymphoma. Histologic features include atypical lymphohistiocytic infiltrates surrounding small and medium-sized arteries and veins, associated with pronounced necrosis of involved organs. The angiocentric pattern, presence of multinucleated giant cells, granulomatous component, and mixed inflammatory cellular infiltrates mimic Wegener's granulomatosis. However, the pronounced cellular atypia resembles a lymphoid malignant disorder (Fig. 13). Clinical manifestations of LYG

are protean. Virtually any organ can be involved, but pulmonary, constitutional, neurologic, and cutaneous manifestations predominate. Glomerulonephritis has only rarely been noted. Aberrations on chest radiographs are almost invariably present (Fig. 14). Multiple nodular lesions are typical, but single mass lesions, alveolar infiltrates, cavitary lesions, or pleural effusions may be found. In early studies, anecdotal responses were noted with regimens employing oral cyclophosphamide and corticosteroids (similar to treatment of Wegener's granulomatosis). Subsequent studies have failed to substantiate benefit from corticosteroids alone or in combination with immunosuppressive or cytotoxic agents. Recent investigations utilizing molecular biologic and immunohistochemical techniques (e.g., T-cell gene rearrangements, monoclonal stains) suggest that most (if not all) cases of LYG represent diverse lymphoreticular disorders, including malig-

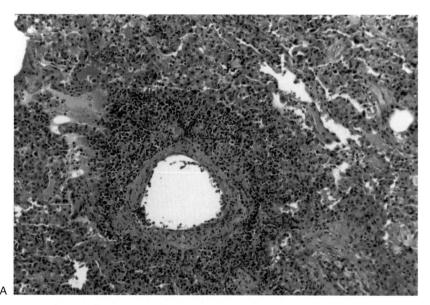

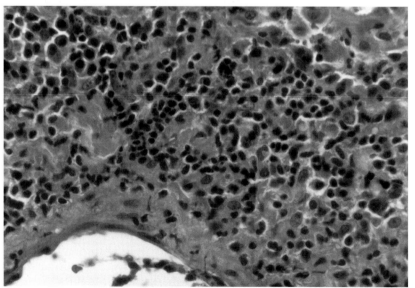

FIG. 13. A: Lymphomatoid granulomatosis. Photomicrograph of open lung biopsy specimen demonstrates intense mononuclear infiltrates surrounding a blood vessel. H&E, high power. (Courtesy of S. Hammar, M.D, University of Washington, Seattle.) **B:** Photomicrograph of specimen from same patient showing polymorphous infiltrate composed of atypical lymphoid and histiocytic cells. Granuloma is not a characteristic histologic abnormality despite the suggestion in the term. H&E, oil immersion. (Courtesy of S. Hammar, M.D, University of Washington, Seattle.)

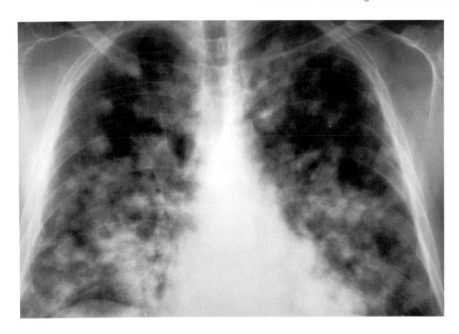

FIG. 14. Lymphomatoid granulomatosis. PA chest radiograph demonstrates multiple nodular mass densities throughout both lung fields. Open lung biopsy specimen demonstrates changes consistent with lymphomatoid granulomatosis.

nant lymphoma, angioimmunoblastic lymphadenopathy, and T-cell lymphomas. LYG should not be classified as a true vasculitis, but rather as a stereotypic response to diverse lymphoreticular disorders. Although optimal therapy has not been clarified, combination chemotherapeutic regimens for malignant lymphoma are appropriate for many patients.

Behçet's Syndrome

Behçet's syndrome is a systemic vasculitis whose major manifestations include oral and genital ulcers, iritis, phlebitis, and nervous system involvement. Recurrent venous thromboses occur in one quarter of patients with Behçet's syndrome. Other possible sites of involvement include skin, gastrointestinal tract, kidneys, heart, joints, and epididymis. Lung involvement occurs in only 1%– 5% of cases. Diverse pulmonary manifestations include transient infiltrates, mass lesions, pleural effusions, hemoptysis, aneurysms of the pulmonary arteries, arterial and venous thromboses, pulmonary infarcts, and pulmonary hemorrhage. Massive, fatal hemorrhage from rupture or erosion of pulmonary arterial aneurysms has been described. Behçet's syndrome is more common in the eastern Mediterranean basin but is worldwide in distribution. The onset of disease is most common in the third through fifth decades of life. Histologic features are nonspecific. A necrotizing vasculitis (composed of lymphocytes, plasma cells, and polymorphonuclear leukocytes) involves arteries, veins, and capillaries. Varying degrees of fibrosis, thrombosis, and necrosis are evident. The etiology is not known, but deposits of immune complexes and complement may be prominent in involved tissues. Because of the rarity of this disease, controlled therapeutic trials have

not been performed. Corticosteroids, combined with cyclophosphamide or azathioprine, are most commonly employed. Colchicine has been advocated as adjunctive therapy for arthralgias or erythema nodosum. When pulmonary arterial aneurysms are documented, prompt resection should be accomplished.

Hughes-Stoven Syndrome

In 1959, Hughes and Stoven described a symptom complex of pulmonary artery aneurysms and recurrent venous thromboses (especially of the vena cava). A review of the literature up to 1981 identified only 12 patients with Hughes-Stoven syndrome; 11 were young males. Symptoms included fever, central nervous system symptoms resulting from increased intracranial pressure, hemoptysis, arthralgias, and skin rash. Nine died of massive hemoptysis caused by rupture of pulmonary arterial aneurysms. Surgical resection of pulmonary aneurysms was accomplished in all three survivors. Cerebral thrombophlebitis was present in 6 of these 12 cases. Histologic features of involved tissue demonstrated a necrotizing vasculitis. Most if not all cases of "Hughes-Stoven syndrome" likely reflect unrecognized pulmonary vasculitis from other causes (e.g., CSS, Behçet's syndrome).

Takayasu's Arteritis

Takayasu's arteritis is a rare vasculitis primarily affecting large vessels (e.g., aorta and its branches). It may cause arterial stenoses, aneurysms, and distal arterial insufficiency. The most common site of involvement is the subclavian arteries, near their junction with the aorta. The absence of radial pulses has given rise to the term *pulseless disease*. Most series have been reported from Japan, the Orient, and Mexico. Takayasu's arteritis is rare in the United States and Europe. Only 32 cases were given the diagnosis at the Mayo Clinic between 1971 to 1983. The incidence among Caucasians has been estimated at 2.6 cases per million per year. Most patients present between ages 20 and 30; the disease is rare in the elderly. There is a striking female predominance.

Clinical Features

Dominant clinical manifestations, which are related to cessation of blood flow in the aorta or its branches, include claudication of arms or legs, dizziness (reflecting occlusion of the carotid or vertebrobasilar arteries), ischemic cardiac disease, visual loss, and back pain (reflecting aortic aneurysms). Multiple vascular bruits or absent or reduced pulses are characteristic findings on physical examination. Fever, malaise, weight loss, and anemia are noted in more than one third of patients and myalgias or arthralgias in nearly 60%. Elevations in the erythrocyte sedimentation rate may be striking and may be a surrogate marker of disease activity. Results of tests for antinuclear antibodies and rheumatoid factor are negative. Renovascular hypertension occurs in approximately 40% of patients. Aortic insufficiency or aneurysms of the root of the aorta, when present, are major causes of death and warrant surgical correction. Pulmonary vasculitis is rarely recognized ante mortem, but pulmonary arterial aneurysms or stenoses have been documented in up to 50% of patients by pulmonary angiography or necropsy. The diagnosis of Takayasu's disease is usually made on the basis of aortic angiographic findings of occlusions, stenosis, luminal irregularities, tortuosity, or aneurysms in a young woman with arterial occlusive symptoms. Dilatation of the aortic root or aortic insufficiency may occur. Similar findings may be observed on pulmonary arteriography. Bypass grafts for aortic occlusive lesions have been successfully performed in some patients. Histopathology is rarely confirmed, except at the time of resection or bypass of arterial lesions. Salient features are a granulomatous, sclerosing arteritis indistinguishable from giant cell (temporal) arteritis.

Therapy

Corticosteroids are the cornerstone of therapy. Most experts initiate therapy with prednisone (1 mg/kg/day) for 4 to 6 weeks, followed by a gradual taper according to symptoms and sedimentation rate. Cyclophosphamide should be considered for severe cases or patients failing corticosteroids. With aggressive medical therapy, survival exceeds 90%, and severe sequelae can be averted. Factors associated with increased mortality include severe systemic hypertension, aortic incompetence, and marked aneurysm formation. Far-advanced stenoses or occlusions caused by inactive, sclerotic lesions are not influenced by immunosuppressive therapy. In these circumstances, when symptoms of vascular compromise are evident, angioplasty, surgical reconstruction, or bypass grafts should be performed.

Henoch-Schönlein Syndrome

Henoch-Schönlein syndrome is a necrotizing vasculitis principally affecting children; major manifestations are palpable purpura, hematuria, and abdominal pain. Lung involvement is exceedingly rare, but extensive alveolar hemorrhage and capillaritis have been described. Henoch-Schönlein syndrome is caused by circulating immune complexes, with IgA reacting to target antigens in the renal glomerulus, skin, or gastrointestinal tract. A small-vessel vasculitis, associated with pronounced deposition of IgA in glomerular capillaries and affected vessels, is pathognomonic. Henoch-Schönlein syndrome is often self-limited and may not require therapy. Corticosteroids should be considered for severe or protracted cases.

ALVEOLAR HEMORRHAGE SYNDROMES

Autoimmune diffuse alveolar hemorrhage (DAH) may occur as a result of diffuse injury to the pulmonary microvasculature (termed *capillaritis* or *endotheliitis*). The course is typically abrupt, associated with bilateral alveolar infiltrates, hemoptysis, hypoxemia, and iron deficiency anemia. Glomerulonephritis is present in the vast majority of cases of DAH with immune-mediated causes (hence the term *pulmonary-renal syndromes*). Etiologies of DAH include antiglomerular basement membrane disease, systemic necrotizing vasculitis, idiopathic glomerulonephritis (immune complex or pauci-immune), collagen vascular disease, bone marrow transplantation, HIV infection, and exposure to exogenous agents or drugs. Idiopathic pulmonary hemosiderosis, a rare cause of recurrent DAH, occurs primarily in children and remains a diagnosis of exclusion.

Diagnostic Evaluation of Diffuse Alveolar Hemorrhage

The clinical features of DAH may be similar, regardless of etiology. Hemoptysis and a fall in the hematocrit support the diagnosis of DAH but are etiologically nonspecific. Nonimmune causes of DAH include endobronchial tumors, ulcerative tracheobronchitis, arteriovenous malformations or aneurysms, hemorrhagic pneumonia, bronchiectasis, congestive heart, failure, uremia, thrombocytopenia, coagulopathy, pulmonary veno-occlusive disease, and massive pulmonary embolism. The nonimmune causes must be excluded in patients with severe DAH. Depending on the clinical scenario, coagulation profiles and ancillary tests (e.g., echocardiogram, pulmonary angiography) may be required to establish a specific diagnosis. Fiberoptic bronchoscopy is useful to look for a site of active bleeding and rule out an infectious etiology. The role of lung biopsies is controversial and will be discussed later. Urinalysis and renal function tests should be performed in cases of suspected DAH, as rapidly progressive glomerulonephritis is a nearly invariable feature of immune-mediated pulmonary-renal syndromes. A battery of serologic studies may disclose an immunologic cause of DAH. These include antinuclear antibody (ANA), antineutrophilic cytoplasmic antibody (ACNA), antiglomerular basement membrane antibody (anti-GBM antibodies), and serum complement. However, the results of tests for anti-GMB antibodies or ANCA may not be available for several days. In this context, biopsy of kidney, lung, or other involved sites (e.g., skin, sinuses) may be required.

The role of open (or thoracoscopic) lung biopsy in the evaluation of DAH is controversial. Lung biopsies are seldom definitive, as gross and histologic findings may be similar irrespective of underlying etiology. Lung biopsies typically demonstrate flooding of alveolar spaces with blood, associated with diffuse injury to the pulmonary microvasculature (capillaritis). Capillaritis is a distinctive histologic lesion characterized by neutrophilic infiltration of capillaries, fragmented neutrophils (leukocytoclasis), and necrosis of the capillary walls. However, this lesion is nonspecific and may be seen in DAH complicating a variety of immune disorders (e.g., systemic necrotizing vasculitis (SNV), systemic lupus erythematosus, anti-GBM disease, idiopathic or immune complex-mediated rapidly progressive glomerulonephritis). Hemosiderin-laden macrophages within the alveolar spaces and interstitium may reflect prior episodes of DAH. Immunofluorescent studies are difficult to interpret in lung tissue and may be misleading. Surgical (open or thoracoscopic) lung biopsy carries significant morbidity, with the potential for prolonged air leak and secondary infections in patients with DAH and marginal pulmonary reserve. Thus, we see no role for surgical lung biopsy in patients with severe or acute DAH. Fiberoptic bronchoscopy with BAL, which can be performed with little morbidity even in intubated patients, is usually adequate to exclude infectious etiologies and may support the diagnosis. Gross blood in the airways, bloody or serosanguinous BAL fluid, and hemosiderin-laden macrophages in BAL fluid strongly suggest DAH in the appropriate clinical setting. Thoracoscopic lung biopsy may have a role in selected patients with a more indolent course, negative serologies, and nondiagnostic renal biopsy and bronchoscopy.

Serologies, renal biopsies (with immunofluorescent stains), or biopsies of extrapulmonary and extrarenal sites (when vasculitis is present) may differentiate the various causes of pulmonary renal syndromes. When urinary sediment or renal function tests suggest glomerulopathy, percutaneous renal biopsy (to include immunofluorescent stains) should be performed. Renal biopsies in immune-mediated DAH demonstrate focal or diffuse glomerulonephritis, with extracellular proliferation (crescents) and necrosis. These findings, although distinctive, are nonspecific. However, the pattern of immunofluorescent staining is pivotal in establishing a specific etiologic diagnosis. A linear pattern of immunofluorescence is pathognomonic for anti-GBM disease. Either a lumpy-bumpy pattern (indicating immune complexes) or negative immunofluorescence (termed *pauci-immune*) can be seen with SNV, systemic lupus erythematosus, or idiopathic rapidly progressive glomerulonephritis. In critically ill patients with severe DAH, percutaneous renal biopsy may be logistically difficult or impractical. In this context, empiric therapy with pulse methylprednisolone (1 g daily for 3 days), possibly combined with cytotoxic agents or plasmapheresis, is reasonable pending results of serologic studies.

Specific Disorders Associated with Diffuse Alveolar Hemorrhage

Antiglomerular Basement Membrane Disease

Antiglomerular basement membrane (anti-GBM) disease, also termed *Goodpasture's syndrome,* is the prototype of pulmonary-renal syndromes, manifested as DAH and rapidly progressive glomerulonephritis (RPGN). Isolated RPGN without DAH may occur, but isolated DAH without RPGN is exceptionally rare. Anti-GBM disease accounted for 18%–32% of immune-mediated DAH syndromes in two recent series. Anti-GBM disease typically presents in patients between 20 and 40 years of age. There is a distinct male predominance. A specific cause has not been elucidated, but exposure to inhaled hydrocarbons and antecedent viral illnesses (particularly influenza) have been cited as risk factors. Cigarette smoking enhances the risk for DAH in patients with circulating anti-GBM antibody.

Clinical Features

Pulmonary manifestations usually dominate in the early phases of the disease. Hypoxemic respiratory failure, with widespread alveolar infiltrates on chest radiographs, is characteristic. Hemoptysis occurs in 70%–80% of patients and anemia in 85%. In 20%–30% of cases, the disease is limited to the kidneys. Organs other than lung or kidney are not involved, but constitutional symptoms (e.g., fatigue, weakness) may be prominent. Gross hematuria has been noted in 10%–41% of patients with anti-GBM disease. Microscopic hematuria or proteinuria are virtually always present. Renal function may be normal in 40%–60% of patients at presentation, but progressive renal failure develops within days to weeks. Oliguria, severe renal failure, or >50% crescents on renal biopsy are associated with a poor prognosis and low rate of recovery of renal function. Early institution of therapy is critical to optimize outcome. Circulating anti-GMB antibodies are detectable by radioimmunoassay or enzyme-linked immunosorbent assay (ELISA) in >95% of patients. These assays are highly specific (95%) but are performed in only a few research laboratories, and results are usually not available for a few days. Prognosis for recovery is related to the severity of the renal lesion. Prompt therapy is mandatory to avert irreversible loss of glomerular function. Thus, percutaneous renal biopsy should be done in any patient with significant abnormalities in urinary sediment or renal function pending the results of serum anti-GMB antibody assays. Identification of the pathognomonic linear immunofluorescent pattern on renal biopsy allows institution of therapy with plasmapheresis and immunosuppressive/cytotoxic therapy (to be discussed later). Serial measurement of serum anti-GBM antibodies is invaluable to monitor the course of the disease. Results of other serologic studies are negative or nondiagnostic.

Histopathology

Renal biopsy with immunofluorescent stains is the preferred method of establishing the diagnosis. Conventional light microscopy demonstrates a proliferative glomerulonephritis with cellular crescents. Foci of interstitial fibrosis or tubular atrophy may be observed but are rarely prominent. These histologic features are nonspecific. However, intense immunofluorescent linear deposits of IgG along glomerular basement membranes are pathognomonic for anti-GBM disease. Linear deposits of IgM or IgA have rarely been described. As was discussed earlier, open (or thoracoscopic) lung biopsies are rarely helpful. Histologic features are dominated by extensive intraalveolar hemorrhage and hemosiderin-laden macrophages. Foci of neutrophilic ''capillaritis,'' hyaline membranes, and diffuse alveolar damage are concomitant features. Extensive necrosis and large-vessel vasculitis are not found. These histopathologic features are nonspecific. Immunofluorescent stains of lung tissue are not reliable. Because of its potential morbidity, we rarely employ open or thoracoscopic lung biopsies in the evaluation of DAH. A diagnosis can usually be substantiated by renal biopsies, BAL, and appropriate serologic studies.

Pathogenesis

Anti-GBM antibodies are directed against the α_3 chain of type IV collagen, an antigen highly expressed in both alveolar and glomerular basement membranes. The stimulus for anti-GBM antibody formation remains speculative, but both environmental and genetic factors may play roles. A genetic susceptibility is plausible, as anecdotal cases of anti-GBM disease have been described in siblings, first cousins, and identical twins, and links between anti-GBM disease and the HLA-DR2 histocompatibility antigen have been noted. Exposure to cigarette smoke, hydrocarbon-containing solvents, hard-metal dust, influenza A2 virus, chlorine gas, and D-penicillamine have been associated with anti-GBM disease. These exogenous factors may injure the basement membrane, resulting in increased capillary permeability and exposure of the Goodpasture antigen (α_3 chain of type IV collagen), which elicits a helper T-cell response. Stimulation of IgG synthesis results in deposits of IgG along the alveolar and capillary basement membranes. Anti-idiotypic (blocking) antibodies and activated suppressor (CD8$^+$) T cells may facilitate resolution of the process, but this is speculative. Pulmonary edema, infection, and cigarette smoking have been associated with an increased risk for DAH in patients with circulating anti-GBM antibody, possibly because of increased lung capillary permeability that allows access of the antibody to the alveolar spaces.

Treatment

Before the availability of therapy, mortality associated with anti-GBM disease exceeded 90%, with mean survival of 6 months. Plasmapheresis, introduced as a therapeutic option for anti-GBM disease in the mid-1970s, was quickly adopted worldwide and is considered as part of standard therapy. Current therapy involves a combination of plasmapheresis (to eliminate circulating anti-GBM antibodies) plus immunosuppressive agents (to suppress antibody synthesis). Prognosis of anti-GBM disease is influenced by the severity of the renal lesion at the outset. In one study, 22 of 23 patients with oliguria or a serum creatinine level of 6 mg% failed to recover, even with aggressive therapy. By contrast, 15 of 17 with nonoliguric renal failure and a serum creatinine level of >6 mg% recovered or improved with plasmapheresis and immunosuppressive/cytotoxic therapy. Thus, prompt diagnosis and initiation of therapy are mandatory to avoid irreversible renal failure. Because of the rarity of anti-GBM syndrome, only one randomized trial has compared immunosuppressive therapy alone versus the combination of immunosuppressive therapy and plasmapheresis. In that study, combined therapy was associated with more rapid disappearance of anti-GBM antibody and improved renal function. End-stage renal disease requiring chronic dialysis developed in 6 of 9 patients treated with immunosuppressive agents alone (compared with 2 of 8 in the plasmapheresis group). The incidence of recurrent pulmonary hemorrhage was similar (4 in each group). Optimal dose and duration of plasma exchange have not been defined. Plasma exchanges have usually been done daily or every

2 to 3 days for the first 10 to 21 weeks, until clinical improvement has occurred and serum anti-GBM antibodies are nondetectable. Less frequent plasmapheresis (every 3 to 5 days) has been used, with purported success. The optimal immunosuppressive regimen has not been delineated. For acute, life-threatening DAH, pulse methylprednisolone (1 g daily for 3 days), following by a corticosteroid taper, is advised. Once the DAH is controlled, oral prednisone (1 mg/kg/day) may be substituted, and oral cyclophosphamide (2 mg/kg/day) or azathioprine (2 to 3 mg/kg/day) are added to suppress continued antibody synthesis. No studies have specifically compared cyclophosphamide with azathioprine, but we favor cyclophosphamide. Immunosuppressive agents should be continued until the clinical syndrome has resolved and anti-GBM antibodies have disappeared. In most cases, symptoms resolve and circulating antibodies clear within 8 weeks, irrespective of the initial titer. Renal function usually recovers in patients with minor functional impairment. Dialysis-dependent patients rarely recover renal function. A 4- to 6-month trial may be adequate in some cases. Long-term survival rates exceed 85%. Late recurrences have been rare.

Systemic Necrotizing Vasculitis

Pulmonary hemorrhage is a well-recognized complication of Wegener's granulomatosis and MPA, and may rarely complicate CSS, Behçet's syndrome, mixed cryoglobulinemia, and other systemic necrotizing vasculitides. Necrotizing vasculitis accounts for 40%–55% of DAH syndromes. Regardless of the specific underlying vasculitic disorder, rapidly progressive glomerulonephritis (RPGN) is a nearly invariable feature. A cardinal feature of DAH complicating vasculitis is diffuse damage to the pulmonary endothelium (capillaritis). The histologic features are nonspecific. Granulomatous or eosinophilic components, geographic necrosis, or vasculitis involving larger vessels (e.g., arterioles) are usually not evident. High-dose intravenous (pulse) methylprednisolone (1 g daily for 3 days) should be given for acute, fulminant DAH. Long-term therapy with oral cyclophosphamide and corticosteroids is appropriate for necrotizing vasculitis. The specific regimens have been discussed in greater detail in the sections on pulmonary vasculitis.

Collagen Vascular Disorders

Collagen vascular disorders, principally systemic lupus erythematosus (SLE), account for 10%–30% of pulmonary-renal syndromes. Pulmonary hemorrhage is a well-recognized, albeit rare, complication of SLE, but only sporadic cases of DAH have been described complicating rheumatoid arthritis, progressive systemic sclerosis, polymyositis, or dermatomyositis. Recently, Schwarz

and colleagues described two patients with polymyositis, progressive respiratory failure, and DAH secondary to pulmonary capillaritis. Management is similar to that for DAH complicating SLE. DAH complicating SLE usually occurs in patients with a prior history of SLE and active disease elsewhere (e.g., fever, arthritis, serositis). However, DAH has been the sole and presenting feature of SLE in some cases. As in other DAH syndromes, results of lung biopsies are nonspecific, showing hemorrhage and foci of capillaritis. Granular deposits of complement (C3) and IgG have been noted in some cases (suggesting immune complex deposits) but this has not been uniform. Intravenous pulse methylprednisolone is the treatment of choice for severe DAH. For less severe cases, high-dose prednisone may be adequate. Plasmapheresis or immunosuppressive/cytotoxic drugs may be required for patients failing to respond to corticosteroids.

Idiopathic Rapidly Progressive Glomerulonephritis

DAH may complicate idiopathic RPGN, a primary renal disorder of unknown etiology. Immune complexes are present in serum or renal tissue in 20% of patients with idiopathic RPGN. When no immune complexes are found, the term *pauci-immune glomerulonephritis* has been used. Clinical features of idiopathic RPGN are similar, irrespective of whether immune complexes are present. Progressive renal failure is the predominant manifestation and major cause of morbidity in this disease. Lung involvement (typically capillaritis) occurs in 20%–50% of cases but is rarely severe. Some patients manifest mild hemoptysis and transient alveolar infiltrates but are otherwise asymptomatic. However, occasional patients manifest life-threatening DAH and require mechanical ventilatory support. Fever, myalgias, malaise, and a flulike illness precede the renal lesion in nearly two thirds of patients. Other organs are not involved and systemic vasculitis is lacking. All ages may be affected, but idiopathic RPGN has a predilection for adults in the sixth and seventh decades; there is a male predominance (2:1 ratio). In untreated patients, progressive renal failure develops within a few weeks to months; nearly 75% require dialysis. The prognosis is poor among patients presenting with serum creatinine levels of >6 mg% or with oliguria. Renal biopsy demonstrates crescentic, rapidly progressive glomerulonephritis (with or without immune complexes). These features are nonspecific. Circulating ANCA (typically p-ANCA) are present in up to 70% of cases with idiopathic RPGN.

Optimal therapy is controversial. A variety of treatment regimens incorporating corticosteroids, immunosuppressive/cytotoxic drugs, and plasmapheresis, alone or in combination, have been tried. In one multicenter, randomized trial, survival and renal function were similar with three treatment regimens utilizing corticosteroids alone, corticosteroids plus oral cyclophosphamide, or corticosteroids plus intravenous cyclophosphamide. Most investigators treat initially with pulse methylprednisolone (30 mg/kg/day for 3 days), followed by high-dose prednisone (2 mg/kg on alternate days) until remission or stability has been achieved. Cytotoxic agents or plasmapheresis can be reserved for fulminant or corticosteroid-refractory cases. A prolonged course of therapy is usually not necessary, as it is in other pulmonary-renal syndromes. Therapy for 4 to 6 months may be adequate in responding patients.

Bone Marrow Transplantation

DAH has been noted in 6%–21% of bone marrow transplant recipients receiving high-dose chemotherapy. Acute respiratory failure and secondary infections are serious, and potentially lethal, complications of DAH. The etiology is likely diffuse injury to the pulmonary microvasculature resulting from the effects of chemotherapy or radiation, compounded by an intense cellular inflammatory response. The onset of DAH frequently coincides with marrow recovery and neutrophils within BAL fluid. High-dose corticosteroids have been associated with improved survival, supporting an immune-mediated mechanism. Methylprednisolone in intravenous doses of 125 to 250 mg every 6 hours for 3 to 5 days, followed by prednisone tapered gradually during 2 to 4 weeks, is suggested. Low-dose prednisone appears to be no better than supportive therapy (approximately 90% mortality).

Human Immunodeficiency Virus (HIV) Infection

DAH may rarely complicate HIV infection. Pulmonary vasculitis has been noted at necropsy in patients with acquired immune deficiency syndrome (AIDS). CMV exhibits tissue tropism for endothelial cells, and CMV pneumonitis has recently been implicated as a cause of DAH. Disseminated viremia, visceral involvement, microangiopathic anemia resulting from intravascular hemolysis, viral giant cells within pulmonary endothelial cells, and pulmonary capillaritis have been noted. Antiviral therapy (e.g., ganciclovir) is usually efficacious.

Exogenous Agents

DAH rarely complicates the administration of exogenous agents (e.g., trimellitic anhydride, isocyanates, lymphangiogram dye) or drugs (D-penicillamine, ''crack'' cocaine). Glomerulonephritis has been observed in DAH associated with D-penicillamine, but not with the other agents. Results of serologic studies (e.g., anti-DNA, ANA, anti-GBM antibody) have been negative. Lung biopsies have revealed nonspecific alveolar hemorrhage with no evidence for vasculitis or immune deposits. Treatment involves discontinuation or avoidance of the implicated agent or drug. For severe cases, a brief course of high-dose corticosteroids is warranted. Plasmapheresis may be considered for fulminant cases refractory to corticosteroids, but data supporting its use are lacking.

Idiopathic Pulmonary Hemosiderosis

Idiopathic pulmonary hemosiderosis (IPH) is a rare cause of recurrent DAH of unknown etiology. It occurs almost exclusively in children. The natural history is variable, but repetitive episodes of DAH for many years is characteristic. Three-year mortality rates of 30%–50% have been cited. Extrapulmonary involvement does not occur, and vasculitis is lacking. Results of serologic studies (including anti-DNA, ANA, ANCA, serum complement) are negative. Because the clinical features of IPH overlap with those of other immune-mediated DAH syndromes, negative renal and lung biopsy findings are required to substantiate the diagnosis of IPH. Many of the reported cases of IPH in adults occurred before the availability of serologic markers (e.g., ANCA, anti-GBM antibody) or immunofluorescent studies. In many cases initially considered ''idiopathic,'' other features of systemic vasculitis or connective tissue disease developed months or even years after the initial presentation. In two studies comprising 85 patients with DAH, only one patient had IPH. The diagnosis of IPH can be made only in individuals with recurrent episodes of DAH, no extrapulmonary involvement, negative lung and kidney biopsy findings, negative serology findings, and no alternative etiology after an exhaustive investigation and long-term follow-up. Because of its rarity, optimal treatment of IPH is not known. Corticosteroids are the mainstay of therapy. Long-term (and possibly indefinite) therapy may be required to prevent recrudescent disease. Alternate-day corticosteroids should be considered after the first 6 to 12 months to minimize long-term side effects. Immunosuppressive or cytotoxic agents may be used in patients refractory to or experiencing adverse effects from corticosteroids. As circulating antibodies have not been identified, we see no role for plasmapheresis.

PULMONARY ALVEOLAR PROTEINOSIS

Pulmonary alveolar proteinosis (PAP), also termed *alveolar phospholipidosis,* is a rare syndrome of unknown cause originally described by Rosen and colleagues in 1958. They reviewed histologic material from 27 patients, referred from across the world, who had undergone lung biopsy or autopsy. The distinctive histologic features included extensive flooding of alveolar spaces with a granular, eosinophilic material; however, an inflammatory component was lacking. It has since been established that the intra-alveolar material is composed primarily of lipoprotein (surfactant apoproteins). This thick, viscid, surfactant-like material fills the alveolar spaces, resulting in cough, dyspnea, and impaired gas exchange. The exact incidence of PAP is unknown. By 1980, only 260 cases had been published. The prevalence has been estimated at one case per million adults per 5-year period. The disease is two to three times more common in male patients, most of whom are between 20 and 50 years of age, but all ages may be affected. The clinical features and course are variable, and spontaneous remissions occur in 20%–30% of cases. Some patients manifest a waxing and waning course for many years.

Clinical Features

Symptoms of cough and exertional dyspnea develop insidiously and typically progress for weeks or months. The cough is usually nonproductive, but some patients expectorate plugs of grayish-yellow viscid sputum. Hemoptysis has been noted in 3%–24% of patients. A sensation of chest tightness or heaviness is present in one third of patients. Constitutional symptoms of weight loss, malaise, and fatigue may be present, but extrapulmonary involvement does not occur. Up to 20% of patients are asymptomatic. Physical examination reveals rales over involved areas; wheezing is unusual. Cyanosis has been noted in up to 20% of cases, and clubbing in 29%–40%. Chest radiographs (discussed in greater detail below) typically reveal bilateral alveolar infiltrates. Serum lactate dehydrogenase (LDH) is increased in approximately 80% of patients; no other distinctive laboratory features exist. Patients with PAP have an increased susceptibility to infections with *Nocardia* species, *S. aureus, Mycobacteria,* and fungi. This heightened susceptibility to infections reflects defects in alveolar macrophage chemotaxis, phagocytosis, and microbicidal activity and obstruction of the alveolar spaces with the thick debris. Defects in alveolar macrophage function reverse following therapeutic whole-lung lavage. Because of the rarity of the disorder and the nonspecificity of symptoms, the mean interval between onset of symptoms and diagnosis often exceeds 1 year. Untreated PAP usually progresses indolently for months to years. Before the availability of therapy, one third of patients died of respiratory failure or infectious complications. Treatment with whole-lung lavage (to be discussed later) is usually efficacious, but relapses occur in 15%–30% of treated patients.

Chest Radiographs

Chest radiographs typically demonstrate symmetric, fluffy, perihilar alveolar infiltrates (a "bat wing" appearance) (Fig. 15A). Asymmetric or even unilateral involvement occurs in 20% of patients. The infiltrates exhibit an alveolar or ground-glass pattern, but reticulonodular patterns or mixed interstitial-alveolar patterns have been noted. Differential diagnosis includes pulmonary edema (cardiac and noncardiac), BOOP, alveolar hemorrhage syndromes, DIP, and a wide spectrum of ILD. Persistent linear interstitial infiltrates have been noted in some patients, which may represent areas of fibrosis. Intrathoracic lymphadenopathy, cavitary lesions, or pleural effusions are not features of PAP. CT more clearly reveals the distinctive alveolar involvement, often with striking air bronchograms (Fig. 15B). However, chest CT is expensive and not required for either staging or follow-up of PAP.

Pulmonary Function Tests

The major physiologic aberration is intrapulmonary shunt, resulting in hypoxemia and a widened $P(A - a)O_2$. DLCO is usually reduced, but pulmonary function tests in PAP may be normal. Vital capacity or lung volumes are only mildly affected. Expiratory flow rates and FEV_1 are usually normal, but airways obstruction may be noted in smokers. These physiologic aberrations typically improve or normalize following treatment with whole-lung lavage.

Histologic Features

Grossly, the lung is consolidated, and alveolar spaces and respiratory bronchioles are filled with a granular, amorphous, acidophilic material (Fig. 16). The alveolar septa are usually normal. Interstitial inflammation and fibrosis are not features of PAP. However, hyperplastic type II pneumocytes may be observed. These histologic features bear some resemblance to those of *P. carinii* pneumonia but lack the interstitial inflammatory component, diffuse alveolar damage, and foamy intra-alveolar exudate seen in that condition. The intra-alveolar material in PAP contains phospholipids (surfactant-like material) that stain bright pink with periodic-acid Schiff (PAS) reagent and negative with alcian blue. The diagnosis of PAP has usually been established by open lung biopsy. However, the diagnosis can sometimes be made by fiberoptic bronchoscopy. The gross characteristics of BAL fluid are distinctive. The lavage effluent reveals thick, viscid, opaque, yellowish-white milky fluid that sediments into multiple layers on standing. Positive PAS and negative alcian blue stains of the foamy BAL fluid may confirm the diagnosis. Large numbers of PAS-positive, eosinophilic acellular bodies, and alveolar macrophages containing granular eosinophilic material within phagocytosomes or cytoplasm, may be found in BAL fluid. High levels of surfactant proteins A (SP-A) and D (SP-D) have been found in BAL fluid from patients with PAP; these

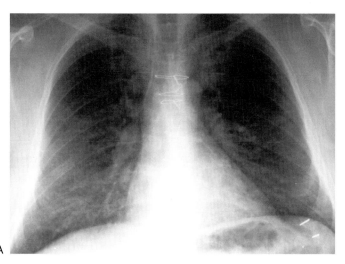
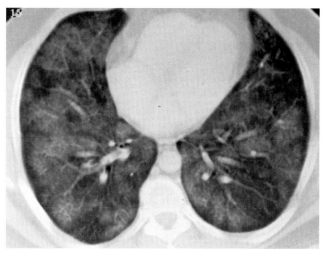

A B

FIG. 15. A: Pulmonary alveolar proteinosis. PA chest radiograph demonstrates bilateral, predominantly basilar infiltrates in a 50-year-old man with progressive exertional dyspnea. **B:** CT in the same patient demonstrates multiple foci of ground-glass opacification throughout through parenchyma. Open lung biopsy demonstrates classic features of PAP.

stain intensely using immunohistochemical methods. These immunohistiochemic techniques are limited to a few research laboratories. SP-A is highly glycosylated, which may account for the positive PAS staining.

BAL or transbronchial lung biopsies may substantiate the diagnosis, provided the typical PAS-positive intraalveolar exudate is evident. Thoracoscopic or open lung biopsies are warranted when bronchoscopic findings are equivocal or nondiagnostic. Electron microscopy and transmission electron microscopy are primarily research techniques. These techniques demonstrate alveolar macrophages engorged with phagolysosomes, complex inclusions, lamellar bodies, cholesterol inclusions, and lipid droplets. Concentric, laminated lamellar bodies containing phospholipids, tubular myelin, and myelin struc-

tures within alveolar spaces or in BAL fluid are pathognomonic for PAP.

Pathogenesis

The pathogenesis of PAP is not known. The massive accumulation of surfactant-like phospholipids within the alveolar spaces suggests that abnormal turnover of phospholipids (e.g., by impaired clearance) or excessive production of surfactant (by type II pneumocytes) is responsible. Defects in the clearance or degradation of surfactant lipoproteins may reflect dysfunction of type II pneumocytes. The inciting signals or stimuli for PAP have not been identified, but a history of exposure to hydrocarbons, chemicals, chlo-

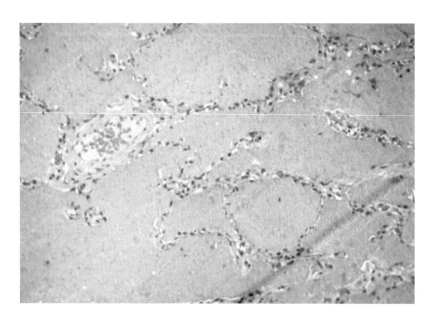

FIG. 16. Pulmonary alveolar proteinosis. Photomicrograph of open lung biopsy specimen demonstrates complete filling of alveolar spaces with a dense proteinaceous exudate. The alveolar architecture is preserved. H&E, high power. (Reproduced with permission from Lynch JP III, Chavis AD. Chronic interstitial pulmonary disorders. In: Victor L, ed. *Clinical Pulmonary Medicine.* Boston: Little, Brown; 1992:250, Fig. 11-15.)

rinated resins, fiberglass, aluminum, cadmium, titanium, silica, asbestos, volcanic ash, or a variety of solvents has been elicited in up to 50% of patients. Exogenous dusts or metals may overwhelm the normal clearance mechanisms of the lung. A variety of animal models resembling PAP have been produced by inhalation of fine dust particles (e.g., silica, crushed fiberglass, volcanic ash, bismuth, nickel, aluminum, antimony, titanium). In these models, inhaled dust particles elicit an influx of macrophages into the alveolar spaces, followed by proliferation of type II pneumocytes and accumulation of phospholipid. The alveolar macrophages ingest and become engorged with the phospholipid material. The alveolar spaces become filled with lipoproteinaceous material from the hyperplastic type II pneumocytes and disintegrating phospholipid-laden macrophages. These pathologic features strikingly resemble the lesion of PAP in humans. Chronic ingestion of certain drugs (e.g., amiodarone, chlorphentermine, and iprindole) induces a PAP-like reaction in animals. Inhibition of phospholipase may be responsible for the excessive accumulation of the lamellar, phospholipid inclusions in alveolar macrophages and within alveolar spaces in these affected animals. Cases of drug-induced PAP in humans have not been described, but these animal models may provide clues to possible mechanisms for PAP. No genetic basis for PAP has been found in humans, but PAP has rarely been reported in siblings. Lesions resembling PAP have been described in mice with severe combined immunodeficiency (SCID mice). These mice exhibit excessive amounts of eosinophilic surfactant-like material in alveolar spaces and BAL fluid and marked increases of SP-A and SP-B in BAL fluid. In animals, distinct forms of spontaneous PAP have been described. In one form, macrophages were unable to digest the phospholipoprotein complex. Other models are consistent with a defect in surfactant homeostasis. In humans, secondary forms of PAP (termed *pseudoproteinosis*) rarely complicate hematologic malignancies, AIDS, solid tumors, tuberculosis, specific infections, and interstitial pneumonitis. In these cases, involvement is usually focal and patchy. The intra-alveolar material in pseudoproteinosis may represent necrotic debris and exudate rather than the surfactant-like material characteristic of PAP. In secondary forms of PAP, remission of the underlying disease is the critical determinant of a successful outcome. Whole-lung lavage, the treatment of choice for primary PAP, is of doubtful value in secondary PAP.

Treatment

Corticosteroids, trypsin, heparin, acetylcysteine, and pancreatic enzymes have been used to treat PAP, but none are efficacious. Whole-lung lavage, introduced by Ramirez and colleagues in 1965, is the treatment of choice for PAP. Whole-lung lavage physically removes the copious, thick viscid material, allowing the alveolar spaces to re-expand and participate in gas exchange. When occupational exposure to solvents, chemicals, or dust is suspected as the cause, withdrawal from that occupation is warranted. Treatment is not required in every patient with PAP, as the disease may be mild and associated with minimal symptoms in some cases. Unilateral lung lavage has potential morbidity and should be performed by individuals who have experience with the technique. This is best accomplished under general anesthesia to ensure adequate control of the airway and optimal ventilatory management. A double-lumen endotracheal tube is placed. The most severely involved lung is allowed to deflate, and the opposite lung is ventilated with oxygen and anesthetic. Unilateral lung lavage is then carried out with successive aliquots (500 to 1000 mL) of sterile isotonic saline solution (warmed to body temperature), and the effluent is immediately suctioned and removed. With repeated instillation, the lavage effluent progressively thins. Chest percussion and rotating the patient during the procedure may enhance clearance of the thick, viscid material. The procedure is terminated after the lavage effluent no longer returns significant viscid material or markedly improves. The volume of fluid instilled is considerable, ranging from 20 to 50 L. The duration of the procedure takes on average 3 to 5 hours. Once it has been completed, the lavaged lung is ventilated. Extubation can usually be accomplished within 1 hour of completion of the procedure. Patients are observed to ensure adequate ventilation. Potential complications of the procedure include pneumothorax, pulmonary edema, spillage of lavage fluid into the contralateral lung, worsening respiratory failure, bronchospasm, and aspiration pneumonia. With proper technique and control of the airway, these adverse events occur in <5% of patients. Most patients can be discharged within 24 hours after lavage has been completed. Gradual improvement in symptoms, arterial blood gases, and chest radiographs occurs during the next few weeks. We prefer to wait 4 to 6 weeks before performing unilateral lavage of the contralateral lung. For more fulminant or severe cases, the contralateral lung can be lavaged immediately or a few days after the initial lavage. Whole-lung lavage is highly efficacious. Symptomatic, physiologic, and radiographic improvement is noted in 75%–95% of patients. Fatalities are rare. Recurrent disease requires repeated lavage in 15%–30% of patients within 1 to 5 years. Serial chest radiographs, oximetry (or arterial blood gases), and LDH should be monitored at 3-month intervals for the first year to rule out relapse. Thereafter, follow-up at 6- to 12-month intervals may be adequate in asymptomatic patients. Recrudescent disease warrants repeated lavage.

EOSINOPHILIC GRANULOMATOSIS

Pulmonary eosinophilic granulomatosis (also termed *histiocytosis X* or *Langerhans' cell granulomatosis*) is a rare granulomatous disease usually seen in smokers. It may present with cough, dyspnea, and interstitial, reticulonodular, or cystic changes on chest radiographs. Eosinophilic granulomatosis (EG) accounts for <4% of chronic ILD. The precise incidence is unknown, but prevalence rates of one to five cases per million population have been suggested. Pulmonary EG is almost exclusively seen in Caucasians, suggesting a genetic predisposition, but a specific genetic defect has not been elucidated. There is a slight male predominance. Pulmonary EG is rare in children and typically affects adults between ages 20 and 50. More than 90% of patients with pulmonary EG are smokers, suggesting an etiologic relationship.

Clinical Features

Clinical features of pulmonary EG are variable. Ten percent to 25% of patients with pulmonary EG are asymptomatic, with incidental findings on chest radiographs. Cough and dyspnea are the most common symptoms, noted in 60%–75% of patients. Symptoms usually develop insidiously during several weeks or months. Physical examination is usually unremarkable, but rales, rhonchi, wheezes, or diminished breath sounds may be present. Clubbing occurs in <5% of patients. Pneumothorax, caused by rupture of subpleural cysts, occurs in 6%–20% of patients and may be the presenting feature (Fig. 17). Pneumothoraces frequently recur and may require surgical pleurodesis. At thoracotomy, numerous subpleural cysts and blebs are usually evident. Low-grade fever, malaise, weight loss, and anorexia are present in 15%–30% of patients. There are no distinctive hematologic or serologic aberrations in pulmonary EG. Blood eosinophil counts are normal. Extrapulmonary involvement (particu-

lar osteolytic bone lesions or diabetes insipidus) occurs in 15%–20% of adults with pulmonary EG. By contrast, EG in children (typically in children under age 10) is characterized by prominent osseous and extrapulmonary manifestations. The incidence of bronchogenic carcinoma is increased in smokers with pulmonary EG. In one study of 93 patients with pulmonary EG, five cases of bronchogenic carcinoma were noted, for an annual risk of 1040/100,000. Cigarette smoking amplifies the cancer risk.

Chest Radiographic Features

Conventional chest radiographs typically reveal diffuse reticular, reticulonodular, or cystic lesions that preferentially involve the middle and upper lung zones, sparing the costophrenic angles (Fig. 18). Cystic radiolucencies, 5 to 15 mm in diameter, reflect dilated bronchi and bronchioles, with peribronchial thickening or areas of destroyed lung parenchyma. Nodules (typically 2 to 5 mm in size) are centered around bronchioles and reflect cellular granulomatous lesions (Fig. 19). The combination of pneumothorax, upper lobe cysts, and finely nodular lesions strongly suggests the diagnosis of pulmonary EG. Other CILD with a predilection for upper lobe involvement include sarcoidosis, granulomatous infections, silicosis, ankylosing spondylitis, and chronic eosinophilic pneumonia. Pleural effusions and intrathoracic adenopathy are not features of EG.

High-Resolution Thin-Section Computed Tomography

High-resolution thin-section CT is far more accurate than conventional chest radiographs in defining the nature and extent of the parenchymal lesions. Numerous thin-walled cysts are observed in >90% of patients with pulmonary EG (Fig. 18B). Peribronchiolar nodules (typically 1 to 4 mm in diameter) are present concomitantly in 60%–78% of patients. The nodules, which correspond to cellular granulomatous lesions around small bronchioles, may be missed on conventional chest radiographs. Coalescence of nodules may result in lesions exceeding 10 mm. This nodular component rarely occurs in the absence of the cystic lesions. Foci of cavitation (resulting from necrosis within the peribronchiolar inflammatory nodules) have been noted on high-resolution CT in up to 20% of patients with pulmonary EG but are rarely evident on plain chest radiographs. As the disease progresses, the nodules are replaced by cysts, some of which become confluent. The cysts or nodules are usually associated with areas of intervening normal lung tissue. Shadows that appear reticular on chest radiographs actually represent the walls of cysts. The cystic lesions correspond to dilated small bronchi and bronchioles or destroyed lung parenchyma. In the early phases, cysts are round and

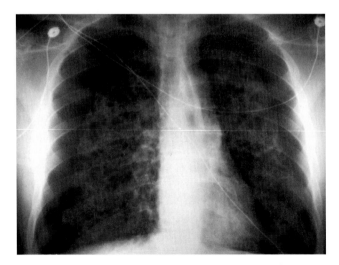

FIG. 17. Eosinophilic granulomatosis. PA chest radiograph demonstrates far-advanced cystic changes throughout lung parenchyma and bilateral pneumothoraces in a patient with pulmonary EG.

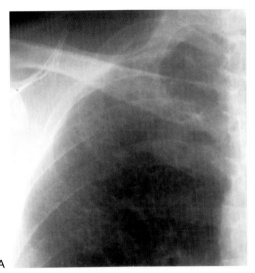

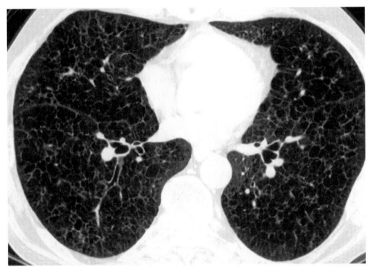

FIG. 18. A: Eosinophilic granulomatosis. Coned-down view of PA chest radiograph demonstrates finely nodular and cystic densities throughout lung parenchyma in a 56-year-old man with progressive cough and dyspnea. Transbronchial lung biopsies demonstrated typical histologic features of EG. S-100 stains were also positive. **B:** CT in the same patient demonstrates multiple, well-defined cystic spaces with walls measuring 1 to 2 cm in size. A few ill-defined, scattered interstitial nodules are also present but are subtle.

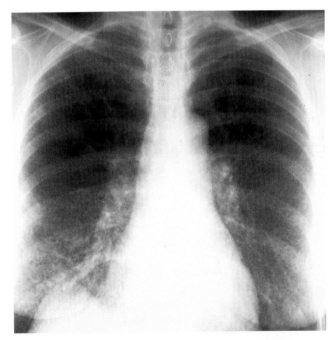

FIG. 19. Eosinophilic granulomatosis. PA chest radiograph demonstrates finely nodular densities throughout lung parenchyma in a 52-year-old woman with progressive cough and dyspnea. Transbronchial lung biopsies demonstrated typical histologic features of EG. S-100 stains were also positive.

small (<4 mm), but they may enlarge and assume distorted shapes. Confluence of cysts may result in bullous lesions exceeding 2 to 3 cm in diameter. Both the cystic and nodular lesions have a predilection for the upper and middle lung zones, with relative sparing of the costophrenic angles. There is no central or peripheral predominance. Cystic radiolucencies may be seen in other pulmonary disorders, but the nature and anatomic distribution of the cystic lesions in pulmonary EG are distinctive. The cysts in pulmonary EG are thin-walled, often regular in size, and are associated with nodules.

Numerous parenchymal cysts are the hallmark of lymphangioleiomyomatosis (LAM). In LAM, the cysts are distributed evenly throughout all lobes and lack the nodular component characteristic of EG. Honeycomb cysts are characteristic features of IPF or UIP. In contrast to cysts in pulmonary EG, honeycomb cysts in UIP have a distinctive affinity for subpleural, peripheral, and basilar regions of the lungs. Ground-glass opacities or septal bands are evident in IPF or UIP but are rarely a prominent feature of pulmonary EG. In chronic obstructive pulmonary disease, emphysematous "cysts" may be seen, but these are more irregular in size and have a thicker wall than the cysts of pulmonary EG. The combination of cysts and nodules strongly suggests the diagnosis of pulmonary EG, particularly when the lesions preferentially affect the middle and upper lung zones.

Pulmonary Function Tests

Aberrations in pulmonary function tests are noted in >80% of patients with pulmonary EG. Reduction in

DLCO occurs in 70%–80% of patients. Severe impairment in DLCO is associated with more extensive honeycombing and a worse prognosis. Reductions in VC and/or TLC occur in 50%–80% of cases. Pure restrictive and mixed obstructive-restrictive patterns may be observed. The mean FEV_1 is often reduced, but the FEV_1/FVC ratio is usually normal or increased. Air trapping (increased RV) is noted in nearly 50% of patients with pulmonary EG, but hyperinflation (TLC >110% of predicted) is rare. Pulmonary function tests are normal in 15%–20% of patients with pulmonary EG. Pulmonary function tests may not correlate with symptoms or chest radiographs. Serial pulmonary function tests are advised to monitor the course of the disease. Cardiopulmonary exercise tests in patients with pulmonary EG usually show reductions in exercise tolerance, maximal workload, oxygen consumption ($\dot{O}_{2max}$), and anaerobic threshold, and worsening gas exchange and increased ratio of dead space to tidal volume (VD/VT) with exercise. Several factors may limit exercise tolerance, including obliteration or loss of the pulmonary microvasculature, impaired pulmonary mechanics, air flow obstruction, and hypoxemia.

Histopathology

Histologically, pulmonary EG is characterized by inflammatory, cystic, nodular, and fibrotic lesions distributed in a bronchocentric fashion. The diagnosis of pulmonary EG usually requires thoracoscopic lung biopsy, but TBB may be adequate provided the salient features are present. The disease appears to evolve in distinct phases. Early in the course, proliferation of atypical histiocytes (i.e., Langerhans' cells) dominates. Later, granulomatous inflammation ensues, followed by destruction and fibrosis of lung parenchyma. In individual patients, all phases of the disorder may be seen concomitantly. Pulmonary EG may be strongly suspected by the distinctive distribution and pattern of lesions on low-power light microscopy. The combination of numerous peribronchiolar nodules and cysts, accompanied by intervening zones of normal lung parenchyma and a stellate pattern of fibrosis, is highly characteristic. Numerous discrete, focal nodules, representing cellular inflammatory lesions, may be seen under low-power magnification. The nodules are centered around bronchioles or may be distributed in subpleural regions. These lesions extend by fingerlike extensions into the adjacent alveolar interstitium, resulting in a distinctive star-shaped or stellate pattern (Fig. 20). High-power light microscopy may show intensely cellular granulomatous lesions involving bronchioles and alveolar walls. In some cases, plugs of immature connective tissue within bronchioles, alveolar ducts, and alveolar spaces may resemble BOOP. The granulomatous lesions are comprised of aggregates of Langerhans' cells (the cornerstone of the diagnosis) admixed with lymphocytes, plasma cells, eosinophils, macrophages, and neutrophils.

The cardinal histologic feature of pulmonary EG is the finding of aggregates of Langerhans' cells (also termed *histiocytosis X cells*) within the peribronchiolar nodules, air spaces, or alveolar interstitium (Fig. 21). Langerhans' cells are moderately large, ovoid histiocytes with pale eosinophilic cytoplasm, indented (grooved) nuclei, inconspicuous nucleoli, and finely dispersed chromatin. Langerhans' cells can usually be recognized under high-power light microscopy and may comprise >50 % of cells in the active cellular lesions in some patients. Langerhans' cells may be found in normal lung but rarely constitute >3% of cells. Eosinophils may be conspicuous, but the number of eosinophils is variable and is not a reliable diagnostic criterion. When light microscopic features are

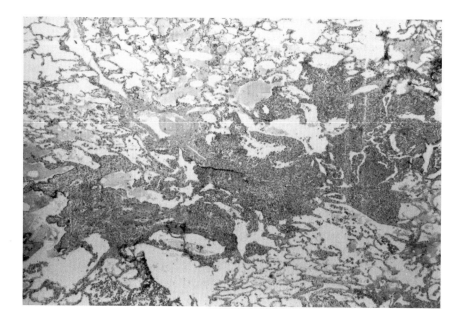

FIG. 20. Eosinophilic granulomatosis. Low-power photomicrograph of open lung biopsy specimen demonstrates stellate pattern of fibrosis. H&E stain. (Reproduced with permission from Lynch JP III and Chavis AD. Chronic interstitial pulmonary disorders. In: Victor L, ed. *Clinical Pulmonary Medicine.* Boston: Little, Brown; 1992:243, Fig. 11-14C.)

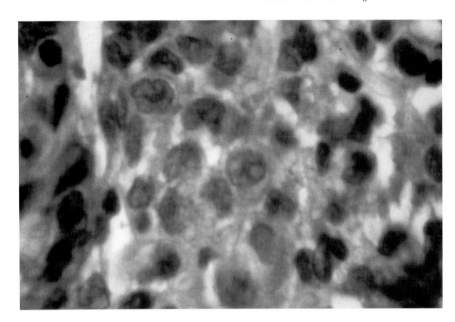

FIG. 21. Eosinophilic granulomatosis. Photomicrograph of open lung biopsy specimen demonstrates an intense cellular infiltrate with multiple Langerhans' cells exhibiting the characteristically clefted nuclei. H&E, high power.

nondiagnostic, immunohistochemical stains [e.g., S-100 protein and common thymocyte antigen (OKT6)] or electron microscopy may substantiate the identity of Langerhans' cells. These ancillary techniques are discussed later. It should be emphasized that neither S-100 nor OKT6 stains are required to diagnose pulmonary EG, provided the light microscopic features on hematoxylin-eosin stains are distinctive.

As the inflammatory process evolves, bronchioles and alveolar interstitium may be destroyed or replaced by fibrotic connective tissue, resulting in dilated, distorted bronchioles and alveolar parenchymal cysts. Blebs, subpleural cysts, and interstitial and intraluminal fibrosis may be prominent. The pulmonary microvasculature may be infiltrated or destroyed, even in areas remote from the bronchocentric nodular lesions. In late phases of pulmonary EG, the distinctive Langerhans' cells and inflammatory cells may no longer be present, and the lung may take on the appearance of an end-stage honeycomb lung, indistinguishable from that of other CILD. The retention of a nodular or stellate configuration may be a clue to the diagnosis.

Ancillary Diagnostic Techniques

Historically, electron microscopy was used to identify Langerhans' cells when light microscopy was not definitive. Langerhans' cells contain distinctive intracytoplasmic rod- or racquet-shaped inclusions (termed *Birbeck granules* or *X-bodies*), 42 to 45 nm in thickness, that have trilaminar membranes and a central line (Fig. 22). Because of the complexity and expense of electron microscopy, immunohistochemical staining for S-100 protein or OKT6 has supplanted this technique. Immunostains for S-100 protein may distinguish Langerhans' cells

from other histiocytes. This technique can be performed in paraffin-embedded biopsy specimens and is less time-consuming and avoids the sampling problems associated with electron microscopy. Large aggregates of S-100-positive histiocytes within stellate nodules or granulomatous lesions are virtually pathognomonic of EG. Staining for S-100 is most intense in the active cellular lesions and diminishes in fibrotic or acellular areas. Langerhans' cells may be found in open lung biopsy specimens or BAL fluid in other ILD but are distributed randomly and in small numbers (rarely exceeding 2% of cells). Lung endocrine cells may also stain for S-100 protein but can be distinguished from Langerhans' cells by histologic criteria or counterstains (e.g., with chromogranin).

Langerhans' cells also express OKT6, whereas lymphocytes and monocytes do not. Intense staining for OKT6 may establish the diagnosis in equivocal cases, but this technique requires fresh or frozen tissue and so is less practical than S-100 staining. In addition, rare OKT6-positive cells may be observed in BAL fluid or lung tissue in patients with diverse pulmonary disorders. Chollet et al. analyzed BAL fluid from 131 patients with various pulmonary diseases. All 18 patients with pulmonary EG had OKT6-positive cells on BAL (mean, 5.6% cells). By contrast, the mean number of OKT6-positive cells in other conditions was only 0.20% (none exceeded 2.8%). Thus, >3% of cells staining for OKT6 is relatively specific for EG.

Langerhans' cells also express other markers, including HLA-DR, Fc receptor, CD4 antigen, CD1a and CD1c (markers of a family of antigen-presenting molecules), and leucyl-B-naphthylamidase. These latter techniques are limited to research laboratories.

It should be emphasized that the diagnosis of pulmonary EG can usually be established by conventional histo-

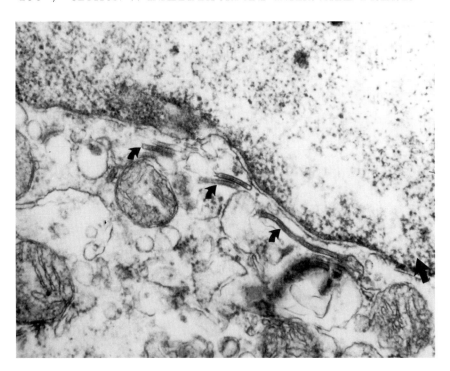

FIG. 22. Eosinophilic granulomatosis. Electron microscopy. Langerhans' histiocyte. *Curved arrows* depict Birbeck granules in the cytoplasm. *Straight arrow* points to the nucleus. (Courtesy of Theodore F. Beals, M.D., Department of Pathology, Veterans Affairs Medical Center, Ann Arbor, Michigan 48109.)

logic stains (e.g., hematoxylin-eosin) and light microscopy. Because of the heterogeneous distribution of the lesions, surgical (e.g., open or thoracoscopic) lung biopsy is usually required to confirm the diagnosis. However, transbronchial lung biopsies may be adequate provided the salient histologic or immunohistochemical features are present. Because of the potential for sampling error associated with transbronchial lung biopsies, we obtain multiple (four to six) specimens from both the upper and lower lobes and employ S-100 stains when the diagnosis is suspected. When features are not definitive, thoracoscopic biopsy should be done.

Pathogenesis

The pathogenesis of pulmonary EG is unknown, but it probably represents an uncontrolled immune response initiated or regulated by Langerhans' cells. Langerhans' cells are prominent in the early inflammatory lesions and may act as accessory cells that drive the immune/inflammatory response. Proliferation of these atypical histiocytes (Langerhans' cells) may be a reactive or neoplastic process. Recent studies using X-linked polymorphic DNA probes in female patients with disseminated, osseous, or extrapulmonary forms of Langerhans' histiocytosis (histiocytosis X) were consistent with a clonal neoplastic disorder. The pathogenesis of these nonpulmonary forms of Langerhans' histiocytosis probably differs from that of pulmonary EG, a disease that differs markedly in clinical expression and prognosis. Pulmonary EG likely represents an exuberant immune (reactive) response to inhaled irritants or allergens. Tobacco smoke has been strongly implicated as a causative factor, as 90%–97% of patients with pulmonary EG are smokers. The peribronchiolar (bronchocentric) distribution of lesions is consistent with a response to inhaled stimuli. Cigarette smoke may stimulate and recruit Langerhans' cells to the lung. Replication of Langerhans' cells in the alveolar structures may perpetuate an alveolitis. Tobacco glycoprotein, a potent immunostimulant isolated from cigarette smoke, acts as a T-cell mitogen and may stimulate macrophage cytokine production (i.e., interleukin-1 and interleukin-6). The relevance of tobacco glycoprotein to pulmonary EG has not been elucidated, but altered peripheral blood lymphocyte responses to tobacco glycoprotein in vitro have been noted in patients with pulmonary EG. Cigarette smoking has been associated with hyperplasia of pulmonary neuroendocrine cells and increased levels of bombesin-like peptides in the lower respiratory tract. Bombesin is chemotactic for monocytes and mitogenic for fibroblasts, and it may play a role in inflammatory or fibrotic responses. Immunohistochemical stains have noted large numbers of bombesin-positive neuroendocrine cells in the lungs of patients with pulmonary EG (particularly within the airways). Open lung biopsies revealed a >10-fold increase in bombesin-like peptides in specimens from patients with pulmonary EG compared with specimens from normal smokers or patients with IPF. Although neither neuroendocrine cells nor bombesin-like peptides are specific for EG, these findings may provide clues to pathogenic mechanisms. Hyperplasia of neuroendocrine cells may recruit and activate mononuclear phagocytes and Langerhans' cells to the lung. Other immune effector cells (e.g., lymphocytes, monocytes, plasma cells, eosinophils) or humoral factors (e.g., immune complexes) may play contributory roles in the pathogenesis of pulmonary EG.

Course and Prognosis

The prognosis of pulmonary EG is variable. The disease stabilizes or becomes less severe in more than two thirds of patients, usually within 6 to 24 months of onset of symptoms. In 15%–31% of patients, the disease progresses, resulting in destruction of lung parenchyma and irrevocable loss of pulmonary function. Severe late sequelae include pulmonary fibrosis, cor pulmonale, and respiratory failure. Fatalities have been noted in 6%–25% of patients. Rarely, the course is rapid, progressing to respiratory failure within a few weeks. Multisystemic disease, honeycombing on chest radiograph, severe reduction in diffusing capacity (DLCO), and multiple pneumothoraces have been associated with a poorer prognosis.

Therapy

Because of the rarity of pulmonary EG and its highly variable natural history, the role of therapy is controversial. Cessation of cigarette smoking is mandatory. Corticosteroids, vinca alkaloids (vinblastine or vincristine), D-penicillamine, and a variety of immunosuppressive and cytotoxic drugs have been associated anecdotally with claims for success, but data affirming their efficacy are lacking. Prognosis for adults with localized pulmonary EG is generally excellent, so therapy should be reserved for patients with severe, progressive, and debilitating disease. Although controlled trials have not been performed, Schonfeld and co-workers cited improvement in 12 of 14 patients with progressive pulmonary EG following institution of prednisone (initial dose of 40 mg/day). Others have failed to confirm the efficacy of corticosteroids. Given the lack of firm data, we are skeptical about the benefit of corticosteroids. However, an empiric trial for 3 to 6 months is reasonable in selected patients with fulminant or severe disease. Prolonged therapy should be continued only for patients manifesting objective and unequivocal responses. Alternative agents (e.g., vinblastine, cyclophosphamide, or D-penicillamine) can be considered for corticosteroid-recalcitrant cases, but their efficacy has not been proved. We are reluctant to use these agents for pulmonary EG, because the potential for adverse effects (including oncogenesis) may outweigh the benefit. Single-lung transplantation has been successfully accomplished in patients with EG and end-stage pulmonary fibrosis.

LYMPHANGIOLEIOMYOMATOSIS

Pulmonary lymphangioleiomyomatosis (LAM) is a rare, idiopathic fibrocystic lung disorder almost exclusively affecting premenopausal women. LAM has very rarely been described in postmenopausal women. Anecdotal case reports of LAM in male patients likely represented tuberous sclerosis or diffuse pulmonary lymphangiomatosis, disorders that share clinical and histologic features with LAM. There is an understandable confusion in acknowledging the terms as representing separate clinical entities because of phonetic similarities. Several authors have previously used the term *lymphangiomyomatosis* rather than *lymphangioleiomyomatosis*. Diffuse pulmonary/intrathoracic lymphangiomyomatosis is characterized by dilated lymphatic vascular lesions; the condition occurs in male or female patients and is not associated with smooth-muscle proliferation. This variceal condition is clinically and histologically distinct from LAM.

LAM is exceptionally rare. Published data is derived from a few series (often extracted from consulting pathologists' files) and anecdotal case reports. In 1990, Taylor and colleagues reported 32 patients with LAM followed at Stanford and the Mayo Clinic. The largest clinical series, reported by Kitaichi et al. in 1995, described 46 patients with LAM from Japan, Korea, and Taiwan. Based on an informal consensus among experts, an estimated 200 to 300 patients have been accumulated through personal files and publications. Interested patients and/or family members recently compiled a list of an additional 100 to 150 affected patients and formed an LAM organization with the support of the National Institutes of Health in the United States. Owing to the nonspecificity of clinical findings and lack of awareness of LAM, the prevalence may be underestimated by historical analyses. Data from the Mayo Clinic suggest an apparent increase in the incidence of LAM in the last decade. This apparent increase could simply reflect an increased awareness of the disorder. Very rough estimates suggest a prevalence ranging from no to three cases per 100,000 population in the United States.

Clinical Features

The classic clinical presentation of LAM is quite distinctive. Women of childbearing age present with spontaneous pneumothorax, hemoptysis, slowly progressive exertional dyspnea, or chylothorax. The mean age at onset of symptoms is approximately 30 years. Dyspnea is nearly invariably present, beginning in the third or fourth decade of life, and progresses inexorably for years. Pneumothoraces occur in 50%–80% of patients with LAM. Chylous effusions occur in 7%–39%, and hemoptysis or focal alveolar hemorrhage in 28%–40%. The clinical course of LAM is heterogeneous. In early reports, most patients died of progressive respiratory failure within 5 to 10 years of onset of symptoms. The life expectancy appears to be highly variable, and prolonged survivorship has been noted in some patients. In the cohort of LAM patients from Stanford and the Mayo Clinic, 25 of 32 patients (78%) were alive 8.5 years after the diagnosis; mean survival was 10.0 years. Kitachi and colleagues cited a lower survival (38% at 8.5 years after the diagnosis) in a cohort of 46 patients with LAM in Asia. Studies assessing the impact of specific therapeutic modalities are lacking but are discussed later.

Pulmonary Function Tests

Pulmonary function tests in LAM typically demonstrate air flow limitation (often with air trapping), impaired DLCO, and hypoxemia. Lung volumes are usually preserved and may be increased. In the series reported from Stanford and the Mayo Clinic, obstructive or mixed obstructive-restrictive defects were noted in 78% of patients. Reductions in DLCO were noted in 96% and hypoxemia was present in 77%. In the series reported by Kitaichi et al., 29% exhibited a pure obstructive air flow limitation; restrictive defects or mixed obstructive-restrictive defects were noted in 26% and 36%, respectively. TLC was increased (>120% of predicted) in 30%. Reductions in DLCO (<80% of predicted) and PaO_2 (<80 torr) were observed in 97% and 81% of patients, respectively. Resting arterial blood gases may be normal in the setting of mild disease, but decreases in PaO_2 and widened $P(A - a)O_2$ are typical as the disease progresses. Exercise performance is impaired; an excessive ventilatory response and increased dead space ventilation are characteristic features on formal exercise testing. Air flow obstruction and impairments in diffusing capacity, exercise capacity, and gas exchange correlate primarily with the extent of airway cystic lesions. However, muscular proliferation in small airways, destruction of pulmonary microvasculature, loss of alveolar support, and loss of parenchymal interdependence may be important contributory mechanisms of physiologic aberrations.

Chest Radiographs

Conventional chest radiographs demonstrate a wide spectrum of abnormalities. These include pneumothoraces; bilateral interstitial, reticulonodular, or cystic radiolucencies; pleural effusions; or hyperinflation (Fig. 23). Early in the course of the disease, chest radiographic findings may be normal. With disease progression, cystic lesions, reticulonodular infiltrates, or pneumothoraces invariably develop. Pneumothoraces have been noted at the time of presentation in 39%–53% of patients with LAM, and reticulonodular infiltrates in 47%–85%. As the disease progresses, both these features are present in >80% of patients. The reticulation actually represents the walls of the numerous alveolar cysts. In some cases, well-defined cystic or bullous lesions may be evident. Hyperinflation develops as the disease worsens and is seen in up

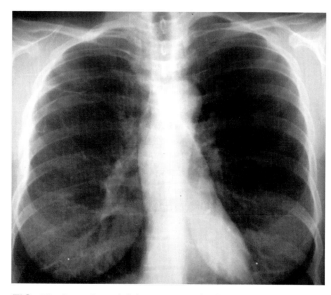

FIG. 23. Lymphangioleiomyomatosis. PA chest radiograph from a 39-year-old woman with LAM demonstrates severe hyperinflation and large cysts and bullous changes. Surgical clips are present on the right from a previous thoracotomy and pleurodesis for recurrent pneumothoraces.

to two thirds of patients in the late phases of the disease. Pleural effusions (typically chylous) occur in 11%–29% of patients. Mediastinal or hilar lymphadenopathy is not a feature of LAM.

High-Resolution Computed Tomography

High-resolution CT findings are highly distinctive in LAM. The cardinal feature is numerous thin-walled cysts (usually <20 mm in diameter) distributed diffusely throughout both lungs; the intervening lung parenchyma is normal (Figs. 24, 25, and 26). Nodules, interstitial fibrosis, cavitary lesions, and intrathoracic lymphadenopathy, features that may be observed in other CILD, are not features of pulmonary LAM. Focal ground-glass opacities have been noted in up to 59% of patients with LAM in some series, and may reflect focal alveolar hemorrhage, pulmonary hemosiderosis, or diffuse proliferation of smooth-muscle cells. However, the cystic lesions predominate. Cystic lesions may be seen on high-resolution CT in other pulmonary disorders (e.g., pulmonary EG, IPF, emphysema), but the distribution of cysts differs among these disorders. In LAM, the cysts are distributed throughout the lung fields, without a predilection for specific regions or lobes. By contrast, in pulmonary EG, the cysts are preferentially distributed in the upper or middle lung zones and are usually associated with a nodular component (which is lacking in LAM). In IPF, areas affected by the disease are patchy and heterogeneous, and cysts are preferentially distributed in the peripheral, subpleural, and basilar regions of the lungs. In addition, reticular or

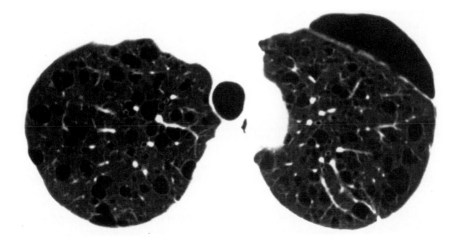

FIG. 24. Lymphangioleiomyomatosis. CT in a 41-year-old woman with LAM demonstrates multiple, thin-walled cystic radiolucencies in upper lobes bilaterally with large zones of intervening normal lung parenchyma, consistent with LAM.

ground-glass opacities are usually prominent associated features in IPF. Cystic or bullous lesions seen in smokers with emphysema do not have well-formed walls and tend to be more extensive in the upper lobes. Tuberous sclerosis, an autosomal dominant disorder associated with mental retardation and cutaneous manifestations, is associated with pulmonary cystic lesions indistinguishable from those of LAM in approximately 1% of patients. Tuberous sclerosis can be distinguished from LAM on clinical grounds, as neurologic or cutaneous manifestations are not observed in LAM.

Histopathologic Features

At thoracotomy, innumerable small cysts are seen on the lung surface, ranging from a few mm to 3 cm (Fig. 27A). Light microscopy demonstrates diffuse proliferation of immature/atypical smooth muscle in the walls of the cysts and throughout the peribronchial, perivascular, and perilymphatic regions of the lungs (Fig. 27B,C). These proliferating

smooth-muscle cells may form highly organized nodules or fascicles but are not considered malignant. The smooth-muscle cells are heterogeneous, and phenotypically they may exhibit features of either spindle cells or epithelioid cells. Electron microscopy shows myofilaments in the smooth-muscle cells of the lung lesions and dense deposits of collagen fibers. Extension of these smooth-muscle proliferations may destroy surrounding lung parenchyma, forming the characteristic cysts. The diffuse distribution of the muscular and cystic lesions explains the clinical manifestations of LAM. Compression of the conducting small airways results in air flow obstruction and alveolar disruption. Pneumothoraces result from rupture of subpleural cysts. Obstruction of pulmonary vessels may cause venular congestion and disruption, resulting in hemoptysis and hemosiderosis. Lymphatic obstruction may cause chylothorax. The extent of cystic LAM lesions on open lung biopsy is an important determinant of prognosis; predominantly cystic lesions sug-

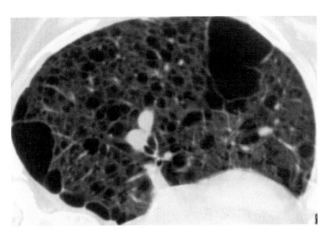

FIG. 25. Lymphangioleiomyomatosis. CT in a 44-year-old woman with LAM demonstrates multiple, thin-walled cystic radiolucencies bilaterally. Note the two large lesions, representing confluent cysts.

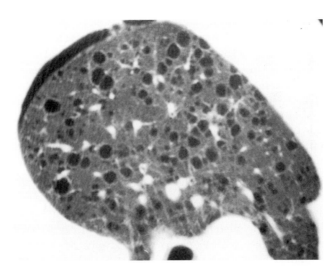

FIG. 26. Lymphangioleiomyomatosis. CT demonstrates multiple, thin-walled cystic radiolucencies throughout lung parenchyma. Note small associated pneumothorax, a typical finding in LAM. (Courtesy of R. Schmidt, M.D, Ph.D., University of Washington, Seattle.)

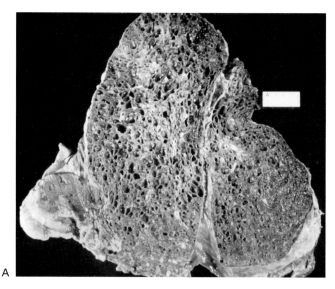

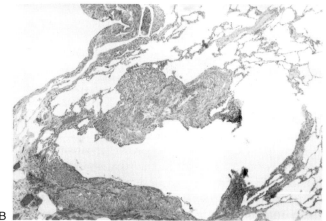

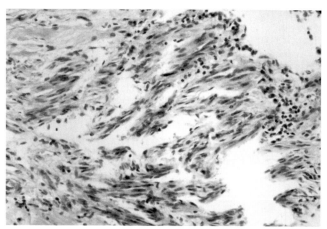

FIG. 27. A: Lymphangioleiomyomatosis. Gross appearance of lung removed from a patient with LAM. Note the numerous cysts throughout the lung parenchyma. **B:** Photomicrograph of lung biopsy specimen demonstrates aggregates of characteristic smooth-muscle bundles in the walls of cysts and in the peribronchial areas. H&E, low power. **C:** Photomicrograph of lung biopsy specimen demonstrates aggregates of characteristic smooth-muscle bundles with a spindle appearance. H&E, high power.

gest a worse prognosis and survival. The extent of smooth-muscle proliferation or hemosiderosis does not correlate with survival.

Immunohistochemical stains of the proliferating smooth-muscle cells in LAM are positive for muscle-specific actin, desmin, and melanoma-related marker (HMB-45). HMB-45 is never found in normal smooth muscle. In the absence of melanoma or clear-cell tumor of the lung (which also stains for HMB-45), positive staining for HMB-45 in the lung is highly specific (>95%) for LAM. Progesterone and estrogen receptors have been demonstrated in the nuclei of proliferating smooth muscle in some patients with LAM, but these findings are not consistently present.

Extrapulmonary lymphangioleiomyomas or cysts may involve the spleen, kidney, liver, abdominal or retroperitoneal lymph nodes, uterus, and ovaries in patients with LAM. Renal angiomyolipomas have been noted in 15%–47% of patients with pulmonary LAM and may give rise to local pain, bleeding, or compression of renal parenchyma.

Differential Diagnosis

The diagnosis of LAM is strongly suggested by the constellation of spontaneous pneumothorax, preserved or increased lung volumes, chylous pleural effusions, and air flow obstruction in women in the third or fourth decade of life. Hemoptysis may be an associated feature (noted in up to 40% of patients). When the clinical presentation is typical, the diagnosis can be strongly suspected based on the radiologic findings (particularly high-resolution CT). Other clinical entities that may be confused with LAM include pulmonary EG, metastatic low-grade sarcomas, tuberous sclerosis, emphysema, and small-airways disease with smooth-muscle proliferation. The diagnosis of LAM needs to be substantiated by lung biopsy. Transbronchial lung biopsy may be diagnostic in some cases, but surgical lung biopsy is warranted when TBB findings are nondiagnostic or equivocal.

Treatment

Given the rarity of LAM, controlled therapeutic trials have not been performed and optimal therapy is controversial. Although a specific hormonal abnormality has not been identified, LAM is exclusively a disease of women and may be exacerbated by estrogens (endogenous or exogenous) or pregnancy. Proliferation of uterine smooth-muscle cells is also regulated by estrogen. Treatment of LAM is directed toward reducing estrogens, either by surgical oophorectomy or anti-estrogen regimens (e.g., progesterone, tamoxifen, androgens, luteinizing hormone-releasing agonists). Exogenous estrogens are strongly contraindicated. Oophorectomy has been considered "gold standard" therapy by some, but results have generally been disappointing. In the retrospective review from Stanford and the Mayo Clinic, oophorectomy was ineffective in all 16 patients. Despite anecdotal responses of improvement or stabilization following oophorectomy, oophorectomy alone was never associated with improvement in the group of patients reported by Kitaichi and colleagues. Medroxyprogesterone acetate has been tried, either alone or combined with oophorectomy, as therapy for LAM. Intramuscular medroxyprogesterone acetate (400 to 800 mg monthly) alone was associated with stabilization or improvement in 2 of 19 and 4 of 8 patients in two series. This form of therapy appears to be more effective in managing chylous effusions; its efficacy in alleviating the airway or cystic lesions is less clear. Tamoxifen has been advocated by some, but data justifying its use are lacking. In four series, tamoxifen, given alone or in combination with other agents, was associated with improvement in only 2 of 31 treated patients. Tamoxifen has partial estrogen-agonist activity, so we believe this agent should not be used in LAM. Anecdotal responses have been cited with synthetic analogues of luteinizing-releasing hormone, but data are sparse. Interferon-α has been tried, but results have been unimpressive. Unfortunately, current therapeutic regimens for LAM are of limited efficacy. In the review by Kitaichi and colleagues, diverse therapeutic options were evaluated in 40 patients. Only two improved; nine stabilized, and the remaining patients deteriorated. In this cohort of patients, factors associated with a poor prognosis included worsening air flow obstruction at 2 years after the initial examination; increase in percentage of predicted TLC at 2, 3, and 5 years after the initial exam; predominantly cystic LAM lesions (compared with predominantly smooth-muscle proliferation) on open lung biopsy; and higher grades of histologically abnormal areas and cystic lesions on open lung biopsy.

Despite the lack of firm evidence that treatment reverses the course of the disease, the course of LAM in the absence of therapy is poor, with inexorable progression. The rate of progression of LAM varies widely among patients regardless of therapy. LAM has been known to continue even after menopause. Given the poor prognosis of untreated LAM, an empiric trial with intramuscular medroxyprogesterone acetate, oophorectomy, or both is reasonable. The influence of pregnancy on the outcome is unknown, but anecdotal cases have documented progression or acceleration of LAM during pregnancy. We believe pregnancy should be avoided, but this

is best left to the informed patient's wishes. Unilateral lung transplantation is an established mode of therapy for far-advanced disease. Three-year survival following lung transplantation for LAM approximates 60%–70%. Recurrence of LAM has been reported in transplanted lung allografts in two patients with LAM, raising questions regarding the long-term outcome of transplantation in this patient population. It is hoped that ongoing research efforts and future studies will shed further light on the pathogenesis of LAM and provide new strategies for curative therapy.

PULMONARY AMYLOIDOSIS

Intrathoracic amyloidosis may rarely complicate primary or secondary amyloidosis in which systemic involvement is evident. In addition, primary pulmonary amyloidosis, lacking extrapulmonary or systemic components, may occur. Amyloidosis comprises a heterogeneous group of diseases characterized by deposition of an insoluble β-pleated fibrillar protein in the extracellular matrix of involved tissues. Amyloid protein takes up Congo red stain and exhibits apple-green birefringence under polarized microscopy (Fig. 28). Primary amyloidosis, the most common variant, can be idiopathic or associated with plasma cell dyscrasias (such as multiple myeloma). This is associated with deposition of the immunoglobulin light-chain fragment (amyloid AL). Secondary amyloidosis (amyloid AA) may complicate diverse chronic inflammatory conditions (e.g., bronchiectasis, tuberculosis, malaria, chronic infections, and diverse collagen vascular disorders or inflammatory disorders). Amyloid AA protein is an apolipoprotein associated with HDL-3 that is produced by proteolysis of serum amyloid A proteins. Familial amyloidosis has also been described. Amyloid protein may also be found with advanced age (senile amyloidosis). Prealbumin has been associated with familial and senile forms of amyloidosis. Clinically significant pulmonary involvement occurs in more than one third of patients with primary systemic amyloidosis but only rarely complicates secondary forms of amyloidosis. Primary or secondary forms of systemic amyloidosis differ from primary pulmonary amyloidosis, a disorder localized to the lungs, tracheobronchial tree, pleurae, and/or mediastinal lymph nodes.

Pulmonary Amyloidosis Associated with Primary Systemic Amyloidosis

Although it has long been recognized that primary systemic amyloidosis tends to involve the lung, reports of lung involvement have been infrequent. Although the prevalence of pulmonary involvement in primary systemic amyloidosis has not been elucidated, diffuse amyloid deposits in an alveolar septal pattern may occur. A recent review of the Mayo

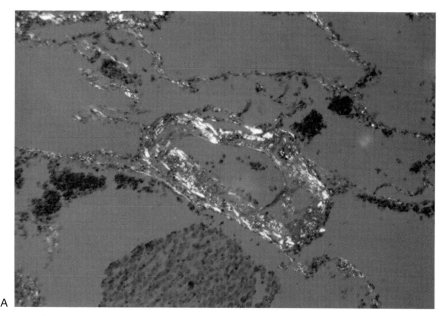

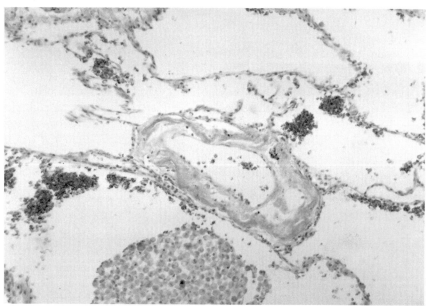

FIG. 28. A: Amyloidosis. Photomicrograph of open lung biopsy specimen demonstrates amyloid deposition within the wall of a pulmonary vessel. H&E. **B:** Photomicrograph of open lung biopsy specimen demonstrates amyloid deposit displaying apple-green birefringence under polarized microscopy following staining with Congo red.

Clinic experience from 1980 to 1993 identified 35 patients with primary systemic amyloidosis, of whom 20 had pulmonary involvement manifesting as diffuse interstitial infiltrates; four had coexisting pleural effusions. The median survival in this series was 16 months. Because cardiac amyloidosis is a frequent concomitant feature, it is difficult to determine the influence of pulmonary amyloidosis on prognosis. However, the presence of pulmonary amyloidosis in patients with primary systemic amyloidosis is generally considered a harbinger of a poor outcome.

Localized or Primary Pulmonary Amyloidosis

Primary or localized pulmonary amyloidosis is characterized by amyloid deposits limited to the lungs and associated structures (i.e., tracheobronchial tree, lung parenchyma, pleurae, and hilar or mediastinal lymph nodes). Most patients with localized tracheobronchial amyloidosis are in the fifth to sixth decade of life. Amyloid deposition in the lung resulting from secondary or familial amyloidosis is not included in this category. In 1983, Thompson and Citron identified 126 published cases of primary pulmonary amyloidosis in the world literature (67 tracheobronchial, 59 lung parenchymal). Of the 67 patients with tracheobronchial disease, 57 had multifocal submucosal plaques and 10 had amyloid tumorlike masses. A review of three recent series cited involvement of the tracheobronchial tree in 23 of 89 patients with pulmonary amyloidosis.

Tracheobronchial amyloidosis is generally localized to the airways and spares the lung parenchyma. Relatively flat submucosal plaques of amyloid protein or tracheo-bronchial nodules may be seen. These may be single, diffuse, or multifocal and are not associated with systemic amyloidosis. Patients may be asymptomatic or may have hoarseness, wheezing, dyspnea, hemoptysis, cough, atelectasis, recurrent pneumonia, or chronic infections. Respiratory symptoms may be related to airway narrowing or stenosis or involvement of the nasopharynx, sinuses, or larynx. Tracheobronchial amyloidosis has been associated with tracheobronchopathia osteoplastica, a rare disorder of unknown cause characterized by the presence of calcified or cartilaginous submucosal nodules within the tracheobronchial tree. Localized tracheobronchial amyloidosis is not associated with primary systemic amyloidosis, but its course may not be benign. In a study by Hui and colleagues at the Armed Forces Institute of Pathology, three of the seven patients for whom follow-up data were available died of respiratory failure or recurrent pneumonia. Management has included observation, intermittent bronchoscopic resection, surgical resection, and laser therapy. Resection or biopsy may be complicated by severe bleeding (see below).

Nodular Amyloid Lesions (Amyloidomas)

Localized pulmonary amyloid nodules (amyloidomas) are uncommon lesions that may be seen in older patients (on

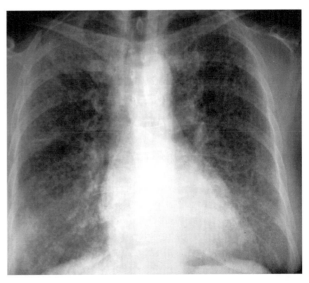

FIG. 30. Amyloidosis. PA chest radiograph demonstrates diffuse bilateral reticulonodular infiltrates in a patient with pulmonary amyloidosis. Small bilateral pleural effusions are also present. (Courtesy of D. Godwin, M.D., University of Washington, Seattle.)

average in the sixth decade) and are generally not associated with primary systemic amyloidosis. Lesions may be single or multiple, ranging in size from 0.4 to 15 cm (average, 3 cm) (Fig. 29). Amyloidomas occur most frequently in the lower lobes and may be asymmetric when multiple nodules are present. Amyloidomas may calcify and rarely cavitate. Metaplastic bone or cartilage formation may occur. Amyloidomas are usually asymptomatic and present as incidental findings on chest radiographs (Fig. 29) or autopsy. However, cough or hemoptysis may occur. For solitary nodules causing symptoms, resection is usually curative. However, biopsy or resection of nodular mass lesions may cause significant bleeding (see below).

Diffuse Interstitial Infiltrates

Amyloid deposits in the alveolar septa and interstitium may appear as reticulonodular or micronodular lesions on chest radiographs or CT scans and cause physiologic aberrations, including restrictive defects, decreased DLCO, widened $P(A - a)O_2$, and pulmonary hypertension (Fig. 30). Alveolar septal amyloidosis is most commonly seen in primary systemic amyloidosis and is relatively uncommon in primary pulmonary amyloidosis. Although diffuse interstitial infiltrates were noted in 6 of 48 patients with primary pulmonary amyloidosis reported by Hui and colleagues from the Armed Forces Institute of Pathology, none of 17 patients with primary pulmonary amyloidosis recently reviewed by the Mayo Clinic group exhibited this radiographic pattern. Some authors have suggested that patients with interstitial pulmonary infiltrates likely represent a subset of patients with primary systemic amy-

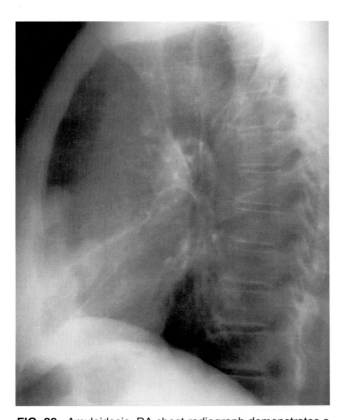

FIG. 29. Amyloidosis. PA chest radiograph demonstrates a solitary pulmonary nodule in the retrosternal space. Open lung biopsy specimen demonstrates typical features of amyloidosis. (Courtesy of D. Godwin, M.D., University of Washington, Seattle.)

loidosis and have unrecognized amyloid deposits in other organs. As the amyloid deposits and infiltrative process in the alveolar septa often involve the pulmonary vasculature, biopsy or resection of pulmonary lesions may be associated with an increased risk for bleeding.

Other Manifestations of Amyloid Deposits

Hilar and mediastinal adenopathy resulting from amyloid deposition may occur in conjunction with tracheobronchial amyloidosis and either primary or secondary forms of amyloidosis. The adenopathy may be unilateral or bilateral (with or without calcification). Pulmonary amyloidosis occurring in elderly patients has been termed *senile pulmonary amyloidosis.* Autopsy studies have detected senile pulmonary amyloidosis in approximately 10% of patients older than 80 years and in 50% of patients older than 90 years. These deposits are usually incidental findings and are not associated with primary systemic amyloidosis or specific symptoms. Pleural effusions (caused by amyloid deposits along the pleural surface) may occur in primary systemic amyloidosis or as a complication of primary pulmonary amyloidosis. Amyloid effusions are exudative and may be hemorrhagic. Transudative pleural effusions may reflect cardiac amyloidosis. Other rare pulmonary manifestations include obstructive sleep apnea (secondary to involvement of the tongue) and respiratory muscle weakness (caused by amyloid infiltrating the diaphragm).

Bleeding Manifestation with Amyloidosis

Hemoptysis may complicate any form of pulmonary amyloidosis (including alveolar septal or tracheobronchial involvement). Focal or diffuse hemorrhage may occur when amyloid deposits involve vessels. In one retrospective review by Yood and colleagues, 41 of 100 patients with amyloidosis experienced one or more episodes of bleeding (three of which were fatal). Manifestations included petechiae, ecchymoses, gastrointestinal bleeding, hematuria, hemoptysis, and bleeding after biopsy. Hemoptysis occurred in only two patients. Although the excessive bleeding associated with amyloidosis is most often caused by amyloid infiltration of blood vessels, isolated deficiency of factor X has been cited as a cause of the bleeding diathesis in some patients with amyloidosis. The risk for pulmonary hemorrhage following lung biopsy is of concern, but firm data assessing risks are not available.

Treatment of Amyloidosis

Unfortunately, no proven therapy for amyloidosis is available. In secondary forms of amyloidosis, aggressive treatment of the underlying disease may delay or reverse the deposition of amyloid protein. Alkylating agents may be effective in amyloidosis associated with plasma cell dyscrasias (e.g., multiple myeloma) but are of unproven efficacy in other forms of amyloidosis and may increase morbidity. Colchicine has been used in both primary and secondary forms of amyloidosis, but its value is doubtful. Interferon-α has been tried but appears to be ineffective. Anecdotal responses have been reported with dimethylsulfoxide and 4'-iodo-4'-deoxydoxorubicin (a new anthracycline), but data are sparse. No proven effective treatment is available for diffuse amyloid infiltrating the tracheobronchial tree or lung parenchyma. Resection of localized amyloid deposits surgically or by laser may be beneficial in symptomatic foci involving the trachea, larynx, or bronchi. In rare cases, laryngeal dilation or tracheostomy have been required. It is hoped that ongoing and future studies will provide strategies for new therapeutic approaches.

ACKNOWLEDGMENT

Dr. Lynch is supported in part by National Institutes of Health Grant IP50HL46487.

REFERENCES

Acquino SL, Webb WR, Gushiken BJ. Pleural exudates and transudates: diagnosis with contrast-enhanced CT. *Radiology* 1994;192:803–808. *Parietal pleural thickening usually indicates the presence of a pleural exudate. In this study, all cases of empyema and approximately half the cases of parapneumonic effusion demonstrated pleural thickening.*

Benacerraf BR, McLoud TC, Rhea JT, Tritschler V, Libby P. An assessment of the contribution of chest radiography in outpatients with acute chest complaints: a prospective study. *Radiology* 1981;138:293–299. *A prospective study designed to identify selective indications, including symptoms, physical findings, and demographics, for adult chest radiography in an ambulatory clinic and an emergency room setting.*

Bessis L, Callard P, Gotheil C, Biaggi A, Grenier P. High-resolution CT of parenchymal lung disease: precise correlation with histologic findings. *Radiographics* 1992;12:45–58. *A review illustrating and correlating high-resolution chest CT and histologic specimens obtained at autopsy.*

Brown LR, Aughenbaugh GL. Masses of the anterior mediastinum: CT and MR imaging. *AJR Am J Roentgenol* 1991;157:1171–1180. *A review article discussing the indications, techniques, and findings as well as the relative merits of CT and MRI in the evaluation of anterior mediastinal masses.*

Brown MJ, Miller RR, Muller NL. Acute lung disease in the immunocompromised host: CT and pathologic examination findings. *Radiology* 1994;190:247–254. *CT pattern of parenchymal abnormalities closely resembles the gross morphologic features identified on pathologic specimens. A nodular pattern is very suggestive of an infectious etiology in immunocompromised patients. The same etiology can appear as a nodular, ground-glass, and/or consolidative pattern.*

Buckley JA, Scott WW Jr, Siegelman SS, Kuhlman JE, Urban BA, Bluemke DA, Fishman EK. Pulmonary nodules: effect of increased data sampling on detection with spiral CT and confidence in diagnosis. *Radiology* 1995;196:395–400. *A study demonstrating one of several advantages of spiral over conventional chest CT. The rate of detection of pulmonary nodules was increased and the false-positive detection rate was decreased in less experienced interpreters.*

Butcher BL, Nichol KL, Parenti CM. High yield of chest radiography in walk-in clinic patients with chest symptoms. *J Gen Intern Med* 1993;8:114–119. *A prospective study of adult men in an ambulatory care setting with chief symptoms of cough, dyspnea, or pleuritic chest pain demonstrating clinically important new radiographic abnormali-*

ties in approximately 35% of patients regardless of past medical history, vital signs, or smoking history.

Corcoran HL, Renner WR, Milstein MJ. Review of high-resolution CT of the lung. *Radiographics* 1992;12:917. *The anatomy of the secondary pulmonary lobule is detailed and the patterns of findings on high-resolution chest CT are illustrated.*

Erdman WA, Peshock RM, Redman HC, Bonte F, Meyerson M, Jayson HT, Miller GL, Clarke GD, Parkey RW. Pulmonary embolism: comparison of MR images with radionuclide and angiographic studies. *Radiology* 1994;190:499–508. *An investigation demonstrating accurate detection of large and medium-sized pulmonary emboli using MRI.*

Forman HP, Fox LA, Glazer HS, McClennan BL, Anderson DC, Sagel SS. Chest radiography in patients with early-stage prostatic carcinoma. *Chest* 1994;106:1036–1041. *A retrospective study of routine preoperative chest radiographs in patients with prostate carcinoma, demonstrating a significant medical impact in a small number of patients. Cost effectiveness could not be confirmed because of, among other factors, sample size.*

Fortier M, Mayo JR, Swensen SJ, Munk PL, Vellet DA, Muller NL. MR imaging of chest wall lesions. *Radiographics* 1994;14:597–606. *The appearance of both benign and malignant lesions of the chest wall is illustrated.*

Friedman PJ. Lung cancer staging: efficacy of CT. *Radiology* 1992; 182:307–309. *A recent editorial discussing the current role of chest CT in the management of mediastinal disease in patients with non-small-cell lung cancer.*

Grover FL. The role of CT and MRI in staging of the mediastinum. *Chest* 1994;106:391S–396S. *A recent review of the literature discussing the sensitivity and specificity of CT and MRI in staging non-small-cell lung cancer in the mediastinum and the implications for surgical management.*

Harris JH (report from the chairman of the board). Referral criteria for routine screening chest x-ray examinations. *Am Coll Radiol Bull* 1982; 38:17. *A useful review.*

Hayabuchi N, Russell WJ, Murakami J. Problems in radiographic detection and diagnosis of lung cancer. *Acta Radiol* 1989;30:163–167. *Errors in detecting lung cancer within a screening population (an abnormality was identified but thought to be some disease other than cancer) were related equally to perception and decision making. A higher index of suspicion would reduce decision-making errors.*

Heckerling PS, Tape TG, Wigton RS, Hissong KK, Leikin JB, Ornato JP, Cameron JL, Racht EM. Clinical prediction rule for pulmonary infiltrates. *Ann Intern Med* 1990;113:664–670. *A study demonstrating that a prediction rule based on clinical findings accurately discriminates between patients with and without radiographic pneumonia.*

Heiken JP, Brink JA, Vannier MW. Spiral (helical) CT. *Radiology* 1993;189:647–656. *The technical details of helical CT and their application to clinical CT scanning are reviewed.*

Henschke CI, Yankelevitz DF, Wand A, Davis SD, Shiau M. Accuracy and efficacy of chest radiography in the intensive care unit. *Radiol Clin North Am* 1996;34:21–31. *A review of the technical aspects as well as the accuracy and efficacy of portable chest radiography in intensive care units. The diagnosis of specific conditions, such as pneumonia and pulmonary edema, and the utility of radiographic monitoring and therapeutic devices are considered.*

Hubbell FA, Greenfield S, Tyler JL, Chetty K, Wyle FA. The impact of routine admission chest x-ray films on patient care. *N Engl J Med* 1985;312:209–213. *In a population with a high prevalence of cardiopulmonary disease, routine admission chest radiography had a very small impact on patient care.*

Jochelson MS, Altschuler J, Stomper PC. The yield of chest radiography in febrile and neutropenic patients. *Ann Intern Med* 1986;105:708–709. *A helpful review.*

Klein JS, Schultz S, Heffner JE. Interventional radiology of the chest: image-guided percutaneous drainage of pleural effusions, lung abscess, and pneumothorax. *AJR Am J Roentgenol* 1995;164:581–588. *The role of percutaneous interventional procedures in a variety of chest abnormalities is reviewed.*

Kuhlman JE, Bouchard LM, Fishman EK, Zerhouni EA. CT and MR imaging evaluation of chest wall disorders. *Radiographics* 1994;14: 571. *The advantages of each modality in detecting and characterizing abnormalities of the chest wall is addressed. CT more readily demonstrates small calcifications and cortical bone destruction. MRI more*

accurately depicts bone marrow invasion and infiltration of soft tissues by masses.

Leung AN, Staples CA, Muller NL. Chronic diffuse infiltrative lung disease: comparison of diagnostic accuracy of high-resolution and conventional CT. *AJR Am J Roentgenol* 1991;157:693–696. *Only a few high-resolution CT scans obtained at three different levels are necessary to arrive at a level of accuracy comparable with that of complete conventional CT scans in evaluating chronic diffuse infiltrative disease.*

Line BR. Scintigraphic studies of inflammation in diffuse lung disease. *Radiol Clin North Am* 1991;29:1095–1114. *Review of the mechanism of uptake and selective use of gallium 67 in the evaluation of diffuse lung disease.*

Link KM, Samuels LJ, Reed JC, Loehr SP, Lesko NM. Magnetic resonance imaging of the mediastinum. *J Thorac Imaging* 1993;8:34–53. *A review of the applications of MRI in the mediastinum, including evaluation of solid and cystic masses, vascular applications, and assessment of lymphadenopathy.*

Mayo JR. Magnetic resonance imaging of the chest. *Radiol Clin North Am* 1994;32:795–809. *A review of the indications for MRI, not only in the mediastinum but also in the cardiovascular system, chest wall, and lung parenchyma.*

McLoud TC, Bourgouin PM, Greenberg RW, Kosiuk JP, Templeton PA, Shepard JO, Moore EH, Wain JC, Mathisen DJ, Grillo HC. Bronchogenic carcinoma: analysis of staging in the mediastinum with CT by correlative lymph node mapping and sampling. *Radiology* 1992;182:319–323. *A prospective study demonstrating that chest CT is an important adjunct in staging non-small-cell lung cancer in the mediastinum but does not eliminate the use of mediastinoscopy or thoracotomy.*

McLoud TC, Flower CDR. Imaging the pleura: sonography, CT, and MR imaging. *AJR Am J Roentgenol* 1991;156:1145–1153. *Use of the three different imaging modalities in evaluating pleural abnormalities is reviewed.*

Mirvis SE, Bidwell JK, Buddemeyer EU, Diaconis JN, Pais SO, Whitley JE, Goldstein LD. Value of chest radiography in excluding traumatic aortic rupture. *Radiology* 1987;163:487–493. *A retrospective review of 205 patients with blunt chest trauma, 45 of whom had proven aortic rupture. Although certain findings on conventional chest radiography were suggestive of aortic rupture, no single sign or combination of signs had a very high positive predictive value, but normal findings on examination did have a high negative predictive value.*

Muller NL. Differential diagnosis of chronic diffuse infiltrative lung disease on high-resolution computed tomography. *Semin Roentgenol* 1991;26:132–142. *A review describing and illustrating the basic radiologic features and signs used in interpreting high-resolution CT.*

Muller NL. Computed tomography in chronic interstitial lung disease. *Radiol Clin North Am* 1991;29:1085–1093. *A review discussing the CT appearance of a variety of common chronic interstitial lung diseases.*

Muller NL. Imaging of the pleura. *Radiology* 1993;186:297–309. *A review article summarizing the typical appearances of clinically important pleural abnormalities and the role of interventional radiology in their diagnosis and management.*

Naidich DP. Helical computed tomography of the thorax. *Radiol Clin North Am* 1994;32:759–774. *A review and illustration of the important applications of helical chest CT.*

Naidich DP, Marshall CH, Gribbin C, Arams RS, McCauley DI. Low-dose CT of the lungs: preliminary observations. *Radiology* 1990;175: 729–731. *A preliminary study suggesting that low-dose CT of the lung parenchyma provides images of diagnostic quality.*

Padley SG, Brendan A, Muller NL. High-resolution computed tomography of the chest: current indications. *J Thorac Imaging* 1993;8:189–199. *The current indications for high-resolution CT, including acute and chronic lung disease, pneumoconiosis, emphysema, and bronchiectasis, are addressed.*

Padovani B, Mouroux J, Seksik L, Chanalet S, Sedat J, Rotomondo C, Richelme H, Serres JJ. Chest wall invasion by bronchogenic carcinoma: evaluation with MR imaging. *Radiology* 1993;187:33–38. *The sensitivity of MRI was 90% and the specificity was 86% to detect invasion of the chest wall by bronchogenic lung cancer.*

PIOPED Investigators. Value of the ventilation-perfusion scan in acute pulmonary embolism. *JAMA* 1990;263:2753–2759. *Classic article reporting the findings of a multicenter trial to determine the sensitivity and specificity of ventilation-perfusion lung scans in the detection of pulmonary embolus.*

Potchen EJ, Bisesi MA. When is it malpractice to miss lung cancer on chest radiographs? *Radiology* 1990;175:29–32. *A commentary examining the elements of negligence, sources of errors, and observer performance.*

Quint LE, Francis IR, Wahl RL, Gross BH, Glazer GM. Preoperative staging of non-small-cell carcinoma of the lung: imaging methods. *AJR Am J Roengenol* 1995;164:1349–1359. *A review of the use of CT, MRI, and nuclear medicine in staging non-small-cell lung cancer, not only in the mediastinum and hilum but also in the chest wall and pleural space.*

Ralph DD. Pulmonary embolism. The implications of prospective investigation of pulmonary embolism diagnosis. *Radiol Clin North Am* 1994;32:679–687. *A coherent and thoughtful review of the PIOPED results and a cogent consideration of the implications for the diagnostic and therapeutic management of a patient with suspected pulmonary embolus.*

Remy-Jardin M, Duyck P, Remy J, Petyt L, Wurtz A, Mensier E, Copin MC, Riquet M. Hilar lymph nodes: identification with spiral CT and histologic correlation. *Radiology* 1995;196:387–394. *Review of the location and varying appearance of hilar lymphadenopathy and possible causes of misinterpretation of CT images.*

Rucker L, Frye EB, Staten MA. Usefulness of screening chest roentgenograms in preoperative patients. *JAMA* 1983;250:3209–3211. *In a retrospective study, a routine preoperative chest radiograph was not indicated for a select population <60 years of age having no significant risk factors and essentially negative findings on medical history, review of symptoms, and physical examination. However, 60% of the study population had at least one risk factor.*

Sagel SS, Evens RG, Forrest JV, Bramson RT. Efficacy of routine screening and lateral chest radiographs in a hospital-based population. *N Engl J Med* 1974;291:1001–1004. *A prospective study analyzing >10,000 examinations identified a lack of efficacy of routine (chest disease not considered associated with the patient's clinical condition) screening chest radiographs before hospital admission or scheduled surgery in patients <20 years of age and a lack of utility of the lateral projection in patients between 20 and 39 years of age.*

Samuel S, Kundel HL, Nodine CF, Toto LC. Mechanism of satisfaction of search: eye position recordings in the reading of chest radiographs. *Radiology* 1995;194:895–902. *A very intriguing investigation into the psychology of perception. Among the important conclusions is that obvious abnormalities capture visual attention and that their presence decreases the rate of detection of more subtle abnormalities.*

Shepard JO. Complications of percutaneous needle aspiration biopsy of the chest. *Semin Intervent Radiol* 1994;11:181–186. *A review discussing the variety of complications associated with percutaneous chest biopsy as well as possible techniques to reduce complication rates.*

Sostman HD, Coleman RE, DeLong DM, Newman GE, Paine S. Evaluation of revised criteria for ventilation-perfusion scintigraphy in patients with suspected pulmonary embolism. *Radiology* 1994;193:103–107. *With the more accurate, revised PIOPED criteria, experienced interpreters of ventilation-perfusion lung scans can increase their accuracy by using subjective judgment after applying formal criteria.*

Su WJ, Lee PY, Perng RP. Chest roentgenographic guidelines in the selection of patients for fiberoptic bronchoscopy. *Chest* 1993;103:1198–1201. *The positive diagnostic yield of fiberoptic bronchoscopy in patients with abnormal chest radiographic findings demonstrating lobar collapse, hilar abnormalities, pericardial effusion, pleural effusion, or a mass lesion >4 cm was significantly greater than in patients with a mass lesion <4 cm, suggesting that a diagnosis should be made by percutaneous biopsy in these subjects.*

Swenson SJ, Aughenbaugh GL, Douglas WW, Myers JL. High-resolution CT of the lungs: findings in various pulmonary diseases. *AJR Am J Roentgenol* 1992;158:971–979. *The technical aspects of high-resolution CT and the appearances of commonly identified pulmonary diseases are reviewed.*

Touliopoulos P, Costello P. Helical (spiral) CT of the thorax. *Radiol Clin North Am* 1995;33:843–861. *A current review discussing the important advances provided by helical chest CT in the evaluation of solitary pulmonary nodules, metastatic lung disease, aortic dissection, pulmonary embolus, and the airways.*

Trerotola SO. Can helical CT replace aortography in thoracic trauma? *Radiology* 1994;197:13–15. *An editorial discussing the diagnostic controversies related to traumatic thoracic aortic injury.*

Tsai TW, Gallagher EJ, Lombardi G, Gennis P, Carter W. Guidelines for the selective ordering of admission chest radiography in adult obstructive airway disease. *Ann Emerg Med* 1993;22:1854–1858. *An unselected, nonconsecutive study population of patients requiring admission for exacerbation of chronic obstructive pulmonary disease classified as uncomplicated did not benefit from routine admission chest radiography.*

vanSonnenberg E, Casola G, Ho M, Neff CC, Varney RR, Wittich GR, Christensen R, Friedman PJ. Difficult thoracic lesions: CT-guided biopsy experience in 150 subjects. *Radiology* 1988;167:457–461. *The authors obtained diagnostic material in approximately 83% of their patients, with a pneumothorax complication rate of approximately 43%.*

vanSonnenberg E, D'Agostino HB, Casola G, Wittich GR, Varney RR, Harker C. Lung abscess: CT-guided drainage. *Radiology* 1991;178:347–351. *The clinical indications for percutaneous drainage of lung abscess are addressed, along with technical considerations.*

Wandtke JC. Bedside chest radiography. *Radiology* 1994;190:1–10. *The issues of efficacy, film quality, standards of practice, and potential for improvement through the use of computed radiology (CR) are considered.*

Webb WR. High-resolution lung computed tomography. *Radiol Clin North Am* 1991;29:1051–1063. *An analysis of normal lung anatomy and abnormal lung pathology, with emphasis on their appearance on high-resolution CT.*

Wernly JA, Kirchner PT, Oxford DE. Clinical value of quantitative ventilation-perfusion lung scans in the surgical management of bronchogenic carcinoma. *J Thorac Cardiovasc Surg* 1980;80:535–543. *The importance of preoperative (pneumonectomy) quantification of expected postoperative pulmonary function values in patients with marginal (1-second forced expiratory volume <2.0L) preoperative pulmonary function values is addressed, and the ability of perfusion lung imaging to predict postoperative pulmonary function accurately is demonstrated.*

Worsley DF, Alvai A, Aronchick JM, Chen JTT, Greenspan RH, Ravin CE. Chest radiographic findings in patients with acute pulmonary embolism: observations from the PIOPED study. *Radiology* 1993;189:133–136. *Westermark's sign, Fleischner's sign, Hampton hump, and a variety of other findings on conventional chest radiographs were all poor predictors of pulmonary embolus.*

Zerbey AL, Dawson SL, Mueller PR. Pleural interventions and complications. *Semin Intervent Radiol* 1994;11:187–197. *A discussion of the management of pleural disorders using interventional techniques.*

Zerhouni EA, Boukadoum M, Siddiky MA, Newbold JM, Stone DC, Shirey MP, Spivey JF, Hesselman CW, Leo FP, Stitik, Siegelman SS. A standard phantom for quantitative CT analysis of pulmonary nodules. *Radiology* 1983;149:767–773. *The ability to distinguish between benign and malignant solitary pulmonary nodules is enhanced with use of a phantom.*

Textbook of Pulmonary Diseases, 6th ed.
edited by G.L. Baum, J.D. Crapo, B.R. Celli, and J.B. Karlinsky,
Lippincott–Raven Publishers, Philadelphia, © 1998.

CHAPTER

Drug-Induced Pulmonary Disease

22

Raed A. Dweik · Muzaffar Ahmad

Stephen L. Demeter

INTRODUCTION

Drug-induced disease is one of the most common iatrogenic illnesses. In the last decade, the lung has been recognized increasingly often as a target organ. Fewer than 25% of drug reactions are truly allergic in origin; the mechanisms of overdose, side effects, and drug interaction are predictable with most drugs. On the other hand, idiosyncratic and allergic or hypersensitivity reactions are unpredictable and are estimated to occur in about 5% of patients receiving any drug. In drug-induced pulmonary disease, an abnormality on the chest x-ray film or a symptom complex is the most common form of presentation. Drug-induced pulmonary disease is diagnosed by maintaining a high index of suspicion in the appropriate clinical setting.

In this chapter, we provide a brief overview of drug-induced pulmonary disease. There are many isolated case reports of drugs that are believed to have caused an adverse pulmonary reaction, but these are vague and doubtful and are excluded from the review. In the first part of the chapter, we discuss various pleuropulmonary patterns of response to drugs. The second part addresses the pulmonary effects of different categories of drugs, including anti-inflammatory, antimicrobial, and antineoplastic agents.

Table 1 summarizes the more common clinical presentations of pulmonary toxicity induced by noncytotoxic medications, including illicit drugs, and Table 2 does the

R. A. Dweik: Department of Pulmonary and Critical Care Medicine, Cleveland Clinic Foundation, Cleveland, Ohio 44195.

M. Ahmad: Department of Medicine, Cleveland Clinic Foundation, Cleveland, Ohio 44195.

S. L. Demeter: Division of Pulmonary Medicine, Northeastern Ohio Universities College of Medicine, Rootstown, Ohio 44195.

same for pulmonary toxicity induced by cytotoxic agents, including radiation. Some unusual manifestations of drug-induced pulmonary toxicity are listed in Table 3. Not all the medications listed in the tables are discussed in the text.

PATTERNS OF RESPONSE

Hypersensitivity Reactions

Pulmonary responses to some drugs may be best thought of in terms of a hypersensitivity reaction (Table 1). Typically, the symptoms consist of cough, dyspnea, and fever, with the appearance of an infiltrate on the chest x-ray film. Occasionally, a pleural effusion is seen. In some instances, there may be laboratory manifestations characteristic of hypersensitivity responses, such as peripheral eosinophilia or, more specifically, a positive lymphocyte transformation test response to the offending drug. The adverse response usually remits after cessation of the drug. Corticosteroids may hasten the recovery, although they are generally not needed.

Noncardiogenic Pulmonary Edema

Several factors are responsible for the transvascular flow of fluid. One factor, the filtration coefficient of permeability of the vascular endothelium, is believed to be altered in cases of noncardiogenic pulmonary edema. Overdoses of sedatives and narcotics are most commonly associated with altered permeability of the pulmonary vasculature. Most patients with noncardiogenic pulmonary edema also display some degree of central nervous system depression; it is unclear whether the response represents a drug effect, ''neurogenic pulmonary edema,'' or a combination of the two. Other drugs that cause non-cardiogenic pulmonary edema characteristically produce an idiosyncratic response within minutes to hours after absorption.

Interstitial Pneumonitis or Fibrosis

A number of drugs have the potential for causing either an interstitial pneumonitis or an interstitial fibrosis. In some cases, the interstitial pneumonitis has many of the features of a hypersensitivity state, and the difference may be semantic rather than real. In other cases, few features of a hypersensitivity state are seen, and the interstitial pneumonitis represents only the precedent inflammatory state of a fibrosing process.

Pleural Effusions

An acute pleural effusion in association with drugs has been reported to be part of a hypersensitivity reaction.

TABLE 1. *Clinical presentation of pulmonary toxicity induced by noncytotoxic drugs*

	PIE	Noncardiac pulmonary edema	IP-F	Acute pleural effusion	Chronic pleural effusion	PVD	Parenchymal Hge	DI-SLE	BOOP	Asthma
• Antiinflammatory										
Acetylsalicylic acid		+								+
Colchicine		+								
Corticosteroids						+				+
Cromoglycate	+		+			+				
Gold			+					+	+	
Methotrexate	+		+	+	+				+	
NSAID				+						+
Phenylbutazone								+		
Penicillamine			+				+		+	
• Antimicrobial										
Amphotericin B (with WBC transfusion)		+	+							
Isoniazid	+							+		
Nitrofurantoin: acute	+		+	+			+			+
chronic			+							
Para-aminosalicylic acid	+			+				+		
Pentamidine										+
Sulfasalazine	+	+							+	+
Streptomycin								+		
Sulfonamides	+							+		
• Cardiovascular										
Alpha-methyldopa								+		
Amiodarone			+	+					+	
Anticoagulants				+			+			
Beta blockers										+
Digitalis								+		
Dipyridamole										+
Flecainide			+							
Hydralazine								+		
Hydrochlorothiazide		+						+		
Procainamide								+		
Propafenone										+
Protamine		+								+
Tocainamide			+							
• Illicit drugs										
Cocaine		+	+			+	+		+	+
Heroin		+	+			+				
Methadone		+	+			+				
Methylphenidate			+			+				+
• Psychotropic/antiepileptic										
Carbamazepine	+		+							
Chlordiazepoxide		+								
Diphenylhydantoin	+		+					+		
Phenothiazines		+								
Trazodone	+									
Tricyclics		+								

TABLE 1. *Continued.*

	PIE	Noncardiac pulmonary edema	IP-F	Acute pleural effusion	Chronic pleural effusion	PVD	Parenchymal Hge	DI-SLE	BOOP	Asthma
• **Miscellaneous**										
Bromocriptine					+					
Chlorpropamide	+									
Contrast media										+
Esophageal variceal sclerotherapy agents				+						
Estrogen						+	+	+		
Methysergide			+		+					
Mineral oil			+				+			
Propylthiouracil									+	
Timolol (ophthalmic)										+
Tocolytic agents		+		+						

Parts of Tables 1 through 3 and portions of related text have been reproduced or adapted with permission from Demeter SL, Ahmad M, Tomashefski JF. Drug-induced pulmonary disease. *Cleve Clin Q* 1979;46:89–124.

BOOP, bronchiolitis obliterans organizing pneumonia; DI-SLE, drug-induced systemic lupus erythematosus; Hge, hemorrhage; IP-F, interstitial pneumonitis or fibrosis; NSAID: nonsteroidal anti-inflammatory drugs; PIE, pulmonary infiltrate with eosinophilia; PVD, pulmonary vascular disease; WBC, white blood cell.

Anticoagulants cause effusion by leading to a pleural hemorrhage. A chronic pleural effusion develops after long-term use of a drug. In some instances, this is a manifestation of a retarded hypersensitivity-like response (methotrexate and procarbazine) or is associated with an interstitial fibrosis (busulfan and methotrexate).

Pulmonary Vascular Responses

Busulfan and cromoglycate are included as possible causes of pulmonary vascular responses because biopsy specimens from patients who display hypersensitivity reactions to these drugs may show an inflammatory vascular response as well. It is unclear what role the angiitis *per se* plays in the development of these disease processes. Illicit drugs are capable of causing angiitis and hypertension; the drugs and their diluents are given intravenously and are filtered by the pulmonary capillaries, where they incite their untoward effects. Heroin-induced pulmonary edema is frequently encountered in urban medical centers. An overdose of methadone and propoxyphene (Darvon) can cause a similar reaction. Corticosteroids are men-

TABLE 2. *Clinical presentation of pulmonary toxicity induced by cytotoxic drugs and radiation*

	Hypersensitivity infiltrate	PIE	Noncardiac pulmonary edema	IP-F	Acute pleural effusion	Chronic pleural effusion	PVD	Parenchymal Hge	BOOP	Asthma
Azathioprine	+			+						
Bleomycin		+		+	+				+	
Busulfan	+			+		+	+			
Chlorambucil				+						
Cyclophosphamide				+					+	
Cytosine arabinoside			+							
Etoposide		+								
Interleukin-2					+					+
Melphalan				+						
Mercaptopurine				+						
Methotrexate		+		+	+	+			+	
Mitomycin C			+	+		+			+	
Nitrogen mustard	+		+	+						
Nitrosoureas				+			+			
Procarbazine		+		+	+	+				
Taxol (with castor oil base)										+
Tumor necrosis factor			+							
Vinblastine (with mitomycin)			+	+						+
Radiation, acute	+	+			+		+	+	+	

BOOP, bronchiolitis obliterans organizing pneumonia; Hge, hemorrhage; IP-F, interstitial pneumonitis or fibrosis; PIE, pulmonary infiltrate with eosinophilia; PVD, pulmonary vascular disease.

TABLE 3. *Unusual manifestations of drug-induced pulmonary toxicity*

Presentation	Causative agent(s)
Alveolar proteinosis	Bulsufan
Bronchial necrosis	Radiation therapy, brachytherapy
Bronchospasm (paradoxical)	Nebulized β_2-adrenergic agonists
	Intravenous hydrocortisone
Calcification (parenchymal)	Antacids, calcium, phosphorous
	Vitamin D
Cough	ACE inhibitors
Goodpasture's syndrome	Penicillamine
Lung mass(es) ± cavitation	Amiodarone, bleomycin
Mediastinal widening	
Lymphadenopathy	Diphenylhydantoin, methotrexate
	Potassium iodide
Lipomatosis	Corticosteroids
Mediastinitis	Esophageal variceal sclerotherapy
Panlobular emphysema	Methylphenidate
Pneumothorax	Nitrosoureas, bleomycin
Pseudosepsis syndrome	Chronic salicylate intoxication

ACE, angiotensin-converting enzyme.

tioned as causing pulmonary vasculitis, but evidence is at best suggestive. In an autopsy review of patients with rheumatoid arthritis, pulmonary vasculitis was found to occur in 29% of patients receiving corticosteroids but in none of the patients who were not taking them.

Alpha-adrenergic nasal sprays have been associated with interstitial fibrosis and obliterated pulmonary vessels on histologic examination. This response, seen in patients who abuse the sprays on a long-term basis, may be caused by the effects of repeated vascular constriction. The chest roentgenogram shows normal parenchyma with prominent pulmonary vasculature. Pulmonary function testing reveals a drop in the DLCO (diffusing capacity) that is proportional to the degree of pulmonary hypertension.

Estrogen-containing drugs are also capable of causing pulmonary hypertension. Affected patients fall into two distinct categories: those with congenital heart disease and those without. In the first group, the relationship between estrogen and pulmonary hypertension appears to be well established, although uncommon; in the second group, the relationship remains only suggestive. Case reports have implicated oral contraceptives as a cause of "primary" pulmonary hypertension in patients who have taken the drug for 6 months to 5 years. In one study, predisposing factors for pulmonary hypertension were found in three of six patients (family history, corrected ductus, and connective tissue disease); the other three were apparently normal.

Pulmonary Parenchymal Calcification

Drug-related calcium deposition in the lungs is very rare. It is usually associated with the soft-tissue calcifica-

tion seen in the milk-alkali syndrome or with hypercalcemic states of other causes. Drugs known to have precipitated calcium deposition include antacids, calcium, phosphorus, and high doses of vitamin D (Table 3).

Parenchymal Hemorrhage

Hemoptysis as the manifestation of an adverse drug effect is most frequently caused by a drug-related pulmonary embolus leading to pulmonary infarction. Pulmonary hemorrhage and hemoptysis can be a manifestation of penicillamine-induced Goodpasture's syndrome, lipoid pneumonia, or chronic radiation pneumonitis.

Spontaneous pulmonary hemorrhage has been reported in patients who were taking oral anticoagulants for 13 days to 3 years. Initial symptoms were dyspnea, hemoptysis, and cough. The presenting feature was either hemoptysis or an infiltrate on the chest roentgenogram. Anticoagulants also may cause a hemothorax, manifested as a pleural effusion associated with a decreasing hematocrit.

Mediastinal Manifestations

Although not necessarily representing a pulmonary disease, adverse mediastinal responses appear initially as an abnormality on the chest x-ray film. Diphenylhydantoin occasionally produces a pseudolymphoma syndrome, manifested as peripheral lymphadenopathy (Table 3). It produces mediastinal lymphadenopathy only rarely, however. The enlarged nodes regress 1 to 2 weeks after cessation of the drug. Potassium iodide has been reported to produce fever, cough, and pruritus, with hilar and mediastinal lymphadenopathy that cleared on discontinuance of the drug. Transient hilar adenopathy may accompany a hypersensitivity-like response to methotrexate. Mediastinal lipomatosis resulting from corticosteroid use is a well-recognized entity.

Drug-Induced Lupus Erythematosus

A number of drugs have been implicated as causative factors in the systemic lupus erythematosus (SLE) syndrome, and it is estimated that they play an activating role in 5%–12% of cases (Table 1). It is still controversial whether the drug exposes a latent case of lupus or actually causes the disease. Animal experiments have not helped to clarify this issue. Acetylator status may be important, for cases of hydralazine- and isoniazid-related SLE are noted more frequently in slow acetylators of these drugs.

The lungs and pleurae are involved in 50%–75% of cases of spontaneous SLE, whereas they are involved in 80% of cases of drug-induced SLE. Patterns of response include the following: (1) pleural effusion with or without pleuritic pain, (2) pleuritic chest pain with or without effusion, (3) atelectatic pneumonitis, (4) diffuse interstitial pneumonitis, and (5) alveolar infiltrates. Positive biochemical markers of SLE are found more frequently than are systemic signs, and the pleuropulmonary manifestations usually regress with removal of the agent.

It is estimated that >90% of cases of drug-induced SLE are caused by diphenylhydantoin, hydralazine, isoniazid, or procainamide. Sulfonamides that have been implicated include acetazolamide, sulfadiazine, sulfamethoxypyridazine, sulfasalazine, and sulfisoxazole.

Hydralazine differs from most drugs in this category in that only 25% of patients have pleuropulmonary symptoms. In one review, the percentages of symptomatic patients found to have chest roentgenographic abnormalities were as follows: (1) pleural thickening (57%), (2) pleural effusion (36%), (3) pulmonary fibrosis (21%), (4) elevated hemidiaphragm (7%), (5) segmental atelectasis (7%), and (6) migratory pneumonitis (7%). Hydralazine-induced SLE is seen in 10%–20% of patients receiving prolonged therapy with doses of 400 mg/d or greater (although it has been reported in patients who received therapy for <1 month and those who received <100 mg/d). It is more common in women (50%–90%), Caucasians, and slow acetylators.

Procainamide-induced SLE is a time- rather than dose-dependent phenomenon. For example, in one study clinical SLE developed in 50% of patients by 3 months, and by 1 year all had a positive test for antinuclear antibodies (ANA). Resolution of the syndrome within a few days to weeks after discontinuance of the drug is the rule; occasionally, corticosteroids are necessary to control symptoms.

Drug-induced bronchospasm/asthma

Drug-induced bronchospasm is caused by a variety of agents (Tables 1 and 2). Mechanisms are diverse and poorly understood. Acetylsalicylic acid produces worsening bronchospasm in about 4% of asthmatic patients. Other nonsteroidal anti-inflammatory agents (NSAIDs) can produce a similar reaction and should be avoided in aspirin-sensitive patients. Dipyridamole increases the concentration of the bronchoconstrictor adenosine, which can cause significant bronchospasm in some patients with underlying obstructive lung disease. Theophylline is the drug of choice for treatment and/or prophylaxis in these patients. Vinblastine appears to act synergistically with mitomycin to produce bronchospasm. Administration of nebulized medications, such as pentamidine, or propellants can further irritate already hyperreactive airways. Paradoxical bronchospasm (Table 3) has been reported with the use of nebulized beta agonists as well as intravenous hydrocortisone (not reported with other steroid preparations).

Bronchiolitis Obliterans Organizing Pneumonia

Bronchiolitis obliterans organizing pneumonia (BOOP) has been described as a response to a variety of medications (Tables 1 and 2). Patients frequently have isolated or patchy air space opacities indistinguishable from those of idiopathic BOOP. This reaction is usually reversible with discontinuation of the drug and sometimes requires treatment with corticosteroids.

EFFECTS OF DRUGS AND RADIATION

Anti-inflammatory Agents

Sodium cromoglycate has been associated with a hypersensitivity-like response, accompanied by fever, eosinophilia, and pulmonary infiltrates.

Overdoses of acetylsalicylic acid (ASA) can produce central respiratory stimulation and noncardiogenic pulmonary edema. Therapeutic serum levels are in the range of 10 to 20 mg/dL. At levels of 35 mg/dL, respiratory alkalosis is seen. Severe hyperpnea is manifested at levels of 50 mg/dL. At a serum level of 45 mg/dL, noncardiogenic pulmonary edema is seen. The pulmonary capillary wedge pressure is normal. Abnormalities on chest x-ray films take 3 to 8 days to clear.

The ASA triad is a syndrome characterized by asthma, nasal polyposis, and drug sensitivity. It was initially described following the use of ASA, but other anti-inflammatory drugs can also produce this reaction (Table 1). The first manifestation of the syndrome is vasomotor rhinitis with a watery discharge. Typically, this develops in the second or third decade in a person who is not atopic and who has previously taken ASA. The reaction is at first intermittent, later perennial. It is followed by the appearance of nasal polyps, and by midlife most patients demonstrate an asthmatic response.

The syndrome is not a hypersensitivity response, despite the asthma and angioedema that may be seen following absorption of the drugs. Results of skin and immunologic tests are negative. Furthermore, other forms of salicylic acid (such as sodium salicylate) do not produce a response in the ASA-sensitive patient. The mechanism of action is postulated to be an inhibition of prostaglandin (PG) synthetase and a disruption in the balance between naturally occurring bronchoconstrictor ($PGF_{2\alpha}$) and bronchodilator (PGE series) prostaglandins. The usual response to this disruption is bronchoconstriction, but bronchodilation also has been reported. Most of the drugs that produce this response fall into the broader category of anti-inflammatory nonsteroidal analgesics, and it is for this reason that the ASA triad has been called *analgesic asthma* by some authors.

The frequency of the syndrome in asthmatic patients is approximately 4%. Patients may or may not be atopic

(3% vs. an expected 10% in one series). Family studies reveal rare clusterings.

Treatment starts with avoidance of the offending drug. Beta-adrenergic agonists reverse the airways response. Corticosteroids diminish the recovery time, but even pretreatment does not prevent the response. Nasal polypectomy is reserved for symptoms of nasal obstruction only; it does not alter the response to ASA, and the polyps usually recur.

Tartrazine (FD&C yellow dye No. 5) is not an analgesic, and it is not known to affect PG biosynthesis. However, it can provoke symptoms of the ASA triad in a small number of ASA-sensitive patients. As a dye, it is contained in a number of medications and food products.

Methotrexate is increasingly being used in low doses (lower than the usual chemotherapeutic dose) as an anti-inflammatory drug for a few conditions, especially rheumatoid arthritis and Wegener's granulomatosis. Typically, the patient is given 10 to 15 mg once a week. Pulmonary reactions develop in about 5% of these patients, most commonly in the form of granulomatous pneumonitis. The onset is insidious and associated with cough, dyspnea, and low-grade fever. Histologically, weakly formed granulomas are seen in most patients. In a recent prospective evaluation of 124 patients receiving low-dose methotrexate, pneumonitis occurred in 3.2% of patients. Pulmonary function tests did not allow detection before clinical symptoms. Methotrexate pneumonitis also seems to predispose patients to *Pneumocystis carinii* pneumonia.

Penicillamine can cause unique pulmonary complications, including BOOP, SLE, and Goodpasture's syndrome (Table 3).

Gold is widely used orally and intramuscularly for the treatment of rheumatoid arthritis. The intramuscular preparations can cause interstitial pneumonitis and fibrosis that is almost always reversible by discontinuation of the gold injections, but sometimes additional treatment with corticosteroids may be required.

Antimicrobial Agents

Griseofulvin, isoniazid, para-aminosalicylic acid, penicillin, streptomycin, the sulfonamides, and tetracycline are all capable of producing a drug-induced SLE syndrome. In addition, isoniazid has been reported to cause a hypersensitivity-like pneumonitis with peripheral eosinophilia. Penicillin has been reported as generating a hypersensitivity pneumonitis distinct from systemic anaphylaxis, with peripheral eosinophilia (as high as 80%), alveolar infiltrates, pleural effusions, and positive skin test results. Sulfonamides can cause a true Loeffler's syndrome, with fever, cough, dyspnea, migratory infiltrates, and peripheral eosinophilia. A hypersensitivity pulmonary response also has been reported following the use of a sulfonamide-containing vaginal cream.

Para-aminosalicylic acid is estimated to produce a hypersensitivity-like response in approximately 0.3%–5.0% of patients receiving the drug. Common adverse responses include fever (up to 10°F), rash, malaise, headache, dry cough, eosinophilia, alveolar infiltrates, and lymphadenopathy. Pleural effusion and hepatomegaly have been seen. The symptoms usually start during the third week of treatment and gradually disappear within 2 to 3 weeks after discontinuance of the drug. Cases of angioneurotic edema with laryngeal edema, cough, and wheezing also have been reported.

Of all the antimicrobial drugs, nitrofurantoin is perhaps the most commonly reported as causing an adverse pulmonary reaction. To gain an appreciation of the relative risk, the manufacturer collected data during a 16-year period. During that time, 237 cases of adverse pleuropulmonary reactions were reported in an estimated 44 million courses of the drug. Reactions to nitrofurantoin are classified as acute or chronic, with no definite relationship between the two types, although both can be fatal.

Lymphopenia is seen during the acute reaction, with a decrease in both the B- and the T-cell population. Results of the lymphocyte transformation test against nitrofurantoin need not be positive for a patient to display an adverse reaction. The following acute reactions are seen: (1) acute asthma (rare), (2) acute tracheobronchitis with a normal chest roentgenogram (very rare), (3) pleural effusions (usually seen in association with hypersensitivity pneumonitis), and (4) hypersensitivity pneumonitis (the most common response).

The onset of symptoms of the hypersensitivity pneumonitis usually occurs within 2 hours to 10 days after start of the medication (although onset has been known to be delayed as long as 1 year). Typically, the patient has fever, chills, dyspnea, and cough. This response is seen much more quickly after subsequent uses of the drug. Physical examination often suggests more diffuse involvement than is seen on the chest roentgenogram. Pleuritic pain and pleural rubs may be present.

The roentgenogram reveals diffuse alveolar or alveolar-interstitial infiltrates. Pleural effusions may be present. Various degrees of peripheral eosinophilia can be seen, as well as eosinophils in the sputum.

Treatment is based on discontinuance and avoidance of the drug. Corticosteroids and antihistamines provide symptomatic relief. The infiltrates clear spontaneously within a 24- to 48-hour period.

The chronic reactions occur less commonly and are estimated to represent 3% of all pleuropulmonary reactions to nitrofurantoin. There is no relationship to the acute response, and deaths are more frequently encountered in this type. Two patterns of response occur—interstitial fibrosis and a desquamative interstitial pneumonitis.

The interstitial fibrosis starts insidiously after 6 months to 6 years of therapy. Symptoms are cough and dyspnea without fever, eosinophilia, or pleural effusion. Desquamative interstitial pneumonitis was described in three patients who received the drug for 2 to 5 years. In contrast to the symptoms of interstitial fibrosis, which show only a variable response to corticosteroid therapy, the symptoms of desquamative interstitial pneumonitis reversed well with treatment.

Sulfasalazine is an effective antibiotic for the treatment of inflammatory bowel disease. It has been reported to cause several pulmonary reactions, including BOOP, pulmonary infiltrates with eosinophilia, pulmonary fibrosis, and asthma. Some overlap may exist in these pathologic presentations. Treatment consists of discontinuing sulfasalazine and the administration of corticosteroids. Although most of the side effects of sulfasalazine are considered to be caused by sulfapyridine (the carrier component), mesalamine (the clinically beneficial component without the carrier sulfapyridine) has also been reported to cause pulmonary toxicity.

Pentamidine given intravenously or by nebulizer can cause bronchospasm. Pretreatment with nebulized albuterol or ipratropium may prevent this adverse effect.

Amphotericin B can be associated with impaired pulmonary function, particularly if administered with granulocyte transfusion. This has also been reported with the liposomal form of amphotericin B. The treatment is to stop the medication and administer corticosteroids. Concomitant granulocyte transfusion and administration of amphotericin B should be avoided.

Cardiovascular Agents

Amiodarone hydrochloride, an antiarrhythmic drug, can cause pulmonary toxicity in about 6% of patients receiving the drug. The clinical features include dyspnea, chest pain, cough, elevated sedimentation rate, and diffuse interstitial and patchy alveolar infiltrates in the roentgenogram. Histologically, an accumulation of foamy macrophages in the alveolar spaces, hyperplasia of type II pneumocytes, and widening of alveolar septa are noted. Increased levels of cytosolic free calcium may cause injury. Cessation of the drug and administration of corticosteroids lead to radiographic resolution in about 2 months.

Amiodarone pneumonitis rarely occurs in patients who have been taking the drug in doses of <400 mg/d for <2 months. The diagnosis of amiodarone pneumonitis is really one of exclusion. Pulmonary embolism, congestive heart failure, and pneumonia are the main differential diagnoses in patients suspected of having amiodarone pulmonary toxicity, and they should be excluded first. Computed tomography (CT) of the lung (without the administration of contrast) may be helpful, because amiodarone is an iodinated compound and appears more dense than usual infiltrates of other etiologies. Bronchoalveolar lavage may be helpful in excluding infection. Results of a gallium scan are positive in almost all patients with

amiodarone pneumonitis. A positive gallium scan can help differentiate amiodarone pneumonitis from pulmonary embolism or congestive heart failure (in which the gallium scan is negative) as long as infection has been excluded as a cause for the positive scan. In patients receiving amiodarone, a picture suggestive of adult respiratory distress syndrome (ARDS) may develop when they are exposed to a high FiO_2 (fraction of inspired oxygen), as during anesthesia for surgical procedures. In an unusual presentation, amiodarone pulmonary toxicity may take the form of parenchymal mass lesion(s), which may show cavitation (Table 3).

Angiotensin-converting enzyme (ACE) inhibitors can produce an irritating cough in about 10%–25% of patients receiving them. The cough occurs with all ACE inhibitors, and changing from one to another does not help. Cough usually resolves within 1 to 2 weeks of stopping the medication, which is both diagnostic and therapeutic.

Beta blockers can exacerbate chronic obstructive lung disease and precipitate bronchospasm. Some examples, in decreasing order of likelihood to cause bronchoconstriction, are propranolol, timolol, nadolol, atenolol, and labetolol. They should be used with extreme caution in patients with a potential for bronchospasm.

Hydrochlorothiazide can cause noncardiac pulmonary edema. Patients present with dyspnea, cough, and a low-grade fever within a few hours of taking the medication. The chest roentgenogram shows changes of pulmonary edema; in cases in which the wedge pressure has been measured, it has always been normal. Treatment is supportive, and the patient should avoid the medication thereafter.

Psychotropic Medications

Overdose of tricyclic antidepressants may be associated with pulmonary complications in about a third of cases, usually in the form of noncardiac pulmonary edema or aspiration. Treatment is supportive and may include mechanical ventilation.

A series of three cases of phenothiazine-induced pulmonary edema has been reported. The authors hypothesized that it is neurogenic in origin, caused by hypothalamic dysfunction.

Trazodone overdose has been reported to cause eosinophilic pneumonia and respiratory failure.

Illicit Drugs

The use of illicit drugs has reached epidemic proportions, resulting in an increased incidence of pulmonary toxicity. The pulmonary manifestations relate not only to the substance used, but also to the route of administration. Narcotic addiction remains a major health problem, with noncardiogenic pulmonary edema occurring as a complication of heroin, methadone, and cocaine abuse.

Pulmonary edema develops within a few hours of use, and the patient appears with constricted pupils and depressed respiration. The chest radiograph shows alveolar infiltrates, usually in "bat wing" distribution. Pathologic studies reveal congested, enlarged lungs with an influx of neutrophils and pigmented macrophages. The therapy is supportive, with administration of oxygen, narcotic antagonism, and mechanical ventilation if needed.

Cocaine is a highly addictive substance. Pulmonary complications are related to all forms of administration. Noncardiogenic pulmonary edema can occur with cocaine regardless of the route of administration. Increased membrane permeability probably occurs as a result of alveolar capillary injury. Pulmonary edema has been reported with freebase inhalation, intravenous freebase, and even "body packing" (smugglers swallowing packets of cocaine, which leak into the gastrointestinal tract). Other reported complications of smoking freebase cocaine include barotrauma, massive hemoptysis with diffuse alveolar hemorrhage, interstitial pneumonitis, recurrent pulmonary infiltrates with bronchospasm, and BOOP. Reduced diffusing capacity, decreased expiratory flow rates, and bronchial asthma have also been associated with smoking of freebase cocaine.

An acute pulmonary syndrome temporally related to inhalation of crack cocaine has also been described and is characterized by fever, hemoptysis, alveolar infiltrates, and respiratory failure. The lung tissue in this entity ("crack lung") reveals alveolar hemorrhage, interstitial and intra-alveolar inflammatory cells, and deposition of IgE in lymphocytes and macrophages. The patients tend to respond to systemic corticosteroids.

Snorting cocaine causes cartilaginous ischemia and can lead to nasal septal perforation. Burns of the oropharynx and larynx can also occur from inhaling hot gases during smoking of freebase cocaine.

Miscellaneous Agents

Estrogens may produce an adverse pulmonary response through a number of mechanisms: pulmonary embolus, drug-induced SLE syndrome, and pulmonary hypertension. It has been estimated that the risk for development of thromboembolic disease in age-matched patients taking oral contraceptives is increased from 5 to 47/100,000. Some associated variables shown to increase the risk include advancing age, obesity, and prolonged bed rest. Thrombogenic risk is directly proportional to the estrogen content of the oral contraceptives.

Pleural thickening is the most common pleuropulmonary side effect of long-term use of methysergide or bromocriptine. A ground-glass appearance on the chest x-ray film can clear spontaneously with cessation of the drug. A pleural effusion may be seen. Onset may be acute, with pleuritic pain and a rub, or may be more insidious. The effusion may be unilateral or bilateral. Pulmonary fibrosis also has been seen with long-term methysergide use. Onset is slow (6 months to 6 years), with cough and dyspnea. The fibrosis may be diffuse; alternatively, localized areas of pleuropulmonary fibrosis may resemble a mass lesion. The fibrosis may reverse on discontinuance of the drug.

Administration of contrast media is an underestimated cause of drug-induced bronchospasm. Most patients receiving intravenous contrast media show a subclinical reduction in FEV_1 (forced expiratory volume in 1 second) within 5 minutes; this returns to normal within 30 minutes. Severe reactions can occur but are relatively rare.

Esophageal variceal sclerotherapy with either sodium tetradecylsulfate, ethanolamine, or sodium morrhuate can cause changes on chest roentgenograms in up to 85% of patients, but these are rarely of clinical significance. Mediastinal widening resulting from noninfectious mediastinitis occurs in 33% of patients. Pleural effusion occurs in 25% of patients, atelectasis in 10%–15%, and pulmonary infiltrates in 10% of patients. Self-limited fever and chest pain are common in the first 24 hours after the procedure. Serious complications, including ARDS, occur in <2% of patients undergoing esophageal sclerotherapy, and these should be suspected if the fever and chest pain last for >24 hours.

Tocolytic medications (albuterol, terbutaline, ritodrine), used to inhibit uterine contractions during premature labor, can cause noncardiac pulmonary edema in 0.5%–5% of cases. These beta-mimetic drugs produce peripheral vasodilation and an increase in the intravascular fluid volume. When the drug is stopped, the vasomotor tone returns to normal, pushing excess fluid out into the tissues, including the lungs.

Antineoplastic Drugs

The adverse pulmonary responses most often produced by antineoplastic drugs are interstitial pneumonitis and interstitial fibrosis (Table 2). The distinction between these two patterns of response is not sharp, and there may be progression from one state to another. In general, the presentation of interstitial pneumonitis tends to be a systemic hypersensitivity response, with fever, malaise, and a rapid decline in respiratory function. Although both entities can emerge from days to years after a medication is started and resolve during days to months, interstitial pneumonitis is more likely to present earlier and resolve quickly. The pathologic differences are also not profound. Interstitial pneumonitis presents with evidence of larger numbers of inflammatory cells and less fibrosis than does interstitial fibrosis. Of the two, interstitial pneumonitis is the more likely to resolve on discontinuation of the drug.

Common symptoms include dyspnea and cough of insidious onset. The cough is usually dry, although a thick white sputum may be present at times. Malaise, fatigue, and fever are occasionally found. Physical examination generally reveals tachypnea and fine crackles that are heard best in the bases. An interstitial infiltrate is the most common roentgenographic abnormality. Pulmonary function testing is consistent with a restrictive ventilatory defect (low vital capacity or total lung capacity) and a reduced DLCO; the flow rates are usually preserved. The DLCO is the most sensitive parameter and can be used to follow the patient as a predictive test. Hypoxemia is common.

Diagnosis is made by lung biopsy. The list of causes of pulmonary infiltrates in the immunocompromised host always includes infection, and infiltrates should be sought with appropriate stains and cultures. Treatment is discontinuance of the agent. Steroids may or may not help but probably should be tried. The response may be followed by serial determinations of PaO_2 (partial pressure of arterial oxygen) and DLCO and by chest roentgenograms.

Occasionally, factors such as total cumulative dosage, patient age, or prior use of agents that may act synergistically (e.g., radiation) can be used to anticipate an untoward response.

The manifestations of drug-induced pulmonary toxicity caused by antineoplastic agents are listed in Table 2.

Azathioprine

At least six cases of azathioprine hypersensitivity pneumonitis have been reported, but the incidence remains well below 1%.

Bischloroethylnitrosourea

Bischloroethylnitrosourea (BCNU) has been reported to cause interstitial pulmonary infiltrates. One report suggested a dose-related phenomenon; a hacking cough developed in 4 of 28 (14%) patients. The mean cumulative dose in patients with symptoms was 2030 mg/m^2; for those without symptoms, it was 710 mg/m^2. Interstitial infiltrates were seen on the chest roentgenogram in three of the four patients, but all four had interstitial fibrosis on lung biopsy. Symptoms progressed despite cessation of therapy, and one patient died of respiratory failure. Another study could find no dose-dependent relationship but suggested that interstitial infiltrates were more common when BCNU was used concomitantly with cyclophosphamide. Of the 10 patients, nine had received other agents capable of causing interstitial fibrosis. In both studies, the pulmonary function tests commonly showed a decreased DLCO, PaO_2, and vital capacity. The projected incidence varied from 1.1% to 14%.

Another peculiar complication of nitrosoureas is pneumothorax (Table 3).

Bleomycin

Interstitial fibrosis is the most commonly mentioned adverse pulmonary response to bleomycin. An acute response consisting of cough and dyspnea has been reported, however. These symptoms may occur separately or together, and were found in 6% of 274 patients in one study. The cough may be so severe as to limit use of the drug. The response usually occurs shortly after injection, but a response did not develop in one patient until the eighth month of treatment. Tracheitis also has been described, although infrequently.

Bleomycin is deposited in the skin and lungs, and not unexpectedly, the two organs displaying the most serious side effects are the skin (ulcerations) and the lung (interstitial fibrosis). The pulmonary manifestation appears to be a result of toxic accumulation, although cases have been reported of a hypersensitivity reaction.

Four patients have been described in whom a reversible interstitial pneumonitis developed after they received total doses ranging from 133 to 1000 mg. Two of the four displayed peripheral eosinophilia (12%–16%), and biopsy of one showed eosinophilic infiltration of the distal air spaces. Pleural effusions, interstitial infiltrates, and alveolar infiltrates all appeared on the roentgenograms. Results of immunofluorescence studies for immunoglobulins, complement, and fibrinogen were negative. Corticosteroids were given to three of the four patients, and all four showed resolution of the infiltrates and symptoms.

Interstitial fibrosis occurs in approximately 11% of patients receiving the drug. The incidence is reported to be only 3%–5% when the total dose is below 450 mg, but 35.3% when the level of 500 mg is exceeded. In a histologic study of 37 patients (34 of 37 specimens were obtained at autopsy), 12 of 37 were found to have interstitial pneumonitis at different stages of development. Total doses ranged from 115 to 800 mg/m^2. Histologic changes consisted of fibrinous exudate, atypical proliferation of alveolar cells, hyaline membranes, squamous metaplasia, epithelial dysplasia of distal air spaces, and interstitial and intra-alveolar fibrosis. Alveolar septa were broadened, with edematous fluid and mononuclear inflammatory cell infiltration, and showed signs of extensive fibrosis. Work on animal models indicates that bleomycin-induced lung injury is characterized by an increase in collagen synthesis in the interstitium.

Bleomycin-induced pulmonary toxicity may therefore be seen as a spectrum of changes. The drug is accumulated in the lungs. There may be an initial toxic inflammatory response that later becomes fibrotic. The earlier the response is identified, the more amenable the lung is to full recovery. Fibrotic states are quite resistant to reversibility, even after cessation of the drug and with the use of corticosteroids. The DLCO may be the most sensitive parameter for following the patient. Factors that appear to increase the toxic potential include (1) advancing age, (2) total cumulative dose (high FiO$_2$), and (3) prior radiation to the thorax. The histologic changes of bleomycin-induced interstitial fibrosis resemble those of busulfan lung as well as desquamative interstitial pneumonitis. The chest roentgenogram shows a nonspecific interstitial pattern. The most severe changes in both the histologic picture and the radiographic appearance are in the lung bases and subpleural areas (as opposed to busulfan toxicity, in which the roentgenographic abnormalities are more pronounced near the hilum). Symptoms include dry cough and dyspnea. Physical examination reveals tachypnea, basilar crackles, and concomitant hyperpigmentation of the skin. Diagnosis is by lung biopsy (Fig. 1), although sputum cytology may be of assistance (Fig. 2). Treatment is discontinuance of the drug. Steroids have been effective in some cases. If the patient's condition demonstrates reversibility, the roentgenographic findings (Fig. 3) and pulmonary function test results usually improve.

A more recently recognized pulmonary complication of bleomycin is BOOP presenting as nodular lesions mimicking metastasis.

Busulfan

Busulfan is considered the prototypic drug for cytotoxic drug-induced pulmonary damage. The usual case is one of long-term toxic damage to the lungs, with an insidious onset of symptoms after the patient has taken the drug for 3 to 4 years.

Abnormalities are found in pulmonary function tests or on the roentgenogram, or else symptoms are present in 2.5%–11.5% of patients treated with busulfan. Histologic

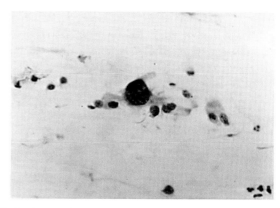

FIG. 2. An atypical cell from bronchial washings of a patient with bleomycin lung. The cell exhibits nuclear enlargement and hyperchromasia. Normal respiratory epithelium is also present. Papanicolaou's stain, x400. (Photomicrograph courtesy of Dr. G. Gephart, Department of Pathology, Cleveland Clinic Foundation.)

evidence of toxicity can be seen in 12.5%–42.8% of all patients treated.

Histologic changes include organizing fibrinous edema with bizarre atypical cells (probably a type II pneumocyte). Alveolar lining cells and bronchiolar epithelial cells can both appear abnormal and may be dysplastic or neoplastic on sputum cytology. There may be evidence of edema or inflammatory cells in the interstitium or, more commonly, fibrotic changes.

The pulmonary function tests show hypoxemia, restriction, and a decrease in diffusing capacity. The DLCO can be used to follow patients. Diffuse interstitial and alveolar infiltrates are typically seen on the chest x-ray film, but nodular densities, pleural effusions, or a normal picture may be seen as well.

Symptoms include cough, dyspnea, and fever. Diagnosis is made by sputum cytology or lung biopsy in the appropriate setting. Treatment is discontinuance of the drug and administration of corticosteroids. The damage is not commonly reversible.

Alveolar proteinosis has been reported in a number of patients receiving busulfan (Table 3). Unlike the usual type of alveolar proteinosis, busulfan-induced disease does not respond to therapeutic lavage.

Chlorambucil

Chlorambucil has been implicated as causing interstitial fibrosis in <5.1% of patients. Symptoms include the insidious onset of cough and dyspnea. Physical examination reveals fine basilar crackles and fever. Histopathology reveals alveolar lining cell dysplasia, interstitial round-cell infiltration, and interstitial fibrosis. Signs and symptoms show good reversibility following discontinuance of the drug and use of corticosteroids.

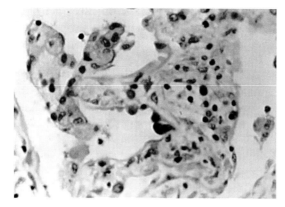

FIG. 1. Bleomycin lung. Hyperplastic alveolar epithelium, septal edema, septal fibrosis, and lymphocytic infiltrates are demonstrated in this open lung biopsy specimen. H&E, x400. (Photomicrograph courtesy of Dr. G. Gephart, Department of Pathology, Cleveland Clinic Foundation.)

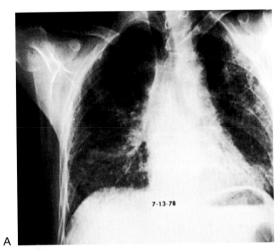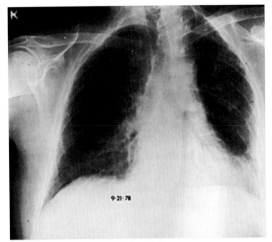

A

B

FIG. 3. Bleomycin pneumonitis. **A:** Posteroanterior chest x-ray film showing bilateral interstitial infiltrates. Total dose of bleomycin was 360 mg during 8 weeks. **B:** Marked clearing after steroid therapy. (Reproduced with permission from Brown L, et al. Successful treatment of bleomycin lung. *Cleve Clin Q* 1980;47:99.)

Cyclophosphamide

The pulmonary response to cyclophosphamide is similar to that seen with busulfan, although it is less common. The pulmonary function tests show hypoxemia, a decreased DLCO, and restriction. Interstitial infiltrates are seen on the chest roentgenogram. Symptoms start insidiously; they include fever, cough, and dyspnea, and may develop after the patient has received the drug for many months. Diagnosis is by lung biopsy. Histologic study shows proliferation of atypical alveolar lining cells. Signs and symptoms may remit with discontinuance of the drug and the administration of corticosteroids.

Melphalan

Pulmonary toxicity is seen in <5% of patients receiving melphalan. Manifestations include interstitial fibrosis, plasma cell interstitial infiltration, and proliferation of bronchiolar and alveolar lining cells.

Methotrexate

An interstitial response to methotrexate may be acute or chronic, and is one of the more reversible of the cytotoxic drug-induced pulmonary reactions. This response has been described following the oral, intravenous, intramuscular, and intrathecal routes of administration.

In some patients, the reaction more closely resembles a hypersensitivity response, with the acute onset of transient hilar lymphadenopathy, eosinophilia, and defervescence with corticosteroids. In other cases, it is more characteristic of a direct toxic action, with fibrosis occurring while the patient is taking corticosteroids and the disability progressing to respiratory failure and death.

In one series, the incidence was 7 of 92, and in another it was approximately 2.5%. The incidence appears to be related to the frequency of dosing rather than to total dose (range, 40 to 6500 mg); the condition is rare, however, in patients receiving 20 mg/week.

There may be synergism with cyclophosphamide, especially in adrenalectomized patients, with an increased frequency and severity of response.

The histologic changes resemble those of desquamative interstitial pneumonitis or busulfan lung (but with fewer abnormal cells). There is alveolar damage, with hyaline membranes and prominent, sometimes atypical, alveolar lining cells; interstitial infiltrates with lymphocytes, plasma cells, and eosinophils; and occasionally, granulomas and giant cells or interstitial fibrosis.

The pulmonary function tests show restriction, hypoxemia, and a decreased DLCO. There may be significant residual abnormalities following clinical recovery. The diffusing capacity is the most sensitive factor but does not allow detection of toxicity before clinical symptoms appear. The chest roentgenogram may be normal or show nodular or reticular nodular infiltrates in the bases and midlung zones, diffuse alveolar infiltrates, pleural effusions, or hilar lymphadenopathy. There may be permanent changes of pulmonary fibrosis.

The onset of symptoms usually occurs 10 days to 4 months after treatment starts. Typically, symptoms include cough, fever, and dyspnea. Headache and malaise are common prodromal symptoms. The differential diagnosis includes leukemic infiltrates (however, the patient is usually in remission when a methotrexate-induced reaction develops) and opportunistic infection. Diagnosis is by biopsy.

Treatment is cessation of the drug. Corticosteroids may hasten recovery. Approximately 7% of patients progress to interstitial fibrosis, and 8% die of respiratory failure.

Methotrexate also has been implicated as causing a pulmonary reaction that histologically resembles bronchiolitis obliterans.

Mediastinal and hilar adenopathy have also been described in patients receiving methotrexate.

Mitomycin

The incidence of pulmonary toxicity with mitomycin C is about 5%. The D$_L$CO declines by >20% in approximately one fourth of patients after they have received three cycles of chemotherapy. Unfortunately, the use of serial D$_L$CO measurements in patients receiving mitomycin cannot predict pulmonary toxicity. Typically, symptoms of cough, fatigue, and dyspnea develop insidiously during several months. The chest x-ray picture shows diffuse reticulonodular infiltrates, and physical examination reveals basilar crackles. Biopsy shows alveolar septal edema and fibrosis, alveolar lining cell hyperplasia, interstitial infiltration with mononuclear and plasma cells, and some atypia of the type II pneumocytes. Prednisone therapy can result in prompt clearing of both symptoms and roentgenographic abnormalities.

Nitrogen Mustard

Unilateral pulmonary edema was seen following instillation of nitrogen mustard into the pleural cavity for control of a recurrent pleural effusion in a patient with breast cancer. Other signs and symptoms included fever, cough, and rales. The reaction was self-limited and was believed to represent a local toxic reaction.

Procarbazine

A hypersensitivity response has been described following the use of procarbazine. It may start within hours of the first dose or may develop after the patient has received the medication for months. Diffuse interstitial infiltrates are seen on the chest roentgenogram. The reaction may terminate in respiratory failure. Pleural effusions and eosinophilia arise. Biopsy shows mononuclear and eosinophilic cell infiltrates and interstitial fibrosis. Diagnosis is by biopsy. Treatment is cessation of the drug and use of corticosteroids. The chest roentgenographic abnormalities may resolve within a month.

Common manifestations of pulmonary toxicity of the various antineoplastic medications are listed in Table 2. Table 3 lists some of the unusual manifestations.

Radiation

The effects of radiation on the lungs are shown in Table 2. Acute radiation pneumonitis can histologically mimic the effects of cytotoxic medications. Changes caused by radiation can resolve completely or progress to become subacute or chronic. Recent studies describe a pulmonary hypersensitivity reaction to radiation, with evidence of lymphocytosis in bronchoalveolar lavage fluid from areas outside the field of radiation. More recently, necrosis of the bronchus (Table 3) has been described following external beam radiation and brachytherapy.

BIBLIOGRAPHY

General

Cooper JAD, White DA, Mathay RA. Drug-induced pulmonary disease. Part 1: cytotoxic drugs. *Am Rev Respir Dis* 1986;133:321–140.
Cooper JAD, White DA, Mathay RA. Drug-induced pulmonary disease. Part 2: noncytotoxic drugs. *Am Rev Respir Dis* 196;133:488–505.
Rosenow EC. Drug-induced pulmonary disease. *Dis Mon* 1994;40 (May):255–310. *In-depth reviews of the topic.*
Demeter SL, Ahmad M, Tomashefski JF. Drug-induced pulmonary disease. Parts 1, 2, and 3. *Cleve Clin Q* 1979;46:89–124. *An early comprehensive report on drug-induced pulmonary disease.*
Hunt LW, Rosenow EC. Asthma-producing drugs. *Ann Allergy* 1992; 68:453–462.
Meeker DP, Wiedemann HP. Drug-induced bronchospasm. *Clin Chest Med* 1990;11:163–175. *Two reviews of drug-induced asthma.*
Meyers JL. Pathology of drug-induced pulmonary disease. In: Katzenstein AL, Askin F, eds. *Surgical Pathology of Non-neoplastic Lung Disease.* 2nd ed. Philadelphia: WB Saunders; 1990:97–127. *A good review of the pathology of drug-induced pulmonary disease.*
Miller WT. Drug-related pleural and mediastinal disorders. *J Thorac Imaging* 1991;6:36–51. *A good general review of drug induced pleural disease.*

Anti-inflammatory agents

Carson CW, Cannon GW, Egger MJ, Ward JR, Clegg DO. Pulmonary disease during the treatment of rheumatoid arthritis with low-dose pulse methotrexate. *Semin Arthritis Rheum* 1987;16:186–195. *An extensive review of 168 patients with rheumatoid arthritis receiving low-dose methotrexate. Methotrexate pneumonitis developed in 5% of these patients.*
Cottin V, Tebib J, Massonnet B, Souquet PJ, Bernard JP. Pulmonary function in patients receiving long-term low-dose methotrexate. *Chest* 1996;109:933–938. *A prospective evaluation of 124 patients receiving low-dose methotrexate. Pneumonitis occurred in 3.2%. Pulmonary function tests did not allow detection before clinical symptoms.*
Evans RB, Ettensohn DB, Fawaz-Estrup F, Lally EV, Kaplan SR. Gold lung: recent developments in pathogenesis, diagnosis, and therapy. *Semin Arthritis Rheum* 1987;16:196–205. *An extensive review of gold-induced pneumonitis. The author reviews 60 cases in the literature.*
Thisted B, Krantz T, Strom J, et al. Acute salicylate self-poisoning in 177 consecutive patients treated in ICU. *Acta Anaesthesiol Scand* 1987;31:312–316.
Leatherman JW, Scmitz PG. Fever, hyperdynamic shock, and multiple system organ failure. A pseudosepsis syndrome associated with chronic salicylate intoxication. *Chest* 1991;100:1391–1396. *Two original articles describing the spectrum of acute and chronic salicylate intoxication.*
Zitnick RJ, Cooper JA Jr. Pulmonary disease due to antirheumatic agents. *Clin Chest Med* 1990;11:139–150. *Good general review of pulmonary effects of anti-inflammatory medication used mainly in the treatment of rheumatic diseases.*

Antimicrobial medications

Gearhart MO, Bhutani MS. Intravenous pentamidine-induced broncho-spasm. *Chest* 1992;102:1891–1892.

Katzman M, Meade W, Iglar K, et al. High incidence of bronchospasm with regular administration of aerosolized pentamidine. *Chest* 1992; 101:79–81. *Reports of bronchospasm caused by pentamidine administered intravenously and in nebulized form.*

Hamadeh MA, Atkinson J, Smith LJ. Sulfasalazine-induced pulmonary disease. *Chest* 1992;101:1033–1037. *A review of the topic.*

Reinoso MA, Schroeder KW, Pisani RJ. Lung disease associated with orally administered mesalamine for ulcerative colitis. *Chest* 1992; 101:1469–1471. *A case report of lung toxicity with oral mesalamine.*

Antineoplastic agents

General

Cherniack RM, Abrams J, Kalica AR. NHLBI Workshop summary. Pulmonary disease associated with breast cancer therapy. *Am J Respir Crit Care Med* 1994;150:1169–1173.

Kreisman H, Wolkove N. Pulmonary toxicity of antineoplastic therapy. *Semin Oncol* 1992;19:508–520.

Lund MB, Kongerud J, Nome O, et al. Lung function impairment in long-term survivors of Hodgkin's disease. *Ann Oncology* 1995;6: 495–501.

McDonald S, Rubin P, Phillips TL, Marks LB. Injury to the lung from cancer therapy: clinical syndromes, measurable end points, and potential scoring systems. *Int J Radiat Oncol Biol Phys* 1995;31:1187–1203. *Several comprehensive recent reviews of cytotoxic drug- and radiation-induced pulmonary toxicity.*

Schwartz CL. Late effects of treatment in long-term survivors of cancer. *Cancer Treat Rev* 1995;21:355–366.

Specific Drugs

Andersson BS, Luna MA, Yee C, Hui KK, Keating MJ, McCredie KB. Fatal pulmonary failure complicating high-dose cytosine arabinoside therapy in acute leukemia. *Cancer* 1990;65:1079–1084. *In this review, 13 of 103 patients receiving cytosine arabinoside (13%), noncardiac pulmonary edema developed in and nine patients died (69% mortality).*

Castro M, Veeder MH, Mailliard JA, Tazelaar HD, Jett JR. A prospective study of pulmonary function in patients receiving mitomycin. *Chest* 1996;109:939–944. *A recent prospective evaluation of 133 patients receiving mitomycin. The diffusion capacity is significantly reduced in many patients, but serial measurement is not a helpful predictor of toxicity.*

Jules-Elysee K, White DA. Bleomycin-induced pulmonary toxicity. *Clin Chest Med* 1990;11:1–20. *A good review of the topic.*

Kuei JH, Tashkin DP, Figlin RA. Pulmonary toxicity of recombinant human tumor necrosis factor. *Chest* 1989;96:334–338. *The authors studied pulmonary function in 27 patients receiving tumor necrosis factor. All patients showed statistically significant decline in DLCO that reached a nadir 2 weeks after initiation of therapy.*

Massin F, Fur A, Reybet-Degat O, Camus P, Jeannin L. Busulfan-induced pneumopathy. *Rev Mal Respir* 1987;4:3–10. *A review of the literature estimated the incidence of busulfan-related pulmonary disease at 6%. The disease begins on average at 41 months after initiation of therapy at an average cumulative dose of 2900 mg.*

Wolkowicz J, Sturgeon MB, Rawji M, Chan CK. Bleomycin-induced pulmonary function abnormalities. *Chest* 1992;101:97–101. *The authors found that total lung capacity was a more specific indicator of bleomycin pulmonary toxicity than the carbon monoxide diffusing capacity.*

Radiation

Mehta AC, Dweik RA. Necrosis of the bronchus: role of radiation. *Chest* 1995;108:1462–1466. *The first report to describe necrosis of the bronchus complicating external beam radiation and/or brachytherapy in four patients.*

Roberts CM, Foulcher E, Zaunders JJ, et al. Radiation pneumonitis: a possible lymphocyte-mediated hypersensitivity reaction. *Ann Intern Med* 1993;118:696–700. *A recent report providing bronchoalveolar lavage evidence for pulmonary hypersensitivity reaction to radiation.*

Cardiac Agents

Chang YC, Patz EF, Goodman PC, Granger CB. Significance of hemoptysis following thrombolytic therapy for acute myocardial infarction. *Chest* 1996;109:727–729. *A recent review of 2634 patients who received thrombolytic therapy. Hemoptysis developed in only 0.4%.*

Faire AE, Gunmpalli KK, Greenberg SD, et al. Amiodarone pulmonary toxicity: a multidisciplinary review of current status. *South Med J* 1993;86:67–77.

Kennedy JI Jr. Clinical aspects of amiodarone pulmonary toxicity. *Clin Chest Med* 1990;11:119–129. *Two good reviews of the clinical presentation, radiographic and histopathologic findings, and management of amiodarone pulmonary toxicity.*

Greenspon AJ, Kidwell GA, Hurley W, et al. Amiodarone-induced postoperative adult respiratory distress syndrome. *Circulation* 1991;84: 407–415.

Hem Don JC, Cook AO, Ramsay MAE, et al. Postoperative unilateral pulmonary edema: possible amiodarone pulmonary toxicity. *Anesthesiology* 1992;76:308–312.

Saussine M, Colson P, Alauzen M, et al. Postoperative acute respiratory distress syndrome. A complication of amiodarone associated with 100% oxygen ventilation. *Chest* 1992;102:980–981. *Three reports of acute amiodarone pulmonary toxicity mediated or enhanced by oxygen administration.*

Israili ZH, Hall WD. Cough and angineurotic edema associated with angiotensin-converting enzyme inhibitor therapy. A review of the literature and pathophysiology. *Ann Intern Med* 1992;117:234–242. *A good review of ACE inhibitor cough clinical presentation, pathophysiology, and management.*

Kavaru MS, Ahmad M, Amirthalingam KN. Hydrochlorothiazide-induced acute pulmonary edema. *Cleve Clin J Med* 1990;57:181–184. *A case report and extensive review of the literature of hydrochlorothiazide-induced noncardiac pulmonary edema.*

Illicit drugs

Albertson TE, Walby WF, Derlet RW. Stimulant-induced pulmonary toxicity. *Chest* 1995;108:1140–1149. *This recent review describes the pulmonary toxicity of amphetamines in addition to those of cocaine.*

Haim DY, Lippmann ML, Goldberg SK, Walkenstein MD. The pulmonary complications of crack cocaine: a comprehensive review. *Chest* 1995;107:233–240. *A recent and comprehensive review of the topic.*

O'Donnell AE, Pappas LS. Pulmonary complications of intravenous drug abuse: experience at an inner city hospital. *Chest* 1988;94:251–253. *This report reviews the spectrum of pulmonary complications of intravenous drug abuse. Pulmonary embolism and infection remain the most frequent problems.*

Pare JP, Cote G, Fraser RS. Long-term follow-up of drug abusers with intravenous talcosis. *Am Rev Respir Dis* 1989;139:233–241. *A long-term follow-up of 10 years of six patients with talcosis showed that despite discontinuation of intravenous use, severe respiratory insufficiency developed in all, and three died of this complication.*

Schmidt RA, Glenny RW, Godwin JD, Hampson NB, Cantino ME, Reichenbach DD. Panlobular emphysema in young intravenous Ritalin abusers. *Am Rev Respir Dis* 1991;143:649–656. *Autopsy review of seven Ritalin abusers. All cases showed severe panlobular emphysema that was most severe in the lower lobes. Most cases were associated with microscopic talc granulomas.*

Psychotropic agents

Li C, Gefter WB. Acute pulmonary edema induced by overdosage of phenothiazines. *Chest* 1992;101:102–104. *The authors describe three cases of phenothiazine-induced pulmonary edema and hypothesize that it is neurogenic in origin, caused by hypothalamic dysfunction.*

Roy TM, Ossorio MA, Cipolla LM, Fields CL, Snider HL, Anderson

WH. Pulmonary complications after tricyclic antidepressant overdose. *Chest* 1989;96:852–856. *These authors report the need for mechanical ventilation for an average of 46 hours in about three forths of patients with tricyclic overdose.*

Salerno SM, Strong JS, Roth BJ, Sakata V. Eosinophilic pneumonia and respiratory failure associated with a trazodone overdose. *Am J Respir Crit Care Med* 1995;152:2170–2172. *The first report of trazodone-associated eosinophilic pneumonia causing respiratory failure.*

Miscellaneous medications

Edling JE, Bacon BR. Pleuropulmonary complications of endoscopic variceal sclerotherapy. *Chest* 1991;99:1252–1257. *This report reviews the significance and management of a newly recognized entity. The authors also provide criteria for the diagnosis of chemical mediastinitis.*

Kinnunen E, Viljanen A. Pleuropulmonary involvement during bromocriptine treatment. *Chest* 1988;94:1034–1036. *A review of the topic. Chronic pleural effusion is associated with lymphocytic pleuritis.*

Nicklas RA. Paradoxical bronchospasm associated with the use of inhaled beta agonists. *J Allergy Clin Immunol* 1990;85:959–964. *A report from the Center for Drug Evaluation and Research of the Food and Drug Administration. Between 1974 and 1988, 126 incidences of paradoxical bronchospasm with the use of beta agonist metered-dose inhalers and 58 incidences with nebulized beta agonists were reported to the FDA.*

Pisani RJ, Rosenow EC III. Pulmonary edema associated with tocolytic therapy. *Ann Intern Med* 1989;110:714–718. *A review of 58 cases of this entity reported in the literature. The report describes the clinical presentation and provides advice for recognition and management.*

Zeller FA, Cannon CR, Prakash UBS. Thoracic manifestations after esophageal variceal sclerotherapy. *Mayo Clin Proc* 1991;66:727–732. *A report describing the Mayo Clinic experience with pulmonary manifestations of esophageal variceal sclerotherapy. Radiographic changes were seen in 85% of patients but were rarely of clinical significance.*

Textbook of Pulmonary Diseases, 6th ed.
edited by G.L. Baum, J.D. Crapo, B.R. Celli, and J.B. Karlinsky,
Lippincott–Raven Publishers, Philadelphia, © 1998.

CHAPTER

Upper Respiratory Tract Infections

23

Richard J. Blinkhorn, Jr.

INTRODUCTION

The goals of this chapter are threefold:

1. To present the anatomic, microbiologic, pathophysiologic, clinical, diagnostic, and therapeutic aspects of infections of the upper respiratory tract, which comprises the oral cavity, nose, pharynx, retropharyngeal tissues, paranasal sinuses, epiglottis, larynx, trachea, and bronchial tree down to the level of the bronchioles.
2. To clarify the relationship of infections in these areas to other diseases affecting the lungs, and the effects of such infections on ventilatory function in general.
3. To describe the complications of infections of the upper respiratory tract, including the syndromes with which they are associated, and methods of diagnosis and treatment.

INFECTIONS OF THE ORAL CAVITY

Infections of the oral cavity most commonly are odontogenic in origin, and, although rare, local spread to the deep fascial spaces may occur, with subsequent life-threatening parapharyngeal, retropharyngeal, or pleuro-pulmonary extension. It is beyond the scope of this chapter to describe all potential intraoral infections; only those infections with complications commonly involving the upper respiratory tract are reviewed.

Although the microbiologic aspects of abscesses of odontogenic origin are not fully elucidated, the evidence available suggests that anaerobes are involved at least as frequently as aerobes. The anaerobes involved most often are fusobacteria, *Bacteroides* species, and anaerobic

R. J. Blinkhorn.: MetroHealth Medical Center, Cleveland, Ohio 44109.

streptococci, whereas the aerobic organisms most frequently isolated are streptococci. Except in hosts compromised by leukemia or diseases in which therapy has resulted in profound neutropenia, facultative gram-negative bacilli and *Staphylococcus aureus* are rarely isolated.

The parapharyngeal space is shaped like an inverted cone, with its base at the skull and its apex at the hyoid bone. Infections of this space may result from peritonsillar abscess, parotitis, mastoiditis, and molar tooth infection. Parapharyngeal abscess may invade the carotid artery or jugular vein, resulting in thrombosis and/or intravascular sepsis, sometimes with metastatic hematogenous spread and development of septic pulmonary emboli. The latter condition is referred to as *Lemierre's postanginal sepsis; Fusobacterium necrophorum* is the leading etiologic agent. Infection may spread to the mediastinum along the carotid sheath or extend into the retropharyngeal space. Appropriate treatment consists of antibiotics, surgical drainage, and emergency ligation of the carotid artery or jugular vein when involved.

The retropharyngeal space is located between the pharynx and prevertebral fascia extending from the base of the skull into the mediastinum. Infection of this space usually results from lymphatic spread to the retropharyngeal lymph nodes with subsequent suppuration and abscess. Afferent drainage to these nodes arises from the nasopharynx, adenoids, and sinuses. Retropharyngeal abscess is mainly a disease of young children, as these lymph nodes atrophy by 3 or 4 years of age. Common causative organisms include *Streptococcus pyogenes* and anaerobic bacteria. Spontaneous rupture into the pharynx may result in aspiration with pneumonia and empyema.

Ludwig's angina is a term that has been loosely applied to a heterogeneous array of infections involving the submandibular and sublingual spaces. First described in 1836, this is a diffuse, bilateral cellulitis of the floor of the mouth and upper cervical areas characterized by toxicity, fever, brawny indurated swelling of the submandibular space, tongue elevation, and dysphagia. A dental source of infection is found in 50%–90% of reported cases, with the second and third mandibular molars most commonly involved. Rapid progression of infection may result in edema of the neck and glottis, thereby precipitating asphyxiation. Treatment requires high-dose parenteral penicillin, airway monitoring, early intubation or tracheostomy when necessary, soft-tissue decompression, and surgical drainage.

RHINITIS

Acute rhinitis is a nonspecific term for infections of the internal nose and may represent the sole or main manifestation of the "common cold." The common cold is a mild, self-limited, catarrhal syndrome that is the leading cause of acute morbidity and of visits to physicians in the United States. Annual epidemics of upper respiratory tract disease occur in the colder months in temperate areas, with a peak incidence from late August until spring in the United States. The major respiratory viruses causing colds include rhinoviruses, coronaviruses, parainfluenza viruses, and respiratory syncytial viruses. Influenza virus and adenovirus may produce the common cold syndrome but tend to be associated with more severe illness often involving the lower respiratory tract.

The incubation period is variable, averaging 48 to 72 hours. Cardinal symptoms are nasal discharge, nasal obstruction, sore throat, and cough. Median duration of illness is 1 week, although almost one quarter of colds last up to 2 weeks. Diagnosis of the specific virus involved is usually not possible on clinical grounds. Influenza and pharyngoconjunctival fever (adenovirus), however, when seen in a typical epidemiologic setting, can be recognized without benefit of viral culture or serologic tests. The main challenge to the physician is to distinguish the uncomplicated cold from the approximately 0.5% of cases with secondary bacterial sinusitis and the 2% with otitis media. Antibiotics have no place in the management of uncomplicated colds, but decongestants and cough suppressants may be beneficial. Although intranasal recombinant human interferon-α has been effective both as therapy and prophylaxis against rhinovirus infection, local nasal irritation has complicated long-term use, and activity against viruses other than rhinovirus has not been demonstrated.

SINUSITIS

The frontal, ethmoid, maxillary, and sphenoid sinuses are paired cavities, lined with mucosa, in the anterior portion of the skull. Predisposing factors to sinus disease can be categorized as local, regional, or systemic. The most common local predisposing cause of suppurative sinusitis is a viral upper respiratory tract infection. Inflammation and edema in the ostial-meatal complex can obstruct the sinus ostium, leading to hypoxygenation of the sinus, disturbed ciliary and mucous blanket function, and diminished local resistance. Other local nasal factors that cause obstruction in the ostial-meatal complex are nasal polyps, allergic rhinitis, foreign bodies, and nasal septal pathology. In hospitalized patients, nasogastric tubes may functionally obstruct sinus ostia, thereby predisposing to nosocomial sinusitis. The immotile cilia syndrome is another local factor predisposing to sinus disease, but it does not involve structural obstruction of sinus ostia. Regional factors include maxillary dental infections, and predisposing systemic factors include malnutrition, diabetes mellitus, long-term corticosteroid therapy, hypogammaglobulinemia, blood dyscrasias, and chemotherapy.

Although normal paranasal sinuses have long been thought to be sterile, transient colonization with organisms normally populating the upper airway may occur. Overgrowth of this transient resident flora may produce infection when local clearance mechanisms are impaired. In all studies of acute community-acquired maxillary sinusitis, >50% of isolates are either *Streptococcus pneumoniae* or unencapsulated *Haemophilus influenzae,* with *S. pyogenes, Branhamella catarrhalis,* and gram-negative bacilli accounting for the rest. Specimens for culture should be obtained by direct sinus aspiration, because nasal swabs and/or irrigation correlate with aspiration <65% of the time. When appropriate anaerobic cultures are performed, anaerobes can be isolated in at least 10% of acute cases, with a higher isolation rate of approximately 50% in chronic sinusitis. A mixed anaerobic infection with *Bacteroides* and anaerobic streptococci would suggest infection of odontogenic origin. Viruses have been isolated in approximately 15% of cases, usually in conjunction with or preceding bacterial infection. Invasive aspergillosis and rhinocerebral phycomycosis occur in immunocompromised patients with granulocytopenia or uncontrolled diabetes mellitus with ketoacidosis, respectively.

Symptoms and signs suggesting acute sinusitis include purulent nasal discharge, facial pain or tenderness, nasal congestion, cough, fever, and a history of recent upper respiratory tract infection. In sphenoid sinusitis, headache is the most common initial symptom. Patients with chronic sinusitis often present with protracted nasal congestion, purulent nasal discharge, and facial pain. Because the typical complaints of acute sinusitis overlap with those of a prolonged but uncomplicated common cold, it may be difficult to make a diagnosis of sinusitis on clinical grounds. Valuable information may be obtained from transillumination of the maxillary and frontal sinuses. The finding of complete opacity of the sinus is strong evidence for the presence of active infection; conversely, the finding of normal light transmission is equally good evidence that no infection is present. Dullness, but not complete opacity, is less helpful. The most sensitive routine test for the diagnosis of acute sinusitis is radiologic examination of the sinuses; opacification, an air-fluid level, or mucosal thickening is strong evidence of active infection. The value of sinus radiology in patients with chronic sinusitis is limited, because radiographic abnormalities are persistent in such patients. Computed tomography (CT) and magnetic resonance imaging (MRI) are particularly useful in the examination of the ethmoid and sphenoid sinuses and for evaluation of suspected intracranial or orbital extension of infection.

Nasal decongestants should be used in the supportive treatment of acute sinusitis, but antihistamines are to be avoided, as they may thicken purulent sinus fluid and impair drainage. Because sinus aspiration to determine a specific microbial etiology is not routinely indicated, empiric antimicrobial therapy should be primarily effective against *S. pneumoniae* and *H. influenzae*. Ampicillin or amoxicillin is recommended for the initial treatment of uncomplicated acute sinusitis. Sinusitis caused by β-lactamase-producing bacteria, including some strains of *H. influenzae* and *B. catarrhalis,* requires treatment with β-lactamase-resistant antimicrobial agents, such as amoxicillin/clavulanate, second-generation cephalosporins, trimethoprim/sulfamethoxazole, and the newer macrolides, azithromycin and clarithromycin.

Patients with cystic fibrosis or immotile cilia syndrome are predisposed to *Pseudomonas aeruginosa* and *Staphylococcus aureus* infection, whereas immunocompromised patients and patients with nosocomial sinusitis have a higher incidence of aerobic gram-negative bacterial infections, which are often polymicrobial. As mentioned earlier, cultures from patients with chronic sinusitis are often polymicrobial, and at least half harbor anaerobes. Empiric antimicrobial therapy in these unique clinical settings must be adjusted accordingly.

The principal goals of sinus surgery are to oxygenate, establish drainage, and remove diseased mucosa. Candidates for surgical intervention include those patients who have failed empiric therapy, who have rhinocerebral complications, or who have nosocomial infections or immunodeficiency. In addition, most patients with ethmoid or sphenoid disease or chronic sinusitis require corrective surgery. Therapy for fungal sinusitis requires immediate surgical debridement coupled with administration of systemic amphotericin B.

PHARYNGITIS

Acute pharyngitis is an inflammatory condition of the pharynx, and its principal symptom, sore throat, is a frequent accompaniment of many other respiratory illnesses. Many of the known microbial causes of pharyngitis are listed in Table 1, with the most common being group A streptococci, various respiratory viruses, and the Epstein-Barr virus associated with infectious mononucleosis. For the clinician, it is most important to differentiate viral from streptococcal pharyngitis, because of the latter's response to penicillin therapy and its potential sequelae of acute rheumatic fever and acute glomerulonephritis.

Viruses account for the majority of cases of pharyngitis in adults; mild-to-moderate pharyngeal discomfort frequently accompanies common colds. Sore throat is a major complaint in some patients with influenza, and the accompanying myalgia, headache, fever, and cough readily suggest the diagnosis. Adenoviral pharyngitis is usually more severe than the illness typical of the common cold, and conjunctivitis is a distinguishing feature present in one third to one half of cases. The presence of vesicles or shallow ulcers of the palate is characteristic of primary infection with herpes simplex virus, although gingivostomatitis is a more common presentation than acute pharyngitis. During the summer and fall months, pharyngitis caused by coxsackievirus, so-called herpangina, can be distinguished by the presence of small vesicles on the soft palate, uvula, and anterior tonsillar pillars. Exudative tonsillitis, fever, cervical adenopathy, and fatigue are characteristic features of infectious mononucleosis caused by Epstein-Barr virus, and approximately half of cases have associated generalized adenopathy or splenomegaly. Febrile pharyngitis has now been described as a characteristic feature of primary infection with human immunodeficiency virus, and it may mimic the mononucleosis syndrome.

Approximately 15% of all cases of pharyngitis are caused by group A streptococci, the bacterial pathogen most commonly isolated from patients of school age. It is not clear whether non-group A β-hemolytic streptococci, such as groups C and G, cause pharyngitis in nonepidemic settings. The severity of infection varies considerably, but generally there is marked pharyngeal pain, dysphagia, tender cervical adenopathy, and fever. In the majority of cases, an etiologic diagnosis is not possible on clinical grounds alone. For patients with mild illness, a throat culture should be obtained, with treatment dependent on a positive result. For patients with more severe clinical presentations, in whom prompt antimicrobial therapy would be beneficial, a rapid streptococcal antigen test should be performed. A positive result establishes the diagnosis of streptococcal pharyngitis, whereas a negative test result should be substantiated by a simultaneous throat culture.

The incidence of diphtheria has fallen dramatically in the past 50 years, but outbreaks still occur in unvaccinated populations in the United States. Most cases occur in the Southwest among blacks, Mexican-Americans, and American Indians. Pharyngeal diphtheria is characterized by small areas of exudate that coalesce to form a light- to dark-gray membrane that becomes progressively

TABLE 1. *Microbial agents associated with pharyngitis*

Agent	Clinical syndrome	Frequency of occurrence
Viral		
Respiratory[a]	Common cold	Common (winter)
Adenovirus	Pharyngoconjunctival fever	Common (winter)
Influenza virus	Flu, pneumonia	Common (winter)
Coxsackievirus A	Herpangina	Occasional (summer, fall)
Epstein-Barr virus	Infectious mononucleosis	Common
Cytomegalovirus	Infectious mononucleosis	Occasional
Human immunodeficiency virus	Primary HIV infection	Uncommon
Herpes simplex virus	Gingivostomatitis	Occasional (immunosuppressed)
Bacterial		
Streptococcus group A	Tonsillitis, scarlet fever	Common
Mixed anaerobes	Gingivitis, Vincent's angina	Occasional
Corynebacterium diphtheriae	Membranous pharyngitis	Rare
Corynebacterium hemolyticum	Scarlatiniform rash	Occasional (young adults)
Neisseria gonorrhoeae	Sexually transmitted disease	Occasional
Treponema pallidum	Chancre, syphilis	Rare
Francisella tularensis	Pharyngeal ulcer, tularemia	Rare
Yersinia enterocolitica	Exudative pharyngitis, enterocolitis	Rare
Fungal: *Candida albicans*	Thrush, esophagitis	Occasional
Chlamydial		
C. psittaci	Pneumonia	Rare
C. trachomatis	Sexually transmitted disease	Occasional
C. pneumoniae	Hoarseness, pneumonia	Occasional
Mycoplasmal: *M. pneumoniae*	Pneumonia, bronchitis	Occasional

[a] Rhinovirus, coronavirus, parainfluenza virus.

thicker and more difficult to remove. The condition usually involves little toxicity and only modest temperature elevation. Membranous spread to the larynx and trachea can cause life-threatening respiratory obstruction, characterized by inspiratory stridor and cyanosis. Secondary infection with streptococci or other bacteria may occur, and in such cases, toxicity, fever, and local pain may increase markedly. Lymphadenitis and subcutaneous swelling may result in a "bull neck" appearance. *Corynebacterium haemolyticum* has been increasingly identified as a cause of exudative pharyngitis in adolescents and young adults, and such infection may be associated with an erythematous, maculopapular, sometimes pruritic skin rash. Effective antimicrobial agents for either *C. diptheriae* or *C. haemolyticum* include penicillin, erythromycin, and tetracycline.

Pharyngitis accompanying sexually transmitted disease caused by *Neisseria gonorrhoeae, Chlamydia trachomatis,* and *Treponema pallidum* is not uncommon, but these agents would be rare causes of pharyngitis in an unselected general population. Gonococcal pharyngitis is being detected with increasing frequency, probably because of improved microbiologic isolation techniques and changes in patterns of sexual behavior. Asymptomatic gonococcal throat colonization is much more common than pharyngitis, as various series have shown that no more than 30% of those with positive pharyngeal cultures have any clinical manifestations. Ceftriaxone, administered intramuscularly in a single dose of 250 mg, is the

drug of choice. Although *C. trachomatis* has been isolated from patients with pharyngitis, asymptomatic throat colonization occurs more often. Rarely, syphilis may present as a primary pharyngeal chancre.

Although exudative pharyngitis with cervical lymphadenopathy may complicate infection with *Yersinia enterocolitica* and *Francisella tularensis,* other manifestations of these systemic diseases usually dominate the clinical picture, and isolated pharyngeal disease would be quite rare. Similarly, when *Chlamydia psittaci, C. pneumoniae,* and *Mycoplasma pneumoniae* are associated with pharyngitis, the pharyngeal disease generally tends to accompany tracheobronchitis or pneumonia rather than occur as an isolated event.

EPIGLOTTITIS

First described in an adult, epiglottitis is a life-threatening disease observed most frequently in 1- to 6-year-old children, most often during the fall and winter. It is important to emphasize, however, that epiglottitis has been increasingly reported in adults during the past three decades. *Supraglottitis* may be the preferred term, as the infection involves the arytenoids, the aryepiglottic folds, and the epiglottis while sparing the pharynx, true vocal cords, and trachea. The infection can be primary or secondary to adjacent infections or trauma, and can result in acute diffuse inflammation, acute ulcerative inflammation, or epiglottitis with abscess formation on the free edge, laryngeal surface, or lingual surface.

Acute epiglottitis develops in two distinct forms: gradually, within days, usually following an upper respiratory tract illness; or accelerated, within hours. The characteristic early symptoms are sore throat and dysphagia. Odynophagia thereafter becomes the predominant symptom and may be so severe that the patient would rather not eat or drink. The voice tends to be muffled rather than hoarse, and the temperature is usually strikingly elevated. Respiratory distress with tachypnea, dyspnea, and cyanosis occurs late and heralds acute airway obstruction. In this setting, the patient will be observed drooling, sitting up, leaning forward, and breathing quite deliberately. Examination should not be performed with the patient in the recumbent position. Despite the prominence of pain, the pharynx is usually normal in appearance. Attempts to visualize the epiglottis must be carried out with great caution, as even the slightest trauma can provoke acute respiratory obstruction. Auscultation of the chest may reveal inspiratory stridor. Cervical lymphadenopathy is present in about 25% of cases.

Roentgenograms of the chest often show hyperinflation, and there may be areas of atelectasis or pneumonitis. The epiglottic swelling can be seen on a lateral x-ray film of the neck. Laboratory examination shows an elevated white blood cell count with an increase in mature polymorphonuclear leukocytes and band forms.

Complications include septic arthritis, meningitis, empyema, and mediastinitis. Asphyxia and cardiopulmonary arrest are dreaded complications, and several factors contribute to the pathogenesis of respiratory tract obstruction. Edema of the lingual mucosa of the epiglottis causes curling of the epiglottis posteriorly and inferiorly, narrowing the air space, and edema of the aryepiglottic folds worsens the obstruction. During inspiration, these swollen structures are drawn downward into the airway, further reducing the size of the lumen. Inflammation of the supraglottic structures inhibits swallowing, leading to an accumulation of secretions and saliva that further compromises the airway.

Acute epiglottitis is a bacterial infection, as viruses have not been conclusively linked to the disease. In 80% of cases in children, *H. influenzae* type b can be isolated from the epiglottis and/or bloodstream. In adults, however, the etiologic agent is not always obvious, and blood cultures are negative in 70%–85% of cases. *H. influenzae* type b accounts for 20%–25% of cases in adults, with *Streptococcus pneumoniae*, β-hemolytic streptococci, viridans streptococci, nonencapsulated *H. influenzae, Moraxella catarrhalis,* and *Staphylococcus aureus* occasionally implicated. No etiologic agent can be recovered in up to 40% of adult cases.

The diagnostic and therapeutic approach depends on the clinical presentation. Unstable patients with ''classic'' epiglottitis (stridor, drooling, dyspnea, and fever) should be taken immediately to the operating room for direct laryngoscopy and nasotracheal or endotracheal intubation. Preparation should be made for emergency cricothyrotomy if intubation is not possible. The majority of adults and a large number of children, however, do not have classic presentations, and their management is less straightforward. In adults, indirect laryngoscopy or flexible nasal endoscopy is safe in the initial assessment, as no complications have been reported with this approach. Radiography, however, remains useful in differentiating other upper airway pathology (e.g., foreign body or abscess) from epiglottitis. In children, manipulating the upper airway is more hazardous, and radiography should be the initial procedure performed when suspicion of epiglottitis is low to moderate. The epiglottis of a stable child with normal radiographic findings should be visualized to rule out normal radiograph epiglottitis. Whereas intubation or tracheostomy is virtually mandatory in children with epiglottitis, whether this is appropriate in the management of adults remains a point of ongoing controversy. It is reasonable in adults to defer airway intervention as long as close follow-up by individuals specifically skilled in emergency airway control can be ensured. Stridor and infection with *H. influenzae* type b appear to increase the likelihood of acute airway obstruction.

Antimicrobial therapy should be directed against the common etiologic agents, and ampicillin/sulbactam, chloramphenicol, and second- or third-generation cephalosporins are reasonable choices until bacteriologic data are available. Although often administered in the hope of diminishing supraglottic edema, corticosteroids have not been conclusively shown to alter the course of the disease. Immunization against *H. influenzae* should reduce the incidence of childhood epiglottitis. The risk for development of invasive *H. influenzae* infection is considerably increased in both siblings and parents of patients with epiglottitis, and rifampin prophylaxis should be administered to these household contacts.

LARYNGOTRACHEOBRONCHITIS

Unlike epiglottitis, which is a bacterial disease, laryngotracheitis (croup) is usually the result of a viral infection. Peak incidence is in late fall, with a smaller peak in late spring; a pattern related to the prevalence of parainfluenza viruses in the community has been observed. The subglottic area and trachea are involved, whereas the area above the true vocal cords is spared. In children, croup usually occurs in the first half-decade of life and begins with rhinorrhea. The first sign of spread to the larynx is the gradual development of a harsh, barking cough and hoarse voice. Fever is variable. The major clinical features of croup are related to inflammatory edema and fibrinous exudate in the subglottic area, which narrows the airway and causes inspiratory stridor. Inflammation and edema

TABLE 2. *Distinguishing features of croup and epiglottitis*

Feature	Croup	Epiglottitis
Patient age	Younger (6 mo–3 y)	Older (3–6 y)
Season	Late spring, late fall	All year
Antecedent illness	Rhinorrhea	Uncommon
Clinical appearance	Child is lying down	Child is sitting
	Nontoxic condition	Toxic condition
	Not drooling	Drooling
Cough	Barking in quality	Absent
Voice	Hoarse	Muffled
Fever	Variable	High-grade
Leukocytosis	Absent	Present
Progression	Usually slow	Rapid
Causative agent	Parainfluenza virus type 1	*Haemophilus influenzae* type b

commonly extend down the trachea and bronchi, producing thick, viscid secretions and ventilation-perfusion mismatch. Involvement of these lower airways, superimposed on the already-narrowed subglottic area, results in increased work of breathing and hypoxemia. As many as 3% of patients admitted with acute laryngotracheobronchitis may require an artificial airway for relief of obstruction, and this chance may reach 6% if sternal and chest wall retractions are present.

The findings on chest roentgenograms vary from normal to evidence of hyperaeration and sometimes areas of atelectasis. The white blood cell count is usually normal, and there may be a predominance of lymphocytes. Parainfluenza virus types 1 through 3 has been implicated most frequently, but influenza virus, respiratory syncytial virus, coronavirus, rhinovirus, adenovirus, enterovirus, and coxsackievirus are all capable of producing the disease. Measles is an infrequent cause.

For the clinician, the initial step in management is to distinguish croup from epiglottitis (Table 2). Treatment of croup in children consists of creating an atmosphere of cool, moist air and administering oxygen in a humidified milieu to avoid drying of the respiratory tract. Antibiotics ordinarily are not necessary. The use of adrenal glucocorticoids and/or racemic epinephrine is controversial, particularly the latter.

Laryngotracheitis is more complex etiologically in adults and in both children and adults compromised by hematologic malignancy or neutropenia. In noncompromised adults, laryngotracheitis is often manifested by hoarseness and substernal pain, frequently of a burning quality. Influenza virus, parainfluenza virus, and adenovirus are the likely offending agents, but in addition, bacteria (particularly *H. influenzae*) and *M. pneumoniae* can produce the syndrome. If the patient is compromised and neutropenic, opportunistic organisms such as *P. aeruginosa* and species of *Klebsiella, Serratia,* and *Enterobacter* can be responsible. If the individual has defective delayed immune mechanisms and oral thrush is present, the *Candida* infection may move from the oropharynx to the larynx and trachea. In patients who are receiving immuno-suppressive agents for severe underlying disease, herpesvirus 1 or 2 may cause laryngotracheitis, and the use of multiple antibiotics in a compromised host may encourage candidal superinfection.

In healthy adults with laryngotracheitis, failure to improve with supportive therapy mandates obtaining a tracheal culture for both viruses and bacteria. In the compromised host, if cough specimens or blood cultures do not show a presumed etiologic agent, it is necessary to obtain proper cultures by laryngoscopy, tracheal intubation, or bronchoscopy. These procedures may be difficult in such persons if thrombocytopenia is present; sometimes broad antimicrobial therapy must be given in the absence of a precise microbial diagnosis, but this is obviously undesirable, and whenever possible, therapy should be guided by proper Gram's stains and cultures.

Bacterial tracheitis in infants and older children has features of both epiglottitis and croup. Clinically, it is characterized by fever, toxicity, brassy cough, and often inspiratory stridor. In most cases, chest roentgenograms show patchy or focal infiltrates. The epiglottic and aryepiglottic folds appear normal on direct examination, but subglottic edema is present. Purulent secretions that are often profuse and thick can be seen, and these can produce tracheal obstruction. The isolated organism is often *S. aureus,* and there is a satisfactory response to appropriate antimicrobial agents. Endotracheal intubation is usually required to maintain a patent airway and handle copious secretions.

ACUTE BRONCHITIS (OR TRACHEOBRONCHITIS)

Acute inflammatory disease of the trachea and bronchi can be caused by a variety of stimuli, including constituents of tobacco and cannabis; ammonia; trace metals, such as vanadium and cadmium; air pollutants, such as sulfur dioxide; nitrogen dioxide; vegetable substances, such as bagasse, cotton, flax, hemp, and paprika; and a farrago of infectious agents, including viruses, mycoplasmas, bacteria, and parasites.

The role of viruses in bronchial disease has been defined best by the Tecumseh studies of respiratory illness. Infectious agents include respiratory syncytial virus, rhinovirus, echovirus, parainfluenza types 1, 2, and 3, herpesvirus, coxsackievirus, influenza, coronavirus, and adenovirus. It is virtually impossible to separate one virus from another clinically. All those capable of producing pharyngeal and nasal disease also can cause bronchitis. Some assumptions can be made on the basis of age and season of the year. In the very young, respiratory syncytial virus, parainfluenza types 1 through 3, and coronavirus are most frequently isolated. Among patients from 1 to 10 years of age, parainfluenza types 1 and 2, enterovirus, respiratory syncytial virus, and rhinovirus predominate. Above that age, influenza A and B, respiratory syncytial virus, and adenovirus are found most frequently. Parainfluenza types 1 and 3 and rhinovirus are found most frequently in the fall; influenza, respiratory syncytial virus, and coronavirus cause infections for the most part in winter and early spring, whereas enterovirus induces infections in summer and early fall. There are differences in the capability of the different viruses to produce lower respiratory tract disease; for example, the disease caused by parainfluenza virus is likely to be more severe than that caused by rhinovirus.

The bacteria most often recovered in acute purulent bronchitis are *H. influenzae, Streptococcus pneumoniae,* and *Moraxella (Branhamella) catarrhalis.* Acute bronchitis and transient mild pneumonitis are sometimes early manifestations of *Salmonella typhosa* infection. *Bordetella pertussis* is responsible for whooping cough in children; it is less well appreciated that it also may cause acute and subacute bronchitis in adults, as may *Legionella* infections.

There is increasing evidence that yeasts and fungi may produce bronchitis in the absence of parenchymal disease. This is true of *Candida albicans* and *C. tropicalis, Cryptococcus neoformans, Histoplasma capsulatum, Coccidioides immitis,* and *Blastomyces dermatitidis.* In the older literature, candidal bronchitis has been described in otherwise healthy hosts, but more recently it appears to be restricted to compromised hosts. *Geotrichum candidum* is also occasionally a cause of acute and subacute bronchitis.

As serologic analyses are performed more regularly, it has become clear that both *M. pneumoniae* and *C. pneumoniae* not infrequently cause acute bronchitis. Bronchitis also can occur during the migration of *Strongyloides* and *Ascaris* larvae, and a few cases of paroxysmal cough caused by the parasite *Syngamus laryngeus* have been reported either in residents of or visitors to Brazil, the Philippines, the West Indies, Puerto Rico, and British Guiana.

Cough is uniformly found in acute bronchitis, and it may be productive of mucoid or purulent sputum. The nature of the sputum may be helpful diagnostically. Except for adenovirus infections, the sputum in viral infections is almost always characterized by marked predominance of mononuclear cells on Gram's or Wright's stain. In contrast, in bacterial infections the sputum shows a predominance of polymorphonuclear leukocytes. *Mycoplasma* infections, like adenovirus infections, are usually associated with mononuclear cells, but there may be a striking predominance of polymorphonuclear leukocytes.

The cough may be accompanied by variable amounts of hemoptysis and/or substernal pain that is often described as being of a burning quality; it is usually accentuated on inspiration. Usually, the temperature is only minimally to moderately elevated; physical examination often shows harsh breath sounds, rhonchi, and variable amounts of expiratory wheezing.

Wheezy bronchitis is a specific clinical entity occurring for the most part in children who have a tendency to wheeze and a family history of atopy. Viruses appear etiologically related in only a minority of cases; rhinovirus and respiratory syncytial virus are the agents that have been most often isolated. The syndrome of intermittent, recurrent wheezy bronchitis in children also may result from reduced esophageal sphincter tone with reflux.

The organisms responsible for bronchitis in the compromised host may be quite different from the agents affecting the uncompromised individual. In older persons and immunocompromised hosts, herpes simplex virus type 1 may cause tracheobronchitis that may be manifested primarily by bronchospasm. Intravenously administered acyclovir is the treatment of choice. Such patients are also susceptible to gram-negative infections caused by species of *Klebsiella, Serratia, Enterobacter,* and *Pseudomonas.* If these gram-negative superinfections occur during antibiotic treatment of infections elsewhere, the organisms may be markedly resistant to antibiotics. The pharynx of alcoholics is colonized more frequently than the pharynx of nonalcoholics by enteric gram-negative organisms, particularly *Enterobacter* species and *Escherichia coli.* Pharyngeal colonization may be followed by aspiration and acute bronchitis.

The treatment of acute tracheobronchitis depends on the clinical setting in which it arises, the Gram's stain of expectorated sputum, the appearance of the sputum, and the findings on physical examination of the chest. If there are myriad polymorphonuclear leukocytes in the sputum, this suggests a bacterial etiology, and antibiotic administration can be predicated on the predominant organisms seen on smear. The bronchitis is not usually so severe as to mandate immediate therapy, and antimicrobial agents can be withheld until culture results are available. If no likely etiologic agent is recovered in culture and there are many polymorphonuclear cells in the sputum, the possibility of *M. pneumoniae* infection should be strongly considered. This usually responds to treatment with erythromycin or tetracycline.

If on routine culture no pathogenic micro-organisms are found and the sputum shows a polymorphonuclear predominance, acid-fast stains also should be obtained, and in appropriate geographic areas, potassium or sodium hydroxide preparations of sputum should be used to search for fungi and parasites.

The presence on physical examination of focal areas of diminished breath sounds suggests that inspissated mucus has caused atelectasis. This may be relieved by the use of humidifiers, bronchodilators, vigorous coughing, and, if needed, tracheal suction. Occasionally, there is diffuse diminution of air intake and/or inspiratory stridor; these findings indicate obstruction of major bronchi or the trachea, which requires sequentially vigorous coughing, suctioning, and intubation or even tracheostomy if needed.

The choice of antibiotic depends on the pathogen involved. There are striking differences in the penetration of antimicrobial agents into the bronchial secretions. However, it is still unclear whether the degree of antibiotic penetration can be related to clinical outcome. For empiric treatment of community-acquired acute purulent bronchitis, amoxicillin, second-generation cephalosporins, erythromycin, or tetracycline would be a reasonable choice. The newer macrolide antimicrobial drugs, clarithromycin and azithromycin, are very attractive agents for this indication, as their spectrum of activity includes the usual bacterial etiologic agents as well as *Mycoplasma* and *Chlamydia*. The choice of antimicrobial agent in nosocomial or ventilator-associated tracheobronchitis should be tailored to the specific organism isolated.

Acute bronchitis is ordinarily not a life-threatening disease. This permits an orderly search for a microbial etiology, careful assessment of environmental exposures, and evaluation for foreign body or esophageal reflux (or a tracheoesophageal fistula in infants). In most cases, supportive therapy, including adrenergic bronchodilators by aerosol if needed, suffices. If the bronchitis persists, fiberoptic bronchoscopy may be advisable. The disease may last for 6 to 8 weeks. A specific diagnosis can often be made only by the study of paired sera for rises in antibody titers against specific viruses. Exacerbations of chronic bronchitis in patients with chronic obstructive pulmonary disease are discussed in Chapter 43.

BRONCHIOLITIS

In the strictest sense, bronchiolitis, a disease of small airways, should be considered an illness of the lower respiratory tract; it is so frequently preceded by an infection of the upper respiratory tract, however, that it is included in the present chapter. Bronchiolitis is a disease of children. The annual incidence is six to seven cases per 100 children, with most cases occurring during the first 2 years of life.

Bronchiolitis was first described as a complication of measles and mumps, but in more recent years, it has been associated with most of the respiratory viruses, especially the respiratory syncytial virus. Although most cases of bronchiolitis are caused by viruses, *H. influenzae* type b and *M. pneumoniae* have been implicated in some cases. Outbreaks usually occur in winter and spring in temperate climates, epidemics usually being associated with respiratory syncytial virus, adenovirus, influenza, or parainfluenza virus.

Airways from 75 to 300 mm in diameter are involved. Following invasion by microorganisms, cellular infiltration and edema occur together with bronchiolar epithelial proliferation and necrosis. Mucous secretion is increased, after which mucus, inflammatory exudate, and cell debris obstruct the bronchioles. Adenoviruses cause a more severe disruption of the mucosa than do respiratory syncytial viruses and produce a necrotizing bronchiolitis, with a resultant higher mortality.

The initial symptoms of nasal discharge and cough are indistinguishable from those of the common cold. Within 1 to 2 days, fever and cough become prominent and are soon followed by tachypnea and suprasternal, substernal, and subcostal retraction. To prevent coughing and reduce the work of breathing, infants and children take rapid, shallow breaths. Deep breaths are accompanied by fine rales and diffuse expiratory wheezing and usually trigger a paroxysm of coughing. Hypercapnia and cyanosis commonly occur as the work of breathing increases, and infants under 6 months of age may present with apnea.

The peripheral white blood cell count may be normal or moderately elevated. Blood gas analysis typically shows profound hypoxemia. Chest roentgenograms reveal hyperinflation, increased bronchial markings, and frequently areas of atelectasis or infiltrate. Densities on chest films may be more striking than the degree of clinical or radiographic evidence of small-airway obstruction, and thereby they may be misinterpreted as pneumonia. It should be emphasized, however, that these pulmonary densities represent predominantly areas of atelectasis.

A specific diagnosis often can be made retrospectively by study of paired sera for antiviral or antimycoplasmal antibodies. Nasopharyngeal secretions can be obtained for viral culture, but growth may require up to 14 days. Respiratory syncytial viral infection can be diagnosed rapidly by antigen detection using immunofluorescence techniques or ELISA (enzyme-linked immunosorbent assay).

In children under 2 years of age, the disease may be life-threatening, and therapy consists of oxygen and supportive treatment, with particular attention to proper ventilation. Corticosteroids are not effective. The value of aminophylline or β_2-adrenergic agents has not been established, although bronchodilators are frequently employed in the management of severely ill children. Ribavirin delivered by small-particle aerosol has been shown to hasten the clinical recovery and decrease virus shedding, although these effects are not dramatic. However, because it may cause irritation of the mucous membranes in caretakers, it is often delivered via an endotracheal tube in a closed system. Although antibiotics are not indicated in most children with bronchiolitis, nosocomial bacterial infections can occur in children receiving intensive supportive care. If the bronchiolitis occurs in fall and early winter, erythromycin should be considered for the possibility of *M. pneumoniae* infection. The incidence of nosocomial spread of respiratory syncytial viral infections is high, and preventive precautions should be implemented.

There is a high frequency of residual lung disease after an acute episode of bronchiolitis. In one series, most children studied 10 years after the disease showed some abnormality, including hyperinflation, small-airway disease, or abnormal gas exchange.

BIBLIOGRAPHY

Caplan ES. Nosocomial sinusitis. *JAMA* 1982;247:639. *During a 24-month period, 34 cases of nosocomial sinusitis associated with nasopharyngeal instrumentation were identified. Gram-negative bacilli were the most frequently isolated pathogens, and polymicrobial infections were common.*

Carenfelt C. Etiology of acute infectious epiglottitis in adults: septic versus local infection. *Scand J Infect Dis* 1989;21:53. *Adult cases of acute epiglottitis hospitalized between 1975 and 1988 were retrospectively analyzed. Among 43 patients from whom adequate bacteriologic specimens were obtained, the most common pathogens identified were Haemophilus influenzae, β-hemolytic streptococci,* Streptococcus pneumoniae, *and* Staphylococcus aureus. *(Cultures were negative in 53%.)*

Chow AW. Infections of the oral cavity, neck, and head. In: Mandell GL, Douglas RG, Bennett JE, eds. *Principles and Practice of Infectious Diseases.* 3rd ed. New York: Churchill Livingstone; 1990:516. *This chapter provides an in-depth review of the pathogenesis, microbial etiology, and management of infections of the deep fascial spaces and orofacial regions.*

Denny FW, et al. Infectious agents of importance in airways and parenchymal diseases in infants and children, with particular emphasis on bronchiolitis. *Pediatr Res* 1977;11:234. *The epidemiology of bronchiolitis in a private pediatric practice was reviewed from 1966 through 1975; during this period, >6000 cases of lower respiratory tract infection were observed, 22% of which were given a diagnosis of bronchiolitis. In the population of children under 2 years of age, six to seven cases of bronchiolitis per 100 children were observed annually.*

Dingle JH, Badger GF, Jordan WS Jr. *Illness in the Home: Study of 25,000 Illnesses in a Group of Cleveland Families.* Cleveland: The Press of Western Reserve University; 1964:1. *This study details the epidemiology, clinical presentation, etiologic agents, and complications of upper respiratory tract infections, especially colds. Specific viral etiology could rarely be ascertained on clinical grounds, and as <1% of cases were complicated by bacterial sinusitis, antibiotic therapy was ineffective.*

Dobie RA, Robey DN. Clinical features of diphtheria in the respiratory tract. *JAMA* 1979;242:2197. *Forty-four cases of culture-confirmed diphtheria involving the respiratory tract were reviewed. Airway obstruction was the most common cause of death in this series, and the authors recommend prompt tracheotomy when a laryngeal membrane is observed by indirect laryngoscopy.*

Douglas RM, et al. Prophylactic efficacy of intranasal alpha₂-interferon against rhinovirus infections in the family setting. *N Engl J Med* 1986;314:65. *Intranasal alpha₂-interferon was administered daily to household contacts when respiratory symptoms developed in another family member in a prospective, double-blinded trial of alpha₂-interferon prophylaxis against naturally acquired respiratory infection. A*

protective effect was demonstrated against illness associated with rhinovirus, but not against coronavirus or influenza A and B.

Ellis EF. Prevention and treatment of respiratory infectious diseases, particularly bronchiolitis. *Pediatr Res* 1977;11:263. *The author reviews the roles of supplemental oxygen, antimicrobial agents, intravenous hydration, aerosolized adrenergic bronchodilators, intravenous aminophylline, and corticosteroids in the management of acute bronchiolitis.*

Flannery MJ. Radiographs in the diagnosis of epiglottitis (Letter). *Ann Emerg Med* 1991;20:438. *Radiography should be the initial procedure performed in stable children when suspicion of epiglottitis is low or moderate. The epiglottis of a stable child with normal radiographic findings should be visualized by a skilled physician to exclude "normal radiograph" epiglottitis.*

Gwaltney JM Jr, Sydnor A, Sande MA. Etiology and antimicrobial treatment of acute sinusitis. *Ann Otol Rhinol Laryngol* 1981;90 (Suppl 84):68. *Prospective evaluation by an otolaryngologist of 113 patients with suspected bacterial sinusitis included puncture and aspiration of the maxillary antrum. The most common bacterial isolates were the pneumococcus and* H. influenzae, *and the response rate to appropriate antimicrobial therapy was 90%.*

Hall CB, et al. Aerosolized ribavirin treatment of infants with respiratory syncytial viral infection. *N Engl J Med* 1983;308:1443. *Ribavirin or placebo was administered to 33 infants in a double-blinded manner by continuous aerosol for 3 to 6 days. By the end of treatment, infants receiving ribavirin showed a significantly greater improvement in their overall severity-of-illness score, reduction in lower respiratory tract signs, and increase in arterial oxygen saturation.*

Hutt DM, Judson FN. Epidemiology and treatment of oropharyngeal gonorrhea. *Ann Intern Med* 1986;104:655. *Sixty patients with untreated pharyngeal gonorrhea were studied. The most effective treatment regimens were aqueous procaine penicillin G and oral tetracycline.*

Jones R, Santos JI, Overall JC Jr. Bacterial tracheitis. *JAMA* 1979;242:721. *The authors reviewed eight cases of infants and children who were managed for an acute, infectious, upper airways obstructive disease with features common to both croup and epiglottitis, coined "bacterial tracheitis." Copious respiratory tract secretions were common, and six of the cases required endotracheal intubation.*

Kessler HA, et al. Diagnosis of human immunodeficiency virus infection in seronegative homosexuals presenting with an acute viral syndrome. *JAMA* 1987;258:1196. *Acute HIV infection was diagnosed in four individuals with negative HIV antibody tests presenting with fever, rash, myalgias-arthralgias, and pharyngitis by obtaining an HIV antigen test (all of which were positive).*

Komaroff AL, et al. Serologic evidence of chlamydial and mycoplasmal pharyngitis in adults. *Science* 1983;222:927. *In a study of 763 adult patients with pharyngitis, the authors found serologic evidence of infection (a fourfold increase in antibodies) with* Chlamydia trachomatis *in 20.5% and with* Mycoplasma pneumoniae *in 10.6% of the patients.*

Mayosmith MF, et al. Acute epiglottitis in adults. An eight-year experience in the state of Rhode Island. *N Engl J Med* 1986;314:1133. *Fifty-six cases of acute epiglottitis in adults were retrospectively reviewed. Indirect laryngoscopy was performed without complications and proved to be more reliable in making a diagnosis than were x-ray films of the neck.*

McGill TJ, Simpson G, Healy GB. Fulminant aspergillosis of the nose and paranasal sinuses: a new clinical entity. *Laryngoscope* 1980;90:748. *Fulminant aspergillosis of the nose and paranasal sinuses represents a new clinical entity occurring in immunocompromised individuals. It is marked by a rapidly progressive gangrenous mucoperiostitis. Control of the disease process requires radical sinus ablation, debridement of nasal structures, and antifungal chemotherapy.*

Miller RA, Brancato F, Holmes KK. Corynebacterium haemolyticum as a cause of pharyngitis and scarlatiniform rash in young adults. *Ann Intern Med* 1986;105:867. *During an 8-year period, 33 cases of* C. haemolyticum *pharyngitis were reviewed. In 20, a diffuse, erythematous, macular skin rash, often with a fine papular component, was present on the extremities and trunk. Rapid clinical improvement was seen with either penicillin or erythromycin therapy.*

Mitchell I, Inglis H, Simpson H. Viral infection in wheezy bronchitis and asthma in children. *Arch Dis Child* 1976;51:707. *Viruses were isolated in almost 15% of 360 children with wheezy bronchitis or asthma admitted to the hospital during a 3-year period. Isolation of viruses, the most common being respiratory syncytial virus and rhinovirus, was significantly more likely during February or August and for readmissions.*

Monto AS, Cavallaro JJ. The Tecumseh study of respiratory illness. II. Patterns of occurrence of infection with respiratory pathogens. *Am J Epidemiol* 1971;94:280. *During the first 3 1/2 years of the study of respiratory infections in Tecumseh, Michigan, certain repetitive, temporal patterns of isolation of infectious agents were found. For instance, rhinoviruses most commonly infected the upper respiratory tract, and such infection was associated with a low frequency of restricted activity; in contrast, parainfluenza and influenza A viruses most commonly infected the lower respiratory tract, and infection was associated with a high frequency of restricted activity.*

Seidenfeld SM, Sutker WL, Luby JP. *Fusobacterium necrophorum* septicemia following oropharyngeal infection. *JAMA* 1982;248:1348. *Anaerobic septicemia frequently is associated with an oropharyngeal source of infection, and fusobacteria are the organisms isolated most often. Proper treatment requires recognition of the oropharyngeal source of the septicemia and differentiation from endocarditis.*

Sherry MK, et al. Herpetic tracheobronchitis. *Ann Intern Med* 1988;109: 229. *In nine patients with bronchospasm unresponsive to standard therapy, bronchoscopic, cytologic, and virologic studies confirmed the presence of necrotizing and exudative tracheobronchitis caused by herpes simplex virus. All patients were successfully treated with intravenous acyclovir.*

Su WY, et al. Bacteriological study in chronic maxillary sinusitis. *Laryngoscope* 1983;93:931. *The bacterial findings from 73 maxillary sinuses in 48 patients with chronic maxillary sinusitis, obtained by intraoperative culture of the antral mucosa, were reported. Anaerobic bacteria were never isolated from sinuses that were not inflamed, but they were the most important pathogen in chronic maxillary sinusitis.*

Trollfors B. Invasive *Haemophilus influenzae* infections in household contacts of patients with *Haemophilus influenzae* meningitis and epiglottitis. *Acta Paediatr Scand* 1991;80:795. *This study showed an increased risk for invasive* H. influenzae *infections in both siblings and parents of children with invasive disease. Although rifampin prophylaxis is effective, <1% of all cases of invasive* H. influenzae *infection would be prevented.*

Wolf M, et al. Conservative management of adult epiglottitis. *Laryngoscope* 1990;100:183. *During a 10-year period, 30 adult cases of acute epiglottitis were reviewed. Two clinical forms of onset were noted (gradual and accelerated), and none of the patients required tracheotomy or intubation.*

Textbook of Pulmonary Diseases, 6th ed.
edited by G.L. Baum, J.D. Crapo, B.R. Celli, and J.B. Karlinsky,
Lippincott–Raven Publishers, Philadelphia, © 1998.

CHAPTER

24 Community-Acquired Pneumonia

Richard J. Blinkhorn, Jr.

INTRODUCTION

Community-acquired pneumonia affects almost 4 million adults annually in the United States, and as much as one fifth of these require hospitalization. Pneumonia is the sixth leading cause of death, and the No. 1 cause of death from infectious diseases. In addition, community-acquired pneumonia accounts for 1% of all patient visits to primary care providers who treat adults. In the outpatient setting, the mortality rate of pneumonia is <5%, but among patients with pneumonia who require hospitalization, mortality rates approach 25%, especially if the individual requires admission to the intensive care unit.

ETIOLOGY

No specific causative organism can be established in 30%–65% of patients with community-acquired pneumonia, despite vigorous bacteriologic and serologic testing for specific pathogens. The incidence of pneumonia attributable to individual pathogens varies considerably and depends on factors such as age, presence or absence of underlying disease, integrity of the immune response, and residence in long-term care facilities (Table 1). It is important to remember that 70%–80% of patients in whom community-acquired pneumonia develops are older than 60 years or have a coexisting medical condition. Those patients are more likely to be colonized with enteric gram-negative bacilli, staphylococci, and *Moraxella catarrhalis*

R. J. Blinkhorn, Jr.: MetroHealth Medical Center, Cleveland, Ohio 44109.

than are young, otherwise healthy persons (Table 2). These epidemiologic differences mandate using individualized diagnostic and treatment strategies based on age and the presence or absence of coexisting medical conditions. At the same time, the therapeutic approach may of necessity be largely empiric, as determination of the specific etiologic pathogen is frequently impossible.

DIAGNOSTIC STUDIES

The diagnosis of pneumonia is based on clinical findings that include respiratory symptoms (cough, sputum production, dyspnea, pleurisy), fever, abnormal sounds on chest auscultation, leukocytosis, and an infiltrate on chest film. These findings, however, may not be present in all persons with depressed immunity, in the elderly, or in individuals with so-called atypical pneumonia. Findings suggestive of pneumonia may also be seen in patients with noninfectious illnesses (e.g., pulmonary embolism, certain autoimmune diseases, and malignancy). The diagnostic confusion created by varying clinical signs is further complicated by the inherent limitations of diagnostic testing. No single test reliably establishes the presence of pneumonia. Nevertheless, the benefit of establishing the infectious cause of pneumonia early in the course of the illness is undisputed, and certain standard tests should be considered (Table 3).

A standard posteroanterior and lateral chest radiograph should be performed in all patients whose symptoms and physical examination suggest pneumonia. This test can be useful in assessing for the presence of pleural fluid, for differentiating pneumonia from conditions that may mimic it, and for demonstrating coexisting pulmonary

TABLE 1. *Prevalence of micro-organisms that cause community-acquired pneumonia*[a]

Pathogen	Percentage of cases (range)
Streptococcus pneumoniae	39 (9–76)
Haemophilus influenzae	10 (0–46)
Legionella species	5 (0–15)
Chlamydia species	5 (0–16)
Aerobic gram-negative bacilli	4 (0–20)
Viruses, including influenza virus	4 (0–18)
Staphylococcus aureus	3 (0–10)
Unknown	30 (0–49)

[a] Literature review of selected community-acquired pneumonia studies.

diseases, such as sarcoidosis or bronchiectasis. Certain radiographic findings may lead to specific diagnoses—for example, cavitation suggestive of lung abscess, apical cavitation in tuberculosis, pneumatoceles in *Staphylococcus aureus* infection, and interstitial infiltrates in mycoplasmal, viral, or *Pneumocystis carinii* infections. The finding of multilobar involvement on chest films would also be helpful in identifying individuals at risk for more severe illness.

The acquisition of expectorated sputum for Gram's stain and culture is widely recommended for the initial evaluation of community-acquired pneumonia. To be of benefit, the specimen must be obtained carefully (admixed with as few oral secretions as possible), transported and processed quickly, confirmed as cytologically adequate (>25 white blood cells and <5 epithelial cells at x100 magnification), and obtained before institution of antimicrobial therapy. The sensitivity and specificity of routine bacterial cultures of sputum are poor, and these should generally be reserved for hospitalized patients. Inability

TABLE 2. *Epidemiologic conditions related to specific pathogens in patients with community-acquired pneumonia*

Condition	Commonly encountered pathogens
Alcoholism	Oral anaerobes, gram-negative bacilli, *Streptococcus pneumoniae*
COPD	*S. pneumoniae, Haemophilus influenzae, Moraxella catarrhalis*, gram-negative bacilli
Influenza season	*S. pneumoniae, Staphylococcus aureus*, influenza virus
Nursing home residency	*S. pneumoniae*, gram-negative bacilli, oral anaerobes, *H. influenzae, S. aureus*
HIV infection	*Pneumocystis carinii, S. pneumoniae, H. influenzae, Mycobacterium tuberculosis*

COPD, chronic obstructive pulmonary disease; HIV, human immunodeficiency virus.

TABLE 3. *Diagnostic procedures for the evaluation of suspected community-acquired pneumonia*

All patients

Posteroanterior and lateral chest radiograph
Gram's stain and routine bacterial culture of sputum
Complete blood cell count

Hospitalized patients

Arterial blood gas analysis
Blood cultures
Metabolic profile (including electrolytes, renal and liver function tests)
Serologic tests (acute and convalescent)[a]
    Complement fixation (*Mycoplasma pneumoniae*)
    ELISA (IgM and IgA) (*M. pneumoniae*)
    Indirect fluorescent antibody test (*Legionella pneumophila*)
    Microimmunofluorescence (IgM and IgG) (*Chlamydia pneumoniae*)
    Specific tests for viruses, fungi, *Coxiella burnettii, C. psittaci*
    HIV antibody
Special tests[a]
    Urinary antigen test (*L. pneumophila*)
Special stains[a]
    Specific for acid-fast bacilli, *L. pneumophila, Pneumocystis carinii*
Invasive techniques
    Thoracentesis for pleural fluid analysis and culture

Severely ill patients

Invasive techniques
    Bronchoalveolar lavage
    Lung biopsy

ELISA, enzyme-linked immunosorbent assay.
[a] As determined by clinical circumstances.

to demonstrate a probable pathogen in an adequate respiratory tract sample may prompt consideration of legionellosis or infection with acid-fast bacilli, *Mycoplasma, Chlamydia, Pneumocystis,* or fungi in appropriate circumstances. Moreover, the identification on sputum Gram's stain of such virulent organisms as *S. aureus* or *Pseudomonas aeruginosa* should prompt consideration of inpatient care.

A number of invasive diagnostic techniques to obtain lower airways specimens, uncontaminated by oropharyngeal flora, have been described but are not indicated in most patients with community-acquired pneumonia. It may be useful, however, to have an early accurate diagnosis in patients who are severely ill and require admission to the intensive care unit, who are immunocompromised, or who are suspected of having HIV infection. In such patients, bronchoscopy with a protected specimen brush or bronchoalveolar lavage have reasonable sensitivity and specificity with low attendant risk and should be considered.

Routine laboratory tests are of little value in determining the etiology of pneumonia. These tests, however, may have prognostic significance, may influence the decision to hospitalize, and may affect the choice and dosing of antimicrobial therapy. Serologic testing is not useful in the initial management of pneumonia, but acute and convalescent serologic testing may help in the retrospective confirmation of a suspected diagnosis or in epidemiologic studies. Special serologic tests and stains are addressed later in the chapter as they pertain to specific etiologic agents.

HOSPITALIZATION AND SEVERE ILLNESS

The decision to hospitalize individuals with community-acquired pneumonia has historically been left to the experience and discretion of the admitting physician, as there are no firm guidelines. A series of well-recognized risk factors are indicative of an increased risk for death or

TABLE 4. *Factors that may increase morbidity and mortality in community-acquired pneumonia*

Patient

Age >65 years
Homeless
Hospitalized in past year

Coexisting illness

Alcohol abuse
Tobacco abuse
Diabetes mellitus
Immunosuppression
Neoplastic disease
Renal failure
Heart failure
Chronic lung disease
Chronic liver disease
Functional asplenia

Physical findings

Respiratory rate >30/min
Temperature >100.9°F (38.3°C)
Systolic blood pressure <90 mmHg
Diastolic blood pressure <60 mmHg
Altered mental status
Extrapulmonary disease (e.g., meningitis)

Diagnostic test results

White blood cell count <4000/μL or >30,000/μL
Anemia
PaO_2 <60 mmHg (on room air)
$PaCO_2$ >50 mmHg (on room air)
Abnormal renal function
Chest roentgenograms showing bilateral or multiple-lobe involvement or rapid progression of infiltrate within 48 hours of admission

PaO_2, partial pressure of arterial O_2; $PaCO_2$, partial pressure of arterial CO_2.

TABLE 5. *Severe community-acquired pneumonia: clinical findings and common pathogens*

Clinical findings

Respiratory rate >30/min
Severe respiratory failure (PaO_2/FIO_2 ratio <250 mmHg)
Requirement for mechanical ventilation
Chest radiograph showing bilateral or multilobar involvement, or increase in size of opacity by 50% or more within 48 h
Shock
Requirement for vasopressors for >4 h
Abnormal urine output <20 mL/h, or <80 mL in 4 h, or acute renal failure requiring dialysis

Likely causative organisms

S. pneumoniae
Legionella species
Aerobic gram-negative bacilli
Respiratory viruses

PaO_2, partial pressure of arterial O_2; FIO_2, fraction of inspired O_2.

a complicated course, and hospitalization should be strongly considered when multiple risk factors coexist (Table 4).

Multicenter prospective studies have validated these risk factors and identified five factors predictive of short-term mortality. These include age >65 years, altered mental status, abnormal vital signs, identification of a high-risk pathogen, and presence of neoplastic disease.

Although there is no universally accepted definition of severe community-acquired pneumonia, the presence of at least one of several recognized clinical findings justifies defining the illness as severe (Table 5). Severity of illness correlates well with likely etiologic pathogens. If severe pneumonia is identified, initial management in the intensive care unit is advised despite the lack of evidence that such support affects outcome.

In the remainder of this chapter, the specific pathogens most commonly encountered in patients with community-acquired pneumonia are reviewed, with an emphasis on the epidemiology, clinical presentation, diagnosis, and therapy for each. Certain pathogens may cause both community- and hospital-acquired infection, and those features unique to the hospital setting are reviewed in the following chapter.

PNEUMONIA CAUSED BY GRAM-POSITIVE BACTERIA

Pneumococcal Pneumonia

The incidence of pneumonia caused by *Streptococcus pneumoniae* has decreased sharply in many areas of the world. Surveillance studies now suggest an incidence of 20 cases of pneumonia per 100,000 young adults, as contrasted with an incidence of 700 cases per 100,000 young adults in the preantibiotic era. This reduction can be attributed in part to better hygiene and in part to the administration of antimicrobial agents to patients with upper respiratory tract infections before the onset of lower respiratory tract involvement. There is no evidence to suggest that the micro-organism is less prevalent in the community, that it has lost its virulence, or that natural host defenses have improved. Nevertheless, *S. pneumoniae* is still the most common cause of community-acquired pneumonia in patients of all ages, accounting for 15%–76% of cases in representative series.

Micro-organism

The pneumococcus, cultivated and isolated by Pasteur in 1881, is a gram-positive round, ovoid, or lanceolate coccus found in pairs or short chains. The distal ends of the paired cocci are usually pointed, and the organism has a capsule that is readily demonstrable on routine staining. More than 80 pneumococcal serotypes have been identified based on antigenic differences in their capsular polysaccharides. Serotypes are numbered in the order in which they have been identified, and virulent strains causing human disease were the earliest to be studied, identified, and assigned numbers. As a result, the lower-number serotypes are more likely to be implicated in human infection, and type 3 is considered the most virulent of the pneumococci. Unfortunately, the characteristic susceptibility of pneumococci to many antibiotic agents and the success of treatment regardless of the type involved have resulted in diminished interest in the antigenic structure of pneumococci, so that in most hospitals pneumococcal typing is no longer performed routinely. Serotyping may be useful, however, in areas experiencing an increasing incidence of penicillin-resistant pneumococcal disease. Certain serotypes (especially 6, 9, 19, and 23) have tended to be highly penicillin-resistant, and early recognition of their presence would facilitate empiric antimicrobial selection.

Susceptibility to Infection

The pneumococcus is the prototypic extracellular pathogen, capable of causing disease only as long as it remains outside phagocytes. Its rapid demise once ingested is largely the consequence of its inability to degrade its own hydrogen peroxide. The propensity for pathogenicity relates to the polysaccharide capsule that impairs phagocytosis. Effective clearance of the organism in the normal host, therefore, depends primarily on opsonization with immunoglobulin and complement. Pneumococcal infection is most prevalent in the extremes of life, with peak incidence rates occurring in newborns and infants up to 2 years old and adults in their 70s. Rates of

disease in these groups appear related to lower reservoirs of antibody or to relatively weak immunoglobulin synthesis. A healthy adult is susceptible to pneumococcal pneumonia only if antibody to the capsular polysaccharide of the infecting serotype is lacking. In contrast, pneumococcal disease is greatly increased in people who have alterations in mucociliary clearance, defects of phagocytic function, defects in humoral immunity, alcohol or narcotic intoxication, malignancy, acquired immunodeficiency syndrome, and many other specific diseases (Table 6). A peculiar relationship between exposure to extreme cold and pneumococcal pneumonia has been observed for centuries, and the putative mechanism includes alterations in mucosal metabolism with impaired ciliary activity and depressed antibody secretion.

Pathogenesis

S. pneumoniae can be recovered from the nasopharynx of almost 40% of healthy adults, and an individual may

TABLE 6. *Defects in host defense mechanisms that predispose to pneumococcal infection*

Defects of humoral systems

Immunoglobulin deficiency
   Hypogammaglobulinemia
   IgA deficiency
   IgG subclass deficiency
Inadequate immunoglobulin production
   Multiple myeloma
   Chronic lymphocytic leukemia
   Lymphoma
   Human immunodeficiency virus infection
   Sickle cell hemoglobinopathy
   Bone marrow/renal transplantation
   Chronic hemodialysis
   Trisomy 21
C2, C3, or factor I deficiency

Defects of phagocyte function

Neutropenia
Hyposplenia, splenectomy
Alcoholism

Defects of mucociliary clearance

Viral respiratory infection
Chronic pulmonary disease
Asthma
Cigarette smoking

Chronic disease

Congestive heart failure
Renal failure, nephrotic syndrome
Cirrhosis

Autoimmune disease

Immunosuppression

carry up to four different serotypes. In both adults and children, most infections occur after the recent acquisition of a new serotype rather than after prolonged carriage. Binding to the nasopharynx is affected by interconversion between two phenotypes distinguished by colonial morphology—opaque and transparent. Transparent, but not opaque, variants adhere to nasopharyngeal epithelial cells.

Pneumococci gain access to the lung via aspiration of infected mucus and can be seen lining the alveolar walls early in disease, presumably via adherence to type II pneumocytes. Progression to pneumonia, however, requires additional events, as suggested by the association of pneumonia with pre-existing viral respiratory infection and the observation that the adherence of pneumococci in vitro is enhanced by viruses and cytokines. Pneumococci, especially transparent variants, bind avidly to interleukin-1-activated pneumocytes. This may involve an interaction between phosphorylcholine of the cell wall and platelet-activating factor (PAF) receptors, the latter upregulated by cytokine stimulation. Although pneumococci are generally not considered invasive for naive endothelial cells, cytokine activation leads to prompt entry. Again, PAF receptors appear to be the target and mechanism of entry.

The lung lesion of pneumococcal lobar pneumonia evolves in four overlapping stages: engorgement, red hepatization, gray hepatization, and resolution. Initially, alveolar capillaries become intensely congested, bacteria and edematous fluid are present in alveolar spaces, and the organism multiples without inhibition (engorgement). The edema-provoking factor consists of a pneumococcal cell wall complex of peptidoglycan and teichoic acid that binds to epithelia and endothelia. It elicits the production of interleukin-1 and the accumulation of a serous exudate.

Activation of procoagulant activity on the surface of endothelial cells leads to further capillary engorgement and diapedesis of erythrocytes into the alveoli (red hepatization). Endothelial activation also leads to accentuated PAF receptor expression, which is the major effector in the lung signaling leukocyte migration. Leukocytes move into the alveolar space by two mechanisms. Half are recruited by the CD18 family of leukocyte-adhesion molecules, and the remainder by a less well-understood CD18-independent pathway that is unique to pneumococcus-induced pulmonary inflammation. As exudate accumulates in the alveoli, capillaries are compressed and leukocyte content increases, giving "gray hepatization." This leukocyte-rich exudate constitutes the first obstacle to further microbial multiplication. Before the appearance of antibody, extensive phagocytosis is achieved by a phenomenon (surface phagocytosis) in which polymorphonuclear leukocytes compress bacteria against the surface of alveoli or other leukocytes to facilitate ingestion. This defense is markedly enhanced by the appearance of specific antibody, present in detectable amounts between the fifth and tenth days, although more recent findings suggest that smaller amounts of opsonizing antibody may be pres-

ent as early as 1 or 2 days after initiation of infection. If the patient's defense mechanisms have succeeded in destroying the pneumococci, the stage of resolution is reached, and macrophages can be seen within the alveolar spaces along with cellular debris. There is typically no necrosis of alveolar walls or interstitium, and the architecture of the lung returns to normal.

Traditionally, the capsule of the pneumococcus has been considered its most important virulence factor, in that it protects the organism from phagocytosis. The capsule itself, however, is not toxic to the host, and at present pneumolysin, an intracellular protein, is the best candidate for a pneumococcus-derived toxin. Pneumolysin is not secreted but is released during bacterial lysis. It has not been identified free in the serum, but serum antibody to pneumolysin has been found after bacteremic pneumococcal pneumonia. The exact mechanism by which this toxin contributes to the virulence of the organism is unclear, but pneumolysin-negative pneumococcal mutants are significantly less virulent in mice. In addition, pneumolysin disturbs the structure and function of ciliated respiratory epithelium in vitro and is capable of inducing the salient histologic features of pneumococcal pneumonia.

Clinical Manifestations

Approximately half the patients give a history of upper respiratory tract infection followed in 2 to 14 days by evidence of lower respiratory tract involvement. The three most common early manifestations of pneumococcal pneumonia are fever, cough, and chest pain. Temperature is variable, ranging from 100°F to 106°F. Maximal fever is observed in the afternoon or evening, or it may be sustained with little diurnal change. The cough, which occurs in almost every case, is associated with the production of sputum in approximately 75% of patients. The sputum may have the classic rusty appearance, but just as often it is green (purulent). Frequently, streaks of blood are found in the sputum, and occasionally the cough is productive of frank blood. The chest pain is usually pleuritic, increasing in intensity during inspiration or cough. The pain is least severe when the patient is at rest, but the most comfortable position varies, with some patients preferring to lie with the painful side downward and others noting relief when the involved area is not in contact with any firm surface. Patients commonly feel chilly, and about half experience teeth chattering and shaking chills. Although a single shaking chill is characteristic, it is not uncommon for the patient to experience two to four such chills during a 48-hr period. Myalgia is commonly observed and may extend to tenderness of the thighs and calves. Severe myalgia, particularly that accompanied by vomiting, should strongly suggest the possibility of bacteremia. In approximately 10% of patients, herpes simplex lesions develop during the course of pneumococcal pneumonia.

Classically, physical examination reveals an acutely ill, perspiring patient who describes chest pain and splints on one side of the thorax. Tachycardia is usual in young patients, but in older patients heart rates are frequently between 70 and 100 beats/min. Examination of the chest reveals one of three findings in most patients. In some individuals, especially early in the course of the disease, bubbling rales and dullness to percussion may be the only abnormalities detected, perhaps correlating with the period of outpouring of fluid into the alveoli. A second group of patients shows the classic signs of consolidation: flatness to percussion, egophony, bronchophony, whispered pectoriloquy, and bronchial breathing. In patients with frank consolidation, frequently no rales or only a few crackling inspiratory rales are detected, and they increase as the pneumonia abates and the consolidation diminishes. In this group, a leathery pleural friction rub, heard throughout inspiration or only at the end of inspiration and expiration, may be associated with striking tenderness in the involved area of the chest. Finally, some patients may have one or more areas in which there is moderate dullness to percussion, inspiratory rales, and suppression of the breath sounds, which, although decreased in intensity, still appear harsh. As these patients presumably have mucous plugs in the smaller bronchial radicles and usually produce only scant amounts of sputum, pneumococci may not be detected in sputum cultures but found only in blood cultures. If pneumonia affects the lower lobes, abdominal pain may be a major manifestation and may be of such severity that the patient is admitted to the surgical service with a diagnosis of acute abdominal disease. In such cases, there may be considerable rigidity of the upper abdominal wall.

Laboratory Findings

The majority of patients with pneumococcal pneumonia have leukocytosis, although in 25% of cases the white blood cell count is normal. Leukopenia may be seen in overwhelming infections, and this poor prognostic factor generally occurs in alcoholic, malnourished, or elderly patients. The serum bilirubin may be increased to levels not exceeding 3 to 4 mg/dL. Levels of lactate dehydrogenase may be elevated. Hyponatremia resulting from inappropriate secretion of antidiuretic hormone has been reported. Measurement of arterial blood gases often reveals hypoxemia and occasionally hypocapnia.

Roentgenograms of the chest usually reveal dense homogeneous shadows involving all or part of one or more lobes (Fig. 1) and corroborate the findings of physical examination. If pneumococcal pneumonia is not apparent clinically, it is infrequently detected roentgenographically in an individual without chronic lung disease; however,

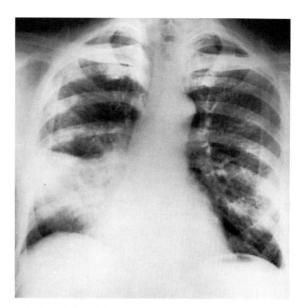

FIG. 1. Right middle lobe pneumococcal pneumonia.

in those with chronic lung disease, roentgenograms may show infiltrates that are undetectable on physical examination. In some cases, infiltrates are more patchy and less homogeneous. Those over the age of 65 may show more subtle manifestations early in the course of the disease, including less pleuritic pain and a lower incidence of shaking chills. Nevertheless, they are more likely to have multilobar involvement, and the chest x-ray film may show extensive coalescing infiltrates.

Diagnostic Microbiology

A careful study of the sputum is the most important laboratory examination. In pneumococcal pneumonia, unlike most types of viral pneumonia, many polymorphonuclear leukocytes can be readily seen in sputum smears stained with Wright's or Gram's stain. Attempts to make a diagnosis based on an inadequate sputum specimen are largely responsible for studies claiming that sputum Gram's stain and culture are not reliable. To be reliable, sputum specimens must contain areas with at least 15 to 20 white blood cells and no epithelial cells in a standard microscopic field under ×1000 magnification. The characteristic gram-positive diplococci are generally seen in abundance (Plate 1). Results of a Gram's stain of the sputum can be used to guide therapy with considerable confidence, but Gram's stains alone without confirmatory cultures are not adequate. Results of blood cultures are positive in one fourth to one third of patients hospitalized with pneumococcal pneumonia.

Therapy

In the pre-antimicrobial era, the "lysis-by-crisis" phenomenon of lobar pneumonia was one of the most dra-

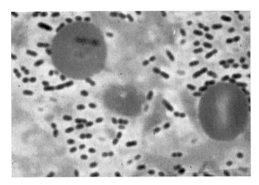

PLATE 1. *Streptococcus pneumoniae* in Gram's stain of sputum. x900. *See color plate 12.*

matic events of clinical medicine. The crisis usually occurred 6 to 10 days after infection. The patient experienced profuse sweating, the temperature could drop 5°F to 6°F, dyspnea and tachypnea disappeared, and dramatic improvement ensued. Currently, this sequence is virtually never seen, because patients are treated with antibiotics as soon as the diagnosis is seriously entertained.

Penicillin remains the drug of choice, with the overwhelming majority of strains of pneumococci being sensitive to small concentrations of the antibiotic. Uncomplicated pneumococcal pneumonia responds to intramuscular penicillin procaine (600,000 units twice daily) or to intravenous aqueous penicillin G (500,000 units every 4 hours), each administered for 7 to 10 days. There is no evidence to suggest that the administration of larger amounts of penicillin effects clinical improvement more rapidly or that larger doses are needed if associated bacteremia or multilobar involvement is present. The administration of higher doses of penicillin or broad-spectrum antimicrobial agents has been shown to increase the likelihood of colonization and superinfection with other pathogens, usually gram-negative bacilli. In patients with meningitis, endocarditis, or arthritis, 20 million units of intravenous aqueous penicillin should be given daily, whereas 5 to 10 million units daily should be adequate for patients with empyema. Oral regimens, including penicillin phenoxyethyl or phenoxymethyl (250 mg every 6 hrs) and amoxicillin (500 mg every 8 hours), are also adequate. Erythromycin, chloramphenicol, vancomycin, imipenem, and many cephalosporins have been shown to be effective in pneumococcal pneumonia, although the response to treatment may be somewhat slower than with penicillin. Tetracycline should be avoided, as 5%–15% of strains are resistant. Pneumococcal meningitis is a well-recognized complication, especially in bacteremic pneumococcal pneumonia, and antimicrobial agents that have good penetration into cerebrospinal fluid should generally be chosen. The optimal duration of therapy is unknown, but therapy for 7 to 10 days, not to exceed 5 days after defervescence, seems appropriate.

Drug-Resistant Streptococcus Pneumoniae

During the past two decades, pneumococci moderately and highly resistant to penicillin alone and pneumococci multiply resistant to various antibiotics have been found throughout the world. By definition, strains with minimal inhibitory concentrations (MICs) of <0.06 μg/mL are regarded as susceptible, those with MICs of 0.1 to 1.0 μg/mL as intermediately resistant, and those with MICs of >1.0 μg/mL as highly resistant. About 2%–25% of strains isolated in the United States show intermediate resistance. The mechanism of resistance involves alterations in penicillin-binding proteins, as the organism does not produce β-lactamase. Mutation to high-grade resistance is thought to involve the acquisition of a packet of genetic material, because resistance to other antibiotics, such as chloramphenicol, erythromycin, and clindamycin, may be present. Of importance, these multiply resistant strains have remained susceptible to vancomycin. Notably, the serotypes accounting for the majority of resistant isolates are included in the currently available pneumococcal vaccine. Serotype 23F has been significantly associated with penicillin-cefotaxime resistance. Most clinical laboratories routinely test pneumococcal isolates for resistance to penicillin using a 1-μg oxacillin disk. As this does not discriminate between intermediately and highly resistant strains, penicillin MICs are required for these oxacillin-resistant pneumococci to determine the appropriate therapeutic agents. Intermediately resistant strains are readily treatable with increased doses of penicillin (150,000 to 250,000 units per kilogram per day), cefotaxime or ceftriaxone, or vancomycin. Ceftazidime is considerably less active and should be avoided. For highly resistant pneumococci, vancomycin should be considered the drug of choice. It is uncertain whether the prognosis of pneumococcal pneumonia is affected by the finding of penicillin resistance.

Prognosis

The mortality associated with pneumococcal pneumonia in a single lobe remains at approximately 1% despite appropriate antibiotic therapy. The majority of deaths are in patients who have severe underlying, concomitant illnesses or who are in the older age groups. The presence of bacteremia, leukopenia, or involvement of two or three lobes is said to increase the mortality to approximately 10%. In older patients with bacteremia, mortality ranges from 30%–60%. Pneumococcal pneumonia in four or five lobes remains a fearful disease, with a mortality rate that approaches 50%. It should be noted that 40% of all deaths caused by pneumococcal pneumonia occur within 24 hours of admission, and antimicrobial therapy does not alter this outcome.

Complications

Empyema

Empyema is now a relatively infrequent clinical complication of pneumococcal pneumonia, but effusions can be found by diligent search in about a third of cases. In patients with empyema, pleural pain continues; fever, which may have diminished initially after penicillin treatment, persists or recurs; and the patient remains toxic. Roentgenograms, especially lateral decubitus films, aid in confirming the diagnosis (Fig. 2).

In all patients in whom empyema is strongly indicated, a diagnostic thoracocentesis should be performed. Fluid obtained shortly after the onset of empyema is cloudy and may contain 1000 to 600,000 leukocytes per milliliter, virtually all of which are polymorphonuclear cells. If the fluid is infected, its pH is usually <7.30. If empyema is untreated, the fluid subsequently assumes the appearance of frank pus. Initially, treatment may be conservative, consisting of repeated thoracocentesis. If the fluid does not become progressively thinner or if adequate drainage is not achieved, closed or preferably open thoracotomy should be performed.

Collection of sterile fluid. Although the cell count of this fluid may be high, ranging up to 300,000/mm^3, the percentage of mononuclear cells is usually considerably greater than that observed in empyema and the pH is >7.30. Even small effusions of this nature are causes for prolonged fever, and such fluids should be drained by needle aspiration.

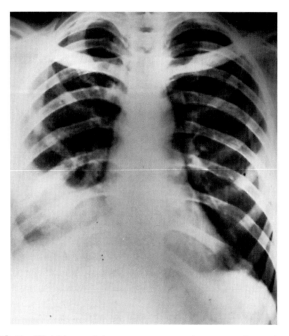

FIG. 2. Right lower lobe pneumococcal pneumonia and empyema in a 34-year-old man.

Pericarditis

Precordial chest pain, persistent fever, or hypotension suggests the possibility of spread to the pericardium, an infrequent but dangerous complication of pneumococcal pneumonia. The three most reliable early signs in acute purulent pericarditis are the presence of a pericardial friction rub, the development of retrosternal dullness to percussion, and the appearance of Ewart's sign posteriorly at the angle of the scapula on the left or in the left basilar paravertebral area. Cardiac tamponade may develop in patients with pericarditis. Treatment of pericardial effusion is in general similar to that for empyema: aspiration and, if necessary, open pericardial drainage. If only a small effusion is present, no drainage may be needed.

Lung Abscess

Lung abscess following lobar pneumonia is extremely rare and occurs most frequently after infection with type 3 pneumococcus, which has a large capsule that inhibits phagocytosis. Prolonged antibiotic therapy (2 to 4 weeks) is usually required, and lung destruction may be so extensive that subsequent surgical intervention is necessary. There is no evidence that an abscess heals more quickly if the penicillin dose is increased or if multiple antibiotics are administered, but the risk for superinfection is great (Fig. 3). Occasionally, the abscess occurs because of a concomitant aerobic or anaerobic infection; in such cases, a change in the therapeutic regimen is mandatory.

Atelectasis

Persistent fever and increasing dyspnea suggest atelectasis, which can usually be confirmed roentgenographically (Fig. 4). Vigorous tracheal suction and forced coughing may clear the mucous plugs, but if these procedures are not successful, bronchoscopy should be undertaken.

Delayed Resolution

Continued low-grade fever, rales, moderate dullness to percussion, and roentgenographic infiltrate may persist as long as 4 to 6 weeks in the absence of evidence of underlying bronchiectasis, obstructing neoplasm, or pulmonary superinfection (Fig. 5). This delayed resolution occurs primarily among older patients, in those suffering from malnutrition or alcoholism, and in some patients with chronic bronchitis, emphysema, and fibrosis. As the healing process cannot be hastened, it is fortunate that this common complication is benign. Repeated bacteriologic studies of sputum should be undertaken, and a single antibiotic agent may be continued at conventional dosage.

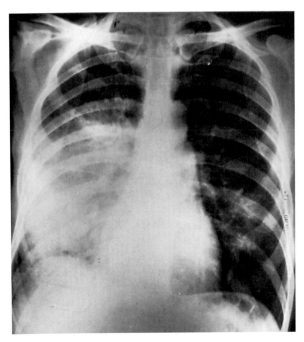
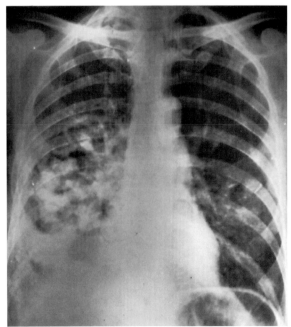

FIG. 3. Right lower lobe pneumococcal pneumonia (*left*) in a 46-year-old alcoholic, with abscess formation (*right*).

In addition, bronchoscopy and cytologic examination of the sputum should be performed, as a small but significant number of these patients have obstructing neoplasms.

Endocarditis

In the course of bacteremia, pneumococci may light on normal or damaged heart valves, chordae tendineae, or papillary muscles. Endocarditis may occur concomitantly

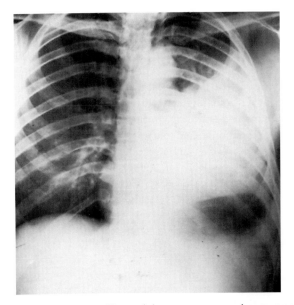

FIG. 4. Left upper and lower lobe pneumococcal pneumonia and atelectasis.

with the pneumonia, or there may be an excellent response to treatment of the pulmonary infection, followed by a period without fever and then a recurrence of fever after antibiotics have been discontinued. If endocardial involvement is associated with fever and other evidence of active infection, vigorous treatment should be undertaken: a minimum of 6 million units of penicillin per day for at least 4 weeks. However, when these cardiac complications occur in the absence of fever or evidence of active infection, they probably represent late rupture of a valve, chorda, or papillary muscle that was damaged by infection acquired during the bacteremia accompanying the pneumonia but was bacteriologically sterilized by treatment of the pneumonia. In these patients, a trial of antibiotics is warranted, but there is no evidence that the disease will be modified by such therapy. Surgical intervention may be necessary. Patients in whom pneumococcal endocarditis develops following pneumonia not infrequently have simultaneous evidence of pneumococcal meningitis.

Meningitis

One third to one half of adult patients with pneumococcal meningitis have concomitant or pre-existing pneumococcal pneumonia. Any patient with pneumococcal pneumonia who evidences disorientation, confusion, or somnolence should have a lumbar puncture to evaluate the possibility of pneumococcal meningitis. Although involvement of the meninges is usually apparent clinically, the manifestations can be extremely subtle.

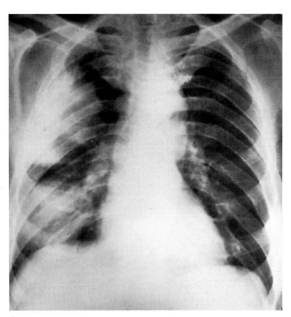
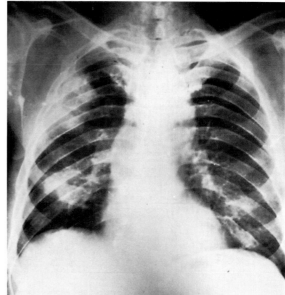

FIG. 5. Pneumococcal pneumonia (*left*) in a 40-year-old alcoholic with slow resolution within a 1-month period (*right*).

There is some controversy as to the most effective treatment of pneumococcal meningitis, but it is unanimously agreed that an adequate regimen is large amounts of aqueous penicillin administered intravenously (minimal daily adult dose being 10 million units). Alternatives to penicillin include ampicillin, chloramphenicol, and a cephalosporin (cefuroxime, cefotaxime, or ceftriaxone). If moderately resistant strains of *S. pneumoniae* infect the meninges, penicillin is usually not effective.

Gangrene

On rare occasions, pneumococcal sepsis is followed by gangrene involving fingers, toes, nose, lips, and earlobes. In such cases, there is usually evidence of disseminated intravascular coagulation. This complication is particularly prevalent in those who have had a splenectomy.

Jaundice

Modest increases in serum bilirubin concentrations may occur in patients with pneumococcal pneumonia. Transaminase concentrations may be markedly elevated. The mechanisms underlying the jaundice are not adequately defined, and the bilirubinemia ordinarily disappears in a few days. Physicians often forget that pneumococcal pneumonia may be associated with jaundice; the incorrect diagnosis most often made is Legionnaires' disease, because of the combination of pneumonia and liver dysfunction.

Prevention

The role of polyvalent pneumococcal vaccine is still unsettled. In some studies, it seems to be reasonably effective; in others, it does not. It is not entirely clear who should be vaccinated, although those with gamma globulin deficiencies, alcoholics, those over the age of 60 in institutions for long-term care, patients with sickle cell disease, HIV-infected patients, and those who have undergone splenectomy are certainly prime candidates. Some advocate the vaccine for all persons over the age of 60.

Streptococcal Pneumonia

In the pre-antimicrobial era, pneumonia resulting from group A β-hemolytic streptococci (*Streptococcus pyogenes*) was not uncommon in children after measles or pertussis or in adults after influenza. During the influenza pandemic of 1918–1919, severe streptococcal pneumonia, often culminating in death, assumed epidemic proportions in many areas of the world. The incidence of streptococcal pneumonia and bacteremia decreased markedly after the discovery and use of penicillin, but in recent years there has been an unexplained recrudescence of serious streptococcal disease. Currently, the total number of cases reported still is small, occurring for the most part in the very young, the very old, and the debilitated. Numerous epidemics have been reported in military recruit populations.

Clinical Manifestations

The onset is typically abrupt, with shaking chills, fever, and cough productive of purulent sputum. Hemoptysis and pleuritic chest pain are commonly observed. Cyanosis is noted in more severe cases. Rales and dullness are found on examination, but signs of frank consolidation are detected less frequently. The radiographic picture is that of bronchopneumonia, although one or more focal areas of pneumonitis may be seen. Empyema develops in 30%–40% of cases, and rapid pleural involvement is considered characteristic of this type of pneumonia.

Laboratory Findings

The leukocyte count is characteristically elevated, with a preponderance of mature and immature polymorphonuclear cells. Gram's stain of the sputum shows many polymorphonuclear leukocytes and gram-positive cocci in chains. An increasing percentage of streptococcal pneumonias are caused not by group A organisms, but rather by organisms belonging to groups B through G. Although specific clinical patterns have not been adequately defined for each group, it appears that *Streptococcus agalactiae* (group B) and *Streptococcus milleri* have the greatest propensity for abscess formation. Additionally, microaerophilic or anaerobic streptococci can cause pneumonia; in these cases, necrotizing pneumonia with empyema is frequently found.

In neonates, group B streptococci cause sepsis and diffuse pneumonitis. These infants, who become sick shortly after birth, are frequently very ill, with marked tachypnea and cyanosis. Roentgenograms usually show bilateral alveolar and interstitial infiltrates; in some cases, focal pneumonitis may be seen. Maternal vaginal colonization is the major risk factor for such infections.

Therapy

Penicillin is clearly the antibiotic of choice. Approximately 25% of group A β-hemolytic streptococci are no longer susceptible to tetracyclines. A penicillin dosage of 600,000 units two to four times a day is usually adequate, but some anaerobic streptococci are more resistant, requiring 3 to 6 million units per day. Cephalosporins, semisynthetic penicillins, erythromycin, and vancomycin can be used as alternatives to penicillin. If the infection is caused by group B, C, or G, therapy must depend on in vitro studies. Once severe streptococcal pneumonia is established, it may become a fulminating disease even if adequate amounts of antibiotics are administered. This is particularly true in group B infections in neonates, with mortality in these infants being about 30%. In adults, this characteristic is undoubtedly related in part to its frequent occurrence in persons whose antimicrobial defenses are impaired. In patients with empyema, conservative therapy with repeated thoracocentesis should be tried, especially while the fluid is still thin. Closed or open chest tube drainage may be needed for loculated fluid.

Staphylococcal Pneumonia

In previously healthy, young adults, *S. aureus* rarely causes pneumonia. Local pulmonary or systemic defenses of the host must be compromised before the organism can produce progressive disease. *S. aureus* accounts for 2%–9% of community-acquired pneumonias in the elderly or in patients with concomitant conditions, such as diabetes mellitus, chronic renal failure, bronchiectasis, lung carcinoma, defective polymorphonuclear leukocyte phagocytosis or killing, and intravenous substance abuse, or who are residents in a facility for long-term care. Infections may also occur in previously healthy adults following viral influenza with resultant impairment in bronchopulmonary clearance mechanisms.

Clinical Manifestations

The clinical manifestations of staphylococcal pneumonia vary considerably, depending on the setting in which it occurs. In the majority of patients who acquire the disease outside the hospital, especially those in whom staphylococcal pneumonia develops after viral influenza, the onset is sudden. Fever occurs uniformly and may be remittent or sustained in type. Most patients have pleuritic chest pain, shaking chills, and cough productive of sputum that is usually purulent and on occasion may also be blood-streaked. Gross hemoptysis occurs in a small number of patients. In infants and young children, cough and chest pain may be minimal, and the major manifestations are fever, dyspnea, and cyanosis.

On physical examination, the majority of patients appear extremely ill, with tachypnea, tachycardia, and commonly pleuritic pain. Cyanosis is often found, but hypotension is recorded infrequently. The findings on examination of the chest are generally indistinguishable from those already described for pneumococcal pneumonia. A pleural friction rub may be heard, accompanied by evidence of pleural fluid.

Laboratory Findings

Gram's stain of the sputum shows many polymorphonuclear leukocytes with intracellular and extracellular large, round cocci arranged in clusters. Specimens obtained from patients with staphylococcal pneumonia almost invariably show a heavy and virtually pure growth of *S. aureus*. If only small numbers are present, or if staphylococci are not clearly predominant, then staphylococcal pneumonia is an unlikely diagnosis.

For most adults with staphylococcal pneumonia, blood culture results are negative, the incidence of bacteremia being higher in infants. Leukocyte counts of $1000/mm^3$ or less in individuals whose counts were previously normal are associated with a poor prognosis.

Chest roentgenograms typically show consolidation in a lobe or in smaller segments of one or more lobes. In some patients, patchy infiltrates in several areas of the lung suggest diffuse bronchopneumonia, and occasionally what appears to be an interstitial infiltrate is observed. Pleural or interlobar fluid may be detected. Single or multiple radiolucencies are often found in the areas of infiltration. In infants, pneumatoceles occur as frequently as abscesses, whereas in adults the radiolucencies almost invariably represent abscess formation. As cyst and abscess formation are not complications of staphylococcal pneumonia but rather an intrinsic part of the natural history of the disease, their presence does not imply a poor prognosis. Furthermore, the appearance of these lesions on the roentgenogram does not indicate failure of antibiotic therapy and does not necessitate a change in the antistaphylococcal regimen. In successfully treated patients, the vast majority of the abscesses and cysts disappear spontaneously and do not require adjunctive surgical treatment (Fig. 6). The x-ray film should ordinarily distinguish between upper respiratory tract-acquired and embolic staphylococcal pneumonia.

Treatment

The mortality among patients who have been treated for staphylococcal pneumonia varies from 15%–50% in different series. Because mortality depends on the virulence of the micro-organism, the ability of the host to mobilize defenses, and the severity of the underlying disease, it is difficult to predict the outcome in any one individual, but it is clear that the presence of leukopenia and the demonstration of bacteremia are ominous prognostic signs.

Therapy should be initiated with large, parenterally administered doses of a penicillinase-resistant semisynthetic penicillin (methicillin, nafcillin, cloxacillin, or oxacillin) or a first-generation cephalosporin. Primarily bacteriostatic agents, including tetracycline, erythromycin, and chloramphenicol, are not advised as initial treatment in seriously ill patients. Clindamycin has significant antistaphylococcal activity but should not be considered a first-line agent. Imipenem also may be effective.

An increasing percentage of both community-acquired and nosocomial cases of staphylococcal pneumonia are caused by methicillin-resistant strains; for these, vancomycin given alone or together with either rifampin or an aminoglycoside is the agent of choice.

In vitro and in vivo animal studies suggest that in severely ill patients, the addition of an aminoglycoside to an agent such as oxacillin or nafcillin results in more rapid killing of the staphylococci. Although convincing clinical data are not now available, the current recommendation is that gentamicin or tobramycin be added to the semisynthetic penicillin for 5 to 7 days if the staphylococcal infection is overwhelming or life-threatening. Rifampicin is an effective intracellular antistaphylococcal agent and may be a useful addition to the antimicrobial regimen in recalcitrant cases.

Treatment should be continued for a minimum of 14 days. Even if adequate and appropriate therapy is given immediately, defervescence may be slow. Persistence of a moderately elevated temperature for 1 to 2 weeks does not in itself necessitate a change in the therapeutic regimen.

Complications

Meningitis

Staphylococcal meningitis with or without clinical evidence of brain abscess may complicate staphylococcal pneumonia. Cerebrospinal fluid examination reveals a variable cell count with a preponderance of polymorphonuclear leukocytes. The protein is elevated, but the glucose level may or may not be reduced. Treatment depends on in vitro susceptibility studies.

Empyema

Empyema develops in 15%–40% of patients with staphylococcal pneumonia, and *S. aureus* still accounts

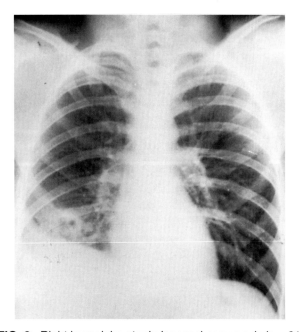

FIG. 6. Right lower lobe staphylococcal pneumonia in a 21-year-old man with prior viral influenza. Note two abscesses in the pneumonic area. These resolved completely in 2 weeks without a change in antistaphylococcal therapy. (Reproduced with copyright permission of The American Society for Clinical Investigation from Louria DB, et al. Studies on influenza in the pandemic of 1957–1958: II. Pulmonary complications of influenza. *J Clin Invest* 1959;38:213.)

for about one third of all cases of pleural empyema. Acute empyema usually arises by direct extension from pneumonia or lung abscess, and therapy is similar to that described for empyema in pneumococcal pneumonia. Insertion of a chest tube, however, is usually necessary, and the presence of very thick pus makes open surgical drainage advisable early in the course of this disease.

Large Abscesses

Lung abscesses (Fig. 7) or pneumatoceles may become large enough to impair pulmonary function, or they may become secondarily infected. Under such conditions, drainage or excision by lobectomy is necessary.

Pneumothorax

A not uncommon complication, especially in infants and children, pneumothorax is not usually of grave prognostic import. Treatment depends on the size; a small pneumothorax will resolve spontaneously, but if a large pneumothorax or a tension pneumothorax is present, tube drainage should be used.

Bronchopleural Fistula

This complication usually occurs in patients who have underlying pulmonary diseases. It may be treated by surgical drainage of the empyema and prolonged antimicrobial therapy, but persistent fistulas should be excised surgically.

Miscellaneous Causes of Gram-Positive Pneumonia

Bacillus species can cause severe pneumonia in the compromised host. Only a small number of cases have been reported; most of the patients have had acute or subacute leukemia. However, in one case lethal grampositive *Bacillus* pneumonia occurred in a previously healthy individual. The organism usually isolated is *Bacillus cereus,* but lethal pneumonia also has been caused by *Bacillus subtilis. B. cereus* multiplies within blood vessels, and as a result wedge-shaped, infarctlike lesions may be seen roentgenologically. Abscesses, cavities, and pneumonic infiltrates also may be found. The sputum is usually bloody, and pleural effusions are found frequently. The antibiotic regimen of choice depends on in vitro sensitivity patterns. The *Bacillus* species isolated from patients with pneumonia have been inhibited by tetracycline, erythromycin, aminoglycosides, and chloramphenicol.

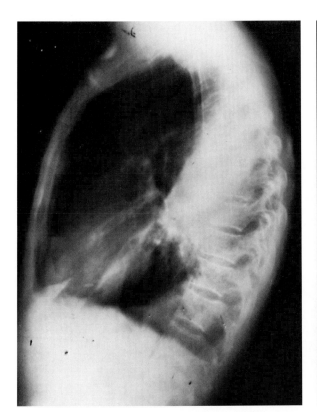 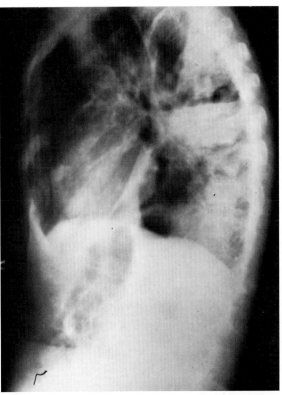

FIG. 7. Staphylococcal pneumonia (*left*) in a 47-year-old man. A large abscess (*right*) developed 1 week later.

Corynebacterium (Rhodococcus) equi is a gram-positive coccobacillus responsible for suppurative bronchopneumonia in horses. In patients who are immunosuppressed, either because of an underlying disease or medications, the organism can cause severe pneumonia, with lobar or lobular infiltrates, infarctlike lesions, abscesses, or cavities. Manifestations include cough, chest pain, and hemoptysis. Pleural effusion may be present, and the organism may be recovered from the sputum or only from bronchial washings and/or pleural fluid. Erythromycin is thought to be the antimicrobial agent of choice (the isolates are also likely to be sensitive to vancomycin, gentamicin, tetracycline, and kanamycin), but too few cases have been reported to make a judgment about an optimal antimicrobial regimen.

Necrotizing pneumonia and empyema may be caused by *Clostridium perfringens*. Some cases follow trauma, surgery, or thoracocentesis, but in others no precipitating event has been noted. Pleural gas may be noted. Hemolysis, renal failure, and profound mental confusion are not present, as they are systemic clostridial infections, and the disease ranges from surprisingly mild to life-threatening. Penicillin, clindamycin, metronidazole, and chloramphenicol appear to be the agents of choice.

PNEUMONIA CAUSED BY GRAM-NEGATIVE BACTERIA

Community-acquired pneumonia is virtually never caused by enteric gram-negative bacilli in previously healthy, young adults. However, these organisms, predominantly Enterobacteriaceae, have been implicated in 3%–15% of cases. This relatively high prevalence of gram-negative bacillary pneumonia in large part reflects the inclusion of debilitated or elderly patients with serious pre-existing diseases. On the other hand, *Haemophilus influenzae* and *Moraxella (Branhamella) catarrhalis* have been increasingly recognized as pulmonary pathogens and account for 8%–20% and 1%–3%, respectively, of cases of community-acquired pneumonia.

Hemophilus influenzae Pneumonia

Because *H. influenzae* is part of the commensal oral flora, this organism was largely unappreciated as a significant pulmonary pathogen until recently. In recent years, there has been a clear increase in the occurrence of *H. influenzae* pneumonia, and it is second only to pneumococcal pneumonia as the most common community-acquired pneumonia in adults. *H. influenzae* pneumonia occurs in perfectly healthy people; in persons with chronic lung disease or other severe, underlying disease; in patients who have undergone splenectomy; and among chronic heavy abusers of alcohol. There is also an increased incidence in patients with disorders of gamma globulin synthesis, including those with chronic lymphocytic leukemia, multiple myeloma, human immunodeficiency virus infection, and the various IgG deficiencies. During epidemics of viral influenza, the incidence of *H. influenzae* pneumonia increases.

Kaplan and Braude, noting that severe infections with bacteremia occurred among adults primarily in alcoholics, performed studies suggesting that serum factors active against *H. influenzae* were less effective in patients with cirrhosis. Reduced effectiveness also was observed immediately after the ingestion of alcohol. These authors postulated that this relationship might be responsible for the enhanced susceptibility of these individuals.

Micro-organism

H. influenzae is a pleomorphic, gram-negative, coccobacillary organism. When grown under unfavorable conditions, it may appear filamentous and elongated and be mistaken for enteric gram-negative rods. It is a fastidious organism requiring special media that supply both X and V factors, such as chocolate or Levinthal agar. It may be recognized in sputum by Gram's stain (Plate 2) or by detection of specific capsular antigen. The encapsulated serotypes of *H. influenzae* (types a through f) can be differentiated by a variety of methods, including slide agglutination, counterimmunoelectrophoresis, and fluorescent antibody techniques. Each method is based on the use of antibodies directed against the capsular polysaccharide, a polymer of ribose and ribitol-5-phosphate.

Pathogenesis

The development of invasive disease caused by *H. influenzae* follows colonization of the upper respiratory tract. The nasopharyngeal carriage rate for nontypeable strains varies from 50%–80%, in contrast to the carriage rate for type b *H. influenzae*, which is estimated at 3%–5%. Type b *H. influenzae* is responsible for 95% of systemic disease in children and a significant percentage of

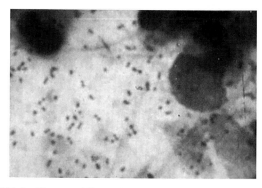

PLATE 2. *Haemophilus influenzae* in Gram's stain of sputum. X900. *See color plate 13.*

invasive bacteremic infections in adults. In contrast, non-typeable *H. influenzae* strains generally cause less severe local infection that spreads in a contiguous fashion within the respiratory tract, and these are the most common isolates causing pneumonia in adults.

Clinical Presentation

Two distinct presentations of *H. influenzae* pneumonia are recognized. The first occurs in infants or in patients with alcoholism or underlying immunodeficiency. In these individuals, the onset is typically rapid, with chills, fever, cough productive of purulent sputum, and pleural pain; the clinical features are indistinguishable from those of pneumococcal or other bacillary pneumonias. Bacteremia is common (up to 75% of cases in children), and the causative organism is almost always type b. Type b strains are responsible for about 10%–15% of pneumonias in adults. In contrast, adults with chronic lung disease usually experience a gradual onset, with low-grade fever, cough, increasing sputum production, worsening dyspnea, and occasionally myalgias and arthralgias. Bacteremia is rare in this setting, and the causative strain is invariably nontypeable.

Roentgenograms frequently show segmental lobar consolidation, but patchy bronchopneumonia and multilobular infiltrates may be seen. In patients with chronic lung disease, the initial chest radiographic findings may not be considered abnormal until after therapy, when improvement occurs in an area previously interpreted as chronic interstitial disease. Cavitary disease and empyema occur rarely, but parapneumonic effusions may occur in up to half of patients.

Diagnosis cannot be based solely on isolation of *H. influenzae* from the sputum, because nasopharyngeal carriage rates are so high. In addition, *H. influenzae* can be recovered from the sputum of most patients with chronic bronchitis if serial cultures are performed. Unless the organism is isolated from the bloodstream or pleural space, the diagnosis of *H. influenzae* pneumonia remains probable at best. Serologic methods, measuring antibodies against nonencapsulated *H. influenzae* strains by ELISA (enzyme-linked immunosorbent assay) from paired sera, may increase the ability to diagnose true *Haemophilus* infections. The sensitivity of this specific approach, however, is low.

Therapy

Until the early 1970s, *H. influenzae* was nearly uniformly susceptible to ampicillin, but during the past two decades, plasmid-mediated, β-lactamase-producing, ampicillin-resistant strains have been noted with increasing frequency. These organisms now constitute the majority of isolates in many centers. Chloramphenicol susceptibility has been preserved, however, as very few chloramphenicol-resistant strains have been reported. Ampicillin is not recommended as initial therapy, unless drug-susceptibility profiles confirm sensitivity. Type b *H. influenzae* has a propensity for invading the meninges, and empiric therapy ideally should have good cerebrospinal fluid penetration. Reasonable choices for initial therapy of invasive *Haemophilus* infections would therefore include ampicillin/sulbactam, chloramphenicol, second- or third-generation cephalosporins, and trimethoprim/sulfamethoxazole. Alternative agents include imipenem/cilastatin, azithromycin or clarithromycin, and the fluoroquinolones, but the cerebrospinal fluid penetration may not be as reliable.

Active immunization against type b *H. influenzae* is now possible, as a vaccine composed of purified type b polysaccharide (PRP) is available. One of these commercially available PRP-conjugated vaccines should be routinely administered to children over the age of 15 months and to adults with conditions predisposing to invasive *Haemophilus* infection.

Outcome

Complications of *Haemophilus* pneumonia include empyema, meningitis, and septic arthritis. All are more likely to occur in the setting of bacteremia, alcoholism, splenectomy, or immunoglobulin deficiency. Mortality rates associated with *Haemophilus* pneumonia are <5% in young, healthy adults, but may be as high as 20%–30% among debilitated, elderly patients.

Moraxella (Branhamella) catarrhalis Pneumonia

Since Osler's time, when the organism was referred to as *Micrococcus catarrhalis,* this gram-negative coccobacillary organism has undergone several name changes. The designation *Neisseria catarrhalis* reflected its resemblance to *Neisseria* in appearance, but DNA homology suggested the genus be transferred to *Moraxella.* In 1970, in honor of Dr. Sarah Branham (for her contributions to the taxonomy of *Neisseria* species), the organism was assigned the genus *Branhamella.* At present, many prefer the designation *Branhamella,* as *Moraxella* implies limited pathogenicity.

This organism has long been recognized as an oropharyngeal commensal, and several studies have established that *B. catarrhalis* colonizes the nasopharynx of up to 7.4% of adults and 30% of children. *B. catarrhalis* is one of the three most common bacteria responsible for exacerbations of chronic bronchitis, and recent studies suggest it is responsible for 1%–3% of community-acquired pneumonias.

Micro-organism

B. catarrhalis is a gram-negative diplococcus shaped like a kidney bean, with its long axes paired side to side. The resemblance of a sputum Gram's stain from a patient with *B. catarrhalis* respiratory tract disease to the urethral smear from a patient with gonorrhea is striking. The organism readily grows on blood agar and can be easily distinguished from *Neisseria* species on the basis of sugar fermentation reactions. At present, 80%–90% of stains produce β-lactamase.

Clinical Manifestations

Chronic obstructive pulmonary disease is the most consistently reported underlying illness associated with *B. catarrhalis* respiratory tract infection, and the mean age of patients exceeds 60 years. Almost three fourths of infected patients are immunocompromised as a consequence of corticosteroid use, diabetes mellitus, or malignancy. Immunoglobulin deficiency is a quantitatively less important risk factor, but the clinical course appears more severe in this setting. More than 85% of cases occur from October through May.

Most cases of *B. catarrhalis* pneumonia are mild and present in a fashion suggesting an exacerbation of chronic bronchitis. There generally is minimal change in the patient's chronic cough, weakness, or dyspnea. In one fourth of patients, chills occur; in one third, pleuritic chest pain is present. Bacteremia, high fever, myalgias, pleural effusion, and empyema are rare. Patchy bronchopneumonia and interstitial or mixed interstitial-alveolar infiltrates are characteristic radiographic features. Lobar consolidation occurs in fewer than one third.

Diagnosis based on the traditional criterion of isolating the organism from blood or pleural fluid is difficult, as bacteremia and empyema are uncommon. A presumptive diagnosis of *B. catarrhalis* pneumonia is suggested by the clinical and radiographic signs of pneumonia, a good-quality sputum Gram's stain showing a predominance of gram-negative diplococci, and heavy growth of the organism on culture. It should be recognized that *B. catarrhalis* is frequently cocultured with other pathogens, especially *S. pneumoniae* and *H. influenzae*.

Therapy

Although 80%–90% of strains of *B. catarrhalis* produce β-lactamase, most of these strains have MICs to ampicillin of 2 μg/mL or less and are not labeled ampicillin-resistant. Clinical evidence suggests that all β-lactamase-producing strains of *B. catarrhalis* be considered ampicillin-resistant. Fortunately, these *B. catarrhalis* β-lactamases are inactivated by clavulanic acid and sulbactam, and have only moderate activity against second-

or third-generation cephalosporins. Alternative, non-β-lactam antimicrobial agents include tetracycline, erythromycin, trimethoprim/sulfamethoxazole, and fluorinated quinolones.

Mortality directly attributable to pneumonia caused by *B. catarrhalis* is rare. Recent studies, however, have shown that up to 45% of patients die within 3 months, usually as a result of the underlying disease.

Neisseria meningitidis Pneumonia

Neisseria meningitidis was first reported as a respiratory pathogen after the influenza pandemic of 1918 and 1919. Thereafter, almost half a century elapsed before a renewed interest in the meningococcus as a cause of lower respiratory tract infection emerged in the 1970s. A majority of cases of meningococcal pneumonia have occurred in military populations, but this may only be a consequence of the ongoing surveillance of meningococcal disease by the armed forces. The association of meningococcal disease with antecedent influenza or adenoviral infection is well-known. Although spread of meningococcal infection beyond the nasopharynx almost exclusively requires bloodstream invasion, an inhalational rather than hematogenous pathogenesis is likely for meningococcal pneumonia.

There is nothing distinctive about its clinical presentation, and the onset may be sudden or more indolent. Patchy, lobular, or lobar infiltrates may be found, and in some cases, the pleura is involved. Bacteremia occurs in 15%–26% of cases. The presence of *N. meningitidis* in expectorated sputum may be easily overlooked unless it is specifically sought, and the use of selective culture media, such as Thayer-Martin medium, is helpful.

Confirmation of the meningococcus as the causative organism in bacterial pneumonia can be difficult. *N. meningitidis* can be recovered from the nasopharynx of 7%–13% of asymptomatic outpatients, and up to 30% of patients with acute respiratory infections but no clinical or radiographic signs of pneumonia have meningococcus-positive sputum. Therefore, to assign a causative role for the organism in pneumonia with confidence, it is necessary to isolate it from blood, pleural fluid, or lung aspirate.

The meningococci have remained broadly antibiotic-sensitive, and rapid clinical improvement on therapy is the rule. It should be noted that the administration of antibiotics (as opposed to sulfonamides) does not usually eliminate the carrier state. Rifampin and sulfonamides are effective agents for eradication of the carrier state and for prophylaxis of close contacts, but because of increasing reports of sulfonamide resistance, susceptibility studies should be performed.

Klebsiella pneumoniae (Friedländer's) Pneumonia

Micro-organism

In 1882, Friedländer discovered the organism that came to bear his name. It is a pleomorphic, encapsulated, fat, gram-negative rod that grows rapidly and aerobically on ordinary bacteriologic media. Four years later, in 1886, Escherich described *Aerobacter aerogenes*. Classified as separate species until recently, the two organisms are antigenically so similar that they have been combined into a single *Klebsiella* genus. *Klebsiella* types 1 through 6 are identical to Friedländer's bacillus types a through f, and *Klebsiella* types 7 through 80 are probably members of the old *A. aerogenes* group.

There are certain striking differences between Friedländer's bacillus (*Klebsiella* types 1 through 6) and higher *Klebsiella* serotypes: (1) Colonies of Friedländer's bacillus are far more mucoid and sticky because of their much larger capsules. (2) Differences in virulence for mice are marked. Friedländer's bacillus produces death within 24 to 48 hours after the intraperitoneal inoculation of small numbers of organisms, frequently <100 per mouse. Deaths after intraperitoneal infection with higher *Klebsiella* serotypes, on the other hand, rarely occur even at an inoculum size of a million organisms per mouse; indeed, many strains produce death only irregularly after an injection of 100 million to a billion bacteria per mouse. (3) The settings in which these two organisms cause pulmonary disease are not similar. Friedländer's bacillus characteristically produces pneumonia in men who are >40 years old and who are alcoholics or have chronic underlying disease, usually pulmonary in nature. Most patients with Friedländer's pneumonia enter the hospital with the disease. In contrast, pneumonia resulting from higher *Klebsiella* serotypes is usually acquired within the hospital environment, occurring in patients who are extensively treated with antibiotics and in whom pneumonia subsequently develops.

In the following discussion, the term *Friedländer's pneumonia* refers only to that caused by *Klebsiella* serotypes 1 through 6, most commonly types 1 and 2. Pulmonary infections caused by higher *Klebsiella* serotypes are discussed with pulmonary disease caused by *Escherichia coli*.

Clinical Manifestations

Friedländer's pneumonia, which accounts for <2% of patients hospitalized with bacterial pneumonia, is usually sudden in onset, with fever, cough, and pleuritic chest pain. In a minority of individuals, the cough is productive of the typical thick, gelatinous, red sputum. Most patients expectorate thick, greenish, purulent material that is frequently streaked with blood, whereas in some patients the cough is productive of frankly bloody sputum. On admission, patients may be seriously ill, with severe dyspnea, tachypnea, striking cyanosis, and hypotension, although many persons have considerably milder forms of the disease. Physical examination generally reveals the classic signs of consolidation, but sometimes only dullness to percussion, inspiratory rales, and diminished breath sounds are observed, the latter apparently because of obstruction of the smaller bronchi by plugs of gelatinous material. In some series, as many as one fifth of the patients have visible icterus.

Laboratory Findings

Gram's stain of the sputum shows many polymorphonuclear leukocytes and a myriad of short, fat, gram-negative, heavily encapsulated rods. The pleomorphism of the organism is frequently marked, and it may be so gram-variable that on examination of the sputum smear, a diagnosis of pneumococcal pneumonia may be made, especially by inexperienced observers. The leukocyte count is extremely variable. Although leukocytosis, sometimes with a count of up to 40,000/mm^3, is the rule, normal leukocyte counts or leukopenia may be observed. Frequently, normocytic, normochromic anemia either is present on admission or develops with startling rapidity after hospitalization. Blood culture results are positive in 20%–50% of cases.

The pneumonia more often affects the right side, with a predilection for the lower lobes and the posterior segment of the upper lobes, which suggests that the organisms have been aspirated from the mouth. Roentgenograms characteristically show massive consolidation with a fissure that bulges outward; this is apparently related to the extensive edema observed histologically (Fig. 8). Although the outward-bulging fissure is found frequently in Friedländer's pneumonia, this sign is by no means pathognomonic of infection with the organism that causes Friedländer's pneumonia, as it also may be observed in pneumonia caused by many other organisms. In 25%–50% of patients with acute Friedländer's pneumonia, one or more abscesses, usually not evident by physical examination, appear on the roentgenogram. The presence of abscesses and periodontal disease may tempt the physician to make a diagnosis of primary putrid lung abscess. The separation of the two diseases can often be made by smelling the sputum, which is not foul in Friedländer's disease.

Treatment

The micro-organism usually is susceptible in vitro to tetracyclines, chloramphenicol, cephalosporins, aminoglycosides, trimethoprim/sulfamethoxazole, the newer penicillins, such as piperacillin and mezlocillin, and the

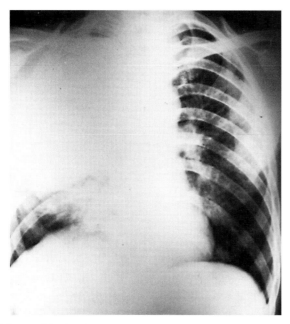

FIG. 8. Friedländer's pneumonia and empyema in a 52-year-old alcoholic. Note the bulging fissure.

fluoroquinolones. The treatment of choice consists of a cephalosporin or β-lactam plus an aminoglycoside. Although this combination seems reasonable, there are no satisfactory data showing the advantages of giving both drugs rather than either one alone. Treatment should be continued for a minimum of 2 weeks.

Complications

Complications include empyema, pneumothorax, chronic pneumonia, spread to contiguous tissues, such as the pericardium, and hematogenous dissemination, especially to the meninges. In patients with empyema, open drainage usually is necessary because of the toxemia and thickness of the pus. Chronic Friedländer's pneumonia, which may follow the acute process, is characterized by progressive inanition, abscess formation, and anemia. It usually responds to prolonged antimicrobial therapy combined with careful supportive measures, but in some patients, lobectomy has to be performed for residual abscesses.

Escherichia coli Pneumonia

E. coli ranks after *K. pneumoniae* as the second most common cause of community-acquired gram-negative bacillary pneumonia. The "colon bacillus," isolated in 1885 by Escherich, is a gram-negative, nonencapsulated bacillus. *E. coli* pneumonia may develop after a bacteremia originating from the genitourinary or gastrointestinal tract

or by endogenous aspiration of the organism from a colonized oropharynx.

Patients with community-acquired *E. coli* pneumonia are usually middle-aged to elderly persons with underlying diseases, such as diabetes mellitus, cirrhosis, cardiac disease, and chronic lung disease. Several days of fever, chills, cough productive of purulent sputum, and pleurisy are generally reported. Alcoholics may present after a binge with pneumonia and meningitis. Tachycardia may be out of proportion to fever. Patchy lower lobe bronchopneumonia is typical, but occasionally lobar consolidation with abscess is seen. Parapneumonic effusion is common. The organism is generally readily recovered from blood, sputum, urine, and pleural fluid. Mortality rates vary from 29%–60%, and in survivors, fever ends by lysis.

Pneumonia Caused by *Proteus* Species

Proteus organisms are highly motile, gram-negative bacilli, notable for their characteristic swarming on agar. Patients acquire *Proteus* pneumonias after endogenous aspiration of pharyngeal secretions, and the typical patient is an elderly, alcoholic man with chronic lung disease. Worsening of bronchitic symptoms for several weeks culminates in an acute episode of fever, rigors, cough productive of purulent sputum, chest pain, and dyspnea. Signs of upper lobe consolidation are generally present. Radiographs show dense infiltrates in the posterior segments of the right upper lobe or superior segments of the right lower lobe, frequently with abscess formation. Pleural effusion is unusual, and healing results in a contracted fibrotic lobe. Species of *Proteus* may be cultured from the sputum as the predominant organism for long periods despite the use of antimicrobial agents.

Acinetobacter calcoaceticus Pneumonia

Acinetobacter is a gram-negative coccobacillus that can be easily misinterpreted as *Neisseria, Haemophilus,* or *Branhamella.* Patients with community-acquired *Acinetobacter* pneumonia are usually middle-aged to elderly persons with antecedent alcoholism and tobacco abuse. Occupational exposure to silica particles appears to be an additional risk factor. Patients have been ill for several days before admission with cough, fever, pleurisy, and bloody sputum. They typically present in severe respiratory distress, often sitting "bolt upright," and half are in shock. Lower lobe consolidation and pleural effusion are common. Leukopenia with an absolute granulocytopenia is present in a majority of cases. Measurement of arterial blood gases shows profound hypoxemia. Blood, sputum, and empyema cultures yield *Acinetobacter.* Pneumonia progresses rapidly despite antimicrobial therapy, and death occurs in <72 hours.

Pseudomonas aeruginosa Pneumonia

Community-acquired *Pseudomonas aeruginosa* pneumonias are rare, accounting for <10% of gram-negative bacillary pneumonias in this setting. Although most patients are elderly with severe, chronic cardiopulmonary disease or malignancy, cases occasionally occur in normal hosts. At presentation, patients are toxic, apprehensive, and confused, and exhibit chills, fever, and coughs productive of greenish sputum. Relative bradycardia and a reversal of the usual diurnal temperature curve (with elevation primarily in the morning) are typical.

Pulmonary infiltrates may be focal or diffuse, the latter mimicking cardiogenic pulmonary edema. The focal form may involve any part of the lungs, often with roentgenologic evidence of cavitation. Nodular infiltrates may be observed.

The diffuse form is a fearsome disease characterized by necrotizing pneumonia, vasculitis, frequent pulmonary hemorrhage, and abscess formation. Bacteremia is common and often accompanied by marked neutropenia. The nonbacteremic, focal form of *Pseudomonas* pneumonia carries a case fatality rate of 30%–60%. The bacteremic variety, which resembles pulmonary edema, is associated with a case fatality rate in excess of 80% unless treated promptly.

In *Pseudomonas* pneumonia, piperacillin, mezlocillin, ceftazidime, aztreonam, or imipenem combined with aminoglycoside should be adequate therapy.

Miscellaneous Causes of Gram-Negative Pneumonia

Evidence of pulmonary involvement may occur in typhoid fever. Indeed, cough is one of the early manifestations of the disease in as many as 25% of patients. Pulmonary infiltrates in typhoid fever are typically small and fleeting, and the pulmonary involvement is not a significant part of the disease process in the vast majority of patients. However, *Salmonella typhi* infection may be manifested by lobar pneumonia and/or empyema. Pneumonia also may be found in infections caused by *Salmonella* species other than *S. typhi*, especially *Salmonella choleraesuis*, which is the most invasive of the *Salmonella* species. Pneumonia, lung abscesses, and empyema may be the predominant manifestations of this disease.

Melioidosis, an acute, often lethal, disseminated infection acquired from rodents, cats, and dogs, is found primarily in Southeast Asia and the West Indies. The causative organism, *Pseudomonas pseudomallei*, is closely related antigenically to the agent responsible for glanders. Although the acute form of the infection is frequently fatal, there have been a small number of cases of chronic disease. These patients may have systemic disease without pulmonary parenchymal involvement, disseminated disease with secondary involvement of the lung, or primary pulmonary infection. In the lung, focal areas of pneumonic involvement rapidly form abscesses and cavities, followed sometimes by chronic empyema. The onset of the disease may be abrupt or the course may be indolent. Abscesses may appear in virtually any tissue of the body, and osteomyelitis with draining sinuses is observed frequently. Ceftazidime is the drug of choice. Extensive surgical drainage and debridement of diseased areas are also helpful.

Nodular infiltrates and pneumonia, occasionally with cavitation, also have been found in patients with *Yersinia enterocolitica* sepsis.

Legionellosis

In the summer of 1976, an epidemic of pneumonia occurred among persons attending a Legionnaires' convention in Philadelphia, Pennsylvania. In this predominantly older population, the case fatality rate was 16%. Approximately 6 months later, investigators from the Centers for Disease Control identified the causative agent as an aerobic gram-negative rod, *Legionella pneumophila*. It is now known that this organism caused epidemic pneumonia some 30 years before the Philadelphia epidemic. Species of *Legionella* account for 1%–4% of community-acquired pneumonias and rank among the top three microbial causes in several large-scale studies.

Micro-organism

Legionella is a pleomorphic bacillus that stains faintly gram-negative. There are at present >30 species, 20 of which have been implicated in human disease. The two most important are *L. pneumophila* and *Legionella micdadei* (the Pittsburgh agent). Within the species *L. pneumophila*, there are 10 serotypes, and most cases of legionellosis are caused by serotypes 1, 4, and 6. The organism can be seen by special tissue stains (modified Giemsa, Brown-Hopps, or Dieterle's stain), and *L. micdadei* can stain weakly acid-fast. *Legionella* organisms are nutritionally fastidious, and charcoal yeast extract agar is the medium of choice. The organism grows slowly; it takes up to 5 days for macroscopically visible colonies to appear. Aquatic environments are the natural habitat of *Legionella*, and this includes man-made habitats such as cooling towers, evaporative condensers, and potable-water distribution systems.

Epidemiology

Legionnaires' disease occurs in sporadic, endemic, and epidemic forms. Most epidemic Legionnaires' disease is caused by exposure to *L. pneumophila* aerosols in the workplace or in industrial or nosocomial settings. Hospital tap water has been frequently reported as contaminated with *Legionella* organisms—hence the current proscription against the use of tap water for irrigation of nasogastric tubes or any activity related to respiratory therapy. Several epidemics have been associated with retail stores or shopping malls.

Sporadic disease and miniclusters of Legionnaires' disease have been associated with proximity of patients residences to cooling towers. Recent interest has been focused on the home as a source of sporadic legionellosis, as 1%–30% of home heaters harbor *Legionella* organisms. The extent of bacterial colonization varies inversely with tank temperatures in this setting. As the water required to reduce *Legionella* colonization is quite high (55°C to 60°C), the potential risk for scald injuries likely outweighs the benefit in reducing disease.

Susceptibility to Infection

The incidence of legionellosis depends on the degree of contamination of the organism in the aquatic reservoir. Risk factors for the acquisition of disease include cigarette smoking, alcoholism, chronic obstructive pulmonary disease, and age. Immunosuppression is a major risk factor, and corticosteroid use is frequently reported. Transplant recipients appear to be at highest risk. The role of polymorphonuclear leukocytes in host defense is unclear, but patients with granulocytopenia are not at increased risk. Humoral immunity plays only a secondary role. Intracellular multiplication of *L. pneumophila* occurs within human monocytes, and cell-mediated immunity appears to be the primary host defense against *Legionella,* as is true for other intracellular pathogens.

Pathogenesis

Pathogenic organisms can enter the lung by aspiration, direct inhalation, and hematogenous dissemination from another focus. Oropharyngeal colonization with *Legionella* has not been demonstrated, so that subclinical aspiration of contaminated water or direct inhalation of aerosols is the likely mode of entry. The organisms probably are cleared by the mucociliary process, and this would be supported by the consistent epidemiologic association of increased risk for disease with conditions characterized by impaired mucociliary clearance (i.e., cigarette smoking, chronic lung disease, alcoholism). *Legionella* readily undergoes phagocytosis by resident alveolar macrophages, but phagosome-lysosome fusion is inhibited, allowing the organism to multiply and escape the microbicidal mechanisms of this cell. Cell-mediated immunity is the primary host defense against *Legionella,* and lymphocyte proliferation and cutaneous delayed hypersensitivity to *Legionella* antigens develop within the first 2 weeks of infection. Mononuclear cells respond to *Legionella*

with the generation of monocyte-activating cytokines, but although the activated monocytes and alveolar macrophage inhibit intracellular multiplication of *Legionella,* killing is not enhanced.

Clinical Manifestations

Legionella infections may vary considerably in presentation, from an acute, self-limited, influenza-like illness (Pontiac fever) to a fulminant pneumonia syndrome with high mortality (Legionnaires' disease). The initial symptoms of Pontiac fever are predominantly malaise, myalgias, headache, and dry cough. The appearance of the chest radiograph is normal, and recovery within a week is the rule.

The incubation period for Legionnaires' disease is apparently 2 to 10 days, and the clinical manifestations vary from mild cough and fever to coma with diffuse pulmonary infiltrates and multiorgan system failure. An antecedent upper respiratory tract infection is reported only infrequently. The respiratory manifestations range from acute, subacute, or even chronic bronchitis to consolidating lobular or lobar pneumonia. Symptoms include malaise, muscle aches, headache, confusion, high fever, chills, and cough that is usually accompanied by some sputum production, with the sputum ranging in quality from serous and thin to thick and purulent. Hemoptysis occasionally may be a prominent manifestation. Pleuritic pain is not infrequent. Early in the course of the disease, there is often a pulse-temperature dissociation with relative bradycardia. This finding may be enormously helpful diagnostically and should not be ignored. Physical examination of the lungs may reveal only a few rales, or there may be more prominent findings, even evidence of frank consolidation.

Pleural effusion occurs in 24%–63% of patients; the fluid may show either a predominance of polymorphonuclear leukocytes or lymphocytes and on rare occasions may be hemorrhagic. Chest x-ray patterns are nondiagnostic. The initial involvement is unilateral in most patients, and the infiltrate is typically alveolar and segmental-lobar or diffuse and patchy. Interstitial infiltrates were described in 25% of patients in the Philadelphia outbreak in 1976. The initial area of infiltration often progresses to more widespread consolidation during the ensuing few days, even in the face of appropriate therapy. The extent of radiographic involvement does not correlate with the severity of illness or ultimate outcome, but it does correlate with the presence of *L. pneumophila* in sputum. Cavitation of infiltrates occurs almost exclusively in immunocompromised patients. Hilar adenopathy and pneumatocele formation are rare.

The many extrapulmonary manifestations include mild to moderate liver dysfunction, hyponatremia, hypophosphatemia, diarrhea, abdominal pain, splenomegaly, renal dysfunction, pericarditis (with or without effusion), and myocarditis. There is a particular propensity for involvement of the central nervous system, including both the brain and spinal cord. Abnormalities of mentation without focal neurologic findings and aseptic meningitis are the most frequent findings.

It is important to stress that extrapulmonary manifestations suggest but do not document a diagnosis of *Legionella* pneumonia. Although they are common (gastrointestinal, neurologic, and laboratory abnormalities, including liver dysfunction, hyponatremia, hypophosphatemia, and hematuria), such clinical manifestations do not occur more frequently in Legionnaires' disease than in pneumonias of other etiology.

Laboratory Diagnosis

Five techniques are currently available for the specific diagnosis of Legionnaires' disease (Table 7). Sputum findings are variable; there may be few or many polymorphonuclear leukocytes. The organism does not stain well by Gram's method. Culture of the organism on selective media remains the definitive method of diagnosis, and maximal yield depends on specimen collection before antimicrobial therapy. The sensitivity of specimens obtained by bronchoscopy is essentially the same as that for sputum, and bronchoalveolar lavage gives higher yields than bronchial wash specimens. Blood culture results may be positive in up to 20% of cases.

No test is generally available to detect *Legionella* antigens in sputum, but a test to detect antigen in the urine is commercially available. Advantages include its sensitivity (75%–90%), specificity (99%), and relatively low cost, and the fact that test positivity persists for days, even during antibiotic therapy. The drawback is that only serogroup 1 of *L. pneumophila* is detected. This shortcoming is relatively minor, as this serogroup causes at least 70% of *L. pneumophila* infections.

Antibody estimation is probably the most widely used diagnostic tool. Maximal sensitivity requires both IgM and IgG determinations. Fourfold seroconversion is the definitive criterion, but this may take up to 9 weeks to be detected. In the first week of disease, 25%–40% of patients may have elevated titers.

Immunofluorescence microscopy, more commonly referred to as direct fluorescent antibody (DFA) testing, is an excellent method for detecting *Legionella* species in laboratory tract specimens. The DFA test is more likely to show positive results when multilobar infiltrates are present on chest films. Cross-reactivity with other gram-negative bacilli can give false-positive results.

The DNA probe methods are about as accurate as DFA testing. The DNA probe test may be preferable in high-volume laboratories, as interpretation requires less technical expertise. The polymerase chain reaction has been used experimentally to detect *L. pneumophila* DNA in clinical specimens, but its role is yet to be defined.

Therapy

There are three methods to determine the susceptibility of *Legionella* species to antimicrobial agents: extracellular testing, intracellular testing, and treatment studies of *Legionella*-infected guinea pigs. All three methods have been used to evaluate promising antimicrobial agents, as no controlled trials of treatment for Legionnaires' disease have been performed.

Erythromycin has historically been considered the treatment of choice based on retrospective analysis of outcomes of Legionnaires' disease. The Philadelphia epidemic fatality rates were twofold lower in erythromycin-treated patients than in those who were not treated with erythromycin. Doses of 2 to 4 g/d are advocated, preferably administered intravenously initially. Both clarithromycin and azithromycin are more active in vitro than erythromycin and have been successfully used in the treatment of Legionnaires' disease. They represent attractive agents for the oral treatment of legionellosis. Therapy should be continued for 3 weeks.

Rifampin is active against both intracellular and extracellular *Legionella* organisms. The use of rifampin as sole therapy for Legionnaires' disease has not been reported, and legionellosis has developed in individuals receiving rifampin for tuberculosis. Rifampin may have a synergistic effect when administered with erythromycin, but this benefit may be limited to the initial 3 to 5 days of treatment. Rifampin in doses of 600 mg twice daily should be considered for individuals with more serious disease.

Tetracycline was equivalent to erythromycin in lowering the case fatality rate in the Philadelphia outbreak. Doxycycline and minocycline appear to be more active in vitro than tetracycline, and they would be reasonable alternative agents for patients who cannot tolerate macrolides.

Increasing evidence now exists that fluoroquinolone an-

TABLE 7. *Specialized laboratory tests for the diagnosis of legionellosis*

Test	Sensitivity, %	Specificity, %
Culture		
Sputum	75	100
Transtracheal aspirate	90	100
Bronchial washings	75	100
Blood	20	100
Serology (IgG and IgM, acute and convalescent)	30–40	96
Direct fluorescent antibody	40–80	99
Urinary antigen	75–90	100
DNA probe	50–65	99

timicrobial agentss (ciprofloxacin, pefloxacin, ofloxacin) are superior in activity to erythromycin, and they have been successfully used for the treatment of Legionnaires' disease. There are no clinical data to demonstrate that combining a fluoroquinolone with either rifampin or erythromycin is more effective than the fluoroquinolone alone. Fluoroquinolones have no adverse effect on cyclosporine metabolism and should be considered the drug of choice for immunocompromised patients taking that agent.

Mycoplasma (Primary Atypical) Pneumonia

Micro-organism

The term *atypical pneumonia* was first used in 1938 to describe an unusual form of "tracheobronchopneumonia and severe symptoms." The organism was first isolated in 1944 by Eaton, Meiklejohn, and von Herick from the sputum of patients who had cold agglutinin-positive, atypical pneumonia. Thereafter, the organism was called *Eaton's agent* until 1961, when Chanock identified it as belonging to the genus *Mycoplasma.*

The organisms contain both RNA and DNA, lack a cell wall, and can be identified by direct isolation on highly enriched artificial media. *Mycoplasma pneumoniae* has distinctive properties among human mycoplasmas in that it ferments glucose and causes β-hemolysis of guinea pig red cells, but the final identification is still by serology or specific growth-inhibition tests.

Clinical Manifestations

M. pneumoniae accounts for 2%–15% of all community-acquired pneumonias, but up to 30% of the pneumonias in adolescents and adults younger than 30. Mycoplasmas are of relatively low virulence; pneumonia develops in only 5%–15% of exposed persons.

The onset of the illness may be either insidious or acute. More than 80% of patients have cough and a temperature above 101°F. A persistent, racking, usually nonproductive cough is the hallmark of the disease; before fluorescent antibody techniques were developed, many observers stated that this cough was a uniform finding. More recent evidence, however, suggests that at least 10% of patients with pneumonia and elevated titers of specific antibody do not experience cough. The majority of patients notice pounding headache, usually frontal or generalized, that may be so severe as to be the dominant symptom. Myalgia is common, and coryza, sore throat, and shaking chills all occur in approximately 25% of patients. Although chest discomfort is reported frequently, frank pleuritic pain occurs in 5% of patients. The pain usually is retrosternal and may be quite severe.

On physical examination, the patient usually appears moderately ill and frequently complains of either cough or headache, the latter markedly accentuated during periods of coughing. The heart rate often appears slow in relation to the degree of pyrexia. The frequent paroxysms of nonproductive cough may at times make the patient virtually incapable of carrying on a prolonged conversation. In patients with extensive pulmonary involvement, moderate or even marked cyanosis may be observed. A clue to the pulmonary diagnosis may be obtained by finding an inflamed tympanic membrane on otologic examination. Bullous myringitis, a frequently emphasized feature of this disease, actually occurs in 5% of patients. Examination of the lungs characteristically reveals fine to medium rales heard early or at the very end of the inspiratory cycle. Early in the course of the disease, physical examination of the lungs may reveal normal findings despite considerable infiltration shown roentgenographically. This discrepancy is notable, especially in the upper lobes, whereas in the lower lobes, which are more commonly involved, physical examination usually shows some abnormality and may give more evidence of pulmonary disease than the roentgenogram. As the disease progresses, dullness to percussion is observed, and the number and intensity of the rales increase so that rales, rhonchi, and wheezes of either a coarse or musical nature are readily detected. Evidence of frank consolidation, pleural friction rubs, and pleural effusion are less frequently found.

Roentgenographic and Laboratory Studies

Roentgenographic study of the chest shows nodular, patchy, or perihilar infiltrates that cannot be distinguished from those of various types of viral pneumonia and on occasion may simulate bacterial lobar pneumonia (Fig. 9). Rarely, *M. pneumoniae* infection has been associated

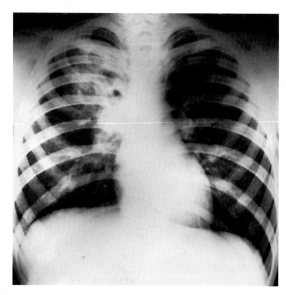

FIG. 9. *Mycoplasma* pneumonia in a 23-year-old man who seemed normal on physical examination.

with parenchymal lung abscesses. One or two lobes are involved in the majority of patients, but occasionally pneumonia may occur in four or five lobes. Hilar adenopathy can be found in up to 22% of cases. Roentgenographic findings suggest pleural fluid in <5% of patients. Because stained smears of the sputum show a marked predominance of mononuclear cells, the presence of large numbers of polymorphonuclear leukocytes should suggest another etiology for the pneumonia. However, in a small percentage of cases, the cellular response in the sputum is predominantly polymorphonuclear. During the first week of the disease, the blood leukocyte count is usually <12,000, but in approximately 10% of patients, the count is as high as 20,000/mm³. During the second to third week of the disease, mild to moderate leukocytosis is common, and on occasion profound leukocytosis has been reported.

Cold agglutinins appear in the blood 1 to 4 weeks after the onset of illness. Maximum titers are found in the second to sixth week of disease and may persist for several months. Cold hemagglutinins are helpful in the diagnosis of *Mycoplasma* pneumonia but are not diagnostic. Cold agglutinins do not develop at any time during the course of illness in 15%–30% of the patients who have pneumonia and a rising titer of antibody specific for *M. pneumoniae*. Furthermore, a considerable number of patients who have positive results on cold hemagglutinin tests do not show a rise in *M. pneumoniae*-specific antibody, the percentage ranging from 15%–65% in different series. Many other pulmonary and extrapulmonary diseases may produce elevation in the cold agglutinin titers; these diseases include influenza, rubella, cirrhosis, lymphatic leukemia, trypanosomiasis, leishmaniasis, relapsing fever, acute hemolytic anemia, pernicious anemia, paroxysmal cold hemoglobinuria, infectious mononucleosis, and psittacosis. In addition, a small number of patients have persistently high titers for unknown reasons. It has also been shown that certain individuals chronically have low cold agglutinin titers, which may rise to diagnostic levels with virtually any acute infection. Significant titers are at least 1:80, and it is not unusual to see levels of 1:1000 or more. Antibody to streptococcus MG also appears in the blood of 40%–60% of patients with *Mycoplasma* pneumonia. However, both cold agglutinins and streptococcus MG titers are negative in at least 20% of patients with pneumonia caused by *M. pneumoniae*.

Specific serologic tests include growth inhibition, ELISA, radioprecipitation, and complement fixation; a fourfold rise in complement-fixing titers is used most often for establishing a firm diagnosis.

Complications

The major complications of *Mycoplasma* pneumonia are related to the central nervous system and to the effects of cold agglutinins. On the third to thirtieth day of illness,

manifestations of nervous system involvement develop in a small number of patients, including papilledema, disorientation, coma, neck stiffness, abnormal reflexes, and transverse myelitis. Lumbar puncture specimens may be entirely normal or may show elevation of the protein to as much as 300 mg/dL and pleocytosis to a maximum of several hundred cells. These may be predominantly polymorphonuclear leukocytes or, more commonly, predominantly mononuclear cells. Central nervous system involvement may be serious. Either meningitis or encephalitis may predominate clinically and result in death or be associated with permanent neurologic residua. Postmortem examination has shown focal hemorrhages, perivascular mononuclear infiltration, and less frequently glial proliferation. Nervous system involvement by *Mycoplasma* also may be expressed as cerebellar ataxia, peripheral neuropathy, or Guillain-Barré syndrome. Cold hemagglutinins in low titer represent no danger to the patient. On the other hand, when titers exceed 1:512, cold hemagglutinemia is potentially dangerous. Peripheral thrombophlebitis, which develops in some patients, may be associated with secondary pulmonary embolism. High-titer cold hemagglutinemia also may be associated with acute hemolysis related either to increased mechanical fragility of antibody-coated cells or to the simultaneous presence of a cold hemolysin. If intravascular hemolysis is rapid, hemoglobinuria may be observed. Occasionally, the use of ice packs, cold oxygen tents, or the administration of cold blood has been associated with arterial occlusion and gangrene, presumably related to intravascular thrombosis induced by cold agglutinins. Dermatologic manifestations usually consist of an erythematous maculopapular or vesicular rash, but the Stevens-Johnson syndrome may occur. Cardiac involvement is infrequent, but myocarditis, pericarditis, and complete heart block have been reported.

Course and Treatment

The course of *M. pneumoniae* pneumonia is variable, although recovery is the rule. Fever may last from 2 days to 2 weeks; it usually subsides by lysis. The cough does not usually subside until at least several days after the fever has disappeared. Malaise, cough, and radiographic abnormalities frequently persist for 2 to 6 weeks. Secondary bacterial infection occurs infrequently in patients with *Mycoplasma* pneumonia. Uncomplicated disease is not fatal in patients who have an inflammatory process in one or two lobes, but it is not generally appreciated that more extensive pulmonary involvement can be associated with some mortality.

In addition to careful supportive therapy, current evidence strongly favors the administration of tetracyclines or macrolides. These antibiotics inhibit the etiologic agent in tissue culture, and well-controlled studies have now demonstrated prompt clinical improvement, defervescence, and more rapid resolution of roentgenographic infiltrates after treatment with one of these drugs. Even after clinical improvement, *M. pneumoniae* may be found in throat cultures for a considerable period.

Chlamydia Infections

Chlamydia pneumoniae *Pneumonia*

C. pneumoniae has only recently been recognized as a pulmonary pathogen. This organism was initially referred to as the TWAR agent, after the laboratory designation of the first two isolates: TW-183 and AR-39.

Serologic studies have demonstrated that *C. pneumoniae* is the most common chlamydial species infecting humans. The prevalence of antibody to *C. pneumoniae* starts to rise in residents of industrialized countries at school age and steadily increases throughout life. Longitudinal studies suggest that only about 10% of infections lead to overt pneumonia. It is estimated that the organism accounts for 2%–10% of community-acquired pneumonias, depending on age and geographic locale.

Micro-organism

C. pneumoniae is an obligate intracellular bacterium having 10% genetic homology with the other *Chlamydia* species. Details of the pathogenesis of *C. pneumoniae* pneumonia are unknown. The agent multiplies in human alveolar macrophages, smooth-muscle cells, and endothelial cells and rapidly induces ciliostasis. Infection with *C. pneumoniae* leads to partial immunity, as reinfections generally do not take the form of pneumonia. When the reinfecting strain, however, is sufficiently different to escape immunologic defense mechanisms, the outcome can be more severe than the illness observed in primary infection. Little is known about the cellular immune response. An IgM response to protein antigens is seen in primary infections but is usually lacking in reinfections. There is also a marked IgA response in reinfections.

Clinical Manifestations

Clinical features of pneumonia attributable to *C. pneumoniae* are similar to those caused by *M. pneumoniae*. The illness is generally mild, but the course may be protracted, with symptoms persisting for 3 to 6 weeks. Severe pharyngitis, hoarseness, and upper respiratory tract symptoms are present in 40%–70% of patients. Fever and cough are common. A biphasic illness is frequently seen; patients seek medical attention with pharyngitis, recover, and then pneumonia develops 1 to 3 weeks later. Rales are almost always present on auscultation. Sputum production is scant and not purulent. In some series, up to 20% of individuals with chlamydial pneumonia are coinfected with other pathogens, such as influenza virus or *S. pneumoniae*. The peripheral blood leukocyte count and differential counts are usually normal, although an elevated erythrocyte sedimentation rate is found in 80% of cases. There are no characteristic radiologic findings. Single, subsegmental alveolar opacities appear frequently, although interstitial infiltrates may be more common in reinfections. Lobar consolidation, hilar adenopathy, and pleural effusion are uncommon.

Diagnosis

Definitive diagnosis requires isolation of *C. pneumoniae* or demonstration of an appropriate antibody response. Cultivation of the organism is difficult, and sensitivity of culture is only 50% in serologically verified cases. Direct antigen detection or fluorescent antibody staining of respiratory tract samples is insensitive. The two primary serologic tests for *C. pneumoniae* are complement fixation and micro-immunofluorescence. Complement fixation is genus-specific and measures antibody against all three *Chlamydia* species (*psittaci, pneumoniae, trachomatis*). The complement fixation test, however, may be useful only in primary infection, as results remains negative in 90% of reinfections. On the other hand, micro-immunofluorescence is specific for *C. pneumoniae* and can distinguish between IgM and IgG antibody. Circulating antibody may not be detectable, however, for 3 to 6 weeks. Criteria for diagnosis using micro-immunofluorescence have been established: a fourfold rise in antibody response, IgM titer $\geq$1:16, or IgG titer $\geq$1:512.

Complications

C. pneumoniae rarely causes life-threatening pneumonia, and most patients do not require hospitalization. Chronic *C. pneumoniae* infection of the lungs has been associated with chronic bronchitis, asthma, and sarcoidosis. Extrapulmonary manifestations include reactive arthritis and erythema nodosum. Dissemination via the bloodstream may explain the recent association of the organism with coronary artery disease and atherosclerotic lesions.

Treatment

Although no clinical studies of efficacy have been performed, tetracyclines, erythromycin, and fluoroquinolones have shown excellent in vitro activity. Tetracycline appears to be the drug of choice, at a dose of 2 g/d. Treatment should be administered for 2 to 3 weeks.

Ornithosis (Psittacosis)

Pathogenesis

Ornithosis is an acute pulmonary infection caused by *Chlamydia psittaci*. These obligate intracellular parasites are larger and more complex organisms than viruses, contain both DNA and RNA, have a cell wall similar in composition to that of some gram-negative organisms, and are stained by Giemsa but not by Gram's stain. Ornithosis is acquired by contact with both psittacine and nonpsittacine birds, including parrots, parakeets, lorikeets, cockatoos, chickens, pigeons, ducks, pheasants, and turkeys. Although the birds are sometimes sick, the disease is frequently acquired from animals that appear to be well. Infection follows inhalation of dried excreta and occurs most often in persons who care for the birds; it is uncommon in persons who visit people with psittacine birds but have no intimate contact with the birds. At least 25% of cases occur without a history of bird contact, and in a small number of cases, human-to-human spread of the disease has occurred.

Clinical Manifestations

After an incubation period, which is usually 7 to 15 days but may occasionally be considerably longer, the patient becomes acutely ill with a mild to moderate cough productive of small amounts of sputum, occasionally blood-streaked. Fever and myalgia are common, and approximately a third of patients experience shaking chills. Pleuritic chest pain occurs relatively infrequently. Hemoptysis also has been described.

The findings on physical examination are extremely variable. In severe cases, consolidation involving several lobes may be accompanied by a pleural friction rub, or examination may show only diffuse, moderate to coarse inspiratory and expiratory rales. In less severe cases, one or two lobes are involved and there are inspiratory rales but no frank consolidation. In some patients with pulmonary involvement, no abnormalities can be detected on physical examination. A few patients have moderate pleural effusion. Not infrequently, the heart rate is slower than expected in a patient with marked elevation in temperature. Splenomegaly is present in 10%–30% of patients. Severe lymphadenopathy, intense pharyngitis, pericardial friction rub, jaundice, evidence of meningoencephalitis, or any combination of these is found occasionally.

Roentgenographic and Laboratory Findings

The variable findings detected on physical examination are reflected in roentgenographic abnormalities. Focal areas of consolidation are seen in 10%–20% of cases. In others, there are small peribronchial or peripheral infiltrates or diffuse, bilateral, confluent pneumonia that is indistinguishable from overwhelming influenza virus pneumonia. Rarely, cavitation may be seen in areas of pneumonia. Mediastinal lymphadenopathy also has been described.

Examination of stained sputum smears usually shows few polymorphonuclear leukocytes, and there is rarely evidence on smear or in culture of secondary bacterial infection. The blood leukocyte count is commonly normal but may be elevated or low. Occasionally, serum titers of cold hemagglutinins rise during the course of ornithosis. The organism can readily be isolated from the sputum or the lungs, and frequently from other tissues at postmortem examination using tissue culture cells or embryonated chicken eggs. Complement-fixing antibodies appear in the serum in the second to fourth week of the disease, but their appearance may be delayed until the fourth to sixth week when patients are treated with antibiotics.

Complications

Complications arising from contiguous or hematogenous spread are reported with increasing frequency; these include pericarditis, myocarditis, hepatitis, meningitis, and encephalitis. If the central nervous system is affected, delirium, stupor, severe headache, and lymphocytic meningitis may be noted, but seizures are extremely uncommon. Hepatic involvement varies from mild to lethal and is characterized by striking hepatocellular abnormalities on liver function studies. Peripheral thrombophlebitis is a not infrequent complication and may cause death by pulmonary embolism.

The mortality associated with ornithosis is currently 2%–10%, with most of the patients dying of respiratory involvement, including the respiratory distress syndrome. In patients who die of ornithosis, the bronchial mucosa is ulcerated.

Treatment

The tetracyclines are the antibiotics of choice and are usually effective in modifying the course of the disease when given in a dosage of 1 to 2 g/d for 10 to 14 days. Chloramphenicol is an equally effective agent, and erythromycin also may be useful. The patient should be placed in strict isolation in view of the well-documented cases of human-to-human spread.

Other Chlamydia Infections

Chlamydia trachomatis usually causes conjunctivitis, trachoma, and urethritis. It also can cause interstitial pneumonia in infants. The infection, which usually appears in infants 2 weeks to 3 months old, is characterized by staccato cough, tachypnea, and variable degrees of cyanosis. There is little or no fever. Roentgenograms show alveolar and interstitial infiltrates. The course of the cases is generally protracted, lasting from several weeks to many months. Arterial oxygen saturations are often markedly reduced. The diagnosis is usually made by isolation of the organism from tracheal aspirations and by serologic tests. Genus-specific complement fixation and immunofluorescent antibody tests using lymphogranuloma venereum antigens are available, and there are now specific immunofluorescent antibody tests for *C. trachomatis.* Eosinophilia occurs frequently. In some instances, prolonged erythromycin therapy has appeared to be beneficial, but similar improvement has occurred with supportive therapy alone. If *C. trachomatis* infection is acquired *in utero,* lethal pneumonia can result. *C. trachomatis* also can cause pneumonia in adults, in both compromised and noncompromised persons, usually characterized by patchy infiltrates without frank consolidations. Mediastinal and supraclavicular lymphadenitis also has been described.

VIRAL RESPIRATORY TRACT INFECTIONS

Viruses may account for 5%–15% of community-acquired pneumonias. Viral respiratory illnesses are caused by >200 serologically distinct viruses, and the clinical manifestations of these illnesses, including rhinitis, tracheobronchitis, bronchiolitis, and pneumonia, are dictated by the principal sites of anatomic involvement. In contrast to bacterial respiratory tract infections, viral infections are transmitted primarily via aerosols or hand-to-hand contact. Although most patients have self-limited symptoms and do not require any specific treatment, some patients, particularly after an influenza illness, have serious secondary bacterial infections.

Influenza

Influenza was undoubtedly known to antiquity. In 1580 and 1782, ravaging epidemics occurred, but the damage therefrom was insignificant in comparison with that observed in the terrifying pandemic of 1918–1919, which struck in three waves, attacked an estimated 20 million persons, and killed 850,000 in the United States alone. Throughout the world, the number of deaths was estimated at 20 million. There is no better or more concise description of the illness produced by influenza viruses than that recorded by Short in 1580:

> "It began with a roughness of the jaws, small cough, then a strong fever with a pain of the head, back, and legs. Some felt as though they were corded over the breast and had a weight at the stomach, all of which continued to the third day at farthest; then the fever went off with a sweat or bleeding at the nose. In some few, it turned to a pleurisy or fatal peripneumony."

Before 1950, it was never clear whether the pulmonary infection was related to the virus itself or to secondary bacterial invasion. This uncertainty was in large part caused by the absence of a defined etiologic agent, as influenza virus was not recovered from humans until 1933. The first opportunity for accurate assessment of the relative roles of the virus and bacteria in pulmonary complications came during the pandemics of 1957–1958 and 1968–1969. It is now clear that the following pulmonary syndromes may arise in patients infected with an influenza virus.

Lower Respiratory Tract Involvement Without Roentgenographic Evidence of Pneumonia

Within 48 hours after the onset of typical influenza, characterized by fever, dry cough, headache, myalgia, and prostration, the patient notes increased cough, which is at times productive of greenish or blood-tinged sputum. In some patients, this is associated with dyspnea and/or pleuritic chest pain of mild to moderate severity. Physical examination of the lungs reveals unilateral or bilateral inspiratory rales, which may be accompanied by diminished or harsh breath sounds. Occasionally, end-inspiratory wheezes and rales suggest bronchiolitis, and rarely a pleural friction rub can be detected. There is no evidence of consolidation, and roentgenographic findings either appear normal or show accentuation of bronchial markings in the lower lung fields. No evidence of concomitant bacterial infection is obtained. This benign complication of influenza is of importance only in that the patient should be observed closely for development of the more serious pulmonary syndromes detailed below, as well as, rarely, marked stridor resulting from virus-induced laryngitis.

The administration of antibiotics to patients having influenza with no evidence of lower respiratory tract involvement or to those with rales but no evidence of pneumonia is not of benefit and encourages colonization with antibiotic-resistant micro-organisms. These resistant organisms may subsequently be responsible for secondary bacterial pneumonia.

Secondary Bacterial Pneumonia

Secondary bacterial pneumonia is the most common pulmonary complication of influenza. This is not surprising, as the influenza virus damages cilia, delays leukocyte mobilization, promotes adherence of certain bacteria, and interferes with bacterial killing by polymorphonuclear phagocytes. In the majority of patients, the diagnosis can be established by history alone. The patient experiences typical influenza followed by a definite period of improvement. Indeed, such persons may feel well enough to return to their usual occupation. Then, 3 to 14 days after the initial influenza symptoms, the patient's condition worsens precipitously: Recurrence of fever is usually accompanied by shaking chills, pleuritic chest pain, and cough productive of bloody or purulent sputum. In approximately a third of the cases of secondary bacterial pneumonia there is no diphasic course, and pulmonary symptoms blend with the initial influenza.

Physical examination reveals focal involvement of the lung, often with the classic signs of consolidation, and physical findings are confirmed by roentgenogram. Gram's stains of sputum smears show many bacteria and polymorphonuclear leukocytes. Large numbers of bacterial pathogens, most frequently pneumococci, are recovered from cultures. Staphylococci, a rare cause of bacterial pneumonia in healthy adults, are also frequently isolated and are responsible for 15%–30% of bacterial pneumonias in patients who have pre-existing influenza. *Haemophilus influenzae* and *Streptococcus pyogenes* are the responsible micro-organisms in a small number of patients, as are *Escherichia coli;* strains of *Enterobacter, Serratia,* and *Klebsiella;* anaerobic cocci; and species of *Bacteroides.* In these individuals, there is no evidence of serious viral invasion of the lung, and the course and prognosis of this type of pneumonia are related completely to the nature and severity of the bacterial infection.

Primary Viral Pneumonia

A significant number of the deaths related to influenza can be ascribed not to concomitant bacterial infection, but rather to viral invasion of and multiplication within the lungs. These patients have a readily recognized clinical illness. Most have underlying cardiopulmonary disease or are pregnant. The initial symptoms are those of typical influenza, but within 12 to 36 hours the patient notes increasing dyspnea, usually accompanied by a cough productive of scant amounts of bloody sputum. On rare occasions, massive hemoptysis has been noted. Pleural pain is uncommon. At the time of hospitalization, respiratory distress is profound and is accompanied by striking tachypnea, tachycardia, and cyanosis. Abnormalities found on physical examination of the lungs vary with the stage of the disease process. Early in the course of the illness, inspiratory rales and occasional wheezes are heard primarily in the lower lung fields, but as the disease progresses, these findings spread to the entire chest. Evidence of consolidation is uncommonly found, and breath sounds are heard relatively well in the early phases of the infection. Thereafter, as dyspnea and cyanosis increase, breath sounds are suppressed throughout. When the pneumonia reaches its terminal phases, unbearable air hunger is the predominant symptom. Diffuse inspiratory rales, marked expiratory wheezes, and progressive prolongation of the expiratory phase of respiration are observed. The dyspnea and air hunger are frequently so intense and agitation so marked that patients cannot tolerate masks.

Laboratory studies reveal leukocytosis in the majority of patients. The cell count may be as high as 20,000/mm^3, with an increase in the number of polymorphonuclear leukocytes and band forms. Despite the increase in the number of polymorphonuclear cells in the peripheral blood, the sputum shows only a relatively small number, the majority of cells being mononuclear. This relationship in itself serves to distinguish this syndrome from the bacterial complications of influenza. Chest roentgenograms show extensive bilateral infiltrates that radiate from the hilum and simulate the findings in pulmonary edema of cardiac origin (Fig. 10). Occasionally, small pleural or interlobar effusions may be observed.

During the pandemic of 1957–1958, the mortality from primary influenza virus pneumonia approached 80%; it was also high in the pandemic of 1968–1969. At postmortem examination, there was evidence of tracheitis, bronchitis, and bronchiolitis, with loss of normal ciliated epithelial cells. The alveolar spaces were frequently filled with edematous fluid, and both mononuclear and neutrophilic infiltrates were found, often accompanied by intra-alveolar hemorrhage. A characteristic finding was the presence of an acellular hyaline membrane lining the alveoli. The virus was readily isolated from these lungs, usually in high titer. There usually was no evidence of congestive heart failure or concomitant bacterial infection.

There is no effective treatment for influenza virus pneumonia. There have been no controlled studies of amantadine treatment, so its use in this setting is based on anec-

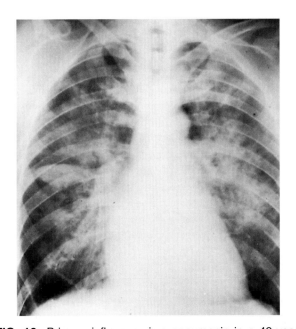

FIG. 10. Primary influenza virus pneumonia in a 49-year-old man with mitral stenosis. Infiltrates radiating from the hilum simulate the findings in cardiogenic pulmonary edema. (Reproduced with copyright permission of The American Society for Clinical Investigation from Louria DB, et al. Studies on influenza in the pandemic of 1957–1958: II. Pulmonary complications of influenza. *J Clin Invest* 1959;38:213.)

dotal reports of a beneficial effect on peripheral airway resistance in uncomplicated influenza. There is currently no evidence that adrenal glucocorticoids are beneficial. Influenza virus pneumonia can be complicated by renal failure and disseminated intravascular coagulation.

In some cases, the pulmonary disease process produced by influenza viruses has been far milder than that observed during pandemics. Focal pneumonitis and lobular or even lobar consolidation have evidently been caused by the viral infection alone. Consequently, influenza virus infection should be considered in the differential diagnosis of any nonbacterial pneumonia.

Concomitant Influenza Virus and Bacterial Pneumonia

In the disease of combined etiology, there may be an interval as long as 4 days between the initial symptoms of influenza and evidence of pulmonary involvement; during this period, considerable improvement may be noted. In many patients, however, the pulmonary disease blends with the original influenza. Cough productive of bloody or purulent sputum, shaking chills, and pleuritic chest pain are reported in most cases. At the time of admission to the hospital, respiratory distress is usually severe, and most patients are cyanotic. Physical examination of the lungs reveals variable findings. The majority of patients have signs of local consolidation involving one or more lobes, and most of these in addition have manifestations of more extensive disease, evidenced by diffuse inspiratory rales and inspiratory or expiratory wheezes. In a minority of individuals, diffuse inspiratory rales or wheezes are present without evidence of focal consolidation. Roentgenograms show diffuse infiltrates similar to those observed in patients with primary influenza virus pneumonia, or a combination of diffuse infiltrates and areas of focal consolidation may be found.

Blood leukocyte counts vary from <1000 to 30,000/ mm^3. If the leukocyte count is normal or elevated, adult and immature polymorphonuclear leukocytes predominate, whereas leukopenia is characteristically accompanied by granulocytopenia. Stained smears of the sputum show a large number of polymorphonuclear leukocytes even in patients who have profound peripheral leukopenia; in addition, myriad bacteria are observed.

In contrast to patients with secondary bacterial pneumonia, in whom the pathogen is usually the pneumococcus, approximately half the patients with combined viral and bacterial pneumonia are infected with *S. aureus* (Fig. 11). This frequency makes it mandatory that initial treatment be directed against the staphylococcus in patients in whom clinical evidence of influenza is followed by pneumonia that, on the basis of physical examination, roentgenograms, and Gram's stains of the sputum, is suggestive of combined viral and bacterial infection. Even

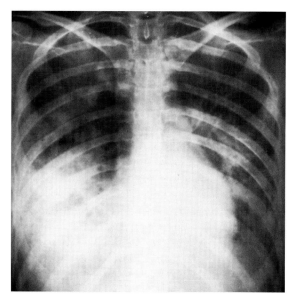

FIG. 11. Chest roentgenogram of a 21-year-old woman with combined staphylococcal and influenza virus pneumonia. (Reproduced with copyright permission of The American Society for Clinical Investigation from Louria DB, et al. Studies on influenza in the pandemic of 1957–1958: II. Pulmonary complications of influenza. *J Clin Invest* 1959;38:213.)

with immediate and appropriate antibiotic therapy, the mortality approximates 50%. The combination of mixed influenza virus and bacterial pneumonia and leukopenia usually indicates staphylococcal infection, and a majority of these patients die. At postmortem examination, both pathogenic bacteria and influenza virus can be cultivated from the lungs. The diagnosis of staphylococcal infection in these patients is so likely, the mortality so high, and the time between initial pulmonary symptoms and death so short that antistaphylococcal therapy should be instituted immediately with antibiotics effective against penicillin-resistant staphylococci, such as nafcillin, oxacillin, or a cephalosporin; in communities where methicillin-resistant strains are common, it would be safer to start treatment with vancomycin.

Several studies have produced additional information on three aspects of influenza infection. First, it has been demonstrated that viremia does occur in influenza, although the data currently available suggest it is infrequent. The virus has been isolated from visceral organs, including the spleen and liver, and has been recovered from the brain. Second, interesting epidemiologic evidence from Great Britain suggests that patients in whom staphylococcal complications of viral influenza develop either have active staphylococcal disease themselves (usually furunculosis) or have close contact with others having active staphylococcal lesions. Third, influenza viruses may cause hospital epidemics in which typical manifestations of influenza occur or in which the disease is manifested primarily by lung involvement in patients compromised by a variety of underlying diseases.

Interferon, arising from virus-exposed cells, appears in the lungs of experimental animals before specific antibody can be detected, but its role in recovery from human influenza is unclear. Amantadine hydrochloride prevents the entry of adsorbed influenza A virus into cells. It is useful prophylactically; it can prevent the clinical manifestations of influenza in about 70% of a population exposed to influenza type A viruses. In patients with influenza A and mild pulmonary involvement, amantadine may result in more rapid return of pulmonary function to normal, but this in itself probably does not justify the use of the drug in such cases. To be effective, amantadine must be given within 48 hours after the onset of clinical illness. Amantadine may be helpful in aborting influenza epidemics within hospitals.

Influenza can be prevented in most cases by immunization with appropriate vaccines. These must be changed constantly to include antigens from newly discovered strains of epidemiologic importance. During periods in which influenza is prevalent, older persons and those with underlying cardiopulmonary disease should be immunized. One problem of growing concern is that the major target group for immunization comprises persons <60 to 65 years old, but this group may show suboptimal antibody response to standard influenza immunization schedules.

Varicella

Epidemiology

Varicella is complicated by pulmonary involvement in the newborn, in approximately 10% of normal adults, in both children and adults who acquire the disease during therapy with adrenal glucocorticoids for another illness, in patients suffering from hematologic malignancy, and in pregnant women. The pulmonary manifestations may be overwhelming. The mortality in adults who are hospitalized ranges from 10%–24%, and in children receiving steroids and in neonates it is even higher. Death in children is often associated with secondary bacterial infection of the lung, especially staphylococcal infection, whereas in adults secondary bacterial infection is unusual and death occurs because of severe hypoxia secondary to the extensive viral pneumonitis. Figure 12 shows the roentgenogram of a 36-year-old woman who died 48 hours after hospitalization despite intensive respiratory care.

Pulmonary involvement is characteristically found 2 to 5 days after onset of the rash. Three types may be distinguished clinically: (1) mild or subclinical disease characterized only by cough; (2) moderate to very severe pneumonia with marked cough and dyspnea, which is usually accompanied by both cyanosis and hemoptysis; and (3) overwhelming and fatal disease with profound cyanosis and shortness of breath. The only findings on physical examination in the patients with milder disease

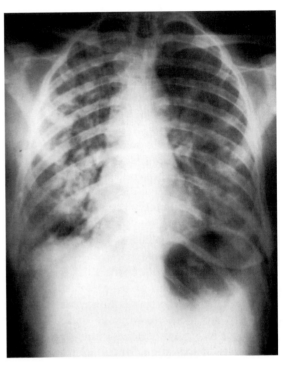

FIG. 12. Fatal varicella pneumonia in a 36-year-old woman. Note the coalescing nodular infiltrates.

are fine rales and some roughening of the breath sounds. In more severely ill patients, rhonchi, inspiratory and expiratory wheezes, and striking suppression of breath sounds may be detected. In each of the three types, roentgenograms of the chest show diffuse bilateral nodular infiltrates, which in the patients with more severe disease may be coalescent. A small number of patients have pleuritic chest pain, which may be associated with pleural effusions that are occasionally massive. Roentgenographic infiltrates may clear rapidly, but not infrequently they resolve slowly, sometimes persisting for 2 to 4 weeks or longer. Late calcification may occur, and diffusion defects may be demonstrated for a prolonged period following clinical improvement. Examination of sputum smears shows predominantly mononuclear cells and giant cells; characteristic type A intranuclear inclusion bodies can sometimes be seen with Giemsa stain. The blood leukocyte count varies from normal to moderately elevated, usually with a predominance of polymorphonuclear leukocytes. Postmortem examination reveals hemorrhagic, edematous lungs with an interstitial mononuclear infiltrate, alveolar hemorrhage, and sometimes hyaline membranes lining the alveoli. There also may be hemorrhagic pleural blebs and, in the liver, spleen, and occasionally the kidneys, focal necrosis and hemorrhage.

Treatment

Acyclovir given intravenously appears to be effective therapy for varicella pneumonia. Reports documenting the safety and efficacy of acyclovir for varicella pneumonia complicating pregnancy have also appeared. Famciclovir would be a reasonable oral alternative to acyclovir, but its safety in pregnancy has not been established (category B). For individuals intolerant of acyclovir or suspected of having acyclovir resistance, intravenous foscarnet may be used. The safety of foscarnet in pregnancy has not been established (category C). Although varicella pneumonia may be excessively severe in patients receiving adrenal glucocorticoids, these drugs are advocated by many in the treatment of overwhelming pulmonary varicella infection. There are no adequate data to indicate whether such treatment is beneficial. Secondary bacterial infection should be suggested by the sudden appearance in the sputum of large numbers of polymorphonuclear leukocytes. Not only have prophylactic antimicrobial agents failed to prevent the secondary bacterial complications, but there is reason to believe that the bacterial invaders in patients receiving antimicrobial agents prophylactically are more likely to be antibiotic-resistant staphylococci and gram-negative organisms, which are currently considerably more difficult to treat. Antibiotics should therefore be withheld until there is evidence of bacterial superinfection. Patients with varicella pneumonia should be maintained in strict isolation, and special care should be taken to keep them separated from patients who are receiving adrenal steroids or who have hematologic malignancies.

Rubeola (Measles)

Rubeola is associated with three types of pulmonary complications. First, especially if the patient is very young or very old, the virus itself may produce interstitial pneumonia in the absence of bacterial infection. This type of pneumonia is acute and occurs concomitantly while, before, or more often shortly after the rash has reached its peak. Cough and dyspnea are found frequently, but only small amounts of sputum are produced and pleuritic pain is unusual. Roentgenograms show infiltrates radiating from the hilar areas. The blood leukocyte count is characteristically normal or reduced. Although the prognosis is usually good, measles virus pneumonia continues to carry a significant mortality, approximating 5%. In children it may be followed by bronchiectasis.

Second, bacterial pneumonia may complicate rubeola, usually occurring 1 to 7 days after the onset of rash. If the patient has typical measles, improves, and then begins to exhibit pulmonary symptoms, this is virtually pathognomonic of a bacterial superinfection. The bacteria most commonly involved are *Streptococcus pneumoniae, Streptococcus pyogenes, Staphylococcus aureus,* and *Haemophilus influenzae.*

Third, when it is grown in human and monkey renal cell cultures, the measles virus produces multinucleated giant cells with characteristic inclusions. Giant-cell pneumonia apparently caused by the measles virus may follow overt measles in previously healthy children. Furthermore, in children with underlying disease, the measles virus may produce subacute or chronic, usually fatal, giant-cell pneumonia, which may occur with or without clinical evidence of typical measles preceding the pneumonia. Pathologically, giant-cell pneumonia is characterized by an interstitial mononuclear infiltrate, alveolar cell proliferation, and giant cells with intranuclear and intracytoplasmic inclusions.

No treatment other than supportive therapy is available for measles virus invasion of the pulmonary parenchyma. Treatment of secondary bacterial complications depends on the antibiotic susceptibility of the bacterial pathogen.

An additional form of pulmonary disease may occur in patients who have previously received killed measles vaccine and subsequently are given a live measles vaccine or are exposed to wild virus. Rash, lymphadenopathy, and pneumonitis may follow. The pulmonary infiltrate, which may not be accompanied by rash, may be interstitial, locular, lobar, or nodular. Nodular or interstitial infiltrates may persist for weeks or even months.

Adenovirus Infection

These viruses infect 8% of children and 1%–3% of adults annually. Adenovirus infections occur throughout the year, with a peak incidence of respiratory infections occurring in late winter to early spring. Adenoviruses are spread by intimate contact or aerosolization of infected secretions, and serotypes 3, 4, and 7 are more frequently associated with lung disease. The first isolation of adenoviruses from diseased patients occurred in a study of military recruits in 1954; these individuals had a variety of influenza-like syndromes, referred to as *acute respiratory disease.* In that report, one fifth of infected individuals required hospitalization.

Fever, headache, nasal congestion, hoarseness, and paroxysms of cough are the most common symptoms and usually last 3 to 5 days. On examination, cervical lymphadenopathy, laryngitis, and rales are common. Sputum examination may reveal either mononuclear cells or a predominance of polymorphonuclear leukocytes. The appearance of the latter does not in itself connote secondary bacterial infection, but bacterial superinfection does occur in a significant percentage of patients with adenovirus pneumonia. Although patchy or lobular infiltrates are found most frequently, there may be extensive consolidation. There are no specific drugs or therapeutic measures available for the treatment of adenovirus infections.

Hantavirus Infection

Hantaviruses are RNA viruses belonging to the family *Bunyaviridae.* Rodents are the primary reservoir for all hantaviruses and shed the virus in their saliva, urine, and feces. Humans acquire infection most often by inhalation of aerosols from rodent excreta. Person-to-person transmission does not occur. Hantaviral disease first became a public health concern in the United States in the 1950s, when soldiers serving in Korea were afflicted with an illness referred to as *Korean hemorrhagic fever* or *hemorrhagic fever with renal syndrome*. Only rarely have there been prominent pulmonary signs or symptoms. However, a new hantavirus was isolated in the southwestern United States in 1993 that caused hantavirus pulmonary syndrome. The deer mouse (*Peromyscus maniculatus*) has been determined to be the vector for this syndrome.

The mortality of hantavirus pulmonary syndrome is 10 times higher than that associated with Korean hemorrhagic fever. The syndrome is manifested by (1) a febrile illness (temperature ≥101°F) occurring in a previously healthy person, characterized by unexplained adult respiratory distress syndrome *or* bilateral interstitial pulmonary infiltrates developing within 1 week of hospitalization with respiratory compromise requiring supplemental oxygen, *or* (2) an unexplained respiratory illness resulting in death in conjunction with an autopsy examination demonstrating noncardiogenic pulmonary edema without an identifiable, specific cause of death. The agent of the syndrome is the first hantavirus to cause disease in North America. Now named *sin nombre virus,* it closely resembles a Prospect Hill strain of hantavirus that is found in voles but is not pathogenic in humans.

The diagnosis is largely based on epidemiologic circumstances and a clinical triad of interstitial infiltrates with adult respiratory distress syndrome, hemoconcentration, and marked elevation of lactate dehydrogenase. Anecdotal evidence suggests ribavirin may be beneficial.

Respiratory Syncytial Virus Infection

Perhaps the most frequently involved virus in young children is the respiratory syncytial virus. Respiratory syncytial virus infection is seasonal, occurring from November through March. The frequency with which infant pneumonia or bronchiolitis is related to this agent obviously depends on the prevalence of the virus in the environment, but current data suggest that respiratory syncytial virus is responsible for 10%–40% of lower respiratory tract disease in infants and children. During epidemics, it may account for 50% of all pediatric hospital admissions.

The virus is most likely spread by aerosol or direct contact with infected specimens, and inoculation routes include the eyes, nasopharynx, and oropharynx. Incubation lasts 2 to 8 days. Respiratory syncytial virus may cause croup, bronchiolitis, or pneumonia, and the latter is more frequent with primary infection. Respiratory syncytial virus infection among adults is usually mild, but

severe disease may be seen among institutionalized persons, the elderly, and patients with underlying cardiopulmonary disease. Abnormal roentgenographic findings may include interstitial infiltrates, bronchopneumonia, and diffuse pneumonia. A specific diagnosis can be made by obtaining nasopharyngeal secretions for viral culture. In addition, respiratory syncytial virus infection can be diagnosed rapidly by antigen detection using immunofluorescence techniques or ELISA. Although aerosolized ribavirin showed promise for respiratory syncytial virus pneumonitis in children, there is no convincing evidence for its benefit. Most authorities now recommend ribavirin only for severe respiratory syncytial virus disease in immunocompromised patients, but experience is anecdotal and efficacy has been dismal.

RICKETTSIAL DISEASE

Q Fever

Q (query) fever was first described in 1937 by Derrick, who detailed an acute febrile illness involving abattoir workers in Brisbane, Australia. Subsequently, Burnet in Australia and Cox in the United States isolated the causative organism and demonstrated that it was one of the rickettsiae. In honor of these investigators, the microorganism is called *Coxiella burnetii. C. burnetii* is worldwide in distribution, the most common reservoirs being sheep, goats, cattle, and ticks. The organism is frequently shed in cows' milk, and the disease may spread by consumption of raw milk, by inhalation of contaminated dust, and occasionally by tick or animal bites. Recent outbreaks have been associated with infected parturient cats. Human-to-human transmission has been reported.

Clinical Manifestations

After an incubation period that ranges from 2 to 4 weeks, clinical evidence of disease appears, usually abruptly. Fever occurs in almost all patients, is frequently of considerable degree, and in untreated cases usually persists for a period of 10 days to 3 weeks, but it may remain for as long as 3 months. It then resolves by lysis. Severe headache, marked sweats, shaking chills, and diffuse myalgia are found in the majority of patients. One third to two thirds of patients report cough that, in contradistinction to that observed in primary atypical pneumonia, is usually not severe. It is typically nonproductive, although occasionally a small amount of sputum is expectorated, infrequently blood-tinged. From 10%–40% of patients experience mild to moderate chest pain that may be pleuritic in nature. Dyspnea is noted in a minority of cases, and vomiting, confusion, and abdominal pain occur uncommonly.

Although the patient usually appears acutely ill on

physical examination and is markedly febrile, the pulse is relatively slow. The abnormalities in the lungs, ordinarily consisting of unilateral or bilateral fine inspiratory rales, are often confined to the lower lobes. On occasion, dullness to percussion, evidence of frank consolidation, a pleural friction rub, and signs of pleural effusion are noted. Splenomegaly occurs in 5%–10% of cases, and hepatomegaly, cyanosis, a maculopapular rash, and stiffness of the neck with resistance to flexion may be observed in a small number of individuals.

Roentgenographic and Laboratory Findings

The leukocyte count is usually normal or slightly elevated, with a moderate increase in the number of polymorphonuclear leukocytes. Stained smears of the sputum show predominantly mononuclear cells. The radiographic picture is variable. Segmental and subsegmental pleurabased opacities are common. Multiple rounded opacities have been reported following inhalational exposures. Pleural effusions are usually small but may be present in up to one third of cases. Hilar adenopathy may occur. Time of resolution ranges from 10 to 90 days. By injection of infected material into the peritoneal cavity of guinea pigs, *C. burnetii* can be isolated from the blood, sputum, or pleural fluid during the acute phase of the illness. Specific complement-fixing and agglutinating antibodies appear in the blood during the second to third week of illness and in most cases establish the diagnosis. The Weil-Felix reaction is invariably negative.

Complications

The pulmonary lesions heal without residua, and the complications of Q fever are found in extrapulmonary sites. The hepatitis may be severe and prolonged, even fatal, with marked icterus and derangement of liver function. Arthritis, iritis, pericarditis with pericardial friction rub, myocarditis, otitis, epididymitis, esophagitis, neuropathy, and radiculitis have all been reported. Although the lumbar puncture usually yields normal results despite the severe headache, the micro-organism has been isolated from the spinal fluid, and on rare occasions spinal tap has revealed lymphocytic meningitis. A small number of cases of endocarditis caused by *C. burnetii* have been described, most of them in the United Kingdom; in 80%, the aortic valve is involved with aortic regurgitation. Perhaps the most frequent complication is thrombophlebitis, which may be accompanied by pulmonary emboli. A significant number of patients in whom well-documented Q fever develops have persistent, vague aches and pains and fail to return to their original state of health for a substantial period of time. The mechanisms underlying these prolonged and at times incapacitating features have not been established, but they are not associated with demonstrable persistence of the micro-organism.

Treatment

Q fever is rarely a fatal disease. The micro-organism is susceptible in vitro to tetracyclines and chloramphenicol, and administration of one of these antibiotics in a dosage of 2 g/d in adults is usually associated with rapid defervescence and clinical improvement. However, in some patients treated with a tetracycline or chloramphenicol, improvement may be surprisingly slow, and relapse may occur after the antibiotics have been discontinued. These relapses usually respond promptly to reinstitution of the same antimicrobial regimen.

Scrub Typhus

Scrub typhus, a rickettsial disease caused by *Rickettsia tsutsugamushi,* is endemic in Japan, Southeast Asia, the southwestern Pacific, and Australia. It is transmitted to humans by mites, and after a 4- to 10-day incubation period a primary eschar appears at the site of the mite bite. The eschar and regional adenitis are found in at least 60% of patients with scrub typhus.

There are three potentially severe complications of the disease: myocarditis, encephalitis, and pneumonitis. Lung involvement, which varies considerably in its manifestations, is said to occur in 40%–50% of patients. Cough, the most frequent pulmonary symptom, may be productive of small amounts of blood-streaked sputum. Extensive pulmonary disease may cause dyspnea and cyanosis. The pneumonia is primarily interstitial in nature, and may be either localized or diffuse. Chest radiographs usually show patchy infiltrates, but lobar consolidation may be seen.

The average mortality is approximately 5% in untreated patients. Tetracyclines are the treatment of choice.

Rocky Mountain Spotted Fever

In Rocky Mountain spotted fever, chest complaints may be the presenting manifestations. Lung involvement is at first characterized by patchy pneumonitis or pleural effusion accompanied by nonspecific symptoms, including chest pain and cough. As the disease progresses, the local vasculitis and systemic thrombocytopenia may result in lung edema and/or hemorrhage. In some cases, the respiratory distress syndrome supervenes. Additionally, Rocky Mountain spotted fever myocarditis can result in congestive heart failure. Roentgenograms vary depending on the pathophysiology: There may be focal infiltrates, dense consolidation from hemorrhage or secondary bacterial infection, or diffuse bilateral infiltrates. In some cases, the lack of a rash and the prominence of pulmonary manifestations result in a substantial delay in establishing a correct diagnosis. Occasionally, myalgias involving thoracic muscles are so severe that a diagnosis of bacterial pneumonia or pulmonary embolus is mistakenly made.

ZOONOTIC PNEUMONIAS

Bacteria associated with domestic and wild animals are often capable of producing disease in humans, and spread may occur by direct contact, inhalation or ingestion, or animal bites or insect intermediates. These zoonotic bacterial infections have few unique clinical characteristics, and the diagnosis is often first considered after a provocative interrogation including travel history, occupation, hobbies, and contact with animals and insects. Although the diseases reviewed here are rare causes of respiratory infections in the United States, they can be severe, life-threatening, and contagious illnesses for which effective antimicrobial therapy is available.

Anthrax

Micro-organism

Bacillus anthracis, a large, aerobic, gram-positive, sporule-forming micro-organism, has played a major role in the history of microbiology. Isolated by Robert Koch in 1877, it consistently produced fatal infections in laboratory animals, and Koch's now famous postulates for determining whether an organism is a pathogen were based on his studies with anthrax.

Epidemiology

Pulmonary anthrax has never been a common disease. Some 200 cases were reported before 1900, and only a small number of cases have been reported since that time, with most of the patients having some contact with wool and wool processing. However, direct contact with wool or hides during processing procedures is not necessary; anthrax has occurred in persons who lived or frequently walked near tanneries but never had direct contact with such procedures. It should be emphasized that finished rugs and carpets are not a source of the infection.

The thoracic form of the disease is not ordinarily pneumonia. After spores have been inhaled, they are carried to the pulmonary parenchyma, where they undergo phagocytosis by macrophages and then are transported to regional lymph nodes, where they germinate. The germination of the spores produces a violent reaction in the host: Necrosis, hemorrhage, and edema lead to acute hemorrhagic mediastinitis. Subsequent pulmonary involvement is secondary to hematogenous spread of the bacteria.

Like mediastinitis, this type of pneumonia is characteristically hemorrhagic. Although parenchymal lung involvement usually follows bloodstream dissemination, there have been reports of pneumonia with necrosis of alveolar walls that apparently occurred as a primary phenomenon following spore inhalation.

Clinical Manifestations

The course of the disease is usually diphasic. The patient initially experiences chills, fever, and myalgia. These symptoms are followed by a 1- or 2-day period during which there is either no change or some improvement; then, progressive disease ensues abruptly and is characterized by tachypnea, dyspnea, cyanosis, and cardiovascular collapse. Rales, and at times rhonchi and wheezes, may be heard in focal areas or diffusely throughout the lung fields. In some patients, dullness to percussion and altered breath sounds suggest consolidation. Chest roentgenograms show congestion, patchy infiltrates, areas of consolidation, and mediastinal widening. While the disease is fulminating, pleural effusion, subcutaneous edema of the chest and neck, splenomegaly, and meningitis may be observed. Most of the patients reported have died.

Therapy

As the anthrax bacillus is susceptible to penicillin and streptomycin, the treatment of choice for adults is 3 to 10 million units of penicillin per day. Some give streptomycin together with penicillin. Erythromycin, chloramphenicol, and tetracycline are alternate agents.

Brucellosis

Brucellae are small, gram-negative, coccobacillary aerobes that can be separated into four major species: *Brucella abortus, Brucella melitensis, Brucella suis,* and *Brucella canis.* Brucellosis occurs in susceptible individuals who deal with animals and animal products, veterinarians, farmers, and persons ingesting unpasteurized dairy products. The organism is acquired through ingestion or, rarely, contact. No human-to-human transmission has been reported.

The clinical presentation of brucellosis involves a variety of nonspecific constitutional symptoms, including relapsing fever and headache. Cough occurs in one fourth of cases, but other respiratory symptoms are notably absent. The most characteristic radiographic findings include perihilar thickening and peribronchial infiltrates, although nodular lesions and miliary infiltrates may be seen.

No data are available on sputum bacteriology, and blood culture findings are rarely positive. Cultures of biopsy specimens of granulomas are frequently positive, and the *Brucella* agglutination test is confirmatory. The most effective therapy is with tetracycline (1.5 to 2.0 g orally) and streptomycin (1.0 g intramuscularly) daily for 1 month.

Pasteurella multocida Pneumonia

Pasteurella multocida is the causative agent of hemorrhagic septicemia in animals and can be isolated from the respiratory tracts of a variety of domestic and wild animals. The organism is a small, gram-negative, bipolar-staining, nonmotile rod that grows well on blood agar, but its growth is inhibited on MacConkey media. In humans, three clinical patterns of disease are observed: (1) local suppuration or cellulitis following a bite or scratch; (2) meningitis or bacteremia; and (3) acute or subacute lung infection, sometimes accompanied by empyema. Although respiratory disease is rarely reported, sputum is the most common source of isolates in cases of animal-bite cellulitis.

Most cases of *Pasteurella* pneumonia occur in individuals with underlying chronic lung disease, including bronchiectasis, emphysema, and carcinoma. Spread to humans is probably from animals, but in only half the cases is there an exposure history. Lung involvement is probably initiated by aspiration of the oropharyngeal flora. Radiographic findings include lobar, multilobar, or diffuse patchy infiltrates with a tendency to spare the upper lobes. Pleural effusions are found in 20% of cases. Empyema and abscess formation occasionally occur. Diagnosis depends on isolation of the organism from sputum, pleural fluid, or blood. Penicillin is the drug of choice, as the majority of strains are exquisitely sensitive. Alternative choices include chloramphenicol, cephalosporins, and tetracycline.

Tularemia

Francisella tularensis is a tiny, gram-negative, pleomorphic, coccobacillary organism that grows poorly on artificial medium unless supplemented with serum, glucose, and cystine. There are approximately 150 cases of tularemia per year in the United States, and pulmonary disease occurs in 10%–15% of these cases. Tularemia can be transmitted to humans by wood ticks, dog ticks, the deer fly, and a variety of wild animals, notably the rabbit. Punched-out skin lesions with secondary lymph node involvement, the so-called ulceroglandular type, is the most common form of the disease; although pneumonic tularemia often arises from hematogenous dissemination from cutaneous foci, as many as 50% of patients with pleuropulmonary tularemia have no demonstrable disease of the skin or lymph nodes.

Respiratory disease often begins with a poorly produc-

tive cough, chest pain, and dyspnea. In airborne tularemia, sore throat has been observed in about one third of patients, and a similar proportion exhibit a skin rash, either erythema nodosum or erythema multiforme. The roentgenographic appearance varies from small areas of bronchopneumonia to extensive lobar or lobular consolidation, often with hilar adenopathy. Extension to the pleura is common. Only rarely are organisms seen on sputum Gram's stain, and because of the potential for laboratory-acquired infection, isolation should be reserved for special reference laboratories. The diagnosis can be established by demonstrating a rise in serologic agglutinations. The micro-organism is susceptible to streptomycin (or gentamicin), tetracycline, and chloramphenicol. Streptomycin remains the mainstay of therapy, with a dramatic response usually being observed within 24 to 48 hours of initiation of the antibiotic, in a dosage of 1.5 to 2.0 g/d.

Plague

Yersinia pestis remains a problem in China, India, Vietnam, and certain areas of the Middle East and Africa. In the past 15 years, a very small number of cases have been reported in the United States, most of these in California and New Mexico; in one case, a domestic cat was the source. Although the bacillus, first isolated by Yersin in 1894, has now been relegated to secondary importance among organisms parasitic to humans, its importance in medical history and perhaps in the course of our civilization is undeniable. During the plague epidemic of the fourteenth century, when many cases were pneumonic, the disease acquired its macabre figurative name, the Black Death. During that epidemic, it is estimated that one half to two thirds of the people in Great Britain died of this infection. In the sixteenth century, *Y. pestis* ravaged the world for 30 to 60 years, "depopulated towns, turned the country into a desert, and made the habitations of men to become the haunts of wild beasts," and during this period it is said to have killed some 100 million persons. During the seventeenth to nineteenth centuries, there was a striking decline in the incidence of the disease, and subsequently, because of higher standards of living, greater attention to personal hygiene, and vigorous efforts to control rat populations, plague virtually disappeared from many areas of the world.

Pneumonic plague is not the natural form of the infection in humans. Ordinarily, plague acquired from wild rodents through infective fleas occurs initially in the bubonic form. Progressive bubonic disease is associated with bacteremia in as many as 70%–85% of patients, and secondary lung involvement ensues in some. As in the epidemic of the fourteenth century, these individuals may spread the disease by the airborne route to other persons, in whom the lungs may become the initial site of invasion. Such patients usually have shaking chills and high fever.

Their sputum varies from gelatinous to rusty, and on occasion there is profuse hemoptysis. Most striking in these patients is profound dyspnea and air hunger. Physical examination and chest roentgenograms show lobar pneumonia or diffuse involvement simulating pulmonary edema. The lung may be heavy, mimicking the roentgenogram of Friedländer's pneumonia. The disease is characteristically fulminating. The average survival time among untreated patients is 1.8 days. Postmortem examination of the lungs shows severe hemorrhage, coagulation necrosis, and infiltration by large numbers of polymorphonuclear leukocytes.

Treatment, which must be immediate if the patient's life is to be saved, consists of oxygen and antibiotics. The micro-organism is usually susceptible to streptomycin, other aminoglycosides, tetracyclines, and chloramphenicol, and the therapeutic regimen of choice appears to be one of the last two in combination with streptomycin or gentamicin. Patients with bubonic plague should probably be isolated, as some may have throat cultures positive for *Y. pestis*. Strict isolation precautions should be observed in cases of pneumonic plague, as the dangers to those attending such patients are great.

PARASITIC DISEASE

Three types of pulmonary disease are associated with protozoal or helminthic infection:

1. Loeffler's syndrome with no evidence of invasion of the pulmonary parenchyma
2. Parasitic disease with direct lung invasion
3. Pulmonary involvement resulting from direct spread from subdiaphragmatic lesions

Loeffler's Syndrome

In 1936, Loeffler described a series of cases characterized by pulmonary infiltrates and mild illness lasting for 3 to 8 days and accompanied by striking peripheral eosinophilia, with the peak of the increase in eosinophils usually following the maximal pulmonary infiltration. Roentgenographic abnormalities were patchy and fleeting. Moderate cough was noted, but most of the patients remained afebrile and sputum was ordinarily not produced. A great number of infections and drugs have been associated with the syndrome. Pulmonary eosinophilia has been observed in patients with certain bacterial and mycotic infections, including tuberculosis, brucellosis, coccidioidomycosis, aspergillosis, and histoplasmosis; in patients with allergic asthma; in individuals exposed to certain drugs, especially antibiotics; and in patients with intestinal parasitism by the following protozoa, nematodes, and trematodes: *Entamoeba histolytica, Trichinella spiralis, Trichuris trichiura, Enterobius vermicularis, Fasciola he-*

patica, Necator americanus, Taenia saginata, Ancylostoma braziliense, Ancylostoma duodenale, Toxocara canis, Toxocara mystax, Ascaris lumbricoides, and *Strongyloides stercoralis.* The last four perhaps do not belong in this category, as there is considerable evidence to suggest that the pulmonary disease with eosinophilia is related to direct invasion of lung tissue. Because Loeffler's syndrome is benign, no specific therapy is required.

Parasitic Disease with Direct Lung Invasion

Schistosomiasis

Micro-organism

Pulmonary schistosomiasis, which may be caused by *Schistosoma mansoni, S. japonicum,* or *S. haematobium,* is a problem of considerable magnitude in areas of the Middle East, Asia, Africa, and Latin America. Free-swimming cercariae infect humans by penetrating the skin. The larvae (schistosomulae) gain access to the circulation, pass through the lungs, and eventually reach the portal and mesenteric vessels. During the period in which the larvae pass through the pulmonary vasculature, asthmatic symptoms may occur, but the major pulmonary involvement occurs later and is related to metastatic spread of ova produced by the adult worms through the systemic circulation to pulmonary vessels. The ova obstruct the arterioles, penetrate the arteriolar walls, and become the focus of obliterative granulomatous arteritis.

Clinical Manifestations

During the larval migration phase, symptoms include wheezing, dyspnea, and nonproductive cough. In a small number of cases, acute pneumonic schistosomiasis occurs 3 weeks to 3 months after the initial cercarial penetration. This is apparently related to an intense inflammatory response to invasion by ova. In such cases, schistosomiasis may be manifested as overwhelming, diffuse disease characterized by severe respiratory distress, productive cough, hemoptysis, cyanosis, and bilateral rales on physical examination of the chest, or there may be signs of focal consolidation. Pulmonary involvement in those in whom symptoms develop is usually chronic and accompanied almost uniformly by extensive extrapulmonary schistosomal involvement, including hepatosplenomegaly. Dyspnea is the most common symptom, and the majority of patients also have a cough that is ordinarily nonproductive. Both cyanosis and hemoptysis are rare.

Roentgenographic and Laboratory Findings

In those with symptoms related to larval migration, the chest roentgenogram appears normal or shows some nonspecific increase in markings. Some degree of eosinophilia is usually found, and this may be marked. In patients with acute pulmonary schistosomiasis, areas of consolidation or coalescing nodular infiltrates are found. The lung fields may appear normal roentgenographically, or there may be a diffuse fibrotic or nodular infiltrate. The vascular dilatation may be marked, as shown in Fig. 13, the roentgenogram of a 16-year-old girl with schistosomal cor pulmonale. Many, but not all, patients with acute pulmonary schistosomiasis have significant peripheral eosinophilia, but eosinophilia is ordinarily absent in patients with chronic obliterative arteritis. The stools of most are positive for *Schistosoma* ova. In addition, in as many as a third of patients who have a productive cough, *Schistosoma* ova may be demonstrated in the sputum.

Once cor pulmonale has appeared, antischistosomal therapy is ineffective. If ova are found in the sputum or if the patient has acute pulmonary schistosomiasis, praziquantel in a single oral dose of 40 mg/kg is now considered to be the drug of choice. It is uncertain whether therapy actually alters the natural course of acute schistosomal pneumonia.

Echinococcosis

Epidemiology

Hydatid disease of the lung is caused by infection with the larval form of *Echinococcus granulosus,* a small tapeworm of the dog. Human infection is especially prevalent in the Middle East, Australia, New Zealand, central Europe, and parts of Latin America, areas in which sheep are an important part of the economy. Hydatid disease is uncommon in North America, except in certain areas of Canada and Alaska.

The incidence of lung involvement in human echinococcosis ranges from 5%–25% in different series. Although pulmonary infection usually arises from primary hematogenous dissemination, it may be secondary to metastatic spread from a ruptured abdominal cyst. Almost all the pulmonary cases are caused by *E. granulosus (unilocularis)*; only rarely is a case caused by the more malignant *E. multilocularis.* There is a clear predilection for the lower lobes, especially the right lower lobe. Approximately one third of patients with pulmonary echinococcosis also have clinical evidence of extrapulmonary hydatid disease.

Clinical Manifestations

Initial symptoms consist most commonly of cough, hemoptysis, and pleuritic pain. Sputum production is usually sparse, and characteristically there is little fever. Physical examination is frequently unrewarding. Clubbing of the fingers and toes is detected infrequently. Chest roentgenography shows one or more discrete, round lesions that typically are sharply defined with little surrounding inflammatory response and are sometimes calcified. These lesions are frequently mistaken for metastatic carcinoma.

Hydatid involvement of the thoracic cavity also may take the form of primary mediastinal disease (Fig. 14), which occurs most commonly in the posterior mediastinum. Anterior mediastinal involvement may be associated with Horner's syndrome (miosis, ptosis, and diminished sweating ipsilaterally).

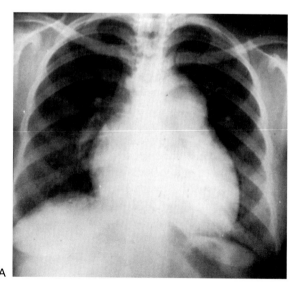
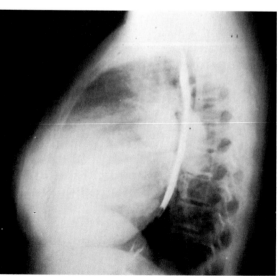

FIG. 13 (A,B). Schistosomal cor pulmonale in a 16-year-old girl. Note the marked dilatation of the pulmonary artery segment.

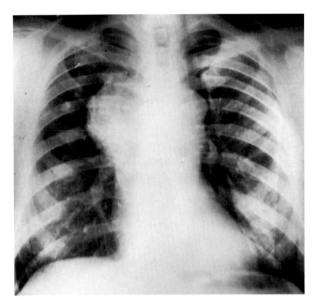

FIG. 14. Mediastinal echinococcosis. Note the thin rim of calcium in the cysts.

Laboratory Findings

Laboratory analysis in patients with echinococcosis reveals a normal total leukocyte count. Eosinophilia, generally moderate, is found in 50% of patients. Careful examination of sputum or of the sediment from material aspirated from the thoracic cavity may reveal hooklets or scoleces. Precipitin, complement fixation, indirect hemagglutination, and bentonite flocculation tests are available, and the results are positive for the majority of patients with echinococcal disease. The most reliable test is an enzyme immunoassay utilizing partially purified hydatid antigen.

Treatment

Surgical removal of the cyst, the treatment of choice, is often not technically feasible, and chronic disease is frequent even after apparently complete extirpation of the cyst. However, despite the persistence of chronic hydatid disease of the lungs or abdomen for many years, the patient may lead a relatively normal life. Secondary infection of the cyst should be treated with appropriate antimicrobial agents and surgical drainage. Medical therapy with mebendazole or albendazole may be effective.

Ascariasis

Ascariasis is a common intestinal nematode infection caused by *A. lumbricoides*. It is worldwide in distribution, and in the United States is found particularly in the southeastern section of the country. After ingestion, the embryonated ova hatch into larvae that penetrate the intesti-

nal wall, reach the circulation, and subsequently arrive in the lungs. During pulmonary migration, fever is commonly of considerable magnitude. Cough, hemoptysis, inspiratory rales, and evidence of focal consolidation are the other common manifestations, but on rare occasions the lesions can be diffuse and produce death either directly or through the development of severe, superimposed bacterial infection. Peripheral eosinophilia is often found during pulmonary migration but may not become evident until late in the course of the pulmonary disease. In addition to pneumonitis with fever, cough, and hemoptysis, there is considerable evidence to suggest that migration of the larvae through the lungs produces a milder illness that is consistent with Loeffler's syndrome.

The diagnosis of pulmonary ascariasis may be established by finding the larvae in the expectorated sputum or in gastric aspirates. The role of *A. lumbricoides* also should be suspected in patients with pneumonitis or Loeffler's syndrome if ova or adult worms are found in the stool. Serologic tests, including agar gel diffusion and immunoelectrophoresis, are available. Treatment of the pulmonary disease is usually not necessary, and in any case it is not known whether any of the currently available antihelminthic agents are beneficial in lung ascariasis. If pulmonary disease persists, a trial of mebendazole might be considered.

Visceral Larva Migrans

Visceral larva migrans results from the ingestion of embryonated ova of the dog or cat roundworm *T. canis* or *T. cati*. The disease occurs predominantly in young children who have close contact with dogs or cats and eat dirt. The larvae hatching from the ova penetrate the intestinal wall and migrate widely. Hepatomegaly is noted frequently. During pulmonary migration, wheezing, cough, cyanosis, or dyspnea may occur in association with roentgenographic evidence of diffuse or focal pneumonitis. The diagnosis can be established best by liver biopsy, with histologic sections of the specimen showing eosinophilic granulomas with larvae. The blood leukocyte count is usually markedly elevated, often reaching 40,000/mm^3 or higher, and eosinophilia of >30% is present in 85% of patients. The available serologic tests, indirect fluorescent antibody and indirect hemagglutination, are sensitive but lack specificity. The prognosis is usually good. Thiabendazole, the present drug of choice, can be given orally in a dosage of 25 mg/kg of body weight twice a day for 5 days (maximal daily dose, 3.0 g).

Strongyloidiasis

An estimated 35 million persons in the world suffer from infection with *Strongyloides stercoralis*. The majority of cases in the United States are confined to the southern parts of the country. Pneumonitis may occur during pulmonary migration of larvae, characterized by fever, wheezes, productive cough, and patchy or diffuse infiltrates on chest roentgenogram. Blood and sputum eosinophilia are found frequently, and typical larvae may be detected in the expectorated sputum.

Pulmonary manifestations are usually transient but may be chronic or recurrent. Recurrence is perhaps related to repeated bouts of endogenous dissemination to the lungs from established foci in the small intestines.

In the normal host, rhabditiform larvae are passed in the stool but can reinvade through the perianal area. This is called *exoautoinfection.* In patients with immunologic defects, in particular resulting from hematologic malignancies, large numbers of filariform larvae may penetrate the intestinal wall and invade various tissues, including the lungs (*endoautoinfection*). In almost all cases, corticosteroids and/or immunosuppressive agents have been administered. As a consequence of the penetration, gram-negative septicemia may occur, involving one or more enteric organisms. Larval meningitis may occur, and the pulmonary involvement varies from small pneumonic patches to massive infiltrates of five lobes. Larvae can usually be seen in expectorated sputum. Findings on stool examination are usually positive but in some cases may be negative, and jejunal intubation is necessary to establish the diagnosis. In the hyperinfection syndrome, eosinophil counts range from normal to markedly elevated. Immunofluorescence, complement fixation, and indirect hemagglutination tests for antibody determination are available, but more data are needed to define their usefulness.

Thiabendazole is the drug of choice in intestinal strongyloidiasis. Whether it is beneficial in acute or chronic pulmonary disease caused by *S. stercoralis* is unknown.

Paragonimiasis

Pulmonary paragonimiasis is found commonly in Southeast Asia, the Philippines, and less frequently in the South Pacific, Africa, India, and Latin America. The etiologic agent is the oriental lung fluke *Paragonimus westermani.*

The pulmonary manifestations vary considerably and depend on the number of parasites involved. Most patients have little fever or prostration. Cough is usually not marked but may be productive of thin sputum with globules of tenacious gelatinous material, or there may be small amounts of blood-stained sputum. Occasionally, the symptoms may be more severe, consisting of prostration and dyspnea. Pleuritic pain is noted infrequently. In most patients, the only findings are inspiratory rales, sometimes accompanied by dullness to percussion and roughened breath sounds. Less frequently, areas of focal consolidation or pleural effusion or pneumothorax may be detected.

Roentgenograms of the chest usually reveal linear or patchy infiltrates in the lower lung fields or nodular densities in which there may be areas of rarefaction. Cystlike lesions may be found and may be as large as several centimeters, and on rare occasions thick- or thin-walled cavities may be present. Pleural effusion and pneumothorax are each observed in <10% of cases.

In most cases of paragonimiasis, the blood leukocyte count is normal and eosinophilia is inconstant. The diagnosis can be made only by finding the characteristic ova, which can usually be seen readily on examination of the sputum or stool.

Paragonimus westermani infection frequently produces chronic disease that is sometimes incapacitating, and occasionally, in patients experiencing very heavy infestation, it is fatal. The treatment of choice is 25 mg of praziquantel per kilogram of body weight, given three times in a 1-day course.

BIBLIOGRAPHY

Anstey NM, Currie BJ, Withnall KM. Community-acquired *Acinetobacter* pneumonia in the Northern Territory of Australia. *Clin Infect Dis* 1992;14:83. *The authors report 11 cases of bacteremic* Acinetobacter *pneumonia and review the literature. Multiple clinical risk factors were noted in all cases and contributed to a high mortality (64%). In all cases, pneumonia was clinically fulminant, and fatal outcomes were associated with inappropriate initial antimicrobial therapy.*

Austrian R, Gold J. Pneumococcal bacteremia with especial reference to bacteremic pneumococcal pneumonia. *Ann Intern Med* 1964;60:759. *During a 10-year period (1952–1962), the authors reviewed 529 instances of pneumococcal bacteremia developing among 2000 cases of pneumococcal pneumonia. Increased risk for mortality was associated with age over 60 years, leukopenia, serotype 3 isolate, and an extrapulmonary form of infection.*

Brook I, Frazier EH. Aerobic and anaerobic microbiology of empyema. *Chest* 1993;103:1502. *A retrospective review of the microbiology and clinical features of empyema in 197 patients hospitalized between 1973 and 1985 in two military hospitals. Most patients with staphylococcal empyema had associated pneumonia, aspiration, or lung abscess.*

Broussard RC, Payne K, George RB. Treatment with acyclovir of varicella pneumonia in pregnancy. *Chest* 1991;99:1045. *After reviewing the literature regarding acyclovir therapy for varicella pneumonia in pregnancy, the authors concluded that acyclovir decreased case fatality rates compared with untreated historical controls and that no adverse effect(s) to mother or fetus had been reported.*

Burman LA, Leinonen M, Trollfors B. Use of serology to diagnose pneumonia caused by nonencapsulated *Haemophilus influenzae* and *Moraxella catarrhalis. J Infect Dis* 1994;170:220. *Antibodies against nonencapsulated* H. influenzae *and* M. catarrhalis *were measured by ELISA in paired sera from 158 adult patients with pneumonia. Specificity of the serologic methods was high, but sensitivity was low.*

Collazos J, Ayarza R. *Moraxella catarrhalis* bacteremic pneumonia in adults: two cases and review of the literature. *Eur J Clin Microbiol Infect Dis* 1992;11:237. *All patients with* Moraxella *bacteremic pneumonia had a serious underlying illness, and the mean age exceeded 60 years. The seasonal recovery of* M. catarrhalis *was significantly increased during late fall through early spring. Overall mortality rate was 13%.*

Cundell D, Masure HR, Tuomanen EI. The molecular basis of pneumococcal infection: a hypothesis. *Clin Infect Dis* 1995;21(Suppl 3):S204. *A review of new insights into the tissue tropism and inflammation of pneumococcal infection. The role of pneumococcal cell wall constit-*

uents in promoting cellular activation and the generation of inflammation is highlighted.

Duchin JS, et al. Hantavirus pulmonary syndrome: a clinical description of 17 patients with a newly recognized disease. *N Engl J Med* 1994; 330:949. *The authors analyzed clinical, laboratory, and autopsy data in 17 persons with confirmed infection from this newly recognized strain of hantavirus. The case fatality rate exceeded 75%, and hemoconcentration and abnormal partial thromboplastin time were predictive of death.*

Edelstein PH. Antimicrobial chemotherapy for Legionnaires' disease: a review. *Clin Infect Dis* 1995; 21:S265. *The author provides an indepth review of in vitro susceptibility testing of promising antimicrobial agents for Legionnaires' disease and combines this with in vivo/ clinical results.*

Edelstein PH. Legionnaires' disease. *Clin Infect Dis* 1993; 16:741. *A state-of-the-art clinical review article emphasizing historical aspects, epidemiology, clinical presentation, diagnosis, and therapy of Legionnaires' disease.*

Enders JF, et al. Isolation of measles virus at autopsy in cases of giant-cell pneumonia without rash. *N Engl J Med* 1959; 261:875. *The authors review the clinical and pathologic findings from three children succumbing to measles (giant-cell) pneumonia. They emphasize the immunocompromised status of the patients and the lack of signs of typical measles (no rash) during their illness.*

Erasmus LD. Friedländer bacillus infection of the lung: with special reference to classification and pathogenesis. *Q J Med* 1956; 25:507. *This classic article dealing with Friedländer's pneumonia shows evidence for the role of aspiration in the pathogenesis of infection.*

Fang G, et al. New and emerging etiologies for community-acquired pneumonia with implications for therapy: a prospective multicenter study of 359 cases. *Medicine* 1990; 69:307. *This prospective multicenter study involved 359 consecutive patients admitted with community-acquired pneumonia. Nearly 70% of the individuals studied had comorbid illnesses, and C. pneumoniae and Legionella species were more commonly encountered than previously recognized.*

Fine MJ, et al. Prognosis and outcomes of patients with community-acquired pneumonia. A meta-analysis. *JAMA* 1996; 275:134. *This meta-analysis, based on 127 study cohorts involving more than 33,000 patients, identified clinical findings predictive of short-term mortality: age 65 years, altered mental status, abnormal vital signs, high-risk pathogen, and neoplastic disease.*

Fraser DW, et al. Legionnaires' disease: description of an epidemic of pneumonia. *N Engl J Med* 1977; 297:1189. *The classic description of the epidemiology and clinical features of an epidemic of pneumonia that came to be called* Legionnaires' disease.

Graysten JT, et al. A new *Chlamydia psittaci* strain, TWAR, isolated in acute respiratory tract infections. *N Engl J Med* 1986; 315:161. *The initial report of acute respiratory disease attributed to* C. pneumoniae, *which at the time was morphologically classified as* C. psittaci, TWAR *strain.*

Graysten JT, et al. Community- and hospital-acquired pneumonia associated with *Chlamydia* TWAR infection demonstrated serologically. *Arch Intern Med* 1989; 149:169. *Retrospective analysis of serum specimens from 198 patients hospitalized with pneumonia revealed 10% of cases with serologic evidence of* C. pneumoniae *infection. Criteria for the interpretation of serologic testing were proposed.*

Guidry GG, et al. Respiratory syncytial virus infections among intubated adults in a university medical intensive care unit. *Chest* 1991; 100: 1377. *The authors report a prospective study of the incidence of respiratory syncytial virus infection among intubated adults in a university intensive care unit during a community outbreak.*

Hammerschlag MR. Antimicrobial susceptibility and therapy of infections caused by *Chlamydia pneumoniae*. *Antimicrob Agents Chemother* 1994; 38:1873. *The results of in vitro susceptibility testing indicate that* C. pneumoniae *has a pattern of susceptibility similar to that of* C. trachomatis, *except for resistance to sulfonamides. Tetracyclines, macrolides, and quinolones are all active against* C. pneumoniae *in vitro.*

Henderson A, Kelly W, Wright M. Fulminant primary *Pseudomonas aeruginosa* pneumonia and septicemia in previously well adults. *Intensive Care Med* 1992; 18:430. *The authors report two cases and review the literature. They emphasize failure to recognize the infection ante mortem and the high subsequent mortality.*

Hoffman J, et al. The prevalence of drug-resistant *Streptococcus pneu-*

moniae in Atlanta. *N Engl J Med* 1995; 333:481. *From January to October 1994, pneumococcal isolates from 431 patients with invasive disease were serotyped and tested to determine susceptibility. Results showed penicillin resistance in 25% (7% highly resistant), 26% resistant to trimethoprim/sulfamethoxazole, 15% resistant to erythromycin, 9% resistant to cefotaxime, and 25% resistant to multiple drugs.*

Irwin RS, Woelk WK, Coudon WL. Primary meningococcal pneumonia. *Ann Intern Med* 1975; 82:493. *The authors discuss the clinical features of primary meningococcal pneumonia. The organism may be easily overlooked in respiratory secretions unless it is specifically sought, there is no distinct presentation, and rapid improvement on therapy is to be expected.*

Jacobs MR. Treatment and diagnosis of infections caused by drug-resistant *Streptococcus pneumoniae*. *Clin Infect Dis* 1992; 15:119. *The author reviews the diagnosis of drug-resistant pneumococcal infection, emphasizing laboratory methods for susceptibility testing of clinical isolates.*

Johnston RB Jr. Pathogenesis of pneumococcal pneumonia. *Rev Infect Dis* 1991; 13(Suppl 6):S509. *This review article summarizes the current understanding of the pathogenesis of pneumococcal pneumonia, including virulence factors, host defense mechanisms, pathologic changes, and mechanisms of inflammatory tissue injury.*

Jonas M, Cunha BA. Bacteremic *Escherichia coli* pneumonia. *Arch Intern Med* 1982; 142:2157. *The findings of this study indicate that* E. coli *pneumonia most often occurred in elderly or chronically debilitated persons and was often localized to lower lobes. The mortality rates approached 90%.*

Kaplan NM, Braude AI. *Haemophilus influenzae* infection in adults: observations on the immune disturbance. *Arch Intern Med* 1958; 101: 515. *The authors report three cases of H. influenzae pneumonia in alcoholic adults and emphasize the role of alcohol in causing immunosuppression and propensity to infection.*

Kauppinen M, Saikku P. Pneumonia due to *Chlamydia pneumoniae*: prevalence, clinical features, diagnosis, and treatment. *Clin Infect Dis* 1995; 21:S244. *A review of the history, pathogenesis, clinical features, diagnostic tools, and therapy of this newly recognized respiratory pathogen.*

MacFarlane JT, et al. Comparative radiographic features of community-acquired Legionnaires' disease, pneumococcal pneumonia, *Mycoplasma* pneumonia, and psittacosis. *Thorax* 1984; 39:28. *Radiographic features of adults with a variety of types of community-acquired pneumonia were compared. Radiographic deterioration was a feature of Legionnaires' disease and bacteremic pneumococcal pneumonia, whereas clearing was more prompt with Mycoplasma. Lymphadenopathy was seen only in* Mycoplasma *pneumonia.*

Marrie TJ. *Coxiella burnetii* (Q fever) pneumonia. *Clin Infect Dis* 1995; 21:S253. *An extensive review of the history, microbiology, epidemiology, clinical features, diagnosis, and treatment of coxiellosis (89 references).*

Mundy LM, et al. Community-acquired pneumonia: impact of immune status. *Am J Respir Crit Care Med* 1995; 152:1309. *This cross-sectional prospective study evaluated 305 adults admitted with community-acquired pneumonia, stratified as immunocompetent, HIV-infected, and non-HIV-infected immunosuppressed.*

Murray HW, et al. The protean manifestations of *Mycoplasma pneumoniae* infection in adults. *Am J Med* 1975; 58:229. *The authors provide an in-depth review of the clinical features of M. pneumoniae infection, emphasizing the extrapulmonary manifestations.*

Niederman MS, et al. Guidelines for the initial management of adults with community-acquired pneumonia: diagnosis, assessment of severity, and initial antimicrobial therapy. *Am Rev Respir Dis* 1990; 148: 1418. *This publication represents the official American Thoracic Society statement on community-acquired pneumonia as prepared by an expert panel of members of the Scientific Assembly on Microbiology, Tuberculosis, and Pulmonary Infections.*

Pallares R, et al. Resistance to penicillin and cephalosporin and mortality from severe pneumococcal pneumonia in Barcelona, Spain. *N Engl J Med* 1995; 333:474. *A review of the results of a 10-year prospective study to examine the effect of resistance to penicillin and/or cephalosporin on mortality in adults with pneumococcal pneumonia.*

Putsch RW, Hamilton JD, Wolinsky E. *Neisseria meningitidis*, a respiratory pathogen? *J Infect Dis* 1970; 121:48. *The authors prospectively sought evidence for meningococcal infection in hospitalized patients* with suspected pneumonia and concluded that the meningococcus should be considered as a potential respiratory pathogen.

Rebhan AW, Edwards HE. Staphylococcal pneumonia: a review of 329 cases. *Can Med Assoc J* 1960;82:513. *One of the largest reported series of staphylococcal pneumonia, with a major emphasis on the clinical features of the disease.*

Schaffner W, et al. The clinical spectrum of endemic psittacosis. *Arch Intern Med* 1967;118:433. *Experience with nine cases of psittacosis pneumonia, emphasizing its clinical variability, the frequency with which it mimics bacterial pneumonia, and its occasional failure to respond promptly to tetracycline therapy.*

Shinzato T, Saito A. The *Streptococcus milleri* group as a cause of pulmonary infections. *Clin Infect Dis* 1995;21:S238. *The* S. milleri *group, encompassing the oral species* S. anginosus, S. constellatus, *and* S. intermedius, *has been increasingly recognized as a cause of pleuropulmonary infections.* S. milleri *is frequently isolated along with oral anaerobes, indicating a synergistic interaction in the pathogenesis of infection.*

Tilloston JR, Lerner AM. Characteristics of pneumonias caused by *Escherichia coli. N Engl J Med* 1967;227:115. *Clinical characteristics of 20 cases of community-acquired* E. coli *pneumonia, which generally followed bacteremia with a source of infection in the gastrointestinal or genitourinary tract. Lower lobe bronchopneumonia was typical, and mortality was 60%.*

Verghese A, et al. Group B streptococcal pneumonia in the elderly. *Arch Intern Med* 1982;142:1642. *A review of clinical features of group B streptococcal pneumonia. Coinfection with staphylococci or gram-negative bacilli was frequent and mortality was high (30%–85%).*

Wallace RJ Jr, Musher DM, Martin RR. *Haemophilus influenzae* pneumonia in adults. *Am J Med* 1978;64:87. H. influenzae *pneumonia was diagnosed in 41 adult patients in this series. Patients over the age of 50 years appeared at greatest risk for bacteremia and death and almost always had serious underlying diseases.*

Wright PW, Wallace RJ Jr, Shepherd JR. A descriptive study of 42 cases of *Branhamella catarrhalis* pneumonia. *Am J Med* 1990;88(5A):2S. *A largely descriptive review of the clinical and radiologic features of* Moraxella *pneumonia. Although mortality attributable to* Moraxella *was low, almost half the patients reviewed died of underlying diseases within 3 months.*

Yu VL. *Legionella pneumophila* (Legionnaires' disease). In: Mandell GL, Douglas RG, Bennet JE, eds. *Principles and Practice of Infectious Diseases.* 3rd ed. New York: Churchill Livingstone; 1990:1764–1774. *The author provides a review of legionellosis, emphasizing microbiologic, clinical, and therapeutic aspects of the disease.*

Textbook of Pulmonary Diseases, 6th ed.
edited by G.L. Baum, J.D. Crapo, B.R. Celli, and J.B. Karlinsky,
Lippincott–Raven Publishers, Philadelphia, © 1998.

CHAPTER

25 Hospital-Acquired Pneumonia

Richard J. Blinkhorn, Jr.

INTRODUCTION

Hospital-acquired pneumonia is the second leading cause of nosocomial infection, accounting for 13%–18% of all nosocomial infections. It is the leading cause of death among patients with hospital-acquired infections, and the cost of therapy for this problem exceeds $2 billion annually. This chapter focuses on the epidemiology, risk factors, pathogenesis, diagnostic strategies, and preventive measures related to hospital-acquired pneumonia. As many of the infective etiologies of pneumonia are reviewed in other chapters, only those organisms and/or features unique to the hospital setting are discussed here. The chapter concludes with a section on pneumonia in the immunocompromised host.

EPIDEMIOLOGY

Lower respiratory tract infection is not a reportable illness, but available data suggest it occurs at a rate of 5 to 10 cases per 1000 hospital admissions. This incidence may be 6 to 20 times higher in patients who are being ventilated mechanically. Nosocomial pneumonia has occurred in as many as 70% of patients with the adult respiratory distress syndrome (ARDS). Crude mortality rates for hospital-acquired pneumonias of 20%–50% have been reported, but they may be as high as 90% when pneumonia occurs in patients with ARDS. Although all these deaths are not the direct result of infection, the attributable mortality of hospital-acquired pneumonia is estimated to account for one third to one half.

RISK FACTORS

Although many of the variables predisposing to the development of hospital-acquired pneumonia are likely to be interrelated, several studies using regression analysis have identified independent risk factors. These include the following: (1) host factors, such as extremes of age and underlying disease; (2) conditions favoring aspiration; (3) surgical procedures, especially thoracic or upper abdominal surgery; (4) colonization of the oropharynx with gram-negative bacilli; and (5) continuous mechanical ventilation. More than 85% of patients in whom a nosocomial pneumonia develops have a serious underlying disease. Patients with chronic lung disease may have altered mucociliary clearance, and those with neurologic disorders may be predisposed to aspiration because of an impaired gag reflex.

Colonization of the oropharynx with gram-negative bacilli is an important risk factor because most cases of nosocomial pneumonia result from aspiration of contaminated oropharyngeal secretions into the tracheobronchial tree. Approximately 45% of healthy adults aspirate during sleep, and aspiration is even more frequent in patients with altered consciousness, abnormal swallowing, depressed gag reflexes, delayed gastric emptying, or decreased gastrointestinal motility. Intubation compromises the natural barrier to aspiration, and the entry of bacteria into the lung may also be facilitated through pooling and leakage of secretions around the endotracheal tube cuff. In the normal respiratory tract, the oropharynx is colo-

R. J. Blinkhorn, Jr.: MetroHealth Medical Center, Cleveland, Ohio 44109.

nized, but not with enteric gram-negative bacilli. When serious illness of any type is present, enteric gram-negative bacilli can replace the normal flora and become the colonizing bacteria in the oropharynx. Patients receiving antibiotics or acid-neutralizing medications also have a higher incidence of colonization. When the time course of colonization was examined, most patients had acquired gram-negative bacteria by the third hospital day.

Gastric colonization as a source of oropharyngeal and tracheal colonization in mechanically ventilated patients has been suggested by studies dating from 1978 and later. These studies have emphasized gastric overgrowth with aerobic gram-negative bacilli and increased rates of pneumonia in patients who have received agents that alter gastric pH. Several meta-analyses found that administration of sucralfate (which does not increase gastric pH) was associated with a reduced incidence of pneumonia when compared with the use of either antacids alone or in combination with H_2 antagonists. In all studies, gastric colonization has correlated best with gastric pH (increasing as pH exceeds 4.0), and rates of pneumonia increase accordingly.

The lower respiratory tract is ordinarily sterile in healthy nonsmokers. Smoking increases the likelihood that the tracheobronchial tree has lost its sterility, and half of patients with chronic bronchitis have a colonizing tracheobronchial microflora, but enteric gram-negative bacilli are not present. Oropharyngeal and tracheobronchial colonization patterns in intubated patients reveal that gram-negative bacteria usually enter the trachea after first colonizing the oropharynx. The exception to this finding is *Pseudomonas aeruginosa,* which can colonize the tracheobronchial tree as a primary event without first becoming established in the oropharynx. Colonization of gram-negative bacteria in the tracheobronchial tree occurs in 50%–100% of intubated patients, and more than one potential pathogen may be present. The relationship of airway colonization to the subsequent development of pneumonia is well-known, as respiratory infection develops in 13%–23% of colonized patients.

In addition to aspiration and colonization, one of the most important risk factors is tracheal intubation and mechanical ventilation, with the incidence of pneumonia rising as the duration of intubation increases. The risk for pneumonia is seven to 21 times greater in intubated patients than in other hospitalized patients, and pneumonia develops in as many as two thirds of patients with tracheostomy who require mechanical ventilation. The relationship of nosocomial pneumonia to the duration of mechanical ventilation was demonstrated by Fagon and colleagues; the risk for pneumonia was found to be 6.5% after 10 days of ventilation, 19% at 20 days, and 28% at 30 days. The endotracheal tube itself is not routinely changed. In one report, 95% of the tubes examined by scanning electron microscopy had partial bacterial colonization, and 84% were covered by bacteria in a biofilm or

glycocalyx. Whether this is clinically relevant remains to be seen.

PATHOGENESIS

Nosocomial pneumonia develops when organisms reach the lung and overcome the pulmonary host defenses. Illness results if the inoculum is sufficiently large, if the organism is virulent, or if host defenses are malfunctioning. Organisms may reach the lung via aspiration of oropharyngeal secretions colonized with pathogenic bacteria, aspiration of esophageal/gastric contents, inhalation of contaminated aerosols, hematogenous spread from a distant infected site, exogenous penetration from a pleural infection, or by direct inoculation into the airways of intubated patients. Not all routes, however, are equally effective in precipitating infection. Of these routes of entry, aspiration of oropharyngeal flora is recognized as the predominant mechanism in both intubated and nonintubated patients. Although microaspiration is a frequent event, reportedly occurring in as many as 45% of healthy adults during sleep, the critical event is the presence of pathogenic bacteria that are able to overwhelm the lower respiratory tract defenses. If organisms reach the lung as a liquid bolus, fewer organisms are needed to cause infection than if they are delivered as an aerosol. In the mechanically ventilated patient, sources of a liquid bolus of organisms include aspiration from a previously colonized oropharynx, aspiration from a colonized stomach to the oropharynx and then to the lung, leakage of pooled subglottic secretions above the inflated endotracheal tube cuff, or direct instillation of colonized ventilator tubing condensate into the lung via the endotracheal tube.

The aerosol route is an effective method for the spread of *Legionella* species, certain viruses, *Mycobacterium tuberculosis,* and fungi, such as *Aspergillus* species. Hematogenous spread from distant sites of infection is especially noted in postoperative patients and in patients with indwelling intravenous or genitourinary catheters.

The initial step in oropharyngeal colonization is the adherence of bacteria to mucosal cells, an interaction dependent on both host and microbial factors. The usual local respiratory tract chemical (salivary proteases, secretory IgA) and physical (mucociliary escalator) barriers to infection may be overcome by bacteria after tracheal intubation or large-volume aspiration. Systemic illness can result in an increase in the number of airway cell receptors and in a loss of surface fibronectin, thereby promoting bacterial adherence. Mucous glycoproteins that trap bacteria may act as actual surface receptors for these gram-negative organisms if they are not cleared as a result of faulty ciliary function. If the airway has been injured, underlying connective tissue and basement membrane, to which bacteria readily bind, can be exposed. Pili or fimbriae act as bacterial adhesions for many enteric gram-negative bacilli; other bacteria secrete exoproducts that promote airway colonization by impairing ciliary function, degrading fibronectin, stimulating excessive mucin production, or degrading mucin. Bacterial adherence has been shown to mediate tracheobronchial colonization and correlate with the subsequent development of pneumonia in mechanically ventilated patients in the intensive care unit (ICU).

It is unlikely that an increase in adherence by itself leads to colonization and infection unless other host defenses are impaired. However, many of the same clinical factors that can cause a rise in adherence can also impair mucociliary clearance and interfere with the cellular and humoral immune functions of the lung. For instance, malnutrition is associated with airway colonization, and this is likely the result of increased buccal and tracheal cell adherence, impaired cell-mediated immunity, decreased neutrophil migration, impaired recruitment of alveolar macrophages to the lung, complement deficiency, and diminished airway levels of IgA.

DIAGNOSIS

Several criteria have been used to establish a clinical diagnosis of nosocomial lower respiratory tract infection; these include fever, leukocytosis, purulent tracheobronchial secretions, and the radiographic appearance of a new or progressive pulmonary infiltrate. The development of these clinical manifestations in a previously healthy individual without underlying lung disease almost invariably indicates pneumonia. When these criteria have been applied to mechanically ventilated patients, however, they have been quite sensitive but not very specific, as a variety of noninfectious causes may lead to pulmonary infiltrates in this setting. Fagon and colleagues prospectively evaluated 147 consecutive patients suspected of having ventilator-associated pneumonia, and three of the usual clinical criteria were met in 93% of the patients and all four criteria were present in 51%. The diagnosis was definitely excluded in 49% of the patients, and no combination of 16 clinical variables was useful in distinguishing patients with bacterial pneumonias. In studies of patients with ARDS, pneumonia was falsely diagnosed using these clinical criteria in 19%–36% of patients but was unrecognized in up to 62%. Whereas overdiagnosis of pneumonia is the problem in mechanically ventilated patients in general, those with ARDS have not only the problem of overdiagnosis but also that of underdiagnosis. The remainder of this section reviews the diagnostic tools that may be useful in the diagnosis of both hospital- and ventilator-associated pneumonia.

General Evaluation

All patients with suspected hospital-acquired pneumonia require certain diagnostic evaluations. A careful history and physical examination can identify the presence of specific risk factors or conditions that may suggest the likely etiologic pathogens (Table 1). Chest radiography is imperative and can be used to define the presence and location of infiltrates, cavitation, and complications such as pleural effusion, and the severity of the process. Diagnostic thoracocentesis should be performed in individuals with parapneumonic effusions, especially if the effusion is 10 mm thick on a lateral decubitus chest x-ray film, if the individual has had chest trauma, or if a chest tube has been placed previously. A complete blood cell count and serum electrolyte levels should be determined, and arterial blood gas analysis and renal and liver function tests should be routinely performed. Although these do not contribute to the identification of a specific etiology, the tests help to define severity of illness and guide appropriate antimicrobial dosing. Serologic studies are of little use in the initial evaluation and should not be routinely performed.

Blood Cultures

Blood cultures can isolate the causative organism in almost one fourth of all cases of hospital-acquired pneumonia. In patients with ARDS, bacteremia has been documented in 27% of those with pneumonia and 67% of those with an abdominal focus of infection. A positive blood culture result in patients with respiratory failure, the appearance of a new pulmonary infiltrate, and the presence of purulent tracheal secretions are not necessarily conclusive evidence of pneumonia, as an additional source of infection may be present in up to 50% of these patients.

Sputum/Tracheal Aspirate

Gram's stain and culture of the respiratory tract secretions are the time-honored methods of microbiologic evaluation but are of limited diagnostic value in ventilator-associated pneumonia. Cultures of expectorated sputum

TABLE 1. *Hospital-acquired pneumonia: pathogens associated with specific patient risk factors*

Organism	Risk factor
Anaerobes	Abdominal surgery, poor dentition, witnessed aspiration
Staphylococcus aureus	Antecedent influenza, coma, head trauma, diabetes mellitus, renal failure
Legionella	Corticosteroids
Pseudomonas aeruginosa, Acinetobacter	Prolonged ICU stay, prior antimicrobial therapy, chronic lung disease

in patients with nosocomial pneumonia in whom the etiologic diagnosis was based on cultures from uncontaminated specimens (blood, transtracheal aspirate, pleural fluid) yielded the implicated bacterial pathogen in up to 80% of patients if *Staphylococcus aureus* was involved. On the other hand, gram-negative bacilli were recovered from sputum in 45% of patients who did not have these organisms as the etiologic agent. The absence of gram-negative bacilli in purulent secretions usually excludes their presence in the lower airways. Quantitative culture of expectorated sputum specimens is of no value diagnostically.

Microscopic examination of respiratory tract secretions is of limited usefulness. Grading of Gram's stains for neutrophils, bacteria, and percentage of intracellular organisms has correlated with quantitative tracheal aspirate colony counts, but overlap with results from patients who do not have infection makes this method less reliable.

The presence of elastin fibers in sputum or tracheal aspirates after digestion with potassium hydroxide is a very reliable indication of the diagnosis of hospital- or ventilator-associated pneumonia (Plate 1). The microscopic finding of elastin fibers is indicative of pulmonary parenchymal destruction or necrosis and was first described in 1846 as pathognomonic for tuberculosis. The demonstration of elastin fibers has subsequently been associated with necrotizing bacterial pneumonia, with a sensitivity of 52% and specificity and positive predictive value of 100% for infection. Recovery of elastin fibers from bronchial aspirates of patients with ARDS has a lower positive predictive value (50%), as noninfectious lung necrosis may occur in that setting. Elastin fibers are more likely to be seen in nosocomial pneumonia caused by gram-negative bacilli than in that caused by gram-positive bacteria, and the presence of elastin fibers may actually precede radiographic evidence of pulmonary infiltrates by a few days.

Qualitative cultures of tracheal aspirates have a high false-positive rate, frequently contain more than one potential etiologic pathogen, and are the least reliable method of diagnosis. Studies evaluating quantitative cultures of tracheal aspirates have yielded inconsistent results, with thresholds for the diagnosis of pneumonia ranging from 10^5 to 10^7 colony-forming units (CFU) per milliliter. The specificity of quantitative culture of tracheal aspirates has been best at higher cutoff points, but at the expense of decreasing sensitivity.

Transthoracic Lung Aspiration

Transthoracic lung aspiration for the diagnosis of bacterial pneumonia is of limited applicability for patients in the ICU, and it is contraindicated in patients receiving mechanical ventilation. Sensitivities as high as 79% have been reported in community-acquired pneumonias, but series dealing with more complex pneumonias have revealed sensitivities of 35%–56%. Because of the high incidence of pneumothorax associated with this procedure and its limited sensitivity, transthoracic lung aspiration is not recommended as a diagnostic procedure for patients in the ICU.

Bronchoscopy

Fiberoptic bronchoscopy has become an increasingly valuable tool for the diagnosis of lower respiratory tract infection. To reach the bronchial tree, however, the bronchoscope must traverse the oropharynx or the endotracheal tube, and colonization of these sites with pathogenic bacteria has been reported in up to 90% of patients receiving mechanical ventilation. Bronchoscopic aspirates in patients undergoing bronchoscopy are frequently contaminated by oropharyngeal bacteria, and as a result routine bacterial cultures obtained through the bronchoscope are unreliable for the diagnosis of pneumonia.

Two diagnostic techniques that have been recently described make it possible to acquire lower respiratory tract specimens for bacterial culture without oropharyngeal contamination. One technique uses a double-sheathed protected specimen brush (PSB), and the second involves bronchoalveolar lavage (BAL) of radiographically involved portions of the lung. Both methods rely on quantitative bacterial cultures to differentiate between infection and colonization.

Accordingly to a meta-analysis, the use of a predetermined threshold concentration for either PSB or BAL may not be appropriate in all clinical settings. Quantitative cultures of PSB and BAL specimens should be interpreted according to the pretest likelihood of pneumonia and how information gained from the procedure will influence management. Because pretest probability, risks of therapy, and likelihood of benefit vary widely among patients, a single value that defines an abnormal PSB or BAL culture result for all patients cannot be defined.

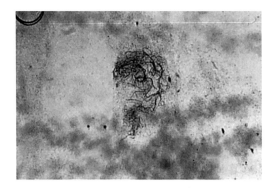

PLATE 1. Elastin fibers in a potassium hydroxide preparation of sputum. *See color plate 14.*

Bronchoalveolar Lavage

BAL refers to the sequential instillation and aspiration of a physiologic solution into the lung through a bronchoscope that has been wedged into an airway and so is subject to contamination with oropharyngeal flora. Quantitative cultures of BAL fluid have yielded growth in excess of 10^5 CFU/mL in the majority of patients with pneumonia, and the presence of 1% squamous epithelial cells in the BAL sample accurately predicts the presence of heavy contamination by oropharyngeal flora. A growth of 10^5 CFU/mL in a BAL specimen with at most 1% squamous epithelial cells has a diagnostic sensitivity of 88% and a specificity of 100%. Unprotected BAL, however, does not discriminate pneumonia from acute bacterial bronchitis. More recently, the technique of protected BAL has been described for diagnosing ventilator-associated pneumonia. Using a threshold of 10^4 CFU/mL, quantitative bacterial cultures of protected BAL samples had a sensitivity of 92% and a specificity of 97%, with a positive predictive value of 97% and a negative predictive value of 92%.

Microscopic analysis of cytocentrifuged BAL fluid may be useful in the diagnosis of pneumonia. Whereas total and differential cell counts are not helpful, the presence of intracellular organisms in 7% of cells (sensitivity of 86%, specificity of 96%) and the presence of bacteria on BAL specimen Gram's stain correlate closely with the results of both BAL and PSB quantitative cultures.

Protected Specimen Brush

The feasibility of obtaining uncontaminated specimens from the lower respiratory tract through a contaminated bronchoscope with a double-sheathed catheter was demonstrated in 1979. The technique has been described in detail and requires that a catheter containing a PSB be passed under direct visualization into the area of lung involvement as defined radiographically. Using a cutoff of 10^3 CFU/mL, quantitative cultures of samples obtained by PSB can separate patients with lower respiratory tract infection from those with airway colonization. Quantitative PSB cultures correlate well with histologic and bacteriologic features of tissue obtained at autopsy in mechanically ventilated patients and have a positive predictive value of 75% in ventilated patients who meet the standard clinical criteria for nosocomial pneumonia. Antecedent use of antibiotics diminishes the diagnostic efficacy of PSB cultures. In general, the sensitivity and specificity of PSB quantitative cultures are cited as 70%–90%. Studies comparing the efficacy of PSB and BAL quantitative cultures for the most part support the concept that these techniques are complementary. In patients with clinically suspected pneumonia in whom quantitative culture of PSB samples yields organisms in a concentration of 10^2 CFU/mL but $<10^3$ CFU/mL, PSB sampling should be repeated if pneumonia continues to be suspected clinically. In one third to one half of these patients, follow-up PSB quantitative culture will yield organisms in a concentration exceeding the diagnostic cutoff of 10^3 CFU/mL.

Plugged Telescoping Catheters

Because the routine use of the PSB technique is time-consuming and requires the use of a fiberoptic bronchoscope, an alternative, simpler technique using a plugged telescoping catheter (PTC) has been presented. Blind PTC sampling is as accurate as directed sampling via the bronchoscope, with a sensitivity of 100% and specificity of 82%. The accuracy of undirected PTC sampling is not unexpected. Pathologic examination of the lungs of intubated patients dying with nosocomial pneumonia has shown that bronchopneumonia is predominantly found in the lower and posterior parts of the lung, and chest radiographs taken during blind BAL via PTC have shown that 95% of catheters are lodged in the distal airways of the lower lobes. PTC sampling thus appears to be a useful tool for the diagnosis of ventilator-associated pneumonia as long as the radiographically defined area of involvement is limited to the lower lung fields.

PROPHYLAXIS

Given the fact that nosocomial pneumonia is the most common fatal nosocomial infection, an effective prophylactic regimen could have a significant impact on survival of hospitalized patients. To date, no single specific measure for pneumonia prevention has been proved to be beneficial, but several techniques currently under investigation may emerge as useful in the future.

Conventional Infection Control

Conventional infection control strategies have focused on identifying reservoirs of infection, interrupting transmission among patients, preventing progression from colonization to infection, and improving host defenses. Conventional infection control practices may fail to prevent nosocomial infection in the ICU, because many patients arrive already colonized with nosocomial bacteria; hand washing and barrier precautions are abandoned during crisis situations; and health care personnel may fail to adhere to traditional measures aimed at preventing infection in colonized patients, such as changing intravenous catheters routinely, discontinuing bladder catheters, suctioning with careful aseptic techniques, and removing ventilator circuit tubing condensate frequently to minimize exposure to the patient. The use of gloves by health care workers, as advocated under universal precautions guidelines, can lead to inadvertent transmission of pathogens (*Acinetobacter, Pseudomonas*) if they are not changed between patients.

Enteral Nutrition

Enteral nutrition is the method of choice for nutrient administration, as it is less invasive, more physiologic, and less expensive than total parenteral nutrition. In one study of patients with abdominal trauma, enteral feeding with a jejunostomy tube was not accompanied by pneumonia in any of the 29 patients treated in this manner, whereas pneumonia occurred in 6 of the 30 patients receiving parenteral nutrition. Although nutrition is an important therapeutic modality used to counteract the adverse effects of malnutrition on lung defense mechanisms, enteral feeding produces a definite risk for infection. The most significant risk of enteral feeding results from gastric colonization and the subsequent transmission of gastric organisms to the trachea, with resultant nosocomial pneumonia. Pingleton and colleagues evaluated simultaneous daily gastric, tracheal, and oropharyngeal cultures in mechanically ventilated patients not receiving antacids or H_2 antagonists, and they demonstrated that the number of gastric gram-negative isolates increased significantly after enteral feeding began. In their study, 36% of patients had gram-negative bacilli recovered first in the stomach that were later recovered in the trachea. The mechanism of transfer of gastric organisms into the trachea appears to be aspiration. Important factors implicated in aspiration associated with enteral feeding are the size and location of the feeding tube. Clinically significant aspiration is infrequent when enteral feeding is administered continuously via a small-bore nasoenteral tube in intubated patients. Feedings delivered directly to the stomach, as opposed to distal enteral feeding, increase the likelihood of aspiration and pneumonia, especially if the patient is being kept supine rather than semi-erect.

Antimicrobial Prophylaxis

Antibiotic prophylaxis of nosocomial pneumonia can be administered systemically, topically, by aerosol, or by a combination of these methods.

Systemic Antibiotic Prophylaxis

Systemic antibiotic prophylaxis has clearly been unsuccessful. In the 1950s, trials of systemic antibiotic prophylaxis involving patients with poliomyelitis who have undergone tracheotomy, comatose patients in the ICU, and patients with congestive heart failure failed to demonstrate a significant reduction in tracheal colonization or

frequency of pneumonia. Furthermore, prophylaxis actually increased the risk for resistant gram-negative bacillary pneumonia, cutaneous infection, and bacteremia. Based on data that 50% of pneumonias appear within 4 days of ICU admission, a more recent multicenter survey readdressed the issue of systemic prophylaxis. In that study of 570 patients in 23 ICUs, antibiotic prophylaxis did not result in a statistically significant decline in rates of early-onset pneumonia or death.

Aerosolization

The delivery of aerosolized antibiotics directly into the tracheobronchial tree has had minimal success as prophylaxis for ventilator-associated pneumonia. Polymyxin B was selected in several studies because it is bactericidal against a broad range of gram-negative bacilli, including *P. aeruginosa,* and it adsorbs well to epithelial surfaces without being absorbed systemically. Although aerosol polymyxin B can clearly reduce the occurrence of *P. aeruginosa* colonization and pneumonia when it is administered for prolonged periods, it results in the emergence of resistant organisms, and overall mortality rates have not been improved. Similarly, the endotracheal administration of gentamicin has been shown to decrease the rate of pneumonia, but overall mortality and infection-related mortality were unchanged. In addition, patient colonization with gentamicin-resistant organisms increased.

Selective Decontamination

Selective decontamination of the oropharynx is a prophylactic technique in which nonabsorbable antibiotics are applied directly to the oropharynx, in either a liquid or paste form. Parenteral antimicrobial agents are not administered. Prospective trials comparing topical nonabsorbable antibiotics with placebo have demonstrated decreased incidence of nosocomial pneumonia, but overall mortality rates were unchanged. Despite promising early results of selective oropharyngeal decontamination trials, flaws in study design have made these results largely unreliable.

Selective digestive decontamination as a method of pneumonia prevention was initially investigated in Europe. It is based on the use of orally administered, nonabsorbable antibiotics that eliminate aerobic gram-negative bacteria from the gut while sparing anaerobes. With time, selective digestive decontamination has been gradually modified. Fungal overgrowth often followed prophylaxis with polymyxin E and tobramycin, so amphotericin B became a standard part of the regimen. Because lower respiratory tract infection occurring within 5 days after ICU admission cannot be prevented solely by the topical administration of antibiotics to the oropharynx and stomach, intravenous cefotaxime given for several days was added to the regimen. Early nonblinded trials of selective digestive decontamination demonstrated reductions in rates of pneumonia, but for the most part no improvement in overall mortality or length of stay. More recent prospective, randomized, double-blinded, placebo-controlled studies using invasive methods to define the presence of pneumonia, however, have failed to demonstrate a benefit of selective digestive decontamination in decreasing the incidence of nosocomial infections (including pneumonia), length of stay, duration of mechanical ventilation, or mortality rates.

Gastric pH and Bacterial Overgrowth

Many studies have correlated high levels of gastric pH with logarithmic increases in the concentrations of gram-negative bacteria in the stomach and demonstrated the development of retrograde colonization from the stomach to the oropharynx and trachea. Several investigators reported increased rates of pneumonia in patients who received agents that alter gastric pH. Meta-analysis has consistently demonstrated that sucralfate (which does not alter gastric pH) is associated with a reduced incidence of pneumonia in comparison with antacids alone or combined with H_2 antagonists. There is disagreement, however, about whether the use of H_2 antagonists alone is associated with a higher rate of pneumonia in comparison with sucralfate or placebo. Nevertheless, it is overly simplistic to say that any intervention that raises gastric pH is undesirable. Other factors, especially gastric volume and the route of enteral feeding (gastric vs. distal) influence gastric bacterial growth, and analyses have not consistently considered the impact of these concomitant risk factors.

Management of Equipment Used for Respiratory Therapy

Bacteria can proliferate in the equipment used during respiratory therapy, and the incidence of pneumonia is increased if the tubing is manipulated frequently rather than infrequently. When tubing is handled, the condensate should always be drained away from the patient, as it can contain large concentrations of bacteria. Although many hospitals have a policy to change ventilator tubing every 48 to 72 hrs, there are no data showing that any particular frequency of circuit changes, compared with no circuit changes, lessens the incidence of pneumonia. The use of heat and moisture exchangers to lessen ventilator tubing contamination may decrease bacterial colonization of the circuit but has no effect on the incidence of pneumonia.

Aspiration of subglottic secretions is achieved with the use of a special endotracheal tube, designed with a suction port above the endotracheal tube cuff, in the subglottic area. The removal of contaminated respiratory secretions pooling above the endotracheal tube cuff reduces the incidence of some forms of ventilator-associated pneumonia. Once endotracheal tubes allowing the aspiration of subglottic secretions become more widely available, this approach may be used more regularly.

Continuous Postural Oscillation

Many years ago, it was recognized that prolonged recumbency increases the risk for pulmonary complications after operation, and for that reason early ambulation after surgery has become standard practice. For many critically ill patients in the ICU, however, ambulation is impossible, and the use of oscillating beds has been advocated as a means of avoiding the adverse pulmonary consequences of prolonged immobilization. Continuous postural oscillation (CPO) has been studied in patients bedridden with acute stroke, immobilized head-injured patients in traction, and victims of blunt trauma, and pneumonia occurred in significantly fewer patients randomized to CPO than to a conventional bed. Other studies, however, have not supported the benefit of CPO. Postoperative chest physiotherapy has failed to affect the incidence of pneumonia after gastric bypass surgery, and the use of CPO in medical patients in the ICU did not reduce overall mortality or the incidence of pneumonia. Although CPO may have a valid role in the care of certain critically ill patients, studies to date can be faulted for relying on clinical criteria for the diagnosis of pneumonia, and future trials are warranted.

MICROBIAL ETIOLOGIC AGENTS

Most reported cases of nosocomial pneumonia are caused by bacteria, and the time of onset of pneumonia after hospitalization is related to the bacterial etiology. Early-onset pneumonia, defined as pneumonia developing within 2 to 4 days after admission, occurs in anywhere from 8%–60% of patients requiring prolonged intensive care and accounts for up to 50%–60% of all cases of nosocomial pneumonia in some series. Early-onset pneumonia may be caused by community-acquired flora, including S. aureus, Streptococcus pneumoniae, and Haemophilus influenzae. After this initial time period, gram-negative bacteria become the major etiologic agents, coinciding with the time frame of oropharyngeal and tracheal colonization described earlier. Gram-negative bacilli account for 50%–80% of all nosocomial pneumonias, and 10%–20% of cases are polymicrobial.

Among the gram-positive bacteria, S. aureus is by far the most common, accounting for at least 10% of all nosocomial pneumonias. S. aureus is the gram-positive organism most often responsible for bacteremic nosocomial pneumonia. Staphylococcal pneumonia is more common in individuals with recent influenza, head injury, coma, a history of injecting drug use, chronic renal failure, or diabetes mellitus. Chest radiographs usually reveal multilobar infiltrates, predominantly in the lower lobes, often bilaterally. Pleural involvement is common, but cavitation and abscess formation infrequently occur. Infection caused by methicillin-resistant organisms is more likely in persons who have previously received antibiotics.

Although *S. pneumoniae* is the most common bacterial cause of community-acquired pneumonia, it accounts for less than 3% of all nosocomial pneumonias but up to 12% of bacteremic nosocomial pneumonias. Pneumococcal nosocomial pneumonia usually occurs within the first few days of hospitalization. Enterococcal nosocomial pneumonia has been associated with antecedent cephalosporin therapy and enteral alimentation.

Pseudomonas, Klebsiella, Enterobacter, Escherichia coli, and *Serratia* species are the most commonly reported causes of gram-negative bacillary pneumonias. *Pseudomonas* and *Serratia* are the most common pathogens causing bacteremic nosocomial pneumonia, whereas *E. coli, Klebsiella,* and *Enterobacter* are more frequently associated with nonbacteremic cases. Patients with ventilator-associated pneumonias who have received antibiotics before the onset of pneumonia are especially likely to be infected by *P. aeruginosa* or *Acinetobacter* species. Bacteremic nosocomial pneumonia caused by gram-negative bacteria is more likely to occur in elderly patients with debilitating underlying diseases, and mortality rates of 58%–82% are typical. *P. aeruginosa* is the most common pathogen, accounting for almost 17% of all nosocomial pneumonias. Oropharyngeal colonization by the organism with subsequent spread to the lower respiratory tract, as is typical for most gram-negative bacillary pneumonias, commonly occurs with *P. aeruginosa* but is not the sole mechanism of pathogenesis. Primary tracheal colonization with *P. aeruginosa* without antecedent oropharyngeal colonization has been described, and for this reason attempts at topical oropharyngeal decontamination would be unlikely to prevent primary colonization of the lower respiratory tract. In addition, hematogenous or bacteremic *Pseudomonas* pneumonia, with a presentation that mimics cardiogenic pulmonary edema, can occur and is nearly universally fatal.

Bacteremic *Pseudomonas* pneumonia is more common in patients with leukemia, lymphoma, solid tumor neoplasms, or chemotherapy-induced granulocytopenia (Plate 2), whereas nonbacteremic disease is seen more frequently in debilitated elderly patients with underlying cardiopulmonary disease. Radiographically, *Pseudomonas* pneumonia may be focal or diffuse. The focal form characteristically involves a lower lobe, although multilobar involvement has been the usual finding in patients with terminal infection. Infiltrates are usually alveolar, often with radiologic evidence of cavitation or abscess formation. Occasionally, a peculiarly nodular broncho-

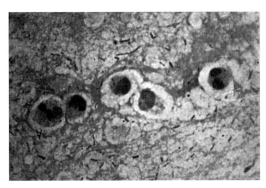

PLATE 2. *Pseudomonas* in sputum of a neutropenic patient. ×900. *See color plate 15.*

pneumonia of the lower lobes, with multiple small, thin-walled radiolucent cystic lesions, is seen. The diffuse form is a fearsome disease having an early radiographic presentation that mimics cardiogenic pulmonary edema. Bacteremia and leukopenia are common. If the patient survives beyond 48 hours, the chest radiograph demonstrates evolution into a necrotizing bilateral bronchopneumonia, often with pleural effusion and abscess formation. Histologically, this form is characterized by necrotizing pneumonia, vasculitis, pulmonary hemorrhage, and abscess formation. Mortality rates of 30%–60% have been reported for nonbacteremic *Pseudomonas* pneumonia, whereas the bacteremic variety is associated with case fatality rates invariably exceeding 80%. Treatment, which depends on in vitro sensitivities, is ordinarily with ceftazidime, aztreonam, imipenem, ciprofloxacin, or extended-spectrum penicillins plus an aminoglycoside. In many series, mortality has been independent of the effectiveness of the antimicrobial regimen applied, correlating mostly with the underlying disease process and degree of immunosuppression.

E. coli is the third most frequently isolated gram-negative organism responsible for hospital-acquired pneumonia, following *Pseudomonas* and *Klebsiella*. Pneumonia caused by *Klebsiella* is discussed in chapter 24. *E. coli* may colonize the oropharynx and subsequently invade the lower respiratory tract, but bacteremic invasion may occur from a distant focus in the genitourinary or gastrointestinal tract. The presence of serious underlying disease is a major factor leading to *E. coli* pneumonia, and two thirds of the patients have had been receiving broad-spectrum antibiotics, corticosteroids, or cytotoxic chemotherapy before the onset of pneumonia. Multilobar involvement is as common as disease localized to one lobe, and parapneumonic pleural effusion occurs frequently. Bacteremic *E. coli* pneumonia is associated with a normal or elevated white blood cell count, unlike bacteremic *Pseudomonas* pneumonia, in which leukopenia is a major predisposing factor. Mortality rates of 60%–80% are reported, with the worse outcomes associated with bacteremia.

Legionellosis may account for up to 30% of nosocomial

pneumonias in hospital settings where potable water is contaminated, but because the diagnosis requires special serologic and microbiologic techniques, the true incidence is unknown. The presentation of nosocomial *Legionella* pneumonia may be sporadic or epidemic. Clinical diagnosis in an outbreak setting is not difficult; however, differentiating *Legionella* pneumonia from other types of pneumonia in a nonepidemic setting can be troublesome. Risk factors for nosocomial legionellosis include malignancy, renal failure, neutropenia, cytotoxic chemotherapy, and corticosteroid therapy. Factors such as altered consciousness, prior antibiotic therapy, and intubation, which are known to be associated with other types of pneumonia, have a negative association with *Legionella* infection. There are no pathognomonic radiologic findings. Initial infiltrates are usually patchy, alveolar, and unilobar, with a predilection for the lower lobes. Generally, the infiltrate spreads locally within a lobe and then to contiguous lobes (Fig. 1). Pleural effusion may occur, and cavitation is seen in 10% of patients, usually in an immunosuppressed host receiving corticosteroids. Diagnosis and therapy are similar to those previously described for community-acquired disease.

Nosocomial viral lower respiratory tract infections are particularly common in children, and in one survey viral agents accounted for 20% of all hospital-acquired pneumonias. Respiratory syncytial, influenza, and parainfluenza viruses are important causes of viral nosocomial pneumonia, but only with prospective monitoring using specialized virologic diagnostic methods can the true incidence of nosocomial disease be determined. Nosocomial viral pneumonias are dissimilar to bacterial infections in several respects. Whereas bacterial nosocomial pneumonias tend to reflect the environmental flora of the hospital, nosocomial viral disease generally parallels activity of these agents in the community. Transmission of respiratory viruses involves active infection of hospital personnel in addition to passive transfer of virus on fomites or hands. Finally, whereas nosocomial bacterial infections are most likely to occur in individuals at high risk, viral diseases may occur in any exposed, nonimmune individual.

Herpes simplex virus (HSV) has been identified as a cause of nosocomial lower respiratory tract infection, but because endogenous reactivation is the likely mechanism leading to disease, the term *hospital-acquired* may be

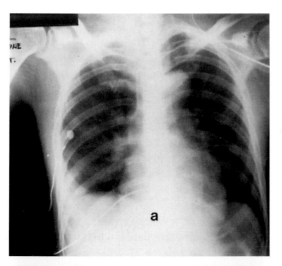

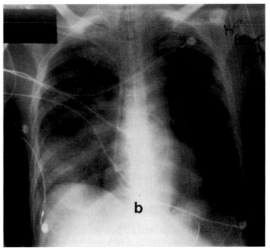

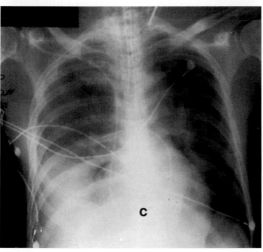

FIG. 1. A,B,C: Nosocomial legionellosis appearing as a patchy infiltrate in the right lower lobe with rapid progression during a period of 4 days.

inaccurate. Most of the cases reported to date have involved patients with alterations of cell-mediated immunity, severe underlying disease, or diffuse lung injury, including ARDS. It should be borne in mind, however, that HSV infection of the lower respiratory tract has occurred in apparently normal, immunocompetent hosts. Chronic lung disease and tobacco abuse have been reported by some authors as predisposing factors. Aspiration or contiguous spread from the oropharynx to the respiratory tract is the predominant pathogenic mechanism, but hematogenous seeding may occur in cases characterized with diffuse interstitial infiltrates (Plate 3). Aspiration as a mechanism is supported by the fact that in most patients, HSV infection of the lower respiratory tract is accompanied by oral or pharyngeal sores.

Clinically, the disease process is variable, and in its mildest form nothing more than the extension of an oropharyngitis occurs. HSV infection can be localized to the trachea and large bronchi, or a more generalized tracheobronchitis with extension into the bronchioles and alveoli can occur. HSV tracheobronchitis usually presents acutely with substernal pain, bronchospasm, and bloody respiratory secretions, and it may progress to respiratory failure, with the need for intubation and mechanical ventilation. When HSV tracheobronchitis arises in the intubated patient, it may manifest as bronchospasm, and weaning from mechanical ventilation is difficult. Localized or diffuse pneumonia can also be seen. Bacterial and fungal superinfections occur frequently.

HSV can be cultured from the mouth of 1%–5% of asymptomatic adults, and with any respiratory illness, the carriage rate rises to 2.7%–11.5%. For this reason, viral cultures of respiratory secretions are nondiagnostic unless supported by cytologic or histologic evidence of infection. Cytologic preparations typically reveal multinucleated giant cells and Cowdry type A intranuclear inclusions in patients with HSV infection of the lower respiratory tract. Bronchoscopy has been particularly useful in the diagnosis of HSV tracheobronchitis, as it allows for direct visualization of the characteristic punctate mucosal ulcerations

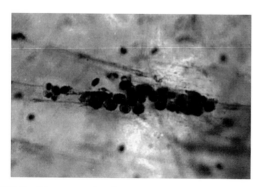

PLATE 3. Giemsa stain of endotracheal secretions showing intranuclear inclusions of HSV. Fever and diffuse interstitial pneumonia developed in this patient after coronary bypass surgery. *See color plate 16.*

and fibrinopurulent tracheal membrane. Direct immunofluorescent staining of HSV-infected tissue may be useful in obtaining a rapid diagnosis.

Acyclovir is the drug of choice, administered in a dose of 5 mg/kg intravenously every 8 hours for 10 days. In patients who fail to respond, an acyclovir-resistant HSV strain may be present, and intravenous foscarnet should be substituted. Mortality rates of 30%–70% have been reported.

PNEUMONIA IN THE IMMUNOCOMPROMISED PATIENT

Pulmonary infiltrates occurring in the immunocompromised host may have a myriad of causes, both noninfectious and infectious (Table 2). The differential diagnosis in any given patient can be narrowed by employing a systematic approach in which the clinician categorizes the nature of the underlying immunodeficiency, the onset of disease relative to hospitalization or immunosuppressive therapy, the tempo of the disease process, and the radiographic pattern of involvement. This section focuses on the diagnostic approach to the infectious etiologies, and only those etiologic agents unique to a particular clinical situation are discussed. Pulmonary infections complicating the acquired immunodeficiency syndrome (AIDS) are reviewed in Chapter 26. This chapter concludes with a discussion of the pulmonary infectious complications of transplantation.

The differential diagnosis of pulmonary pathogens in a particular patient is influenced in part by the nature of the immunologic defect (Table 3). Patients with abnormalities of immunoglobulin synthesis, hyposplenism, or complement deficiencies are uniquely predisposed to infections with encapsulated bacteria, especially *S. pneumoniae, H. influenzae,* and *Branhamella catarrhalis.* Quantitative or qualitative defects in neutrophil function primarily predispose patients to both bacterial and fungal pathogens, whereas cellular immune dysfunction can lead to infection by a variety of opportunistic organisms. The clinical situation is seldom so easily defined, and coexistent immune defects may be present. For example, although Hodgkin's disease is classically associated with cell-mediated immune dysfunction, both humoral and granulocytic immune dysfunction may also develop in these patients secondary to cytotoxic chemotherapy, radiation therapy, and splenectomy.

The time of onset of the pulmonary illness relative to the underlying immunodeficiency or immunosuppressive therapy may help to focus the differential diagnosis (Table 4). A retrospective review of patients with acute leukemia found that focal infiltrates occurring before initiation of therapy were likely to represent bacterial infections, whereas diffuse infiltrates were never caused by opportunistic pathogens and were usually noninfectious in etiol-

TABLE 2. *Pulmonary infiltrates in the immunocompromised host*

Infectious	Noninfectious	Unknown cause
Bacterial	Pulmonary edema	Nonspecific interstitial pneumonia (or organizing pneumonia)
Staphylococcus aureus	Cytotoxic drug-induced lung injury	
Gram-negative bacilli		
Legionella species	Radiation pneumonitis/fibrosis	
Nocardia		
Viral	Leukostasis	
Measles virus	Leukoagglutinin reaction	
Cytomegalovirus		
Herpes simplex virus	Spread of underlying neoplasm	
Adenovirus		
Respiratory syncytial virus		
Varicella-zoster	Leukemic cell infiltration	
Fungal		
Cryptococcus	Leukemic cell lysis	
Aspergillus		
Phycomycosis	Pulmonary hemorrhage	
Histoplasmosis	Pulmonary infarction	
Candida		
Mycobacterial		
Mycobacterium tuberculosis		
Mycobacterium avium complex		
Parasitic		
Strongyloides		
Protozoal		
Pneumocystis		
Toxoplasma		

TABLE 3. *Immunologic defects and associated pathogens*

Immunologic defect	Primary condition	Pathogens
Humoral (B-cell) defect	Hypogammaglobulinemia	*Streptococcus pneumoniae*
	Agammaglobulinemia	*Haemophilus influenzae*
	Lymphoma	*Branhamella catarrhalis*
	Lymphocytic leukemia	
	Multiple myeloma	
	Cytotoxic chemotherapy	
	Corticosteroid therapy	
	Severe burns	
Cell-mediated (T-cell) defect	Lymphoma	*Pneumocystis*
	Solid tumors	*Legionella*
	Organ transplantation	*Nocardia*
	Cytotoxic chemotherapy	*Mycobacterium*
	Corticosteroid therapy	Cytomegalovirus, herpes simplex virus
	Uremia	
	Acquired immunodeficiency syndrome	*Cryptococcus*
		Endemic fungi
	Radiation therapy	*Toxoplasma*
		Strongyloides
Hyposplenism	Splenectomy	*S. pneumoniae*
	Sickle cell hemoglobinopathy	*H. influenzae*
		B. catarrhalis
Granulocyte defect	Neutropenia	*Staphylococcus aureus*
	Myelogenous leukemia	Gram-negative bacteria
	Aplastic anemia	*Aspergillus*
	Corticosteroid therapy	Phycomycosis
	Chronic granulomatous disease	*Candida*
Complement defect	Primary deficiency	*S. pneumoniae*
	Systemic lupus erythematosus	*H. influenzae*

TABLE 4. *Time of onset of pulmonary infiltrate in relation to etiology*

Before immunosuppressive therapy	Bacterial, viral
	Pulmonary hemorrhage
	Neoplasia
	Primary bronchogenic carcinoma
	Metastatic carcinoma
	Lymphangial spread
	Leukemic cell infiltration
During chemotherapy	Opportunistic pathogen
	Leukoagglutination reactions
	Leukemic cell lysis pneumonopathy
	Pulmonary edema
Late or delayed	Cytomegalovirus
	Radiation pneumonitis/ fibrosis
	Cytotoxic drug-induced

ogy. In contrast, once patients had received chemotherapy, the occurrence of pulmonary infiltrates was usually secondary to opportunistic infections. Nodular or patchy alveolar infiltrates developing after prolonged periods of granulocytopenia are likely to represent invasive pulmonary aspergillosis. Lastly, pulmonary infectious complications of organ transplantation commonly follow characteristic temporal patterns, and this is discussed at the end of the chapter.

The rate of disease progression varies according to etiology and helps in narrowing the differential diagnosis (Table 5). Acute illnesses of 24 hours' duration suggest a bacterial pneumonia, whereas subacute presentations spanning several days are more consistent with infectious processes such as cytomegalovirus (CMV), *Pneumocystis carinii,* nocardiosis, or fungi. Lastly, chronic illnesses occurring during a period of weeks are more typical of mycobacterial or endemic fungal pathogens.

The radiographic pattern of involvement is rarely pathognomonic, but classification into diffuse, nodular, or focal infiltration is useful (Table 6). A definitive diagnosis cannot be established on the basis of the radiographic

presentation alone, as more than one etiology may be present and progression of infiltration from a focal to a diffuse pattern may occur. The air-crescent sign, however, is virtually pathognomonic of invasive pulmonary aspergillosis and is perhaps the only diagnostic radiographic pattern (Fig. 2). In addition, a characteristic halo sign, or zone of lower attenuation surrounding a pulmonary mass, has been observed on computed tomography in patients with invasive pulmonary aspergillosis.

Diagnostic techniques, including sputum examination and fiberoptic bronchoscopy with BAL, are similar to those described for the diagnosis of hospital-acquired pneumonia. In addition, transbronchial biopsy may be necessary for the diagnosis of pulmonary infiltrates in the immunocompromised host. Unfortunately, a significant number of transbronchial biopsies fail to establish a definitive diagnosis. For example, a specific diagnosis was made in only 45% of nearly 600 procedures reported in 18 studies. Furthermore, at least 11% of the transbronchial biopsy results in those studies were falsely negative, largely attributable to sampling error. It should also be borne in mind that the addition of transbronchial biopsy to fiberoptic bronchoscopy increases the risk of the procedure 20-fold, with a resultant 14% complication rate. Open lung biopsy remains the definitive diagnostic procedure. In the critically ill immunosuppressed patient, frequently with a bleeding diathesis, it offers the additional advantage of direct control of complications resulting from the tissue biopsy. Complication rates vary from 8%–20%, with 3% of them major. Procedure-related mortality is estimated at 1%. The highest diagnostic yield of open lung biopsy in general is in patients with pulmonary nodules, masses, and cavities. It has been useful in patients with diffuse infiltrates who have had previous bronchoscopic evaluation. Overall diagnostic yields range from 44%–94%, and the incidence of missed diagnoses is about 6%.

Lower respiratory tract infection in the immunocompromised host may be caused by a variety of microbes, including bacteria, *Legionella,* viruses, and opportunistic

TABLE 5. *Time course of pulmonary disease in immunocompromised patients*

Rapid	Subacute	Insidious
Infectious		
Bacterial	Cytomegalovirus	*Nocardia*
Gram-negative organisms	Fungal	Fungal
Staphylococcus aureus	*Aspergillus*	*Cryptococcus*
Legionella	*Cryptococcus*	Histoplasmosis
Viral	Phycomycosis	Mycobacterium
Herpes simplex virus	*Pneumocystis carinii*	
Measles virus		
Noninfectious		
Pulmonary edema	Leukemic cell infiltration	Cytotoxic drug-induced
Leukoagglutination reaction		Radiation pneumonitis/fibrosis
Pulmonary hemorrhage		
Leukemic cell lysis pneumonopathy		

TABLE 6. *Radiographic patterns of pulmonary infiltrates in immunocompromised patients*

Diffuse	Nodular or cavitary	Focal
Common		
Bacteremia	Bacterial lung abscess	Bacteria
Pneumocystis carinii	*Nocardia*	*Nocardia*
Cytomegalovirus	*Staphylococcus aureus*	*Cryptococcus*
Herpes simplex virus	*Cryptococcus*	*Aspergillus*
	Aspergillus	Phycomycosis
Uncommon		
Candidemia	Tuberculosis	Tuberculosis
Miliary tuberculosis	*Legionella*	Histoplasmosis
Disseminated histoplasmosis	*Pneumocystis carinii*	*Legionella*
	Septic emboli	

fungi. The clinical manifestations of these etiologic agents have been reviewed earlier in this chapter, as well as in Chapters 24, 26, and 27. The reader is referred to the respective sections for details. *P. carinii* and CMV, however, are uniquely pathogenic to the immunocompromised host and warrant further discussion.

P. carinii has been recognized as a cause of pneumonia for 30 years, and through the 1970s the majority of cases occurred in patients with lymphocytic leukemia, lymphoma, or congenital T-cell deficiencies, or those receiving chronic corticosteroid therapy. In the 1980s, *P. carinii* emerged as the most common cause of pneumonia in patients with human immunodeficiency virus (HIV) infection, accounting for thousands of cases annually in the United States (Chapter 26). Nevertheless, *P. carinii* continues to cause considerable morbidity and mortality in non-HIV-infected immunocompromised patients, and this discussion focuses on such individuals.

Not all patients with neoplastic disease are at risk for *P. carinii* infection. Attack rates of 20%–40% have been reported in children with acute lymphocytic leukemia, and patients with underlying hematologic neoplasm, especially lymphoma, account for the majority of cases. Cases in patients with underlying solid tumors have become more common, now accounting for approximately 40% of the cases complicating neoplastic disease. Treatment with corticosteroids represents the main chemotherapeutic risk in most series, a risk factor noted in 80%–90% of all cases. Interestingly enough, in 80% of patients, the corticosteroid dose was being tapered at the time of diagnosis.

The clinical presentation is marked by fever, dry cough, and dyspnea of several days' duration. Chest radiographs disclose bilateral interstitial infiltrates, and arterial blood gas determination shows hypoxia. Serum lactate dehydrogenase levels may be elevated. There are dissimilarities in the clinical presentation of *P. carinii* pneumonia between patients with AIDS and those without AIDS (Table 7). The onset of illness is typically more acute in the non-HIV-infected host, and a more fulminant presentation mimicking that of bacterial pneumonia may be seen. The *Pneumocystis* cyst burden seen on microscopic examination of the respiratory tract secretions is generally much lower than that encountered in AIDS patients. Recurrence is rare, as is the development of extrapulmonary pneumocystosis in the non-AIDS host. Although adverse reactions to trimethoprim/sulfamethoxazole are uncommon in patients without AIDS, the overall mortality rate is consis-

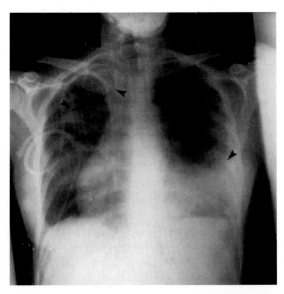

FIG. 2. Multiple air-crescent signs (*arrowheads*) in the lingula, right upper lobe, and right lower lobe in a patient with refractory acute myelogenous leukemia and invasive pulmonary aspergillosis.

TABLE 7. *Clinical features of* Pneumocystis carinii *pneumonia: AIDS versus non-AIDS patients*

Clinical feature	AIDS	Non-AIDS
Mean duration of symptoms, days	28	5
Cyst load in secretions	High	Low
Recurrences	Common	Rare
Side effect to trimethoprim-sulfamethoxazole	Common	Rare
Mortality rate, %	10–15	50

tently higher than in patients with AIDS (50% vs. 10%–15%, respectively). The diagnostic methods, therapeutic aspects, and prophylactic strategies are similar to those in AIDS patients (Chapter 26). It should be noted, however, that no trials have assessed the utility of adjunctive corticosteroid therapy for *P. carinii* pneumonia in non-AIDS patients.

CMV is ubiquitous among organ transplant recipients and has been referred to as the "troll of transplantation." CMV infection is associated with increased susceptibility to bacterial, fungal, and protozoal superinfection; increased risk for chronic transplant rejection; and increased overall mortality. CMV-seronegative recipients of marrow or granulocyte infusions or organs from seropositive donors are at the greatest risk for development of serious CMV disease. CMV infection typically occurs 2 to 12 weeks after transplantation, with a mean time to diagnosis of primary disease of 3 to 4 weeks and to discovery of reactivation/reinfection of 6 weeks. Fever occurs in 90% of patients and is frequently prolonged. Headache, arthralgias, myalgias, fatigue, and diarrhea may antedate the onset of pneumonitis. Neutropenia, anemia, and hepatitis are frequent accompanying abnormalities. Diffuse interstitial and/or alveolar infiltrates are the most common radiographic findings, although focal infiltrates, nodules, discoid atelectasis, and normal findings have been reported.

The diagnosis of CMV pneumonitis requires cytologic or histologic confirmation of positive CMV cultures, titers, or antigen detection. Conventional culture of BAL fluid has a high sensitivity and negative predictive value; however, the cultures must be incubated for several weeks, and a positive culture lacks specificity. The BAL fluid may also be cultured in the shell-vial method and stained after 24 to 48 hours of incubation for expression of early CMV antigen. Although more rapid than conventional culture techniques, an analogously high sensitivity and low specificity are expected. Standard cytologic examination of BAL fluid for cells with viral inclusions has had a low sensitivity (21%) but a high specificity (98%). Immunocytochemical staining of BAL cells to detect the presence of CMV antigen has a higher sensitivity (86%), lower specificity (84%), and a good negative predictive value (96%). The sensitivity of transbronchial biopsy for the diagnosis of CMV pneumonia cannot be readily ascertained; it remains the diagnostic procedure of choice, however, and open lung biopsy is rarely necessary. Coinfection with other opportunistic pathogens, particularly *P. carinii,* is common. Ganciclovir or foscarnet is the drug of choice, and outcome is much better in recipients of solid organ transplants than in bone marrow transplant recipients.

ORGAN TRANSPLANTATION

Largely as a result of improvements in immunosuppressive therapy, 1-year survival rates among recipients of livers, kidneys, hearts, and lungs now approach 70%–80%, and in 1990 it was estimated that 9560 kidney, 2656 liver, 2085 heart, 262 lung, 50 heart-lung, and 2200 allogeneic bone marrow transplantations were performed in the United States. Transplantation of any organ is often followed by a variety of complications, prominent among which are pulmonary disorders, both noninfectious and infectious. This section reviews the pulmonary infectious complications as they pertain to the specific organ transplanted.

Liver Transplantation

Orthotopic liver transplantation was first performed by Starzl in 1963, and 1-year survival rates now exceed 70%. The early postoperative course is marked by the development of pleural effusions, atelectasis, and diaphragmatic dysfunction. Infection is the most important postoperative pulmonary complication, and it is the principal source of morbidity and mortality from pulmonary disease in orthotopic liver transplant recipients. Risk factors for infection after transplantation include prolonged operating time, prolonged postoperative antibiotic therapy, renal failure, and gastrointestinal or vascular complications, and overall, the incidence of bacteremia and fungemia is 70%. The critical time period for the development of infection after orthotopic liver transplantation is the first 2 months.

Bacterial pneumonia occurs in 2%–25% of recipients and accounts for almost 50% of all pulmonary infections. The majority of cases of bacterial pneumonia develop in intubated patients and are not usually associated with bacteremia. A decline in the incidence of pneumonia has been reported when selective bowel decontamination is employed, although gram-positive organisms then become more frequent etiologic agents. Case fatality rates approach 40%.

CMV is the most common infectious agent in this patient population, with an incidence 60%. Symptomatic disease occurs in 20%–70% of infected individuals, and augmentation of immunosuppression for treatment of allograft rejection often precedes the onset of CMV disease. In particular, treatment of allograft rejection with OKT3 has been associated with an increased incidence of disseminated disease. Ganciclovir is effective therapy, with complete clearing of virus occurring in 75%–100% of patients.

The majority of fungal pneumonias occur within the first month of transplantation, and are usually caused by *Candida* species and *Aspergillus*. Disseminated infection with these organisms is associated with 70%–100% mortality. *P. carinii* pneumonia usually occurs 3 to 5 months after transplantation, and prophylaxis with trimethoprim/sulfamethoxazole is recommended.

Renal Transplantation

Both patient and renal allograft survival rates have improved during the past decade, such that transplantation now compares favorably with dialysis as a therapeutic modality for end-stage renal disease. More than 95% of renal transplant patients are alive at 1 year, and graft survival rates of 70%–90% are expected. Infections account for 65% of all pulmonary complications after renal transplantation, and the incidence of pneumonia has ranged from 8% to 16% in recent surveys.

Bacterial nosocomial pneumonias usually develop within the first month of transplantation, and the clinical presentation may be quite fulminant. The administration of steroid boluses for the treatment of allograft rejection is associated with an increased risk for hospital-acquired pneumonia. The incidence of fungal pneumonia may be directly related to the number of treated rejection episodes, and fungal infections that are superimposed on CMV infection have an especially poor prognosis. *Aspergillus* is the most frequent and most serious of the pulmonary mycoses described, and infection usually occurs within the initial 4 months. Amphotericin B is the treatment of choice, and the response is variable. The presence of copathogens significantly affects outcome. Eighty percent of those with primary *Aspergillus* infection respond to therapy, whereas none of those with *Aspergillus* infection superimposed on another pulmonary infection survive.

The incidence of mycobacterial infection in renal transplant patients is several times higher than that in the general population, occurring in 0.6%–2.3% of patients. Pulmonary involvement is the most frequent clinical manifestation, although an increased incidence of joint and skin disease occurs. The onset of infection is usually late, often developing a year or more after transplantation. Respiratory symptoms are often minimal, and an unexplained fever or abnormal-appearing chest radiograph may be the only clue to the infection. Dissemination is common, and ARDS has occurred. Response to standard antituberculous therapy is good.

The incidence of *P. carinii* pneumonia was 5% in the early experience with renal transplantation, but a striking increase in incidence of disease followed the introduction of cyclosporine. The onset of illness is typically acute, with fever and respiratory symptoms evolving within several days. Illness usually develops 2 to 4 months after transplantation, and prophylaxis with trimethoprim/sulfamethoxazole for 12 months after transplantation is recommended.

CMV infection is the most common infectious complication after renal transplantation, with an incidence of 75% consistently reported. Overall, symptomatic disease develops in 20%–40% of infected patients. The majority of patients have either asymptomatic or mildly symptomatic disease that usually appears within the first 2 months

after transplantation. Before the availability of ganciclovir, CMV pneumonia in the renal transplant patient carried a 48% mortality, and 90% of patients requiring mechanical ventilation died. Ganciclovir is effective therapy for CMV pneumonia in renal transplant patients, and the survival rate approaches 78%, including a 39% survival rate in patients requiring mechanical ventilation. Complete virologic clearing is seen in 70%–90% of treated patients.

Bone Marrow Transplantation

Bone marrow transplantation has been successfully applied to a growing list of hematologic and malignant diseases, and 2-year, disease-free survival rates exceed 60% for some forms of leukemias and aplastic anemia. Pulmonary complications occur in 40%–60% of marrow recipients, and particularly prominent among the infectious pulmonary complications are the respiratory viral and fungal infections.

Bacterial pneumonia is infrequently diagnosed during the early period after marrow transplantation, primarily because of the early empiric use of broad-spectrum antibiotics during episodes of fever. Nevertheless, a recent publication reported a 12%–60% incidence of bacterial pneumonia in this population, with gram-negative organisms as the predominant cause. Most of the late bacterial infections occurring after marrow transplantation involve the respiratory tract, are associated with chronic graft-versus-host disease, and are caused predominantly by gram-positive organisms, including *S. pneumoniae*.

The incidence of CMV infection after allogeneic bone marrow transplantation ranges from 50%–70%, and CMV pneumonia develops in one third of infected patients. Overall, CMV pneumonitis occurs in 15% of all bone marrow recipients, and an increased incidence has been observed among older patients, seropositive patients, those who have received total-body irradiation, those with severe graft-versus-host disease, and seronegative recipients of marrow from seropositive donors. The single feature that distinguishes CMV pneumonia in bone marrow recipients from CMV pneumonia in recipients of solid organ transplants is the high mortality. Despite the significant antiviral action of ganciclovir in vitro, its clinical efficacy for CMV pneumonia in bone marrow recipients has been variable. When used alone, ganciclovir has resulted in 17%–48% survival rates. The combination of ganciclovir with high-titer, CMV-specific immune globulin has proved beneficial, with survival rates ranging from 52%–70%. Relapses occur, however, in nearly one third of these patients.

Recent studies have demonstrated the efficacy of antiviral agents for the prophylaxis of CMV infection. In one study, high-dose, intravenously administered acyclovir reduced the incidence of both CMV infection (from 75%

to 59%) and pneumonia (from 31% to 19%). In addition, survival was greater in the acyclovir-treated patients. Even better results have been found with ganciclovir. Schmidt and co-workers randomized recipients of allogeneic bone marrow who had CMV detected in BAL fluid at day 35 after transplantation to receive full-dose ganciclovir versus observation. The incidence of CMV pneumonia or death was reduced from 70% in the control group to 25% in the prophylaxis group. Based on these findings, ganciclovir should be considered for prophylaxis in asymptomatic bone marrow recipients shedding CMV in BAL fluid or blood.

In the absence of acyclovir prophylaxis, HSV is excreted by 80% of seropositive bone marrow recipients, usually between the second and third week after transplantation. Most of these infections represent viral reactivation and involve the oropharyngeal mucosa. The clinical features are nonspecific, and two forms of HSV pneumonitis exist. Focal or multifocal pulmonary involvement usually arises from direct, contiguous spread from the oropharynx, whereas diffuse pulmonary involvement represents hematogenous dissemination from oropharyngeal or genital sites. Virtually all patients have mucocutaneous involvement, and copathogens are frequent.

Respiratory syncytial virus may cause interstitial pneumonitis in bone marrow recipients. Patients present with fever, cough, and signs of ear or sinus involvement before the onset of clinical and radiographic pulmonary disease. The majority of cases occur during the winter and spring. Therapy with aerosolized ribavirin and intravenous immunoglobulin has been advocated. Mortality rates exceed 80%.

Although pulmonary infection with *Candida, Cryptococcus, Histoplasma,* and *Coccidioides* are described, *Aspergillus* species are the most common cause of invasive fungal disease in bone marrow transplant recipients. Recipients of bone marrow are the most susceptible of all transplant patients to invasive pulmonary aspergillosis because of the nature of their immunosuppression. The duration of granulocytopenia and the administration of high-dose corticosteroids are well-recognized risk factors for the development of invasive pulmonary aspergillosis, and these factors concomitantly exist in the majority of bone marrow transplant patients. Treatment of invasive pulmonary aspergillosis is unsatisfactory, and outcome is best determined by the recovery of the granulocyte count. Mortality rates are high, approaching 80%–90%.

The incidence of *P. carinii* pneumonia has dropped significantly since the routine introduction of prophylaxis with trimethoprim/sulfamethoxazole, and cases are now limited to those patients who either cannot tolerate sulfa drugs or are noncompliant. The median time to onset of *P. carinii* pneumonia is 2 months after transplantation. Response to therapy is good if it is started early.

Heart Transplantation

In the United States, approximately 2500 heart transplantations are performed annually, with a 5-year actuarial survival rate of 72%. Pulmonary infections are by far the leading infectious complication after heart transplantation, occurring in 40%–60% of patients in the era before cyclosporine and in 24%–40% of patients in recent years. The majority of infections occur within the first 3 to 4 months, and multiple pathogens are present in 20%–25% of patients.

Most episodes of bacterial pneumonia occur within the first few weeks after transplantation and are usually caused by the aerobic gram-negative bacteria present in the hospital environment. *Legionella pneumophila* may cause up to 5% of bacterial pneumonias after heart transplantation, and unlike immunocompetent patients, organ transplant recipients may present with nodular infiltrates that progress to necrotizing pneumonia with cavitation. Treatment with erythromycin is usually successful, but 6 to 12 months of therapy may be required, because relapse is common. The incidence of nocardial pulmonary infection varies from 0–6% following cardiac transplantation. Fever and cough are the most common clinical features, and in 80% of patients the radiographic presentation is a solitary nodular lesion. The lung is the only site of involvement in about 80% of patients; the remainder, with disseminated disease, often exhibit skin or bone involvement. Treatment with trimethoprim/sulfamethoxazole is universally successful.

In approximately 30% of heart transplant recipients, invasive fungal disease develops, and the reported incidence of *Aspergillus* infection ranges from 0–24%. The clinical presentation is similar to that previously described, and mortality rates of 50%–86% are typical.

The use of prophylactic trimethoprim/sulfamethoxazole has reduced the incidence of *P. carinii* infection substantially. Mortality rates of 34% in heart transplant recipients have been reported, but outcome is generally good if the disease is diagnosed and treated early.

CMV infection after heart transplantation occurs in 67%–100% of patients, and CMV pneumonia develops in up to 16% of infected patients. Before the advent of effective antiviral therapy, mortality ranged from 46%–75%. Ganciclovir has proved to be effective in this patient population, and mortality rates have been reduced to 14% with this antiviral agent.

Of special concern to the heart transplant recipient is pulmonary infection by *Toxoplasma gondii*. Twelve percent to 17% of heart transplant recipients have had no previous exposure to this organism and receive a heart from a seropositive donor. A symptomatic primary infection develops in more than half of these patients. The most frequent clinical manifestations include fever, chorioretinitis, encephalitis, myocarditis, and pneumonitis. The diagnosis of toxoplasmosis requires the demonstration of tachyzoites in body fluids or tissues. Serologic studies may be useful, and titers begin to rise 4 to 12 weeks after transplantation. Prophylaxis with pyrimethamine or trimethoprim/sulfamethoxazole is recommended for patients at risk for primary infection.

Heart-Lung Transplantation

Infection is the leading cause of mortality after heart-lung transplantation, accounting for 48% of early postoperative (30 days) deaths and 73% of the late deaths. The lung as an allograft is more vulnerable to infection, as ischemia, handling, preservation, and reimplantation alter local pulmonary defenses. In addition, the normal cough reflex has been ablated by denervation, and mucociliary clearance has been markedly reduced.

Bacterial pneumonia is common after heart-lung transplantation. An overall incidence of 66% during the early experience with heart-lung transplantation has been reduced to only 13% by administering antibacterial prophylaxis with ceftazidime and clindamycin and by promptly adjusting the drug regimen to treat any bacteria isolated from airway secretions during the first 7 to 10 days. As with most hospital-acquired infections, gram-negative organisms, *S. aureus,* and *L. pneumophila* have been the most frequent causes.

CMV pneumonitis poses a special problem, as its clinical presentation is similar to that of acute rejection. Fiberoptic bronchoscopy with BAL and transbronchial biopsy, as described earlier in this chapter, have a good diagnostic yield and a low complication rate in this setting. There are no controlled trials evaluating the efficacy of ganciclovir in such patients; however, other treatment modalities have been disappointing. Therefore, ganciclovir should be considered the treatment of choice, and immune globulin can be considered in refractory or severe cases.

Before the routine administration of prophylactic therapy, *P. carinii* pneumonia developed in 75% of heart-lung transplant recipients at risk, although the majority of cases were subclinical. The diagnosis, therapy, and prophylactic regimen are similar to those already described.

Deep-seated fungal infections have been uncommon following heart-lung transplantation. *Candida* infection has been the most frequent, and these infections are usually disseminated. Although isolation of *Candida* species from respiratory tract specimens is not unusual, true *Candida* pneumonitis occurs infrequently. Only a few cases of *Aspergillus* infection after heart-lung transplantation have been reported, and mortality rates have been high.

BIBLIOGRAPHY

Baker AM, Bowton DL, Haponik EF. Decision making in nosocomial pneumonia. An analytic approach to the interpretation of quantitative bronchoscopic cultures. *Chest* 1995;107:85. *The authors reviewed the literature comparing PSB and BAL quantitative cultures for the diagnosis of ventilator-associated pneumonia. Current data do not suggest that either culture technique offers an advantage over the other.*

Bell RC, et al. Multiple organ system failure and infection in adult respiratory distress syndrome. *Ann Intern Med* 1983;99:293. *The authors evaluated the role of multiple organ system failure and infection in 37 consecutive survivors and 47 consecutive nonsurvivors on whom autopsies were performed.*

Bryan CS, Reynolds KL. Bacteremic nosocomial pneumonia: analysis of 172 episodes from a single metropolitan area. *Am Rev Respir Dis* 1984;129:668. *The authors retrospectively reviewed 172 episodes of bacteremia attributed to nosocomial pneumonia during a 5-year period. Mortality for these patients was 58% and occurred almost exclusively in those with serious and largely irreversible underlying disease.*

Campbell GD Jr, et al. Hospital-acquired pneumonia in adults: diagnosis, assessment of severity, initial antimicrobial therapy, and preventive strategies. *Am J Respir Crit Care Med* 1995;153:1711. *This article represents a consensus statement of the American Thoracic Society on the clinical approach to hospital-acquired pneumonia. As the title implies, the focus is predominantly on the diagnosis, therapy, and prevention of this nosocomial infection (110 references).*

Carratala J, et al. Risk factors for nosocomial *Legionella pneumophila* pneumonia. *Am J Respir Crit Care Med* 1994;149:625. *The authors prospectively studied 300 episodes of nosocomial pneumonia from 1985 to 1990 to determine risk factors for nosocomial legionellosis compared with other infectious etiologies.*

Chastre JY, et al. Diagnosis of nosocomial bacterial pneumonia in intubated patients undergoing ventilation: comparison of the usefulness of bronchoalveolar lavage and the protected specimen brush. *Am J Med* 1988;85:499. *The authors compared the usefulness of specimens recovered using a PSB and those recovered by BAL in the diagnosis of ventilator-associated pneumonia.*

Chastre JY, et al. Evaluation of bronchoscopic techniques for the diagnosis of nosocomial pneumonia. *Am J Respir Crit Care Med* 1995;152:231. *A comparison of specimens obtained by BAL and PSB in the diagnosis of nosocomial pneumonia was made by performing both procedures just after death in a series of 20 ventilated patients in whom pneumonia had not developed before the terminal phase of their illness.*

de Castro FR, et al. Reliability of the bronchoscopic protected catheter brush in the diagnosis of pneumonia in mechanically ventilated patients. *Crit Care Med* 1991;19:171. *Quantitative cultures of PSB specimens were used in a prospective study of 103 ventilated patients with suspected pneumonia. The technique was safe, sensitive, and specific, and the results led to modification of treatment in almost half the patients.*

Dreyfuss D, et al. Clinical significance of borderline quantitative protected brush specimen culture results. *Am Rev Respir Dis* 1993;147:946. *The authors prospectively evaluated 30 ventilated patients with clinically suspected pneumonia; initial PSB quantitative cultures yielded organisms in concentrations that were ≥10² CFU per milliliter but 10³ CFU per milliliter. In 12 instances (40%), a diagnosis of pneumonia was confirmed by a second PSB culture yielding organisms in a concentration of 10³ CFU per milliliter or higher.*

Dreyfuss D, et al. Mechanical ventilation with heated humidifiers or heat and moisture exchangers: effects on patient colonization and incidence of nosocomial pneumonia. *Am J Respir Crit Care Med* 1995;151:986. *The authors found that bacterial colonization in ventilator tubing was considerably reduced with the use of a heat and moisture exchanger.*

Ettinger NA, Trulock EP. State of the art: pulmonary considerations of organ transplantation. Part 1. *Am Rev Respir Dis* 1991;143:1386. Part 2. *Am Rev Respir Dis* 1991;144:213. Part 3. *Am Rev Respir Dis* 1991;144:433. *The authors provide an in-depth, state-of-the-art review of pulmonary considerations of organ transplantation (530 references).*

Fagon JY, et al. Detection of nosocomial lung infection in ventilated patients: use of a protected specimen brush and quantitative culture techniques in 147 patients. *Am Rev Respir Dis* 1988;138:110. *The authors prospectively studied 147 ventilated patients suspected of having nosocomial pneumonia. Among patients with a new pulmonary infiltrate and purulent tracheal secretions, positive cultures of PSB specimens (defined by concentrations 10³ CFU per milliliter) were found in only 45 patients (31%).*

Fagan JY, et al. Nosocomial pneumonia in patients receiving continuous mechanical ventilation: prospective analysis of 52 episodes with use of a protected specimen brush and quantitative culture techniques. *Am Rev Respir Dis* 1989;139:877. *The authors prospectively studied 567 mechanically ventilated patients with suspected pneumonia using bronchoscopy and PSB. The actuarial risk of ventilator-associated pneumonia was 6.5% at 10 days, 19% at 20 days, and 28% at 30 days.*

Ferrer M, et al. Utility of selective digestive decontamination in mechanically ventilated patients. *Ann Intern Med* 1994;120:389. *In this prospective, randomized, placebo-controlled, double-blinded study involving 80 mechanically ventilated patients, selective digestive decontamination had no effect on the incidence of nosocomial infections (including pneumonia) or mortality rate.*

Gastinne H, et al. A controlled trial in intensive care units of selective decontamination of the digestive tract with nonabsorbable antibiotics. *N Engl J Med* 1992;326:594. *A randomized, double-blinded, multicenter study including 445 mechanically ventilated patients. Selective digestive decontamination had no effect on incidence of pneumonia or survival.*

Johanson WG Jr, et al. Nosocomial respiratory infections with gram-negative bacilli: the significance of colonization of the respiratory tract. *Ann Intern Med* 1972;77:701. *The authors performed a prospective study of 213 patients admitted to a medical ICU to determine the frequency of colonization of the respiratory tract with gram-negative bacilli and the relation of such colonization to nosocomial infection.*

Kaye MG, et al. The clinical spectrum of *Staphylococcus aureus* pulmonary infection. *Chest* 1990;97:788. *The authors retrospectively reviewed 31 cases of staphylococcal nosocomial pneumonia. In contrast to findings in previous reports, chest radiographs showed multilobar infiltrates, often bilateral, and a lower incidence of abscess formation. Mortality rate was 32%.*

Mandelli M, et al. Prevention of pneumonia in an intensive care unit: a randomized, multicenter clinical trial. *Crit Care Med* 1989;17:501. *A randomized, multicenter trial of the efficacy of systemic antibiotic administration in the prevention of early-onset pneumonia. One thousand three hundred nineteen patients in 23 ICUs were enrolled, and no statistically different rates of pneumonia or death were found among the groups.*

Meduri, GU, et al. Protected bronchoalveolar lavage. A new bronchoscopic technique to retrieve uncontaminated distal airways secretions. *Am Rev Respir Dis* 1991;143:855. *The authors tested the effectiveness of protected BAL, performed through a protected transbronchoscopic balloon-tipped catheter, in collecting distal airways secretions with a minimal degree of contamination. Using a threshold of 10⁴ CFU per milliliter, quantitative protected BAL cultures had a diagnostic efficiency of 96%.*

Pennington SE, Reynolds HY, Carbone PP. *Pseudomonas* pneumonia. A retrospective study of 36 cases. *Am J Med* 1973;55:155. *Review of the clinical course in 36 cases of Pseudomonas pneumonia collected from 1956 to 1970. Mortality was 81% and not influenced by type of antibiotic therapy. No patient with positive findings on blood culture survived.*

Pham LH, Brun-Buisson C, Legrand P, et al. Diagnosis of nosocomial pneumonia in mechanically ventilated patients. Comparison of a plugged telescoping catheter with the protected specimen brush. *Am Rev Respir Dis* 1991;143:1055. *A prospective study of 55 ventilated ICU patients with suspected nosocomial pneumonia, comparing quantitative culture results of PSB, bronchoscopic PTC, and blind PTC samples. Blind or directed PTC sampling (sensitivity 100%, specificity 82%) was at least as accurate as PSB.*

Pingleton SK, Hinthorn D, Luci C. Enteral nutrition in patients receiving mechanical ventilation: multiple sources of tracheal colonization include the stomach. *Am J Med* 1986;80:827. *Multiple sources of tracheal colonization exist in patients receiving enteral nutrition. The stomach is an important source of tracheal colonization. Enteral*

nutrition can be associated with gastric flora colonizing the trachea and causing nosocomial respiratory infection.

Rello J, et al. Ventilator-associated pneumonia by *Staphylococcus aureus*. Comparison of methicillin-resistant and methicillin-sensitive episodes. *Am J Respir Crit Care Med* 1994;150:1545. *Persons infected with methicillin-resistant* S. aureus *were more likely to have received antibiotic previously, to have received steroids before infection developed, to have been ventilated 6 days, to have been older than 25 years, and to have had preceding chronic obstructive pulmonary disease (COPD).*

Rose HD, Heckman MG, Unger JD. *Pseudomonas aeruginosa* pneumonia in adults. *Am Rev Respir Dis* 1973;107:416. *In 19 patients with Pseudomonas pneumonia, prior multiple or broad-spectrum antimicrobial drug therapy was usual, multilobar involvement that included a lower lobe was characteristic, and mortality rate was 90%.*

Rouby JJ, et al. A prospective study of protected bronchoalveolar lavage in the diagnosis of nosocomial pneumonia. *Anesthesiology* 1989;71:679. *Protected BAL not requiring bronchoscopy is of value for the diagnosis of nosocomial pneumonia.*

Salata RA, et al. Diagnosis of nosocomial pneumonia in intubated, intensive care unit patients. *Am Rev Respir Dis* 1987;135:426. *In 51 intubated ICU patients prospectively studied by serial examinations of tracheal aspirates, the presence of elastin fibers frequently preceded the appearance of pulmonary infiltrates, had a positive predictive value of 100%, and had a sensitivity of 52% for infection.*

Schmidt GC, et al. A randomized, controlled trial of prophylactic ganciclovir for cytomegalovirus pulmonary infection in recipients of allogeneic bone marrow transplants. *N Engl J Med* 1991;324:1005. *The authors demonstrate the effectiveness of ganciclovir in preventing the development of CMV interstitial pneumonia in recipients of allogeneic bone marrow.*

Schuller D, et al. Herpes simplex virus from the lower respiratory tract: epidemiology, clinical characteristics, and outcome in immunocompromised and nonimmunocompromised hosts. *Am Rev Respir Dis* 1992;145(Suppl):A110. *A retrospective study of the hospital course of 42 patients with HSV recovered from the respiratory tract showed that nonimmunocompromised patients, in comparison with the immunocompromised group, had a more severe course, with increased lengths of stay, days of ventilation, and mortality rate.*

Seidenfeld JJ, et al. Incidence, site, and outcome of infections in patients with the adult respiratory distress syndrome. *Am Rev Respir Dis* 1986;134:12. *A prospective study of 108 infections in 129 patients with ARDS. Bacteremia was more common in abdominal infections than in infections at other sites. Survival was better in patients with abdominal infections than in patients with lung infections.*

Sepkowitz KA, et al. Pneumocystis carinii pneumonia among patients without AIDS at a cancer hospital. *JAMA* 1992;267:832. *The authors retrospectively reviewed 142 cases of* P. carinii *pneumonia occurring in patients without AIDS. Virtually all patients had previously established predisposing factors, including corticosteroid use in 87%.*

Shelhamer JH, et al. Respiratory disease in the immunosuppressed patient. *Ann Intern Med* 1992;117:415. *A summary of a National Institutes of Health consensus conference on pulmonary disease in immunocompromised patients, emphasizing predisposing immunologic factors, differential diagnosis, diagnostic procedures, therapy, and prevention.*

Tenholder MF, Hooper RG. Pulmonary infiltrates in leukemia. *Chest* 1980;78:468. *In 98 episodes of pulmonary infiltrates developing in hospitalized patients with leukemia, infiltrates appearing before treatment or within 72 hours of initiation of therapy were not opportunistic. Local disease during treatment was infectious in 74%, diffuse disease was noninfectious in 65%, and opportunistic infection was more likely if diffuse rather than local infiltrates were seen.*

Whimbey E, et al. Respiratory syncytial virus pneumonia in hospitalized adult patients with leukemia. *Clin Infect Dis* 1995;21:376. *Among hospitalized adult patients with leukemia who experienced an acute respiratory illness, 10% of cases were attributed to respiratory syncytial virus infection, and 75% of these progressed to pneumonia. Mortality rate, despite therapy with ribavirin and intravenous immunoglobulin, was 83%.*

Textbook of Pulmonary Diseases, 6th ed.
edited by G.L. Baum, J.D. Crapo, B.R. Celli, and J.B. Karlinsky,
Lippincott–Raven Publishers, Philadelphia, © 1998.

CHAPTER 26

Pulmonary Complications of HIV Infection

Mark J. Rosen · Roslyn F. Schneider

INTRODUCTION

The AIDS epidemic, now in its second decade, is one of the most important global health problems of the twentieth century. In many urban communities in the United States, AIDS-related disorders are the leading causes of death among adults 25 to 44 years of age. By June 1996, 548,000 cases of AIDS had been reported in the United States, about half of them since 1993, and 343,000 had died. The worldwide impact is even more devastating: some sub-Saharan countries could lose a quarter of their adult population to AIDS, and without a cure, an estimated 10 million Asians will die of AIDS-related illnesses before the year 2015.

Since the beginning of the epidemic, lung diseases have been among the most important causes of illness and death. The first cases of AIDS were described in homosexual men in Los Angeles who had *Pneumocystis carinii* pneumonia (PCP) without a known reason for immunodeficiency. Lung diseases were later recognized not only in HIV-infected patients with full-blown AIDS, but in others with less severe immune compromise. Over the years, shifts in the demographics of HIV-infected populations and advances in the prophylaxis of HIV-associated infections have profoundly influenced the types of lung diseases in these patients.

PATHOGENESIS

Human immunodeficiency virus type 1 (HIV-1), the etiologic agent of AIDS, is a cytopathic RNA virus in the lentivirus subfamily of retroviruses. HIV-2, a retrovirus endemic in West Africa, also causes an immunodeficiency syndrome. In almost all cases, the virus is transmitted by sexual contact, by exposure to blood or blood products (most often among injection drug users), or from mother to child during childbirth.

The pathogenesis and immunologic effects of HIV infection involve a complex interplay of persistent viral replication, immune activation, and dysregulation of cytokine secretion. After primary infection, HIV disseminates widely through the blood. The virus is initially contained within follicular dendritic cells in the germinal centers of lymphoid tissue, and the number of $CD8^+$ T lymphocytes increases, opposing the progression of infection. Humoral responses, with antibodies directed against HIV proteins, may also reduce the severity of viremia. However, proinflammatory cytokines (interleukin-1β, interleukin-6, tumor necrosis factor, granulocyte-macrophage colony-stimulating factor) are overexpressed, upregulating HIV expression.

HIV causes disease mainly by infecting cells that express the CD4 molecule. Infection of $CD4^+$ (helper) T lymphocytes usually leads to progressive depletion of this cell line and immunosuppression, but some nonprogressors remain well, with stable CD4 cell counts for at least 10 years. $CD4^+$ T lymphocytes also regulate immune responses mediated by B cells, suppressor T cells, natural killer cells, monocytes, and macrophages, so the effects of HIV infection on immune responses are far more profound than simple T-cell depletion.

HIV may be identified in alveolar macrophages and lymphocytes early in the course of HIV infection, and the function of these cells may become impaired. Initially, the $CD8^+$ alveolitis may protect against immune killing of HIV-infected cells. Release of proinflammatory cytokines may be directly toxic to pulmonary epithelium, activate neutrophils, or facilitate HIV replication.

M. J. Rosen and R. F. Schneider: Department of Medicine, Albert Einstein College of Medicine, New York, New York 10461.

DEFINITION OF AIDS

In 1983, the Centers for Disease Control (CDC) established a case definition of AIDS to track the epidemic. AIDS was defined by the presence of specific opportunistic infections and neoplasms that occurred with advanced immunosuppression, and PCP was the most common AIDS-defining disorder. Since the purpose of surveillance is to describe the affected populations so as to anticipate trends and guide public health planning and responses, the case definition was revised in 1987, and again in 1993. The current definition includes recurrent pneumonia, pulmonary tuberculosis, and carcinoma of the cervix in HIV-infected persons. Advanced immunosuppression, defined as a CD4 count of $200/\mu L$, was also included in the case definition, even in the absence of opportunistic infections or neoplasms. The expanded case definition of AIDS led to a 111% increase in reported cases from 1992 to 1993, and new case reports increased disproportionately in women, racial/ethnic minorities, and injection drug users.

Knowledge of the types of pulmonary disorders that are associated with HIV infection are reflected in the updated case definitions. In October 1983, the National Heart, Lung, and Blood Institute Workshop on Pulmonary Complications of HIV Infection found that 41% of the 1067 patients in whom AIDS was diagnosed in the participating institutions had serious pulmonary disorders, and PCP was by far the most common, occurring in 85% of the patients with lung disease. For years, PCP was considered the predominant pulmonary disease in HIV-infected patients. However, the early reports of pulmonary disorders associated with HIV infection considered only patients who met the case definition for AIDS, and almost all had advanced immunosuppression. We now recognize that other common respiratory illnesses develop in patients with less severe immunologic impairment, and the full range of pulmonary disorders associated with HIV infection is wide. Table 1 lists the infectious, neoplastic, and inflammatory diseases that occur in patients with HIV infection, and their typical radiographic patterns are summarized in Table 2.

RISK FACTORS FOR SPECIFIC PULMONARY DISEASES

The pulmonary disorders associated with HIV infection range from mild abnormalities in pulmonary function unaccompanied by respiratory symptoms to fatal opportunistic infections. The risk for each of these disorders is strongly influenced by the severity of immunosuppression, the patient's demographic characteristics and place of current or prior residence, and whether the patient is using prophylaxis against common HIV-associated infections. Genetic factors are probably also important but less precisely defined.

TABLE 1. *HIV-associated respiratory disorders*

Bacterial infections
Streptococcus pneumoniae
Haemophilus influenzae
Chlamydia pneumoniae
Pseudomonas aeruginosa
Staphylococcus aureus
Moraxella catarrhalis
Rhodococcus equi
Mycobacterium tuberculosis
Mycobacterium avium-intracellulare
Other nontuberculous mycobacteria

Protozoal infections
Pneumocystis carinii (fungus?)
Strongyloides stercoralis
Toxoplasma gondii

Viral infections
Cytomegalovirus
Adenovirus
Herpes simplex virus
Measles virus

Fungal infections
Cryptococcus neoformans
Histoplasma capsulatum
Aspergillus fumigatus
Coccidioides immitis
Blastomyces dermatitidis

Malignancies
Kaposi's sarcoma
Non-Hodgkin's lymphoma
Carcinoma of the lung

Other disorders
Sinusitis
Bronchitis/bronchiectasis
Lymphocytic interstitial pneumonitis
Nonspecific interstitial pneumonitis
Bronchiolitis obliterans organizing pneumonia
Primary pulmonary hypertension

Influence of Immune Function

The severity of the abnormality in host defense is a primary determinant of the risk for specific pulmonary disorders. Early in the course of HIV infection, when the immune system is not severely compromised, respiratory disorders may occur that are similar to those in the general population; opportunistic infections occur only with severe immunodeficiency. The CD4-lymphocyte count is used most often as a surrogate marker for severity and progression of HIV disease, and the probability of specific diseases developing can be estimated by this measurement. Assessment of HIV load by measurement of the number of HIV-1 viral RNA copies in the blood also correlates strongly with disease progression.

The spectrum of disease in patients with severe immuno-

TABLE 2. *HIV infection: chest radiographic patterns and common etiologies*

Focal opacification	Mediastinal lymphadenopathy
Bacteria	*M. tuberculosis*
Mycobacterium tuberculosis	*M. avium-intracellulare*
Pneumocystis carinii	Kaposi's sarcoma
	Lymphoma
	Fungi
Diffuse opacification	**Pleural effusion**
P. carinii	Bacteria (parapneumonic effusion, empyema)
M. tuberculosis	*M. tuberculosis*
Kaposi's sarcoma	Kaposi's sarcoma
Bacteria	Lymphoma
Fungi	Fungi
Cytomegalovirus	Cardiomyopathy
	Hypoproteinemia
Diffuse nodules	**Cavitation**
Kaposi's sarcoma (large nodules)	*M. tuberculosis* (high CD4)
M. tuberculosis (miliary)	*P. carinii* (low CD4)
Fungi (small nodules)	*Pseudomonas aeruginosa* (low CD4)
	Rhodococcus equi
Pneumothorax	Fungi
P. carinii	Lymphoma
	Cytomegalovirus

suppression was well-described early in the epidemic, but more recent studies have confirmed the relationship of immune function to the risk for common problems like upper respiratory infection, bacterial pneumonia, and pulmonary tuberculosis. In the Pulmonary Complications of HIV Infection Study, 1353 subjects were followed prospectively in six U.S. cities to determine the prevalence, incidence, and types of lung diseases that occur in persons in selected HIV transmission categories. To describe the types of disorders that occur in early HIV infection, patients with an AIDS-defining diagnosis (1987 case definition) were excluded from enrollment. After 18 months of follow-up, the most frequent respiratory diagnoses in the HIV-seropositive subjects were upper respiratory infection (33.4%), acute bronchitis (16%), and acute sinusitis (5.3%). Although these disorders were also common in a control group of HIV-seronegative homosexual men and injection drug users, the incidence of acute bronchitis and sinusitis was significantly higher in the HIV-infected subjects. Surprisingly, upper respiratory infection (defined as a mild, self-limited illness with coryza and sometimes sore throat and cough) occurred less frequently in subjects with a baseline CD4 count of 250/μL than in those with higher lymphocyte counts. The reason for this is not known, but it is possible that patients with severe immunosuppression may have a less vigorous immune response and milder symptoms with this self-limited illness. In the same study, bacterial pneumonia and PCP occurred more frequently in subjects with baseline CD4 lymphocyte counts of 250/μL than in those with higher counts.

The association between reduction in the CD4 lymphocyte count and the risk for specific diseases was explored in a survey of the medical records of more than 18,000 HIV-infected subjects who received care at more than 100 sites in 10 U.S. cities (Table 3). Common disorders like sinusitis, bronchitis, and pharyngitis occurred at all strata of CD4-cell counts. With lower counts, different pulmonary infections occurred with increasing frequency: 80% of cases of bacterial pneumonia and pulmonary tuberculosis occurred with CD4 counts of 400/μL; recurrent pneumonia and nontuberculous pulmonary mycobacterioses at CD4 counts of 300/μL; and PCP, Kaposi's sarcoma (KS), and disseminated *Mycobacterium tuberculosis* infection at CD4 counts of 200/μL. More than 80% of cases of disseminated nontuberculous mycobacteriosis, including *M. avium-intracellulare* infection, disseminated fungal infection, central nervous system toxoplasmosis, and cytomegalovirus (CMV) disease occurred in patients with the most severe immunosuppression (CD4 count of 100/μL).

Therefore, common respiratory problems like sinusitis and bronchitis may occur at any CD4 count, and bacterial pneumonia and tuberculosis often occur before AIDS-defining opportunistic infections and neoplasms. Declining immune function increases the risk for all HIV-associated respiratory disease, except for mild upper respiratory tract infections.

Demographic Factors

The demographic characteristics of persons with HIV infection also have a major impact on the incidence of specific pulmonary disorders, and demographic shifts were accompanied by a changing spectrum of disease. Persons who acquired HIV infection through injection drug use and heterosexual contact represent an increasing proportion of new cases of AIDS. From 1981–1987, 64% of cases of AIDS were in homosexual men, compared

TABLE 3. *Treatment of* Pneumocystis carinii *pneumonia*

Drug	Dose	Comments
Moderate-to-severe disease (PaO$_2$ ≤ 70 mm Hg, or P(A-a)O$_2$ ≥ 35–45 mm Hg breathing room air)		
Trimethoprim/sulfamethoxazole	15–20 mg/kg/75–100 mg/kg IV or PO in 3 divided doses	Drug of choice, but toxicity (rash, fever, nausea) is frequent
Pentamidine isoethionate	3–4 mg/kg IV daily	Toxicity: dysglycemia, renal failure, neutropenia, QT prolongation, arrhythmias, pancreatitis, orthostatic hypotension
Trimetrexate/folinic acid	45 mg/m^2 IV daily 20 mg/m^2 IV or PO q6h	Not as effective as trimethoprim/ sulfamethoxazole, but better tolerated
Prednisone	40 mg PO bid, days 1–5 20 mg PO bid, days 6–10 20 mg PO daily, days 11–21	Recommended as adjunctive therapy, along with an anti-*Pneumocystis* agent for all patients with PCP who meet criteria for moderate-to-severe disease
Mild-to-moderate disease (PaO$_2$ ≥70 mm Hg, or P(A-a)O$_2$ ≤ 35 mm Hg breathing room air)		
Trimethoprim/sulfamethoxazole	Same as above	Most likely to cause hepatotoxicity of all oral regimens
Dapsone/trimethoprim	100 mg PO daily 5–6 mg/kg PO tid	Methemoglobinemia and hemolysis in patients with G6PD deficiency
Clindamycin/primaquine	600 mg IV or PO tid	Rash, leukopenia, nausea, diarrhea
	15 mg base PO daily	Methemoglobinemia and hemolysis in patients with G6PD deficiency
Atovaquone suspension	750 mg bid	Less effective than trimethoprim/ sulfamethoxazole, but better tolerated

PaO$_2$, partial pressure of arterial O$_2$; P(A-a)O$_2$, alveolar-arterial difference in partial pressure of O$_2$; PCP, *Pneumocystis carinii* pneumonia; G6PD, glucose-6-phosphate dehydrogenase.

with 45% of new cases from 1993–1995. In the early years of the epidemic, most patients with AIDS were white. Now, the majority are black and Hispanic.

These demographic trends are reflected in the recognition of bacterial pneumonia and pulmonary tuberculosis as important HIV-associated infections. CDC surveillance data in the 1980s showed a doubling of mortality rates for pneumonia among persons ages 25 to 44 years in cities with a high prevalence of injection drug use and AIDS. Selwyn et al. found that the incidence of bacterial pneumonia was five times greater in HIV-infected than non-HIV-infected injection drug users, and that bacterial infections accounted for substantial mortality. In the cohort followed in the Pulmonary Complications of HIV Infection Study, bacterial pneumonia occurred more frequently than PCP, and the risk for bacterial pneumonia was significantly higher in injection drug users than in others.

Race and ethnicity may also influence the risk for bacterial pneumonia and tuberculosis, but these associations are confounded by differences in access to health care, the higher prevalence of tuberculosis in minority communities, and the disproportionately high numbers of injection drug users who are black or Hispanic. Nevertheless, the risk for tuberculosis is higher in blacks and Hispanics than in whites, whereas whites have a higher risk for HIV-associated malignancies and CMV disease.

Residence

A person's place of residence strongly influences the risk for acquiring specific infections. The high incidence of PCP in the United States and Europe contrasts sharply with that in Africa, where it is much less common. It is still unknown whether genetic or environmental factors account for the lower incidence of PCP in Africa. In the United States, the incidence of HIV-associated tuberculosis is highest in the Northeast. The geographic distribution of endemic fungi is a strong determinant of risk for those infections; disseminated histoplasmosis and coccidioidomycosis are common in patients with AIDS who live in endemic areas. These infections may also occur as reactivation disease after HIV-infected persons move to other areas and become immunocompromised.

Use of Prophylaxis

The risk for specific opportunistic infections declines with the use of prophylaxis. This is reflected in studies that document a declining incidence and mortality of PCP and a declining case rate for tuberculosis despite the relatively constant number of persons in the United States who are immunocompromised by HIV infection.

PULMONARY FUNCTION TESTS

Pulmonary function tests are usually not performed in the evaluation of patients with suspected HIV-associated pulmonary disorders, as no pattern of abnormality is specific for any disease and precise measurement of severity of physiologic derangements in patients with acute illnesses is usually not helpful in management. The common disorders (PCP, pulmonary KS) may reduce the vital capacity (VC), and they consistently reduce the single-breath carbon monoxide diffusing capacity (DLCO). Measurement of DLCO is sometimes used in the diagnostic evaluation of patients with normal chest radiographic findings who are suspected of having PCP; a normal value is interpreted as strong evidence against this infection.

Persons with HIV who have no apparent lung disease may also have abnormalities in pulmonary function. Values for forced vital capacity (FVC), forced expiratory volume in 1 second (FEV_1), and FEV_1/FVC are usually normal, but FVC and FEV_1 may be reduced in injection drug users compared with other HIV-infected persons, perhaps related to their high prevalence of cigarette smoking. The DLCO is often reduced in asymptomatic persons with HIV infection, especially in those with advanced immunosuppression. In the Pulmonary Complications of HIV Infection Study, asymptomatic HIV-infected subjects with CD4-lymphocyte counts of $400/\mu$L and/or HIV-associated symptoms had small but significant reductions in DLCO compared with HIV-infected persons with higher CD4 counts. Perhaps subclinical inflammatory pulmonary processes such as nonspecific interstitial pneumonitis and lymphocytic interstitial pneumonitis occur in asymptomatic HIV-seropositive patients, reflected by a reduction in DLCO. In many patients, DLCO may be reduced by factors unrelated to HIV infection, including race, cigarette smoking, and injection drug use.

PNEUMOCYSTIS CARINII PNEUMONIA

Despite the development of effective prophylaxis against *P. carinii,* PCP remains the most common AIDS-defining infection. Until recently, *P. carinii* was assumed to be a protozoan, but recent molecular studies classify it as a fungus. Whether the organism is acquired from an environmental source or by person-to-person transmission is unknown.

Clinical, Radiographic, and Laboratory Features

The presenting features of PCP are nonspecific; they include dyspnea, dry cough, and fever that usually progress gradually during several weeks. However, it may occasionally present as an acute illness with rapid deterioration within a few days. The chest radiograph usually reveals diffuse granular opacities, which strongly suggests the diagnosis (Fig. 1), but sometimes patients with PCP have nodular densities, lobar consolidation, or normal radiographic findings. All of these radiographic patterns may also occur with other infections and neoplasms. Cystic abnormalities and spontaneous pneumothorax in patients with known or suspected HIV infection are usually caused by PCP (Fig. 2).

The diagnosis of PCP may be supported by adjunctive testing. This infection is unlikely in a patient who had a CD4-cell count of $200/\mu$L in the preceding 2 months in the absence of other HIV-associated symptoms. Approximately 90% of patients with PCP have an elevated serum lactic dehydrogenase level, but this may occur with other pulmonary diseases. Oxygen desaturation with exercise is a relatively sensitive and specific test in patients suspected to have PCP, but it is not diagnostic.

Gallium 67 and indium 111 lung scans are highly sensitive indicators of PCP, but isotope uptake also occurs in

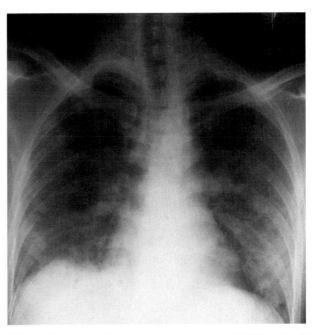

FIG. 1. Typical radiographic appearance of PCP, with diffuse granular opacifications.

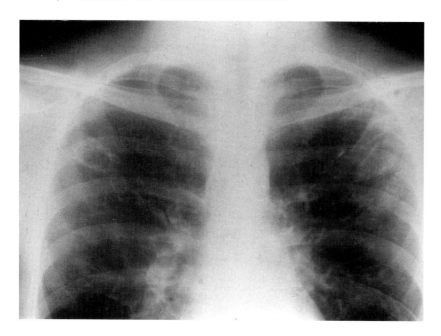

FIG. 2. Chest radiograph of a patient with cystic pulmonary lesions caused by PCP.

other pulmonary infections, so they are seldom useful in a diagnostic algorithm. One of these tests could be used in patients with normal chest radiographic findings in whom an opportunistic infection is suspected. If the scan shows abnormal uptake in the lungs, further diagnostic studies may be appropriate, whereas most patients with a negative scan can be observed. The lesions of KS do not take up gallium 67 or indium 111, and lymphoma does not take up indium 111, so the scans may be useful adjuncts in the noninvasive diagnosis of these malignancies in patients with abnormal chest radiographic findings.

Microbiologic Diagnosis

P. carinii cannot yet be cultured in vitro; therefore, infection and the diagnosis of PCP can be confirmed only by demonstrating organisms in a lung-derived specimen. The least invasive test is the analysis of sputum induced with 3% saline solution delivered by ultrasonic nebulization. By means of modified Giemsa, methenamine silver, or immunofluorescent staining, the organism can be identified in up to 80% of cases, depending on the experience of the laboratory. Other pathogens, especially *M. tuberculosis* and fungi, may also be found in induced sputum by using appropriate staining and culture techniques.

Whether to proceed routinely with fiberoptic bronchoscopy to confirm the diagnosis of PCP in patients suspected of having the disease but whose sputum specimens are nondiagnostic is controversial. Some prefer to treat these patients empirically for PCP and establish a diagnosis only if no clinical response occurs within 5 days. Proponents of empiric therapy hold that a presumptive diagnosis of PCP is usually accurate and that the procedure usually carries unnecessary inconvenience, risk, and discomfort

to patients, as well as expense. A decision analysis supporting initial empiric therapy indicated that the expected 1-month survival rate was identical whether patients received early bronchoscopy or whether the procedure was offered only to nonresponders, and that bronchoscopy was associated with greater costs and effort.

Proponents of early bronchoscopy maintain that routinely using an empiric approach subjects many patients to treatment and its attendant toxicity for a disease that they do not have, and nonresponders may be too ill to undergo bronchoscopy after several days of inappropriate therapy. Coinfection with other pathogens is common and may not be diagnosed in patients treated empirically. Also, adjunctive corticosteroid therapy may transiently improve symptoms in patients with other pulmonary disorders and contribute to the emergence of other opportunistic infections, such as aspergillosis and CMV disease.

In any case, fiberoptic bronchoscopy with bronchoalveolar lavage (BAL) is the next procedure in the diagnostic algorithm for PCP when sputum specimens are nondiagnostic. The complication rate is very low, and the yield is 90% in most centers. This yield is optimized by performing lavage in more than one lobe, and the yield is higher in the upper lobes than the lower. All lavage specimens should be examined for the presence of acid-fast bacilli, fungi, and viral cellular inclusions, as patients with suspected PCP may have another infection or may be coinfected with other pathogens. The use of BAL in the diagnosis of bacterial pneumonia in HIV-infected persons is not generally indicated.

When bronchoscopy with BAL is carried out in patients with HIV-associated pulmonary disorders, it is also controversial whether to perform bronchoscopic lung biopsies routinely. Because the diagnostic yield of BAL in

PCP is so high, some authors recommend that biopsy be omitted initially and performed during a second bronchoscopy if the lavage specimen is nondiagnostic. However, biopsy specimens are occasionally diagnostic of PCP and other pathogens when the lavage result is negative, and it is the least invasive means of diagnosing other pulmonary conditions that require histologic interpretation. Transbronchial biopsies are contraindicated in the presence of bleeding disorders, and the high risk for pneumothorax usually precludes biopsies in patients undergoing mechanical ventilation. Diagnosing PCP by video-assisted thoracoscopy or an open procedure is rarely necessary, as almost all cases are confirmed using sputum induction or bronchoscopy.

Treatment

The drugs used to treat PCP are outlined in Table 3. Trimethoprim/sulfamethoxazole (T/S) is the agent of choice, regardless of the severity of disease. It is consistently the most effective in comparative studies and also inexpensive and available in both oral and intravenous preparations. Although it is usually well tolerated, many patients are unable to tolerate the drug for a full course. The optimal duration of treatment is unknown, but most clinicians treat for 14 to 21 days, followed by prophylaxis for life.

The choice of anti-*Pneumocystis* treatment depends on the severity of disease and how the patient tolerates the medication. Outpatient treatment with oral agents is an option for patients with mild to moderate episodes whose arterial oxygen tension (PaO_2) while breathing room air is 70 mm Hg. In a comparison of oral T/S, trimethoprim/dapsone, and clindamycin/primaquine, all three had similar efficacy and rates of treatment-limiting toxicity. Atovaquone is available as second-line treatment for mild to moderate PCP, defined as a PaO_2 of 60 mm Hg and an alveolar-arterial oxygen difference [$P(A-a)O_2$] of 45 mm Hg, in patients who cannot tolerate T/S. This drug is administered orally and is associated with fewer adverse reactions than T/S, but it is also less effective.

T/S is the treatment of choice of patients with moderate to severe PCP. However, the high rate of toxicity limits or precludes its use in many. Adverse effects include fever, rash, stomatitis, nausea, vomiting, neutropenia, nephritis, and elevated serum aminotransferase concentrations. For unknown reasons, persons with HIV infection are more likely than others to have adverse reactions to T/S.

Patients with PCP who cannot tolerate T/S are usually given intravenous pentamidine isethionate. This drug is as effective as T/S, but severe adverse effects are also common with pentamidine, including nephrotoxicity, pancreatitis, hyperglycemia, hypoglycemia, leukopenia, hypotension, and ventricular arrhythmias. Trimetrexate/leucovorin is also an alternative for patients who cannot tolerate or who do not respond to T/S. It not as effective as T/S but is associated with fewer side effects. Whether trimetrexate should replace pentamidine as second-line treatment of moderate to severe PCP is unknown, because comparative trials of these two drugs have not been performed.

Adjunctive therapy with corticosteroids at the start of anti-*Pneumocystis* treatment reduces the likelihood of respiratory failure, deterioration of oxygenation, and death in patients with moderate to severe infection. The precise mechanisms of the beneficial effects of corticosteroids in patients with PCP are unknown. An inflammatory response in the lung occurs at the start of anti-*Pneumocystis* treatment in patients who do not receive corticosteroids, probably in response to components of killed organisms and manifested by deteriorating gas exchange. Corticosteroids modify this inflammatory response, prevent the initial worsening of gas oxygenation, and allow the patient to receive more antimicrobial treatment.

The patients with PCP most likely to benefit from adjunctive corticosteroids have a PaO_2 of 70 mm Hg or a $P(A-a)O_2$ of 35 mm Hg. Patients with less severe abnormalities of gas exchange usually do not benefit, mainly because their outcomes are very good with anti-*Pneumocystis* treatment alone. Benefit is also questionable when corticosteroids are administered 72 hours after anti-*Pneumocystis* treatment has begun.

The optimal dosage and duration of corticosteroid treatment are unknown, but the largest controlled trial that showed benefit used oral prednisone in the following regimen: on days 1 through 5, 40 mg was given twice daily; on days 6 through 10, 40 mg was given daily; on days 11 through 21, 20 mg was given daily. Adverse reactions occur infrequently, and although life-threatening superinfections have been described, they are uncommon. Patients in whom pulmonary disorders develop shortly after apparently successful treatment of PCP should be evaluated for another opportunistic infection, especially CMV disease.

Prophylaxis

The prevention of PCP with drugs has reduced its incidence, and PCP-associated mortality in HIV-infected persons has fallen dramatically (Fig. 3). Although anti-*Pneumocystis* prophylaxis may prevent this infection and prolong life, longevity is usually accompanied by progressive immunosuppression, rendering patients susceptible to other potentially fatal infections. While the percentage of HIV-related deaths in the United States caused by PCP declined, deaths caused by nontuberculous mycobacteriosis, CMV disease, bacterial infections, non-Hodgkin's lymphoma, and tuberculosis increased. In an analysis of 844 HIV-infected homosexual men enrolled in the

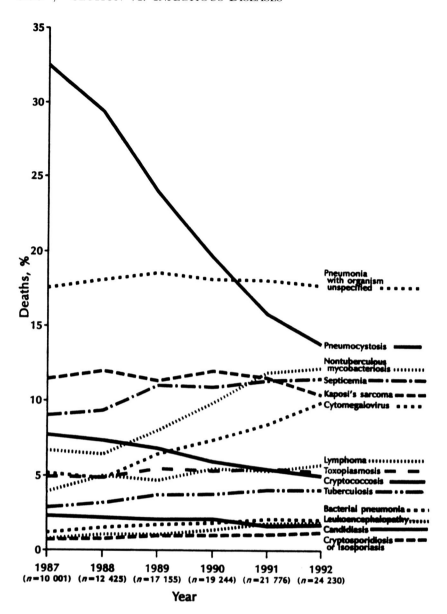

FIG. 3. Trends in the prevalence of infectious diseases and cancers reported among persons dying of HIV infection in the United States from 1987 to 1992. (Reproduced with permission from Selik RM, Chu SY, Ward JW. Trends in infectious diseases and cancers among persons dying of HIV infection in the United States from 1987 to 1992. *Ann Intern Med* 1995;123:933–936.)

Multicenter AIDS Cohort Study, those who received prophylaxis for PCP before being given a diagnosis of AIDS had a lower incidence of PCP and lower mean CD4 count at the time of the AIDS diagnosis than those who did not. However, they had a higher incidence of *M. avium* disease (33.4% vs. 24.8%), wasting syndrome (18.4% vs. 6.4%), and esophageal candidiasis (21.3% vs. 12.8%). PCP prophylaxis also appeared to delay the time to the first AIDS-related illness by 6 to 12 months.

Lifelong prophylaxis against *P. carinii* infection is recommended for all HIV-infected persons with CD4-cell counts of 200/μL, and for patients with HIV-related symptoms, including unexplained persistent fever (100°F) for 2 weeks, oropharyngeal candidiasis unrelated to antibiotic or corticosteroid therapy, and unexplained weight loss. Oral T/S, dapsone, and aerosolized pentamidine are the drugs most extensively studied and used.

The preferred regimen is one double-strength tablet of T/S (160 mg trimethoprim, 800 mg sulfamethoxazole) daily. In addition to its superior efficacy against *P. carinii*, this drug may also prevent toxoplasmosis and bacterial infections. However, the high rate of intolerable side effects limits its application. Lower doses (one single-strength tablet daily, or one double-strength tablet thrice weekly) appear to be almost as effective and more likely to be tolerated. Desensitization to T/S may be attempted in patients allergic to the drug who have not had life-threatening reactions. Failure of T/S prophylaxis is associated with noncompliance and with CD4-lymphocyte counts of 50/μL.

Patients who cannot tolerate T/S should take 100 mg of dapsone daily, in single or divided doses. Fifty milligrams of dapsone daily, along with 50 to 75 mg of pyrimethamine weekly and 25 mg of leucovorin weekly, also confers protection against toxoplasmosis. Pentamidine administered by aerosol has the potential advantages of high drug levels in the lung and minimal systemic absorption and toxicity, but it is less effective than T/S and dapsone. The only aerosolized pentamidine regimen recommended by the CDC is 300 mg administered monthly using the Respigard II nebulizer (Marquest, Englewood, Colorado). Other doses and delivery systems are under investigation.

When PCP occurs in patients using aerosolized pentamidine, it is associated with atypical clinical and diagnostic features. Normal regional differences in ventilation deposit the drug preferentially in the lower lung zones, accounting for a higher rate of predominantly upper lobe involvement. These patients are also more likely to have cystic lung lesions and pneumothorax. Extrapulmonary *P. carinii* infection may occur in patients receiving prophylaxis with aerosolized pentamidine, as the drug is delivered only to the lung.

Other agents have been used to prevent PCP in patients who cannot tolerate standard treatments, or in whom PCP develops despite prophylaxis. These include clindamycin/primaquine, atovaquone, pyrimethamine/sulfadoxine, alternative aerosol pentamidine regimens, and intermittent parenteral pentamidine or trimetrexate. Their efficacy is not known, and they should not be used unless recommended drugs cannot be given.

Respiratory Failure Caused by *Pneumocystis carinii* Pneumonia

Despite the use of prophylaxis and declining mortality rates associated with PCP, the infection is still the most common cause of respiratory failure and admission to intensive care units (ICUs) in patients with AIDS. When treatment of PCP is postponed or ineffective, a clinical syndrome develops that resembles the acute respiratory distress syndrome (ARDS), with severe hypoxemia, intrapulmonary shunt, reduced pulmonary compliance, and the radiographic appearance of diffuse opacities. Just as severe PCP clinically resembles ARDS, the supportive treatment, including intubation, mechanical ventilation, and application of positive end-expiratory pressure, is similar. Continuous positive airway pressure (CPAP) delivered by face mask may improve gas exchange without endotracheal intubation, but its usefulness is limited in patients with severe disease. However, it may afford the patient and physician more time to consider whether mechanical ventilation is desirable.

As changes in therapy modified the prognosis, three distinct eras of critical care for patients with PCP and respiratory failure were identified. Initially, the outlook for survival was dismal. In the 1984 National Institutes of Health Workshop, 88 of the 102 patients with AIDS who received mechanical ventilation died, and nearly all

had PCP. Other studies from individual centers confirmed that survival after respiratory failure was about 15%. In some centers, ICU utilization declined because physicians did not recommend aggressive interventions, and patients were more likely to decline ICU care. After 1986, mortality rates seemed to decrease to about 50%, with the decline attributed to the selection of patients with a better prognosis and the benefits of adjunctive corticosteroid therapy.

We are now in a third era of outcomes, when patients who require mechanical ventilation for PCP again have a very high mortality rate. At San Francisco General Hospital, mortality increased from 61% in the period from 1986–1988 to 76% in the next 2 years. At the same time, the proportion of patients who were injection drug users and who had recurrent episodes of PCP increased. Mortality was strongly associated with a CD4-lymphocyte count of $50/\mu L$ (94%) and with the development of a pneumothorax (100%). Recent patients who require mechanical ventilation for PCP are also more likely to have failed prophylaxis, anti-*Pneumocystis* treatment, or adjunctive corticosteroid therapy and therefore are expected to have a poor prognosis. Recent studies show that when respiratory failure follows several days of appropriate therapy for PCP, the probability of survival is only 10%–20%.

The prospects for long-term survival following PCP and respiratory failure are better than earlier in the epidemic. Prolonged survival is probably related to the selection of patients with a better prognosis for mechanical ventilation, and to improvements in prophylaxis and treatment of subsequent infections.

BACTERIAL PNEUMONIA

The importance of bacteria as HIV-associated pulmonary pathogens was established by investigations in patients who did not have advanced immunosuppression. HIV infection impairs humoral immunity through quantitative and functional defects in CD4 lymphocytes. This increases the risk for bacterial infections, including sinusitis and pneumonia. Although a first episode of bacterial pneumonia usually occurs before the diagnosis of AIDS, the risk for pneumonia increases as the CD4-lymphocyte count declines. Injection drug users are at higher risk than other groups, and neutropenia is an independent risk factor. Prophylaxis with T/S appears to reduce the risk for bacterial pneumonia. Bacterial pneumonia may also accelerate the course of HIV disease, as it is an independent predictor of progression to AIDS and mortality.

In early HIV infection, the pathogens that cause pneumonia are similar to those in the general population. Encapsulated organisms, especially *Streptococcus pneumoniae* and *Haemophilus influenzae*, are the most frequent etiologic agents. Although pneumonia caused by atypical pathogens like *Mycoplasma* and *Legionella* is described, it is relatively uncommon. However, in a careful prospective analysis of 149 episodes of pneumonia in HIV-seropositive former injection drug users, *Chlamydia pneumoniae* was confirmed serologically as the second most common cause of pneumonia (after *S. pneumoniae*), and infection occurred at higher mean CD4-cell counts than infection caused by other pathogens.

Pathogens that rarely cause community-acquired pneumonia in the general population occur more frequently in HIV-infected persons. *Rhodococcus equi*, an aerobic, gram-positive, acid-fast bacillus, may cause focal consolidation, endobronchial disease, and cavitation, usually in patients with advanced HIV disease. Pneumonia caused by *Pseudomonas aeruginosa* was rare in the early years of the AIDS epidemic but is now emerging as an important entity. It usually follows another opportunistic infection or occurs when the CD4-cell count is 50/μL. Although many patients have histories of recent hospitalization, this infection usually presents as community-acquired pneumonia and is not necessarily associated with neutropenia or the use of corticosteroids. Cavitation is common, and the infection is often recurrent or chronic. *Nocardia asteroides* may cause nodules, consolidation, cavitation, pleural effusions, empyema, and intrathoracic lymphadenopathy in patients with HIV infection.

Bacterial pneumonia usually presents in a typical fashion, with fever, chills, productive cough, and localized areas of consolidation on chest radiograph. Although this clinical picture strongly suggests bacterial pneumonia, it may also occur with tuberculosis and fungal infection. Conversely, patients with bacterial pneumonia may have diffuse pulmonary opacities that resemble those of PCP. HIV-infected patients with bacterial pneumonia may be bacteremic and critically ill, but overall mortality is similar to that of HIV-seronegative persons with comparable severity of illness.

The approach to diagnosis and treatment of bacterial pneumonia is the same as that for HIV-negative patients. Because bacterial pneumonia is so common, it should be suspected in any patient with a compatible clinical syndrome and abnormal chest radiographic findings. The routine evaluation includes blood cultures, and if pleural fluid is present, it should be cultured and stained for bacteria, fungi, and mycobacteria. Patients with a productive cough should always have sputum specimens examined for acid-fast bacilli, but the usefulness of sputum Gram's stain and culture in the diagnosis of bacterial infection is controversial.

Empiric coverage for common bacterial pathogens should be started promptly after specimens are obtained. The initial antibiotic regimen should always cover *S. pneumoniae* and *H. influenzae,* and empiric treatment of *P. aeruginosa* should be considered in patients with advanced HIV infection or CD4-lymphocyte counts of 50/μL. Bronchoscopy should be performed in patients who do not respond to empiric therapy without an established diagnosis, to determine whether they have mycobacterial or fungal infection. Occasionally, pulmonary involvement with KS or lymphoma may resemble bacterial infection and can be diagnosed with bronchoscopy.

The polyvalent pneumococcal vaccine is recommended for all HIV-infected people, although persons with low CD4 counts are unlikely to mount an adequate antibody response. A vaccine against *H. influenzae* type b is available, but its usefulness in patients with HIV infection is questionable, as most of these infections are caused by nontypeable strains. Although influenza vaccine is also recommended, there are no data to show that persons with HIV infection are at increased risk for contracting influenza, or that the illness is more severe than in the general population.

TUBERCULOSIS

Modest reductions in cell-mediated immunity increase the risk for reactivation of latent tuberculosis, and the risk increases as CD4-cell counts decline. In HIV-infected persons, tuberculosis often occurs before opportunistic infections, probably because *M. tuberculosis* is more virulent. In patients with mild immunodeficiency, the clinical presentation is similar to that of tuberculosis in HIV-negative patients. Atypical pulmonary presentations, including diffuse infiltrates, miliary patterns, intrathoracic lymphadenopathy, or normal chest radiographic findings, occur more frequently in patients with advanced immunosuppression (Table 3). These patients also have a high incidence of extrapulmonary infection affecting the pleurae, lymph nodes, gastrointestinal tract, bone marrow, and blood.

The diagnosis of tuberculosis may be difficult in HIV-infected persons. Cutaneous anergy is more prevalent as CD4-cell counts decline, making tuberculin skin tests less useful. Radiographic clues to the diagnosis include cavitation, hilar and mediastinal lymphadenopathy, and pleural effusions. When cavitation is present, results of acid-fast smears and cultures of sputum are usually positive. In patients who do not expectorate spontaneously, sputum may be induced with hypertonic saline solution. Results of bronchoscopy with BAL, transbronchial biopsy, and analysis of postbronchoscopy sputum specimens are often diagnostic. Biopsies enhance the immediate diagnostic yield of bronchoscopy in the diagnosis of pulmonary tuberculosis, in comparison with BAL alone.

Despite an appropriate evaluation, results of acid-fast smears of sputum and bronchoscopic specimens may be negative, and cultures may not yield positive results for several weeks. Early treatment of tuberculosis improves the outcome and reduces transmission of the disease to others, so initial empiric therapy is warranted for patients with radiographic abnormalities consistent with tuberculosis unless another disorder is identified.

ATYPICAL MYCOBACTERIAL INFECTION

M. avium-intracellulare causes devastating complications and death in patients with AIDS. In HIV-infected persons with severe immunosuppression, *M. avium-intracellulare* usually causes bacteremia and disseminated infection with fever, weight loss, diarrhea, and anemia. However, *M. avium-intracellulare* is rarely a pulmonary pathogen in patients with AIDS. It is usually isolated from pulmonary specimens in patients with symptomatic pulmonary disease along with another pathogen (such as *P. carinii*) that accounts for the clinical picture. When *M. avium-intracellulare* is isolated from asymptomatic persons, it is strongly predictive of the later development of disseminated infection.

Other nontuberculous mycobacteria may cause pulmonary infection in patients with HIV infection. Like tuberculosis, atypical mycobacterial infections are usually diagnosed first by direct microscopy of smears of any specimen, and the species is then identified by nucleic acid probe or culture. However, if acid-fast bacilli are identified from sputum or bronchoscopic specimens, patients should be treated presumptively for *M. tuberculosis* infection until the species is identified, mainly because tuberculosis is more common and responds better to treatment, and because early treatment of active tuberculosis is an essential public health measure.

CYTOMEGALOVIRUS INFECTION

In patients with CD4-lymphocyte counts of $50/\mu L$, CMV commonly causes retinitis, esophagitis, gastritis, colitis, hepatitis, encephalitis, pneumonia, and death. Patients with AIDS may also have CMV pneumonitis, but uncommonly. Although the virus can often be isolated in cultures of BAL fluid, it is not usually pathogenic. Pulmonary infection can be inferred when typical intranuclear or intracytoplasmic inclusions are found in BAL fluid or biopsy material. The likelihood that CMV is a pulmonary pathogen is also greater when CMV infection is found at other sites.

CMV pneumonitis usually occurs in patients who have had prior AIDS-defining illnesses. They present with a clinical syndrome similar to that of PCP, with dyspnea, nonproductive cough, fever, and diffuse pulmonary opacities. Unilobar radiographic involvement, cavitation, nodules, and pleural effusions are also described. It is treated in the same way as infection in other sites, with intravenous gancyclovir or foscarnet, and the response to therapy is similar to that of CMV retinitis or gastrointestinal disease. As CMV infection occurs only in patients with very severe immunosuppression, the long-term prognosis is very poor.

FUNGAL PNEUMONIA

Life-threatening fungal disease may occur in HIV-infected patients, either by new infection or reactivation of latent disease. The types of fungal infections depend on the severity of immunodeficiency and whether the patient has lived in endemic areas.

Cryptococcosis

Cryptococcus neoformans is distributed throughout the world and is the most common fungus causing life-threatening illness in patients with AIDS. The meninges are the most common site of infection, and cryptococcal meningitis is often the first manifestation of AIDS. With cryptococcal pneumonia, the chest x-ray film usually shows diffuse infiltrates, similar to those of PCP, but localized infiltrates, nodules, cavitation, pleural effusions, miliary patterns, and lymphadenopathy are also seen. Almost all patients with cryptococcal pneumonia have meningitis and disseminated disease, and CD4-lymphocyte counts are typically $100/\mu L$. The diagnosis is established by identification of the organism from sputum, BAL fluid, pleural fluid, or lung biopsy specimens. A high titer of cryptococcal antigen in serum is strongly suggestive, and an antigen titer of 1:8 in BAL fluid is diagnostic of cryptococcal pneumonia.

Because most patients with HIV and cryptococcal pulmonary infection have disseminated disease, 0.5 to 1.0 mg of amphotericin B per kilogram of body weight daily is usually the therapy of first choice. Four hundred milligrams of fluconazole daily is a reasonable alternative in patients who are less ill. After the patient improves and the cerebrospinal fluid is sterilized, lifetime prophylaxis with 200 mg of fluconazole daily is indicated.

Histoplasmosis

Histoplasma capsulatum is endemic in the Ohio and Mississippi River valleys, Central and South America, and the Caribbean Islands. Disseminated disease may develop in patients with HIV infection who come from endemic areas when immunodeficiency permits reactivation of latent infection. The clinical presentation is usually subacute, and the chest roentgenogram typically shows a diffuse or miliary pattern, although localized infiltrates may occur. The diagnosis is established by identification or culture of the organism from blood, lung-derived specimens, bone marrow, or liver.

Amphotericin B is the treatment of choice for most cases of HIV-associated histoplasmosis. An alternative in patients with milder disease is 200 mg of itraconazole daily, and it should be used as suppressive therapy for life after the primary infection has been controlled.

Aspergillosis

Life-threatening pulmonary aspergillosis may develop in patients with advanced immunosuppression. Two common patterns of disease are identified: an invasive parenchymal infection, which is usually fatal, and a predominantly bronchial disease with initial symptoms of dyspnea and airway obstruction. The classic risks for *Aspergillus* infection—namely, prolonged neutropenia and treatment with high-dose corticosteroids—are often absent. Aspergillosis probably develops in patients with advanced AIDS because of defects in neutrophil or alveolar macrophage function. The CD4-lymphocyte count is typically $30/\mu L$, and the prior use of corticosteroids and neutrophil counts of $500/\mu L$ increase the risk. Disseminated disease is common, especially to the brain.

Clues to the diagnosis of invasive pulmonary aspergillosis include upper lobe disease with cavitation and hemoptysis (Fig. 4). Histologic proof has traditionally been required for this diagnosis, because *Aspergillus* is ubiquitous and its presence in nasopharyngeal secretions, sputum, and BAL fluid may represent contamination or colonization. However, recent studies in patients with severe immunosuppression, including AIDS, indicate that the isolation of *Aspergillus* in BAL fluid correlates strongly with histologic proof of tissue invasion.

Invasive aspergillosis is usually treated with amphotericin B, and itraconazole is a reasonable alternative. Despite treatment, most patients die within a few weeks.

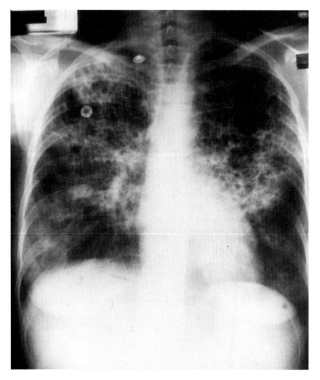

FIG. 4. Chest radiograph of a patient with invasive pulmonary aspergillosis. Diffuse cavitary lesions are present, especially in the upper lung fields.

Other Fungal Infections

In endemic areas, disseminated coccidioidomycosis and blastomycosis may occur in patients with AIDS, usually as a complication of advanced immunosuppression. In some patients, a prior infection may become reactivated after they have moved from an endemic area. These infections usually involve the lung; the presentation includes cough, fever, dyspnea, and the appearance of nodular, focal, cavitary, or diffuse disease. The diagnosis is established by demonstrating the organism by microscopy or culture in respiratory specimens.

Patients with disseminated disease should be treated with amphotericin B, and if they respond, suppressive treatment is indicated for life. Fluconazole is recommended for coccidioidomycosis, and itraconazole for blastomycosis.

NEOPLASTIC DISEASES OF THE LUNG

Kaposi's Sarcoma

KS is the most common malignancy in persons with HIV infection, and the skin is the major site of involvement. KS is believed to be caused by a herpesvirus that infects many healthy adults and may be isolated commonly in saliva, prostate tissue, and semen. The virus is probably transmitted by sexual contact, and it causes disease when activated during HIV-associated immunosuppression. This hypothesis helps to explain why KS is much more common among HIV-infected homosexual men than in other transmission groups.

KS may involve many organs, including the lung. Patients with pulmonary KS usually have obvious mucocutaneous lesions, but the lung may be the only site of disease in up to 15% of cases. Involvement of the airways, parenchyma, pleurae, and intrathoracic lymph nodes causes a diverse range of symptoms and radiographic findings. The majority of patients with pulmonary KS diagnosed ante mortem have cough, dyspnea, and fever.

In the airways, KS lesions are usually asymptomatic, but sometimes cause obstruction or hemoptysis. The finding of typical lesions on inspection of the airways is usually considered diagnostic. Histologic diagnosis may be difficult, because the yield of forceps biopsy is low. Some authors believe that forceps biopsy of KS lesions places the patient at significant risk for bleeding, but this is controversial.

Parenchymal involvement with KS is suggested by bronchial wall thickening, nodules, Kerley B lines, and coexisting pleural effusions, especially in patients with cutaneous disease (Fig. 5). Bronchoscopy may be performed to determine whether diffuse radiographic opacities are caused by KS or an opportunistic infection. The yield of bronchoscopic lung biopsy in the diagnosis of

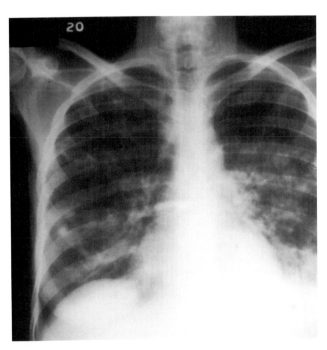

FIG. 5. Chest radiograph of a patient with pulmonary parenchymal KS. The nodular densities suggest this diagnosis, especially in patients with cutaneous disease.

KS is low, and even open lung biopsy is nondiagnostic in approximately 10% of cases because of the focal distribution of lesions. Therefore, the diagnosis of pulmonary parenchymal KS is usually inferred in patients with cutaneous disease, chest radiographs that suggest this disorder, visual confirmation of airway lesions, and no evidence of opportunistic infection on BAL or bronchoscopic lung biopsy. Patients with parenchymal opacities who have typical lesions in the airways and no identified pulmonary infection are assumed to have parenchymal KS.

When KS involves the pleurae, effusions are usually exudative and sanguinous, but the cytologic examination is nondiagnostic. Results of closed pleural biopsy are rarely positive because of the focal nature of pleural lesions and predominant involvement of the visceral, rather than parietal, pleura. Because establishing a diagnosis usually necessitates a thoracoscopic or open pleural biopsy, the presence of pleural involvement with KS is usually inferred in a patient with cutaneous disease and a serosanguinous effusion without any reasonable alternative explanation.

Other Malignancies

Non-Hodgkin's B-cell lymphoma is associated with HIV infection. Although pulmonary involvement is usually clinically innocuous, the lung is a common site of extranodal disease. If symptoms occur, they usually do so late in the course of HIV disease and simulate common opportunistic infections. Even in patients with an established diagnosis of lymphoma, lung involvement is usu-

ally a late feature of disease. It may present with lobar consolidation, nodules, reticular opacities, and masses. The diagnosis is established by bronchoscopic or open biopsy; BAL has a very low diagnostic yield.

Radiographically, intrathoracic lymph node involvement is manifested by lymphadenopathy, pleural involvement by effusions and pleural thickening, and airway involvement by atelectasis. The diagnosis is established by biopsy or cytologic analysis of pleural fluid.

Carcinoma of the lung has been reported in patients with HIV infection. Although reports emphasize the relatively young age of these patients and aggressive nature of their disease, it is not established that HIV infection increases the risk for lung cancer.

OTHER PULMONARY DISORDERS

For unknown reasons, patients with advanced HIV infection may have chronic bronchitis and bronchiectasis, even if they do not smoke. These patients usually have CD4 counts of $100/\mu L$. Standard antimicrobial agents are usually effective, but symptoms are likely to recur, especially when *P. aeruginosa* is isolated from the sputum. The role and efficacy of bronchodilators and anti-inflammatory agents in HIV-associated airway disease have not been studied.

Pulmonary disorders without a defined infectious or neoplastic etiology occur in HIV-infected persons. Lymphocytic interstitial pneumonitis and nonspecific interstitial pneumonitis are believed to comprise a spectrum of inflammatory changes in response to HIV infection of the lung itself. Lymphocytic interstitial pneumonitis is most common in HIV-infected children and African-Americans. It may occur as part of a systemic CD8 lymphoproliferative syndrome, with lymphadenopathy, blood lymphocytosis, and involvement of other organs. Nonspecific interstitial pneumonitis is very common in persons with low CD4 counts but is rarely diagnosed because it usually causes no symptoms. When symptomatic, both lymphocytic interstitial pneumonitis and nonspecific interstitial pneumonitis are treated with corticosteroids.

Bronchiolitis obliterans organizing pneumonia is also described in patients with HIV infection, but the reasons for this association are unknown. The manifestations are similar in patients with and without HIV infection. Lung biopsy is necessary for the diagnosis. This disorder often improves dramatically with corticosteroids.

Pulmonary hypertension occurs more commonly in HIV-infected patients than in the general population. It may occur without a prior AIDS diagnosis or severe immunosuppression, and the clinical and histologic features of this disorder are indistinguishable from those of primary pulmonary hypertension. The etiology is unknown, no effective treatment is available, and the prognosis is dismal.

BIBLIOGRAPHY

Baron AD, Hollander H. *Pseudomonas aeruginosa* bronchopulmonary infection in late human immunodeficiency virus infection. *Am Rev Respir Dis* 1993;148:992–996. *The clinical features and risks for the development of* Pseudomonas *lower respiratory tract infection are analyzed.*

Barre-Sinoussi F, Chermann JC, Rey F, et al. Isolation of a T-lymphotropic retrovirus from a patient at risk for acquired immune deficiency syndrome (AIDS). *Science* 1983;220:868–871.

Gallo RC, Salahuddin SZ, Popovic M, et al. Frequent detection and isolation of cytopathic retroviruses (HTLV III) from patients with AIDS and at risk for AIDS. *Science* 1984;224:500–503. *These studies first identified that the etiologic agent of AIDS is the virus now known as HIV.*

Boschini A, Smacchia C, Di Fine M, et al. Community-acquired pneumonia in a cohort of former injection drug users with and without immunodeficiency virus infection: incidence, etiologies, and clinical aspects. *Clin Infect Dis* 1996;23:107–113. *In a cohort of drug users living in a residential community in Italy, HIV-infected persons had a higher incidence of bacterial pneumonia than did HIV-negative residents. The relative risk for pneumonia caused by* S. pneumoniae, H. influenzae, *and* C. pneumoniae *was significantly higher among the HIV-seropositive persons.*

Centers for Disease Control. *Pneumocystis* pneumonia—Los Angeles. *MMWR Morb Mortal Wkly Rep* 1980;30:250–252. *This is the first published report of AIDS, describing the five cases of PCP in homosexual men with no identifiable cause of immunodeficiency.*

Centers for Disease Control. Update on acquired immune deficiency syndrome (AIDS). *MMWR Morb Mortal Wkly Rep* 1982;31:507–514.

Centers for Disease Control. Revision of the CDC surveillance case definition for acquired immunodeficiency syndrome. *MMWR Morb Mortal Wkly Rep* 1987;36:1S–15S.

Centers for Disease Control and Prevention. 1993 revised classification system for HIV infection and expanded surveillance case definition for AIDS among adolescents and adults. *MMWR Morb Mortal Wkly Rep* 1992;41(No. RR-17):1–19. *These publications present the case definitions of AIDS since the beginning of the epidemic. The current (1993) classification includes pulmonary tuberculosis, recurrent pneumonia, and low CD4-lymphocyte counts as AIDS-defining in HIV-infected persons.*

Centers for Disease Control and Prevention. First 500,000 AIDS cases—United States, 1995. *MMWR Morb Mortal Wkly Rep* 1995;44:849–853.

Centers for Disease Control and Prevention. *HIV/AIDS Surveillance Report*, 1996;8(No. 1):1–33. *Temporal trends in the epidemiology of HIV-infected populations in the United States are described. New cases are represented increasingly by racial/ethnic minorities and by persons who acquired HIV infection through injection drug use or heterosexual transmission.*

Centers for Disease Control and Prevention. USPHS/IDSA guidelines for the prevention of opportunistic infections in persons infected with human immunodeficiency virus: a summary. *MMWR Morb Mortal Wkly Rep* 1995;44(No. RR-8):1–34. *These comprehensive guidelines for the prevention of opportunistic infections in persons with HIV infection emphasize PCP, tuberculosis, toxoplasmosis, and* Mycobacterium avium *complex. Guidelines for general assessment and laboratory tests at initial and subsequent visits are also proposed.*

Daley CL, Mugusi F, Chen LL, et al. Pulmonary complications of HIV infection in Dar es Salaam, Tanzania: role of bronchoscopy and bronchoalveolar lavage. *Am J Respir Crit Care Med* 1996;154:105–110. *Among 95 HIV-infected patients hospitalized with acute respiratory disease in an African hospital, tuberculosis was the most common diagnosis (75%), followed by bacterial pneumonia (14%). PCP was diagnosed in only one case.*

Fauci AS, Pantaleo G, Stanley S, et al. Immunopathogenetic mechanisms of HIV infection. *Ann Intern Med* 1996;124:654–663. *The proceedings of an NIH conference summarize the biology of HIV and the effects of infection on the immune system.*

Hanson DL, Chu SY, Farizo KM, et al. Distribution of CD4⁺ T lymphocytes at diagnosis of acquired immunodeficiency syndrome-defining and other human immunodeficiency virus-related illnesses. *Arch Intern Med* 1995;155:1537–1542. *The severity of immunosuppression, as assessed by the CD4-lymphocyte count, was associated with the development of specific HIV-associated disorders in this large, multicenter study.*

Hawley PH, Ronco JJ, Guillemi SA, et al. Decreasing frequency but worsening mortality of acute respiratory failure secondary to AIDS-related *Pneumocystis carinii* pneumonia. *Chest* 1994;106:1456–1459. *If respiratory failure develops in PCP despite treatment with appropriate antimicrobial agents and adjunctive corticosteroids, the prognosis is dismal.*

Hirschtick RE, Glassroth J, Jordan MC, et al. Bacterial pneumonia in patients infected with human immunodeficiency virus. *N Engl J Med* 1995;333:845–851. *In the Pulmonary Complications of HIV Infection Study, bacterial pneumonia was the most common cause of lower respiratory infection in a cohort followed prospectively. Mortality during the follow-up period and results of prophylaxis with T/S are discussed.*

Hoover DR, Saah AJ, Bacellar H, et al. Clinical manifestations of AIDS in the era of *Pneumocystis* prophylaxis. *N Engl J Med* 1993;329:1922–1926. *In the Multicenter AIDS Cohort Study, subjects who received prophylaxis for PCP before being given a diagnosis of AIDS had a significantly lower incidence of PCP and lower mean CD4 count at the time of AIDS diagnosis than those who did not. PCP prophylaxis appeared to delay the time to the first AIDS-related illness by 6 to 12 months.*

Huang L, Hecht FM, Gruden J, et al. Predicting *Pneumocystis carinii* pneumonia: results of a multivariate analysis. In: *Proceedings of the 11th International Conference on AIDS*, July 9, 1996, Vancouver, BC(abst TuB110). *This study shows that the presence of granular opacities on chest radiographs and the absence of purulent sputum are very strongly predictive of PCP in patients with a CD4 count of 50/μL.*

Huang L, Schnapp LM, Gruden J, Hopewell PC, Stansell JD. Presentation of AIDS-related Kaposi's sarcoma diagnosed by bronchoscopy. *Am J Respir Crit Care Med* 1996;153:1385–1390. *The clinical, laboratory and radiographic, and bronchoscopic features of pulmonary KS are described in a large series of patients.*

Ioannidis JP, Cappelleri JC, Skolnick PR, Lau J, Sacks HS. A meta-analysis of the relative efficacy and toxicity of *Pneumocystis carinii* prophylactic regimens. *Arch Intern Med* 1996;156:177–188. *T/S is more effective than aerosolized pentamidine and dapsone in preventing both PCP and toxoplasmosis, but discontinuing T/S because of adverse reactions is much more likely.*

Jules-Elysee KM, Stover DE, Zaman MB, Bernard EM, White DA. Aerosolized pentamidine: effect on diagnosis and presentation of *Pneumocystis carinii* pneumonia. *Ann Intern Med* 1990;112:750–757. *The presentation of PCP in patients using aerosolized pentamidine prophylaxis is atypical, with a high incidence of cystic disease and reduced diagnostic yield of BAL.*

Kovacs JA, Ng V, Masur H, et al. Diagnosis of *Pneumocystis carinii* pneumonia: improved detection in sputum with use of monoclonal antibodies. *N Engl J Med* 1988;318:589–593. *By means of immunofluorescent staining, PCP was diagnosed in induced sputum specimens in 80% of cases.*

Lortholary O, Meyohas M-C, Dupont B, et al. Invasive aspergillosis in patients with acquired immunodeficiency syndrome. Report of 33 cases. *Am J Med* 1993;95:177–187. *A large series of patients is the basis of this description of the clinical features of invasive aspergillosis in AIDS. The authors demonstrate that a positive culture of BAL fluid is diagnostic of the disease.*

Masur H. Prevention and treatment of *Pneumocystis* pneumonia. *N Engl J Med* 1992;327:1853–1860. *A concise, thorough review of anti-*Pneumocystis *agents.*

Miller RF, Mitchell DM. *Pneumocystis carinii* pneumonia. *Thorax* 1995;50:191–200. *The molecular biology, diagnosis, treatment, and prophylaxis of PCP are discussed thoroughly.*

Monini P, De Lellis L, Fabris M, Rigolin F, Cassai E. Kaposi's sarcoma-associated herpesvirus DNA sequences in prostate tissue and human semen. *N Engl J Med* 1996;334:1168–1172. *By means of the polymerase chain reaction, the virus believed to cause KS was identified in 91% of semen samples from immunocompetent men. HIV-related immunocompromise probably leads to viral activation and emergence of the malignant disease.*

Murray J, Felton CP, Garay SM, et al. Pulmonary complications of the acquired immunodeficiency syndrome: report of the National Heart, Lung, and Blood Institute Workshop. *N Engl J Med* 1984;310:1682–1688. *This historic multicenter survey shows that PCP is the major cause of pulmonary disease and mortality in patients with AIDS.*

Murray J, Mills J. Pulmonary infectious complications of human immunodeficiency virus infection. *Am Rev Respir Dis* 1990;141:1356–1372, 1582–1598. *This authoritative review offers comprehensive descriptions of a wide range of HIV-associated pulmonary diseases and provide extensive references.*

National Institutes of Health–University of California Expert Panel for Corticosteroids as Adjunctive Therapy for *Pneumocystis Pneumonia.* Consensus statement on the use of corticosteroids as adjunctive therapy for *Pneumocystis* pneumonia in the acquired immunodeficiency syndrome. *N Engl J Med* 1990;323:1500–1504. *This consensus conference reviews the studies of adjunctive corticosteroid therapy of PCP and offers recommendations for clinical use.*

Phair J, Munoz A, Detels R, et al. The risk of *Pneumocystis carinii* pneumonia among men infected with human immunodeficiency virus type I. *N Engl J Med* 1990;322:161–165. *Data from the Multicenter AIDS Cohort Study showed that PCP occurred predominantly in persons with a CD4 count of 200/μL within the past 6 months. CD4 levels together with HIV-associated symptoms, including thrush, unexplained fever, and unintentional weigh loss, identified the group most likely to benefit from anti-Pneumocystis prophylaxis.*

Rodriguez-Barradas MC, Stool E, Musher D. Diagnosing and treating cytomegalovirus pneumonia in patients with AIDS. *Clin Infect Dis* 1996;23:76–81. *The diagnosis of CMV pneumonia is difficult to establish with certainty. This study describes the clinical and laboratory features of patients with confirmed CMV pneumonia.*

Rosen MJ, Jordan MC, Kvale PA, et al. Pulmonary function tests in HIV-infected persons without AIDS. *Am J Respir Crit Care Med* 1995;152:738–745. *Patients with HIV infection who do not have AIDS have normal values for FVC and FEV₁. The DₗCO may be slightly reduced in injection drug users and in persons with CD4-lymphocyte counts of 200/μL, but race and cigarette smoking have a greater influence on this measurement.*

Saah AJ, Hoover DR, Peng Y, et al. Predictors for failure of *Pneumocystis carinii* prophylaxis. *JAMA* 1995;273:1197–1202. *In 476 subjects, failure of prophylaxis correlated with the degree of reduction in the CD4-lymphocyte count. More than 85% of the 92 failures of prophylaxis occurred in persons with counts of 75/μL.*

Safrin S, Finkelstein DM, Feinberg, et al. Comparison of three regimens for treatment of mild to moderate *Pneumocystis carinii* pneumonia in patients with AIDS: a double-blind, randomized trial of oral trimethoprim-sulfamethoxazole, dapsone-trimethoprim, and clindamycin-primaquine. *Ann Intern Med* 1996;124:792–802. *In this large, multicenter study, the three oral regimens had similar rates of dose-limiting toxicity and similar efficacy in patients with PCP and a P(A-a)O₂ of 45 mm Hg.*

Salzman SH, Rosen MJ. HIV infection. In: Feinsilver SH, Fein AM, eds. *Textbook of Bronchoscopy.* Baltimore: Williams & Wilkins; 1995. *Comprehensive review of the indications and diagnostic usefulness of bronchoscopy in the diagnosis of pulmonary complications of HIV infection.*

Sarosi GA, Ampel N, Cohn DL, et al. Fungal infection in HIV-infected persons. *Am J Respir Crit Care Med* 1995;152:816–822. *This statement of the American Thoracic Society reviews clinical manifestations, approach to diagnosis, and therapy of fungal infections.*

Selik RM, Chu SY, Ward JW. Trends in infectious diseases and cancers among persons dying of HIV infection in the United States from 1987 to 1992. *Ann Intern Med* 1995;123:933–936. *The percentage of HIV-related deaths caused by PCP declined from 32.5% to 13.8%, whereas the percentage of deaths resulting from nontuberculous mycobacteriosis, CMV disease, bacterial infections, non-Hodgkin's lymphoma, and tuberculosis increased.*

Staikowsky F, Lafon B, Guidet B, Denis M, Mayaud C, Offenstadt G. Mechanical ventilation for *Pneumocystis carinii* pneumonia in patients with the acquired immunodeficiency syndrome: is the prognosis really improved? *Chest* 1993;104:756–762. *In a retrospective analysis of 33 patients who required mechanical ventilation for PCP, there was an 82% mortality rate. However, only one of the 22 patients who started mechanical ventilation after the days of appropriate medical therapy survived.*

Travis WD, Fox CH, Devaney KO, et al. Lymphocytic pneumonitis in 50 adult HIV-infected patients: lymphocytic interstitial pneumonitis versus nonspecific interstitial pneumonitis. *Hum Pathol* 1992;23:529–541. *The clinical and pathologic features of these inflammatory disorders were studied. They probably represent different manifestations of HIV infection of the lung.*

Tu JV, Bien HJ, Detsky HS. Bronchoscopy versus empirical therapy in HIV-infected patients with presumptive *Pneumocystis carinii* pneumonia: a decision analysis. *Am Rev Respir Dis* 1993;148:370–377. *A decision analysis supports the use of initial empiric treatment for patients suspected of having PCP.*

Verghese A, Al-Samman M, Nabhan D, et al. Bacterial bronchitis and bronchiectasis in human immunodeficiency virus infection. *Arch Intern Med* 1994;154:2086–2091. *Recurrent bronchitis and bronchiectasis developed after the diagnosis of HIV infection in patients with a mean CD4-lymphocyte count of 61/μL. Response to antimicrobial therapy was usually prompt when H. influenzae or S. pneumoniae was isolated, but slower with P. aeruginosa.*

Wachter RM, Luce JM, Safrin S, et al. Cost and outcome of intensive care for patients with AIDS, *Pneumocystis carinii* pneumonia, and severe respiratory failure. *JAMA* 1995;273:230–235. *In this third era of mechanical ventilation for PCP, survival at San Francisco General Hospital fell from 39% to 24%, in association with an increased admission rate for injection drug users and patients with recurrent PCP. The cost of each year of life saved was $215,233.*

Wallace JM, Rao AV, Glassroth J, et al. Respiratory illness in persons with human immunodeficiency virus infection. *Am Rev Respir Dis* 1993;148:1523–1529. *The most frequent respiratory diagnoses among HIV-infected subjects who did not have AIDS (1987 definition) at the time of enrollment in the prospective Pulmonary Complications of HIV Infection Study were also common in the general population: upper respiratory infections, acute bronchitis, and sinusitis.*

White DA, Matthay RA. Noninfectious pulmonary complications of infection with the human immunodeficiency virus. *Am Rev Respir Dis* 1989;140:1763–1787. *A comprehensive and authoritative review.*

Textbook of Pulmonary Diseases, 6th ed.
edited by G.L. Baum, J.D. Crapo, B.R. Celli, and J.B. Karlinsky,
Lippincott–Raven Publishers, Philadelphia, © 1998.

CHAPTER

27 ▷ Pulmonary Fungal Infections

Gerald L. Baum · Judith Rhodes

INTRODUCTION

Infection by fungi generally occurs by inhalation. Thus, the lungs are the organs most frequently encountering these microorganisms and the organs that most often demonstrate the pathologic changes of fungal disease. Generalized dissemination of the fungus may cause spread of the infection from the lungs to the rest of the body as part of a process that has been called *primary infection and postprimary dissemination,* in which the immune system is involved in a complicated series of reactions reflecting innate factors as well as humoral and cell-mediated immunity.

In general, the resistance of the body to infection by fungi characterized as saprogphytic is excellent; in fact, these fungi rarely cause significant infection in healthy humans. A group of more aggressive fungi regularly causes primary infection in healthy human subjects, but this infection is limited and not associated with significant disease, even when postprimary dissemination occurs. In this respect, these fungi behave similarly to *Mycobacterium tuberculosis,* but they are considerably less prone to produce active disease. The fungi making up this group include *Histoplasma capsulatum, Coccidioides immitis, Blastomyces dermatitidis, Sporothrix schenckii, Paracoccidioides brasiliensis,* and *Cryptococcus neoformans.* There is also evidence that species of *Nocardia* can cause disease when inhaled.

Special consideration for *Aspergillus* species is warranted, as this genus represents one of the common environmental organisms that rarely, under circumstances not clearly understood, may cause progressive infection in ostensibly normal humans. In addition, this organism may elicit a syndrome of hypersensitivity in the human airways, and it may lodge as a commensal organism in pre-existing cavities and produce a mat of tissue called a *fungus ball* or *mycetoma.* Other fungi have been found to cause fungus balls, but this is rare.

Another special situation relates to organisms normally found within the body, such as *Candida* species and *Actinomyces israelii,* that normally do not produce disease. *Candida* is a normal commensal of the gastrointestinal tract, and it is extremely rare for it to cause progressive systemic disease in immunocompetent persons. *Actinomyces* is likewise a friendly inhabitant of the body but may produce disease in the presence of local trauma to the mouth and throat, where the organism is found, especially in tonsillar crypts and tooth sockets.

When the human immune system is suppressed, any microorganism may cause progressive disease, and fungi are clearly part of this threat. Thus, in any consideration of the impact of fungi on the body in general and the lungs in particular, the state of the immune system must be accounted for.

Although fungi are the subject of this chapter, *Actinomyces* and *Nocardia* species, which are bacteria, are included for two reasons: They have traditionally been dealt with in this manner, and many of the characteristics of diseases caused by these organisms are similar to those of true fungal diseases.

G. L. Baum: Israel Lung Association, Tel-Aviv 63 346 Israel.

J. Rhodes: Department of Pathology and Laboratory Medicine, University of Cincinnati College of Medicine, Cincinnati, Ohio 45267-0529.

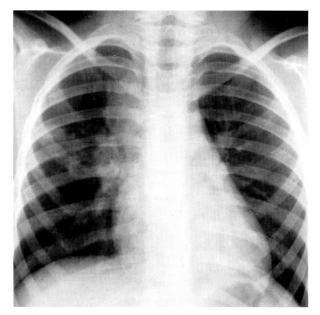

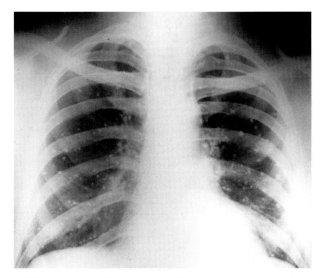

FIG. 3. Healed lesions of pulmonary histoplasmosis.

FIG. 1. Primary histoplasmosis with peripheral pneumonia and hilar adenopathy.

FUNGAL DISEASES

Histoplasmosis (Figs. 1–5)

Originally thought to be a rare, disseminated, tropical disease, infection with *H. capsulatum* has been found to be very common in endemic areas (the Mississippi and Missouri River valleys in the United States, and isolated areas elsewhere in the world), and sporadic but not rare in other areas. The first patients were found in Panama and described by Darling in 1905. Although he was able

to differentiate the organism in tissues from *Leishmania*, which it closely resembles, he nonetheless thought it was a parasite. The fungal nature of the organism was clarified by da Rocha-Lima in 1913. Most infected persons have asymptomatic infections. Humans have excellent resistance to the organism, and despite uniform dissemination in the bloodstream at the time of primary pulmonary infection, progressive disease is uncommon. Healing is associated with massive production of scar tissue and frequently with florid calcification.

Organism

H. capsulatum variety *capsulatum* is a dimorphic fungus that occurs in nature as a mold with septate hyphae

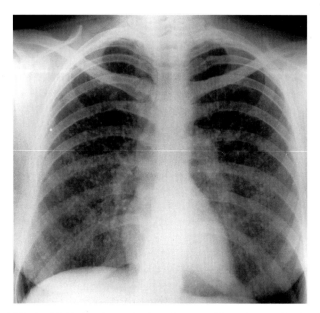

FIG. 2. Multiple primary lesions in acute histoplasmosis simulating hematogenous dissemination.

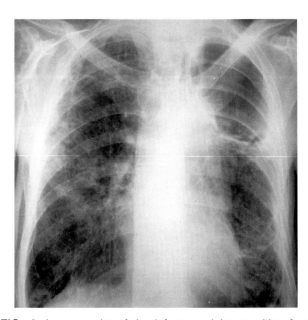

FIG. 4. Large cavity of the left upper lobe resulting from histoplasmosis. Diffuse disease is seen throughout the lung.

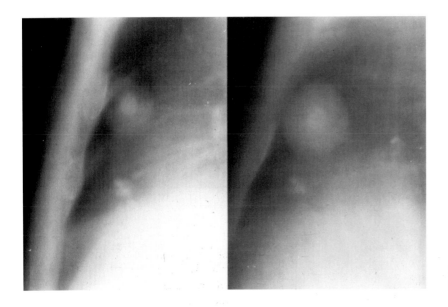

FIG. 5. Enlarging histoplasmoma with central and peripheral laminated calcifications.

bearing tuberculate macroconidia and infectious microconidia. When the microconidia are inhaled, they convert into small budding yeasts (3 to 5 μm) that are found as intracellular pathogens of mononuclear phagocytes.

Pathology

After the microconidia are inhaled and reach the respiratory parenchyma of the lungs, a transient purulent exudate is produced, quickly followed by the sequence of T and B lymphocytes as well as circulating macrophages. This evolution is characteristic of a cell-mediated immune response and is often accompanied by caseous necrosis in the center of the granulomatous focus (or foci) of primary infection. Shortly after infection, a local lymphangitis and lymphadenitis with similar characteristics occur, which may involve the lymph system in progressive fashion until the bloodstream is invaded, with dissemination of the organism throughout the body. The organ most frequently demonstrating foci of infection outside the lungs and thorax is the spleen. This may be a consequence of the large concentration of reticuloendothelial cells found in the spleen. The liver is much less frequently involved. The adrenal glands, bones, gastrointestinal tract, and central nervous system may also host foci of infection. In all, the process is mainly granulomatous in nature.

The healing tendency is remarkable, and the formation of large amounts of scar tissue and calcification, especially in the mediastinal nodes and spleen, may be seen on x-ray films. In fact, scarring and calcification are so prominent that syndromes caused by obstruction and penetration of mediastinal structures, with no evidence of active infection, are part of the clinical spectrum of histoplasmosis. The question of exogenous reinfection occurring in normal hosts is moot, but a few case reports have suggested that it occurs. Much more problematic is whether endogenous reinfection occurs when the primary encounter has ended in clinical healing.

In immunosuppressed humans, primary infection with *H. capsulatum* is associated with much more active dissemination than in immunocompetent hosts. The granulomatous reaction does not develop as well or as typically, and frequently, depending on the degree of lowering of the CD4-lymphocyte count, the reaction to infection may be primarily neutrophilic. Exogenous reinfection almost certainly occurs, and there is evidence to suggest that endogenous reinfection may occur in immunosuppressed hosts.

Immunopathology of *Histoplasma* infection is mainly manifested by activation of the cellular immune system and associated delayed hypersensitivity. The role of humoral immunity is unclear, and the presence of antibodies of both IgG and IgM types appears to be merely a marker of infection.

Epidemiology

The central United States, especially the southern half, is probably the most highly endemic area in the world. Populations of Eastern Europe, South Africa, and parts of South America and China have shown higher than average rates of skin test positivity. Sporadic cases of infection and disease have been found all over the world, which may reflect the increase in worldwide travel. High concentrations of the organism are found in specific regions outside the endemic areas, and persons who travel to these locales may be subjected to massive exposure. Most dramatically, closed areas, such as caves, abandoned chicken houses, and places where common house bats tend to congregate, may contain very large numbers of infectious conidia in the soil. *H. capsulatum* is a normal inhabitant of the bat colon and is expelled in the feces.

Exposure to bat guano is often associated with massive pulmonary infection. Association with starling roosts has been reported.

Clinical Manifestations

Primary histoplasmosis of the lungs is usually clinically silent. If the dose of inhaled conidia is large or if the infection occurs in a young child or weakened adult, there may be flulike symptoms, including fever and chills. These persist for a few days at most unless the host is immunosuppressed from any cause, in which case the symptoms may continue and progress. Cough and scanty sputum production are evanescent. Symptoms clear spontaneously and the diagnosis is usually overlooked. Associated clinical and roentgenographic findings seen in the course of primary infection include pericardial effusion and erythema nodosum. The latter clears spontaneously, as does the former, which rarely persists as chronic constrictive pericarditis. If the infection is massive, the infected person is under 1 1/2 years of age, or immunosuppression is present, blood pancytopenia and more severe signs of systemic organ involvement, affecting the liver and kidneys, may appear. Disseminated infection may be devastating in patients with AIDS, as no effective cell-mediated immunity remains to resist infection.

Healing of the primary infection is almost always associated with massive formation of scar tissue and accompanying calcification. In the lung itself, this leads to a dramatic chest radiographic pattern that has little or no clinical significance. In the mediastinum, however, the results of this process may be devastating. The spectrum includes mild bronchial obstruction (in young patients an enlarged node may cause narrowing from pressure alone); broncholithiasis; esophageal obstruction and formation of diverticula; obstruction of various vascular structures, including the aorta, pulmonary arteries, and most frequently the superior vena cava; bronchiectasis; and lobar or whole-lung collapse. In extreme cases, fibrosing mediastinitis may develop. The signs and symptoms are related only to the anatomic abnormality and usually not to any activity of the infection.

Acute eosinophilic pneumonia caused by *H. capsulatum* has been described with typical clinical characteristics. If indeed this exists, it is a self-limited syndrome; if severe, it responds well to steroid treatment.

Solitary (occasionally multiple) pulmonary nodule may be caused by *H. capsulatum* (histoplasmoma) and appears to be a remnant of the primary focus. It is imperative to differentiate between carcinoma and inactive *Histoplasma* infection as the cause of the nodule. In many instances this requires resection, although the presence on chest x-ray films of a diffuse, ''popcorn'' kind of calcification in the lesion, especially when the patient is asymptomatic, strongly suggests histoplasmosis as the cause.

Chronic granulomatous disease of the lungs may result from *Histoplasma* infection. There are no clinical or roentgenographic criteria to differentiate between mycobacteria, *Histoplasma,* or for that matter *C. immitis* as a cause of the syndrome, which usually occurs in men of middle age or older and is associated with progression to death if not treated. There is disagreement as to the pathogenesis of this form of histoplasmosis. It would appear to develop in patients with an active cell-mediated immune system, as seen in patients with cavitary tuberculosis. On the other hand, it has been suggested that this form of histoplasmosis represents superinfection of previously existing emphysematous areas in the lung. If this is true, it is hard to explain the very typical pathology of chronic granulomatous infection that is routinely seen. The possibility of endogenous reinfection exists.

Epidemic histoplasmosis is an acute, multifocal bronchopneumonia caused by a massive inhalation of conidia of *H. capsulatum.* Such cases frequently occur in clusters, as numbers of persons may be exposed at the same time or in the same area during a prolonged period of time. Such highly contaminated areas are often inhabited by bats. Roosts of starlings have also been associated with these outbreaks. Exploration of caves containing large quantities of bat guano (spelunkers' disease), use of an abandoned chicken house for storage or playing (chicken house disease), and acute exposure to highly contaminated soil in a central city play area have all been associated with such outbreaks. Patients have an acute febrile illness beginning between 7 and 14 days after exposure, characterized by toxemia, dry cough, and often chest muscular pains. Extensive lung involvement may lead to adult respiratory distress syndrome (ARDS). Only in immunosuppressed patients does the infection progress to extrapulmonary dissemination and death if not treated. In immunocompetent patients, respiratory support may be needed but recovery is almost universal. Of interest is the appearance of multiple parenchymal calcifications in the lungs of persons initially exposed to the fungus. In persons previously infected, the multiple lesions usually heal with no or minimal radiographic findings.

In infants under 1 1/2 years of age or persons over the age of 65 to 70, a first encounter with *H. capsulatum* almost always leads to widely disseminated infection that may be accompanied by miliary pulmonary histoplasmosis. This is potentially fatal and requires treatment. In infants the infection progresses rapidly, whereas in the elderly it may progress slowly and be accompanied by painful mucosal ulcerations.

Cases of typical sarcoidosis have been described from which *H. capsulatum* has been isolated. It is assumed that the fungus triggers the massive granulomatous reaction, noted particularly in the lungs and mediastinal lymph nodes. The principles for treating sarcoidosis are generally adhered to in these cases, and the presence of the organism does not change the therapy.

Diagnosis

Chest x-ray films may show the peripheral focus and enlarged regional and hilar nodes of a typical primary complex. The lymph node enlargement may not be as obvious in adults as in children under the age of 16 years.

Chronic granulomatous disease is associated with characteristic radiographic changes in the lungs, details of which are shown best by computed tomography (CT). Although little used currently, classic tomography is also helpful if CT is not available. Histoplasmomas show solitary or multiple well-circumscribed homogeneous densities anywhere in the lung fields, but most typically in the periphery. The presence of single or multiple calcifications strongly suggests a granulomatous etiology, but a single calcification is not totally reliable. In so-called epidemic cases, multiple, poorly defined densities are seen, usually bilaterally, and there may be associated hilar adenopathy. The parenchymal shadows may simulate miliary disease. Again, the x-ray picture is not specific, but with an appropriate history it can be highly suggestive. In true disseminated disease, miliary lesions may be seen in the lungs, and other organs and systems may be involved by inflammatory changes, including liver, kidneys, bones, and central nervous system.

In epidemiologic surveys, the presence of splenic calcifications, especially more than two, has been found to be a reliable indicator of previous infection with *H. capsulatum*. These may also be seen in patients with active lung disease, but their significance in this setting is no greater than that of any other indicator of previous infection.

Except for pancytopenia, seen in disseminated active infection, and nonspecific signs of inflammatory liver involvement, general laboratory findings are not helpful.

Definitive diagnosis of histoplasmosis is made by isolation of the organism from bronchoalveolar lavage (BAL) fluid, bone marrow, blood, or biopsy material. Although the organism may require 7 to 21 days for initial growth, rapid confirmation may be obtained within 24 hours using a commercially available DNA probe for colony hybridization. A presumptive diagnosis of histoplasmosis is frequently made by direct microscopic examination of clinical material using the Grocott silver stain in tissue or a Giemsa stain of bone marrow or buffy coat. Culture of peripheral blood by the lysis-centrifugation technique has been shown to have equivalent sensitivity to bone marrow culture in HIV-positive patients. Serologic tests for antibody include complement fixation, immunodiffusion, and an enzyme-linked immunosorbent assay (ELISA). In immunocompetent patients, a complement fixation titer ≥1:16 is highly suggestive of histoplasmosis. The presence of an M band on immunodiffusion suggests a previous infection with the organism, but the H band is diagnostic of active infection. ELISA has shown promise as a screening test, with greater sensitivity than immunodif-

fusion. Testing for antigenuria and antigenemia is the serologic procedure of choice in immunocompromised patients; the tests are very sensitive for the diagnosis of disseminated disease, and changes in titer in serial specimens appear to be prognostic. Skin testing with the reagent histoplasmin is useful for epidemiologic investigation, but it is not recommended for diagnosis because of the high incidence of skin test positivity in endemic regions and the propensity of a positive response to modulate antibody responses in subsequent tests using mycelium-derived antigens.

Prognosis and Treatment

In immunocompetent patients over the age of 1 1/2 years who are not elderly or otherwise ill, the prognosis in primary infection is excellent without any specific treatment. This is also true in cases of eosinophilic pneumonia caused by *Histoplasma* and histoplasmoma. The prognosis is grave in chronic granulomatous histoplasmosis and in disseminated active infection. Without treatment, almost all such patients die of their disease.

Thus, antibiotic therapy is indicated in these two forms of histoplasmosis. The antibiotic of choice is amphotericin B. The total dose is between 30 and 40 mg/kg of body weight, given as 1.0 mg/kg/dose intravenously. The dose is smaller at first and increased gradually to the maximum. The drug is administered daily in more acutely ill patients and then continued 2 to 3 times per week. There are many side effects, especially retention of urea and creatinine, which is generally completely reversible if the total dose is 45 to 50 mg/kg. Hypokalemia may also develop, as well as mild hematologic abnormalities. The almost uniform chills, fever, and nausea that occur at the time of drug infusion are treated symptomatically but are less troublesome if the daily dose is given within 1 1/2 hours. Liposomal/lipid-complexed drug has been used to avoid side effects. The decreased efficacy of these preparations requires the administration of increased total doses to achieve similar clinical results.

Itraconazole is the one azole antibiotic that has shown significant activity in potentially fatal histoplasmosis. It should be considered as an alternative in patients who cannot tolerate amphotericin B therapy. The dose is 200 to 400 mg/day, and the therapy should be continued for 2 months or more. Use of this drug has been recommended for life to prevent recurrences of active infection in HIV-positive patients. The maintenance dose is 200 mg/day.

Coccidiodomycosis (Figs. 6–9)

Described in South America by the young Posadas and his pathologist teacher Wernicke in 1892, this disease was thought to be exclusively a tropical protozoan disease

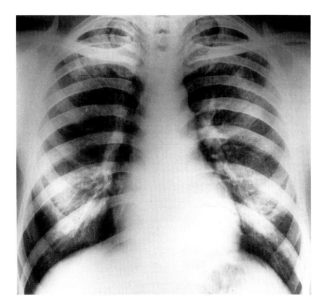

FIG. 6. Acute coccidioidomycosis with bilateral upper lobe infiltrates.

until the work of Dickson and Gifford in the 1930s uncovered a mild pulmonary form of the infection. As with histoplasmosis, natural resistance to the infection is high, but certain ethnic groups appear to have increased susceptibility to the development of active disseminated infection. The clinical spectrum of the disease is broad, and in certain situations curative treatment does not exist.

Organism

C. immitis is another of the dimorphic fungi. It is present in the soil as a mold with septate hyphae that form

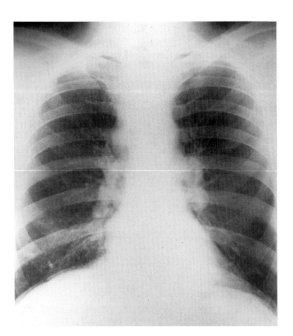

FIG. 7. Acute coccidioidomycosis with bilateral hilar adenopathy.

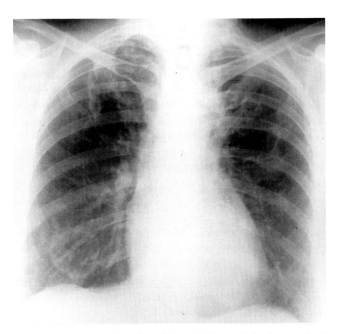

FIG. 8. Thin-walled cavity of the right lower lobe in a patient with chronic coccidioidal infection.

alternating, barrel-shaped arthroconidia. These arthroconidia are easily aerosolized and highly infectious. Following inhalation, the conidia round up and convert into the tissue form, referred to as *spherules*. Spherules are round, thick-walled structures averaging 30 to 60 μm in diameter. When mature, they are filled with 2- to 5-μm endo-

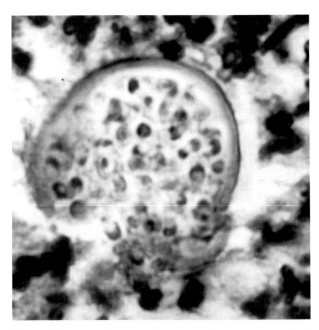

FIG. 9. Spherule of *C. immitis* seen with endospores in tissue section. (Reproduced with permission from Straub M, Schwarz J. Coccidioidomycotic thoracic lesions in dogs in Tucson, Arizona. *Arch Pathol* 1956;62:479. Copyright 1956 by the American Medical Association.)

spores that develop into spherules after being released in the tissue.

Pathology

In most infections, the portal of entry is the lung. After sufficient conidia are inhaled to reach the respiratory tissue, acute inflammation occurs, followed quickly by lymphocyte/macrophage infiltration and the development of a granulomatous process. As in histoplasmosis, caseous necrosis takes place. The lymph system is involved concurrently, with lymphangitis and local lymphadenitis and early dissemination. The pattern is similar to that of other granulomatous infections. The differences are that the degree of scarring and calcification is less than in histoplasmosis, and in a significant fraction of cases the organism clearly remains viable, even if not actively replicating, after the primary infection has healed. This makes subsequent endogenous reinfection a real possibility. Exogenous reinfection has been seen.

In addition to the T lymphocyte/macrophage-associated delayed hypersensitivity response, antibodies of both the IgG and IgM types develop. They may be demonstrated by a variety of techniques, such as complement fixation, immunodiffusion, and latex agglutination. If the cell-mediated immune system fails to react, active dissemination is common. The active role of the antibodies is unknown at present.

Epidemiology

The endemic areas of infection with *C. immitis* are referred to as the *Lower Sonoran Life Zone*, an area encompassing western Texas, New Mexico, Arizona, southern California, and northwestern Mexico. In addition, the disease has been seen in Central America, Venezuela, Colombia, Paraguay, and Argentina. Other regions have been investigated, but the organism has not been found. Support for this localization has come from widespread skin testing programs using spherulin and coccidioidin. A confounding factor has been the increasing number of people who travel.

Because the organism is present in relatively superficial soil layers in its highly infectious mold form, massive exposure may occur during wind storms in endemic areas, especially during dry weather, or when the infected soil is disturbed by digging. Outbreaks have even occurred after the organism was introduced into an air-conditioning system!

Clinical Manifestations

Primary infection with *C. immitis* is usually silent. Occasionally, nonspecific symptoms of a flulike illness may be accompanied by fever, most often in children. On chest x-ray films, a typical primary complex may be seen that includes both peripheral lung infiltrate(s) and accompanying enlarged regional hilar and/or mediastinal lymph nodes. There may be an associated pleurisy with fluid, an event that usually clears spontaneously. This is almost always a self-limited illness, but in certain ethnic groups (nonwhites in general but especially Filipinos) the likelihood of active disseminated disease developing at the time of primary infection is much higher. If dissemination occurs, it is fatal unless treated.

As in histoplasmosis, there may be dramatic occurrences of widespread bronchopneumonia resulting from exposure to high concentrations of fungus in the soil. Many such events have been described, and the associated syndrome, which has been called *desert fever,* is an acute febrile episode with respiratory symptoms that is usually self-limited. It may be associated with erythema nodosum and other allergic skin manifestations as well as migratory arthopathy, known as *desert rheumatism.* All these symptoms may occur with primary coccidioidomycosis, even if not so dramatically. The symptoms spontaneously resolve. The chest x-ray film shows widespread areas of bronchopneumonia that may simulate miliary lung disease. Potentially, this could cause ARDS. The need to treat with antifungal antibiotics is questionable, but in any case careful clinical follow-up is indicated.

Cavitary coccidioidomycosis is seen both as an asymptomatic surprise finding on chest x-ray films or as part of the syndrome of chronic granulomatous disease of the lungs. Although the so-called typical coccidioidal cavity is described as thin-walled, cavities characteristic of any granulomatous disease are the rule rather than the exception. This form of the disease occurs more frequently in adults than in children and has been ascribed to endogenous or exogenous reinfection. In fact, the pathogenesis is not well understood. Whether asymptomatic individuals require treatment is a controversial point, but currently it is felt that antibiotic therapy is indicated. Clinically, a stable cavitary lesion may not progress and appear to represent localized disease. More frequently, there is true progressive disease. In fact, if the so-called stable lesions are followed long enough, clinical and roentgenologic progression is often noted. Complications of a cavity include hemorrhage, pneumothorax, and the development of a fungus ball. Although fungus balls are usually caused by *Aspergillus* species, there have been rare instances of coccidioidal mycetomas. The presence of the mold form of the fungus within a cavity suggests possible person-to-person transmission of the disease, which does not happen in other forms of active coccidioidomycosis.

Other syndromes may occur. Coccidioidomas are seen, often as a direct result of the primary infection. They are often found on a routine x-ray film. Of importance is that within these lesions as well as within cavitary lesions the organism may remain viable for many years. This is in contrast to the rare positive culture from histoplasmomas. Disseminated disease, which may occur as noted above or in immunosuppressed patients, is rapidly progressive and fatal unless treated, and even then the prognosis is guarded. The most dramatic form of disseminated disease is coccidioidal meningitis, which is a chronic and ultimately fatal disease unless treatment is maintained for life!

Diagnosis

Chest x-ray findings in pulmonary coccidioidomycosis are characteristic of the syndrome but not specific. Radiographic features of primary infection include peripheral foci, hilar node enlargement, and occasionally the accumulation of pleural fluid, findings that in no way differ from those associated with a variety of agents, including mycobacteria or other fungi. The same is true for the cavitary form of the disease, except for the suggestive nature of a thin-walled cavity associated with little or no pericavitary infiltrate. This is usually localized to the upper zones. Fluid levels may be seen. When a fungus ball is present, there are no roentgenologic methods to differentiate between the fungi that can cause this entity.

General laboratory findings include leukocytosis, elevated erythrocyte sedimentation rate, and possible mild liver enzyme abnormalities, but in general they are not pathognomonic for this specific infection.

Microbiologic examinations and immunologic testing are critical in diagnosis and prognosis. The large, endosporulating spherules of *C. immitis* are easily visualized in BAL fluid or biopsy tissue specimens with routine hematoxylin and eosin staining or any of the special stains for fungi. Culture of the organism provides definitive diagnosis; the organism grows relatively rapidly, with most cultures becoming positive within 7 to 10 days, often within 48 hours. Confirmation of the identification of cultures is most rapidly made by utilizing the DNA probe hybridization that is commercially available. Serologic diagnosis of coccidioidomycosis is available as a tube precipitin test for early (IgM) response and as a complement fixation test for IgG response. Immunodiffusion screening tests are available that correlate with both the precipitin and complement fixation tests. The titers of complement-fixing antibodies are prognostic. The diagnosis of coccidioidal meningitis is almost always made by the demonstration of complement-fixing antibodies in cerebrospinal fluid; only in highly immunocompromised patients are spherules seen in or organisms grown from cerebrospinal fluid. Two skin-testing reagents are available, coccidioidin and spherulin, for epidemiologic investigations; the latter is a newer reagent of greater sensitivity and specificity.

Prognosis and Treatment

Most cases of primary coccidioidomycosis clear spontaneously and leave minor residua. Calcification of peripheral foci and hilar and mediastinal lymph nodes is much less pronounced than in histoplasmosis. Chronic cavitary disease may persist with no activity for years and then either slowly progress or, if some associated stress to the body occurs, rapidly disseminate. In cases of progressive cavitary or disseminated disease, only extended treatment prevents mortality. Meningitis may persist with many exacerbations and remissions before causing death, and treatment needs to be lifelong for death to be prevented or significantly delayed.

The drug of choice in serious progressive disease is amphotericin B. Treatment needs to be prolonged, and a total dose of about 60 mg/kg is required. This large dose may cause permanent renal damage. Some cases of meningitis have required even larger doses, but such treatment is rarely permanently effective. As an alternative, up to 50 to 60 mg/kg may be given in one prolonged course of 8 to 12 weeks, after which the drug may be given once a year 3 to 5 times during one week in separate doses of 1 mg/kg. This regimen must continue for the life of the patient. In addition, intrathecal amphotericin B is frequently given. There are numerous side effects, and treatment must be continued intermittently for life.

Alternatively, the drug ketoconazole has been used as extended treatment of pulmonary coccidioidomycosis at a dose of 200 mg/d for as much as a year or more in addition to amphotericin B. More recently, both fluconazole and itraconazole have been found effective and show particular promise for the treatment of coccidioidal meningitis. Amphotericin B, however, remains the major drug for treatment of serious, life-threatening disease.

In cases of skin test-negative coccidioidomycosis, treatment was previously given with transfer factor. This substance, the crude extract of polymorphonuclear leukocytes taken from persons with a strongly positive spherulin skin test, seems to increase the body's immune response, but the effect is temporary and repeated injections of the material are required every 4 to 6 weeks. It is not generally used.

There is increasing experience with a vaccine against *C. immitis* infection, and it may be indicated in persons from nonendemic areas who anticipate exposure for significant periods of time or to possibly high concentrations of the organism.

Blastomycosis (Figs. 10–12)

North American blastomycosis was first described by Gilchrist in 1894 as a disseminated skin disease, and it was considered to be mainly an inoculation infection with

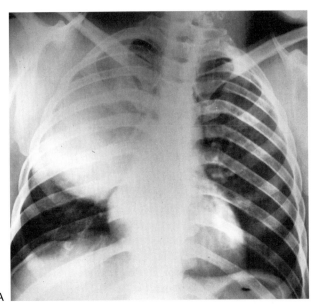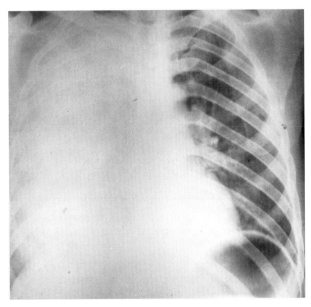

A   B

FIG. 10. A,B: Acute blastomycotic pneumonia with consolidation of most of the right upper lobe.

occasional instances of dissemination to the lungs and the rest of the body. In the early twentieth century, a group of cases was reported from Chicago, which gave the city's name to the disease. In 1951, it was proposed that the primary infection was almost always pulmonary and that skin lesions represented dissemination of the organism. In the late 1940s, the first effective chemotherapeutic agent for blastomycosis, stilbamidine, was reported, soon to be followed by 2-hydroxy-stilbamidine and subsequently amphotericin B.

Organism

B. dermatitidis is the etiologic agent of North American blastomycosis. The septate hyphae of this dimorphic fun-

gus occur transiently in the soil, where they produce small, round to pyriform conidia, the infectious form of the organism. On inhalation, the conidia are transformed into large (8 to 12 μm), thick-walled, budding yeast cells that are characterized by single buds, separated from the mother cell by a wide isthmus.

Pathology

The classic pathology of blastomycotic lesions of the skin is a combination of pseudoepitheliomatous hyperplasia of the epidermis with microabscess formation in the dermis breaking into the epidermis. In the lung, there may be an acute inflammatory response with primarily

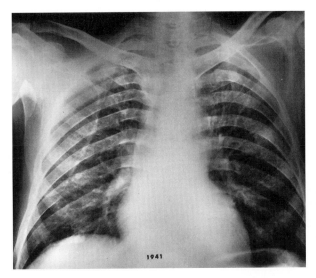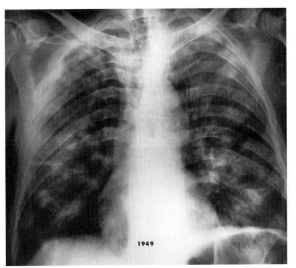

FIG. 11. Chronic pulmonary blastomycosis characterized by linear infiltrates with slow but relentless progression during an 8-year period.

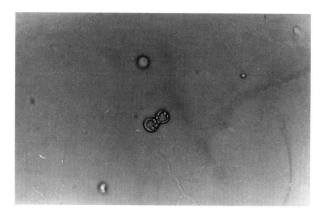

FIG. 12. Yeast-phase *B. dermatitidis* showing characteristic single bud and presenting a "figure 8" appearance.

polymorphonuclear leukocytes and abscess formation. A granulomatous response is seen in blastomycosis, but almost always in combination with a suppurative reaction. Alternate inflammation and scarring are seen in the same areas of involvement in skin, lung, and other organs. All organs in the body may be involved, but the development of pleural lesions is seldom accompanied by fluid formation. Hilar and mediastinal lymph node enlargement can be found, even in the presence of minimal pulmonary parenchymal involvement. This speaks for the primary pulmonary nature of most infections.

Immunopathology has not been well defined, but the development of delayed skin hypersensitivity suggests that the cell-mediated immune system plays a role. This is supported by the combination of suppuration with granulomatous inflammation seen in most cases. Specific antibody formation is not consistent, and the role of this factor is not clear.

Epidemiology

This infection has been mainly localized to North America, cases having been described in Canada as well as the United States and Mexico. Dogs in these areas have been infected, indicating the localization of the fungus in soil. In the latter part of the twentieth century, cases have been described in natives of central Africa.

Although once known as *Chicago disease,* it is now felt that the endemic area of the infection, if indeed one exists, is in Wisconsin. Outbreaks have been described in other areas as well, but in general the infection has been found east of the Mississippi River. Sporadic cases have been found in the southeastern United States especially. The absence of a reliable skin test or other tools useful in widespread testing for symptomless infection has hindered the collection of accurate epidemiologic data.

Ethnic factors do not appear to influence resistance to the infection or its dissemination. Because of the signifi-

cantly higher prevalence of the disease in men than in women, there is a question of some genetic determinant of susceptibility. Immunosuppression from any cause favors more malignant dissemination, but blastomycosis is not a special problem of AIDS patients.

Clinical Manifestations

Few cases of clinically diagnosed primary pulmonary infection have been reported. Most of those appear to have been part of so-called mini-epidemics in which acute bronchopneumonia was seen in association with hilar lymph node enlargement. Isolated cases have been reported and support the presence of a definite hilar lymph node component. These cases have been associated with mild flulike symptoms that clear spontaneously within a week to 10 days. Careful history reveals the critical fact of exposure to *B. dermatitidis.* Only if the possibility of the diagnosis is entertained will the critical diagnostic tests be carried out.

ARDS has been described in 10 patients with blastomycotic pneumonia. It was not clear whether these cases were primary infections, but the clinical picture was one of severe acute pneumonia. No underlying immunosuppression was found in any of the patients. Mortality was high despite amphotericin treatment.

Healed primary infection may be encountered, usually on a chest radiograph taken for other reasons. The pulmonary parenchymal and hilar elements of the primary complex are identifiable on x-ray films in such cases, but in contrast to healed primary histoplasmosis, the scarring rarely causes mechanical problems of mediastinal structures. Solitary pulmonary nodules have been described as being caused by *B. dermatitidis,* and almost certainly these are remnants of healed primary pulmonary parenchymal blastomycosis.

Disseminated blastomycosis may present clinically with isolated, chronic skin lesions that exhibit peripheral extension and central scarring, resemble basal cell or even squamous cell carcinomata of the skin, and are associated with peculiarly characteristic microabscesses, typically at the periphery of lesion. This appearance should alert the physician to the possibility of blastomycosis. Patients may present with chronic cough, production of mucopurulent sputum, weight loss, low-grade fever, and many of the symptoms associated with chronic granulomatous disease of any etiology. Chest x-ray findings are nonspecific but indicate a destructive inflammatory process of the lungs. Involvement of the pleurae may occur but is rarely associated with pleural effusion. Lesions may be found in any organ system but rarely in the gastrointestinal tract. The urinary tract in men and women is a common site. Blastomycotic prostatic abscesses have been seen as a cause of urinary obstruction. Occasionally chronic widely disseminated disease is enountered, and such patients are clearly cachectic.

Acute blastomycotic pneumonia has been described in immunosuppressed patients; the only distinguishing characteristic is the presence of the organism in secretions obtained from the tracheobronchial tree or lungs. The clinical picture is that of an acute lower respiratory tract infection modified by the immune suppression of the patient.

Diagnosis

The chest x-ray film in primary pulmonary blastomycosis may show poorly defined infiltrates associated with lymph node enlargement in the hilar/mediastinal areas, or there may be few findings in the pulmonary parenchyma, with nodal enlargement as the only finding. Rarely, bilateral hilar node enlargement may be seen, suggesting the diagnosis of sarcoidosis. In progressive chronic pulmonary disease, most frequently associated with dissemination, typical changes of chronic granulomatous inflammatory disease with cavitation may be seen. There is nothing to distinguish these changes from those caused by *M. tuberculosis* or other fungi.

Results of general laboratory tests add little other than to confirm the debilitating nature of the chronic disseminated infection. Involvement of liver and kidneys may be expressed by abnormalities of function studies.

The diagnosis of blastomycosis is made by the demonstration of the typical, thick-walled, single-budding yeast in sputum, BAL fluid, or tissue. The organism is easily visualized using any of the special stains for fungi. Definitive identification depends on culture of the organism, and confirmation of the morphologic identification may be made by DNA hybridization with the colonies. The organism often requires 7 to 14 days or longer to grow in culture. Serologic testing for blastomycosis rarely is useful. The immunodiffusion test for antigen A is specific but lacks sensitivity. Recent work with an ELISA to detect antibody to an antigen termed *WI-1* shows promise.

Prognosis and Treatment

Based on experience, particularly with epidemics of blastomycosis, prognosis is excellent for spontaneous remission of primary infections in immunocompetent persons. In cases of progressive disease, mortality is high unless the patient is treated with specific antibiotics. Skin lesions tend to recur even after local therapy has been apparently effective. As noted, the mortality in ARDS, even with treatment, is high.

Amphotericin B given intravenously is effective in all types of cases. The total dose is between 20 to 40 mg/kg given as single doses of 1 mg/kg. Therapy is given daily for acutely ill patients, then 2 to 3 times per week according to the clinical situation. Itraconazole (200 to 400 mg/d) may be used as an alternative to amphotericin B in patients not judged to be critically ill.

Paracoccidioidomycosis (South American Blastomycosis)

This disease was first described by Adolfo Lutz in 1908 and has been identified in areas localized to Central and South America. At first thought to be acquired by extrinsic inoculation into the skin and/or mucosae, it is now recognized to be a primary pulmonary infection in almost all cases. Just how common the asymptomatic infection is has not been clarified, but almost certainly the number of active cases seen represents a small fraction of persons infected with *P. brasiliensis*.

Organism

The dimorphic fungus *P. brasiliensis* is found in the soil as a mold with septate hyphae that produce small, round to pyriform conidia, resembling those of *B. dermatitidis*. The yeast cells of *P. brasiliensis* are extremely variable in size, with an average of 10 to 20 μm and a range of 2 to 30 μm. The yeast cells are characterized by multiple buds separated from the mother cell by a narrow isthmus. A specialized form of the budding cells, called a *mariner's wheel*, features a large, 20- to 30- μm mother cell surrounded by many 2- to 3-μm daughter cells.

Pathology

Grossly, the pathology of this infection is most obvious on skin and mucosal surfaces. The cutaneous lesions seen resemble those of blastomycosis and leishmaniasis. Tumorlike growths of granulomatous tissue frequently involve the gastrointestinal tract, as opposed to the lesions of blastomycosis, which are rarely seen in this area. Areas of localized inflammation may be seen in the lungs; interstitial thickening is found in disseminated disease, and cavities may form. This infection involves the lymph system particularly, and nodes are enlarged and necrotic in all areas of the body, but especially in the mediastinum and hilar areas, when the infection is widespread. Histopathology is characterized by the combination of granulomatous inflammation and suppuration, a similarity with blastomycosis. This is noted in all organs involved.

The presence of delayed hypersensitivity skin reactions and the above noted histopathology suggest that the cellular immune system is an important but not the only element in natural resistance to *P. brasiliensis*. There is little information relating to the impact of AIDS or other causes of immune suppression on this infection.

Epidemiology

Paracoccidioidomycosis is encountered almost exclusively in Central and South America but is not seen in areas of rain forest or desert. Up to a few years ago, no cases had been reported from Chile, Guyana, Surinam, or Nicaragua. Southern Brazil is the area of highest prevalence. The definition of the areas in which the organism is found includes elevation of 500 to 1800 m, 800 to 2000 mm annual rainfall, average yearly temperature of 18° to 23°C, and acid soil.

A skin test has been used to identify endemic areas, and to the extent that it has been used the results correlate with the distribution of active cases and with the area defined above.

Clinical Manifestations

This disease is seen mainly in male patients, the estimate being about 90%. Skin test surveys, however, demonstrate a 50:50 relationship between men and women infected with the organism. This is a rare disease in persons under the age of 10 years but may occur in a fulminant form in childhood.

Generally, the disease presents with mucocutaneous lesions, especially in the oropharynx and gingivae, and also in the gastrointestinal tract. The port of entry is the respiratory tract, the extrapulmonary lesions being metastatic, as in blastomycosis.

Pulmonary disease may be localized to the lung parenchyma and the hilar and mediastinal lymph nodes or be part of progressive disseminated disease. The acute limited disease is manifested by nonspecific symptoms and x-ray findings of multiple foci of infiltrates in both lungs. These may recede spontaneously and the enlarged nodes calcify. The primary infection may occur without symptoms. Minimal parenchymal fibrosis occurs as a residual. Immune factors that determine the outcome of this disease have not been well defined.

A chronic progressive form of the disease seen in adults resembles tuberculosis in all its manifestations. Without effective treatment, it leads to cachexia and death. Cavities are seen in the lungs in only 15% of such cases. Often, extrapulmonary lesions involve the pleurae and all extrathoracic organs.

Diagnosis

A history of residence in the endemic area is the most important diagnostic finding. As the clinical manifestations are nonspecific, awareness of the possibility of this disease is an indication for appropriate diagnostic tests.

Chest x-ray films demonstrate parenchymal infiltrates and hilar node enlargement if the infection is primary. In chronic progressive pulmonary disease, the findings are similar to those of tuberculosis, histoplasmosis, and coccidioidomycosis. Cavities are seen in only 15% of such patients. Geographic prevenience of the patient determines the likelihood of this disease.

Laboratory diagnosis of paracoccidioidomycosis is based on demonstration of the characteristic multiple budding yeast form in respiratory secretions or tissue. The organisms stain readily with any of the special stains for fungi. Confirmation by culture requires patience, as *P. brasiliensis* is one of the most slowly growing of the dimorphic fungi, usually requiring 3 to 6 weeks of incubation. Identification is based on the morphology of the organism and confirmed by in vitro conversion to the yeast forms or an immunologic procedure referred to as the *exoantigen test*. The serologic tests that show the most promise for the diagnosis of paracoccidioidomycosis are the immunodiffusion test for band 1 and an ELISA directed at antigen E2.

Prognosis and Treatment

Most cases of primary pulmonary infection clear spontaneously. Acute pulmonary infection, primary or not, in adults up to about 60 years of age also tends to clear, but chronic pulmonary disease is progressive and fatal unless treated. Disseminated disease, including lesions on skin and mucosae, is progressive and requires treatment; otherwise it progresses, albeit slowly, to a fatal end.

Treatment with sulfadiazine is effective. Other antibiotics have been used also, but sulfadiazine is still considered the drug of choice. Treatment must continue for up to a year at a dosage of 4.0 g/d. Amphotericin B is also effective and used in disseminated cases. The dosage is the same as for chronic histoplasmosis, up to 2 to 3 g per total dose. Ketoconazole has been found effective at a dosage of 200 mg/d for at least 1 year.

Sporotrichosis (Fig. 13)

This disease is much better known as a skin disease than as a pulmonary disease, as the majority of cases have localized skin ulcerations and the route of infection is by direct inoculation. The organism was discovered by a medical student, Schenck, in 1898, and the pulmonary form of the infection was recognized much later. Animal infection was noted for the first time in 1907 in Brazil, and since then the presence of the organism in soil has been demonstrated repeatedly.

Organism

S. schenckii is another of the dimorphic fungi. The mold form of the organism features delicate septate hyphae bearing pyriform conidia arranged like petals on a

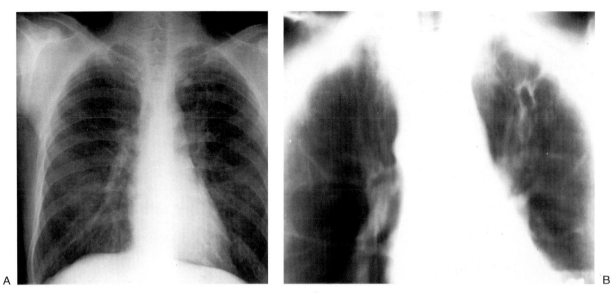

FIG. 13. A: Cavity of the left upper lobe in a young adult with pulmonary sporotrichosis. **B:** Linear tomogram of the cavity. Diagnosis was proved by sputum cultures and by culture of material from resected cavity.

daisy. The yeast cells are small (2 to 5 μm), round to cigar-shaped cells that are difficult to visualize in tissue.

Pathology

Skin lesions appear grossly as induration with or without ulceration, and usually they occur in line with the associated lymphatic channels. Histologically, granulomas and suppuration are seen along with dystrophic changes of the skin that resemble carcinoma. Organisms are rarely demonstrated in tissues, even with the use of special stains.

The lung shows nodular lesions that are occasionally plaquelike and tend to occur in the upper lobes more than in other areas of the lung. Cavities are frequently seen and often are thin-walled. Necrotic lining of the cavities is the best place to look for organisms. Histologically, the lesions are similar to the skin lesions in that both granulomas and purulent exudate are present. The cavities are usually limited by scar tissue, which is also found in the areas of noncavitary pulmonary lesions.

Epidemiology

The organism is found worldwide in soil and on the leaves of a variety of plants. In particular, rose and burberry bushes host the fungus, and it is also found on hedge bark, reeds, potting soil, sphagnum moss, grasses, and tree bark. It has been isolated from timbers used to shore up a mine in South Africa, and this source infected more than 3000 miners in the largest outbreak of the skin dis-

ease that has been reported. The skin disease is an occupational risk for gardeners and soil workers.

The distribution of pulmonary cases is sporadic and probably more related to the interest and diagnostic capability of the involved physicians than to the distribution of the fungus! There is no diagnostic skin test to identify asymptomatic infected persons.

Clinical Manifestations

The disease is best known as a skin problem. The distribution of the lesions tends to follow the lymphatic channels, but lymph nodes are involved infrequently.

Pulmonary sporotrichosis appears to be a separate form of the disease, in which the primary encounter with the fungus is through inhalation. Little is known about early events. The patients usually have cough, sputum production, rarely hemoptysis, and occasionally weight loss and weakness, depending on how long they have been ill. There is nothing to differentiate this chronic lung infection from tuberculosis, histoplasmosis, or coccidioidomycosis.

Dissemination is a rare event and is usually associated with immunosuppression. Lesions may appear in any organs and clinically resemble disseminated infection caused by any fungal organism.

Diagnosis

The history of occupational exposure to potential sources of the fungus may be diagnostically important in evaluating the skin lesions, but not in pulmonary sporotrichosis.

Chest x-ray films reveal localized infiltrates, usually in the upper lobes and often associated with cavities, possibly thin-walled. There may be pericavitary spread of the infection. Findings are nonspecific.

In the laboratory, the organism is readily isolated when cultures are held for at least 2 weeks. The morphologic identification of the mold form is confirmed by in vitro conversion of the organism to its yeast form. The organisms are difficult to see in tissue, even when special stains for fungi are used. Although a number of serologic tests for sporotrichosis have been proposed, none is widely used or commercially available.

Prognosis and Treatment

The skin lesions of sporotrichosis progress slowly but inexorably. Dissemination is rare, as is spontaneous cure of the lesions. The pulmonary lesions progress slowly, and all the reported cases have improved only after treatment.

Iodides are the treatment of choice for skin lesions. Why this very old treatment works is a mystery. It is not because of a direct effect on the fungus. Usually, a saturated solution of potassium iodide is used and continued until all lesions have healed. As a matter of interest, this is the only fungal disease in which iodides are effective, although they have been used in the treatment of all.

Pulmonary sporotrichosis is unaffected by iodides; amphotericin B is required for effective treatment. The exact dose is unknown, but if a total of 1 to 2 g is given according to the usual dosage schedule, results are excellent, with disappearance of pulmonary lesions, conversion of sputum to negative, and clinical improvement. Occasionally, surgery may be necessary to eradicate large cavities.

Itraconazole, which has been successfully used for cutaneous sporotrichosis, has been shown to control systemic disease at a dosage of 600 mg/d for a few weeks and then 400 mg/d for up to a year in patients unable to tolerate amphotericin B.

Cryptococcosis (Fig. 14)

This yeast infection was first described in 1894 by Busse and later by Buschke in a patient with involvement of the tibia. Early on, the organism was considered to be a cause of lymphoma, as it was found as a coexisting infection is such patients. A variety of names was given to the organism, but finally it was recognized as a member of a separate genus and the confusion with *B. dermatitidis* was resolved. The major clinical form of the infection, the one most feared because of its high mortality, is men-

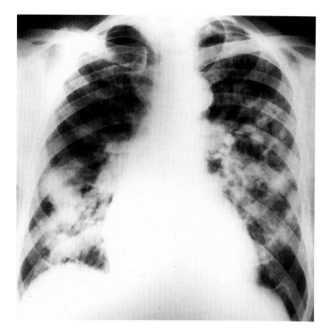

FIG. 14. Chronic pulmonary cryptococcosis in a 66-year-old man with multiple nodular lesions simulating metastatic carcinoma.

ingitis, and to this day the differential diagnosis between cryptococcal and tuberculous meningitis is a challenging one.

Organism

C. neoformans varieties *neoformans* and *gattii* occur as budding yeast cells (2 to 10 μm) with distinctive polysaccharide capsules. The two varieties correspond to the serotypes A/D and B/C, respectively. The yeast cells of variety *neoformans* are typically rounder, whereas those of variety *gattii* tend to be more oval to lemon-shaped. Infrequent isolates of *C. neoformans* have been reported that demonstrate the presence of hyphae in tissue or culture; these are now believed to be the result of failure of haploidization during the sexual reproductive cycle.

Pathology

In humans, this organism may be found in any organ system. Entrance to the body, however, is almost certainly through the respiratory tract. Desiccation of the organism in pigeon fecal material allows for aerosolization of particles of appropriate size to be inhaled and transported to the respiratory areas of the lungs and there cause the initial infection. Dissemination from such primary foci occurs regularly, with special tropism to the central nervous system.

The tissue response to the organism is quite varied, ranging from acute suppuration to practically no response at all. Lesions may display a variety of inflammatory components, including granuloma formation and proliferation of scar tissue. In some cases, significant accumulations of organisms are found with almost no tissue reaction whatsoever. Grossly, such lesions, especially in the skin, look like blisters full of mucus that on microscopic examination demonstrate countless organisms, with the mucinous capsule being responsible for the gross appearance.

The special relationship between infection with *C. neoformans* and immunosuppression, either from lymphomatous disease, AIDS, or immunosuppressive therapy, demonstrates a varied pathology microscopically. There may be a severe, acute, purulent inflammatory response when cell-mediated immunity is suppressed, as in AIDS; there may be granuloma formation (if the T lymphocytes are functional) in lymphomatous disease, or there may be little cellular response in cases in which the immune system has been overwhelmed. Combinations of the above may be seen in a single patient. The clear lack of a granulomatous reaction in patients with AIDS reflects the basic immune pathology of AIDS.

Epidemiology

Infection with *C. neoformans* occurs worldwide, although the occurrence of the various serotypes of the yeast is area-related. Variety *neoformans* is found in Austria, Belgium, Denmark, France, Holland, Switzerland, Italy, and Japan as well as Argentina, Canada, the United Kingdom, and the United States. Variety *gattii* is found in Australia, California, Brazil, Cambodia, Hawaii, Mexico, Paraguay, Thailand, Vietnam, Nepal, and central Africa. The factor that seems to determine the presence of human infection by variety *neoformans* is contamination of the environment by pigeon feces. Variety *gattii* is found in association with the red gum eucalyptus tree.

From early in the history of this infection, clinical disease has been related to the presence of lymphomatous disease, especially Hodgkin's disease. The disease was also described in patients receiving immunosuppressive therapy. Since the early 1980s, cryptococcosis has been identified as the most common life-threatening fungal infection of AIDS patients.

Clinical Manifestations

The most dramatic clinical presentation of cryptococcosis is meningitis, which is very similar in character to tuberculous meningitis. The course is usually protracted in the immunocompetent patient but may be fulminant in the immunosuppressed patient.

Pulmonary cryptococcosis is most frequently encountered as asymptomatic single or multiple pulmonary nodules found by routine chest x-ray examination. The diag-

nosis is most often made in these situations by the histology of the resected lesion.

Acute progressive pneumonia may occur, with symptoms of cough, sputum production, fever, and weakness. The clinical picture is not pathognomonic. The progression to abscess formation is more common than in pneumonias caused by bacteria and viruses. Failure of the patient to respond to routine treatment should lead to a search for the causal fungus.

Rapidly progressive infection is most frequently encountered in the immunosuppressed host, especially the AIDS patient. There is often widespread dissemination with involvement of extrathoracic organs. A unique form of the infection consists of multiple superficial mucosal ulcers in the airways, visible on fiberoptic bronchoscopy.

Pleural involvement may occur in all types of pulmonary cryptococcosis, and the resulting pleural exudate is an excellent source for obtaining a culture of the organism. Chronic pleuritis has not been described.

Diagnosis

In the most common clinical presentation of pulmonary cryptococcosis, chest radiography demonstrates single or multiple nodules, well defined and rarely calcified. These may occur in any location. There is nothing to distinguish these nodules from those caused by other fungi, tuberculosis, or tumor. Frequently, only histology is diagnostic. In acute respiratory infection, there may be infiltrates that resemble those of any acute bronchopneumonia. Cavitation may appear, resembling lung abscess. When the lungs are involved as part of a progressive dissemination, there may be multiple foci of infiltration and involvement of lymph nodes in the mediastinum. In all forms of cryptococcosis, CT adds to the exactness of the anatomic diagnosis but not the specificity. It also may reveal enlargement of mediastinal lymph nodes not seen on regular chest x-ray films.

General laboratory findings in all the above presentations are nonspecific and may indicate an underlying lymphomatous process or suggest AIDS. In the asymptomatic syndromes, usually no abnormalities are present.

The diagnostic findings come from the microbiology and pathology laboratories. Culture of bronchoalveolar fluid, cerebrospinal fluid, blood by lysis centrifugation, or tissue readily yields the organism, usually after 24 to 72 hours of incubation. Presumptive identification of *C. neoformans* is obtained within 24 hours by testing for the presence of the enzyme phenoloxidase in any urease-positive yeasts. Although a DNA probe for colony hybridization is commercially available, the sensitivity and specificity of the tests for phenoloxidase render it a less cost-effective procedure than its counterparts for the dimorphic fungi. Confirmation then depends on traditional biochemical testing, using any of the numerous commercially available systems. Rapid diagnosis of *C. neoformans* may also be obtained by the finding of soluble cryptococcal polysaccharide antigen in cerebrospinal fluid or serum, using either a latex agglutination test or an ELISA. Testing of BAL fluid has shown some promise but has a high false-positive rate. Finally, cryptococci are easily visualized in clinical specimens. The India ink preparation is positive in 50%–75% of cerebrospinal fluid specimens from patients with cryptococcal meningitis. The yeasts are stained well by any of the special stains for fungi; cryptococci may be presumptively identified by the intense staining of their polysaccharide capsules by the mucicarmine stain.

Prognosis and Treatment

Asymptomatic pulmonary cryptococcosis appears to be of little threat to an immunocompetent person. This is said with some hesitation, because prolonged follow-up of a significant number of patients in whom the diagnosis was established by resection of a nodule, even a single one, revealed active cryptococcosis in other locations—either the lung or extrathoracic organs, including the meninges—in almost 20% of a total of 60 patients. This included meningitis in almost 10% of them! Thus, the prognosis must be guarded.

In disseminated disease, the outcome is death, but this may not occur until after a long course. If immunosuppression is present, especially if caused by AIDS, the prognosis is for relatively rapid progression to death. All this is without treatment. Of special concern is cryptococcal meningitis. In the days before effective treatment, it was known that exacerbations and remissions could occur spontaneously. This gave rise to stories of spontaneous cures, which merely represented premature conclusions being drawn about remissions in a uniformly fatal disease.

Treatment is now indicated for all cases given a diagnosis of cryptococcosis, even if the diagnosis has been made by resection of a solitary, asymptomatic pulmonary nodule. In the case of an immunocompetent patient with an asymptomatic nodule, the treatment is 2 to 400 mg of fluconazole per day for a minimum of 6 weeks. The basic regimen used for meningitis is applicable to all other cases of pulmonary cryptococcosis. This includes amphotericin B given intravenously at a dose of 0.3 to 0.5 mg/kg per day to a total of 15.0 mg/kg. Initially, treatment is given daily, but if the patient is not seriously ill, this can be quickly reduced to three times per week. Accompanying treatment may be given with 5-fluorocytosine at a dosage of 150 mg/kg daily in four divided doses for a total of 6 weeks. This treatment is 80% effective in meningitis in immunocompetent patients and even more so in pulmonary disease. In immunosuppressed patients, maintenance therapy is required, and this may take the form of 30 mg of amphotericin B every 2 weeks in one intravenous dose.

This continues for a year or two, and in the experience of several observers, it is effective on condition that response to the active treatment has been good. In addition to this treatment, it is possible to administer amphotericin B intrathecally in patients with meningitis. The side effects of amphotericin B include decreased clearance of urea and creatinine, anemia, fever, electrolyte abnormalities, and nausea. All these clear when treatment is stopped and can be reduced by giving premedication with antihistamines and antipyretics and by limiting the infusion to no more than 1 1/2 hours. 5-Fluorocytosine is cleared by the kidneys and causes very few side effects. If renal function is already restricted, the amount of 5-fluorocytosine administered each day is reduced in relation to the creatinine clearance.

Liposomes have been used to deliver amphotericin B, but it is necessary to increase the dose to achieve adequate coverage. As of this writing, liposomal treatment is not generally accepted.

Fluconazole is now an accepted treatment alternative, especially for maintenance therapy after completion of amphotericin B treatment of the acute disease. Itraconazole shows promise but is not yet recommended. Two hundred milligrams of either drug daily is continued for a year or more and is well accepted by the patients.

Dosages of fluconazole as high as 800 to 1200 mg/d have been used in the treatment of immunosuppressed patients. The success rate is considerably less than the 80%–90% seen in immunocompetent patients, but it is still significant and worth pursuing. In immunosuppressed patients, maintenance therapy is of critical significance, as the primary treatment is not totally fungicidal and the possibility of a relapse is very high.

Candidiasis

In 1839, the German surgeon Langenbeck described *Candida* in mucosal lesions in a patient with typhus. Actually, the clinical manifestations of candidiasis had been described by both Hippocrates and Galen some 2000 years before. Because the orifices of the body, where the organism normally is found, are readily accessible, *Candida* has been accused of causing many diseases, but as our sophistication has grown it has become clear that even though the surface of the body may suffer insults by *Candida*, the internal organs are extremely well protected by an intact immune system. When the internal milieu of the body is upset by antibiotics, steroids, or other factors, then the normally diminutive organism overgrows and clinical problems ensue.

Organism

Candidiasis is caused by numerous species of *Candida*; the most common include *C. albicans, C. tropicalis, C.*

parapsilosis, C. krusei, and *C. (Torulopsis) glabrata.* All species of *Candida* form round to oval budding yeast cells in the size range of 3 to 7 μm. In addition, the first four species listed also form pseudohyphae (elongated yeast cells attached like strings of sausages) in tissue.

Pathology

The normal presence of the yeast *Candida* on mucosal surfaces of healthy persons does not provoke any reaction. When skin surfaces become macerated by moisture or when disease or antibiotic or steroid treatment upsets the ecologic balance of mucosal surfaces, an acute and subacute inflammatory reaction occurs that leads to local irritation. Microscopically, the inflammatory reaction is neutrophilic and lymphocytic. The same basic pathology is found in the esophagus and throat when the infestation progresses to the clinical syndrome of thrush and esophagitis, but a pseudomembrane is added consisting of fungal elements, cell detritus, and fibrin.

Lung involvement almost always occurs in the presence of immunosuppression or cachexia. There may be multiple foci of neutrophilic inflammation with necrosis that may evolve into abscesses. In severely weakened patients, little inflammatory response may be associated with the large collections of yeast cells in lung tissue. Extrathoracic organ tissues are often involved by a similar process, especially the renal cortices. Demonstration of the yeast cells or pseudohyphae of *Candida* is easily done with regular tissue stains or the special fungal stains.

Special consideration must be given to the possibility of *Candida* pneumonia occurring in otherwise normal hosts. *Candida* may undoubtedly gain entrance to pulmonary tissue via contaminated intravenous needles or tubing, and in such situations blood cultures may well be positive for the yeast. It is highly unlikely, however, that the presence of organisms in the lungs on this basis alone is a threat to an otherwise normal person. The body has excellent defenses against this infection, probably because the organism is normally present on body surfaces. Serum from normal persons inhibits growth of *Candida* in culture. The organisms are subjected to efficient phagocytosis and killing by neutrophils, T lymphocytes and macrophages recognize *Candida* yeast cells, and at least three clones of antibodies are found in serum—IgA, IgM, and IgG. Thus, adequate means are available to control the organism. Entrance of *Candida* to the lungs via aspiration of mouth or nose contents may occur in normal persons, but this is probably quite rare. If it does happen, the same efficient defense takes over, so that finding *Candida* in sputum collected from normal persons almost certainly represents a mouth contaminant of the specimen and not active *Candida* infection of the lungs or airways.

One other expression of altered immune responsiveness is the occurrence of chronic mucocutaneous candidiasis, which is characterized by granulomatous lesions on the skin. This pathologic entity, often associated with various endocrine deficiencies in children, has not been described in the lung.

Epidemiology

The occurrence of systemic candidiasis and candidiasis of the lung as a unique entity is related primarily to immunosuppression and neutropenia. Other factors are associated with a higher incidence of systemic candidal disease are prematurity of infants, chronic cachexia, immunosuppressive therapy for any cause, and long-term steroid therapy. Interestingly, although local candidal involvement of the mouth and esophagus is associated with AIDS, true systemic candidiasis is almost never seen.

Clinical Manifestations

Pulmonary candidiasis occurs for all practical purposes only in immunosuppressed patients, and the only open question is whether the disease is part of a generalized systemic candidiasis. The patients are almost always acutely ill and clearly seriously weakened by their underlying conditions. There may be spiking fever, or in the case of a prolonged underlying illness, the fever may be low-grade. The entire clinical picture is one of overall deterioration. In the most confusing situation, a patient has multiple foci of bronchopneumonia and is unresponsive to antibiotic therapy, and *Candida* is found in the sputum. Even more compelling is the concurrent finding of *Candida* in a blood culture. Clinical judgment is difficult, but careful evaluation of all relevant factors in the case, such as the presence of a long-standing intravenous line or chronic ulcerative skin lesions (foci for dissemination of *Candida*) and the underlying status of the immune system, usually leads to a correct assessment of the need to treat.

Of special concern are patients undergoing bone marrow transplantation. These patients are almost completely depleted immunologically and are extremely susceptible to all types of infections. *Candida* is a significant threat in this situation. It is recommended that preventive therapy be given.

If pulmonary and/or generalized candidiasis has been diagnosed, the clinical situation is grave and treatment is urgently indicated.

If an immunocompetent patient presents with a pneumonia that does not respond to the usual treatment and *Candida* is found in sputum, it is unlikely that the presence of *Candida* is significant.

Diagnosis

The most helpful diagnostic tool is awareness of the overall clinical situation of the patient, especially the immune status, and of whether systemic candidiasis is a likely possibility.

Chest x-ray films demonstrate single or multiple foci of bronchopneumonia, in which radiolucencies often develop. This is a highly suggestive finding, but not specific.

The general laboratory findings are a reflection of the overall clinical situation and not diagnostic.

Specific diagnosis of pulmonary candidiasis depends on the demonstration of yeasts and pseudohyphae consistent with *Candida* in tissue, and the diagnosis is confirmed by the subsequent isolation and identification of the organism from the specimen. Because *Candida* is found as a commensal and a colonizer of mucosal surfaces, identification of the organism from sputum or BAL fluid may be suggestive, but mucosal contamination should always be suspected. The organism is easily cultured from blood, tissue, or respiratory tract specimens; identification depends on demonstration of defined morphologic and biochemical properties. Serologic tests for antibody to *Candida,* such as the immunodiffusion test, lack sensitivity and specificity because of the high prevalence of antibodies in the normal population. Tests for circulating antigen, either mannan or enolase, show promise, but the first generation of commercially available antigen assays has been disappointing.

Prognosis and Treatment

Untreated pulmonary or systemic candidiasis is fatal. In an immunocompetent patient with a positive blood culture resulting from a long-standing intravenous needle or cannula that has become contaminated, the prognosis is excellent if the offending needle or cannula is promptly removed. No other treatment is necessary. Otherwise, serious disease is a possibility, although not a certainty.

Amphotericin B is the treatment for life-threatening candidiasis. The total dose in adults is 15 to 20 mg/kg administered daily (at first) and then three times weekly in intravenous infusions of 0.75 to 1.0 mg/kg per dose. Premedication with antihistamine and antipyretic medication is indicated, and the instillation of 50 mg of hydrocortisone in the infusion helps to minimize side effects. Also, the administration of the entire infusion in 1 1/2 hours is advisable. Almost all species of *Candida* are sensitive to amphotericin B, so that resistance is not a problem. Most cases respond to this treatment. If the immunosuppression that so often underlies the problem can be dealt with, the prognosis is improved. The prognosis is not good for cachectic patients who are deteriorating progressively, even with treatment. In cases of bone marrow transplantation, this treatment should be effective.

Use of the imidazoles and triazoles in life-threatening situations is not recommended at this time. These drugs are effective in various forms of skin and mucosal candidiasis and are indicated as prophylaxis in patients undergoing bone marrow transplantation, but they are not effective in life-threatening candidiasis. Fluconazole has been shown to have the same efficacy in treating candidemia in patients who are not neutropenic as amphotericin B. For preventive therapy, fluconazole is the preferred drug; the dose is 200 mg/d and should be continued until all signs of immunosuppression have disappeared.

Aspergillosis (Fig. 15)

Aspergillus species have been observed in nature for several hundred years. The name *Aspergillus* is based on the similarity of the spore head of the fungus, first noted by Micheli in 1792, to an aspergillum, the instrument used for sprinkling holy water on supplicants. The fungus was found to cause disease in jays by Mayer and Emmert in 1815 and was suspected as the cause of human disease later in the nineteenth century. The spectrum of disease caused by this fungus became clear only in the middle of the twentieth century.

Organism

Invasive aspergillosis is caused most frequently by *A. fumigatus* and *A. flavus. A. niger* is often the cause of aspergilloma. Allergic bronchopulmonary aspergillosis (ABPA) is almost always caused by hypersensitivity to *A. fumigatus.* The two species causing invasive disease are heat-tolerant organisms. All species form septate hyphae in tissue; in culture and in nature, millions of conidia, the infectious propagules, are formed on aspergillum-shaped heads produced by the hyphae.

Pathology

The presence of the fungus on the intact skin produces no reaction, and even if there are breaks, there is almost

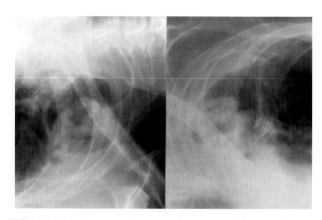

FIG. 15. Cavity in a 68-year-old man containing a fungus ball caused by organisms of a species of *Aspergillus.* Two positions show movement of the ball with change in position of the downward side of the patient.

never any inflammatory reaction. On mucous surfaces, the fungus may induce an immediate allergic reaction in persons previously sensitized. The presence of specific IgE seems to be the mediator of the reaction, which is similar to immediate hypersensitivity caused by any allergen. In the airways, there may be an immune response in sensitive individuals that is mediated by IgM and especially IgG antibodies. An acute inflammatory reaction characterized mainly by lymphocytic exudate, edema, and local vasodilation occurs in response to the presence of antigen-antibody complexes lodged in the mucosa at the site of the *Aspergillus* residence. This in turn may result in necrosis locally in the airway, with the development of local bronchiectasis. If the individual colonized with the fungus is allergic, the resulting exudation is characterized by the presence of eosinophils and neutrophils and the hypersecretion of mucus. In such cases, mucous plugs containing inflammatory cells and often hyphae may obstruct airways. The presence of hyperreactive airways and asthma may be suggested pathologically by hypertrophy and hyperplasia of smooth-muscle cells in the bronchial wall.

In the pulmonary parenchyma, *Aspergillus* is seen in at least three circumstances. In the case of hypersensitivity, as described above, in which the lymphocytic infiltrate predominates in the bronchial wall, similar infiltrates may be seen in the pulmonary parenchyma, characterized also by the presence of macrophages and generally similar to those of typical hypersensitivity pneumonitis.

Disseminated aspergillosis may occur in immunosuppressed patients, especially those with leukopenia (granulocytic leukemia, either in an aleukemic phase or being treated with chemotherapy) who are cachectic. This is characterized by widespread dissemination of the fungus in the body, especially in the lung. The pulmonary lesions may demonstrate a lymphocyte/macrophage exudate with few neutrophils associated with necrosis, or in an overwhelmed patient, there may be almost no cellular reaction whatsoever. The fungi may be demonstrated easily by all stains. Similar pathologic changes may occur in all other organs.

It is not clear whether progressive, necrotizing aspergillosis of the lung can occur in patients who are not immunosuppressed. Cases have been reported with localized, acute inflammatory lesions in the lung, suppurative and necrotic in nature, in patients with no obvious underlying disease. This is rare.

In pre-existing cavities with an underlying cause that is usually not active, *Aspergillus* may enter and grow rapidly. The abundance of nutrients in the cavity and the narrow bronchial exit lead to the development of an aspergilloma (fungus ball). Little or no pericavitary invasion by the fungus is seen, but there may be an intense inflammatory reaction caused by the presence of antigen–anti-*Aspergillus* antibody complexes in the wall of the cavity, with associated dilatation of the blood vessels sup-

plying the cavity. As these usually come from the high-pressure bronchial circulation, bleeding into the cavity occurs and may be identified histologically.

Epidemiology

The presence of *Aspergillus* in the environment is the primary factor in determining where various forms of aspergillosis will be encountered. The fungus occurs more frequently in temperate areas of the world, especially if the annual rainfall is more than 25 in (650 mm). The prevalence of the fungus in the air in any given area is relevant in that it increases or reduces the likelihood of contamination of sputum cultures.

Clinical Manifestations

Disseminated aspergillosis is a ravaging disease, seen especially in neutropenic patients and cachectic patients who have leukopenia. Patients with abnormalities of other branches of the immune system seem less prone to the infection. With the advent of treatment for acute leukemia and the use of bone marrow transplantation in a variety of situations, and the associated therapeutic pan-immunosuppression, the physician must be alert for the development of this specific infection.

Acute necrotizing pneumonia has been diagnosed in immunocompetent patients when there has been no response to routine antibiotic therapy and an invasive procedure has been performed that reveals *Aspergillus* species on culture. These cases are similar clinically to any other acute necrotizing pneumonia and are rare.

A fungus ball may first be revealed on chest x-ray films. On the other hand, hemoptysis may be the symptom that calls attention to the mass. Systemic symptoms of fever and muscle aches may be associated with evanescent pulmonary infiltrates in hypersensitive patients. The cavity may have been caused by histoplasmosis, tuberculosis, coccidioidomycosis, or even sarcoidosis, and the underlying process is usually not active at the time the fungus ball is discovered.

ABPA is characterized usually but not always by severe attacks of asthma, fever, cough with scanty sputum and the production of mucous plugs, the appearance of pulmonary infiltrates in varying locations, and proximal bronchiectasis that may be associated with normal bronchi more peripherally in the same bronchial branch. The serologic and skin test findings are described below. The fungus may be found in the sputum of the patient, but this is not essential to the diagnosis. The sedimentation rate is usually greatly elevated, and values for specific anti-*Aspergillus* IgE are high. The active disease waxes and wanes spontaneously but may ultimately lead to localized pulmonary fibrosis.

The above description relates to pure syndromes, but

in fact cases are encountered in which a fungus ball may be associated with locally invasive, albeit limited, disease, symptoms of ABPA may be appear in association with a "quiet" fungus ball, and a local necrotizing lesion may be associated with dissemination or aggressive local progression.

In AIDS patients, treatment-induced neutropenia is often the predisposing factor for disseminated aspergillosis with pulmonary manifestations. The use of steroids is also associated with the development of widespread disease. Cavities containing fungus balls tend to bleed and thus pose an added threat to patients.

Patients with cystic fibrosis are at greater risk for ABPA than the general population. The reason for the relationship is not clear. The course and treatment are the same as for patients without cystic fibrosis, and the response to therapy is good. The ultimate impact of ABPA on the course of cystic fibrosis is not clear.

Diagnosis

A clinical picture of periodic worsening of underlying asthma is suggestive of the diagnosis of ABPA. The coming and going of pulmonary infiltrates seemingly not related to other events and without the usual allergic seasonal connection is also suggestive of the diagnosis, especially in asthmatic patients. The sudden onset of hemoptysis in a patient known to have a cavity caused by one of the usual granulomatous infections should arouse suspicion of a fungus ball.

In ABPA, the x-ray film demonstrates the infiltrates as noted. Bronchiectasis proximally located may be seen by high-resolution CT and, in rare cases these days, bronchography. The presence of an intracavitary mass, especially one that moves when the patient changes position, is clear evidence of a fungus ball. CT makes the picture even prettier, but no more accurate. In disseminated aspergillosis, poorly defined focal infiltrates may be seen that are nonspecific. Small radiolucencies may be seen.

Diagnosis of ABPA is aided by the demonstration of elevated titers of anti-*Aspergillus* IgE and IgG and the presence of a wheal-and-flare reaction following skin testing with *Aspergillus* antigen. Specificity of these tests has been improved with the introduction of a purified antigen, Asp f1. In cases of aspergilloma, cultures of sputum and BAL fluid are usually positive, and precipitin tests for IgG antibodies often demonstrate numerous positive bands.

Diagnosis of invasive aspergillosis is the most difficult. Because the organisms are ubiquitous, positive cultures of respiratory secretions do not always indicate the presence of invasive disease. Therefore, definitive diagnosis often depends on the demonstration of septate hyphae in biopsy material (easily seen in tissue stained with any of the fungal stains), with the subsequent isolation of the organism in culture. Isolation of the organism is necessary, as many organisms with the same morphology have been described as opportunistic pathogens of profoundly neutropenic patients. The organism is rapidly growing; cultures are positive in 24 to 72 hours. Identification is based on morphologic criteria. Antibody-based serologic tests are of little value in the diagnosis of invasive aspergillosis. Antigen tests show great promise, but those currently available lack sensitivity, in part because of the transient nature of the antigenemia.

Prognosis and Therapy

Disseminated aspergillosis is a fatal disease unless the underlying immunosuppression and/or cachexia can be reversed. Even with antibiotic treatment, death is almost certain. Fungus ball is a benign syndrome and is not threatening to the life of the patient except when hemoptysis is significant. ABPA is very disturbing to the patient but rarely if ever life-threatening unless the asthma that usually accompanies the syndrome becomes very severe. The syndrome does not spontaneously disappear permanently, but it may be in remission for prolonged periods.

Treatment of disseminated disease is ineffective unless the underlying depression of the immune system is repaired. Amphotericin B, which is the antibiotic most frequently used, is relatively ineffective in this situation. There is still a possibility that one of the newer triazole drugs will prove useful against *Aspergillus* species, although itraconazole at a dosage of 600 mg/d for the first few days and then 400 mg/d continued for months has shown limited effectiveness.

It is not necessary to treat a fungus ball unless hemoptysis or recurrent systemic symptoms that have been proved to be caused by the fungus ball are present. If treatment is required, resection is indicated. Inhaled amphotericin B has been suggested for this condition, but it is ineffective as a systemically administered drug. The reason is that the bleeding and other symptoms are caused by the inflammatory reaction in the wall of the cavity, as a consequence of the large quantity of antigen present. Antifungal therapy has no effect on that.

Treatment of ABPA is aimed at two different aspects of the problem. In the first place, the asthma that so frequently accompanies ABPA is usually severe and thus requires the use of β_2-adrenergic agonists, inhaled steroids, and in certain cases oral theophylline. Systemic steroids, usually oral prednisone, may be required on the basis of the severity of the asthma. The other role of steroids is to reduce the immunologic response to the specific fungal immunogen that is the basis of the syndrome. The dose is about 1.0 mg/kg daily at the outset, with slow tapering of the dose guided by both the clinical condition and the level of specific IgE in the serum. In cases with pulmonary infiltrates only and no asthma, steroids are the only therapy indicated.

PULMONARY DISEASE CAUSED BY ACTINOMYCETACEAE

This group of organisms is identified with fungi, although taxonomically they are bacteria closely related to *Mycobacteria*. In some respects they resemble fungi (e.g., staining and behavior within the body), but they resemble bacteria morphologically and in their characteristics on culture. They have traditionally been considered with the fungi, and we shall do so in this chapter.

Actinomycosis (Fig. 16)

This infection was first recognized in cattle in 1826, and in humans in 1845. The localization of the disease to the mouth in both mammalian species was a frequently observed clinical characteristic. The advent of sulfonamides and antibiotics changed the perception of this disease, and also its frequency.

Organism

The most common cause of actinomycosis in humans is *A. israelii,* an anaerobic, non–spore-forming, gram-positive rod. It is catalase-negative, and succinic acid and lactic acid are its two major metabolic products in culture. Its historical inclusion with the fungi can be attributed to its propensity to form filamentous rods, especially in tissue.

Pathology

This organism is found in the mouth normally, and in otherwise healthy persons there is no reaction to its presence. When local trauma or aspiration of mouth contents containing the organism occurs, the body reacts and disease develops. The response under these conditions is acute inflammation with suppuration and necrosis of tissue. The suppurative process is inexorable in its progression unless treated and has the tendency to cross tissue boundaries that usually limit inflammatory processes caused by bacteria, even mycobacteria. This process leads to fistula formation wherever the infection is found: in the facial tissues, in the lung and pleurae, and in the abdominal organs and peritoneum. Pleurocutaneous fistula (empyema necessitatis) may occur. The disease has been identified in all body organs, implying hematogenous spread.

The characteristic tissue finding in this disease is the so-called sulfur granule, which is a collection of filaments radiating out from a central necrotic core. These may be up to 5.0 mm in diameter and can be recognized grossly in pus. In fact, collections of pus should be routinely examined for sulfur granules. They characterize this disease in tissues, although they are not absolutely pathognomonic, as they may be found in nocardiosis and less frequently in pus associated with staphylococcal infection. In tissues, the sulfur granules take the hematoxylin-eosin stain and are dramatic findings.

A chronic form of this infection is seen in which localized, slowly progressive granulomatous lesions are associated with a plethora of scar tissue. These may be seen on skin, in mediastinal lymph nodes, and in other locations of the body.

Epidemiology

The distribution of cases in the world is related more to clinical awareness of the possibility of the disease than to any external characteristic such as climate, terrain, or living conditions. This is because the organism can be found in the mouths of almost everyone in the world! The wide use of sulfonamides and antibiotics has reduced the incidence of this disease, as this organism is exquisitely sensitive to most of them.

Clinical Manifestations

Actinomycosis most commonly appears in a localized, maxillofacial form. Swellings and distortion of tissues in

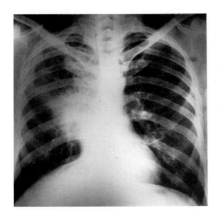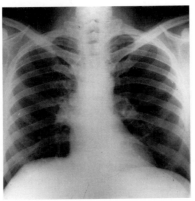

FIG. 16. Acute actinomycosis with focal infiltrates in a 40-year-old man (**A**) before and (**B**) 9 months after initiation of penicillin therapy.

the maxillofacial area result in fistula formation unless the disease is diagnosed and treated. There is often a history of mouth or face trauma before the development of clinical actinomycosis of this type. In the abdomen, fistula formation is disastrous, and the diagnosis is usually made late in the course of the disease.

Pulmonary actinomycosis is almost certainly secondary to aspiration of mouth contents containing the organism. Also, mouth or facial trauma have frequently occurred before the onset of pulmonary disease. The clinical presentation may be acute and characteristic of pneumonia caused by any organism. It may also be more chronic in onset, with a course similar to the development of aspiration lung abscess of any cause. In fact, a diagnosis of actinomycosis should be considered in any case of lung abscess in which aspiration is a possible factor, and the organism should be specifically looked for. The course of the disease is prolonged and downhill if it is not appropriately treated. Suppuration is extensive, with all the associated toxic systemic signs as well as increasing shortness of breath, cough, production of large quantities of purulent sputum, and chest pain if the pleurae become involved. Empyema may develop, and if untreated it may be complicated by the formation of a pleurocutaneous fistula.

Lesions of the chronic form of actinomycosis are quite rare in the pulmonary parenchyma. There are usually no acute symptoms; rather, the patient is chronically mildly ill. The course may be many years long before a specific diagnosis is made.

Diagnosis

A history of mouth trauma or of aspiration should arouse suspicion of this disease. Chest radiography is helpful if pulmonary infiltrates cross natural tissue boundaries, such as pleural borders, or chest wall structures. The picture of lung abscess is nonspecific, but again attention should be paid to the anatomic configuration of the lesions.

Laboratory diagnosis begins with clinical suspicion, so that material for culture is collected and transported to maintain anaerobiosis. Collections of pus may be examined for sulfur granules; if found, these should be rinsed in sterile saline solution before culture. Cultures must be incubated anaerobically and held for at least 7 to 10 days; they should be examined every other day for the presence of the characteristic molar tooth colonies. Identification of the organism depends on demonstration of appropriate morphology on Gram's stain and characteristic reactions to a panel of biochemical tests. Direct microscopic examination of sulfur granules or tissue often provides a presumptive diagnosis. The granules are irregular in size (0.1 to 5 mm) and shape and may have a slightly yellow hue. They are made up of filamentous bacteria in a radial array;

the exterior ends of the rods are coated with eosinophilic material in hematoxylin and eosin. Serologic testing does not play a role in the diagnosis of actinomycosis.

Prognosis and Treatment

All forms of actinomycosis are rapidly or slowly inexorably progressive and potentially fatal if untreated.

Treatment of actinomycosis is preferably penicillin given in doses of 2 to 10 million units, at first systemically and then continued by mouth. The response is usually prompt, but the treatment must be continued for a minimum of 6 to 9 months, preferably a year. The rationale for this is based, in part at least, on the presence of a great deal of necrotic and fibrotic tissue in the lesions and the persistent viability of the organism residing in this tissue. Results with prolonged treatment are excellent, even in the chronic form of the disease.

If the patient is hypersensitive to penicillin, sulfonamides may be given as well as tetracyclines and many other antibiotics. The emphasis is on length of treatment, regardless of which antibiotic is used.

Treatment of empyema with adequate drainage is mandatory. It is important to prevent the spontaneous formation of a pleurocutaneous fistula, as this increases morbidity significantly.

Nocardiosis (Fig. 17)

Infection with this organism was first described by Nocard in 1888. Its place in the spectrum of suppurative

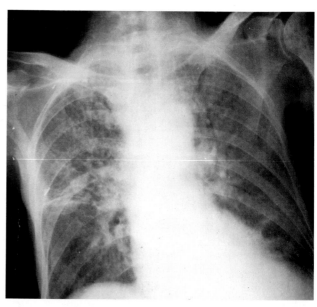

FIG. 17. Acute, fatal pulmonary nocardiosis occurring during steroid therapy in a 73-year-old man with lymphatic leukemia. Note the diffuse infiltrates.

diseases became clearer in the mid-twentieth century, especially when it was noted to be an accompaniment of alveolar proteinosis. This organism has been found in soil all over the world. There are many confusing elements to this infection, not the least being the weak acid-fast nature of the hyphae and their tendency to fragment and resemble bacilli. The organism has many cousins that cause a variety of serious skin lesions.

Organism

Pulmonary nocardiosis is most commonly caused by *N. asteroides; N. brasiliensis, N. otitidis-caviarum,* and *N. farcinica* represent the etiologic agents of the majority of the remaining cases. All are aerobic, non–spore-forming, gram-positive, branching filamentous bacteria that stain weakly acid-fast. The filaments (1.5 mm) tend to break into coccobacillary forms; aerial filaments are formed in culture. The cell wall of the genus is characterized by the presence of meso-diaminopimelic acid.

Pathology

This is a suppurative disease in whatever organ it is found. The lung is the most common site, as the route of infection appears to be by inhalation of the organism, with primary lesions in the lung. Other sites in which the disease may be found include the central nervous system, skin, and urinary system, especially the kidneys. Histologically, the characteristic inflammation is neutrophilic, and only rarely are granulomatous changes seen. There may be scarring, but it is less pronounced than that seen in actinomycosis. The sulfur granules that may be found in actinomycotic pus may also be found in nocardial suppuration. The tendency for crossing tissue barriers noted in actinomycosis is also present in nocardiosis, although it is less dramatic. The frequency of extrapulmonary suppurative and fibrotic lesions is estimated to be close to 50%, but accurate figures are not available.

Epidemiology

Nocardiosis is found all over the world. In the United States, 90% of cases are caused by *N. asteroides* and the rest by the other *Nocardia* species. There is an association with certain underlying conditions, such as malignant disease, cachexia, alveolar proteinosis, and immunosuppression from diseases or treatment, but about 20% of cases have been found in patients with no identifiable predisposing factor. There appears to be no association with occupation, season, sex, or ethnic origin.

Clinical Manifestations

Pulmonary nocardiosis is almost always an acute or subacute pneumonia that progresses to abscess formation. There is nothing specific about the clinical picture, but the frequency of extrapulmonary lesions is high. There may be pleural involvement with empyema. Of the extrathoracic sites, the central nervous system and the skin are most frequently involved. In fact, the syndrome of multiple subcutaneous abscesses, pulmonary lesions, and possibly pleural effusion is very suggestive of nocardiosis. Cases of chronic brain abscess have been seen. The course of the untreated disease is progressively downhill, and death is inevitable. The disease progresses much more rapidly in patients with immunosuppression.

The association between alveolar proteinosis and nocardiosis was reported in the 1960s, but the reason for the association is not known. The course of the combined diseases is more malignant than the course of either one alone. Treatment of the nocardial infection with antibiotics is not hindered by the proteinosis.

There appears to be a chronic form of nocardiosis that resembles cavitary pulmonary tuberculosis; only the microbiologic findings differentiate between disease caused by two different agents.

Diagnosis

The clinical syndrome noted above of subcutaneous and pulmonary lesions is suggestive of the diagnosis, as is a complicated course of alveolar proteinosis. In malignant disease with complicating pulmonary, subcutaneous, or central nervous system lesions, nocardiosis must be considered among other opportunistic infections.

Chest radiography shows focal bronchopneumonia frequently associated with abscess formation. Empyema is present in a significant percentage of the patients. None of these findings is specific, however. The typical lesions of proteinosis, widespread alveolar or interstitial shadows, are not modified by the superinfection by *Nocardia*. The brain abscesses that may develop are well demonstrated by standard radiography, CT, and magnetic resonance imaging (MRI), but the lesions are not diagnostic.

Laboratory diagnosis of nocardiosis depends on the isolation of the organism from BAL fluid, pus, or tissue. Clinical suspicion of the diagnosis must be communicated to the laboratory to ensure appropriate handling of the cultures. The organism grows slowly for a bacterium, requiring 5 to 10 days to become positive on culture; because it is sensitive to many antibiotics, it may not grow on the selective media used for routine isolation of fungi. The organism is identified by morphology, staining characteristics, and biochemical profile; analysis of cell wall components by chromatography may also be used. A presumptive diagnosis based on the appearance of filamentous, branching, gram-positive bacteria in clinical material is strengthened if the filaments are determined to be weakly acid-fast (i.e., require the use of dilute mineral rather than acid alcohol for decolorization). In tissue, the filaments may be stained with Brown and Brenn, Grocott, or the Fite modification of the acid-fast stain. Granules are rarely seen in pulmonary disease but may be present in infections acquired by the direct inoculation of the organism into skin.

Prognosis and Therapy

The disease progresses without treatment, with dissemination throughout the body in immunosuppressed cases especially. A fatal outcome occurs in a large fraction of cases. Even with response to therapy, significant scarring may occur.

Effectiveness of therapy varies based on the sensitivity of various strains of *N. asteroides* and other *Nocardia* species to antibiotics, and on the underlying condition of the patient. The most frequently effective antibiotic or chemotherapeutic agent is trimethoprim/sulfamethoxazole. Other effective antibiotics are amikacin and to some extent the tetracyclines. In any case, treatment should be continued for at least half a year and perhaps longer, depending on the clinical course. In the case of brain abscess, surgery may be necessary, and when collections of pus are present subcutaneously, in the pleurae, or elsewhere in the body, adequate drainage is essential.

In the case of a patient who has AIDS or is HIV-positive, it is especially important to test for drug sensitivity, as the organism is more often resistant to the above-mentioned antibiotics in this situation, possibly because of the use of sulfa drugs as chemoprophylaxis against *Pneumocystis*.

MISCELLANEOUS FUNGAL DISEASES

The following infections are rare indeed and almost always associated with some underlying factor that renders the patient more susceptible.

Trichosporonosis

This infection caused by *Trichosporon* species was extremely rare as a cause of human systemic disease until the advent of immunosuppression as a relatively common clinical situation. Involvement of the lungs is seen almost always as part of disseminated disease. There may be superinfection of chronic inflammatory lesions of the lung caused by other conditions. Treatment with a variety of antibiotics, including 5-fluorocytosine and amphotericin, is not very effective but should be tried.

The majority of cases are caused by *T. beigelii*. Regard-

less of the species involved, infection is characterized the presence of budding yeast cells, hyphae, and arthroconidia in tissue.

Pseudoallescheriasis

Pulmonary involvement includes the formation of a fungus ball, colonization of the tracheobronchial tree, and invasive parenchymal disease. This latter is almost always associated with immunosuppression, and the lesions occur as foci of bronchopneumonia. Treatment is indicated only in the pneumonic form of the infection; the imidazoles have been reported to be effective. Colonization of the airways alone is not a threatening condition, and the fungus ball is dealt with in the same way as an *Aspergillus* fungus ball.

Pseudoallescheria boydii (*Scedosporium apiospermum*) is the most frequent cause of this infection. Rarely, cases are caused by *Scedosporium prolificans*. The organisms appear identical in tissue and must be differentiated in culture.

Zygomycosis

This infection is caused by several fungi belonging to the order Mucorales, including *Mucor, Rhizopus,* and *Absidia* species. Infection with these organisms is associated with diabetes mellitus and neutropenia. Pulmonary disease is rare and is usually seen as a progressive pneumonia that is resistant to usual antibiotic therapy. More frequent is the syndrome of rhinocerebral disease, in which the paranasal sinuses are involved and there may be spread to the major venous sinuses of the head. The pathology in all forms of the infection is acute inflammation associated with a prominent amount of tissue necrosis. Underlying pathology is nonspecific except that the fungi tend to invade blood vessels and thus cause intravascular thrombosis. This phenomenon may be the factor responsible for the prominent necrosis. Treatment is inconsistently effective with amphotericin B. Surgical debridement is often necessary to remove necrotic bone or other tissues.

Rhinocerebral mucormycosis is caused by *Rhizopus* species in 90% of cases. Although *Rhizopus* is also the most common cause of pulmonary disease, species of *Mucor* and *Absidia* are seen more frequently. In tissue, all appear identical, and differentiation is made by identification of the organism in culture.

ABPA Syndrome of Various Causes

Clinically and roentgenographically, typical ABPA has been described infrequently as caused by a variety of fungi, many of them known as saprophytes. These include

Aspergillus species other than *fumigatus, Candida albicans, Pseudoallescheria boydii, Fusarium vasinfectum, Curvularia lunata, Rhizopus, Helminthosporium, Penicillium, Stemphylium, Candida glabrata, Bipolaris,* and *Drechslera hawaiiensis.* The diagnosis is made only by means of serology, skin tests, and finding the specific fungus in culture, the finding of lesser frequency. The treatment is mainly with steroids using the same criteria for length of treatment as in ABPA.

BIBLIOGRAPHY

General

American Thoracic Society Official Statement (Sarosi G, et al.). Fungal infection in HIV-infected persons. *Am J Respir Crit Care Med* 1995; 152:816–822. *Concise summary of the problems of coexistence of HIV infection with each of the following: candidiasis, cryptococcosis, histoplasmosis, coccidioidomycosis, blastomycosis, sporotrichosis, and aspergillosis.*

Chandler FW, Kaplan W, Ajello L. *Histopathology of Mycotic Disease.* Chicago: Year Book Medical Publishers; 1980. *One of two excellent atlases of pathology. Although the older of the two, this one contains beautiful examples of histopathology and special stains for fungi.*

Goodman JL, Winston DJ, Greenfield RA, et al. A controlled trial of fluconazole to prevent fungal infections in patients undergoing bone marrow transplantation. *New Engl J Med* 1992; 326:845–851. *Many of the advantages of fluconazole, the rationale for its use, and results of preventive therapy are presented.*

Kwon-Chung KJ, Bennett JE. *Medical Mycology.* Philadelphia: Lea & Febiger; 1992. *Excellent general textbook dealing with all aspects of fungi and fungal infections.*

Powderly WG, Finkelstein DM, Feinberg J, et al. A randomized trial comparing fluconazole with clotrimazole troches for the prevention of fungal infections in patients with advanced human immunodeficiency virus infection. *New Engl J Med* 1995; 332:700–705. *Fluconazole is shown to be especially effective in preventing cryptococcosis, esophageal candidiasis, and superficial fungal infections. The role of the CD4 count is emphasized.*

Salfelder K. *Atlas of Fungal Pathology.* Dordrecht: Kluwer Academic Publishers; 1990. *The second atlas of pathology. The text represents a somewhat different approach than the Chandler atlas; the illustrations are excellent.*

Segal E, Baum GL. *Pathogenic Yeasts and Yeast Infections.* Boca Raton, FL: CRC Press; 1994. *This book covers both candidal and cryptococcal species, from basic science to clinical manifestations and treatment. It is a succinct but complete source that includes the molecular biology of both organisms.*

Wheat J. Endemic mycoses in AIDS: a clinical review. *Clin Microbiol Rev* 1995; 8:149–159. *Well-referenced review of histoplasmosis, blastomycosis, and coccidioidomycosis in AIDS patients. Both diagnosis and therapy are discussed.*

Actinomycosis and Nocardiosis

Andriole VT, Ballas M, Wilson GL. The association of nocardiosis and pulmonary alveolar proteinosis: a case study. *Ann Intern Med* 1964; 60:266–275. *A summary of seven cases describing the pathology and clinical findings of the association. An excellent clinicopathologic study.*

Hsieh M-J, Liu H-P, Chang J-P, Chang C-H. Thoracic actinomycosis. *Chest* 1993; 104:366–370. *Seventeen patients given a diagnosis of actinomycosis between 1984 and 1990 are reported. Excellent descriptions of clinical, radiographic, and therapeutic aspects.*

Marrie TJ. Pneumonia caused by *Nocardia* species. *Semin Respir Infect* 1994; 9:207–213. *Excellent review of pulmonary nocardiosis. Difficulties in diagnosis and newer species involved are discussed.*

Uttamchandani RB, Daikos GL, Reyes RR, et al. Nocardiosis in 30 patients with advanced human immunodeficiency virus infection: clin-ical features and outcome. *Clin Infect Dis* 1994; 18:348–353. *In 30 patients, 22 with lung disease, AIDS was either present at the time of diagnosis of the infection or appeared shortly after. Clinical description is excellent, and details of immune function are noted. Treatment is effective, but mortality is high.*

Young LS, Armstrong D, Blevins A, Lieberman P. *Nocardia asteroides* infection complicating neoplastic disease. *Am J Med* 1971; 50:356–367. *A detailed description of 22 cases, 13 of which clearly represent nocardiosis in patients with malignancy.*

Aspergillosis

Berenguer J, Allende MC, Lee JW, et al. Pathogenesis of pulmonary aspergillosis: granulocytopenia versus cyclosporine and methylprednisolone-induced immunosuppression. *Am J Respir Crit Care Med* 1995; 152:1079–1086. *Animal work dealing with a central issue in the pathogenesis of disseminated aspergillosis and supporting the concept that the polymorphonuclear leukocyte is the critical cell protecting against this catastrophe.*

Kauffman HF, Tomee JFC, van der Werf TS, et al. Review of fungus-induced asthmatic reactions. *Am J Respir Crit Care Med* 1995; 2109–2116. *Excellent summary of the basic mechanisms responsible for asthmatic reactions to the presence of fungi, especially* Aspergillus, *in the tracheobronchial tree.*

Khoo SH, Denning DW. Invasive aspergillosis in patients with AIDS. *Clin Infect Dis* 1994; 19(Suppl):S41–S48. *This article details the partially successful treatment of aspergillosis in AIDS patients with itraconazole. Worth trying, is the message.*

Miller WT Jr, Sais GJ, Frank I, et al. Pulmonary aspergillosis in patients with AIDS: clinical and radiographic correlations. *Chest* 1994; 105:37–44. *A very clear summary of these correlations and the clinical and radiographic diagnostic findings.*

Mroueh S, Spock A. Allergic bronchopulmonary aspergillosis in patients with cystic fibrosis. *Chest* 1994; 105:32–36. *A review of 236 patients with cystic fibrosis, of whom 60 had colonies of* Aspergillus *species grown from their sputum. ABPA was diagnosed in 15 of them. Risk factors are emphasized.*

Blastomycosis

Kinasewitz GT, Penn RL, George RB. The significance of pleural disease in blastomycosis. *Chest* 1984; 86:580–584. *This article emphasizes how infrequently pleural effusion accompanied pleural inflammation in blastomycosis in the 26 patients carefully studied.*

Klein BS, Vergernt JM, Weeks RJ, et al. Isolation of *Blastomyces dermatitidis* in soil associated with a large outbreak of blastomycosis in Wisconsin. *New Engl J Med* 1986; 314:529–534. *Although this article is not the first report of an epidemic of blastomycosis associated with soil contamination, the material is well presented and provides considerable information on many aspects of the problem.*

Meyer KC, Mc Manus EJ, Maki DG. Overwhelming pulmonary blastomycosis associated with the adult respiratory distress syndrome. *New Engl J Med* 1993; 329:1231–1236. *Presents conclusive evidence that blastomycosis can indeed cause ARDS and needs to be considered in the differential diagnosis of patients with this syndrome.*

Pappas PG, Poltage JC, Powderly WG, et al. Blastomycosis in patients with acquired immunodeficiency syndrome. *Ann Intern Med* 1992; 116:847–853. *A study of 15 patients dealing with therapy, prognosis, and clinical findings.*

Soufleris AJ, Klein BS, Courtney BT, et al. Utility of anti-WI-1 serological testing in the diagnosis of blastomycosis in Wisconsin residents. *Clin Infect Dis* 1994; 19:87–92. *Describes the best new test under development for diagnosing blastomycosis and discusses the shortcomings of the currently available tests.*

Candidiasis

Haron E, Vartivarian S, Anaissie E, et al. Primary *Candida* pneumonia. Experience at a large cancer center and review of the literature. *Medicine* 1993; 72:137–142. *Report of 31 cases and review of 55 cases from the literature. The difficulty of making the diagnosis owing to the protean nature of the disease is stressed.*

Walsh TJ, Merz WG, Lee JW, et al. Diagnosis and therapeutic monitoring of invasive candidiasis by rapid enzymatic detection of serum D-arabinitol. *Am J Med* 1995;99:164–172. *More than 3000 samples from 274 cancer patients were tested by this automated assay. The largest trial of this methodology to date, with the most promising results.*

Coccidioidomycosis

Galgiani JN. Coccidioidomycosis: changes in clinical expression, serological diagnosis, and therapeutic options. *Clin Infect Dis* 1992;14(Suppl):S100–S105. *Discusses changes in the spectrum of clinical disease resulting from coinfection with HIV, newer serologic tests, and therapeutic options provided by the newer azole antifungal agents.*

Pappagianis D, et al. Evaluation of the protective efficacy of the killed *Coccidioides immitis* spherule vaccine in humans. *Am Rev Respir Dis* 1993;148:656–660. *A summary of the results of a large trial with the vaccine. Although an interim report, it suggests definite effectiveness.*

Stevens DA. Coccidioidomycosis. *New Engl J Med* 1995;332:1077–1082. *An excellent statement of all aspects of the disease and its treatment.*

Wack EE, Ampel NM, Galgiani JM, Bronnimann DA. Coccidioidomycosis during pregnancy: an analysis of ten cases among 47,120 pregnancies. *Chest* 1988;94:376–379. *Experience indicating the increased risk for dissemination of infection that exists during pregnancy. An excellent survey.*

Winn WE, Johnson B, Galgiani JN, Butler C, Pluss J. Cavitary coccidioidomycosis with fungus ball formation: diagnosis by fiberoptic bronchoscopy with coexistence of hyphae and spherules. *Chest* 1994;105:412–416. *An important occurrence, albeit infrequent, as it represents a circumstance creating the possibility of person-to-person transmission of infection.*

Cryptococcosis

Currie BP, Casadevall A. Estimation of the prevalence of cryptococcal infection among patients infected with human immunodeficiency virus in New York City. *Clin Infect Dis* 1994;19:1029–1033. *A very large survey population; thus, the numbers resulting from this study are impressive and establish C.* neoformans *as the fourth leading opportunistic (all types of organisms) and the most common fungal infection of HIV-infected persons.*

Mitchell TG, Perfect JR. Cryptococcosis in the era of AIDS—100 years after the discovery of *Cryptococcus neoformans. Clin Microbiol Rev* 1995;8:515–548. *Excellent review of all aspects of the organism and the clinical presentation of cryptococcosis in AIDS, including the immune response to the organism and therapy of the infection.*

Patz EF Jr. Pulmonary cryptococcosis. *J Thorac Imaging* 1992;7:51–55. *Good review of the radiologic aspects of pulmonary cryptococcosis.*

Vechiarelli A, Dottorine M, Pietrella D, Monari C, Retini C, Todisco T, Bistoni F. Role of human alveolar macrophages as antigen-presenting cells in *Cryptococcus neoformans* infection. *Am J Respir Cell Mol Biol* 1994;11:130–137. *Alveolar macrophages from healthy humans were studied in the laboratory and their capability at integrating the immune response to the fungus was demonstrated. Well done and clearly presented.*

Histoplasmosis

Deepe GS Jr. The immune response to *Histoplasma capsulatum:* unearthing its secrets. *J Lab Clin Med* 1994;123:201–205. *An excellent exposition of the human immune response to the fungus. Extremely well written.*

Goodwin RA Jr, Owens FT, Snell JD, et al. Chronic pulmonary histoplasmosis. *Medicine* 1976;55:413–452. *One of the largest collections of cases of chronic pulmonary histoplasmosis cases and valid up to the present, although the theory of pathogenesis is not accepted generally.*

McKinney DS, Gupta MR, Riddler SA, et al. Long-term amphotericin B therapy for disseminated histoplasmosis in patients with the acquired immunodeficiency syndrome (AIDS). *Ann Intern Med* 1989;111:655–659. *Based on experience with 22 patients, the authors suggest that the treatment is effective and relatively well tolerated.*

Schwarz J, Schaen M, Picardi JL. Complications of the arrested primary histoplasmic complex. *JAMA* 1976;236:1157–1161. *A classic paper that is relevant today as the best summary of the topic in print. These reactions are not often thought of.*

Wheat LJ, Connolly-Stringfield P, Williams B, et al. Diagnosis of histoplasmosis in patients with the acquired immunodeficiency syndrome by detection of *Histoplasma capsulatum* polysaccharide antigen in bronchoalveolar lavage fluid. *Am Rev Respir Dis* 1992;145:1421–1424. *An important breakthrough using immunologic techniques on lavage fluid to arrive at a diagnosis quickly.*

Wheat LJ, Hefner R, Wulfsohn M, et al. Prevention of relapse of histoplasmosis with itraconazole in patients with the acquired immunodeficiency syndrome. *Ann Intern Med* 1993;118:610–616. *Promising therapy in a very difficult situation reported in 42 patients.*

Paracoccidioidomycosis

Brummer, E, Castaneda, E, Restrepo, A. Paracoccidioidomycosis: an update. *Clin Microbiol Rev* 1993;6:89–117. *This is a complete review of the disease, the organism and the immunological response to infection. The impact of immunosuppression is noted and details of treatment are updated to include the imid- and triazoles. An excellent resource.*

Sporotrichosis

Baum GL, Donnerberg RL, Stewart D, et al. Pulmonary sporotrichosis. *New Engl J Med* 1969;280:410–413. *Four cases of an infrequently seen form of sporotrichosis are described, and the clinical and radiographic spectrum of the disease presented.*

Winn RE, Anderson J, Piper J, Aronson NE, Pluss J. Systemic sporotrichosis treated with itraconazole. *Clin Infect Dis* 1993;17:210–217. *Reports the successful use of this triazole in place of amphotericin B in six cases of systemic sporotrichosis.*

Miscellaneous Fungal Diseases

Backman KS, Roberts M, Patterson R. Allergic bronchopulmonary mycosis caused by *Fusarium vasinfectum. Am J Respir Crit Care Med* 1995;152:1379–1381. *Case report of a special syndrome caused by an organism other than an Aspergillus species.*

Tedder M, Spratt JA, Anstadt MP, et al. Pulmonary mucormycosis: results of medical and surgical therapy. *Ann Thorac Surg* 1994;57:1044–1050. *Examination of outcome in this infection associated with high morbidity and mortality based on the outcome in 30 patients and a review of 255 case reports.*

Textbook of Pulmonary Diseases, 6th ed.
edited by G.L. Baum, J.D. Crapo, B.R. Celli, and J.B. Karlinsky,
Lippincott–Raven Publishers, Philadelphia, © 1998.

CHAPTER

28 ▶ Tuberculosis

Reynard J. McDonald · Lee B. Reichman

INTRODUCTION

Does it not seem reasonable that if a new infectious epidemic were to emerge that annually infected one third of the earth's population (1.7 billion people), causing sickness in 8 million new victims, striking 20 million people at any one time, and killing 3 million, then scientists and policy makers would work overtime to highlight the problem, identify the cause, and find a cure to eliminate this scourge rapidly?

Tuberculosis is an ancient disease that fulfills all the above descriptions regarding its infection prevalence, incidence of morbidity, and mortality. The disease is quite common, its cause is well characterized, and it is by current state of the art both preventable and curable with inexpensive, nontoxic medications.

Yet, embarrassingly, tuberculosis still kills more people than any other infectious disease. Even though its cause and methods of cure are well established, the global health organizations have never put enough political pressure on governments to apply the practical solutions that would eliminate this disease from the world.

By all rights, when the first edition of Baum's *Textbook of Pulmonary Disease* was published, anybody would have predicted that by the sixth edition tuberculosis would have been considered as a rare, historic curiosity. In the sixth edition, however, we are still considering a disease that now affects and kills more people worldwide than at any time in history.

R. J. McDonald and L. B. Reichman: Department of Medicine, New Jersey Medical School National Tuberculosis Center, University of Medicine and Dentistry of New Jersey, Newark, New Jersey 07107.

This chapter presents a 1997 view of an ancient killer and includes current information regarding its epidemiology, transmission, pathogenesis, prevention, and treatment. The medical community and world governments merely need to exert the political will necessary to ensure that by later editions, tuberculosis will rightfully have become the curiosity it deserves to be.

EPIDEMIOLOGY

Ever since Robert Koch's remarkable discovery of the tubercle bacillus in 1882, many mycobacterial species have been identified. Pulmonary disease caused by atypical mycobacterial infection, which frequently is clinically indistinguishable from tuberculosis, is now recognized as being caused by several different nontuberculous mycobacteria, most often *M. avium* complex and *M. kansasii.*

Tuberculosis in humans is caused by infection with the *Mycobacterium tuberculosis* complex of organisms. *M. tuberculosis, M. bovis,* and *M. africanum* are mammalian tubercle bacilli that are included in this group.

It is estimated that 1.7 billion persons—one third of the global population—are infected with mammalian tubercle bacilli. Annually, on a worldwide basis, 20 million prevalent active cases occur, including 8 million new cases, with an incidence of approximately 160 cases per 100,000 population. This disease is the leading infectious cause of death in the world, with approximately 3 million people worldwide dying yearly of tuberculosis.

It was estimated in 1990 that 3 million people worldwide are coinfected with the tubercle bacillus and human immunodeficiency virus (HIV). More recent estimates (1994) place this figure closer to 5.5 million. Because of

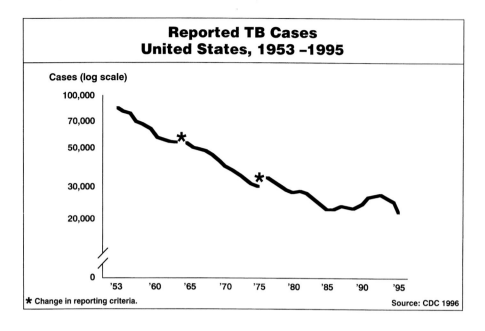

FIG. 1. Reported tuberculosis cases in the United States, 1953–1995.

the increased numbers of tuberculosis cases that will likely occur from this cohort of dually infected patients, it is projected that global rates of tuberculosis will rise in the decade ahead, particularly in sub-Saharan Africa and perhaps most seriously in Southeast Asia.

Tuberculosis has re-emerged as a very important public health problem in the United States. It is estimated that 10 to 15 million people are infected with the tubercle bacillus in this country and that most new cases of tuberculosis come from this infected cohort. It should be pointed out, however, that recently there have been increasingly frequent reports, primarily in persons coinfected with the tubercle bacillus and HIV, of clusters of new tuberculosis cases documented by DNA fingerprinting to have resulted from recent infection.

The number of tuberculosis cases declined approximately 5%–6% per year from 84,304 cases in 1953, when nationwide reporting began, to 22,255 cases in 1984 (Fig. 1). However, from 1985, when the number of reported tuberculosis cases reached its lowest point (22,201), through 1992, tuberculosis morbidity in the United States increased by almost 20%, to 26,673 cases (Fig. 1). Since 1992, largely because of an unprecedented expenditure of resources designed to re-establish the public health infrastructure for tuberculosis prevention and control, the number of reported tuberculosis cases has begun once again to show a downward trend, although sustaining this reduction in an era of budget cuts and health care reform may be difficult.

In 1993 and 1994, and again in 1995, reported tuberculosis cases declined in the United States from 25,287 to 24,361 (3.7% reduction) to 22,812 (6.4% reduction). However, the number of reported cases in 1995 still represents a 2.8% increase over 1985. During the period from 1985 through 1995, it is estimated that >75,000 excess

cases of tuberculosis were reported in this country than would have been reported if the trend of a 5%–6% decline per year, as from 1953 to 1984, had continued.

Of the main factors that contributed to the increase in the number of reported tuberculosis cases in the past decade, first and foremost is the deterioration of the infrastructure of the health care system that was allowed to occur. Other contributing factors include coinfection with tubercle bacilli and HIV, transmission of infection in congregate settings, and immigration from countries where tuberculosis is common. The reason that the infrastructure is so important is that all the other factors can be successfully managed in the presence of a proper infrastructure for tuberculosis control.

In 1994, the number of tuberculosis cases reported in persons born in the United States decreased in all age groups except young children (<15 years of age), in whom a 0.4% increase was noted. In foreign-born persons that year, the number of reported tuberculosis cases increased in all age groups except children <15 years of age, in whom a 7.5% decrease was noted. The number and percentage of tuberculosis cases that have been re-

TABLE 1. *Reported tuberculosis cases in foreign-born persons in the United States, 1986–1994*

Year	Cases, No.	Percentage
1986	4925	22
1987	5025	22
1988	4868	22
1989	5411	23
1990	6262	24
1991	6982	27
1992	7270	27
1993	7354	29
1994	7627	32

TABLE 2. *Tuberculosis cases and case rates per 100,000 population by age in the United States, 1984–1995*

Year	All ages	<5	5–14	15–24	25–44	45–64	≥65
			Age group, No. cases (case rates)				
1984	22,255 (9.4)	759 (4.3)	477 (1.4)	1682 (4.2)	6409 (9.0)	6427 (14.4)	6501 (23.2)
1985	22,201 (9.3)	789 (4.4)	472 (1.4)	1672 (4.2)	6764 (9.2)	6143 (13.7)	6361 (22.3)
1986	22,768 (9.4)	724 (4.0)	490 (1.4)	1719 (4.4)	7321 (9.7)	6119 (13.6)	6395 (21.9)
1987	22,517 (9.3)	674 (3.7)	503 (1.5)	1776 (4.6)	7566 (9.7)	5840 (12.9)	6158 (20.6)
1988	22,436 (9.1)	687 (3.7)	447 (1.3)	1616 (4.3)	7724 (9.8)	5863 (12.7)	6099 (20.1)
1989	23,495 (9.5)	810 (4.3)	511 (1.5)	1742 (4.8)	8553 (10.7)	5778 (12.4)	6101 (19.7)
1990	25,701 (10.3)	936 (5.1)	660 (1.9)	1867 (5.1)	9740 (12.1)	6371 (13.7)	6127 (19.6)
1991	26,283 (10.4)	1007 (5.2)	656 (1.8)	1973 (5.4)	10,269 (12.5)	6303 (13.5)	6076 (19.1)
1992	26,673 (10.5)	1074 (5.5)	633 (1.8)	1975 (5.5)	10,453 (12.7)	6496 (13.4)	6042 (18.7)
1993	25,287 (9.8)	1075 (5.5)	643 (1.7)	1841 (5.1)	9615 (11.6)	6225 (12.5)	5847 (17.8)
1994	24,361 (9.4)	1024 (5.2)	671 (1.8)	1825 (5.1)	9106 (11.0)	6141 (12.1)	5546 (16.7)
1995	22,812 (8.7)	—	—	—	—	—	—

ported in the United States since 1985 in foreign-born persons have progressively increased, and in 1994 they represented almost one third of the cases of tuberculosis reported in this country (Table 1).

Tuberculosis occurs across racial and ethnic lines and among all age groups. However, case rates are higher among racial and ethnic minorities in the United States than among non-Hispanic whites. In 1994, the risk for

tuberculosis was eightfold greater for blacks, sixfold greater for Hispanics, fivefold greater for Native Americans, and 13-fold greater for Asian and Pacific Islanders than for non-Hispanic whites in this country.

Among all age groups, regardless of sex, race, or ethnicity, tuberculosis case rates are highest in the elderly, but they have been declining for several years (Table 2). The largest increase in the number of reported cases of

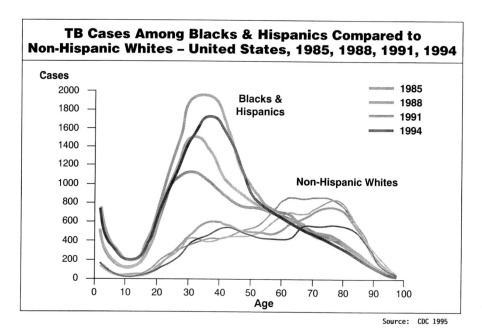

TB Cases Among Blacks & Hispanics Compared to Non-Hispanic Whites – United States, 1985, 1988, 1991, 1994

Source: CDC 1995

FIG. 2. Cases of tuberculosis among blacks and Hispanics compared with non-Hispanic whites in the United States: 1985, 1988, 1991, and 1994.

tuberculosis occurred primarily in the younger groups, particularly the 25- to 44-year-old age group; this is in large part a consequence of the increase in tuberculosis morbidity in persons who are coinfected with HIV.

In a general sense, in the non-Hispanic white population in the United States, tuberculosis is primarily a disease of the elderly ($\geq$65 years of age), whereas among minorities, tuberculosis morbidity primarily affects younger age groups (Fig. 2). In 1989, the Centers for Disease Control and Prevention (CDC) reported that the median age of members of minority groups with tuberculosis was 39 years, compared with 61 years in non-Hispanic whites.

Between 1989 and 1992, multiple outbreaks of multidrug-resistant tuberculosis (MDRTB) were reported. These outbreaks were associated with HIV infection, high mortality rates, and evidence of transmission to health care workers. In response to this threat of MDRTB, the CDC began to monitor the number of reported cases of MDRTB each year. For the first quarter of 1991, the percentage of tuberculosis cases that were reported to be resistant to both isoniazid (INH) and rifampin (RIF) was approximately 3.4%. This represented approximately a sevenfold increase over the percentages in 1984, when only 0.5% of reported cases were resistant to both INH and RIF.

One of the most constant aspects of tuberculosis epidemiology has been the dictum that 90% of cases arise in persons previously infected. Recent studies utilizing DNA fingerprinting for tracking infection by the same strain reveal that 33% or more of tuberculosis cases in several areas represent recent infection. By the same technique, HIV-infected patients have been shown to be at high risk for reinfection with new organisms that may be responsible for apparent relapses.

TRANSMISSION AND IMMUNOPATHOGENESIS

Tuberculosis in humans is caused by infection with one of four closely related mycobacterial species that collectively make up the *M. tuberculosis* complex of organisms, which includes *M. tuberculosis, M. bovis, M. africanum,* and the bacillus Calmette-Guérin (BCG), which is a modified strain of *M. bovis. M. microti,* the vole bacillus, is an infrequently encountered mycobacterial species that is also included in the *M. tuberculosis* complex by some mycobacteriologists but does not cause disease in humans.

In the United States, tuberculosis caused by the *M. tuberculosis* complex of mycobacteria is almost always caused by infection with *M. tuberculosis.* However, in this country *M. bovis* has not been completely eliminated as a cause of tuberculosis, and in third world nations, where the pasteurization of milk is less common, *M. bovis* is a prominent source of tuberculosis morbidity. In rare

instances, the administration of BCG to victims of bladder cancer and HIV-infected persons has led to reported tuberculosis outbreaks. Cases of tuberculosis in patients from equatorial Africa caused by *M. africanum* were initially reported in 1969 and are presumed to be spread via airborne transmission.

Infection with *M. tuberculosis* is almost exclusively spread from person to person by airborne transmission. The studies of Riley clearly demonstrated airborne transmission of *M. tuberculosis* from humans to guinea pigs, and Houk's studies of an airborne tuberculosis outbreak on the USS Richard E. Byrd strongly support this principle.

Tiny particles containing tubercle bacilli (droplet nuclei), 1 to 5 μm in size and enveloped in an aerosol droplet, are expelled into the air primarily when someone with pulmonary or laryngeal tuberculosis coughs or sneezes. These microscopic infectious particles can remain suspended in air for extended periods of time (several hours). If a new host inhales the air contaminated by these droplet nuclei, transmission may occur. Larger particles fall out of suspension and are deposited on the mucociliary escalator lining the airways and are simply expectorated or swallowed. Smaller droplet nuclei are not deposited on the airway mucosa but are transported by air currents primarily to the periphery of the lower lung zones and deposited on the surfaces of alveoli, where they may be ingested by alveolar macrophages and destroyed, or, as happens in certain instances, the tubercle bacillus may multiply.

Following inhalation, any one of several outcomes is possible. The tubercle bacillus can be eliminated immediately (no infection) or can remain dormant in the host indefinitely (infection without disease), as occurs in the majority (90%) of persons, who are free of disease but remain infected with *M. tuberculosis* for the rest of their lives. The organism can immediately or rapidly cause tuberculosis (primary tuberculosis), as occurs in approximately 5% of persons, in whom tuberculosis develops in the first or second year following infection. Finally, the tubercle bacillus can cause disease many years after infection has occurred (recrudescent tuberculosis), as occurs in approximately 5% of patients. Thus, disease develops at some point during their lifetime in only about 10% of persons infected with *M. tuberculosis.*

Despite recent advances in molecular biology that have greatly increased our knowledge of the immunopathogenesis of tuberculosis, the complex interactions (checks and balances) that occur between the tubercle bacillus and the human immune system remain incompletely understood. Lurie's studies on the histopathology of tuberculosis using immune-competent and immune-incompetent rabbit models were seminal. Dannenberg's subsequent observations, based on Lurie's work, pointed out the importance of the interaction between delayed-type hypersensitivity (DTH) and cell-mediated immunity (CMI) in determining what form tuberculosis takes and greatly aided our understanding of these complex events. Dannenberg proposed that both CMI and DTH inhibit growth of *M. tuberculosis.* CMI enhances the ability of macrophages to destroy tubercle bacilli, causing little tissue damage, whereas DTH destroys nonactivated macrophages that are laden with tubercle bacilli, causing tissue damage. Nardell, in a review of Dannenberg's analysis of the pathogenesis of tuberculosis, outlines four stages (Fig. 3): onset, logarithmic growth, immunologic control, and liquifaction.

Stage 1: Onset

Following ingestion of droplet nuclei by nonspecifically but highly activated alveolar macrophages, the mycobacterial inoculum is either destroyed (90%) or inhibited or may multiply, depending on the innate mycobacteridal ability of the macrophage and the innate resistance of the tubercle bacilli to the defenses of the host.

Stage 2: Logarithmic Growth

Intracellular multiplication of tubercle bacilli occurs when the innate mycobactericidal ability of the macrophage is inadequate to destroy the initial inoculum of mycobacteria. *M. tuberculosis* organisms not destroyed by alveolar macrophages are released when the macrophages die and lyse, attracting inactivated monocytes from the bloodstream to form an early primary tubercle

(initial granuloma formation). Although these monocytes are capable of ingesting the released tubercle bacilli, they do not have the ability to destroy them or inhibit their growth, which increases logarithmically during this stage (7 to 21 days).

Stage 3: Immunologic Control

By 3 weeks, CMI and DTH have developed, as can be demonstrated by intradermal injection of purified protein derivative (PPD), resulting in tuberculin reactivity at 48 to 72 hours. During stage 3, tubercle bacilli have multiplied in many of the inactivated macrophages to a number far in excess of what can be destroyed by immune cellular mechanisms (CMI), and only cytotoxic lymphocytes carrying the CD8 marker (DTH) can limit further logarithmic growth by killing the *M. tuberculosis*-laden macrophages. The destruction of these tubercle bacilli results in the formation of the caseous necrotic center of the granuloma. This necrotic, soft, cheeselike center is surrounded by an accumulation of partially and highly activated macrophages and lymphocytes that have organized to form a granuloma.

The tubercle bacillus is an obligate aerobe and is unable to multiply in solid necrotic granulomas, which contain toxic fatty acids and are very acidic and anoxic. The organism either dies or becomes dormant. Tubercle bacilli that are released from destroyed macrophages within the granuloma are also ingested and destroyed during stage

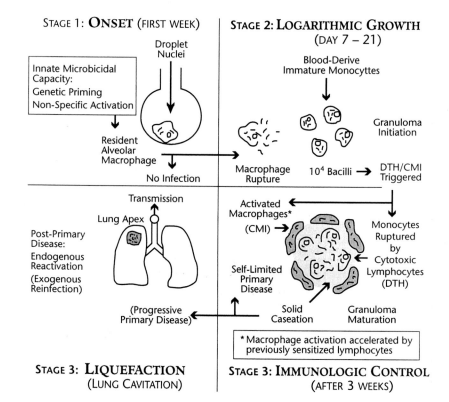

FIG. 3. Four stages in the pathogenesis of tuberculosis in the normal host. See text for detailed description. (From Nardell 1993, with permission. Based on Dannenberg 1991.)

3 by highly activated macrophages that are specifically activated by helper T lymphocytes (Th1 subset).

Released tubercle bacilli as well as those in infected macrophages are transported via peribronchial lymphatic channels to regional lymph nodes. If infection is not contained (stage 4), ultimately it spreads to the hilar and mediastinal lymph node chains, from which entrance to the systemic circulation via the thoracic duct is possible.

Stage 4: Liquifaction (Lung Cavitation)

The causes of liquifaction are incompletely understood; however, the release of hydrolytic enzymes that liquefy solid caseum and DTH to tuberculin proteins are thought to be contributing factors. Liquifaction of the solid, necrotic, caseous center of the granuloma kills macrophages but provides a favorable environment for abundant multiplication of tubercle bacilli. The large antigenic load that is created triggers a DTH response, causing extensive tissue damage. Erosion of the liquefied caseous material into adjacent airways, lymphatics, and blood vessels leads to pulmonary spread via the bronchial tree and extrapulmonary spread by lymph and hematogenous dissemination.

Immunologic Mechanisms

Several cell types—including helper (CD4) T cells (subsets Th1 and Th2), cytotoxic (CD8) T cells, and $\gamma\delta$ T cells as well as natural killer (NK) cells, alveolar macrophages, and monocytes—play an important role in regulating CMI and DTH. However, the actual roles that these cells play in producing and regulating the various cytokines, the most important of which include interleukin-2 (IL-2), tumor necrosis factor (TNF), and interferon-γ (INF-γ), is not well understood.

DIAGNOSIS

Clinical Presentation

Important components of a complete diagnostic evaluation for tuberculosis are an accurate medical history and physical examination. Particular care should be taken in determining tuberculosis exposure, prior treatment for the disease, concurrent medical problems, including HIV infection, and use of medications that affect host immunity.

The presenting symptoms of tuberculosis may differ depending on the site affected. In most cases—approximately 85%—the lung is the site of disease, and respiratory symptoms predominate. The clinical presentation of pulmonary tuberculosis may include nonspecific cough, chest pain, and hemoptysis. At its onset, the cough is usually nonproductive but persistent, and it may become productive of mucopurulent or blood-streaked sputum; occasionally hemoptysis can be moderate to severe. Chest pain may occur and often is described as dull and aching or pleuritic in nature. The latter may frequently be associated with the presence of a pleural effusion. Dyspnea is an uncommon feature; when present, it is usually caused by extensive parenchymal disease or a large pleural effusion.

Chills, fever, night sweats, fatigue, and loss of appetite and weight are systemic symptoms consistent with both pulmonary and extrapulmonary tuberculosis. Approximately 15% of tuberculosis cases are extrapulmonary (the percentage is higher when coinfection with HIV is present). The clinical symptoms of extrapulmonary tuberculosis also depend on the site affected. Headache, back pain, swelling of the neck, and blood in the urine may be the presenting symptoms in patients with tuberculosis of the central nervous system, spine, lymph nodes, and kidneys, respectively.

Unfortunately, in elderly patients many of the classic clinical features that many physicians rely on to diagnose tuberculosis may be absent. Frequently in this group, symptoms are nonspecific or atypical. The presence of concurrent illnesses, such as chronic obstructive pulmonary disease (COPD) or lung cancer, in an elderly person may obscure the diagnosis of tuberculosis, delaying therapy, or tuberculosis may be completely missed, only to be found at autopsy. The physical examination may provide important information regarding the patient's overall medical condition and guide the physician in choosing appropriate diagnostic and therapeutic approaches.

Tuberculin Skin Testing

The tuberculin skin test is a useful diagnostic test for evaluating persons who have symptoms of tuberculosis or who are suspected of being infected with *M. tuberculosis*. It is the standard test for detecting tuberculosis infection before progression to disease occurs. The tuberculin test may also be of particular assistance in evaluating patients with extrapulmonary tuberculosis, who may have normal findings on chest roentgenograms.

A negative tuberculin skin test reaction *never* excludes the diagnosis of tuberculosis. Normally, a period of 2 to 10 weeks is required after infection for a DTH response to tuberculin to develop. Infants <6 months of age may have a false-negative tuberculin skin test reaction because their immune systems have not yet fully developed. False-negative tuberculin skin test reactions may occur in persons with severe illness, HIV infection, sarcoidosis, and uremia, and in those receiving therapy with immunosuppressive drugs.

Overall, approximately 10%–25% of person with tuberculosis will have a false-negative reaction when given a tuberculin skin test. Although infected with *M. tubercu-*

losis, 30% of patients who are HIV-seropositive may have false-negative tuberculin skin tests (<5 mm) when tested. Thus, a positive tuberculin skin test reaction supports the diagnostic possibility that a suspected illness is tuberculosis; however, a negative tuberculin skin test reaction by no means excludes the diagnosis of tuberculosis.

Two preparations, purified protein derivative (PPD) and to a much lesser extent old tuberculin (OT), are currently used clinically. Robert Koch in 1890 first used the filtered and concentrated heat-sterilized broth in which tubercle bacilli had been grown as a therapeutic agent, and designated the concentrated extract *old tuberculin.* OT was later adopted as a diagnostic tool but proved to be a crude, nonspecific preparation containing extraneous antigenic substances that caused skin test reactions that were not always diagnostic of infection with *M. tuberculosis.* In the United States, OT is used primarily as an antigen in multiple puncture screening tests, in which the exact antigen dose introduced into the skin cannot be standardized. Therefore, these multiple puncture devices should not be used as diagnostic tests.

In the early 1930s, Florence Siebert isolated a protein from filtrates of OT, which she called *purified protein derivative.* PPD-S (Siebert's lot 49608) has subsequently been adopted as the international standard for purified protein derivative of mammalian tuberculin by the U.S. Public Health Service.

In the United States and Canada, the potency of PPD preparations is measured in tuberculin units (TU); a TU is defined as 0.00002 mg of PPD-S. The dose that best separates true-positives from false-positives is the 5-TU (standard in the United States) dose of prepared PPD, which produces a skin reaction equivalent in size to one produced by using PPD-S, regardless of the actual amount of tuberculin used. Because tuberculin is absorbed by glass and plastics, a detergent, Tween 80, has been added to prevent loss of potency of tuberculin during storage.

The standard for diagnosing infection with mammalian tubercle bacilli is the Mantoux test, performed by the intracutaneous injection of 0.1 mL of Tween-stabilized liquid PPD into the dorsal or volar surface of the forearm. In 48 to 72 hours, the area of induration (not erythema) is measured and recorded in millimeters. If a delay occurs in reading, a positive test reaction, if present, may be valid up to 1 week following placement of a Mantoux test. A negative test reaction must be confirmed by 72 hours.

A Mantoux skin test reaction size of ≥5 mm is interpreted as positive in the following cases:

1. Persons having or suspected of having HIV infection
2. Close contacts of a person with infectious tuberculosis
3. Persons with abnormal chest radiographic findings suggestive of old healed tuberculosis who have not been previously appropriately treated

4. Persons who inject drugs and whose HIV status is unknown

A tuberculin skin test reaction size of ≥10 mm is considered positive in the following cases:

1. Persons with certain medical conditions, excluding HIV infection
2. Persons who inject drugs (if HIV-negative)
3. Medically underserved, low-income populations, including racial and ethnic groups at high risk
4. Residents of long-term care facilities
5. Children <4 years of age
6. Locally identified high-prevalence groups (e.g., migrant farm workers or homeless persons)

A Mantoux skin test reaction of ≥15 mm is considered positive in all persons with no known risk factors for tuberculosis.

Anergy testing, although currently recommended by the U.S. Advisory Council for the Elimination of Tuberculosis (ACET) in the evaluation of immunosuppressed persons suspected of having tuberculosis but whose tuberculin skin test reaction is negative, is a controversial point. Recent studies suggest that anergy is a complex, unstable process that varies dramatically within short periods. A recent study of anergy in HIV-positive persons found that the degree of anergy was best defined by the helper lymphocyte count. Clearly, to recommend routine evaluation of CD4 counts and placement of antigens, such as mumps virus or *Candida,* in all immunosuppressed patients who are suspected of being anergic, adds substantially to patient care cost without evidence of definite benefit. Anergy testing should not be used for individual patient decisions.

Roentgenographic Examination

Historically, the chest roentgenograph has been an important diagnostic tool in evaluating patients, particularly for pulmonary tuberculosis. The chest x-ray film can be used to rule out tuberculosis in a person with a positive tuberculin skin test reaction and no symptoms of tuberculosis. A posteroanterior projection is the standard view needed for the detection of chest abnormalities. Lateral, lordotic, oblique, and decubitus views may be helpful, depending on the location or nature of the suspected lesion.

In some instances, newer imaging techniques, such as computed tomography (CT), may be helpful. CT of the chest is particularly helpful in evaluating hilar and mediastinal adenopathy, pleural effusion, and calcifications of the visceral and parietal pleural surfaces, and may also be helpful in evaluating patients with extrapulmonary tuberculosis. Tuberculosis involving the vertebrae, with paravertebral abscess formation, and lesions of the central nervous system may be evaluated using CT with or without contrast. Magnetic resonance imaging (MRI) may also be helpful in evaluating tuberculous lesions of the central nervous system.

Although certain abnormalities on chest x-ray films are highly suggestive of tuberculosis, it should be remembered that they are *never* diagnostic. Parenchymal infiltration and cavitation changes involving the apical or posterior segments of the upper lobes and less commonly the superior segments of the lower lobes are compatible with postprimary tuberculosis.

The manifestations of primary tuberculosis of the lungs include hilar and mediastinal adenopathy, pleural effusions, and infiltrates in the lower lung fields. However, the lung changes associated with pulmonary tuberculosis can vary and include consolidation (as occurs in endobronchial spread of disease) and miliary nodules, in addition to the previously described changes. Some elderly patients and those with HIV infection may have unusual chest x-ray findings, which may be normal or compatible with primary tuberculosis (adenopathy, lower lung infiltrates).

It has been reported that 60% of patients with advanced AIDS have hilar or mediastinal adenopathy, compared with 3% of non-AIDS patients; 29% have localized middle or lower lung field infiltrates, compared with 3% of non-AIDS controls; and 12% have normal chest x-ray findings, compared with none of the non-AIDS patients. In one study, none of the AIDS patients had chest cavitary lesions, compared with 67% of the non-AIDS patients, and 97% of the non-AIDS patients had upper lobe disease, compared with 18% of the AIDS patients.

Laboratory Evaluation

Specimen Collection

A joint statement of the American Thoracic Society (ATS), the CDC, and the Infectious Disease Society of America states that an important feature in the diagnostic evaluation for tuberculosis is ''. . . to obtain appropriate specimens for bacteriologic and histologic examination.'' Depending on the location of the disease, sputum, bronchial washings, lung tissue, lymph node tissue, bone marrow, liver, blood, urine, stool, and cerebrospinal fluid may be examined.

Because most cases of tuberculosis are pulmonary, examination of sputum is of primary importance. The yield of positive sputum smears in patients with pulmonary tuberculosis when three sputum specimens are collected has varied from approximately 50%–80%, depending on the study. The specificity of a positive smear has remained high (>99%). Some of the variability in studies reporting the sensitivity of positive sputum smears in patients with pulmonary tuberculosis may be explained by differing clinical presentations. In one review, 52% of patients with cavitary tuberculosis and only 32% of patients with local infiltrates had positive smears; similarly, only 45% of AIDS patients (noncavitary disease) with tuberculosis had positive sputum smears, compared with 81% of non-AIDS patients.

Patients who are suspected of having pulmonary tuberculosis should have 10 mL of an early morning sputum specimen submitted to an appropriate laboratory for smear and culture for tubercle bacilli. Several methods exist for obtaining specimens from patients who have difficulty producing sputum spontaneously (i.e., after inhalation of a saline aerosol). Transmission of tuberculosis, especially in HIV-infected populations, may occur in association with sputum induction, so special precautions should be taken by using portable hoods and sputum induction chambers that are appropriately vented. Gastric lavage fluid may be used for culture of tubercle bacilli but not smears as saprophytic mycobacteria are normally found in the stomach. Fiberoptic bronchoscopy with bronchoalveolar lavage (BAL) and/or biopsy has a high yield and may be useful in such patients or in those whose initial sputum specimens are negative for acid-fast bacilli (AFB) on smear. These procedures also may generate hazardous aerosols. The yield of bronchoscopy specimens in the demonstration of AFB is extremely high.

Invasive procedures beyond bronchoscopy to obtain diagnostic specimens are warranted when other techniques fail. Body fluid specimens should always be analyzed for differential cell count and glucose and protein content. In tuberculosis, lymphocytosis and elevated protein and low glucose levels are usually present in infected body fluid. Tissue biopsy (needle aspiration biopsy, transbronchial biopsy, biopsy of bone marrow, lung, liver) specimens should be divided and a portion sent to the laboratory for culture and another sample placed in formalin for histologic examination. Histologic changes characteristic of tuberculosis include granuloma formation and caseation necrosis.

Acid-Fast Bacillus Stains

Although far less sensitive than culture, the AFB smear is an important diagnostic aid for tuberculosis. AFB stains may be done quickly and provide the physician with the first preliminary confirmation of a clinical diagnosis of tuberculosis. AFB smears do not actually confirm tuberculosis, because nontuberculous mycobacteria and nonmycobacterial organisms such as *Nocardia* and some species of *Legionella* may produce positive stains.

The fluorescent staining technique that utilizes fluorochrome dyes (auramine/rhodamine) is now the preferred staining method for AFB. When the fluorochrome stain is viewed with fluorescence microscopy, AFB stain bright against a dark background and are more easily detected than when conventional AFB staining techniques are used. Because of the shortened amount of time needed to review a slide, fluorescent stains are considered more sensitive for detecting AFB. Until recently, the conventional Ziehl-Neelsen stain or one of its modifications, the Kinyoun stain, viewed under a light microscope were the conventional stains of choice for AFB, and positive smears correlated closely with infectiousness.

Mycobacterial Identification

Digestion and Decontamination

Sputum contains numerous microbes and various types of organic debris that interfere with mycobacterial growth on culture medium. Raw sputum specimens, therefore, must undergo a process of digestion and decontamination before being cultured for mycobacteria. The digestion and decontamination method most widely used in the United States utilizes N-acetyl-L-cysteine (NALC) and sodium hydroxide (NaOH). Raw sputum samples contain mucus and other proteinaceous materials that surround microbial contaminants and mycobacteria. NALC is used to liquify the debris that surrounds and protects these microbes from the decontamination effects of NaOH. Liquification of the debris also gives surviving mycobacteria freer access to the nutrients of the medium into which they are subsequently inoculated.

Raw sputum contains numerous bacteria that grow more rapidly (doubling time of <1 h) than tubercle bacilli (doubling time of 18 to 24 h), and these will quickly overgrow the mycobacteria if a raw sputum specimen is inoculated directly onto culture medium. To prevent this occurrence, decontamination of the raw specimen is accomplished by adding NaOH. Because of the high lipid content of the cell wall, mycobacterial growth is less inhibited by NaOH than is the growth of normal bacterial flora. However, some mycobacterial growth is inhibited by the chemical. Normally sterile fluids like blood, cerebrospinal fluid, and pleural fluid should therefore not be decontaminated for fear of further decreasing the small number of mycobacteria present.

Conventional Growth Techniques

Culture of specimens containing tubercle bacilli is a much more sensitive method of detecting mycobacteria than are direct smears. It is estimated that ≥10,000 AFB must be present per milliliter of sputum for a sputum smear to give a positive result, whereas a culture of sputum can detect as few as 10 AFB per milliliter of a digested, concentrated specimen. Culture of AFB also allows speciation of the organism and recognition of its drug susceptibility pattern.

Two types of solid media have traditionally been used:

an egg-based medium (Lowenstein-Jensen) and an agar-based medium (Middlebrook 7H10 and 7H11). A liquid medium (Dubos Oleic-Albumin) that requires incubation in 5%–10% carbon dioxide (CO_2) for 3 to 8 weeks is also available. The principal drawback to the use of solid culture media is that cultures grow slowly, and the process requires highly skilled personnel and is labor-intensive.

Because all mycobacterial strains cannot be grown on a single substrate, it is a common laboratory practice to inoculate both egg and agar media to obtain the initial isolate. Following growth of the mycobacteria, colony morphology, growth rate, and pigment production should be determined and tested biochemically to identify the organism completely. When sufficient mycobacterial growth has occurred, evaluation of colony morphology is helpful. Colonies of *M. tuberculosis* are typically rough with irregular edges when viewed on translucent Middlebrook 7H10 agar with a stereo-optic microscope.

Most mycobacteria, including *M. tuberculosis,* require >1 week for growth. Notable exceptions to this observation are the rapid growers, such as *M. fortuitum* complex, which often produces mature colonies on Lowenstein-Jensen media in 3 to 5 days, and *M. marinum* (5 to 7 days). *M. tuberculosis, M. avium* complex, and *M. fortuitum* usually do not have significant pigment and are buff-colored. This contrasts sharply with the highly pigmented (orange) scotochromogens, such as *M. scrofulaceum,* and the highly pigmented photochromogens, such as *M. kansasii* and *M. marinum,* which become bright yellow when exposed to light. The bacteriology of nontuberculous mycobacteria is discussed in Chapter 29.

Nearly 99% of the strains of *M. tuberculosis* are niacin-positive. However, some strains of *M. simiae* and *M. kansasii* may also be niacin-positive. In biochemical testing, the combination of a positive niacin test, positive nitrate reduction test, and negative heat-stable catalase test is diagnostic of *M. tuberculosis.*

The Bactec system is an automated radiometric culture method, introduced in the late 1970s, that can detect the growth of mycobacteria more quickly than can other conventional culture methods using solid media. The system uses a liquid Middlebrook 7H12 medium containing radiometric palmitic acid labeled with radioactive carbon (^{14}C). Growth of mycobacteria within the system is measured as a daily growth index that represents the production of carbon dioxide ($^{14}CO_2$) by the metabolizing organisms. The detection of ($^{14}CO_2$) allows early recognition of mycobacterial growth, even before there is visible evidence of growth. The growth of *M. tuberculosis* complex is inhibited by p-nitro-L-acetylamino-β-hydroxypropiophenone (NAP), but NAP does not impede the growth of nontuberculous mycobacteria. When an increase in the growth index indicates that AFB are growing in a Bactec system, confirmation by a positive stain of the specimen is usually carried out. Samples of the specimen can then be subcultured in Bactec bottles with and without NAP. If the growth index value of each Bactec bottle is monitored daily, it is easy to tell whether *M. tuberculosis* complex or nontuberculous bacteria are growing in the sample. Results are usually available in 5 to 7 days.

DNA Probe

A significant advancement in the ability to identify mycobacteria rapidly and precisely occurred in the late 1980s, when nucleic acid hybridization assays were introduced. A complementary DNA (cDNA) probe is labeled with acridinium ester as a detector, and most commonly is directed at ribosomal RNA (rRNA) of the target mycobacteria in the sample. When the cDNA probe reacts with the target rRNA, a DNA-RNA hybrid is formed, producing light (chemiluminescent assay) that can be measured with a luminometer. This detection method is very sensitive; chemiluminescence is 10^6-fold more sensitive than fluorescence. Commercially available probes can react specifically with *M. tuberculosis* complex, *M. avium, M. intracellulare, M. kansasii, M. gordonae,* and *M. avium-intracellulare* complex. The sensitivities and specificities of these assays are >95% for these species.

At least 10^5 to 10^6 organisms must be present for best results; thus, the probes require cultures. A DNA probe can be completed in a matter of hours and can be used in combination with the Bactec system. When an increase in the growth index is noted in a Bactec system, a sample of the broth culture medium is stained, and if AFB are observed, a DNA probe is performed on the medium. It is estimated that by using this method the time required for identification of *M. tuberculosis* can be reduced to 1 to 2 weeks.

Both high-performance liquid chromatography (HPLC) and gas-liquid chromatography are used to identify mycobacterial species, with HPLC perhaps enjoying wider use. However, although HPLC provides a rapid and sensitive means of detecting mycobacteria, this technique has been used preferentially in level III reference laboratories because of its high cost. Because substantial growth of the mycobacteria is required for analysis, HPLC is not applicable for direct detection of mycobacteria in clinical specimens. HPLC is based on the observation that each species of mycobacteria produces specific fatty acids in its cell wall. These mycolic acids are extracted from the cell wall and methylated to form a methyl ester; when analyzed by chromatography, the methyl ester produces a characteristic pattern that can be used to differentiate the various species of mycobacteria. This test provides a specific diagnosis for most species in <4 hours. Detection of tuberculostearic acid by gas-liquid chromatography has proved to be a very sensitive and rapid method of detecting *M. tuberculosis* and may be particularly useful in the diagnosis of tuberculous meningitis. However, this test is still in a developmental stage.

Drug Susceptibility Testing

A drug susceptibility test should be obtained for all initial isolates, and whenever patient response to treatment is inadequate or cultures remain positive for ≥2 months after initiation of treatment. Drug susceptibility testing may be performed using the conventional method or Bactec system; both methods have advantages and disadvantages.

Conventional Method

The conventional method for drug susceptibility testing uses solid media (Middlebrook-Cohn 7H10) that can be impregnated with antituberculosis drugs, depending on the desired test. The proportion method is most commonly used in the United States. An isolate of *M. tuberculosis* is considered drug-resistant if the number of colonies on the drug-containing medium is >1% of the number of colonies on the drug-free control plate.

Direct and Indirect Methods

Drug susceptibility tests can be carried out directly or indirectly. A direct test can be performed on a digested and decontaminated specimen with a smear positive for AFB. A direct test provides results faster (21 days) and gives a truer picture of the population of mycobacteria in the isolate.

Indirect tests are usually performed when the smear of the clinical specimen is negative for AFB or when significant contamination with pyogenic bacteria or other non-AFB is present. The inoculum for indirect drug susceptibility tests is obtained from the culture of the initial isolate. When indirect tests are performed, there is a risk of inadvertently selecting a predominant population of susceptible or resistant mycobacteria that are not truly representative of the population of organisms in the isolate that is being subcultured. This bias may be lessened by preparing a dilution of the entire subcultured population of mycobacteria. Because it is more difficult to avoid contamination and adjust the inoculum size when using the Bactec system, conventional drug susceptibility testing using solid media is the suggested method for performing direct drug susceptibility testing. The Bactec system (see above) is more applicable to indirect drug susceptibility testing using solid culture media or Bactec broth media. The Bactec method is best suited for testing first-line drugs and is preferable for pyrazinamide (PZA) testing. PZA susceptibility testing requires a very low pH (5.5) in conventional solid media, which prevents the growth of some strains of *M. tuberculosis*.

Newer Laboratory Methods

Polymerase Chain Reaction

The polymerase chain reaction (PCR) is a laboratory method for amplification of the amount of DNA in a specimen. The technique can be used on raw (uncultured) clinical specimens and theoretically is capable of detecting a single mycobacterium in a biologic sample. The process requires initial denaturation of double-stranded DNA by heating the specimen. Highly specific oligonucleotide primers—synthetic, short, single-stranded DNA probes—are added and attach only to cDNA sequences of the target mycobacteria. A DNA polymerase then enzymatically extends the primers to make a complete strand of cDNA. Multiple cycles of this process repeated sequentially create millions of identical copies of target DNA sequences of mycobacteria. These markers are specific for *M. tuberculosis* complex or other species of mycobacteria and can be detected by gel electrophoresis. If the target mycobacteria are absent from the sample, the primer has nothing to bind to, and amplification of the target DNA sequence does not occur. Although available in many laboratories, PCR is so far not generally used for the routine diagnosis of tuberculosis. It is highly sensitive, and contamination must be rigorously controlled. However, it is a promising tool for the rapid diagnosis of tuberculosis and may prove to be particularly helpful in the diagnosis of smear-negative tuberculosis.

Ligase Chain Reaction

Like PCR, ligase chain reaction (LCR) is a recently developed target amplification system used for the detection of species of mycobacteria. In research laboratories, the test has been demonstrated to have very high sensitivity and specificity and can be performed rapidly. However, it is still in the developmental stage.

Restriction Fragment Length Polymorphism or DNA Fingerprinting

DNA fingerprinting is not a diagnostic test but is a recently developed epidemiologic tool used primarily to evaluate the transmission of tuberculosis and identify cross-contamination of specimens within the laboratory. Restriction fragment length polymorphism (RFLP) subtypes strains of mycobacteria by fragmenting target DNA from *M. tuberculosis* with restriction enzymes (endonucleases) that recognize specific sequences and cut DNA into fragments of varying length. Cloned mycobacterial DNA (IS6110) probes are used to hybridize the fragments, which produce specific electrophoretic patterns and can be compared from strain to strain.

Luciferase Reporter Phages

A functional assay for the rapid assessment of drug-resistant mycobacteria using luciferase reporter phages has been recently developed but has not yet been tested clinically. This system can provide susceptibility results within 18 to 24 hours after a culture containing ≥ 1 million mycobacteria has been obtained.

The assay involves placing the firefly gene for the production of luciferase into mycobacteriophages that then infect *M. tuberculosis*, introducing the firefly luciferase gene into the tubercle bacillus. Luciferin is added to the system and the activity of luciferase is monitored. Luciferase in the presence of adenosine triphosphate oxidizes luciferin to oxyluciferin, resulting in the production of light that can be measured in a luminometer. If an antituberculosis drug is added to the system, drug-resistant strains continue to produce light, whereas drug-susceptible strains do not.

Adenosine Deaminase

Adenosine deaminase is an enzyme produced by macrophages and activated T lymphocytes. Levels of adenosine deaminase have been reported in various studies to be present in increased amounts in several different body fluids infected with *M. tuberculosis*. Clinical value is still not clear.

SCREENING

In the United States, screening is a valuable method for controlling and ultimately eliminating tuberculosis. Screening should be performed only in selected, high-risk populations to identify infected persons who would benefit from therapy to prevent the development of tuberculosis, and to identify persons with active tuberculosis who should be treated to prevent transmission. Table 3 lists high-risk groups of people for whom screening is indicated. Groups not at high risk for tuberculosis should not be routinely screened because of cost and low yield;

TABLE 3. *Groups that should be screened with the tuberculosis skin test*

Persons with or at risk for HIV infection
Close contacts of persons with infectious tuberculosis
Persons with certain medical conditions
Persons who inject drugs
Foreign-born persons from areas where tuberculosis is common
Medically underserved, low-income populations, including high-risk racial and ethnic groups
Residents of long-term care facilities
Locally identified high-prevalence groups (e.g., migrant farm workers or homeless persons)

false-positive reactions may lead to inappropriate preventive treatment.

Screening in most instances is carried out by health departments or health care providers affiliated with drug treatment centers, long-term care facilities, correctional institutions, and hospitals. However, all primary health care providers should be aware of the high-risk persons in their practices and should administer skin tests to these patients as part of their routine medical evaluations.

The Mantoux tuberculin skin test is the preferred method of screening for tuberculosis infection. However, to identify tuberculosis in specific settings where the risk of transmission is very high and/or the stay is short (conjugate settings such as homeless shelters, hospitals, and jails), intake screening with chest roentgenograms or sputum smears may be more appropriate. Tuberculin screening in institutional settings provides baseline information on the tuberculin skin test status of clients and staff, identifies candidates for preventive therapy, and detects whether transmission of tuberculosis is occurring within the facility.

Tuberculosis screening is recommended for residents of long-term care facilities. It is also recommended for staff members, who may be exposed to patients with tuberculosis on the job, or who would pose a significant risk to large numbers of susceptible persons if they became infectious with tuberculosis disease (e.g., staff of AIDS wards or child care centers). These people should be screened on entry or beginning of employment and at least yearly thereafter, depending on the risk for transmis-

TABLE 4. *First-line drugs*

Drug[b]	Dose in mg/kg[a] (maximum dose)					
	Daily		Two times weekly[c]		Three times weekly[c]	
	Children[d]	Adults	Children[d]	Adults	Children[d]	Adults
INH	10–20 (300 mg)	5 (300 mg)	20–40 (900 mg)	15 (900 mg)	20–40 (900 mg)	15 (900 mg)
RIF	10–20 (600 mg)	10 (600 mg)	10–20 (600 mg)	10 (600 mg)	10–20 (600 mg)	10 (600 mg)
PZA	15–30 (2 g)	15–30 (2 g)	50–70 (4 g)	50–70 (4 g)	50–70 (3 g)	50–70 (3 g)
EMB	15–25	15–25	50	50	25–30	25–30
SM	20–40 (1 g)	15 (1 g)	25–30 (1.5 g)	25–30 (1.5 g)	25–30 (1.5 g)	25–30 (1.5 g)

Source: Centers for Disease Control, 1994.
INH, isoniazid; RIF, rifampin; PZA, pyrazinamide; EMB, ethambutol; SM, streptomycin.
[a] Weight-based dosage should be adjusted as weight changes.
[b] Fixed-dose combinations of INH, RIF, PZA, Rifater® or INH, RIF (Rifamate®) should be used when treatment is not directly observed.
[c] All regimens administered two or three times weekly should be used with DOT (directly observed therapy).
[d] Children, <12 years old.

sion in a particular facility. For persons who are screened periodically (e.g., staff of tuberculosis clinics), a two-step Mantoux skin test procedure should be used for initial skin testing.

Two-Step Mantoux Skin Testing

DTH to tuberculin tends to wane with aging. Persons who are given a tuberculin skin test many years after their initial infection with *M. tuberculosis* may have a negative reaction. However, that skin test may boost or recall their DTH response to tuberculin, causing a positive reaction to a subsequent test that may be misinterpreted as a skin test conversion.

A two-step Mantoux skin test should be used for the initial testing of elderly patients and adults who will be retested periodically as follows:

1. If the first test result is negative, give a second test 1 to 3 weeks later.

2. If the second test result is positive, consider that the person is infected with the tubercle bacillus but is not a skin test converter. If the second result is negative, consider the person uninfected with the tubercle bacillus.

3. Any positive reaction to a subsequent test is considered a conversion.

TREATMENT

More than a quarter of a century ago, Dr. Wallace Fox stated that effective chemotherapy and patient coopera-

for tuberculosis

Adverse reactions	Monitoring	Comments
Hepatic enzyme elevation Hepatitis Peripheral neuropathy Mild effects on central nervous system Drug interactions	Baseline measurements of hepatic enzymes for adults Repeat measurements • if baseline results are abnormal • if patient is at high risk for adverse reactions • if patient has symptoms of adverse reactions	Hepatitis risk increases with age and alcohol consumption Pyridoxine can prevent peripheral neuropathy
GI upset Drug interactions Hepatitis Bleeding problems Flulike symptoms Rash	Baseline CBC measurements for adults • CBC and platelets • hepatic enzymes Repeat measurements • if baseline results are abnormal • if patient has symptoms of adverse reactions	Significant interactions with • methadone • birth control pills • many other drugs Colors body fluids orange May permanently discolor soft contact lenses
Hepatitis Rash GI upset Joint aches Hyperuricemia Gout (rare)	Baseline measurements for adults • uric acid • hepatic enzymes Repeat measurements • if baseline results are abnormal • if patient has symptoms of adverse reactions	Treat hyperuricemia only if patient has symptoms
Optic neuritis	Baseline and monthly tests • visual acuity • color vision	Not recommended for children too young to be monitored for changes in vision unless TB is drug-resistant
Ototoxicity (hearing loss or vestibular dysfunction) Renal toxicity	Baseline and repeat as needed • hearing • kidney function	Avoid or reduce dose in adults >60 years old

TABLE 5. *Second-line drugs for tuberculosis*

Drug[a]	Daily dose[b] (maximum dose)	Adverse reactions	Monitoring	Comments[c]
CM	15–30 mg/kg (1 g)	Toxicity • auditory • vestibular • renal	Assess • vestibular function • hearing function Measure • blood urea nitrogen	After bacteriologic conversion, dosage may be reduced to 2–3 times per week
KM	15–30 mg/kg (1 g)	Toxicity • auditory • vestibular • renal	Assess • vestibular function • hearing function Measure • blood urea nitrogen • creatinine	After bacteriologic conversion, dosage may be reduced to 2–3 times per week
ETA	15–20 mg/kg (1 g)	GI upset Hepatotoxicity Hypersensitivity Metallic taste Bloating	Measure hepatic enzymes	Start with low dosage and increase as tolerated May cause hypothyroid condition, especially if used with PAS
PAS	150 mg/kg (12 g)	GI upset Hypersensitivity Hepatotoxicity Sodium load	Measure hepatic enzymes Assess volume status	Start with low dosage and increase as tolerated Monitor cardiac patients for sodium load
CS	15–20 mg/kg (1 g)	Psychosis Convulsions Depression Headaches Rash Drug interactions	Assess mental status Measure serum drug levels	Start with low dosage and increase as tolerated Pyridoxine may decrease CNS effects
Ciprofloxacin	500–1000 mg/d	GI upset Dizziness Hypersensitivity Drug interactions Headaches Restlessness	Drug interactions	Not approved by FDA for TB treatment Should not be used in children Avoid • antacids • iron • zinc • sucralfate
Ofloxacin	400–800 mg/d	GI upset Dizziness Hypersensitivity Drug interactions Headaches Restlessness	Drug interactions	Not approved by FDA for TB treatment Should not be used in children Avoid • antacids • iron • zinc • sucralfate
Amikacin	15 mg/kg	Renal toxicity Vestibular dysfunction Hearing loss Chemical imbalance Dizziness	Assess • hearing function Measure • renal function • serum drug levels	Not approved by FDA for TB treatment
Clofazimine	100–300 mg/d	GI upset Discoloration of skin Severe abdominal pain and organ damage caused by crystal deposition	Drug interactions	Not approved by FDA for TB treatment Avoid sunlight Consider dosing at mealtime Efficacy unproved

Source: Centers for Disease Control, 1994.

CM, capreomycin; KM, kanamycin; ETA, ethionamide; PAS, para-amino salicyclic acid; CS, cycloserine.

[a] These drugs should be used only in consultation with a clinician experienced in the management of drug-resistant TB.

[b] Doses for children are the same as for adults. Weight-based dosage should be adjusted as weight changes.

[c] Other drugs: Rifabutin and clarithromycin are not FDA-approved for the treatment of *M. tuberculosis* complex. However, use as second-line drugs may be helpful in the treatment of multidrug-resistant TB when drug susceptibility tests demonstrate sensitivity of the infecting *M. tuberculosis* strain.

tion in taking prescribed medications were important factors influencing the success of a tuberculosis treatment program. The passage of time has borne out the accuracy of his observations.

Current principles on which recommendations for treatment are based include (1) the use of multiple drugs to which the tubercle bacilli are sensitive, (2) continuation of treatment for a period of time that is sufficient to control and usually eradicate the disease, and (3) regular ingestion of medications by the patient.

Two-Phase Chemotherapy

Multiple drugs are used to treat primary resistance present at the inception of therapy, or to prevent the emergence of acquired drug resistance. The concept of initiating treatment with multiple drugs is based on the fact that tuberculosis may occur from infection with initially resistant strains of *M. tuberculosis*. In addition, at the initiation of treatment of cavitary pulmonary tuberculosis, a large population ($>10^8$ bacilli) of mycobacteria is present, with the potential for spontaneous emergence of resistant strains. These mutants can be resistant to any of the antituberculosis drugs, but resistance occurs more frequently with some drugs than with others.

It is estimated that the frequency of mutations resistant to INH and streptomycin (SM) in populations of *M. tuberculosis* is approximately 1 in 1 million (1 in 10^6), and for mutations resistant to RIF it is 1 in 100 million bacilli (1 in 10^8). Therefore, mutants resistant to both INH and RIF given at the same time would occur approximately once in a population of 10^{14} organisms. By giving initial chemotherapy with two or more drugs, the likelihood of drug resistant bacilli surviving in the bacterial population is extremely small.

Drug Treatment

After multiple drug therapy has been started, the second principle of treatment is to ensure that therapy is continued for a sufficient period of time. Prolonged therapy is necessary to eliminate persistent bacilli and prevent relapse of tuberculosis.

Before the introduction of RIF or currently when RIF is not used in a treatment regimen, 18 to 24 months of treatment are required to ensure a cure of tuberculosis. However, using multidrug regimens currently available that contain INH, RIF, and PZA, treatment can be completed in as short a period as 6 months, and trials for even shorter courses of chemotherapy are under way.

Chemotherapy is divided into an initial bactericidal phase, in which INH is the most effective drug, followed by a sterilizing phase, during which RIF and PZA are the most effective drugs. INH has its greatest effect against actively dividing tubercle bacilli, and PZA exhibits its greatest effect on organisms in an acid environment (tubercle bacilli ingested by macrophages). RIF is noted for the speed with which its bactericidal action starts, resulting in the selective killing of organisms that are largely dormant but have occasional short spurts of growth. Completely dormant mycobacteria are not killed by any drugs but may be eliminated by the host immune response.

Studies initiated by the British Medical Research Council and expanded by the U.S. Public Health Service, using 6 months of therapy with INH and RIF supplemented by PZA for the first 2 months, clearly established that short-course treatment regimens are both safe and effective.

Drugs available for the treatment of tuberculosis have been separated into "first-line" (Table 4) and "second-line" (Table 5) agents. The initial regimen for the treatment of tuberculosis consists of four drugs, including INH, RIF, PZA, and either ethambutol (EMB) or SM in communities where INH resistance is >4%. The treatment regimen can be adjusted as soon as drug susceptibility results are known.

In areas where INH resistance is <4%, an initial regimen of INH, RIF, and PZA may be used; alternatively, in very rare instances, a 9-month regimen containing INH and RIF may be used for those who cannot be treated with PZA. EMB or SM should be included in the treatment regimen until the results of drug susceptibility studies are known.

Patient adherence to a prescribed drug regimen is a major determinant of treatment success. The use of bus passes, vouchers, fixed drug combinations of demonstrated bioavailability, and other treatment incentives and enablers enhance patient adherence to a given drug regimen. Recent publications have emphasized the importance of directly observed therapy (DOT) in reducing tuberculosis case rates. DOT is the standard of care in the United States. Whenever possible, all patients should receive DOT. All intermittent regimens should be administered only under direct observation.

CASE 1: TUBERCULOSIS IN AN HIV-NEGATIVE PATIENT WITH SENSITIVE ORGANISMS

A 43-year-old African-American male bookbinder was admitted to the hospital with a productive cough of 3 months' duration, chest pain, fever, night sweats, easy fatigability, and weight loss of 10 lb. He denied having a known tuberculosis contact, had never had a tuberculin skin test, and stated that a findings on a chest roentgenogram taken 2 years previously were normal.

The patient was febrile (102°F), and crackles were heard over the posterior left lung base.

The admission chest x-ray films (Fig. 4) revealed volume loss with associated tracheal deviation and elevation

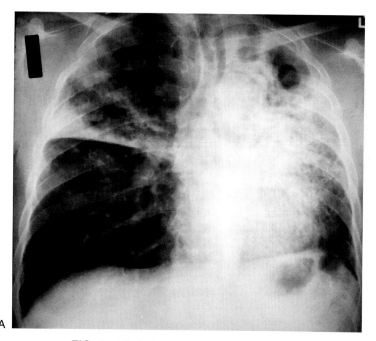
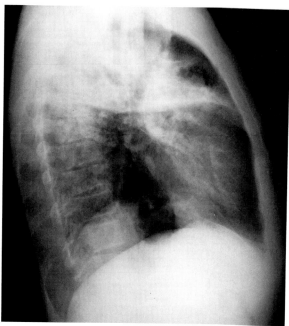

FIG. 4. Admission posteroanterior (**A**) and lateral (**B**) x-ray films of case 1. Note the volume loss and bilateral upper lobe infiltrates with a cavity in the left upper lobe.

of the left diaphragm, bilateral upper lobe infiltrates, and a large left upper lobe cavity. Laboratory findings included a negative HIV serology, a hemoglobin of 11.3 g/dL, and an erythrocyte sedimentation rate of 59 mm/h; three separate sputum specimens were reported positive on smear for AFB.

The patient was started on daily DOT with a four-drug regimen of 300 mg of INH, 600 mg of RIF, 1500 mg of

PZA, and 1200 mg of EMB. He tolerated the regimen well and after 1 week was continued on DOT five times weekly under the supervision of a trained field worker. On weekends he took a fixed-dose combination of INH, RIF, and PZA (Rifater) with EMB. All members of his immediate household (five people) were receiving preventive treatment with INH or therapy for active tuberculosis.

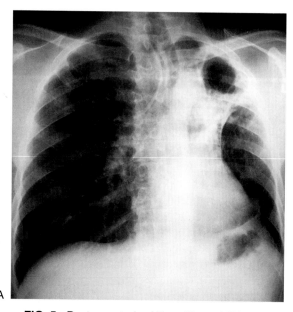
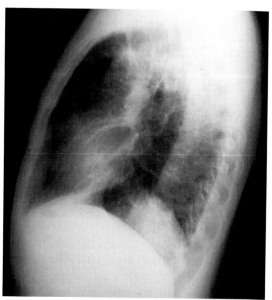

FIG. 5. Posteroanterior (**A**) and lateral (**B**) chest x-ray films of case 1 after the completion of treatment for tuberculosis. Note the clearing of disease in the right lung with residual cavitation and scarring in the left lung with volume loss.

After 8 weeks, *M. tuberculosis* isolated from the patient was reported sensitive to all first-line antituberculosis drugs (INH, RIF, PZA, EMB, and SM). At this point, PZA and EMB were discontinued and he was maintained on twice-weekly oral DOT with 900 mg of INH and 600 mg of RIF for an additional 16 weeks, after which all medications were discontinued. His compliance taking antituberculosis medications approached 100%. On discharge, he noted marked improvement in his symptoms and had regained approximately 25 lb; despite improvement, residual changes persist on his chest roentgenogram (Fig. 5).

COMMENT: This is a case of recrudescent, drug-sensitive tuberculosis in an HIV-seronegative patient that responded well to treatment. Unfortunately, the tubercle bacilli of this patient were transmitted to two of his children and his spouse, documenting the infectiousness of symptomatic cavitary tuberculosis. Despite appropriate treatment, he has significant residual lung damage.

TREATMENT OF SMEAR-NEGATIVE, CULTURE-NEGATIVE TUBERCULOSIS

Patients with smear- and culture-negative tuberculosis who are from areas where INH resistance is <4% and drug resistance is unlikely should be treated with a 4-month regimen of INH and RIF that is supplemented with PZA for the first 2 months. Patients with smear- and culture-negative tuberculosis who are from areas where INH resistance is ≥4% or who have personal risk factors for drug resistance should be treated with a 4-month regimen of 4 drugs including INH, RIF, PZA, and EMB or SM.

TREATMENT OF HIV-SEROPOSITIVE PERSONS

Current recommendations for treatment of tuberculosis in HIV-seropositive patients are the same as those for HIV-seronegative patients, with the caveat that treatment should be prolonged if the response is suboptimal. There have been isolated cases of relapse of tuberculosis in AIDS patients, and when this occurs in AIDS patients with drug-sensitive tuberculosis, malabsorption of medications, new infection with tubercle bacilli, or some other reason for apparent treatment failure should be suspected. We recommend longer treatment and follow-up until clinical studies determine the optimal duration.

TREATMENT OF EXTRAPULMONARY DISEASE

The basic principles that guide the selection and duration of treatment for pulmonary tuberculosis are generally the same as for extrapulmonary tuberculosis, in which 6- to 9-month short-course regimens have proved effective. Some exceptions are miliary tuberculosis, bone and joint tuberculosis, and tuberculous meningitis in infants and children, in whom treatment should be extended for at least 12 months. For diagnostic as well as therapeutic reasons, surgery may be more commonly required in extrapulmonary tuberculosis than in pulmonary tuberculosis. Corticosteroid therapy has also been of benefit in treating some forms of extrapulmonary tuberculosis, and in preventing neurologic problems associated with tuberculous meningitis and cardiac constriction in tuberculous pericarditis.

TREATMENT FAILURE AND RELAPSE

Patients whose sputum remains positive on culture after 4 to 6 months of treatment should be considered treatment failures. Unlike patients undergoing initial treatment, patients requiring retreatment frequently are nonadherent, and their infecting organisms are drug-resistant. Patient motivation to adhere to treatment and selection of effective therapeutic regimens are more difficult to control but extremely important in such a setting. A detailed history, including the duration and frequency of previous treatment and the drugs used, should be obtained, and prior tuberculosis treatment records and chest x-ray films should be reviewed whenever possible.

Most patients who relapse following treatment with short-course chemotherapy have fully sensitive organisms and can be retreated with INH and RIF. However, drug susceptibility testing is of paramount importance when a retreatment program is undertaken. While waiting for results, which are frequently delayed, the original drug regimen may be continued, or new treatment should be started with at least two, but preferably three, drugs to which the patient's organisms have known sensitivity or that the patient has not previously received. *A potentially effective new or previously used single drug should never be added to a failing or failed regimen!* If the susceptibility pattern is known and the addition is highly unlikely to cause resistance, adding a single drug may be considered.

INTERMITTENT TREATMENT

Intermittent therapy is effective and more readily supervised than daily therapy. Several methods of delivering intermittent regimens have been identified and are listed in Table 6. In general, with the exception of the RIF dose, which remains the same, the dose of all the first-line drugs is increased when they are given intermittently.

TREATMENT OF DRUG-RESISTANT TUBERCULOSIS

A 6-month regimen of RIF, PZA, and EMB or SM is adequate for treatment of tuberculosis that is known to

TABLE 6. Regimen options for treatment[a]

Option	Indication	Total duration, mo	Initial phase Drugs	Initial phase Interval and duration	Continuation phase Drugs	Continuation phase Interval and duration	Comments
1	Pulmonary and extrapulmonary TB in adults and children	6	INH RIF PZA EMB or SM	Daily for 8 weeks	INH RIF	Daily or 2 or 3 times per week[b] for 16 weeks[c]	EMB or SM should be continued until susceptibility to INH and RIF is demonstrated. In areas where primary INH resistance <4%, EMB or SM may not be necessary for patients with no individual risk factors for drug resistance.
2	Pulmonary and extrapulmonary TB in adults and children	6	INH RIF PZA EMB or SM	Daily for 2 weeks and then 2 times per week[b] for 16 weeks	INH RIF	2 times per week[b] for 16 weeks[c]	Regimen should be directly observed. After the initial phase, continue EMB or SM until susceptibility to INH and RIF is demonstrated, unless drug resistance is unlikely.
3	Pulmonary and extrapulmonary TB in adults and children	6	INH RIF PZA EMB or SM	3 times per week[b] for 6 months[c]	—	—	Regimen should be directly observed. Continue all four drugs for 6 months.[d] This regimen has been shown to be effective for INH-resistant TB.

Option	Indications		Initial drugs	Initial phase	Continuation drugs	Continuation phase	Comments
4	Smear- and culture-negative pulmonary TB in adults	4	INH RIF PZA EMB or SM	Follow option 1, 2, or 3 for 8 weeks	INH RIF PZA EMB or SM	Daily or 2 or 3 times per week[b] for 8 weeks	Continue all 4 drugs for 4 months. If drug resistance is unlikely (primary INH resistance <4% and patient has no individual risk factors for drug resistance), EMB or SM may not be necessary and PZA may be discontinued after 2 months.
5	Pulmonary and extrapulmonary TB in adults and children when PZA is contraindicated	9	INH RIF EMB or SM[e]	Daily for 8 weeks	INH RIF	Daily or 2 times per week[b] for 24 weeks[c]	EMB or SM should be continued until susceptibility to INH and RIF is demonstrated. In areas where primary INH resistance <4%, EMB or SM may not be necessary for patients with no individual risk factors for drug resistance.

Source: Centers for Disease Control, 1994.

[a] For all patients, if susceptibility results show resistance to any of the first-line drugs or if the patient remains symptomatic or smear or culture positive after 3 months, consult a TB medical expert.

[b] DOT should be used with all regimens administered two or three times weekly.

[c] For infants and children with miliary TB, bone and joint TB, or TB meningitis, treatment should last at least 12 months. For adults with these forms of extrapulmonary TB, response to therapy should be monitored closely. If response is slow or suboptimal, treatment may be prolonged as judged on a case-by-case basis.

[d] There is some evidence that SM may be discontinued after 4 months if the isolate is susceptible to all drugs.

[e] SM should not be prescribed for pregnant women because of the risk of ototoxicity to the fetus.

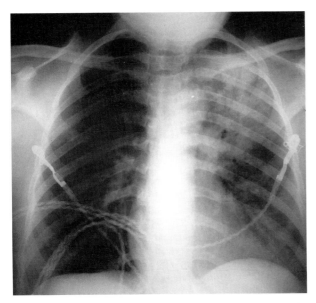

FIG. 6. Posteroanterior chest x-ray film of case 2 reveals a left upper lobe infiltrate.

be only INH-resistant. An acceptable alternative would be to treat with RIF and EMB for a minimum of 12 months. If for any reason RIF cannot be included in a treatment regimen, treatment should be continued for a minimum of 18 months. If resistance to PZA is demonstrated, treatment should be continued for a minimum of 9 months if INH and RIF are included in the regimen. Tuberculosis treatment in the face of resistance to EMB or SM only may not need to be prolonged but may require replacement of these two agents with second-line drugs.

MDRTB (i.e., tuberculosis resistant to at least INH and RIF) may be primary or secondary. Primary resistance is noted particularly in patients who are HIV-positive and have never had antimycobacterial treatment. Secondary resistance occurs in patients who have previously received treatment and whose infecting mycobacteria have acquired resistance to the antituberculosis medications previously given. MDRTB significantly complicates patient management and treatment, and treatment should be individualized based on the results of drug susceptibility tests and the patient's prior medication history.

When treating MDRTB, at least two and preferably three antituberculosis medications to which the organisms are susceptible should be used. Unfortunately, studies are not available that unequivocally establish the effectiveness and duration of various treatment regimens for MDRTB. In general, treatment should be continued with at least two drugs for a minimum of 18 to 24 months following culture conversion. Physicians unfamiliar with treatment of these patients should always seek expert consultation, as these are complicated, perhaps life-threatening situations, often with major significance to public health.

CASE 2: MULTIDRUG-RESISTANT TUBERCULOSIS

A 34-year-old African-American woman came to the hospital with fever and a persistent cough. Four years earlier, she had converted her tuberculin skin test but declined INH preventive treatment. Her chest roentgenogram revealed a left upper lobe pulmonary infiltrate (Fig. 6), and sputum smears were positive for AFB.

Treatment with INH, RIF, PZA, and SM was begun while awaiting identification of the AFB and the results of drug susceptibility tests. The patient's symptoms worsened and sputum cultures obtained monthly remained positive at 12 weeks, when the initial sputum studies identified *M. tuberculosis* resistant to INH, RIF, SM, and ethionamide (ETA). Her chest x-ray film taken at that time is seen in Fig. 7.

Directly supervised therapy during the next 9 months with various drug regimens comprising second-line drugs not previously used was not successful. Treatment failure may have been related to side effects of her medications, particularly gastrointestinal intolerance, that often led to discontinuation of one or another of the drugs, thus raising the possibility of monotherapy. Approximately 1 year after starting treatment, the patient remained stable but unimproved, with positive sputum cultures for *M. tuberculosis* on a drug regimen including PZA, EMB, rifabutin (RBT), cycloserine (CS), and capreomycin (CM).

At this point, the patient came to our center, where

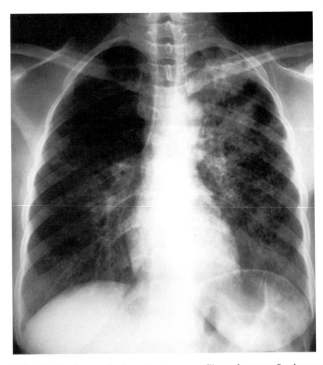

FIG. 7. Posteroanterior chest x-ray film of case 2 shows bilateral infiltrates with worsening of the infiltrate in the left lung.

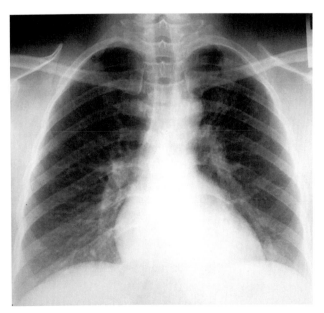

FIG. 8. Posteroanterior chest x-ray film of case 2 reveals residual scarring in the left lung after completion of treatment.

drug susceptibility tests were repeated and chest roentgenograms were taken. A decision was made to discontinue her treatment regimen and substitute a treatment regimen containing at least three drugs that the patient had not previously received and potentially effective drugs that she had previously taken. This was the approach used pending the results of drug susceptibility studies.

Under direct supervision, the patient was started on the following regimen: kanamycin (KM) (new), para-aminosalicylic acid (PAS) (new), clofazimine (new), RBT (previously received), EMB (previously received), ciprofloxacin (previously received). She tolerated the regimen well after slight modifications were made for gastrointestinal intolerance.

After 12 weeks of therapy with the new regimen, her symptoms improved, sputum smears were negative for AFB, and cultures were negative for *M. tuberculosis.* Drug susceptibility studies revealed resistance to KM, ciprofloxacin, INH, RIF, SM, ETA, and CS. The organism was sensitive to PZA, amikacin, PAS, clofazimine, EMB, and CM.

At this point (12 weeks after starting the new regimen), her treatment regimen was modified. KM and ciprofloxacin were discontinued and replaced with CM and PZA; PAS, RBT, EMB, and clofazimine were continued. Six months after starting this treatment, the patient remained culture-negative for *M. tuberculosis* and CM was discontinued. Eighteen months after initiation of treatment, sputum remained culture-negative and RBT and PZA were discontinued, and 24 months after initiation of treatment and sputum conversion, PAS and EMB were stopped. The patient remains clinically well, her chest x-ray find-

ings are improved (Fig. 8), and she has returned to work full-time.

COMMENT: This case illustrates the importance of drug susceptibility tests in the treatment of tuberculosis. The delay in obtaining drug sensitivity information adversely influenced drug selection. It is probable that the drug resistance of the infecting organism was both primary and secondary.

TREATMENT DURING PREGNANCY

Certain precautions must be considered when treating tuberculosis during pregnancy. There is no doubt, however, that untreated tuberculosis represents a far greater hazard to a pregnant woman and her fetus than does any specific treatment.

In general, INH, RIF, EMB, and PAS are drugs that have been used during pregnancy in the United States because they have not been found to have teratogenic effects (Table 7). Although PAS is not associated with teratogenic effects, the frequent associated gastrointestinal side effects preclude its use as a first-line drug either with or without pregnancy.

PZA is approved by international guidelines for routine use during pregnancy; however, in the United States it is not recommended because of insufficient data concerning its teratogenic effects. Therefore, in the United States INH and RIF are the recommended initial treatment regimen. EMB should be included when primary INH resistance in the patient's locale is >4%. If PZA is not included in the initial treatment regimen, a minimum of 9 months of therapy must be given. SM has been demonstrated to have adverse effects on fetal development of the eighth cranial nerve in the third trimester, causing congenital deafness. KM and CM are also aminoglycosides, and all three are not recommended. Because data on the safety of the other second-line drugs and newer antimycobacterial agents, such as the quinolones and macrolides, are limited or suggest toxicity, their use should be avoided if possible during pregnancy.

Breast-feeding should not be discouraged, because the concentrations of drugs in breast milk are not sufficient to cause toxic effects in nursing infants. To prevent peripheral neuropathy, pyridoxine (10 to 50 mg/d) is recommended for pregnant women receiving INH.

TREATMENT OF TUBERCULOSIS IN CHILDREN

Treatment of tuberculosis in infants and children is generally guided by the same basic principles that apply to adults. However, because tuberculosis is more likely to disseminate in infants and younger children (<4 years old), the rapid institution of effective therapy is of the utmost importance. The initial treatment regimens pre-

TABLE 7. *Drugs for tuberculosis in special situations*

Drug	Pregnancy	CNS TB disease	Renal insufficiency
INH	Safe	Good penetration	Normal clearance
RIF	Safe	Fair penetration Penetrates inflamed meninges (10%–20%)	Normal clearance
PZA	Avoid	Good penetration	Clearance reduced Decrease dose or prolong interval
EMB	Safe	Penetrates inflamed meninges only (4%–64%)	Clearance reduced Decrease dose or prolong interval
SM	Avoid	Penetrates inflamed meninges only	Clearance reduced Decrease dose or prolong interval
CM	Avoid	Penetrates inflamed meninges only	Clearance reduced Decrease dose or prolong interval
KM	Avoid	Penetrates inflamed meninges only	Clearance reduced Decrease dose or prolong interval
ETA	Do not use	Good penetration	Normal clearance
PAS	Safe	Penetrates inflamed meninges only (10%–50%)	Incomplete data on clearance
CS	Avoid	Good penetration	Clearance reduced Decrease dose or prolong interval
Ciprofloxacin	Do not use	Fair penetration (5%–10%) Penetrates inflamed meninges (50%–90%)	Clearance reduced Decrease dose or prolong interval
Ofloxacin	Do not use	Fair penetration (5%–10%) Penetrates inflamed meninges (50%–90%)	Clearance reduced Decrease dose or prolong interval
Amikacin	Avoid	Penetrates inflamed meninges only	Clearance reduced Decrease dose or prolong interval
Clofazimine	Avoid	Penetration unknown	Clearance probably normal

Source: Centers for Disease Control, 1994.

Safe: The drug has not been demonstrated to have teratogenic effects.

Avoid: Data on the drug's safety are limited, or the drug is associated with mild malformations (as in the aminoglycosides).

Do not use: Studies show an association between the drug and premature labor, congenital malformations, or teratogenicity.

scribed for the treatment of tuberculosis in adults are also recommended for children (Tables 4–6). EMB is less useful in young children because the ocular toxicity that the drug may cause is difficult to monitor. SM or PZA is an acceptable alternative. Because there is less cavitary disease in children, confirmation of the diagnosis on culture is less likely than in adults. When hilar adenopathy or parenchymal infiltrates are present on chest roentgenograms in a child with a positive tuberculin test, the child should be treated as a case of active pulmonary tuberculosis.

Because the results of sputum culture are often negative in children, the results of culture and drug sensitivity studies from the contact case are very helpful in guiding the selection of treatment regimens. When knowledge of drug susceptibility patterns is critical, as in suspected MDRTB, it may be necessary to obtaining early morning gastric aspirates or BAL fluid. Assessing improvement in children depends more on clinical and x-ray findings than on results of sputum cultures, as noted above. Extrapulmonary tuberculosis in children is treated the same as pulmonary tuberculosis, except for tuberculous meningitis, bone and joint tuberculosis, and disseminated tuberculosis, for which a minimum of 12 months of treatment is recommended.

MONITORING TREATMENT

Adults who are treated with INH and RIF should have baseline measurements of hepatic enzyme, bilirubin, and serum creatinine levels, and a complete blood count and platelet count should be obtained. Serum uric acid should be measured if PZA is included in the regimen, and a baseline test of visual acuity and color vision should be obtained in those receiving EMB. Audiometry should be performed in patients receiving SM or other aminoglycosides. The purpose of these tests is to detect abnormalities that may cause complications or require modification of treatment regimens, and to provide a baseline for comparison if abnormalities develop during therapy. Tables 4 and 5 present guidelines for monitoring during treatment with both first-line and second-line drugs.

All patients should be educated regarding adverse reactions to the medications they are receiving and instructed to stop medications and seek help immediately if these symptoms develop. Patients should be followed by a physician monthly while on treatment and specifically queried regarding symptoms at each visit. Monthly laboratory monitoring for toxicity in adults with normal baseline values is not required. If symptoms develop, laboratory testing should be performed immediately.

PREVENTIVE TREATMENT

INH preventive therapy has been shown to reduce substantially the risk for progression of tuberculous infection to disease. Infected persons at high risk for development of tuberculosis, listed below, should be given INH preventive therapy regardless of their age:

1. Tuberculin-positive reactors (≥5 mm) who are HIV-seropositive; included are positive reactors who have risk factors for HIV infection but whose HIV serologic status is unknown. Tuberculin-negative reactors (<5 mm) who are HIV-seropositive and who live in areas with a prevalence of tuberculosis infection of 10% or greater should be given INH preventive therapy regardless of their age.

2. Tuberculin-positive reactors (≥5 mm) who are close contacts of infectious tuberculosis cases. Tuberculin-negative (<5 mm) children and adolescents in this category should also be started on INH preventive therapy. The tuberculin skin test should be repeated 12 weeks later; if the result is still negative and contact with the infectious case was interrupted when preventive therapy was started, INH can be discontinued.

3. Tuberculin-positive reactors (≥5 mm) who have chest roentgenograms suggestive of old healed tuberculosis and who were inadequately treated or untreated (these individuals can be given INH and RIF for 4 months).

4. Tuberculin-positive persons who have within the past 2 years converted their tuberculin skin test from negative to positive (≥10 mm increase if <35 years of age; ≥15 mm increase if ≥35 years of age).

5. Tuberculin-positive (≥10 mm) persons with certain medical conditions that have been reported to increase the risk for tuberculosis, including silicosis, diabetes mellitus, prolonged corticosteroid therapy (>15 mg of prednisone daily for 2 to 3 weeks), other immunosuppressive therapy, some hematologic and reticuloendothelial diseases, injection drug use in a person known to be HIV-seronegative, end-stage renal disease, and conditions associated with weight loss to 10% or more below ideal body weight or chronic undernourishment (head and neck cancer, intestinal bypass surgery or gastrectomy, chronic malabsorption syndromes).

Tuberculin-positive reactors (≥10 mm) <35 years of age who remain high-priority candidates for preventive therapy but are at somewhat lower risk for development of tuberculosis than persons in the above groups should also receive INH preventive treatment; they include the following:

1. Foreign-born persons from regions of the world with a high incidence of tuberculosis, such as Asia, Africa, and Latin America

2. Medically underserved low-income domestic populations, including high-risk ethnic or racial minorities such as blacks, Hispanics, and Asian-Americans

3. Residents of long-term care facilities such as mental institutions, nursing homes, and correctional institutions

4. Other groups, such as migrant farm workers and the homeless that are locally identified as having an increased prevalence of tuberculosis

Tuberculin positive reactors (≥15 mm) who are <35 years of age and have no risk factors for tuberculosis should also be considered for INH preventive therapy but should be given a lower priority for preventive treatment than the groups previously discussed.

Because the risk for INH-induced hepatitis outweighs the benefits of preventive therapy, INH is not recommended for tuberculin-positive reactors (≥10 mm) who are ≥35 years of age and are not at high risk for development of tuberculosis.

To prevent the progression of tuberculous infection to disease, INH is used alone as preventive therapy in a single dose of 5 mg/kg of body weight per day up to 300 mg/d in adults and 10 to 15 mg/kg of body weight per day in children, not to exceed 300 mg/d.

Clinical trials have demonstrated that the greatest reduction (90%) in the risk for development of tuberculosis occurs with daily administration of INH for 12 months. However, 6 months of daily INH preventive therapy also conveys a high degree of protection and reduces the risk for development of tuberculosis by approximately 70%. Administration of daily INH for <6 months has been shown to reduce the level of protection significantly. Administration of INH for >1 year has not been shown to convey additional protection. Therefore, current recommendations are that every effort should be made to ensure continuation of daily INH preventive therapy for at least 6 months. Children should receive therapy for 9 months and individuals with HIV infection for 12 months.

Data on the effectiveness of intermittent INH preventive therapy are limited; however, studies in which INH is given twice weekly during the sterilizing phase of tuberculosis treatment suggest that this would be an effective preventive treatment. For potentially nonadherent treated persons at high risk, supervised intermittent INH preventive therapy has been recommended twice weekly at a dose of 15 mg/kg. Tuberculin-positive adults who have silicosis or abnormalities on chest roentgenograms as noted above with no evidence of current disease should receive 4 months of therapy with INH and RIF, as they are considered to have sputum-negative, active pulmonary tuberculosis. An acceptable alternative is 12 months of INH therapy, provided that infection with INH-resistant organisms is unlikely.

Pregnant women with positive tuberculin skin test results generally should not be started on INH preventive treatment until after delivery. Exceptions are made when recent skin test conversion has occurred or when high-risk medical conditions such as HIV infection exist. Under these circumstances, INH preventive therapy should be given.

No data are currently available that document the clinical efficacy of any drug other than INH for preventive therapy in any setting. Short-course preventive therapy regimens using RIF and PZA for 2 months and RIF alone for 4 months have shown promise in animal models and are being evaluated in humans.

When the source case has INH-resistant organisms or when treatment candidates cannot tolerate INH, preventive treatment with RIF should be considered. The RIF should be given daily in standard doses for at least 6 months in adults and 9 months in children. Guidelines for preventive treatment of individuals who may be infected with INH- and RIF-resistant organisms are based on the likelihood that the infection is recent and the probability that active tuberculosis will develop (i.e., HIV-seropositive patients). If these circumstances are unlikely, then observation of the patient or the administration of standard preventive therapy has been recommended. For patients with an especially high risk for tuberculosis, as in HIV infection or other immunosuppression, preventive therapy with EMB and PZA or PZA and one of the quinolones (ofloxacin or ciprofloxacin) in the usual standard doses should be considered.

Peripheral neuropathy may result from the use of INH but is extremely uncommon at a daily dose of 5 mg/kg of body weight. We give pyridoxine (10 to 50 mg/d) only in the presence of conditions commonly associated with neuropathies, such as diabetes, alcoholism, anemia, malnutrition, seizure disorders, and pregnancy.

Increasing age, chronic liver disease, and alcohol abuse have been associated with an increased incidence of INH-induced hepatitis in patients receiving preventive therapy. Young women, particularly blacks and Hispanics, have been reported to be at increased risk for fatal hepatitis associated with administration of INH. It is recommended that all patients ≥35 years of age and younger patients at risk for hepatoxicity have liver function tests (measurements of hepatic transaminase, bilirubin, and alkaline phosphatase) before starting INH preventive therapy. If patients report symptoms of adverse reactions after therapy is begun and hepatic transaminase measurements exceed five times the upper limits of normal, INH should be discontinued. Baseline measurements of liver function parameters are not necessary for persons <35 years of age. Patients should be told what the symptoms of hepatitis are and advised to discontinue INH and report immediately if they occur. Patients should be clinically evaluated monthly while receiving INH preventive therapy.

BCG Vaccination

The bacille Calmette-Guérin (BCG) was developed from an attenuated strain of *M. bovis* in 1919 and serially cultured into several different, variable strains. It is used in many countries as a vaccine to protect against tuberculosis and is the most widely used vaccine in the world. Because the potency of the various strains varies, the protection obtained from the vaccine has been reported from none to 80%. A recently conducted meta-analysis by the Harvard School of Public Health attributes an overall 50% protective effect to the vaccine and a 64% protective effect against tuberculous meningitis. A large number of studies have suggested that it protects infants and young children from the more serious forms of tuberculosis, although its ability to prevent disease in adults is much less clear. Thus, its contribution is epidemiologic control of tuberculosis is not great. (Most cases of tuberculosis in children are sputum-negative and thus not infectious.)

BCG is not generally recommended for use in the United States, where most cases of tuberculosis occur in persons who are already infected with *M. tuberculosis* and would not benefit from BCG. Additionally, the use of BCG vaccination causes tuberculin skin test conversion, thus rendering the tuberculin test, the major indicator of new infection, useless. BCG vaccination of tuberculin-negative infants and children may be warranted when they are at high risk for intense, prolonged exposure to untreated or ineffectively treated cases of infectious tuberculosis, contact with the infectious case cannot be broken, and long-term effective preventive therapy is not possible. BCG is contraindicated in patients who are immunosuppressed.

In the United States, all persons who have a positive tuberculin skin test and who have a history of BCG vaccination should be considered infected with *M. tuberculosis* and evaluated for INH preventive therapy.

INFECTION CONTROL

This section briefly discusses selected public health aspects of tuberculosis control and the importance of coordinating the activities of public health departments and facilities that provide health care for tuberculosis patients. Effective tuberculosis control programs are based on the early detection, isolation, and treatment of infectious tuberculosis patients to reduce the risk for exposure to others. Infection control programs utilize various measures to achieve these goals, including administrative, engineering, and personal respiratory protective measures to prevent the transmission of *M. tuberculosis*.

Administrative Controls

The essential components of administrative infection control consist of detecting infectious tuberculosis cases early, isolating them, and providing rapid, effective therapy to reduce the risk for transmitting the organism to others. This requires a high index of suspicion by health care providers, particularly regarding HIV-infected patients with tuberculosis whose presentation may be unusual. Following diagnosis, all infectious tuberculosis patients should be isolated and started on DOT with an appropriate drug regimen (see above).

All facilities that provide health care to tuberculosis patients should have procedures for reporting cases and for coordinating activities between public health departments and other facilities that are involved in patient care.

Administrative controls should focus principally on reducing the risk of exposing susceptible persons to patients with infectious tuberculosis. Such administrative controls include the following:

1. Developing and implementing effective written policies and protocols to ensure rapid identification, diagnosis, isolation, and treatment of individuals who are likely to have tuberculosis
2. Implementing effective work practices among health care workers within health care facilities
3. Educating, training, and counseling health care workers regarding basic concepts of tuberculosis transmission, pathogenesis, diagnosis, treatment, and infection control
4. Screening health care workers for tuberculosis infection and disease

The transmission of the tubercle bacillus has long been a recognized risk in health care facilities, and as a result infection control guidelines were developed by the CDC. Unfortunately, a relaxation of infection control practices occurred with time, which led to several outbreaks of tuberculosis.

In the early 1990s, numerous accounts of institutional outbreaks of MDRTB were reported. These outbreaks occurred primarily in HIV-infected persons and were associated with high mortality rates and a rapid progression from diagnosis to death. The outbreaks occurred most often in clinics or wards where HIV-infected patients received care. Not only was patient-to-patient transmission identified, but the spread of infection from patients to health care workers was reported to be common.

Major factors that contributed to these outbreaks included the comingling of highly susceptible immunocompromised patients with infectious tuberculosis patients, delayed recognition and treatment of both drug-sensitive and drug-resistant tuberculosis, delayed initiation and premature discontinuation of isolation, and delayed implementation of existing infection control measures (adequate respiratory protection during cough-induction procedures).

Recently collected data from several of the health care facilities involved in the outbreaks indicates that once implemented, infection control measures significantly limited or entirely stopped the continued transmission of *M. tuberculosis*.

Engineering Controls

Engineering and personal respiratory protective measures used during outbreaks of MDRTB were proved to be important infection control measures for stopping further spread of MDRTB in institutional settings.

In health care facilities, as part of a tuberculosis infection control plan, rooms for isolation and treatment of infectious tuberculosis patients, in addition to facilities for sputum induction and aerosol-generating procedures, should be available.

Ventilation reduces the concentration of droplet nuclei in room air by diluting and removing contaminated air and directing air flow patterns within a room. Two types of general ventilation systems (single-pass and recirculating) are used for dilution and removal of contaminated air. The preferred choice is the single-pass system, in which the air supply (either outside air or clean air from a central reservoir) is passed through a room or area and completely exhausted to the outside.

For optimal air mixing, the air supply source and exhaust should be located at opposite sides of the room, so that clean air flows from areas where health care workers are located across the infectious source (patients) and out through the room exhaust. It is currently recommended that a minimum of six air changes per hour be required for tuberculosis isolation and treatment rooms.

Air normally flows from an area of higher pressure to one of lower (negative) pressure. Negative pressure can be achieved by exhausting air from a room faster than it is being supplied to the room. Thus, the direction of air flow can be controlled. Preferably, the direction of air flow should be from a less contaminated area to a more contaminated area. A minimum pressure difference of 0.001 inch of H_2O is required to create and maintain adequate air flow.

Ideally, potentially infectious tuberculosis patients should be isolated and treated in a negative-pressure room ventilated by a single-pass ventilation system having at least six air changes per hour and exhausted directly to the outside.

As an interim measure, a small exhaust fan placed in a window or an outside wall will exhaust air to the outside and create a negative room pressure, but it will not provide clean air and thus offers suboptimal dilution. Negative room pressure can be checked visually with smoke tubes or by measuring the pressure difference between a room and its surrounding area.

Booths, hoods, and tents (local exhaust ventilation devices) are useful for preventing the introduction of airborne tubercle bacilli into room air by trapping them near their source; this prevents exposure of health care workers in the area. The use of these devices is especially important during sputum induction procedures.

Of the two types of local exhaust ventilation devices (enclosing and exterior) that are available for use, enclosing devices are preferable because they completely enclose the infectious source. Enclosing-type devices should provide adequate air flow to remove at least 99% of airborne tubercle bacilli. All air from booths, hoods, and tents should be exhausted to the outside; however, if it is recirculated, air should be exhausted through a high-efficiency particulate air (HEPA) filter.

HEPA filtration is a method of removing tubercle bacilli from room air that supplements the previously discussed ventilation control measures. HEPA filters have a minimum efficiency of 99.97% for removing particles ≥ 0.3 μm in size from room air. Although their ability to filter tubercle bacilli from room air has not been studied, the droplet nuclei that contain tubercle bacilli are approximately 1 to 5 μm in size. HEPA filtration can be used to remove droplet nuclei from room air before it is exhausted to the outside or recirculated to other areas, in fixed or portable room air filtration units for recirculating air within a room, or, as previously discussed, in the exhaust of ventilation equipment such as booths and hoods.

Ultraviolet germicidal irradiation (UVGI) kills tubercle bacilli under experimental conditions; it has been shown to reduce transmission of other microbes in hospitals and classrooms and has been recommended as an engineering control measure to supplement other infection controls. UVGI probably kills or inactivates airborne tubercle bacilli, but before its role can be unequivocally defined in preventing tuberculosis transmission, further study is required. Germicidal ultraviolet lamps are low-pressure mercury vapor lamps that emit radiant energy at a wavelength of 253.7 nm.

UVGI can be used to inactivate tubercle bacilli from contaminated room air by placing ultraviolet lamps within ventilation ducts that exhaust air before it is recirculated from tuberculosis isolation or treatment rooms or other areas of general use, including waiting rooms, emergency rooms, or patient rooms where air could be contaminated by undiagnosed cases of tuberculosis. The advantage of using UVGI within ventilation ducts is that patients and other persons are protected from its harmful effects.

UVGI is also used to inactivate tubercle bacilli in contaminated upper room air by placing ultraviolet lamps on an upper wall or suspending them from the ceiling. The lamps are constructed to direct the flow of irradiation upward, which minimizes exposure to individuals in the lower part of the room. UVGI of upper room air is used in tuberculosis isolation and treatment rooms, hallways, and patient, waiting, and emergency rooms.

Short-term exposure to UVGI can cause erythema and keratoconjunctivitis, and long-term exposure is associated with an increased risk for squamous and basal cell carcinomas of the skin. Recent studies have reported an increase in HIV replication caused by ultraviolet radiation. However, in places where UVGI has been used properly, there have been no reports of untoward effects.

Personal Respiratory Protection Controls: Particulate Respirators

From a public health perspective, the use of personal respiratory protective equipment is the least efficient and least effective of all infection control methods, because it protects only the user and must fit well to work well. Such equipment is used primarily when it is likely that high concentrations of tubercle bacilli are contaminating room air, as in tuberculosis isolation and treatment rooms during sputum induction and aerosol-generating procedures, or when administrative and engineering controls are inadequate to remove droplet nuclei from room air.

The Occupational Safety and Health Administration (OSHA) standard for respiratory protection requires certification by the National Institute for Occupational Safety and Health (NIOSH) of all respiratory protective devices used in the workplace.

Until recently, the only particulate respirators used for protection against transmission of *M. tuberculosis* that met NIOSH certification criteria were HEPA filter particulate respirators. Recently, NIOSH developed new regulations that are more stringent, under which nine types of particulate respirators are certified. Three different levels of filter efficiency of 95%, 99%, and 99.97% were classified, and three different categories based on the resistance to filter efficiency degradation, labeled *N, R,* and *P,* were outlined. In health care settings, either N, R, or P respirators may be selected.

All nine classes of particulate respirators certified by NIOSH meet or exceed CDC filtration efficiency performance standards. Several of the newer classes of particulate respirators will be less expensive and easier to wear than the HEPA filter respirators previously certified.

The policy of OSHA with respect to particulate respirators currently allows the use of an HEPA filter particulate respirator or any of the nine classes of particulate respirators for protection against *M. tuberculosis*. OSHA requires that all respirators be properly fit-tested. Manufacturers recommend that users of the respirators follow fit-checking procedures each time the respirator is worn.

Role of the Public Health Department

Tuberculosis is a prime example of the impact that public health policy may have on the diagnosis and treatment of disease. The best trained, most informed clinicians cannot ever hope to have any impact on tuberculosis care and control without dedicated and sustained cooperation from the local public health agency.

Because many tuberculosis patients are beset with a myriad of social problems, a practicing physician cannot treat tuberculosis in isolation. DOT, follow-up of contacts, and investigation of outbreaks are at least three areas in which major interactions are required between the clinician and the public health agency.

In an era of reform of health care delivery strategies, it behooves all treating clinicians not only to forge and sustain relationships with health departments to facilitate a beneficial clinical and public health outcome, but to advocate the proper appreciation and funding of these specialized services.

BIBLIOGRAPHY

American Thoracic Society, Centers for Disease Control, and Infectious Disease Society of America. Control of tuberculosis in the United States. Am Rev Respir Dis 1992;146:1623–1633. *An official statement of the American Thoracic Society, Centers for Disease Control, and Infectious Disease Society of America. The objectives of a tuberculosis control program are discussed, including contact investigation, screening, and treatment.*

American Thoracic Society, Centers for Disease Control. Diagnostic standards and classification of tuberculosis. Am Rev Respir Dis 1990; 142:725–735. *A joint statement of the American Thoracic Society and Centers for Disease Control giving guidelines for the diagnosis and classification of tuberculosis.*

Bass JB. Tuberculosis in the 1990s. Alcohol Clin Exp Res 1995; 19:3–5. *A discussion of epidemiology and the factors contributing to the resurgence of tuberculosis in the United States. The use of a four-drug initial regimen to combat MDRTB is recommended.*

Bass JB, Farer LS, Hopewell PC, O'Brien R, Jacobs RF, Ruben F, Snider DE, Thornton G. Treatment of tuberculosis and tuberculosis infection in adults and children. Am J Respir Crit Care Med 1994; 149:1359–1374. *A joint statement of the American Thoracic Society, Centers for Disease Control and Prevention, and the American Academy of Pediatrics giving the current recommendations for the selection of medications to be used in the treatment of tuberculosis infection and disease in adults and children with and without HIV infection.*

Centers for Disease Control. Tuberculosis morbidity—United States, 1994. MMWR Morb Mortal Wkly Rep 1994;44:387–395. *A summary of tuberculosis surveillance data for 1994, comparing the findings with data for 1992 and 1993.*

Centers for Disease Control. Guidelines for preventing the transmission of Mycobacterium tuberculosis in health care facilities, 1994. MMWR Morb Mortal Wkly Rep 1994;43:1–132. *A brief discussion of the epidemiology, transmission, and pathogenesis of tuberculosis, with guidelines for the evaluation and management of both ambulatory and hospitalized patients in a health care setting.*

Centers for Disease Control. Core Curriculum on Tuberculosis: What the Clinician Should Know. Washington, DC: US Government Printing Office; 1994. *A review of the diagnosis, epidemiology, methods of infection control, prevention, transmission, pathogenesis, and treatment of tuberculosis. The publication is a good reference source for health care providers whose patients have tuberculosis infection or tuberculosis.*

Centers for Disease Control. Reported Tuberculosis in the United States, 1994. Atlanta: US Department of Health and Human Services, Public Health Service, Centers for Disease Control; 1995. *Statistics regarding the demography and epidemiology of tuberculosis in the U.S. population in 1994.*

Chaulk CP, Moore-Rice K, Rizzo R, Chaisson RE. Eleven years of community-based directly observed therapy for tuberculosis. JAMA 1995;274:945–951. *The authors report a significant reduction in reported incidence of tuberculosis in Baltimore compared with the five major U.S. cities having the highest incidence of tuberculosis during an 11-year period, 1981–1992. They attribute the decline to the broad use of community-based directly observed therapy in Baltimore.*

Dannenberg AM. Immunopathogenesis of pulmonary tuberculosis. Hosp Pract 1993;28:33–40. *A discussion of the roles of cell-mediated immunity and delayed-type hypersensitivity in the pathogenesis of tuberculosis.*

Division of Tuberculosis Control, Centers for Disease Control. Screen-ing for tuberculosis and tuberculosis infection in high-risk populations and the use of preventive therapy for tuberculosis infection in the U.S. MMWR Morb Mortal Wkly Rep 1990;39:1–12. *Lists high-risk groups for tuberculosis and gives recommendations for screening for infection and disease.*

Fox W. The John Barnwell Lecture: Changing concepts in the chemotherapy of pulmonary tuberculosis. Am Rev Respir Dis 1968;97:767. *A classic article discussing the concept of drug treatment for tuberculosis.*

Houk VN, Kent DC, Baker JH, et al. The epidemiology of tuberculosis infection in a closed environment. Arch Environ Health 1968;16: 26–35. *One of the first discussions of the airborne transmission of tuberculosis.*

Hudson LD, Sbarbaro J. Twice weekly tuberculosis chemotherapy. JAMA 1973;223:139–143. *One of the first articles to discuss a method of supervised therapy.*

International Union Against Tuberculosis Committee on Prophylaxis. Efficacy of various durations of isoniazid preventive therapy for tuberculosis: five years of follow-up in the IUAT trial. Bull World Health Organ 1982;60:555–564. *A 5-year follow-up confirmed that INH is an extremely effective drug for the preventive treatment of tuberculin reactors with fibrotic lung lesions.*

Iseman MD. Drug therapy: treatment of multidrug-resistant tuberculosis. N Engl J Med 1993;329:784–791. *Discusses the treatment of a group of very ill patients with drug-resistant tuberculosis at the National Jewish Center for Immunology and Respiratory Medicine in Denver.*

Johnston RF, Wildrick KH. "State of the Art" review. The impact of chemotherapy on the care of patients with tuberculosis. Am Rev Respir Dis 1974;109:636–664. *A classic review article that discusses in depth the epidemiology, transmission, diagnosis, prevention, and principles of treatment of tuberculosis, including the use of intermittent and short-course drug regimens.*

Jordan JT, Lewit EM, Montgomery RL, Reichman LB. Isoniazid as preventive therapy in HIV intravenous drug abusers—a decision analysis. JAMA 1991;265:2987–2991. *A decision analysis suggesting that INH can be given to HIV-infected injecting drug users without regard to skin test, because of the high degree of anergy and high risk of dually infected parties.*

Jordan TJ, Lewit EM, Reichman LB. Isoniad preventive therapy for tuberculosis. Am Rev Respir Dis 1991:144:1357–1360. *An analysis of the use of INH preventive therapy in low-risk tuberculin reactors, suggesting that ethnicity, sex, and age should be considered.*

Kopanoff DE, Snider DE, Caras GJ. Isoniazid-related hepatitis. Am Rev Respir Dis 1978;117:991–1001. *One of the first articles to evaluate the relationship between INH preventive therapy and drug-induced hepatitis.*

Law KF, Jagirdan J, Weiden MD, Bodkin M, Rom WN. Tuberculosis in HIV-positive patients: cellular response and immune activation in the lung. Am J Respir Crit Care Med 1996;153:1377–1384. *Report of the findings of a study in which the cellular response in BAL obtained from both infected and uninfected lung segments of HIV-positive and HIV-negative patients was analyzed and compared with the response of normal controls and the response in peripheral blood.*

Malasky C, Jordan T, Potalski F, Reichman LB. Occupational tuberculosis infection among pulmonary physicians in training. Am Rev Respir Dis 1990;142:505–507. *A questionnaire study documenting a very strong risk in pulmonary fellows as opposed to infectious disease fellows with the same demographics. The conclusion is that exposure to infected aerosols carries high risk for tuberculosis infection.*

McDonald RJ, Memon AM, Reichman LB. Successful supervised ambulatory management of tuberculosis treatment failures. Ann Intern Med 1982;96:297–303. *One of the first articles reporting the successful use of directly observed therapy in nonadherent patients, most with MDRTB, using various enhancers and enablers.*

McKenna MT, McCray E, Onorato I. The epidemiology of tuberculosis among foreign-born persons in the United States, 1986 to 1993. N Engl J Med 1995;332:1071–1076. *Reports the effects of immigration on the epidemiology and resurgence of tuberculosis in the United States.*

Mitchison DA. Basic mechanisms of chemotherapy. Chest 1979;76: 771–781. *Discusses the bacterial activity of the first-line tuberculosis drugs and the sterilizing effect of RIF and PZA on mycobacteria.*

Moulding T, Dutt AK, Reichman LB. Fixed-dose combinations of anti-tuberculosis medications to prevent drug resistance. Ann Intern Med

1995;122:951–954. *Discusses the desirability of using fixed-dose combinations of antituberculosis drugs to prevent the development of drug-resistant tuberculosis.*

Moulding TS, Redek AG, Kanel GC. Twenty isoniazid-associated deaths in one state. *Am Rev Respir Dis* 1989;140:700–705. *Report of a series of deaths in young women in California associated with the use of INH preventive therapy.*

National Institute for Occupational Safety and Health. *NIOSH Guide to the Selection and Use of Particulate Respirators Certified Under 42 CFR 84.* Cincinnati: US Department of Health and Human Services, Public Health Service, Centers for Disease Control; 1996. *Certification criteria and types of particulate respirators currently certified by the NIOSH for protection against tuberculosis.*

Passannate M, Gallagher CT, Reichman LB. Preventive therapy for contact of multidrug-resistant tuberculosis. A Delphi survey. *Chest* 1994;106:431–434. *A survey of tuberculosis experts with recommendations for preventive therapy for contacts of MDRTB. No regimen met consensus. The popular regimen was PZA and ciprofloxacin for 4 months.*

Raviglione MC, Snider DE Jr, Koch A. Global epidemiology of tuberculosis. *JAMA* 1995;273:220–226. *Review of the worldwide incidence and mortality rates of tuberculosis, with a discussion of global epidemiology and control strategies. The authors warn of an increase in worldwide cases and deaths in future years if tuberculosis control does not improve.*

Reichman LB. Tuberculin skin testing—the state of the art. *Chest* 1979; 765:7645–7705. *A basic review of the technique of tuberculin skin testing.*

Reichman LB. The U-shaped curve of concern. *Am Rev Respir Dis* 1991;144:741–742. *A description of the focus of government funding for tuberculosis control efforts and how program successes invariably lead to decreases in funding, which lead to increases in case rates.*

Reichman LB. Fear, embarrassment, and relief: the tuberculosis epidemic and public health. *Am J Public Health* 1993;83:639–641. *An editorial lamenting the degree and scope of the recent tuberculosis epidemic, attributing causation to neglect and lack of attention.*

Reichman LB. Multidrug-resistant tuberculosis: meeting the challenge. *Hosp Pract* 1994;29:85–96. *A review of the control and treatment strategies of MDRTB.*

Reichman LB. How to ensure the continued resurgence of tuberculosis. *Lancet* 1996;347:175–177. *An analysis of three areas of global neglect that have promoted the worldwide resurgence of tuberculosis in the 1980s and 1990s.*

Reichman LB, Felton CP, Edsall Jr. Drug dependence. A possible new risk factor for tuberculosis disease. *Arch Intern Med* 1979;139:337–339. *One of the first articles to define injection drug use as an independent risk factor for active tuberculosis.*

Reichman LB, Hershfield ES, eds. *Tuberculosis: A Comprehensive International Approach.* New York: Marcel Dekker; 1993. *A text dedicated to tuberculosis care and control, emphasizing the situation in the developing world.*

Reichman LB, Mangura BT. Use of bacille Calmette-Guerin vaccine in health care workers. *Clin Infect Dis* 1996;22:392. *A hypothetical scheme illustrating how not using BCG in health care workers allows surveillance for new infection and therefore enhanced tuberculosis control.*

Reichman LB, O'Day R. Tuberculosis infection in a large urban population. *Am Rev Respir Dis* 1978;117:705–712. *A study of risk factors related to tuberculosis infection showing race and socioeconomic status as the strongest risk factors.*

Riley RL, Mills CC, O'Grady F, et al. Infectiousness of air from a tuberculosis ward. *Am Rev Respir Dis* 1962;85:511–525. *A classic article supporting the concept of airborne transmission of M. tuberculosis.*

Rom WN, Garay S, eds. *Tuberculosis.* Boston: Little, Brown; 1996. *Covered topics include the history, epidemiology, pathogenesis, diagnosis, treatment, prevention, and control of tuberculosis.*

Rossman MD, MacGregor RR, eds. *Tuberculosis.* New York: McGraw-Hill; 1995. *Covered topics include the epidemiology, pathogenesis, diagnosis, prevention, and treatment of tuberculosis and nontuberculosis mycobacterial infections.*

Schluger NW, Rom WN. Current approaches to the diagnosis of active pulmonary tuberculosis. *Am J Respir Crit Care Med* 1994;149:264–267. *An evaluation of the clinical and laboratory methods used for diagnosing tuberculosis. Besides conventional techniques, newer techniques, including species-specific nucleic acid probes, analysis of cell-wall lipids by gas-liquid chromatography, PCR, RFLP, and a technique employing a luciferase reporter gene within a mycobacteriophage for use in drug-sensitivity testing, are discussed.*

Schluger NW, Rom WN. The polymerase chain reaction in the diagnosis and evaluation of pulmonary infections. *Am J Respir Crit Care Med* 1995;152:11–16. *Reviews the application of a method of DNA-amplification PCR in the early diagnosis of several pulmonary infections, including* Pneumocystis carinii *pneumonia, cytomegalovirus pneumonitis, and tuberculosis.*

Selwyn PA, Hartel D, Lewis VA, et al. A prospective study of the risk of tuberculosis among intravenous drug users with human immunodeficiency virus infection. *N Engl J Med* 1989;320:545–550. *A classic study evaluating the risk for tuberculosis among patients in a methadone clinic who have positive tuberculin skin tests and identifying HIV infection as a high-risk factor for the development of tuberculosis.*

Simone PM, Dooley SW. *Multidrug-Resistant Tuberculosis.* Atlanta: US Department of Health and Human Services, Centers for Disease Control; 1994. *Discusses transmission and treatment and the pathogenesis of drug resistance in tuberculosis. Includes a report of outbreaks of MDRTB.*

Small PM, Shafer RW, Hopewell PC, Singh SP, Murphy MJ, Desmond E, Sierra MF, Schoolnik GK. Exogenous reinfection with multidrug-resistant *Mycobacterium tuberculosis* in patients with advanced HIV infection. *N Engl J Med* 1993;328:1137–1144. *Genetic fingerprinting is used as an epidemiologic tool to show that exogenous reinfection with* M. tuberculosis *may occur during or after treatment for tuberculosis.*

Snider DE, Caras GJ. Isoniazid-associated hepatitis deaths: a review of available information. *Am Rev Respir Dis* 1992;145:494–497. *Reviews the literature related to INH-associated hepatitis deaths and provides guidelines for INH use.*

Sundaram G, McDonald RJ, Moniatis T, Oleske J, Kapila R, Reichman LB. Tuberculosis as a manifestation of the acquired immunodeficiency syndrome (AIDS). *JAMA* 1986;256:362–366. *Early article describing coinfection of tuberculosis and AIDS in injecting drug users, with concomitant preponderance of extrapulmonary tuberculosis.*

US Congress, Office of Technology Assessment. *The Continuing Challenge of Tuberculosis.* Washington, DC: US Government Printing Office; 1993; OTA-H-574. *A report summarizing current activities involving tuberculosis in the United States, with an overview of the role of the federal government in these activities. The epidemiology of tuberculosis and the state of research into new diagnostic, preventive and therapeutic technologies to assist in the control of tuberculosis and the delivery of effective services are also discussed.*

Textbook of Pulmonary Diseases, 6th ed.
edited by G.L. Baum, J.D. Crapo, B.R. Celli, and J.B. Karlinsky,
Lippincott–Raven Publishers, Philadelphia, © 1998.

CHAPTER

29

Nontuberculous Mycobacterial Pulmonary Disease (NTM)

Bonita T. Mangura · Lee B. Reichman

BACTERIOLOGY

After the tubercle bacillus (*Mycobacterium tuberculosis*) was identified as a cause of human disease, identification of other mycobacteria affecting various animals, such as livestock, fowl, and marine creatures, followed. Better and more specific bacteriologic techniques allowed microbiologists to separate and identify various mycobacteria pathogenic for humans.

Early on, *Mycobacterium avium*, pathogenic to fowl, was found not to be pathogenic for humans, but subsequently *M. avium* complex (MAC) was described as pathogenic for humans. Seroagglutination has allowed the identification of 28 types of MAC. It is difficult to distinguish *M. avium* from *M. intracellulare* without seroagglutination; Infection/disease by either one is generally referred to as MAC or *Mycobacterium avium-intracellulare* (MAI) disease. *M. avium* includes serotypes 1 through 11 (except 7) and 21; *M. intracellulare* includes serotypes 7, 12 through 20, and 25.

A wider spectrum of mycobacterial lung disease was recognized following the descriptions of *M. fortuitum* in individuals with chronic obstructive lung disease secondary to aspiration, and of *M. kansasii* in individuals without prior lung diseases.

Timpe and Runyon's classification of nontuberculous mycobacteria (NTM) in the 1950s provided a working algorithm; groups were based on pigment production, colony morphology, and growth rates. The schema in Fig. 1 shows temperature growth preferences; the cutaneous mycobacteria grow best at 30°C to 32°C. At 37°C and above, two growth rates are noted: rapidly growing mycobacteria and slowly growing mycobacteria. *M. chelonei* and *M. fortuitum* are rapidly growing organisms, also classified as Runyon group IV. Runyon groups I through III are slowly growing mycobacteria. The organisms included in Runyon group I are photochromogenic mycobacteria; cream-colored colonies grown in the dark turn yellow on exposure to light. Runyon group II organisms are scotochromogens; yellow-colored colonies change to orange in the dark. Runyon group III mycobacteria produce cream-colored colonies that do not change pigment color on exposure to either light or dark. Pigmentation was eventually found to be related to soluble beta carotene found in mycobacteria and controlled by an oxygen-dependent light-activated enzyme. *M. tuberculosis*, MAC, and *Mycobacterium xenopi* belong to Runyon group III and are differentiated by their reaction to niacin (*M. tuberculosis* is niacin-reactive, whereas MAC does not react to niacin). Arylsulfatase activity differentiates MAC from *M. xenopi*.

The tree in Fig. 1 includes some of the important pathogens and highlights the biochemical reaction (niacin) that differentiates *M. tuberculosis* from the rest of the NTM organisms. The laboratory characteristics of pigment production and growth rate have not contributed to clinical diagnostic or therapeutic decision making. The only clinical correlates were that the organisms were easy to treat or difficult to treat (Bailey classification). Standard antimycobacterial drugs had to be juggled to find an appropriate combination.

More modern techniques are currently available to identify specific mycobacteria rapidly. These include thin-layer chromatography, gas-liquid chromatography, high-pressure chromatography, species-specific DNA probes, and the Bactec NAP (*p*-nitro-L-acetylamino-β-hydroxy-propiophenone) test. These are sensitive and specific tests that may provide identification of species within 4 hours using isolates from broth or agar.

B. T. Mangura and L. B. Reichman: New Jersey Medical School National Tuberculosis Center, University of Medicine and Dentistry of New Jersey, Newark, New Jersey 07107.

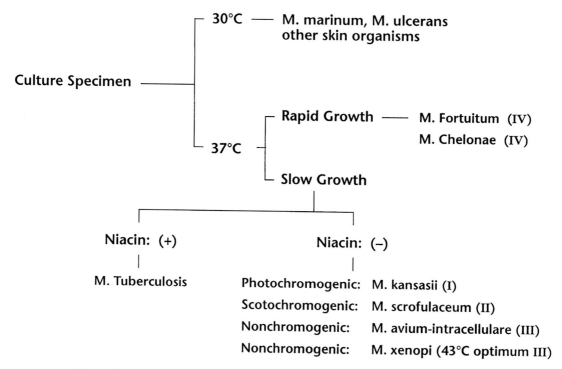

FIG. 1. Temperature growth preferences of NTM (nontubercular myocobacteria).

The geographic distribution of the NTM is wide and variable. Species-specific skin-testing antigens have not been standardized and are not highly specific. Clinically, some patients with NTM disease may have a positive skin test using purified protein derivative-tuberculin (PPD-T), with reactions of <10 mm. The only utility of the tuberculin skin test in the clinical setting in which NTM are suspected is to determine the presence of intact delayed hypersensitivity.

Because many mycobacterial species have similar bacterial wall antigens, cross-reactions are expected and common. However, among a group of patients with cystic fibrosis and documented NTM infection, none responded to PPD-T. All were from the southeastern United States (an endemic area for NTM). The few who reacted to PPD were known to have been exposed to *M. tuberculosis.*

Data from restriction fragment length polymorphic (RFLP) typing, plasmid typing, and serotyping show two populations of *M. avium,* one infecting humans and the other infecting animals. Until more specific skin-testing antigens are available, however, skin-test antigens developed from different geographic locations and strains must be utilized with caution.

The most important NTM pulmonary pathogens are MAC, *M. kansasii, M. fortuitum-M. chelonei,* and *M. xenopi.* Occasional pulmonary pathogens are *M. scrofulaceum, M. szulgai, M. simiae,* and *M. malmoense.* Because NTM disease is not reportable, information regarding its incidence and prevalence is based largely on estimates. In 1979–1980, these diseases were estimated to occur in one third of 32,000 mycobacterial isolates. Of

these, 60% were MAC, 19% were *M. fortuitum-M. chelonei,* and 10% *M. kansasii.* The estimated incidence of NTM disease is 1.8 cases per 100,000 in the U.S. population.

SPECIFIC NONTUBERCULOUS MYCOBACTERIAL DISEASES

Mycobacterium avium-intracellulare Complex Disease

MAC occurs in the environment, notably soil, bodies of water, and water systems, and in animals, such as poultry. The epidemiology of disease, however, has no correlation with the distribution of MAC in the environment, as MAC is found throughout the United States, including the western states. Migration of native residents from primary endemic regions to nonedemic areas after primary infection (not unlike what occurs with *M. tuberculosis*) may contribute to the wide distribution. The clinically predominant serovar types are 1, 4, and 8. Serovar 4 is dominant in northern California and the eastern United States, while serovar 8 is dominant in southern California.

MAC is found in geographically warmer environments and in highly acidic brown swamps of the southeastern coastal plains of the United States. MAC isolates from patients differ from environmental isolates. In addition, MAC isolates from patients with acquired immunodeficiency syndrome (AIDS) differ from environmental isolates and those found in patients without AIDS. In San Francisco, for example, environmental contamination does not account for the high prevalence of MAC cultured from AIDS patients.

Next to *M. tuberculosis,* MAC organisms are the most common mycobacteria in human disease. It traditionally occurs in patients with underlying pulmonary conditions, such as chronic obstructive pulmonary disease (COPD), bronchiectasis, old healed tuberculosis, or currently active tuberculosis. Individuals in occupations associated with heavy exposure to dust are also more likely to be infected.

During the last two decades, attention has been directed to other groups of patients infected with pulmonary MAC or other NTM. Infections have been reported in patients with cystic fibrosis and in women without underlying lung diseases. MAC has also been associated with human immunodeficiency virus (HIV) disease, especially in full-blown AIDS; it is a case-defining pathogen in HIV-infected persons. Pulmonary disease and extrapulmonary involvement occur frequently in the latter group when the CD4-cell count falls to $<100/\mu L$. MAC infection occurs in from 15%–40% of HIV-infected patients.

Pulmonary MAC disease develops in three major groups of patients (Table 1). There may be overlap of the groups (i.e., patients with AIDS may have underlying COPD).

In group 1 (patients with underlying lung disease), the most important underlying disease is COPD. It is fairly evenly distributed among men and women, and generally, the patients are older (>50 years). Chronic alcoholism and cigarette smoking are associated conditions in most patients. Eighty-five percent of patients with MAC disease are white. Upper lobe cavitary changes are a common radiologic feature. Symptoms are usually progressive and include productive cough accompanied by fever and night sweats. Malaise is common. When disease is unilateral initially, clinical progression results in bilateral radiologic involvement.

Because of improvements in the care and treatment of patients with cystic fibrosis, they are living longer but are increasingly vulnerable to a multitude of bacterial organisms, including NTM. MAC appears to be the most important NTM pathogen in adult patients with cystic fibrosis. Patients range in age from 18 to 35 years. As with the other chronic lung diseases, diagnosis and treatment may be confounded by the underlying disease. Although some patients with cystic fibrosis have diabetes mellitus resulting from pancreatic insufficiency, they generally do not have immune dysfunction. Their underlying lung disease is obstructive and their nutritional status is often poor. Clinical deterioration resulting from pulmonary bacterial infection is frequent. It is difficult to distinguish colonization from disease, as bacterial infections (*Pseudomonas* and *Staphylococcus aureus*) are particu-

TABLE 1. *Clinical description of groups with pulmonary MAC infection*

Group 1 (with underlying lung disease)	Group 2 (without underlying lung disease)		Group 3 (immune deficiency disease)	
	a	b	a	b
Age, y 50–75	30–40	52–78	26–40	>66
Male:female 50:50	2:1	19:81	94:6	2:1
Associated conditions	thoracic deformities:	none	immunosuppression with HIV	immunosuppression without HIV:
alcoholism	pectus excavatum,			malignancy
smoking	narrow AP distance,			chemotherapy
heavy exposure to dust	mitral valve prolapse			steroids
gastrectomy				
prior TB				
bronchiectasis				
COPD				
bronchogenic cancer				
chronic aspiration				
cystic fibrosis[a]				
Chest x-ray findings	localized to RML/lingula	localized to RML/lingula	rare changes	nodular
cavitary upper	nodular changes,	nodular changes,	—	—
lobe infiltrate	bronchiectasis	upper lobe	interstitial	interstitial
		involvement	solitary nodule	
Symptoms				
cough: productive	small	productive	rare/absent	nonproductive
fever: common	absent	uncommon	frequent	—
night sweats:	absent	uncommon	—	—
prominent				
malaise: common	prominent	uncommon	frequent	common

From Prince, Kennedy, Iseman. Group 1 patients have underlying lung disease, group 2 patients have no underlying lung disease (subgroups differ in age), and group 3 patients have a common mechanism of immune deficiency with or without HIV.

AP, anteroposterior; RML, right middle lobe; MAC, *Mycobacterium avium* complex.

[a] Generally of younger age group.

larly common causes of radiologic changes and clinical deterioration. Bacterial contamination (i.e., overgrowth of *Pseudomonas*) has been described, often adding to the clinical dilemma of assessing true disease from colonization.

Patients in group 2 have no underlying lung disease. The majority in this group are women, both young and old. In the younger patients (group 2a), associated thoracic deformities, such as narrowing of the anteroposterior diameter of the chest, pectus excavatum, and scoliosis with mitral valve prolapse, have been observed. These abnormalities may occur singly or in combination. Male patients are less frequently affected. Chest x-ray abnormalities are fairly localized, involving predominantly the right middle lobe or lingula. Nodules and bronchiectasis are usually prominently displayed by computed tomogram (CT) of the chest.

The patients in group 2b are elderly women without underlying lung disease. Radiologic changes in the chest are similarly localized to the right middle lobe and/or lingula. Nodular changes as well as bronchiectasis have been observed. Some patients have upper lobe involvement, most commonly of the anterior segment. Symptoms are similar for both subgroups, including productive cough, malaise, fever, and night sweats. Although the disease course is indolent, it can accelerate and become fatal without treatment.

Group 3 comprises patients with immunosuppression. Group 3a has been fairly recently described as a major part of the AIDS epidemic. The main feature is the presence of infection with HIV. MAC infection has occurred together with *M. tuberculosis* disease; the HIV transmission categories are usually homosexual and bisexual men. Extrapulmonary involvement is a prominent feature in these cases. Disseminated MAC infection is associated with pulmonary involvement in 80% of cases. Patients generally present with gastrointestinal symptoms, fever, weight loss, and fatigue. There are usually no pulmonary symptoms or radiologic evidence of pulmonary disease unless another pulmonary disease is present.

Described radiologic abnormalities have included hilar masses, solitary pulmonary nodules, upper lobe changes, diffuse infiltrates, and cysts, with diffuse infiltrates accounting for 85%. Most of the infiltrates are caused by concomitant *Pneumocystis carinii* pneumonia, tuberculosis, cytomegalovirus infection, and other opportunistic infections.

The patients in group 3b have secondary or acquired immunosuppression resulting from malignancy or blood disorders (leukemia and lymphoma) or from therapeutic interventions, such as chemotherapy and steroid therapy. Immunosuppression is not HIV-related. Pulmonary disease is associated with cavitary infiltrates, as in group 1, and often accompanied by constitutional symptoms, such as productive cough, fever, night sweats, and malaise.

The course of the disease is dictated by the underlying malignancy or blood disorder.

Diagnosis of pulmonary MAC infection is made by acid-fast smear of sputum and culture. Diagnostic procedures have included sputum induction, bronchoscopy with lavage, aspiration, and tissue biopsy. Rarely, open lung biopsy is performed. MAC has been identified as a cause of solitary nodules after resection, tissue biopsy, and culture performed as part of the nodule workup. Adenopathy may also require a surgical biopsy (open excision or via mediastinoscopy). CT of the chest has been widely used to detect bronchiectasis and nodules, whereas ventilation-perfusion scan is utilized to determine residual function of a nonresectable lung or the remaining lung.

Treatment

Few clinical trials of the treatment of pulmonary MAC disease were undertaken until 1988, when rifabutin was introduced. Promising responses of combination therapy for MAC infection in AIDS began to be reported. Clearly, monotherapy had no role in MAC disease, because it was associated with rapid relapse, recurrence, and development of bacterial resistance. Treatment results were limited by persistence of MAC and inability to eradicate the infection. The application of this experience using four-drug therapy to treat pulmonary MAC disease has been derived from seemingly successful trials for disseminated MAC infection in AIDS.

Recommendations for the treatment of MAC infection are based on evolving and accumulating experience. Isoniazid and pyrazinamide have no role in the treatment of MAC disease. Susceptibility testing based on *M. tuberculosis* standards is not applicable in MAC infection. In addition, MAC isolates have a broad range of drug susceptibility, so that a standardized regimen may not be useful. For example, MAC isolates from AIDS patients have shown genetic diversity—that is, individuals may be concurrently infected with more than one strain of MAC. Thus, the choice of antimycobacterial agents should be based on quantitative tests for drug susceptibility.

In the treatment of MAC lung disease, regimens are separated into two treatment phases. During the initial phase, at least four drugs are used: clarithromycin (500 mg orally twice daily), ethambutol (25 mg/kg orally once daily), rifabutin (300 mg orally once daily) or clofazimine (200 mg orally once daily), and streptomycin (10 to 12 mg/kg intramuscularly once daily) or amikacin (12 to 15 mg/kg intravenously three times a week). This regimen is given for 2 months and is followed by a continuation phase. The regimen during the continuation phase is clarithromycin (750 mg orally once daily), ethambutol 15 mg/kg orally once daily), and rifabutin (300 mg orally once daily). Treatment should continue for 24 months or at least 12 to 18 months past the last positive sputum culture. There will likely be instances of relapse. For unresponsive localized disease, surgical resection is often indicated. Commonly used antimycobacterial agents for MAC infection are listed in Table 2, along with some of their adverse effects.

Therapeutic goals may include a reduction in symptoms (fever, night sweats, cough), stabilization or diminution of chest radiologic abnormalities, and improvement in pulmonary function. Adverse reactions should be monitored. An incremental dosing strategy or dose staggering has been recommended for non-HIV patients to reduce discontinuation of treatment because of toxicity and intolerance.

Prophylaxis for MAC Disease in HIV-Infected Persons

Rifabutin was approved by the U.S. Food and Drug Administration for prophylaxis of MAC disease based on two cohort studies. The studies reported significant reduction in bacteremia, clinical symptoms, and laboratory abnormalities when rifabutin was used as a prophylactic agent. The drug was found to be safe, effective, and well tolerated, and adverse effects were infrequent. It improved the quality of life, but there was no overall survival benefit from its use. The current recommendation is 300 mg of rifabutin orally once a day for HIV-infected persons having a CD4-cell count of $<100/mm^3$, with the treatment to continue for life. In areas with a high prevalence of tuberculosis, the use of rifabutin may preclude the use of rifampin as part of the standard antimycobacterial treatment for tuberculosis because of high levels of cross-resistance. Rifampin-resistant cases of tuberculosis have been documented as a result of rifabutin use for MAC infection. Rifabutin is not recommended as MAC prophylaxis for non-HIV patients.

Drug Interactions

Absorption and efficacy of the drugs may be affected by drug interactions. Clarithromycin interferes with compounds metabolized by the hepatic P_{450} cytochrome system; azithromycin does not interfere with the P_{450} system. Fluoroquinolones are chelated by aluminum compounds, such as antacids. Iron and multivitamin compounds may also reduce their bioavailability. Rifabutin may interact with zidovudine.

M. kansasii Disease

Most isolates of M. kansasii have been recovered from tap water in cities known to be endemic for M. kansasii. In Texas, where both M. kansasii and MAC occur, M. kansasii infection and disease were noted to be more frequent in urban dwellers with pulmonary disease, whereas MAC infections were noted in rural dwellers. Almost all strains of M. kansasii are susceptible to rifampin and only slightly resistant to isoniazid, ethambutol, and streptomycin. However, rifampin-resistant strains of M. kansasii have been reported among patients with and without AIDS. Patients with rifampin-resistant isolates have clinical profiles showing prior use of one or two antimycobacterial drugs and noncompliance. One third of the resistant isolates were from HIV-seropositive patients.

Clinical features of pulmonary M. kansasii disease are similar to the features of pulmonary MAC infection. Cavitary lung disease is common; M. kansasii disease predominantly occurs in white, middle-aged men; the ratio of men to women affected is 2:1. A greater number of cases are noted among the 30- to 39-year age group in both sexes; upper gastrointestinal disorders, such as prior gastrectomy and peptic ulcer disease, are frequently observed. The majority have previous or existing lung diseases, especially COPD. The presence of underlying lung

TABLE 2. *Antimycobacterial agents commonly used in pulmonary MAC infection*

Agents	Dose (adults)	Side effects/toxicity[a]
Azithromycin	250–500 mg PO od	diarrhea, nausea, abdominal pain, elevated liver enzymes
Clarithromycin	500 mg PO bid; 750 mg PO bid	same as above
Ethambutol	25 mg/kg PO od	optic neuritis, anorexia, nausea, vomiting
Rifabutin	450 mg PO od	similar to those of rifampin
Ciprofloxacin	500 mg PO bid; 750 mg PO od	GI complaints: nausea, diarrhea
Amikacin	12–15 mg/kg three times a week	cranial nerve (auditory/vestibular)
Rifampin	600 mg PO od; 450 mg for <45 kg	orange discoloration of body secretions, flulike illness, hepatitis, low platelet count
Clofazimine	50–200 mg PO od	skin discoloration, GI complaints
Streptomycin	10–15 mg/kg od	cranial nerve VIII and renal toxicity, low potassium and magnesium levels

Adapted from Masur H, and the Public Health Service Task Force on Prophylaxis and Therapy for MAC. Special report: recommendations on prophylaxis and therapy for disseminated *Mycobacterium avium* complex disease in patients infected with the human immunodeficiency virus. *N Engl J Med* 329:898–904.

[a] Patients should be monitored for side effects and toxicity.

disease adversely affects the course of treatment and prognosis. Conversely, the absence of prior lung disease portends a more favorable outcome with treatment.

M. kansasii disease in HIV-infected persons has been extensively described. Clinical features include fever, cough, dyspnea, and rarely hemoptysis. Most diagnoses have been made from spontaneously produced sputum specimens, whereas a third have been based on bronchoscopy specimens. Sputum positive for acid-fast bacilli (AFB) is more likely in patients with pulmonary infiltrates, which range from predominantly upper lobe infiltrates to pulmonary cavitary and reticulonodular types. Concomitant organisms such as *P. carinii, S. aureus,* and cytomegalovirus are more frequent when infiltrates are bilateral, diffuse, and interstitial.

Treatment

A better response to treatment with chemotherapy alone has been reported among patients without prior or existing underlying lung disease. Treatment failures are associated with persistence of cavities in association with isoniazid-resistant organisms. Sputum conversion is generally achieved by 92% of drug-treated patients in the first 6 months of treatment. Consideration of surgical resection of cavities was previously suggested if improvement was not observed after 6 months of treatment. The use of rifampin at a higher dose (600 mg to 900 mg) in the initial therapeutic regimen along with ethambutol and isoniazid has changed this situation, with almost a 100% response rate to chemotherapy.

Treatment for *M. kansasii* disease has been suggested using a triple regimen (isoniazid-rifampin-ethambutol). However, in most instances only smears positive for AFB are available at the onset, and the patient is started on four drugs (including pyrazinamide) to treat conventional tuberculosis empirically. When cultures for *M. kansasii* become available, pyrazinamide can be dropped, as it does not have any activity against *M. kansasii*. At the very least, *M. kansasii* is intermediately susceptible to isoniazid; thus, the raised dose of 600 mg is indicated.

A combination regimen of rifampin and ethambutol for 9 months has been used successfully in Great Britain. Relapse rates (8%) were similar to rates in groups who initially started with combinations of four drugs in the first 2 months. A quadruple regimen is recommended for rifampin-resistant cases. Susceptibility testing using the proportion method may not be reliable in predicting resistance, and minimal inhibitory concentrations (MICs) may differ, especially with isoniazid and streptomycin. Clarithromycin is a promising alternative drug.

M. fortuitum-M. chelonei Complex Disease

M. fortuitum complex includes *M. fortuitum* and *M. chelonei* strains. This is the third most prevalent NTM infection in the United States. Men are likely affected by *M. fortuitum,* whereas women are affected by *M. chelonei*. These mycobacteria are generally cutaneous and pulmonary pathogens.

A rapidly growing organism, *M. chelonei* causes a significant number of pulmonary cases. It is not readily isolated from the environment. As is typical in most NTM disease, bronchiectasis, prior mycobacterial disease, and chronic lung disease from aspiration are found in *M. fortuitum-M. chelonei* complex lung disease.

M. fortuitum was first described in cases of chronic aspiration pneumonia and esophageal achalasia. Bilateral patchy infiltrates are frequent; cavitary disease is not common. A slow, progressive course is characteristic, and response to therapy may be observed with amikacin and cefoxitin. Both isolates (*M. fortuitum, M. chelonei*) are often susceptible to amikacin, cefoxitin, and imipenem, and are partially susceptible to doxycycline. Separately, *M. fortuitum* is also susceptible to ciprofloxacin and sulfonamides, whereas *M. chelonei* is susceptible to tobramycin. Some *M. fortuitum-M. chelonei* isolates have been shown to be susceptible to erythromycin. Both *M. fortuitum* and *M. chelonei* are generally resistant to first-line antituberculosis agents.

M. xenopi Disease

Water is a favorite habitat for *M. xenopi;* it is thermophilic, known to grow at 42°C. It has been reported in outbreaks as a pseudoinfection, mostly in nosocomial settings (contaminated bronchoscopy). Pulmonary disease in AIDS has also been reported. The organism is common in Europe, Asia, and Canada. An outbreak of *M. xenopi* pulmonary disease was described in a Veterans Administration hospital in Connecticut. The nosocomial infection was ascribed to the hospital's hot water system. Predisposing factors were pre-existing lung disease and prior hospitalizations in the same environment. Radiographic findings included nodular/mass lesions, thick-walled cavities, and associated apical pleural changes, singly or in combination. Nosocomially acquired infections were indolent and often asymptomatic. In patients not infected with HIV, sporadic cases have been reported to be asymptomatic, with abnormal chest x-ray findings on routine examination. On the other hand, other *M. xenopi* pulmonary disease has been described accompanied by cough, fever, weight loss, and hemoptysis. It has rarely been reported in the United States among AIDS patients presenting with positive findings on sputum smear and negative radiographic findings. It has also been associated with pre-existing conditions such as alcoholism, gastrectomy, cigarette smoking, and lung cancer. Diagnosis has been made from spontaneous sputum, bronchial washing, and resected lung tissue in a workup to exclude neoplasm. The organism is fairly responsive to antituberculosis agents, especially streptomycin, isoniazid, and para-aminosalicylic acid. The initial recommended regimen is isoniazid, rifampin, ethambutol, and pyrazinamide pending cultures for specific mycobacteria.

DIAGNOSIS OF NONTUBERCULOUS MYCOBACTERIAL PULMONARY DISEASE

A general approach to diagnosis in NTM pulmonary disease was recommended in 1990. Some controversies and disagreements still exist, however. A sputum culture positive for NTM must be assessed by determining and defining transient contamination versus true pulmonary disease versus prolonged colonization, usually in the presence of chronic lung disease. Contamination of specimen culture is defined by a single positive culture among several specimen collections and by absence of clinical features or evidence of NTM disease. True pulmonary infection/disease is more difficult to distinguish from NTM colonization. For colonization, bronchial hygiene has been recommended as the first therapeutic step, with or without antimycobacterial drugs. This has been successfully employed with *M. kansasii* and MAC. It has not been studied in other NTM colonization but would be presumed to work as well. In the evaluation of such situations, fungal, neoplastic, and *M. tuberculosis* disease must be considered in the differential diagnosis.

For patients with a radiologic cavitary infiltrate, contamination must be ruled out. Thus, the presence of mycobacteria must be confirmed in two or more sputum or other respiratory specimens on smear and/or by a moderate or heavy growth on culture. Other reasonable diagnoses must have been excluded.

For patients with radiologic noncavitary infiltrate, the criteria are as follows: (1) Two or more sputum or other respiratory specimens (bronchial washings, endotracheal aspirates) must show a positive stain for AFB and/or moderate to heavy growth on culture; (2) after bronchial hygiene has been attempted with or without 2 weeks of antimycobacterial therapy and the NTM does not clear on smear, disease may be presumed when (3) other causes for the infiltrate have been ruled out.

If a sputum evaluation is nondiagnostic in the presence of either a cavitary or noncavitary infiltrate and other diagnoses cannot be excluded, an invasive procedure such as lung biopsy is recommended. True disease is confirmed by the presence of changes consistent with mycobacterial histopathology (i.e., granulomatous inflammation and/or a positive tissue stain for AFB). When two or more sputum specimens are positive for NTM in low numbers and accompanied by the histologic changes described, the diagnosis is presumptive. Clinically, a symptomatic patient with a single culture positive for NTM and a noncavitary infiltrate may require empiric therapy.

Solitary Nodules in Nontuberculous Mycobacterial Infection

Sixty percent of asymptomatic solitary pulmonary nodules are caused by MAC. This entity is generally discovered during routine chest examination. Excellent outcome is observed following resectional surgery in cases treated preoperatively with a standard antituberculosis regimen (two drugs) for positive AFB smears and compatible histology before culture reports become available. There are generally no postoperative complications or dissemination of infection.

Endobronchial Nontuberculous Mycobacterial Infection

Endobronchial mycobacterial disease is infrequently reported, because the ready availability of sputum for diagnosis in most cases of NTM disease precludes bronchoscopy. A few reports have noted that patients having mycobacterial disease may present with normal lungs and a mediastinal mass mimicking malignancy, seen with MAC, *M. kansasii*, and rarely *M. fortuitum*. In the reports, bronchoscopic findings have included ulcerating mass lesion and submucosal masses obstructing bronchial orifices, with resulting segment collapse.

SURGICAL CONSIDERATIONS

The outcome of surgical resection for NTM pulmonary disease is poorer than that of similar resection for multidrug-resistant *M. tuberculosis* pulmonary disease. Complication rates are high, especially in patients with previous chest irradiation or pulmonary resection, perioperative positive sputum cultures, and multimicrobial lung infection. Bronchopleural fistulas, prolonged air leak, and space problems may be frequent, although the use of muscle flaps has reduced these complications. Consideration of early resection for localized disease is still recommended in NTM. Preoperative treatment for at least 3 months and continuation of drug therapy postoperatively are also recommended.

BIBLIOGRAPHY

Ahn CH, Lowell JR, Onstad GD, Shuford EH, Hurst GA. A demographic study of disease due to *Mycobacterium kansasii* or *M. intracellulare-avium* in Texas. *Chest* 1979;75:120–125. *Review of* M. kansasii *and* M. intracellulare-avium *disease reported during a 9-year period to the Texas Health Department. The incidence of* M. kansasii *infection was twice that of* M. intracellulare-avium *in urban areas.*

Bamberger DM, Driks MR, Gupta MR, O'Connor MC, Jost PM, Neihart RE, McKinsey DS, Moore LA. Kansas City AIDS Research Consortium. *Mycobacterium kansasii* among patients infected with human immunodeficiency virus in Kansas City. *Clin Infect Dis* 1994;18: 395–400. *Description of the clinical characteristics of 35 patients* with AIDS in Kansas City whose presentation differed from those in prior reports. All patients except two had advanced HIV infection, with a median CD4-cell count of 12/μL.

Bennett SN, Peterson DE, Johnson DR, Hall WN, Robinson-Dunn B, Dietrich S. Bronchoscopy-associated *Mycobacterium xenopi* pseudoinfections. *Am J Respir Crit Care Med* 1994;150:254–250. *Report from a Michigan hospital of an increase in recovery of* M. xenopi *isolates (35% of mycobacterial isolates) during a 3-year period.*

British Thoracic Society. *Mycobacterium kansasii* pulmonary infection: a prospective study of the results of 9 months of treatment with rifampicin and ethambutol. *Thorax* 1994;49:442–445. *Report from Great Britain of the results of a prospective multicenter study of a 9-month trial of chemotherapy with rifampin and ethambutol.*

Costrini AM, Mahler DA, Gross WM, Hawkins JE, Yesner R, D'Esopo ND. Clinical and roentgenographic features of nosocomial pulmonary disease due to *Mycobacterium xenopi*. *Am Rev Respir Dis* 1981;123:104–109. *A nosocomial source of* M. xenopi *infection was identified in hot water taps in a veterans' hospital; 12 of 15 cases were successfully treated with antimycobacterial drugs.*

Davidson PT. *M. avium* complex, *M. kansasii, M. fortuitum,* and other mycobacteria causing human disease. In: Reichman LB, Hershfield ES, eds. *Tuberculosis: A Comprehensive International Approach.* New York: Marcel Dekker; 1993:505–530. *Comprehensive overview of NTM pulmonary disease.*

Elston HR, Duffy JP. *Mycobacterium xenopi* and mycobacteriosis: a clinical and bacteriologic report. *Am Rev Respir Dis* 1973;108:944–949. *Case report of* M. xenopi *cavitary lung disease (non-HIV) responsive to streptomycin, isoniazid, and ethambutol.*

Gribetz AR, Damsker B, Bottone EJ, Kirschner PA, Teirstein AS. Solitary pulmonary nodules due to nontuberculous mycobacterial infection. *Am J Med* 1981;70:39–43. *Review of nontuberculous mycobacteria as cause of solitary pulmonary nodules.*

Heifets LB, Iseman MD. Individualized versus standard regimens in the treatment of *Mycobacterium avium* infections. *Am Rev Respir Dis* 1991;144:1–2. *Quantitative drug susceptibility testing is recommended to guide the choice of antimicrobial agents for MAC disease.*

Iseman MD, Buschman DL, Ackerson LM. Pectus excavatum and scoliosis: thoracic anomalies associated with pulmonary disease caused by *Mycobacterium avium* complex. *Am Rev Respir Dis* 1991;144:914–916. *Two thoracic anomalies, pectus excavatum and/or scoliosis, were observed to be more prevalent in patients with MAC than in those with* M. tuberculosis *infection seen at a major referral center for mycobacterial disease.*

Johanson WG, Nicholson DP. Pulmonary disease due to *Mycobacterium kansasii:* an analysis of some factors affecting prognosis. *Am Rev Respir Dis* 1969;99:73–85. *Description of the clinical features of 99 patients with* M. kansasii *pulmonary disease.*

Kennedy TP, Weber DJ. Nontuberculous mycobacteria: an underappreciated cause of geriatric lung disease. *Am J Respir Crit Care Med* 1994;149:1654–1658. *Retrospective 2-year review of 21 cases of mycobacterial lung infection in a middle class setting. MAC infection exceeded* M. tuberculosis *disease.*

Kilby JM, Gilligan PH, Yankaskas JR, Highsmith WE, Edwards LJ, Knowles MR. Nontuberculous mycobacteria in adult patients with cystic fibrosis. *Chest* 1992;102:70–75. *The prevalence of nontuberculous mycobacteria among patients with cystic fibrosis was noted to be high (20%) in a group followed at a center for cystic fibrosis in the southeastern United States.*

Levine B, Chaisson RE. *Mycobacterium kansasii:* a cause of treatable pulmonary disease associated with advanced human immunodeficiency virus (HIV) infection. *Ann Intern Med* 1991;114:861–868. *Descriptive review of the clinical features and response to therapy in 19 cases of* M. kansasii *infection associated with HIV infection.*

Lordi GM, Reichman LB. Pulmonary *Mycobacterium fortuitum* com-

plex infections. *Curr Ther Respir Dis* 1989;3:74–77. *Short review of* M. fortuitum *and* M. chelonei *respiratory infections.*

Mangura BT, Reichman LB. Prevention and treatment of *Mycobacterium avium* complex infection. *Res Microbiol* 1994;145:181–187. *Review of prevention and treatment of MAC in HIV disease. Several earlier combinations of therapy for MAC are cited.*

Masur H, and the Public Health Service Task Force on Prophylaxis and Therapy for MAC. Special report: recommendations on prophylaxis and therapy for disseminated *Mycobacterium avium* complex disease in patients infected with the human immunodeficiency virus. *N Engl J Med* 1993;329:898–904.*A brief summary and report of recommendations for prophylaxis and therapy for disseminated MAC.*

McDonald RJ, Reichman LB. A new classification for some mycobacteria. *Chest* 1983;84:511–512. *Discussion of the nonutility of the existing classification for NTM. The Bailey classification is introduced as a practical tool.*

McSwiggan DA, Collins CH. The isolation of *M. kansasii* and *M. xenopi* from water systems. *Tubercle* 1974;55:291–297. *Increased recovery of* M. xenopi *and* M. kansasii *isolates was traced to several hospitals in northwest London. Cold water taps yielded more* M. kansasii. *Main water system did not yield either.*

Pomerantz M, Madsen L, Goble M, Iseman M. Surgical management of resistant mycobacterial tuberculosis and other mycobacterial pulmonary infections. *Ann Thorac Surg* 1991;52:1108–1112. *Retrospective review of surgical outcome during a 7-year period of patients with resistant mycobacterial tuberculosis and other mycobacterial pulmonary infections.*

Prince DS, Peterson DD, Steiner RM, Gottlieb JE, Scott R, Israel HL, Figueroa WG, Fish JE. Infection with *Mycobacterium avium* complex in patients without predisposing conditions. *N Engl J Med* 1989;321:863–868. *Description of three groups of patients with cultures positive for MAC during 10-year period in two Philadelphia hospitals.*

Reichman LB, McDonald RJ, Mangura BT. Rifabutin prophylaxis against *Mycobacterium avium* complex infection. *N Engl J Med* 1994;330:437–438. *Letter calling attention to potential rifampin resistance through inadvertent rifabutin prophylaxis of undiagnosed pulmonary tuberculosis.*

Rosenzweig DY. Pulmonary mycobacterial infections due to *Mycobacterium intracellulare-avium* complex: clinical features and course in 100 consecutive cases. *Chest* 1979;75:115–119. *Clinical description and follow-up of 100 cases of MAC pulmonary disease.*

Stover DE, White DA, Romano PA, Gellene RA, Robeson WA. Spectrum of pulmonary disease associated with the acquired immune deficiency syndrome. *Am J Med* 1985;78:429–437. *Early clinical description of pulmonary complications of AIDS in a metropolitan center where 21% of patients with infectious pulmonary complications had MAC infection.*

Tellis CJ, Beechler CR, Ohashi DK, Fuller SA. Pulmonary disease caused by *Mycobacterium xenopi*. *Am Rev Respir Dis* 1977;116:779–783. *Two cases of pulmonary* M. xenopi *infection, one presenting as a solid density and the other as an upper lobe infiltrate. Observed accompanying factors were moderate cigarette smoking and neoplasm of lung.*

Wallace RJ, Dunbar D, Brown BA, Onyi G, Dunlap R, Ahn CH, Murphy DT. Rifampin-resistant *Mycobacterium kansasii*. *Clin Infect Dis* 1944;18:736–743. *Rifampin-resistant isolates were characterized during a 5-year period in Texas. The incidence was 3.7% per year, with greatest recovery between 1990 and 1991.*

Wallace RJ, O'Brien R, Glassroth J, Raleigh J, Dutt A. ATS statement: diagnosis and treatment of disease caused by nontuberculous mycobacteria. *Am Rev Respir Dis* 1990;142:940–953. *Diagnostic criteria and treatment of NTM; differentiation between presentations of cavitary and noncavitary infiltrates.*

Wolinsky E. State of the art: nontuberculous mycobacteria and associated diseases. *Am Rev Respir Dis* 1979;119:107–159. *Classic, comprehensive review of nontuberculous mycobacteria, with 592 references. Detailed historical perspective and microbiologic overview.*

Textbook of Pulmonary Diseases, 6th ed.
edited by G.L. Baum, J.D. Crapo, B.R. Celli, and J.B. Karlinsky,
Lippincott–Raven Publishers, Philadelphia, © 1998.

CHAPTER

30

Embolic Infections of the Lungs and Lipoid Pneumonia

Richard J. Blinkhorn Jr.

EMBOLIC INFECTIONS

Embolic infections may result from secondarily infected bland infarcts or from septic emboli. Pulmonary infarction usually arises from thrombotic emboli situated in the deep venous system of the lower extremities (Chapter 66). Secondary infection of the infarcted lung occurs most often as a result of invasion by way of the airway but occasionally via the bloodstream. Autopsy studies indicate that the incidence of secondary infection is between 4.0% and 5.0%, but actual incidence is probably lower, because infection results in a higher case fatality rate. Predisposing factors are cardiac decompensation and oropharyngeal sepsis. Empyema may be the presenting feature.

The diagnosis may be suspected by persistent fever and leukocytosis and the production of purulent or fetid sputum. Chest radiography confirms the presence of an abscess in the previously infarcted area, with or without pleural fluid. Bacteriologic diagnosis is made by the examination of sputum, occasionally from positive blood cultures, and from examination of pleural fluid if it is present. Oropharyngeal anaerobic bacteria are commonly involved, as are *Staphylococcus aureus* and gram-negative bacilli. In the differential diagnosis, cavity formation caused by ischemic necrosis in the center of large infarcts resulting from inadequate bronchial arterial collateral circulation should be considered.

Septic emboli of the lungs most commonly arise in the right side of the heart (endocarditis) or in the peripheral veins, where the underlying process is septic thrombophlebitis. Other, less common sites of origin include the head and neck (postanginal sepsis, mastoiditis, dental in-

fections), the pelvic veins of women post partum (septic pelvic thrombophlebitis), and the central veins when catheters are placed therein for prolonged administration of therapeutic biologic products. The latter site has become more important as the numbers of patients with acquired immunodeficiency syndrome (AIDS) or advanced cancer who require total parenteral nutrition has increased. Similar embolization may accompany suppurative thrombophlebitis of the internal jugular vein from deep infections of the pharynx and tonsils, known as *postanginal sepsis* or *Lemierre's syndrome.*

The presenting clinical picture usually is that of the underlying disease, although occasionally the primary manifestations are related to the lungs. The pulmonary signs are pleuritic pain, cough, and eventually purulent sputum. The radiographic findings have been well characterized. There may be areas of consolidation with subsequent suppuration and necrosis, especially in *S. aureus* infection (Fig. 1). More often, small, localized infiltrates are scattered through both lungs that rapidly break down to form thin-walled cavities (Fig. 2). On occasion, necrosis causes a piece of lung tissue to be sequestered in the centers of such nodules, with the development of an intracavitary loose body simulating a ''target.'' Computed tomography (CT) is useful in diagnosis. Typical CT appearances include multiple peripheral nodules, a feeding vessel sign, cavitation, wedge-shaped lesions abutting the pleurae, and air bronchograms within the nodules.

In Lemierre's syndrome, the common etiologic agent is an anaerobic organism, especially *Fusobacterium.* When pelvic veins are infected, the agent is generally an anaerobe of the *Bacteroides* group. *S. aureus* is the usual culprit from other sites. Treatment should be directed at the underlying condition and may include surgical drainage, removal of infected catheters, and administration of appropriate antibiotics. Progression of the lung disease to

R. J. Blinkhorn Jr.: MetroHealth Medical Center, Cleveland Ohio 44109.

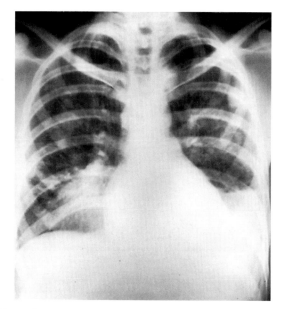

FIG. 1. Embolic lesions of lung associated with submandibular *S. aureus* infection in a 30-year-old man.

empyema requires repeated aspiration, tube drainage, or thoracotomy.

LIPOID PNEUMONIA

The inflammatory reaction associated with the presence of oil or fat in the alveoli is known as *lipoid pneumonia.* The lipid material may originate in the lung itself, or it may be aspirated or inhaled into the lung.

Endogenous Lipoid Pneumonia

In endogenous lipoid pneumonia, the lipid material consists of cholesterol and its esters, released during the breakdown of cell walls in atelectatic pulmonary tissue distal to an obstructed airway. Endogenous lipoid pneumonia may also be seen in association with long-standing tuberculosis, chronic pulmonary abscesses, or bronchiectasis. The usual cause of obstruction in the airway is tumor. In primary or idiopathic endogenous lipoid pneumonia, there is no underlying condition to explain the process. In children, coexisting endogenous lipoid pneumonia and pulmonary alveolar proteinosis have been reported as complicating otherwise benign pulmonary disorders.

The clinical presentation is that of the underlying bronchogenic tumor or chronic infection. Fever, chills, productive cough, and pleuritic chest pain are common. No predisposing conditions that favor aspiration are present, nor is there any history of ingestion of oily substances. The chest radiograph shows a segmental or lobar consolidation with many variations, depending on the underlying

condition (Fig. 3). Neither expectorated sputum nor bronchial washings contain lipid-laden macrophages. Only after open lung biopsy or lobectomy is the diagnosis established. The lung is golden-yellow in appearance, and the bronchial lymph nodes often are enlarged. Under the microscope, a dense infiltrate of foamy macrophages containing homogeneously distributed vacuoles of fat can be seen (Fig. 4). The lipid material may form the cleft-like crystals of cholesterol after extrusion into the parenchyma.

Exogenous Lipoid Pneumonia

Exogenous lipoid pneumonia is an inflammatory reaction to the aspiration or inhalation of oil or fat. The disease is seen mainly in children, elderly debilitated adults, or individuals with underlying conditions predisposing to aspiration (e.g., altered consciousness, difficulties in swallowing resulting from neurologic disease, or disorders of esophageal motility). There is usually a history of prolonged use of mineral oil in laxatives or nose drops. Undoubtedly, exogenous lipoid pneumonia now is less frequent than in the 1930s, when it was seen during almost 9% of autopsies in children and 1.2% in adults. Retrospective studies since the 1950s, nevertheless, indicate that the disease persists. A survey of 389 chronically ill patients showed that 58 (15%) had exogenous lipoid pneumonia, and 87% of them admitted to the ingestion of mineral oil or oil-containing medication or the use of oily nose drops.

It is reasonable to postulate that the oil reaches the lungs because of an incompetent lower esophageal sphincter and aspiration from the esophagus during the night. Radiopaque oily material instilled into the nose of healthy people during sleep often may be detected in chest radiographs the next morning. When instilled intratracheally, oil fails to provoke two important protective responses of the airway: glottic closure and coughing. In addition, it overcomes another defense mechanism, mucociliary transport. Although mineral oil does not affect ciliary beating, it markedly impairs the movement of the mucous blanket by altering the physical properties of the secretions.

The nature of the oil reaching the alveoli determines the pathologic response. Simple vegetable oils provoke little response and may be cleared from the lung largely by expectoration. Animal oils cause inflammation involving mononuclear and giant cells, proliferation of connective tissue, and variable necrosis. Mineral oil is rapidly emulsified and elicits a brisk outpouring of alveolar macrophages, which ingest oil globules. Later, a foreign-body granulomatous reaction is seen, and with time, a proliferative fibrotic reaction develops. Although most of the oil remains within alveoli, some droplets and lipid-laden macrophages may travel via lymphatic vessels to regional bronchial lymph nodes.

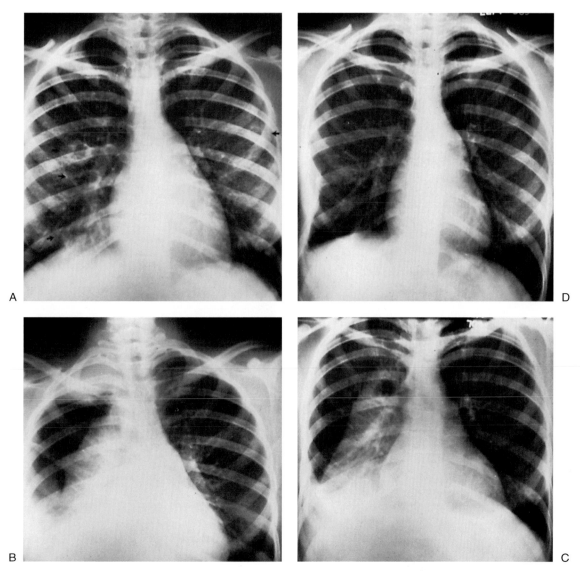

FIG. 2. Serial chest roentgenograms taken during a 6-month period in an 18-year-old girl with pelvic inflammatory disease demonstrate multiple metastatic lung abscesses caused by *Bacteroides* and microaerophilic streptococci (**A**) and paravertebral empyema (**B**) with gas formation (**C**), which eventually resolved following drainage (**D**). Note multiple abscesses (*arrows,* A.)

The clinical presentation may be one of chronic cough, wheezing, dyspnea, and low-grade fever. About half of the patients have no symptoms, their disease being evident only because of abnormal findings on a chest radiograph taken for other reasons (Fig. 5). In early disease, the acinar location of oil causes a homogeneous dense consolidation, often with air bronchograms and a "spun glass" appearance. A pattern of reticular markings can develop as emulsified oil enters the interstitium, and Kerley B lines may be visible. Fibrosis may result in nodules or masses. CT may be useful in detecting areas of consolidation with low attenuation values typical of fat. Although early reports of magnetic resonance imaging (MRI) in lipoid pneumonia indicated that the high signal intensity observed on T_1-weighted images (equal to subcutaneous

fat) were indistinguishable from findings of hemorrhagic infiltrates, recent studies suggest that the use of chemical-shift MRI can differentiate these two conditions.

The diagnosis may be confirmed by the finding of macrophages containing stainable fat in the sputum, bronchial washings, or bronchoalveolar lavage (BAL) fluid (Fig. 6). BAL fluid may be grossly oily. Transbronchial or open lung biopsy may be necessary for cases in which the diagnosis cannot otherwise be established. Stains for oil in tissue must be performed on frozen sections, because routine preparation for paraffin-embedded samples removes the oil.

A careful study of BAL fluid from seven patients with mineral oil pneumonia was recently reported. Increased numbers of polymorphonuclear leukocytes, eosinophils,

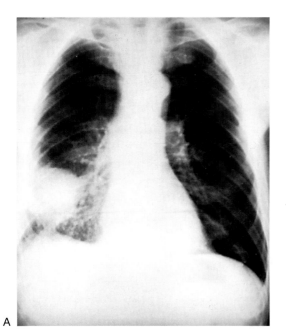

A

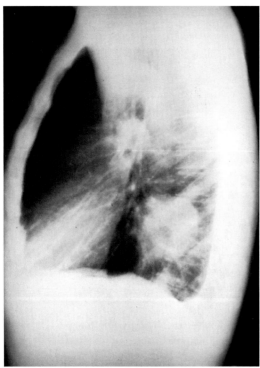

B

FIG. 3. Posteroanterior (**A**) and lateral (**B**) chest roentgenograms showing a well-circumscribed homogeneous infiltrate in a patient with endogenous lipoid pneumonia. (Courtesy of Dr. Robert Pugatch.)

and lymphocytes were indicative of a cell-mediated immune response; the authors postulated that this response accounted for the later appearance of interstitial fibrosis. The alveolar macrophages contained large vacuoles in which liquid paraffin could be identified by thin-layer chromatography and infrared spectroscopy.

Secondary infection may be demonstrable in and around areas of lipoid pneumonia. Especially important is infection with rapidly growing mycobacteria, as discussed in Chapter 29.

The most important aspect of treatment is immediate cessation of use of the oily material. Underlying conditions, such as swallowing dysfunction and disorders of esophageal motility, should be corrected whenever possible. Mycobacterial infection should be treated with appropriate drugs (Chapter 29). Repeated BAL with physical removal of oily material may be helpful in early cases, at least theoretically. Resection may be beneficial for selected patients who have circumscribed areas of disease.

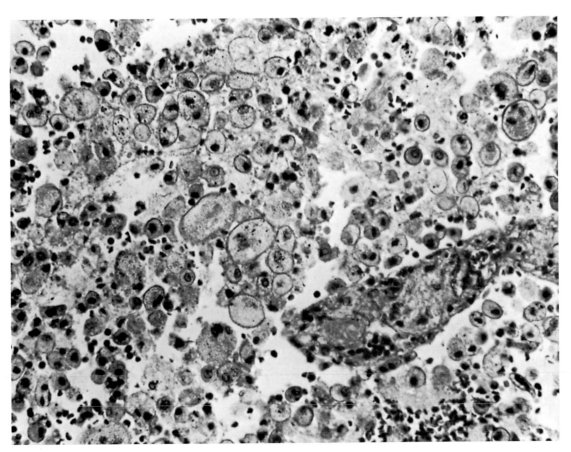

FIG. 4. Microscopic section of lobectomy specimen obtained from patient whose roentgenograms are shown in Fig. 3. Foamy macrophages are consistent with cholesterol pneumonia. (Courtesy of Dr. Y. Jung Legg.)

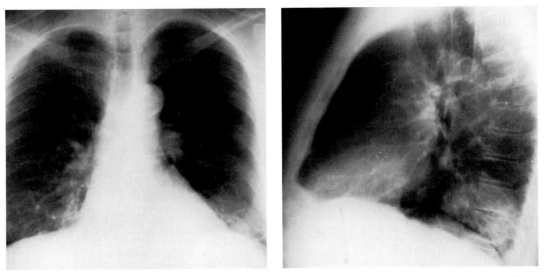

A   B

FIG. 5. Posteroanterior (**A**) and lateral (**B**) chest roentgenograms demonstrating a well-circumscribed homogeneous retrocardiac infiltrate in the left lower lobe. The patient was asymptomatic and initially denied taking any medicines. Repeated questioning revealed daily ingestion of mineral oil using a gulping technique. Results of cytology, stain for acid-fast bacilli, and Sudan stain for fat in specimens of expectorated sputum were negative.

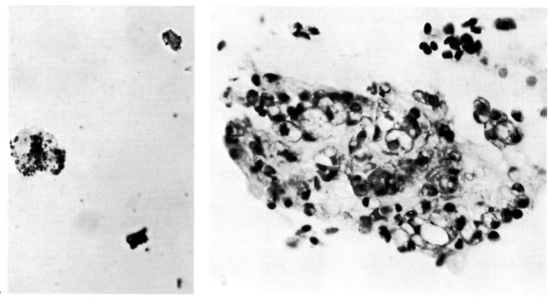

FIG. 6. Bronchial washings from patient whose roentgenograms are shown in Fig. 5. **A:** Hematoxylin and eosin stain shows typical clear areas of lipid-laden macrophages. **B:** Sudan black stain reveals oil. In this setting, such findings are considered diagnostic of exogenous lipoid pneumonia. (Courtesy of Dr. J. Merriam.)

BIBLIOGRAPHY

Brechot JM, et al. Computed tomography and magnetic resonance findings in lipoid pneumonia. *Thorax* 1991;46:738. *Report of a case of exogenous lipoid pneumonia, comparing CT with MRI features. The authors conclude that CT is the best imaging modality for diagnosis.*

Christensen PJ, et al. Septic pulmonary embolism due to periodontal disease. *Chest* 1993;104:1927. *Description of a case of periodontal infection leading to bacteremia, seeding of the lungs, and multiple lung abscesses, including a succinct review of the pathogenesis and radiographic features of septic pulmonary emboli.*

Cox JE, Choplin RH, Chiles C. Chemical-shift MRI of exogenous lipoid pneumonia. *J Comput Assist Tomogr* 1996;20:465. *Description of the use of opposed-phase (chemical-shift) MRI to differentiate exogenous lipoid pneumonia from primary lung carcinoma and hemorrhagic infiltrates.*

DeNavasquez S, Haslewood GAD. Endogenous lipoid pneumonia with special reference to carcinoma of the lung. *Thorax* 1954;9:35. *In reviewing the necropsy results from nine cases of primary lung carcinoma, the authors found a constant presence of fat, maximal in the lung distal to bronchial obstruction, composed of cholesterol and its esters, and felt to have been derived from degenerating lung tissue rather than from the tumor itself.*

Fisher M, et al. Coexisting endogenous lipoid pneumonia, cholesterol granulomas, and pulmonary alveolar proteinosis in a pediatric population: a clinical, radiographic, and pathologic correlation. *Pediatr Pathol* 1992;12:365. *Report of the clinical, radiographic, and morphologic findings in eight patients with diverse pulmonary diseases found to have varying and coexisting degrees of endogenous lipoid pneumonia and pulmonary alveolar proteinosis.*

Hampton AO, Bickham Jr CE, Winship T. Lipoid pneumonia. *AJR Am J Roentgenol* 1955;73:938. *Review of the clinical and pathologic findings in 35 cases of lipoid pneumonia, with an emphasis on the radiographic features of the disease.*

Kuhlman JE, Fishman EK, Teigen C. Pulmonary septic emboli: diagno-sis with CT. *Radiology* 1990;174:211. *Review of the CT features of 18 patients with pulmonary septic emboli. Characteristic findings included multiple peripheral nodules (83%), a feeding vessel sign (67%), cavitation (50%), wedge-shaped lesions abutting the pleurae (50%), air bronchograms within the nodules (28%), and extension into the pleural space (39%).*

Lauque D, et al. Bronchoalveolar lavage in liquid paraffin pneumonitis. *Chest* 1990;98:1149. *The authors evaluated the cells recovered in BAL fluid from seven patients with liquid paraffin pneumonitis. The number and percentage of alveolar macrophages were decreased, whereas the number of neutrophils, eosinophils, and lymphocytes was increased, suggesting that this cell-mediated inflammatory response plays a role in the later development of interstitial fibrosis.*

Lee KS, et al. Lipoid pneumonia: CT findings. *J Comput Assist Tomogr* 1995;19:48. *The authors reviewed chest radiographic and CT findings in six patients with proven lipoid pneumonia. In five of the patients, CT demonstrated areas with low attenuation diagnostic of fat or areas with nonspecific low attenuation of soft-tissue density.*

Sinave CP, Hardy GJ, Fardy PW. The Lemierre syndrome: suppurative thrombophlebitis of the internal jugular vein secondary to oropharyn-geal infection. *Medicine* 1989;68:85. *A beautifully composed article (with 75 references) reviewing the literature on Lemierre's syndrome from the early 1900s through the 1980s.*

Spickard A III, Hirschmann JV. Exogenous lipoid pneumonia. *Arch Intern Med* 1994;154:686. *An in-depth review (91 references) of the history, reported cases, pathologic and clinical features, diagnosis, and treatment of exogenous lipoid pneumonia.*

Volk BW, et al. Incidence of lipoid pneumonia in a survey of 389 chronically ill patients. *Am J Med* 1951;10:316. *The authors found 57 cases of lipoid pneumonia during a prospective survey of 389 chronically ill patients. In 55 of the cases, the diagnosis could be established by examination of the sputum, which demonstrated either lipid-laden macrophages or free lipoid material.*

Zelefsky MN, Lutzker LG. The target sign: a new radiologic sign of septic pulmonary emboli. *AJR Am J Roentgenol* 1977;129:453. *The authors describe the target sign as a radiographic feature of septic pulmonary emboli and discuss a potential pathogenic mechanism.*

Textbook of Pulmonary Diseases, 6th ed.
edited by G.L. Baum, J.D. Crapo, B.R. Celli, and J.B. Karlinsky,
Lippincott–Raven Publishers, Philadelphia, © 1998.

CHAPTER

31

Aspiration Pneumonia, Lipoid Pneumonia, and Lung Abscess

Hugh A. Cassiere · Michael S. Niederman

ASPIRATION PNEUMONIA

Pathogenic organisms can invade and infect the lung through four pathways: aspiration, inhalation, hematogenous seeding, and contiguous spread. Aspiration of pathogens from a previously colonized oropharynx is the primary pathway by which organisms gain entrance to the lungs, and thus in a broad sense, most pneumonias are aspiration-related. However, when the term *aspiration pneumonia* is used, it is meant to refer to the development of a radiographic infiltrate in the setting of either a witnessed episode of gross aspiration or risk factors for aspiration.

Aspiration pneumonia, like other respiratory tract infections, usually occurs in patients with underlying disease. Although normal adults commonly aspirate while sleeping without any obvious health effects, pneumonia can develop after episodes of aspiration in patients with certain underlying diseases that predispose to host defense impairment. Other factors that modify the risk for pneumonia after aspiration, besides host factors, include certain characteristics of the aspirated material. The pH, tonicity, and volume of the aspirate in addition to the frequency of aspiration all contribute to the development of pneumonia.

Not all infiltrates that follow aspiration represent an infectious process. In some patients, depending on the type of material aspirated, a noninfectious inflammatory response develops that results in pulmonary leukocyte sequestration. Most of these noninfectious infiltrates resolve, but 25%–50% progress to infectious pneumonia or fulminant acute lung injury. In a study by Croghan and colleagues of patients in a nursing home who were evaluated for aspiration with videofluoroscopy, pneumonia developed in 50% of patients with documented aspiration during a 12-month period and in 12.5% of patients without aspiration. In that study, the volume of the aspirate was directly related to the risk for pneumonia; pneumonia developed in 43% of patients with mild aspiration (of thin liquids), and in 67% of patients with severe aspiration (of material of all consistencies at almost every swallow). In a study by Bynum and Pierce, 50 patients with significant aspiration were evaluated. Rapid clearing of infiltrates was noted in 62%, and adult respiratory distress syndrome (ARDS) developed in 12%. Infectious pneumonia developed in the remaining 26% of patients, often after initial improvement.

Risk Factors

Risk factors for aspiration pneumonia are numerous and complex. One general way of categorizing these risks is according to whether they are host factors or characteristics of the aspirated material. Host factors lead to impaired host defenses and/or increased exposure to bacteria because of an increased risk for aspiration. Usually, it is the combination of disease-related immune impairments and exposure to large numbers of aspirated bacteria that leads to pneumonia.

H. A. Cassiere: Division of Thoracic and Cardiovascular Surgery, Winthrop University Hospital, Mineola, New York 11501.
M. S. Niederman: Pulmonary and Critical Care Division, Winthrop University Hospital, Mineola, New York 11501.

Host Factors

Host factors that predispose to aspiration pneumonia are numerous (Table 1); they either impair host defenses or enhance the risk for aspiration. A number of conditions, such as diabetes mellitus, congestive heart failure, malnutrition, chronic obstructive lung disease, renal failure, and malignancy, can impair host defenses. Diabetes is associated with neutrophil dysfunction, including diminished chemotaxis and impairment of phagocytosis. In patients with congestive heart failure, clearance of pneumococci and staphylococci from the respiratory tract can be impaired as a result of pulmonary edema. If liver disease is complicated by cirrhosis, atelectasis from pleural effusions and/or ascites can result in stagnation of secretions. Cirrhosis is also associated with diminished leukocyte chemotaxis in response to inflammation, depressed levels of complement, and defects in cellular immunity. Renal failure can increase the rate of colonization of the oropharyx by gram-negative bacteria and *Staphylococcus aureus* and can lead to complement deficiency, impaired cellular immunity, and, in animal models, decreased clearance of staphylococci and *Pseudomonas aeruginosa* along with an increase in the binding capacity of buccal cells for gram-negative bacteria. Neoplastic disease can affect host defenses either directly or as a consequence of therapy. For example, neutropenia, endobronchial obstruction, and impaired cough reflex are common in cancer patients and can all predispose to the development of pneumonia.

Host factors that predispose to aspiration as the result of neurologic, mechanical, and/or contractile dysfunction of the esophagus and upper airway are listed in Table 2. They include stroke, dysphagia, gastroesophageal reflux, altered sensorium, placement of a feeding tube, and the postgastrectomy state. Once material has gained access to the airways, the clinical response depends on the characteristics of the aspirate. If the aspirate is small in volume but highly contaminated with bacteria, then host defenses may be overwhelmed and pneumonia can result. If the aspirate is large in volume but relatively less contaminated, then pneumonia will result only if the aspirated organisms are highly virulent or the host defenses are severely abnormal. Most episodes of aspiration involve

TABLE 1. *Aspiration pneumonia*

Host risk factors	Aspirate risk factors
Underlying serious illness	Fluid pH ⩽ 2.5
Altered sensorium	Large particles
Stroke	Large volume (1 mL/kg)
Dysphagia	Hypertonic fluid
Gastroesophageal reflux	Bacterial contamination
Postgastrectomy	
Xerostomia	
Feeding tube	
Periodontal disease	

TABLE 2. *Conditions that increase the risk for aspiration*

Neurologic	Mechanical	Contractile
Unconsciousness	Obesity	Gastroesophageal
Laryngeal nerve	Head and neck	reflux
damage	surgery	Diabetic
Advanced age	Bowel	gastropathy
Acute stroke	obstruction	Critical illness
Pseudobulbar	Abdominal	Trendelenburg
palsy	surgery	position
Seizures	Enteral feeding	Protracted
Parkinson's	Pregnancy	vomiting
disease	Endotracheal	
General anesthesia	intubation	
Insulin-induced	Tracheostomy	
hypoglycemia		
Alcoholism		
Drug abuse		
Cardiac arrest		
Metabolic		
encephalopathy		

oropharyngeal flora, which can achieve extremely high concentrations in the presence of periodontal disease. Whereas normal saliva contains 10^8 organisms/mL, saliva from a patient with gingivitis may contain 10^{11} organisms/mL. In periodontal disease, anaerobes predominate among the oral flora.

Xerostomia has recently been shown to predispose to aspiration pneumonia, probably reflecting the fact that normal saliva flushes the oral cavity and maintains a bacterial level of $<7 \times 10^8$ organisms per milliliter. With xerostomia, the normal salivary flow rate is diminished and patients are at risk for gingivitis, and these two factors can result in bacterial counts that are higher than normal. When a patient with xerostomia aspirates, the lower respiratory tract is exposed to larger numbers of bacteria than normal, and aspiration pneumonia can result.

When aspiration develops in the hospitalized patient, many of the same host risk factors prevail. However, for patients in an intensive care unit, particular issues to consider in evaluating aspiration risk include patient position, site of enteral feeding (stomach or small bowel), volume of gastric contents, and size of any feeding tube that is used. Studies have suggested a reduced risk for aspirating gastric contents in patients who are maintained in a semi-erect position, in those whose feeding tubes are placed in the small bowel, and in those with small-bore feeding tubes.

Characteristics of the Aspirate

The characteristics of aspirated material play an important role in the pathogenesis of pneumonia. As only 25%–50% of all cases of aspiration progress to pneumonia, infection is particularly likely if the patient aspirates contaminated material. Pneumonia may also develop in patients who aspirate noninfectious material as a result of the lung injury caused by certain types of material.

Aspiration of very toxic, irritant material with high concentrations of hydrogen ion (pH ≪2.5) results in a chemical pneumonitis. This initial type of lung injury is typically noninfectious and characterized by a predominance of neutrophils. The magnitude of lung injury is directly related to the volume and hydrogen ion concentration of the aspirated material. In animal models of aspiration, acid pneumonitis does not occur unless the pH is <2.5. The resulting damage renders the mucosal barrier of the lower respiratory tract incompetent and places the patient at risk for infectious pneumonia as new sites for bacterial binding are created.

Large-volume and large-particle aspirates predispose to pneumonia by a different mechanism. A number of studies have shown that the majority of large-volume and large-particle aspirates are composed of vegetable matter, which can mechanically obstruct the lower airways and cause atelectasis, stagnation of secretions, and thus an increased risk for infection. In addition, aspirates containing particulate matter can be contaminated by bacteria, as oral secretions are often heavily colonized by potentially pathogenic organisms. In hospitalized patients, the stomach can harbor large numbers of enteric gram-negative bacteria if the gastric pH is >3.5 to 4.0. In patients in the intensive care unit, the risk for development of pneumonia is great when morning gastric pH is high (>3.5). Gastric pH may be elevated by enteral feeding, antacids, or H_2 antagonists. The role of prophylaxis for intestinal bleeding in the pathogenesis of pneumonia is uncertain, with continuing controversy about the role of the stomach in causing pneumonia. In addition, H_2 antagonists have not uniformly led to an increased risk for pneumonia in all studies, and their impact must be considered in relation to gastric volume, patient position, and site of enteral feeding.

Classification of Aspiration Syndromes

The aspiration of material into the tracheobronchial tree can result in a number of clinical consequences, ranging from no evident reaction to respiratory failure, ARDS, and/or death. Three different types of aspiration syndromes can result, depending on the type of material entering the tracheobronchial tree. These syndromes, which are not mutually exclusive and can occur in combination, include the irritant-toxic type, the inert-nontoxic type, and the infectious type.

The irritant-toxic syndrome is caused by aspiration of acidic liquids (pH ≪2.5) and/or fine particulate material; it results in acute pneumonitis or, if severe enough, ARDS. The inert-nontoxic syndrome is caused by aspiration of large particulate matter and/or large volumes of fluid; the clinical response ranges from chronic respiratory symptoms (e.g., cough and wheezing) to atelectasis or, if massive enough, sudden death. Infectious aspiration syndromes result from the entry of potentially pathogenic organisms into the lower airways. Although pneumonia is part of the infectious aspiration syndrome, other infectious syndromes can result, including lung abscess, necrotizing pneumonia, and empyema.

As community-acquired aspiration pneumonia usually involves anaerobic bacteria, aspiration pneumonia should be viewed as part of a continuum that can progress to cavitation (lung abscess) or even development of empyema. If aspiration pneumonia is not treated, necrotizing abscess formation follows in 8 to 14 days, usually in a peripheral location, and is characterized by the expectoration of putrid sputum. When anaerobic lung infection occurs, the pleura is commonly involved, being affected alone or in combination with parenchymal tissue in up to half of all patients.

Mendelson's syndrome (acid pneumonitis) is an example of irritant-toxic lung injury; it usually follows a witnessed episode of aspiration of acidic gastric fluid. Initially, an asthma-like reaction occurs, but within 2 hours a patient may exhibit dyspnea, cough with nonpurulent sputum, bronchospasm, bilateral lower lobe infiltrates, hypoxemia, and decreased lung compliance. In Mendelson's original description of this syndrome, no deaths were documented, although subsequent investigators have reported mortality rates as high as 70%, with some patients progressing to ARDS.

Pathogenesis

Aspiration-induced lung injury is believed to be biphasic, with the volume and pH of the material dictating the severity of the response. The first phase of injury is characterized by an acute localized response to the physical effects of the material aspirated, which, in the case of acid-induced lung injury, is a consequence of the chemical burn. This local response is immediate and limited to the areas of direct contact with the acid; the amount of resulting injury is directly related to the acidity and volume of the aspirated material.

The first-phase response results in local inflammation; this triggers a second phase characterized by a generalized neutrophilic infiltration, occurring within 2 to 6 hrs after aspiration. The initial response, although local in nature, causes cell injury and death secondary to the physical insult of the aspirated material. Pathologically, peribronchial hemorrhage, bronchial epithelial cell death, and pulmonary edema can be seen. This in turn can lead to the release of multiple inflammatory cytokines and proteases. Once released, these inflammatory substances set off a cascade of responses that result in microvascular permeability defects, pulmonary leukocyte sequestration, fibrinous alveolar exudation, tissue hypoxia, and hyaline membrane formation, all of which characterize the acute lung injury.

Neutrophils are thought to be the cells primarily responsible for the second-phase response to injury, and several inflammatory mediators have been identified as potential neutrophil chemoattractant agents. In one animal model, acid-induced lung injury was mediated by a mechanism dependent on interleukin-8 (IL-8). IL-8, a potent chemoattractant for neutrophils, also primes neutrophils for activation and upregulates neutrophil adhesion molecules on endothelial cells. Acid-induced abnormalities of oxygenation and enhanced amounts of extravascular lung water did not develop in animals given anti-IL-8 antibodies, either as pretreatment or 1 hr after acid aspiration.

Aspiration-induced neutrophil sequestration in the pulmonary vasculature can lead to lung injury in several ways. In one study, the complement system was shown to play a role; animals pretreated with a complement-receptor inhibitor had reduced lung edema, decreased alveolar protein accumulation, and improved tissue oxygenation after acid aspiration when compared with untreated animals. There was no effect of complement inhibition on pulmonary leukocyte sequestration, possibly indicating that neutrophils activate the complement system and cause lung injury via this mechanism. Another possible mechanism of lung injury in these patients is the release of high levels of neutrophil-derived serine proteases, which can overcome the normal antiprotease defense mechanisms of the lungs. In one study using a model of acid-induced lung injury, high levels of serine proteases were found in the bronchoalveolar fluid of injured animals. This pathophysiologic response can impair both local and systemic lung defense mechanisms and predispose to pneumonia, even if the aspirated material is sterile.

Bacteriology

The bacteriology of aspiration pneumonia is intimately tied to the flora of the oropharyngeal cavity. Under normal circumstances, the saliva of the oral cavity contains 10^8 organisms/mL, with a predominance of anaerobic organisms. Individuals with poor dental hygiene or gingivitis can have anaerobic bacterial levels of 10^{11}/mL of saliva, and patients with underlying illness who are hospitalized for prolonged periods can become colonized by enteric gram-negative bacilli. The majority of cases of aspiration pneumonia are caused by anaerobic organisms originating in the oropharynx and are usually polymicrobial, with at least two anaerobic organisms and sometimes a mixture of aerobic and anaerobic pathogens.

The bacteriology of aspiration pneumonia has not changed much during the last few decades, although the taxonomy of some of the involved pathogens has. For example, some organisms originally classified in the *Pep-*

tostreptococcus genus have now been reclassified in the *Streptococcus* genus, e.g., *S. intermedius*. With this in mind, many studies in the 1970s and 1980s documented anaerobic streptococci, *Fusobacterium nucleatum*, and *Prevotella melaninogenicus* (formerly classified in the genus *Bacteroides*) as the three major pathogens in aspiration pneumonia. It was once thought that *B. fragilis* was a significant pathogen in anaerobic lung infections, although recent data make this seem less likely.

Aerobic bacteria are found as either primary pathogens (approximately 10% of the time) or as coinfectors (approximately 40%); they include *Streptococcus* species, *S. aureus, Klebsiella pneumoniae, Escherichia coli, E. cloacae,* and *P. aeruginosa.* A more recent study examining early aspiration pneumonia in intensive care unit patients has documented a more virulent profile of aerobic pathogens. In this series, no anaerobes were isolated, but in those patients who had community-acquired early aspiration pneumonia, *Streptococcus pneumoniae, S. aureus, E. coli, E. cloacae, Haemophilus influenzae, Streptococcus viridans,* and *P. aeruginosa* were isolated alone or in combination. In those patients who aspirated in the hospital, *S. aureus, H. influenzae, Serratia marcescens, Morganella morganii, Candida albicans, K. pneumoniae, P. aeruginosa,* and *Proteus mirabilis* were isolated alone or in combination by a protected specimen brush. These data suggest that the bacteriology in severely ill patients with underlying medical diseases may differ from that of patients with aspiration pneumonia that is not severe.

Treatment

The two major modes of therapy for aspiration pneumonia are administration of antibiotics and supportive care. In the setting of a witnessed or suspected aspiration, antibiotics should be started if an infiltrate is present. If the infiltrate clears in 24 to 48 hrs, the pneumonitis was likely noninfectious, and therapy can be discontinued. If no infiltrate is present, therapy can be withheld provided that the patient is followed with serial chest radiographs. Antibiotic therapy for patients with aspiration pneumonia should be based on an assessment of the severity of illness (Table 3), where the infection was acquired (community

TABLE 3. *Severe aspiration pneumonia*

Respiratory rate >30 breaths per minute
Need for mechanical ventilation
Chest radiographic findings:
  50% increase in the infiltrate in 48 hours
  Bilateral multilobar involvement
Presence of shock
SIRS (systemic inflammatory response syndrome) or need
  for vasopressors to support blood pressure
Severe lung injury (PaO$_2$/FiO$_2$ ratio $\leqslant$ 250 mmHg)
Urine output $\leqslant$20 mL/h
Acute renal failure requiring dialysis

versus hospital), and the presence or absence of risk factors for gram-negative colonization (Table 4).

If pneumonia is acquired in the community, then an anaerobic pathogen is more likely than if the infection was acquired in the hospital. In community-related aspiration pneumonia, the antibiotic regimen should be directed against the oral anaerobes (e.g., anaerobic streptococci, *F. nucleatum,* and *P. melaninogenicus*). Patients should be treated empirically without collection of sputum for culture by expectoration or invasive aspiration. The initial empiric antibiotic used in this case may be clindamycin, penicillin alone, or a combination of penicillin and metronidazole. Some data show a lower failure rate in patients treated with clindamycin compared with penicillin for anaerobic pleuropulmonary infection, suggesting a primary role for clindamycin in this infection. Recent data from patients with community-acquired lung abscess found resistance rates to penicillin, metronidazole, and clindamycin of 21%, 12%, and 5%, respectively, again supporting a primary role for clindamycin in anaerobic lung infections.

Clindamycin is a bacteriostatic antibiotic that binds to the 50S ribosomal subunit of bacteria and inhibits protein synthesis. Clindamycin potentiates opsonization and phagocytosis of bacteria, and has a prolonged effect that suppresses bacterial growth after concentrations fall below the minimal inhibitory concentration for the target organism. Clindamycin has antibacterial activity against most anaerobes, including *Bacteroides, Prevotella, Fusobacterium, Clostridium,* and *Porphyromas* species, and against aerobic gram-positive cocci, such as group A, B, C, and G streptococci, microaerophilic streptococci, *S. viridans,* most pneumococci, and methicillin-sensitive *S. aureus.*

The route of antibiotic administration is determined by the severity of the pneumonia and whether the patient is treated as an outpatient or inpatient. Treatment may be given orally on an outpatient or inpatient basis, depending on the severity of illness, but initial therapy in severely ill and hospitalized patients is usually by the intravenous route.

The above antibiotic regimen needs be modified if the

TABLE 4. *Risk factors for gram-negative colonization*

Malnutrition
Severe illness
Coma
Intubation
Diabetes
Prior surgery
Lung disease
Renal failure
Prior antibiotic use
Hypotension
Cigarette smoking
Prolonged hospitalization

TABLE 5. *Initial antibiotic regimen for aspiration pneumonia*

Community-acquired infection that is not severe	Hospital-acquired infection or severe community infection
Oral route	**Intravenous route**
Penicillin	Clindamycin plus ciprofloxacin[a]
Penicillin plus metronidazole	Clindamycin plus aminoglycoside[a]
Clindamycin	Ampicillin/sulbactam
Amoxicillin/clavulanate	Cefoxitin
Intravenous route	Piperacillin[a]
Penicillin	Imipenem[a]
Penicillin plus metronidazole	
Clindamycin	
Ampicillin/sulbactam	
Ticarcillin/clavulanate	

[a] If any of the following are present, *P. aeruginosa* infection is possible: prior antibiotic use, prolonged hospital course, and/or severe pneumonia. If *P. aeruginosa* infection is suspected, dual anti-*Pseudomonas* therapy should be initiated with a β-lactam/aminoglycoside or a β-lactam/quinolone combination.

patient has severe infection, hospital-acquired aspiration, or risk factors for gram-negative colonization (Table 4). In this situation, the likelihood of infection with a virulent gram-negative bacillus or an aerobic organism is greater, and therefore additional antibiotic coverage is required. Sputum or tracheal aspirate may be helpful in identifying high-risk pathogens, such as *P. aeruginosa,* in intubated patients. After empiric therapy has been started, culture results can be useful to determine the presence or absence of infection with *P. aeruginosa.* In this patient population, clindamycin plus an antibiotic with activity against gram-negative bacilli is recommended, or a single antibiotic with activity against anaerobes and gram-negative bacteria is adequate (e.g., ampicillin/sulbactam or ticarcillin/clavulonate) (Table 5). If risk factors for infection with *P. aeruginosa* are present, we recommend empiric antibiotic therapy with a dual anti-*Pseudomonas* combination until culture results are known.

LUNG ABSCESS

A lung abscess is defined as a localized (usually >2 cm in diameter), suppurative, necrotizing process occurring within the pulmonary parenchyma. Several processes, either respiratory or systemic, can lead to abscess formation. Most abscesses are primary and result from necrosis in an existing parenchymal process, usually an untreated aspiration pneumonia. Among the causes of necrotizing pneumonitis, infections and neoplasms are the most frequent. A secondary abscess is one that complicates either a septic vascular embolus (e.g., right-sided endocarditis) or a bronchial obstruction (e.g., aspirated foreign body).

Classically, anaerobes have been identified as the most common cause of lung abscess, although aerobic bacilli, fungi, parasites, and mycobacteria may also be responsible. Among neoplastic causes, primary squamous carcinoma of the lung is the most common malignancy associated with abscess formation. Between 8% and 18% of lung abscesses have been associated with neoplasms in all age groups, but in patients whose age is >45 years, the association approaches 30%.

The incidence of lung abscess has declined by as much as 10-fold during the last few decades, presumably as a result of improved treatment regimens for pneumonia. Accompanying this decrease in incidence is a decrease in mortality to between 5% and 10%, with a recent series reporting a mortality rate of 2.4% in community-acquired lung abscess and 66.7% in hospital-acquired abscess. Diagnosis and treatment have changed little through the years, as lung abscesses are uncommon and it is difficult to obtain enough patients to perform controlled clinical trials. As will be discussed, administration of antibiotics is the most important treatment, as in aspiration pneumonia. The role of the newer antimicrobial agents remains controversial, although they may represent an advance over traditional therapeutic agents (penicillin), especially as drug-resistant bacteria become more prevalent.

Pathogenesis

Most lung abscesses are caused by infectious agents, such as bacteria, fungi, parasites, and mycobacteria. In the majority of cases, a mixed bacterial flora can be found, with anaerobes being present in up to 90% of cases. Aerobic bacilli may be present in up to 50% of patients, but in most cases they coexist with anaerobes, and in only 10% of cases are they the sole responsible pathogens.

As in aspiration pneumonia, the basis of lung abscess formation is aspiration of infectious oropharygeal material in a host who cannot adequately clear the infectious challenge. Individuals predisposed to lung abscess formation are those with host defense defects in the setting of risk factors for aspiration (Tables 1 and 2). Aspiration, as described above, is more likely in patients who have neurologic, mechanical, and muscular dysfunction associated with alcoholism, seizure disorders, drug overdose, general anesthesia, protracted vomiting, or neurologic disorders such as cerebrovascular accidents, myasthenia gravis, amyotrophic lateral sclerosis, and other bulbar processes.

In addition to having risk factors for aspiration, patients predisposed to the formation of lung abscess are exposed to large concentrations of potentially pathogenic bacteria, usually orogingival in origin. It appears that the size of the aspirated bacterial inoculum is important, as abscess formation is enhanced by the presence of poor dentition and gingival disease, two conditions that are associated with bacterial counts in saliva in excess of 10^{11}/mL. Approximately 73% of patients with lung abscess have at least one predisposing factor for aspiration, and many have clinically silent gingival disease.

The pathophysiology of lung abscess formation appears to be related to a combination of aspiration, host defense defects, and the size of the infectious inoculum. Experimental data suggest that lung abscess formation occurs 8 to 14 days after aspiration of infectious orogingival material. When aspirated in large amounts, a single species of anaerobic bacteria or a combination of organisms can cause a necrotizing pneumonitis that, if progressive or untreated initially, forms a lung abscess. As expected, the location of the abscess is determined by gravity and body position at the time of aspiration. Lung abscess is typically located in the basal segments of the lower lobes, the superior segment of the lower lobe, or the posterior segments of the upper lobes, analogous to the location of infiltrates found in patients with aspiration pneumonia.

With these pathogenetic principles in mind, it is clear that an abscess arising in an edentulous patient (without oral anaerobes) or in a location other than the ones mentioned should raise suspicion of another pathologic process, involving either a nonanaerobic infection (such as tuberculosis), an esophageal disorder, or an obstructing endobronchial lesion.

Microbiology

Approximately 90% of lung abscesses are associated with anaerobic bacteria, either as the primary pathogens or in combination with aerobic bacteria. This observation may be explained by the fact that anaerobic bacteria commonly cause necrotizing inflammation. Other bacteria associated with lung abscess include *S. aureus, E. coli, K. pneumoniae, P. aeruginosa*, other gram-negative bacilli, *Streptococcus pyogenes, Pseudomonas pseudomallei* (melioidosis), *H. influenzae* (especially type b), *Legionella pneumophila, Nocardia asteroides, Actinomyces* species, and rarely pneumococci. Parasites (*Paragonimus westermani, Entamoeba histolytica*), fungi, and mycobacteria also may cause lung abscess (Table 6).

Anaerobes are usually part of a polymicrobial flora, with the average number of organisms isolated being three, either strictly anaerobes or a combination of aerobic-anaerobic bacteria. The change in bacterial taxonomy has been referred to in the section on aspiration pneumonia.

Classification

Lung abscesses have been categorized using several methods, but the classification into acute versus chronic appears to have the most clinical utility. This distinction is not absolute but can aid the clinician by helping to

TABLE 6. *Cavitary lung lesions*

INFECTIOUS

Bacterial	Fungal	Parastic
Anaerobic abscess	Coccidioidomycosis	Echinococcosis
Aerobic abscess	Histoplasmosis	Amebiasis
Infected bulla	Blastomycosis	
Infected pulmonary infarct	Aspergillosis	
Empyema	Cryptococcosis	
Tuberculosis		
Actinomycosis		

NEOPLASTIC	INFLAMMATORY
Bronchogenic carcinoma	Wegener's granulomatosis
Squamous cell	Sarcoidosis
Metastatic carcinoma	
Colorectal	
Renal	
Lymphoma	
Hodgkin's disease	

formulate treatment regimens and identify patients who may need further diagnostic evaluation, such as bronchoscopy.

A lung abscess is defined as acute if the patient presents with symptoms of <2 weeks' duration. Patients with an acute lung abscess are less likely to have an underlying neoplasm but are more likely to have an infection caused by a virulent aerobic bacterial agent, such as *S. aureus*. In a recent series of patients with acute community-acquired lung abscess, a mean of 2.3 bacterial species per patient was identified, with anaerobes isolated alone in 44% of cases, aerobes alone in 19%, mixed aerobes and anaerobes in 22%, and the remainder caused by an unidentified pathogen or *Mycobacterium tuberculosis*. The most common anaerobic pathogens identified were from the *Prevotella* species, and the most common aerobic pathogens were *S. viridans* and *Staphylococcus* species.

A chronic lung abscess is defined by symptoms lasting for >4 to 6 weeks; patients are more likely to have an underlying neoplasm or infection with a less virulent, anaerobic agent. There may be some overlap in this classification scheme, because it does not take into account host defense factors or serious comorbidity, but this scheme can be useful during initial patient evaluation.

Clinical Features

Most patients with lung abscess have an insidious presentation, with symptoms lasting at least 2 weeks before evaluation. Signs and symptoms include cough, foul-smelling sputum that forms layers on standing, hemoptysis (25% of patients), fever, chills, night sweats, anorexia, pleuritic chest pain (60% of patients), weight loss, and clubbing. Although most of these signs and symptoms

are seen, their specificity for lung abscess is low. On the other hand, putrid sputum is a highly specific sign that is pathognomonic for anaerobic infection, although it is found in only 50%–60% of patients. A history of weight loss is also common, occurring in 60% of patients, with an average loss of between 15 and 20 lb. Historical data usually include risk factors for aspiration, such as alcoholism, drug overdose, seizures, head injury, or stroke, and the absence of such risk factors should prompt a search for a diagnosis other than primary lung abscess.

Laboratory data are also nonspecific. Erythrocyte sedimentation rate is elevated, and anemia of chronic inflammation and leukocytosis are present. Culture and microbiologic information from sputum are generally not helpful unless the abscess is caused by nonanaerobic agents, such as mycobacteria, fungi, or aerobic bacteria. Sputum is contaminated with anaerobes from the oral cavity, so that finding these organisms is not specific. If the abscess is associated with an empyema, as is the case 30% of the time, then culture of the empyema fluid may yield reliable bacteriologic data.

More invasive methods for microbiologic diagnosis (transtracheal aspiration and bronchoscopy) are rarely employed, as the majority of patients are treated empirically. This approach is supported by recent data showing that most lung abscess pathogens are sensitive to conventional antimicrobial therapy. If, on the other hand, the patient presents in an atypical fashion or is not responding to therapy, then invasive techniques are justified (Table 7).

Chest radiography generally shows a solitary cavitary lesion of variable size. Some studies report that the size of the cavity is helpful in distinguishing neoplastic from non-neoplastic lung abscesses, but others have not found such a correlation. A dearth of inflammation seen radiographically surrounding the abscess suggests patients with underlying neoplasm.

Radiographically, empyema and infected bullae are sometimes difficult to distinguish from a lung abscess. Empyema is a purulent infection that in most cases is confined to the pleural space, although it can develop as a complication of, or be a cause of, a lung abscess. An

TABLE 7. *Criteria for fiberoptic bronchoscopy in patients with lung abscess*

Atypical presentation
  Absence of fever
  WBC count ≤ 11,000
  Absence of systemic symptoms
  Fulminant course
  Absence of predisposing factors for aspiration
  Atypical abscess location
  Abscess formation in an edentulous patient
Failure to respond to antibiotics
Presence of mediastinal adenopathy
Suspected underlying malignancy
Suspected foreign body

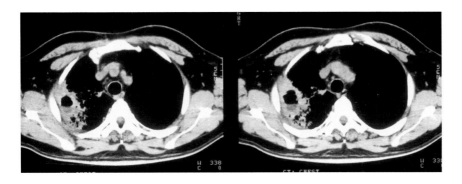

FIG. 1. CT of a patient in whom a lung abscess was diagnosed. Note the cavitary lesion with the characteristic air-fluid level and surrounding inflammation and tissue necrosis.

infected bulla is pneumonia within a pre-existing bullous cavity and does not result from tissue necrosis. Both entities can demonstrate air-fluid levels, but one is parenchymal (infected bulla) and the other is extraparenchymal (empyema). If an empyema contains an air-fluid level, then a bronchopleural fistula is present. When the chest radiograph cannot distinguish these two entities from a lung abscess, computed tomography (CT) suggests a lung abscess if a thick, irregular, walled cavity with no associated lung compression is seen (Fig. 1). Empyema and an infected bulla usually have thin, smooth walls with compression of uninvolved lung and, in the case of the infected bulla, minimal surrounding inflammation (Fig. 2). The real difficulty arises when one tries to differentiate between a lung abscess and an empyema with a bronchopleural fistula. Prior pleural fluid on chest radiograph, extension of the air-fluid level toward the chest wall, extension of the air-fluid level across a fissure, and tapering of the air-fluid collection on the radiograph suggest empyema.

If a lung abscess fails to communicate with a bronchus, the characteristic air-fluid level within a cavity will not be seen radiographically. In this case, the radiographic appearance is one of a focal, ground-glass infiltrate with indistinct borders. Given the history of illness and this radiographic picture, the differential diagnosis includes other chronic pulmonary infections, such as postobstructive bacterial pneumonia, nocardiosis, fungal pneumonia, tuberculosis, and actinomycosis. In addition, a variety of noninfectious pulmonary processes can also be confused with a noncavitary lung abscess. These include BOOP (bronchiolitis obliterans organizing pneumonia), radiation pneumonitis, chronic eosinophilic pneumonia, and allergic bronchopulmonary aspergillosis. When a lung abscess presents in this manner, it is usually necessary to perform a further diagnostic workup, such as bronchoscopy and or lung biopsy. This is also the case if multiple cavities are seen on the radiograph, a rare finding in an anaerobic process not complicated by immunosuppression, recurrent aspiration, or virulent anaerobe(s) causing a necrotizing pneumonitis.

Treatment

In the pre-antibiotic era, three treatment modalities were available for lung abscess. These included supportive care, postural drainage with or without bronchoscopy, and surgery. All three modalities led to the same mortality rate of 30%–35%. Currently, the mainstay of therapy for lung abscess is antimicrobial therapy with either intravenous penicillin alone, penicillin plus metronidazole, or clindamycin. Penicillin has historically been the therapy of choice since its first use in the 1950s, with a cure rate of 95%. With the growing concern over penicillin-resistant anaerobes, two trials compared clindamycin with penicillin in a prospective study design. Both studies found that clindamycin therapy was associated with fewer treatment failures and a shorter time to symptom resolution. When metronidazole was evaluated as a single treatment modality, it was found to have a 43% rate of treatment failure and hence is not recommended for single-agent therapy. Metronidazole in combination with

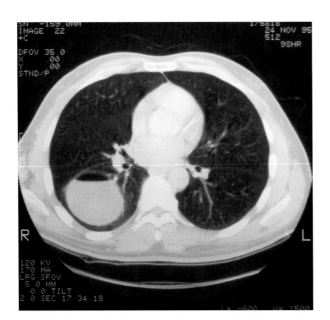

FIG. 2. CT of the chest showing typical findings in an infected bulla. The cavity is thin-walled without surrounding inflammation or necrosis.

penicillin is considered an appropriate treatment regimen for lung abscess, because penicillin has activity against the aerobic and microaerophilic streptococci that are often resistant to metronidazole. Many other antibiotics have *in vitro* activity against oral anaerobes but have never been evaluated in clinical trials to gain FDA approval for use in these infections. These antibiotics include chloramphenicol, imipenem, erythromycin, azithromycin, clarithromycin, and β-lactams with a β-lactamase inhibitor (e.g., ampicillin with sulbactam).

After the appropriate antimicrobial agent has been selected, the next issue is determining the length of therapy. Although there is considerable controversy in the literature, the approach taken by Bartlett seems the most conservative and appropriate. He recommends treating most patients until the pulmonary infiltrates have resolved or until the residual lesion is small and stable. Initially, antibiotics are given intravenously until the patient is afebrile and shows clinical improvement (4 to 8 days). Oral medications are then given, usually for a prolonged period, although the length of time needed varies from patient to patient. Many patients require a total of 6 to 8 weeks of antimicrobial therapy.

In the past, bronchoscopy was part of the standard care of patients with lung abscess. Its uses included helping to promote drainage and ruling out underlying malignancy. Currently, bronchoscopy is reserved for those patients with atypical presentations who are suspected of having an underlying malignancy or foreign body (Table 7). Bronchoscopy is no longer routinely used for abscess drainage, as the majority spontaneously communicate with the airways and drain. There is also a possibility of rupturing an abscess during bronchoscopy and causing contamination of previously uninvolved lung segments.

As for using bronchoscopy to rule out underlying malignancy, several patient characteristics appear to be correlated with underlying carcinoma. Criteria for bronchoscopy in patients with lung cavities are (1) mean oral temperature ≤100°F, (2) absence of systemic symptoms, (3) absence of predisposing factors for aspiration, and (4) mean leukocyte count ≤11,000/mm³. When more than three of these factors are present in a patient with lung abscess, an underlying carcinoma is likely. Other factors that should prompt bronchoscopic evaluation include an atypical clinical presentation (noncavitary lesion or lesions and fulminant time course), atypical abscess location (especially in the anterior half of the lung), abscess formation in an edentulous patient, failure to respond to antibiotics, and lung abscess associated with mediastinal adenopathy, a finding not commonly found in anaerobic lung infection.

Complications of lung abscess include empyema formation resulting from a bronchopleural fistula, massive hemoptysis, spontaneous rupture into uninvolved lung segments, and failure of the abscess cavity to resolve. Although uncommon, these complications often require

TABLE 8. *Factors associated with failure of medical therapy in patients with lung abscess*

Recurrent aspiration
Large cavity size (>6 cm)
Prolonged symptom complex before presentation
Abscess associated with an obstructing lesion
Presence of thick-walled cavities
Underlying serious co-morbidity
Development of empyema

prolonged medical therapy as well as surgical intervention, either with tube thoracostomy in the case of empyema or lung resection in the case of massive hemoptysis.

Surgical treatment of lung abscess is usually reserved for cases with complications such as massive hemoptysis, bronchopleural fistula, and empyema. It is also used in the setting of fulminant infection and in those patients who fail medical therapy. Approximately 10% of lung abscesses require surgical intervention. Prognostic factors associated with failure of medical treatment include recurrent aspiration, large cavity size (>6 cm), prolonged symptom complex before presentation, abscess associated with an obstructing lesion, abscess with a thick-walled cavity, advanced age, neoplasm, and other chronic medical conditions (Table 8). An alternative to surgical drainage is percutaneous catheter placement. At this time, percutaneous drainage should be reserved for patients who are unresponsive to medical therapy and have lung abscesses located peripherally. Placement of a percutaneous catheter can obviate the need for surgery in a significant percentage of patients who have failed medical treatment, with a mean time to abscess resolution of 10 to 15 days and improvement in clinical parameters within 48 hours. These patients should also receive intravenous antibiotics during and after percutaneous drainage of a lung abscess.

LIPOID PNEUMONIA

Lipoid pneumonia is a chronic illness of the lower respiratory tract resulting from the accumulation of lipoid material in the alveoli and/or the interstitium; it is not strictly an infectious syndrome. The clinical characteristics of this disease depend on whether the syndrome is exogenous or endogenous in origin. A noninfectious alveolar filling process causes chronic, nonresolving pneumonia, but lipoid pneumonia can be complicated by secondary infection. An example of this can be seen in patients with postobstructive pneumonia secondary to an endobronchial lesion.

Exogenous lipoid pneumonia, now an uncommon occurrence, was first described by Laughlen in 1925, when he identified lipid deposits in four autopsy specimens from the lungs of patients who had received either oil nose drops or oily laxatives. Experimental studies later confirmed similar findings in animals who had mineral oil artificially instilled in the trachea. Exogenous lipoid pneumonia is the result of aspiration of lipid material such as mineral oil, vegetable oil, and animal fats, with the type of aspirate predicting the underlying pathologic response. As a result of fatty acid production, aspiration of animal fat usually causes a severe inflammatory reaction resulting in hemorrhagic pneumonia. On the other hand, aspiration of vegetable oil results in little to no pathologic response, whereas mineral oils usually cause a foreign body reaction resulting in pulmonary fibrosis. This pathologic response to mineral oil is actually used, in animals, as a model of pulmonary fibrosis.

In exogenous mineral oil lipoid pneumonia (the most common syndrome), the clinical features include cough, dyspnea, sputum production, occasional hemoptysis, and chest radiographic abnormalities consisting of nonspecific infiltrates in the lower lobes, although any pattern can be seen, including cavitary lung lesions. Ordinarily, patients have minimal or no clinical symptoms and seek medical assistance because of abnormal findings on a chest radiograph. Intratracheal aspiration of mineral oil usually occurs subclinically, and patients are usually without cough, other signs associated with liquid aspiration, or acute inflammation.

The typical patient who recurrently aspirates mineral oil-based medicinal aids is an elderly individual who has used oil-based nose drops or an oil-based laxative for several years. The diagnosis can be made by a history of use of mineral oil or other oil in a patient with respiratory symptoms and a chronic nonresolving pneumonia. Not uncommonly, the diagnosis is made on biopsy, as lipoid pneumonia can mimic infectious diseases and lung malignancy. Once the diagnosis of exogenous lipoid pneumonia is made, treatment consists of removal of the cause (e.g., oil-based laxatives) and supportive therapy. Other therapeutic modalities, such as repeated bronchoalveolar lavage and corticosteroids, are available, but their overall clinical usefulness is uncertain.

Endogenous lipoid pneumonia is caused by the accumulation of lipids derived from the breakdown of endogenous products (e.g., cell membranes and surfactant). The material most often associated with this type of lipoid pneumonia is cholesterol, and thus *cholesterol pneumonia* is another name for this entity. The pathologic process is usually localized and limited to an abnormal region of the lung, in contrast to what occurs in exogenous lipoid pneumonia. The most common underlying abnormality resulting in endogenous lipoid pneumonia is an obstructing endobronchial lesion, either lung cancer or a foreign body.

The clinical presentation of patients with endogenous lipoid pneumonia is typically that of the underlying cause. In the case of an obstructing lesion, it is characterized by cough, fever, chills, and a chest radiograph revealing an underlying mass or segmental lesion with a concomitant postobstructive pneumonia. In sharp contrast to exogenous lipoid pneumonia, there is no predisposition to recurrent aspiration or history of use of an oil-based substance. Like the exogenous type, endogenous lipoid pneumonia is not infectious in origin, but secondary infection from the underlying obstructive process can occur.

BIBLIOGRAPHY

Bartlett JG. Antibiotics in lung abscess. *Semin Respir Infect* 1991;6: 103–111. *A review describing the antimicrobial activities of commonly prescribed antibiotics against the typical anaerobes causing lung abscess. The clinical efficacy of antibiotic therapy and other therapeutic modalities are discussed.*

Bartlett JG, Gorbach SL. Treatment of aspiration pneumonia and primary lung abscess. Penicillin G versus clindamycin. *JAMA* 1975;234: 935–937. *Clinical trial evaluating the clinical efficacy of penicillin G and clindamycin in the treatment of anaerobic lung infections.*

Bartlett JG, Gorbach SL. The triple threat of aspiration pneumonia. *Chest* 1975;68:560–566. *A classic review article that discusses the clinical consequences of aspirating material into the lower respiratory tract.*

Bartlett JG, Gorbach SL, Finegold SM. The bacteriology of aspiration pneumonia. *Am J Med* 1974;56:202–207. *A prospective study involving 54 cases of lung infection following aspiration. Anaerobic bacteria were isolated from 93% of specimens, and in 25% of these specimens, they were the only isolate.*

Bynum LJ, Pierce AK. Pulmonary aspiration of gastric contents. *Am Rev Respir Dis* 1976;114:1129–1136. *A retrospective analysis of 50 patients observed to aspirate gastric contents.*

Cassiere HA, Niederman MS. New etiopathogenic concepts of ventilator-associated pneumonia. *Semin Respir Infect* 1996;11:13–23. *A discussion of current concepts in ventilator-associated pneumonia, including the role of aspiration in the development of pneumonia.*

Cesar L, Gonzalez C, Calia FM. Bacteriologic flora of aspiration-induced pulmonary infections. *Arch Intern Med* 1975;135:711–714. *A study of the role of anaerobic and aerobic bacteria in the formation of lung infection in patients with aspiration.*

Croghan JE, Burke EM, Caplan S, et al. Pilot study of 12-month outcomes of nursing home patients with aspiration on videofluoroscopy. *Dysphagia* 1994;9:141–146. *A retrospective review of 40 patients who had videofluoroscopy swallowing studies performed in a teaching nursing home.*

Folkesson HG, Matthay MA, Hebert CA, et al. Acid aspiration-induced lung injury in rabbits is mediated by interleukin-8-dependent mechanisms. *J Clin Invest* 1995;96:107–116. *This animal study shows that IL-8 is necessary for the development of acid-induced lung injury in the rabbit model.*

Ha HK, Kang MW, Park JM, et al. Lung abscesses: percutaneous catheter therapy. *Acta Radiol* 1993;34:362–365. *A series describing catheter treatment of six patients with large, peripherally located lung abscesses that failed medical therapy.*

Hammond JM, Potgieter PD, Hanslo D, et al. The etiology and antimicrobial susceptibility patterns of micro-organisms in acute community-acquired lung abscess. *Chest* 1995;108:937–941. *A prospective survey study that evaluated the antimicrobial sensitivity patterns of pathogens found in acute community-acquired lung abscess.*

Holas MA, DePippo KL, Reding MJ. Aspiration and relative risk of medical complications following stroke. *Arch Neurol* 1994;51:1051–1053. *Prospective, longitudinal cohort study evaluating inpatients treated for stroke rehabilitation.*

Holtsclaw-Berk SA, Berk SL, Thomas CT, et al. Gastric microbial flora in patients with gastrointestinal disease. *South Med J* 1984;77:1231–1233. *Prospective study of 100 consecutive patients undergoing fiberoptic endoscopy for the evaluation of gastrointestinal disease.*

Irwin RS, Garrity FL, Erickson AD, et al. Sampling lower respiratory tract secretions in primary lung abscess. *Chest* 1981;79:559–565. *A prospective comparison of the accuracy of four diagnostic methods used in the evaluation of lung abscess: transtracheal aspiration, expectorated sputum, wire brushing under direct vision using fiberoptic bronchoscopy, and percutaneous needle lung aspiration.*

Kidd D, Lawson J, Nesbitt, et al. Aspiration in acute stroke: a clinical study with videofluoroscopy. *Q J Med* 1993;86:825–829. *In this study of 60 patients with acute stroke examined by means of videofluoroscopy, 42% of the patients aspirated.*

Kikuchi R, Watabe N, Konno T, et al. High incidence of silent aspiration in elderly patients with community-acquired pneumonia. *Am J Respir Crit Care Med* 1994;150:251–253. *Case-control study evaluating the incidence of silent nocturnal aspiration in 14 elderly patients with a recent episode of community-acquired pneumonia and 10 age-matched control subjects.*

Klein JS, Schultz S, Heffner JE. Interventional radiology of the chest: image-guided percutaneous drainage of pleural effusions, lung abscess, and pneumothorax. *AJR Am J Roentgenol* 1995;164:581–588. *Review article discussing the use of percutaneous drainage of lung abscesses that fail medical therapy. The etiology, pathophysiology, and diagnosis of parapneumonic pleural effusions are also reviewed.*

Knight PR, Druskovich G, Tait AR, et al. The role of neutrophils, oxidants, and proteases in the pathogenesis of acid pulmonary injury. *Anesthesiology* 1992;77:772–778. *Study supporting the concept that neutrophils are necessary for acid-induced lung injury, with serine proteases, not leukocyte-derived oxidants, being the source of injury.*

Lee KS, Muller NL, Newell JD, et al. Lipoid pneumonia: CT findings. *J Comput Assist Tomogr* 1995;19:48–51. *Six patients with proven lipoid pneumonia underwent CT evaluation, with the finding that areas of low attenuation were diagnostic for intraparenchymal fat accumulation.*

Levison ME, Mangura CT, Lorber B, et al. Clindamycin compared with penicillin for the treatment of anaerobic lung abscess. *Ann Intern Med* 1983;98:466–471. *A randomized, prospective study. Clindamycin was associated with a shorter febrile period, fewer days of putrid sputum, and no treatment failures versus a 53% treatment failure rate in the penicillin-treated group.*

Lipinski JK, Weisbrod GL, Sanders DE. Exogenous lipoid pneumonitis: pulmonary patterns. *AJR Am J Roentgenol* 1981;136:931–934. *A pictorial essay describing the different radiographic patterns seen in 11 patients with exogenous lipoid pneumonitis.*

Lorber B, Swenson RM. Bacteriology of aspiration pneumonia. *Ann Intern Med* 1974;81:329–331. *Prospective evaluation of 24 cases of community-acquired aspiration pneumonia and 23 cases of hospital-acquired aspiration pneumonia.*

Marina M, Strong CA, Civen R, et al. Bacteriology of anaerobic pleuro-pulmonary infections: preliminary report. *Clin Infect Dis* 1993;16:S256–S262. *A retrospective study examining the bacteriology of anaerobic infections during a 15-year period in a Veterans Administration hospital.*

Martin BJ, Corlew MM. The association of swallowing dysfunction and aspiration pneumonia. *Dysphagia* 1994;9:1–6. *Study showing a significant difference in the incidence of videofluoroscopically confirmed oropharyngeal swallowing defects in patients with aspiration pneumonia versus patients with nonaspiration pneumonia.*

Marumo K, Homma S, Fukuchi Y. Postgastrectomy aspiration pneumonia. *Chest* 1995;107:453–456. *Retrospective chart review of 186 patients who were status post total gastrectomy.*

Mier L, Dreyfuss D, Darchy B, et al. Is penicillin G an adequate initial treatment for aspiration pneumonia? A prospective evaluation using a protected specimen brush and quantitative cultures. *Intensive Care Med* 1993;19:279–284. *Prospective study of 52 patients given a diagnosis of aspiration pneumonia beginning shortly after aspiration, either in the community or the hospital.*

Mori T, Ebe T, Takahashi M, et al. Lung abscess: analysis of 66 cases from 1979–1991. *Intern Med* 1993;32:278–284. *Retrospective study analyzing 66 cases of lung abscess during a 12-year period. The authors found that the prognosis of patients with lung abscess was correlated with the presence of underlying medical diseases and superinfection with aerobes.*

Perlino C. Metronidazole versus clindamycin treatment of anaerobic pulmonary infection. *Arch Intern Med* 1981;141:1424–1427. *Prospective, randomized study evaluating the efficacy of metronidazole and clindamycin in the treatment of 17 patients with anaerobic lung infections. The conclusion of the study was that metronidazole should not be used as a single agent in lung infections caused by anaerobic pathogens.*

Rabinovici R, Neville LF, Abdullah F, et al. Aspiration-induced lung injury: role of complement. *Crit Care Med* 1995;23:1405–1411. *In this animal study, aspiration of acid induced pulmonary leukocyte sequestration, pulmonary edema, tissue hypoxia, and a pulmonary vascular permeability defect.*

Sosenko A, Glassroth J. Fiberoptic bronchoscopy in the evaluation of lung abscesses. *Chest* 1985;87:489–494. *A retrospective study evaluating the records of 52 consecutive patients undergoing bronchoscopy for lung abscess during a 7-year period.*

Spickard A, Hirschmann JV. Exogenous lipoid pneumonia. *Arch Intern Med* 1994;154:686–692. *A review article describing the history, pathology, and clinical presentation of exogenous lipoid pneumonia.*

Terpenning M, Bretz W, Lopatin D, et al. Bacterial colonization of saliva and plaque in the elderly. *Clin Infect Dis* 1993;16:S314–S316. *This preliminary study reports an association between xerostomia and the risk for aspiration pneumonia in an elderly population.*

Wiedemann HP, Rice TW. Lung abscess and empyema. *Semin Thorac Cardiovasc Surg* 1995;7:119–128. *Review article discussing the medical and surgical therapy available for patients with lung abscess and empyema.*

Wynne JW, Modell JH. Respiratory aspiration of stomach contents. *Ann Intern Med* 1977;87:466–474. *Review article discussing the clinical consequences of aspirating gastric contents. The pathophysiology and treatment of each aspiration syndrome are discussed as they relate to the type of material aspirated.*

Wynne JW, Ramphal R, Hood CI. Tracheal mucosal damage after aspiration. A scanning electron microscope study. *Am Rev Respir Dis* 1981;124:728–732. *Animal study evaluating the effects of aspirating fluids of several different types and pHs on the injury induced in large airways.*

VII ENVIRONMENTAL LUNG DISEASE

Textbook of Pulmonary Diseases, 6th ed.
edited by G.L. Baum, J.D. Crapo, B.R. Celli, and J.B. Karlinsky,
Lippincott–Raven Publishers, Philadelphia, © 1998.

CHAPTER

32

Occupational Lung Diseases Caused by Asbestos, Silica, and Other Silicates

Jason Kelley

INTRODUCTION

Lung diseases caused by asbestos, silica, and the other silicates are the most prevalent pneumoconioses. They have produced very significant morbidity and mortality, particularly during the early part of the twentieth century. In the industrialized regions of the world, conditions of exposure increased rapidly during the nineteenth century. Like all major health problems, the pneumoconioses have been easier to recognize in the field at times when exposures of large cohorts of workers have been intense. As the twentieth century draws to an end, the epidemiology of the life-threatening pneumoconioses is undergoing global shifts. Dust-induced diseases are becoming more problematic in emerging nations with rapidly expanding industrial sectors. This has occurred while disease in advanced nations has gradually been reduced through enforcement of strict regulations to control dusts in the workplace.

Typically, cases of pneumoconiosis that continue to accumulate in the advanced nations represent incidental radiographic findings not associated with disability or premature mortality. Under these conditions, the challenge to the diagnostician to recognize subtle but typical radiographic features is more daunting. Characteristic presentations of pneumoconiosis at the end of the twentieth century in nations with effective dust controls in place are complicated by (1) the minimal extent of disease (often apparent only radiographically), (2) a history of multiple dust exposures leading to aberrant radiographic patterns, and (3) the preponderance of cigarette smoke-induced lung disease in the exposed population. Ever increasingly, pneumoconioses are detected as a perplexing radiographic

pattern in an elderly patient undergoing evaluation for an unrelated medical problem. When cases of severe pneumoconiosis do occur, they tend to be limited to small groups of employees receiving intense but often brief exposures not appropriately monitored by regulatory agencies.

OCCUPATIONAL HISTORY

The most important step in the diagnosis of unsuspected pneumoconiosis is to question the subject regarding specifics of the actual job and of the minerals or materials involved. Without an adequate occupational history, scientific principles of risk management cannot be implemented. Often, the subject's past or present occupation may not immediately suggest mineral dust exposure. In an era of a mobile work force, it is always important to seek a detailed account of the subject's past employment. Because some pneumoconioses develop after only brief but intense dust exposures, it is important to inquire about part-time employment. Sometimes, the subject's story must be corroborated by reviewing samples of suspected dusts or materials brought from the workplace. Mixed exposure to silica, talc, or other mineral dusts occurs when multiple minerals are mined in a single region or used in a single factory setting. The type of work done may give clues to the severity of exposure. When the interviewer is unfamiliar with the work-related terms (e.g., bagger, miller, weaver, pipe fitter, fettler, tunneler), it may be easier to seek a description of the actual working habits. Many pneumoconioses are now related to exposures outside the workplace; hence, it is of key importance to ask about hobbies and unusual activities in the home. Subjects should be questioned about whether they worked with a respirator or other protective equipment and whether they were alerted to potential hazards. Given the gender com-

J. Kelley: Department of Medicine, University of Vermont College of Medicine, Burlington, Vermont 05405.

position of the blue collar work force, almost all workers exposed to asbestos have been men. Moreover, because increased regulation of exposure has been a relatively recent development, chronic asbestosis is generally found in the older segment of the work force.

Cigarette smoking can have a particularly devastating impact on workers exposed to mineral dusts. For the clinician/epidemiologist, the coexistence of smoking-related diseases invariably confounds all epidemiologic studies of the pneumoconioses. In those mineral dust diseases causing minimal impairment, the deleterious effects of smoking far overshadow any effects attributable to dust. Rates of smoking as high as 80% have often been recorded among miners and hard rock workers.

ASBESTOS-RELATED DISEASE

Asbestos (from the Greek $\alpha\sigma\beta\epsilon\sigma\tau\sigma\sigma$, "unquenchable") is the collective term for a group of fibrous mineral silicates of the serpentine and amphibole groups that break into fibers when crushed rather than into dust. They share the properties of being nearly indestructible, heat- and acid-resistant minerals. Perhaps no mineral has presented more social and political controversy during the past century than asbestos. During the middle of the twentieth century, an epidemic of asbestos-related disease afflicted many heavily exposed workers.

There is no doubt that asbestos continues to be an important health concern. However, as the disorder has abated in prevalence and severity, concern for other than occupational exposures, particularly among groups such as schoolchildren and office workers, has grown, often without sound basis. Many observers feel that this heightened level of concern with asbestos has inappropriately

TABLE 1. *Mineral forms of asbestos*

Amphiboles	Serpentines
Crocidolite (blue asbestos)	Chrysotile
Amosite (brown asbestos)	
Tremolite	
Actinolite	
Anthophyllite	

drawn public attention from other, potentially more hazardous features of the environment.

Asbestos exists in multiple forms, all of them fibrous silicate minerals. They are variably resistant to heat and to destruction by acids and other chemicals. All asbestos forms have a fibrous structure, which makes them suitable for use in woven fabric. The main elements present in addition to silicon are magnesium, calcium, iron, and sodium in differing proportions. All forms of asbestos can be divided into one of two mineralogic types, the serpentines and the amphiboles. Commercially, chrysotile is the most important serpentine. Long chrysotile fibers have a curled appearance; the amphiboles have more needle-shaped fibers (Fig. 1). Common amphiboles include crocidolite, amosite, anthophyllite, tremolite, and actinolite (Table 1).

Commercial Uses of Asbestos

Chrysotile accounts for the preponderance (>95%) of asbestos mined and used in the world. It has been mined primarily in eastern Canada and New England as well as in Russia. Crocidolite comes primarily from South Africa and was previously mined in western Australia. However, with recognition of its toxicity, demand for crocidolite has greatly decreased.

Asbestos has been widely mined since the end of the nineteenth century. Regulatory efforts by government agencies, such as the Environmental Protection Agency (EPA) in the United States, has greatly cut down on its use. World production of asbestos rose steadily from <0.2 million tons in 1920, peaked at 5 million tons in the late 1970s, and has shown a slight decline since that time. For many years, sheathing and insulation used in the construction of office buildings and houses consisted largely of agents that had been reinforced and rendered heat-resistant with asbestos fibers. Asbestos was used to line furnaces and lag pipes; it was also used as friction material in brakes, as a fire retardant in spray paints, and as a binder and strengthener for cement pipes. It was extensively used in warships as insulation and to prevent fire. In the 1950s, asbestos was even a component of cigarette filters.

Historical Aspects and Effects of Exposure to Asbestos

Asbestos exposure can lead to three serious pulmonary conditions: asbestosis (a diffuse fibrosing disease of the

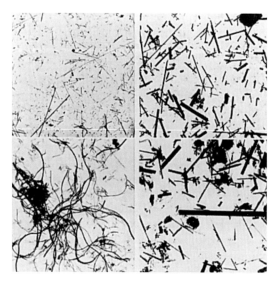

FIG. 1. Various types of asbestos. Anthophyllite (*top left*). Chrysotile (*top right*). Amosite (*bottom left*). Crocidolite (*bottom right*).

lungs), lung cancer, and mesothelioma. Whereas asbestosis can vary from mild to lethal, the latter two disorders are almost invariably fatal.

Asbestosis was first recognized as a distinct disease entity in 1907 by Murray in the United Kingdom. The magnitude of the hazard and the exposure-response relationship were worked out in the subsequent decades. Recommendations for improved industrial hygiene practices grew out of those seminal studies. The risk to users of the finished asbestos products became more generally apparent by the early 1960s. Before that, sporadic case reports of asbestosis occurring in pipe fitters, welders, and others had been reported. Most such instances suggested that the victim had acquired the condition as a result of an exceptional and unusual exposure. Studies in the 1960s made it clear that a significant risk existed in all users of asbestos. Furthermore, it was clear from those studies that the prevailing regulatory statutes were not protecting the work force from asbestosis.

The role of asbestos as a carcinogen was debated during the 1930s and 1940s. However, the issue remained controversial until 1955, when Doll published a classic article presenting the statistical evidence needed to confirm the association with certainty. Doll's study described the increased risk for lung cancer only in subjects with coexisting asbestosis, and did not consider asbestos exposure in the absence of fibrosis as a potential cause of lung cancer.

In the late 1950s, the association between malignant pleural mesothelioma and prior asbestos exposure was made by clinicians in South Africa. The risk for development of mesothelioma, like that for asbestosis and lung cancer, is concentration-related and depends significantly on the type of asbestos fibers inhaled. The prolonged inhalation of asbestos fibers has been said to be associated with an increased risk for laryngeal, ovarian, gastrointestinal, and renal carcinomas. This association is not clear, however, as some cases of mesothelioma may have been incorrectly diagnosed as primary cancers of other organs.

Standards for Asbestos Exposure

Exposure limits for asbestos have been developed and applied throughout the twentieth century in response to epidemic disease and disability. Precise standards vary somewhat between industrialized nations. In the United States, the regulated standard has progressively been reduced to 0.2 fibers per cubic centimeter. To allow for frequent changes in ambient dust levels in the workplace, this standard refers to an 8-hr time-weighted average (TWA). Asbestos fibers 5 μm and larger are responsible for most of the toxicity and are therefore the focus of regulatory standards. To account for the different toxicities of different fiber types, some jurisdictions apply more rigorous standards for the amphiboles.

For many years, asbestos levels were measured as the number of particles present per cubic centimeter of the ambient air. Asbestos content is usually determined by trapping airborne particles on filters. Fiber size and number are then determined by phase-contrast microscopy. Only fibers >5 μm in length are measured, as smaller fibers are cleared from the lungs and are not likely to lead to pulmonary disease or malignancy. When particles and fibers are counted, asbestos is not distinguished from other substances. Although this does not matter much in asbestos textile factories, where most of the airborne fibers are asbestos, in other occupational settings the percentage of asbestos fibers is much smaller and may be as low as 5%–10%. Under such circumstances, optical counts using a microscope can be misleading, and when it is imperative to separate asbestos fibers from other types of fibers, more definitive techniques, such as transmission or scanning electron microscopy, must be used.

As a result of regulatory efforts in the industrialized nations of the world, the incidence of asbestos-related lung disease has become less common during the past several decades. Subjects with established asbestosis are thus becoming an increasingly elderly population. Moreover, as the ambient levels have fallen in the workplace, the latency time between exposure and appearance of asbestos-related disease has lengthened. For example, a report from 1938 showed that asbestosis was present with exposures as short as 5 years. At that time, dust levels could be as high as 400 particles per cubic centimeter. During and after World War II, the average duration of exposure before the development of asbestosis rose from 10 to 12 years to >20 years. Nonetheless, asbestosis still occurred in certain industries. Since then, the regulations have become considerably more stringent; it is highly likely that no new cases of asbestos-related lung diseases will develop under current standards. The reduction in the use of amphiboles makes this prospect even more likely.

Specific Occupational Risks

It has been estimated that as many as 27 million workers in the United States received a significant exposure to asbestos during the middle four decades of the twentieth century. Environmental exposure to asbestos and other minerals can occur at each stage of production and use: extraction (miners), purification and production (weavers), and use of the finished product (plumbers, laggers, insulation layers). Workers involved in removal of the used product from buildings, ships, and other sites may be exposed. This statement applies only to those involved in removal efforts in older buildings and equipment in which the risk of asbestos is not apparent. Somewhat surprisingly, miners of asbestos have generally been found to be at lower risk for disease than millers and weavers. Regardless of the context, exposure to chrysotile carries significantly less risk than exposure to crocidolite and the other amphiboles.

Very close contact is a critical determinant of risk. Examples abound of work forces in which certain jobs carried much higher risks than others. Thus, welders working in the same factory with pipe fitters had little or no increase in asbestos-related lung disease, whereas the latter group was at high risk.

Asbestos-related disease as a result of exposure outside the workplace occurs but is infrequent and requires very substantial exposure. Stories of wives washing their husbands' asbestos-laden clothing may be true but are less frequently documented as regulations have been enforced. Low levels of asbestos fibers are found in ambient air in the urban environment. Sources include demolition of equipment and buildings. These levels continue to drop as regulatory measures have been implemented. People who work or live in older buildings containing asbestos are not at significant risk, as the asbestos is largely immobilized in building materials. One recent study has indicated that public buildings contain as few as 0.002 fibers per cubic centimeter, far below the regulated standard. Finally, asbestos occurs as an air and water pollutant in certain regions of the world where surface deposits are a part of the landscape.

Pathogenesis of Asbestos-Related Disease: Inhalation and Deposition

Inhaled asbestos fibers deposit on airway bifurcations of terminal and respiratory bronchioles. Lesser degrees of deposition occur in the alveoli. Somewhat paradoxically, it is the longer fibers that have the potential to reach the distal lung and exert toxicity. Fibers as long as 60 μm, a size not normally considered to be in the respirable range, evade impaction in the large airways. Their exaggerated length-to-width ratio allows them to penetrate into the small airways, from which they migrate into the lung interstitium. Small fibers (<5 μm in length) are removed by the mucociliary escalator mechanisms of the lungs and therefore represent less of a lasting risk.

On ingestion by macrophages, asbestos fibers undergo a process of chemical leaching and partial dissolution. This phenomenon occurs chiefly with chrysotile asbestos; the amphiboles are more resistant to macrophage ingestion and leaching, and once deposited, they have a much longer half-life. As a result of their different half-lives, the longer-lasting amphiboles tend to become predominant with time in subjects exposed to mixed dusts. Clearance cannot be effected if the length of the fiber is >20 μm. Fibers that cannot be cleared via the mucociliary escalator up the airway lumen move into the interstitium, from which they migrate to the regional lymph nodes.

How might asbestos prove toxic to lung cells? Heintz and colleagues have shown that asbestos increases the expression of certain proto-oncogenes (c-*fos*, c-*jun*) in mesothelial cells and tracheal epithelial cells. Asbestos induces increases in protein factors that bind specifically to the DNA sites that mediate gene expression by the AP-1 family of transcription factors. The persistent induction of transcription factors by asbestos suggests a model of asbestos-induced carcinogenesis involving chronic stimulation of cell proliferation through activation of the early-response gene pathway, which includes c-*jun* or c-*fos*. The inflammatory nature of the evolving asbestos lesions can be seen graphically in workers and in experimental animals using gallium scanning. In workers with positive findings on gallium scanning, the intensity of gallium uptake correlates with the activity of the inflammatory process.

Nuclear factor kappa B (NF-κB), a transcription factor regulating expression of genes intrinsic to inflammation and cell proliferation, may be an important intracellular intermediary in initiating asbestos-associated diseases. Crocidolite asbestos causes protracted and dose-responsive increases in proteins binding to nuclear NF-κB-binding DNA elements in airway epithelial cells. NF-κB induction by asbestos may prove to be a key event in the regulation of multiple genes involved in the pathogenesis of asbestos-related fibrosis and lung cancers.

The issue of variability of susceptibility to asbestosis and other pneumoconioses between workers with comparable exposures has long interested investigators. The best available evidence suggests that the retention and accumulation of dust in the lungs is a more important determinant than absolute exposure levels. Lung and airway size correlate with the presence or absence of disease in workers exposed to asbestos, silica, and other dusts. Airway caliber in particular seems to be a major determinant of person-to-person variation.

The weight of evidence suggests that smokers are at greater risk for the development of asbestos-related disease through similar mechanisms. Smoking has the potential to delay the clearance of particles such as asbestos from the lungs by incapacitating the mucociliary escalator. In line with the hypothesis presented above, cigarette smoking enhances fiber retention in the lungs; the longer residence time and greater burden of fibers in the lungs of smokers allows uptake of fibers by epithelial cells and other structural cells.

Asbestosis

Asbestosis is a diffuse interstitial fibrosis of the lungs caused by inhalation of asbestos. It results from heavy exposure to respirable forms of asbestos. The common presenting symptoms of asbestosis are dyspnea and dry cough, which may initially be ascribed by both subject and physician to heavy cigarette use. As with other pulmonary disorders, the victim often does not seek medical advice until the condition is fairly disabling. Weight loss is an early feature. If the original asbestos exposure was intense, disabling symptoms may continue to progress despite removal from further exposure.

Early in the disease process, the clinician can hear middle- to late-inspiratory crackles, which are most prominent in the bases of the lungs. As the disease progresses, these extend from the bases to the middle zones and become more widespread. Tachypnea is almost always present by the time the disease has reached the symptomatic stage. Cyanosis may be visible. Clubbing of the fingers, when present, usually signals advanced disease and a poor prognosis. Signs consistent with failure of the right side of the heart also become apparent later in the course.

Radiographic Features

Asbestosis is characterized by the development of irregular small shadows on chest x-ray films. To assist in standardization of interpretation of chest radiographs, the International Labor Office (ILO) developed a classification based on plain chest radiography. In the ILO system, small irregular shadows are described as *s, t,* and *u* in increasing size. Rounded shadows (such as are seen typically in silicosis) are termed *p, q,* or *r* shadows. The amount or profusion of small round or irregular shadows is graded as either 0, 1, 2, or 3. When the reader is somewhat uncertain about the grading, intermediate grades can be indicated with a slash mark. For example, a reading between grades 1 and 2 would be 1/2, with the first number given being the one the reader believes to be correct and the second one being also possible. In asbestosis, the smaller *s* and *t* shadows predominate over the larger *u* shadows. Scanty irregular shadows are present on chest radiographs in a significant percentage of smokers who have had no asbestos exposure, making their presence less specific. As in other interstitial lung disorders, these small irregular shadows tend to blur the margins of normal anatomic structures such as the diaphragm and the cardiomediastinal and bronchovascular markings (Fig. 2). Initially, the small irregular shadows appear in the lower zones, the site of most intense asbestos inhalation. With progression of disease, the upper lung zones become more obviously involved. Use of computed tomography (CT) to detect disease in exposed workers with normal chest x-ray findings is controversial. In asbestos-exposed subjects who have normal chest x-ray films, high-resolution CT can identify a group with significantly reduced lung function, indicative of restrictive lung disease, in comparison with a group having normal or near-normal CT scans. Pathologic correlation to indicate what early shadows signify are limited. Because the ILO classification system was set up to categorize disease according to plain chest x-ray features, the chest x-ray remains the widely used diagnostic standard.

Often, the parenchymal shadows are accompanied by pleural thickening with or without calcification (Fig. 3). In this circumstance, the evaluation of the character and profusion of the irregular parenchymal shadows can be

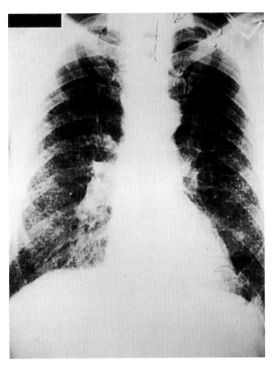

FIG. 2. Radiograph of a worker with category 2/3 asbestosis. He had worked for 30 years as an insulator.

confounded; the pleural changes when viewed *en face* can be mistaken for parenchymal disease. CT is particularly helpful in clarifying this issue. Another clue on the posteroanterior chest x-ray film is that the pleural thickening is most prominent in the middle third of the chest.

With late disease, other radiographic features emerge. As in other forms of interstitial fibrosis, a pattern of honeycombing—radiographically apparent cystic spaces in the lung—develops. In all the interstitial disorders in which it is seen, honeycombing provides incontrovertible evidence of advanced and irreversible lung remodeling and fibrosis. Its appearance, therefore, confirms that the asbestosis is severely disabling. In advanced disease, CT reveals features similar to those of other forms of late interstitial pulmonary fibrosis. Enlargement of the right ventricle and the central pulmonary arteries occurs late in the disease process, when pulmonary hypertension and cor pulmonale develop. Exceptionally large conglomerate masses in upper lung zones, such as are seen in coal workers' pneumoconiosis and silicosis, are rarely seen in asbestosis. These generally occur in subjects with concomitant silica exposure or in conjunction with rheumatoid arthritis (Caplan's syndrome, discussed below).

The presence of irregular shadows in low profusion in the lower zones cannot be considered unique or specific for asbestosis. Exposure to fibrous dusts other than asbestos may cause the appearance of small irregular shadows in the lung bases, particularly in smokers and elderly patients. Irregular shadows are seen in all forms of interstitial fibrosis, after exposure to non-asbestiform fibers,

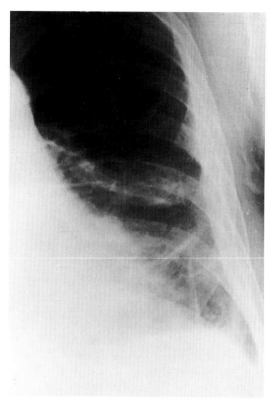

FIG. 3. Lateral wall pleural thickening and pleural plaques. Also evident are calcified pleural plaques viewed *en face.*

and in cigarette smokers. However, in these circumstances the irregular shadows are usually not profuse. Finally, the ILO classification can be used in predicting life expectancy.

Rounded atelectasis is a distinctive radiographic pattern nearly unique to asbestosis. It probably develops as an exuberant focal pleural reaction that entraps subjacent lung tissue in a swirl of pleural inflammation. It is important to recognize this lesion, as it may be mistaken on the plain chest x-ray film for a peripheral lung mass, an error that often leads to an unnecessary search for a lung tumor (Fig. 4). Rounded atelectasis, when suspected, can easily be confirmed by CT, which shows the characteristic atelectatic lung tissue and distorted bronchovascular markings.

Pulmonary Function Studies

Symptomatic asbestosis is associated with changes in mechanical properties of the lungs resembling those seen in other forms of interstitial fibrosis. As remodeling progresses and extracellular matrix proteins are deposited in excess amounts, the lungs become regionally less compliant and all lung volumes are reduced. In consequence, there is a marked increase in the respiratory rate, a decrease in the tidal volume, and an absolute increase in the minute volume as the ventilation-perfusion relationship

becomes less evenly matched. The diffusing capacity may be reduced before lung volumes are overtly lowered. Tests of regional lung function have shown impaired ventilation of the lower zones. As a result of the altered ventilation-perfusion relationship, hypoxemia and hypercapnia may be severe in advanced disease, particularly during exercise.

A number of attempts have been made to detect the disease at a presymptomatic stage and in the absence of overt chest radiographic abnormalities. Most such efforts have focused on measurements of lung mechanics. It has been possible to show a lower maximal expiratory flow for a given transpulmonary pressure in subjects with normal chest x-ray findings but with significant dust exposure. However, because these approaches require invasive studies with particular attention to calibration and are relatively cumbersome, measurements of lung mechanics are not feasible in field studies of exposed populations.

The potential importance of small-airways disease in asbestos exposure remains unclear. Certainly, the early lesions in asbestos exposure are localized to the terminal and respiratory bronchioles, and tests of small-airways function detect flow limitation in small airways before results of other pulmonary function tests become abnormal. However, asbestos-induced small-airways disease may occur independent of the other abnormalities of asbestosis.

Diagnosis of Asbestosis

The diagnosis of asbestosis is based on four criteria: (1) an appropriate history of exposure, (2) compatible radiographic changes (ILO category >1/1), and (3) diffusing capacity and forced vital capacity below the lower limits of normal. These criteria and the evidence supporting their applicability have been published by the American Thoracic Society. It is particularly difficult to diagnose asbestosis in the absence of changes on the chest x-ray film. Lung biopsy via bronchoscopy, thoracotomy, or video-assisted thoracoscopy are only rarely required or justified in making the diagnosis. Biopsy can be occasionally justified to exclude other causes of interstitial fibrosis but should never be carried out merely to provide evidence for litigation.

Pathology of Asbestosis

Visual inspection of lungs from victims of asbestosis usually demonstrates thickened visceral pleural membranes. The cut surfaces of the shrunken lungs display honeycombing and fibrosis identical to those seen in other forms of diffuse interstitial fibrosis.

The microscopic hallmark of asbestosis is the asbestos is body. Asbestos bodies are elongated, golden-brown structures beaded with proteinaceous material; their

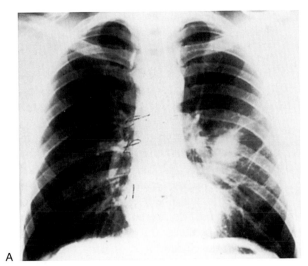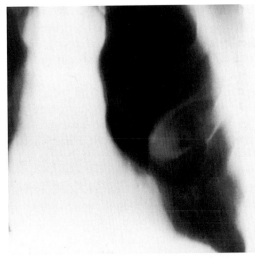

A B

FIG. 4. Rounded atelectasis in a worker who had been an insulator for 15 years. The subject had no chest symptoms and normal lung function. **Panel A:** Posteroanterior film. **Panel B:** Tomographic view.

lengths correspond to the individual asbestos fibers that form their cores (Fig. 5). Because of their high iron content, they stain particularly well with iron stains. Early in the disease process, asbestos fibers are found intracellularly within macrophages recruited to the area of deposition. Within the macrophage, the fiber may become leached and fragmented to a smaller size. The beading represents biologic modification of the fiber and is composed of proteinaceous material rich in ferritin. After the death of the macrophage, the acellular coated fiber can be recognized under the microscope as a mature asbestos body.

The minimal number of asbestos bodies in lung samples needed for a certain diagnosis of asbestosis remains unclear despite considerable research. One study has shown that lungs of urban dwellers with no occupational expo-

sure to asbestos should contain only one asbestos body for every hundred sections of lung tissue examined. To make the diagnosis of asbestosis, there should be evidence of interstitial inflammation (early) and fibrosis (later) in the presence of asbestos bodies.

With a few notable exceptions, asbestos bodies are found regularly in patients with asbestosis; conversely, the absence of asbestos bodies is a reliable sign that the disease is not present. In any case, large tissue samples are required for certain diagnosis; biopsy material obtained by bronchoscopic biopsy is not adequate to identify the occasional asbestos body.

Inhalation of certain other fibrous minerals, such as glass wool, fibrous alumina, or silicon carbide, may induce formation of similar bodies. Because the core of these structures is composed of fibers other than asbestos,

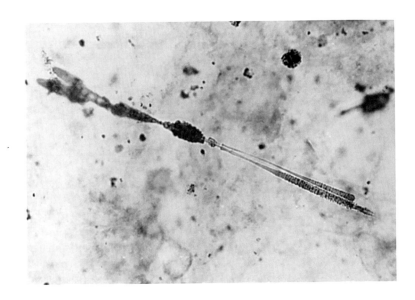

FIG. 5. High-power photomicrograph of asbestos body.

they are more accurately referred to as *ferruginous bodies.* Specific mineralogic identification of the fibers using electron microscopy and x-ray energy spectroscopy may be required to distinguish between asbestos and the other fibrous minerals.

The expectorated sputum of workers exposed to asbestos often contain asbestos and asbestos bodies many years after exposure has ceased. Asbestos bodies can also be found in samples of alveolar lavage fluid recovered by bronchoscopy. These findings confirm the exposure to asbestos but do not indicate the diagnosis of asbestosis. Most residents of industrialized areas have some asbestos bodies in their lungs. However, their presence is not diagnostic of asbestosis in the absence of clinical manifestations of disease.

When ferruginous bodies are detected in lungs or respiratory secretions of subjects who report no occupational exposure, the types of asbestos most often found are chrysotile and tremolite. Tremolite may be inhaled during the use of facial powder composed of talc contaminated with small amounts of the nonasbestiform mineral tremolite.

Chrysotile is particularly susceptible to the leaching process; with time the number and size of chrysotile fibers decline notably. In contrast, amphiboles are more resistant to chemical leaching and tend to persist in the lungs. The intracellular production of asbestos bodies may inactivate the fiber and prevent further toxicity. In chrysotile-induced asbestosis, numerous asbestos bodies and uncoated fibers may be found for prolonged periods despite the leaching process.

From the above discussion, it is apparent that the numbers of fibers and ferruginous bodies found in respiratory secretions and lung tissue at postmortem examination can vary considerably, depending on exposure history and other factors. Urban dwellers without specific occupational exposure have relatively few fibers; much greater numbers of fibers are seen in subjects with clear occupational exposure and clinical manifestations of asbestosis.

The hazards of asbestos exposure—namely, asbestosis, pleural thickening and plaques, bronchogenic carcinoma, and mesothelioma—can be related to the extent of exposure. The density of fibers found in the dried lung samples of various population groups depends on the intensity of exposure and shows an enormous range. Although subjects with no occupational exposure have detectable fiber counts, it is important to keep in mind that the numbers of coated and uncoated fibers are hundreds of times lower than in exposed healthy workers and thousands of times lower than in workers with apparent lung disease. Urban dwellers without occupational exposures have <1000 fibers per gram of dry lung tissue. Fiber counts in lung samples from established cases of asbestosis and mesothelioma usually exceed 80 million per gram of dried tissue. In subjects with lung cancer, fiber counts are more diffi-

cult to relate to disease risk because of the dominant carcinogenic effect of cigarette smoke.

Measuring Asbestos Fibers in Tissues

Most of the asbestos present in the lungs of exposed workers is in the form of short (<5 μm) translucent fibers that do not take up histologic stains. Hence, most of the asbestos burden in lung tissue is invisible by standard light microscopy but can be seen by phase-contrast or electron microscopy techniques. Only a very small minority of the longer fibers evolve into more conspicuous asbestos bodies. To overcome this problem, standardized scientific approaches for evaluating the asbestos burden have been developed.

The Pneumoconiosis Committee of the American College of Pathologists has specified that the minimal criteria for the histologic diagnosis include the identification of peribronchiolar fibrosis and at least two asbestos bodies in tissue sections. Fiber counting can be done on a digest of tissue. However, enumerating asbestos bodies in tissue sections is the usual approach for general pathologists. Because the segmented coating of asbestos bodies is rich in iron, the use of iron staining is a particularly sensitive method for detecting asbestos bodies. It turns out that agreement is excellent between the numbers of asbestos bodies seen in tissue sections and those present in digests of tissue. An average of two asbestos bodies on 2 × 2-cm sections of lung tissue is equivalent to approximately 200 asbestos bodies per gram of wet fixed tissue.

Pathogenesis of Asbestosis

Little is known about the earliest tissue responses to inhaled asbestos in humans. Experimental studies in animals exposed to asbestos in relatively high concentrations show that the first lesions are inflammatory in nature and are localized to bifurcations of small airways, the sites of most intense deposition of inhaled fibers. With further exposure, a macrophage-dominant inflammatory process involves the lumina of small airways and extends into alveoli. Because the macrophage is central to dust phagocytosis, it can be assumed to modulate many of the subsequent pathologic events. It is important to note that activated macrophages release a number of inflammatory mediators and proinflammatory cytokines. These include chemotactic cytokines and peptides, growth modulators such as insulin-like growth factor-1, platelet-derived growth factor, interleukin-1α, and tumor necrosis factor-α. Also produced are enzymes allowing rapid generation and release of active oxygen species, such as peroxides, hydroxyl radicals, and superoxide anions. These in turn directly oxidize lipids of cellular membranes and damage DNA and proteins. The proteolytic enzymes such as elastases and cathepsins induce injury and death of adjacent structural lung cells, such as epithelial cells, endothelial cells, and interstitial fibroblasts.

A second step in the pathogenesis of asbestos lesions involves fibers interacting directly with epithelial cells and fibroblasts. Undegraded asbestos fibers enter epithelial cells by endocytosis and are transported along the intracellular microtubular network. From the basolateral surfaces of the cells, the fibers migrate into the interstitium and can directly interact with interstitial fibroblasts.

With time, pathologic amounts of extracellular matrix proteins such as collagen, elastin, and proteoglycans are deposited. The lungs lose air space volume and elasticity. The lesions are found more in the lower lung zones, reflecting the proportionally greater ventilation (and hence particle burden).

Clinical Course of Asbestosis

Severe asbestosis advances to physiologic deterioration, disability, and death. Death is the result of respiratory failure, failure of the right side of the heart, and respiratory malignancies. The major reductions in deaths caused by asbestos during recent years can be traced to the relatively milder disease present in the population of aging workers. Efficacious therapy for asbestosis does not exist. Treatment of the symptoms—bronchodilators if obstruction is present, cardiac medications if right-sided heart failure is present—probably have little effect. Whether continuous low-flow oxygen therapy is helpful in hypoxemic patients has not been proved.

Pleural Effusion and Diffuse Pleural Thickening

Benign pleural effusions often appear during or after asbestos exposure. Effusions usually occur within the first decade of exposure. The chief symptoms are dyspnea and pleuritic pain. The radiographic appearance is no different from that of other effusions. Because the majority of such effusions are not associated with signs of established asbestosis, diagnostic thoracocentesis is often required. Systemic signs of inflammation, including an elevated white blood cell count and elevated sedimentation rate, may be present. The pleural fluid is an exudate and may contain both polymorphonuclear leukocytes and mononuclear cells. Only infrequently is the fluid overtly bloody. Asbestos fibers are hard to find, and usually biopsy of the pleura shows only a chronic, nonspecific reaction. The effusion tends to linger for several months and frequently leads to diffuse pleural thickening and a fibrothorax. In some instances, the fibrothorax leads to appreciable restrictive impairment. When a substantial fibrothorax develops, there is a tendency to consider surgical decortication; however, asbestos-induced pleural thickening and fibrothorax generally improve during the course of several years and should be observed without interven-

tion. Pleural effusions and thickening do not portend the development of mesothelioma.

Pleural Plaques

Pleural plaques are a characteristic feature of prolonged asbestos exposure. Plaques, often calcified, are usually located on the lower lateral chest wall and on the central portion of the diaphragm; radiographically discernible plaques usually do not develop until after more than a decade of exposure. Their pathogenesis is distinct from the development of effusion and fibrothorax. They represent markers of asbestos exposure but do not by themselves constitute a disease process, nor do they portend later pulmonary impairment. In many instances, such plaques may extend around the lateral curvature of the chest. Sometimes they are seen on the anterior or posterior chest wall only. Pleural plaques, usually on the diaphragm, can be found at autopsy in most subjects who have worked for >5 years with asbestos. Although diffuse pleural thickening is often associated with fibrothorax and restrictive ventilatory impairment, pleural plaques probably have no adverse effect on lung function. Plaque formation and calcification may also involve the pericardium (Fig. 6).

When viewed *en face* on the posteroanterior chest film, plaques can be mistaken for parenchymal shadows and disease (Fig. 3). In such cases, absence of parenchymal

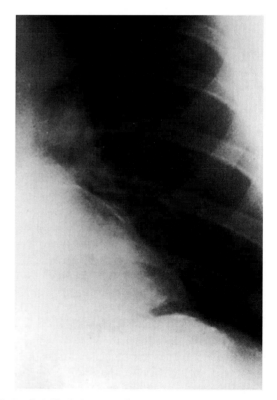

FIG. 6. Calcified plaques of pericardium and left diaphragm.

disease on the lateral chest film should alert the interpreter that pleural disease has obscured the interpretation of the posteroanterior film. Also, CT has proved to be a sensitive and definitive method for defining plaques and distinguishing them from parenchymal disease, but it is not required except in complex cases.

It is a mistake to assume that the presence of plaques portends the development of mesothelioma or lung cancer. Pleural plaques are seen more frequently after exposure to the amphiboles than to the serpentine chrysotile. Calcification usually appears in the plaque that has been present for more than a decade. However, calcification is seldom noted on the plain film until two decades after first exposure to asbestos.

Asbestos as a Carcinogen

No aspect of asbestos is more controversial than the issues surrounding its association with malignancy. That there is an association between exposure to asbestos and risk for malignancy has been clear for the past 40 years. Moreover, at intense exposure levels there is an approximately linear dose-response relationship. What remains difficult to pin down is the precise risk of asbestos exposure relative to other carcinogens, and the precise mechanisms of tumor induction. One analysis suggested that lung cancer may account for as many as 26% of deaths in some groups of asbestos workers, a risk three to five times higher than that expected in other workers. The excess mortality is detectable after at least a decade of exposure and climbs progressively thereafter. The risk depends somewhat on the type of industrial exposure, as asbestos textile workers exhibit a higher incidence of lung cancer than cement workers, who in turn have more malignancies than asbestos miners. In most of these studies, the populations were exposed to chrysotile fibers only; the amphiboles are considered more carcinogenic than chrysotile.

With control of asbestos exposure in the workplace, cigarette smoking may be a more important determinant of lung cancer risk in exposed workers than asbestos itself. In this regard, lung cancer has developed in relatively few nonsmoking workers with significant asbestos exposures. Moreover, the very high incidence of smoking among industrial workers increases the risk for lung cancer in nonsmoking co-workers through secondhand exposure to smoke. Certainly, the risk of smoking in the induction of lung cancer was considerably underestimated in early population studies.

The minimal level of asbestos exposure or disease that puts an individual at risk for malignancy remains uncertain. Back extrapolation of the concentration response that applies for workers with heavy exposures cannot be scientifically justified; there are too few reliable data among subjects with lower levels of exposure. One analysis sug-

gested a threshold level of exposure rather than a finite but decreasing risk at low exposure levels. This threshold is close to the threshold for development of asbestosis. Studies in asbestos cement workers in the United States and miners exposed to amosite in South Africa both provide support for the notion of a threshold value for asbestos-induced lung cancer.

Malignant Mesothelioma

Pleural mesotheliomas can occur as either benign or malignant tumors. The benign form, which is not associated with asbestos exposure, is frequently accompanied by hypertrophic pulmonary osteoarthropathy. In contrast, malignant mesothelioma is an aggressive, uniformly fatal, diffuse cancer arising from the pleura and sometimes the peritoneum (Figs. 7–9). Most malignant mesotheliomas can be traced to previous exposure to asbestos or the non-asbestiform fibrous mineral erionite. As mentioned previously, asbestos-induced mesotheliomas develop only after intense exposure; they do not occur following the minimal exposures experienced by urban dwellers.

Malignant mesothelioma remains a rare cancer. It typically appears several decades after the first exposure to asbestos, although shorter incubation periods have been recorded following particularly intense exposures. In certain instances, however, the intense exposure may have

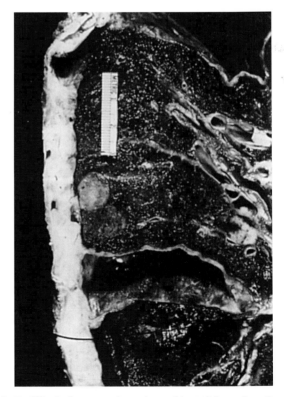

FIG. 7. Whole-lung section of a subject dying of malignant mesothelioma. The lung is encased in white tumor tissue, and a secondary deposit is apparent in the lung parenchyma.

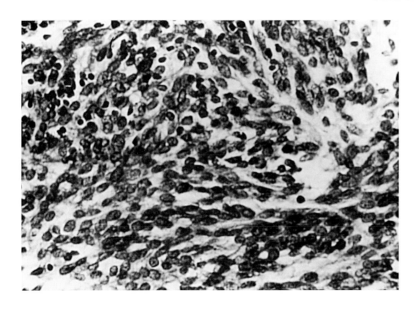

FIG. 8. Photomicrograph showing the histologic features of a sarcomatous type of mesothelioma.

ceased several decades before the mesothelioma becomes clinically apparent. Treatment options for this resistant neoplasm, which remain limited, are discussed in Chapter 70.

DISEASES ASSOCIATED WITH EXPOSURE TO SILICA

Silicosis is the disease induced by the inhalation of free crystalline silica (silicon dioxide). Silicon is the second most abundant element and forms the greater part of the earth's crust. It is therefore ubiquitous in the human environment, and some exposure to silicon dioxide and the salts of silicic acid is a fact of life. Silicosis probably occurred in paleolithic times, as soon as humans began to make stone tools. Indeed, the term *silicosis* derives from the Latin word *silex,* meaning

"flint." Intense exposure leading to disease occurs in mining and in those industries in which the mineral is used, such as the manufacture of ceramics, pottery, and bricks. However, as with asbestos, public health regulations have significantly reduced the numbers of silicosis cases in the industrialized world.

Silicon can exist free, that is, not chemically combined with other elements, or it may form silicates by combining with various elements. Silicon dioxide exists in crystalline and amorphous forms, as well as mixed forms. The crystalline forms include cristobalite, tridymite, and quartz. All can produce fibrotic pulmonary disease, with quartz being somewhat less potent in this respect than the others. The amorphous silicas include diatomite, derived from the skeletons of oceanic diatoms, and vitreous silica, a manufactured product of heated silica. The amorphous

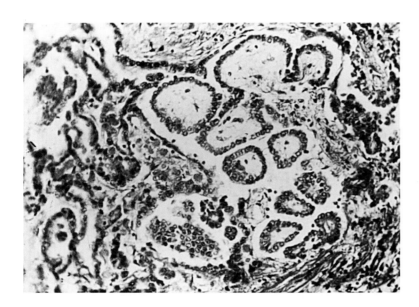

FIG. 9. Photomicrograph of a section of a tubo-papillary mesothelioma. This histologic variant bears a close resemblance to a papillary carcinoma of the thyroid.

forms are generally not fibrogenic. Mixed forms, deposits containing crystalline and amorphous features, include chert and flint.

Many of the silicates, salts of silicic acid, are also variably fibrogenic. With the obvious exception of asbestos, the silicates tend to be less toxic than the free crystalline forms of silica. Sandstone and flint are composed of almost pure quartz; granite contains from 15%–70% of free silica by weight, slate 30%–45%, and shales around 10%.

Sources of Exposure

The harmful effects of hard rock mining have been known for millennia. Pliny the Elder wrote about them but may not have associated them with the respirable dusts. In the sixteenth century, Agricola correctly associated most of the lung disease of metal miners with the continued inhalation of mine dust in *De Re Metallica.* Later, Ramazzini pointed out that many diseases originated from workers' occupations and that mining was particularly dangerous. He noted that stone cutters were particularly at risk for the development of lung disease. In the nineteenth century, grinding, the manufacture of pottery, and trades using flint and slate emerged as particularly hazardous.

Definitive regulatory efforts in the industrialized nations have resulted in a major decrease in silicosis during the past half-century. New cases of silicosis tend to be sporadic rather than epidemic. In contrast, the pneumoconioses present a growing problem in the emerging industrial nations. Silicosis persists as a public health menace in coal and metal mines, sandblasting, ceramics refractories, and foundries. Silica flour, finely ground silica used as filler for cosmetics, abrasives, and paint extenders, represents a particularly hazardous form of silica.

Sandblasting is a particularly high-risk occupation, generating large amounts of airborne silica. The use of silica for this purpose has ceased under regulatory pressure in many advanced nations. In nations such as the United States, where its use persists, it remains the most frequent cause of acute silicosis.

Exposure-Response Relationships

As many as a million Americans may be exposed to silica in the workplace. Precise figures of the prevalence and incidence of silicosis are not available. It is certain, however, that the prevalence of silicosis has fallen very significantly in recent decades. This drop has been best documented in the small but well-studied Vermont granite industry.

Although large groups of workers exposed to free silica have undergone surveillance for many years, few attempts have been made to derive an exposure-response relationship. Currently, studies are under way in the United States, South Africa, and Canada to establish the relationship between the development of silicosis and cumulative dust levels. The current evidence suggests that an air quality standard for free silica of 0.1 mg/m^3 should protect the vast majority of the work force. Chronic forms of clinically important silicosis are seldom seen before a decade of moderately intense exposure.

Silicosis

Clinical Features

For clinical purposes, silicosis has traditionally been divided into chronic, subacute, and acute forms (Table 2). Classic or chronic silicosis, the usual type, can be further divided into simple and complicated forms based on the radiographic appearance. Simple silicosis is characterized by the presence of small rounded shadows that usually appear in the upper lobes and later are noted throughout all lung zones (Fig. 10). Complicated silicosis is said to be present when shadows on the chest x-ray film expand to >1 cm in diameter (conglomerate masses).

Simple silicosis is not associated with respiratory symptoms. Typically, simple silicosis is discovered during radiographic screening. The chest x-ray film shows a striking profusion of small rounded shadows, not associated with symptoms. If any respiratory symptoms, such as cough or dyspnea, are present at this stage, they are more likely the results of an associated respiratory illness other than silicosis. Given the high prevalence of cigarette smoking among workers exposed to mineral dusts, smoking-related lung disorders must also be considered as a cause of symptoms at this stage.

In general, simple silicosis does not progress after cessation of exposure, and the patient can be assured that disability will not occur. In complicated silicosis, however, the large shadows on the chest x-ray film slowly enlarge during a period of years. This can occur even without further exposure. Subjects with massive fibrosis, high relative levels of exposure to dust, or tuberculosis are most likely to progress to complicated silicosis. The

TABLE 2. *Clinical classification of silica-induced syndromes*

Chronic silicosis
Simple silicosis
Complicated silicosis
Conglomerate shadows ("progressive massive fibrosis")
Caplan's syndrome (rheumatoid pneumoconiosis)
Acute silicosis (silicoproteinosis)
Other syndromes
Irritant bronchitis
Small-airways disease
Emphysema

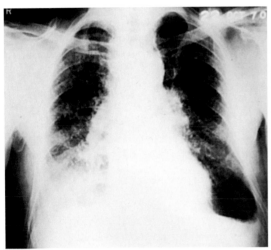

FIG. 10. Chest radiograph of a worker with simple silicosis. Note the evidence of a resolved pleural effusion in the right hemithorax.

earlier the onset of complicated silicosis, the greater the likelihood that the disease will progress and become disabling. When complicated disease reaches more advanced stages, symptoms of breathlessness, cough, and sputum production appear. As the size of the conglomerate masses increases, the symptoms worsen, and pulmonary function tests demonstrate a worsening restrictive pattern. When cor pulmonale develops, it is not related as much to hypoxia as to a generalized decrease in the vascular bed. Thus, pulmonary hypertension and overt cor pulmonale occur late in the disease course.

Irritant Bronchitis and Emphysema in Silicosis

Productive cough in victims of silicosis is usually a consequence of smoking; less frequently, cough may be a result of silica exposure. Silica-induced bronchitis would appear to be limited to severe cases of silicosis. The possibility that it is caused by other substances in the workplace (industrial bronchitis) cannot be ruled out. Pulmonary function tests show somewhat reduced flow rates. Correlation between these abnormalities and the radiographic evidence of advanced silicosis is poor.

The airways obstruction appears to be a result of torsion and distortion of the large airways and is usually associated with some bullous emphysema and marked overdistension. Questions have been raised as to whether silicosis might be associated with an increased incidence of emphysema. This issue has been difficult to study, given the very high incidence of smoking among workers exposed to silica. A recent Canadian study based on CT analysis suggests a significant excess of emphysema in both smokers and nonsmokers working with silica. Radiographically evident emphysema was associated with abnormal pulmonary function both in those with established pneumoconi-

oses and in smokers with silica exposure but no radiographic changes of silicosis. In nonsmokers, radiographic evidence of emphysema was detected by CT only when there was evidence of established pneumoconiosis. Not surprisingly, smokers in this study had emphysema even without evidence of overt pneumoconiosis.

Acute Silicosis

Intense exposure to very high ambient concentrations of silica within a short period leads to the characteristic syndrome of acute silicosis. Because acute silicosis shares pathologic features with alveolar proteinosis, it has also been referred to as *silicolipoproteinosis.* Certain exposed workers, including sandblasters, ceramic workers, and surface coal miners who drill holes to place explosives, are at particular risk for acute silicosis. The production of silica flour may be associated with intense exposure and lead to the development of acute silicosis. The duration of exposure to silica is usually a matter of only months. In the United States, the most notorious epidemic of acute silicosis involved miners constructing a hydroelectric tunnel through a sandstone mountain, the Hawk's Nest Tunnel at Gauley Bridge, West Virginia, in 1933. In what was the United States' worst industrial disaster, nearly 500 miners died of acute silicosis within several years, and many more were severely disabled.

The clinical features of acute silicosis include severe dry cough, fever, intense dyspnea, and weight loss. Hypoxemia may be profound. Pulmonary hypertension and cor pulmonale rapidly develop. The chest x-ray findings may resemble those of classic silicosis; alternately, it may show coalescent shadows in the lower lung zones (Fig. 11). Once acute silicosis becomes established, hypoxic respiratory failure develops inexorably. Patients who survive for more than a few months with acute silicosis have been thought to be particularly susceptible to infection with various intracellular respiratory pathogens, such as mycobacteria and *Histoplasma capsulatum.* Use of antifibrotic and antiinflammatory drugs such as corticosteroids has proved ineffective; lung transplantation or heart-lung transplantation may prove to be the only effective therapy.

Pulmonary Function in Silicosis

Altered pulmonary function accounts for much of the disability and death in severe cases of silicosis. However, in the early stages of simple silicosis, pulmonary function is usually not impaired. Spirometric values, gas exchange, and lung volumes and mechanics are normal or minimally altered. Perhaps because of their focal nature, the silicotic nodules present throughout the lung parenchyma have surprisingly little effect on lung function. The pathways of removal of silica particles into the pulmonary interstitium and regional nodes bypass the distal airways and

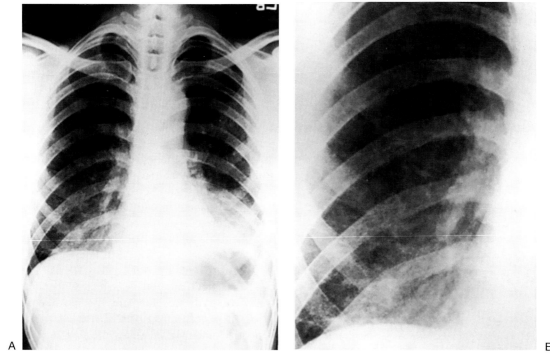

FIG. 11. Chest radiograph of a subject with acute silicosis. **Panel A:** Acinar filling pattern in both lower zones and in the left lateral chest. The extensive soft shadowing seen in acute silicosis is more often seen in the upper zones. **Panel B:** Detail of a right lower lung zone containing an acinar filling pattern with scanty irregular opacities.

alveoli, minimizing any deleterious effects on gas flow or mechanics. In this regard, silicosis differs importantly from asbestosis, in which extensive bronchiolar and alveolar inflammation and scarring of the gas exchange surface takes place.

In simple silicosis, a small but statistically significant decrement in the forced vital capacity can be detected when exposed population groups are studied and compared with control subjects without exposure. These changes have no clinical significance and are not associated with symptoms. Because these changes are small, they cannot routinely be detected in individual subjects. The lung volumes in simple silicosis are nearly always normal. Indices of gas exchange, such as the diffusing capacity and arterial oxygen concentration, are generally normal. Pulmonary compliance may be reduced even though spirometric values are normal. The extent of the mechanical changes, although somewhat more sensitive than the spirometric measurements, can only roughly be related to radiographic score.

Studies defining the rate of decrement of pulmonary function among exposed workers have been used to justify current standards for ambient dust levels. Cross-sectional studies of workers in the Vermont granite industry have provided the most comprehensive picture of the impact of any respirable dust on pulmonary function and indicate that granite dust exposure leads to a loss of vital capacity of 2 mL/y. This compares with a decline of 30 mL/y attributable to aging and of 9 mL/y to smoking. This study served as the basis for the National Institute of Safety and Health criteria document recommending that the permissible exposure limit be halved from 0.10 to 0.05 mg/m^3. An additional longitudinal study in the same workers found no difference in the rates of decline in function and no difference in the changes between granite workers and unexposed blue collar workers from the same region. At this time, there is no compelling evidence that exposures to quartz at levels at or below the current standard of 0.1 mg/m^3 result in loss of pulmonary function.

Without a doubt, declines in pulmonary mechanics and volumes occur more rapidly in workers with complicated silicosis. In subjects with simple silicosis in an Asian study, most of whom continued to smoke, the FVC (forced vital capacity) and FEV$_1$ (forced expiratory volume in 1 second) declined by 59 and 64 mL/y, respectively.

The presentation of the patient with acute silicosis is that of rapidly progressing respiratory insufficiency. Both the lung volumes and the diffusing capacity are markedly reduced. The reduction is generally proportional to the extent of the conglomerate shadows. Lung compliance is markedly reduced, and marked hypoxemia results from ventilation-perfusion mismatch.

Radiographic Features

In uncomplicated early silicosis, the chest x-ray film shows multiple small round shadows, usually developing in the upper zones first. These represent the summation of multiple small silicotic nodules superimposed on one another. High-resolution CT demonstrates the individual nodules.

In complicated silicosis, larger rounded nodules (type *r*) become more profuse than the *p* and *q* shadows. However, these radiographic changes resemble those of many other advanced nodular pneumoconioses, including coal workers' pneumoconiosis (Chapter 33). Eggshell calcification in the hilar nodes occurs fairly frequently, and peripheral shadows themselves may also become calcified. Volume loss in the upper lobes results in overdistension of the lower lobes and retraction upward, with migration of the hila. The conglomerate shadows that form in complicated silicosis are not specific to silicosis and resemble those seen in coal workers' pneumoconiosis. They typically appear in the periphery of the upper lobes first, later appearing to migrate toward the hilum. High-resolution CT allows their detection before they are apparent on the chest x-ray film. However, the prognostic significance of such findings is unknown. Hence, it is rarely necessary to perform CT in the initial evaluation or follow-up of silicosis.

Cavitation of conglomerate shadows may occur and in some cases indicates superinfection with tuberculosis. Pleural plaques can develop in silicosis but are infrequent. Single conglomerate shadows often represent a diagnostic dilemma, as malignancy and tuberculosis must be ruled out. Acute silicosis, as already mentioned, presents as a bilateral alveolar filling process, often in the absence of small rounded shadows.

Pathology

The lungs of silicotic subjects are adherent to the chest wall, and the pleural surfaces are thickened. There may be calcified pleural plaques on the visceral pleural surfaces. The cut surfaces of the lungs are studded with rounded grayish nodules, usually more numerous in the upper lobes; calcification may be present. In some instances, individual nodules may have aggregated into conglomerate masses. These masses may form cavities as a result of ischemic necrosis or superinfection with tuberculosis.

Under the microscope, the hallmark of simple pulmonary silicosis is the silicotic nodule, a pathognomonic feature. The nodule begins as an aggregation of dust-laden macrophages within the interstitium, particularly near respiratory bronchioles, pulmonary vessels, and pleura. The mature nodule has a central area that gradually becomes acellular and is composed of connective tissue arranged in a concentric onion skin pattern. The central area may eventually become necrotic. The periphery is populated with inflammatory cells, particularly lymphocytes and dust-laden macrophages. The nodules may actually assume a granulomatous appearance. Accompanying these changes may be some interstitial thickening in the alveolar wall and a proliferative response of type II pneumocytes in areas of epithelial denudation.

As simple disease progresses to complicated silicosis, the small nodules enlarge and coalesce into large masses of hyalinized tissue. One sees a whorled nodule consisting of an acellular center, through which course fibers of hyalinized collagen. More peripherally, there is granulation tissue and some palisading of epithelioid cells (Fig. 12). The nodules are most prominent around pulmonary arterioles and respiratory bronchioles. The pulmonary vascular bed is slowly obliterated as the nodule increases

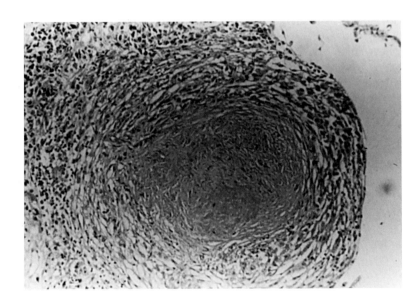

FIG. 12. Photomicrograph of silicotic nodule. Note the typical whorled appearance.

in size. Smaller vessels become incorporated into the evolving nodule. Expanding conglomerate masses eventually envelop larger segmental and lobar arteries, which then undergo thrombosis and gradually become engulfed by the fibrotic tissue mass. The center of the silicotic nodules, when viewed microscopically under polarized light, contains birefringent silica particles. These tend to be located at the periphery of the nodule, away from the acellular center.

Complicated silicosis usually develops in the upper lobes, which become fibrotic and atelectatic. The lower lobes in turn become overdistended (Figs. 13 and 14), and the hila shift upward. A variant of the classic conglomerate mass is the even larger rheumatoid silicotic nodule. As its name implies, it is seen in subjects with obvious rheumatoid arthritis or those with high circulating levels of rheumatoid factor.

In acute silicosis, the alveoli are diffusely filled with a homogeneous pinkish exudate; the interstitium is infiltrated with mononuclear cells (Fig. 15). The alveoli are lined with degenerating pneumocytes and abundant quantities of birefringent material. The interstitium is thickened and fibrosis is apparent. Mixed pathologic patterns containing features of both acute and chronic silicosis are occasionally seen and have been dubbed *subacute silicosis*.

Cellular Pathogenesis of Silicosis

Free silica is not biodegradable and presents a toxic burden to a wide variety of lung cells; it is not surprising

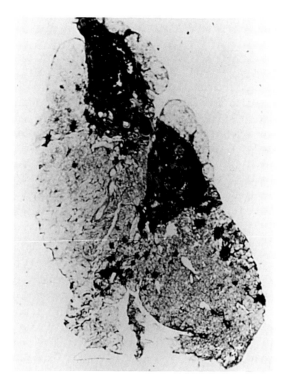

FIG. 14. Whole-lung section of complicated silicosis.

then that all cellular constituents of the lung may be involved in silicosis. However, the precise mechanisms by which silica exerts its toxic effects are poorly understood. Because ingestion of silica particles by macrophages is such a prominent feature of the disease, their possible role in pathogenesis has been well studied. Ingested silica particles appear in the phagosomes of macrophages; the phagosomes fuse with and damage lysosomal membranes, which then rupture. When this occurs, the macrophage dies and disgorges the silica particles. Along with the released silica particle (which is available to be ingested by another phagocyte), the macrophage releases cytokines, oxidant species, proteolytic enzymes, and other mediators of cellular toxicity.

Alveolar lining cells (type I pneumocytes) are also major targets of silica toxicity. Death of type I cells denudes the alveolar wall, exposing interstitial cells, such as fibroblasts, to contact with fibrogenic mediators, such as growth-promoting cytokines. Proliferation of these cells and their migration into the damaged alveolar space may result in effacement of the distal air spaces by extracellular matrix components.

Plausible and comprehensive hypotheses regarding the exact mechanisms of toxicity of inhaled silica have been put forward by Ghio and colleagues. Biophysical and biochemical interactions between the negatively charged surfaces of silica particles may be a central event. It has been proposed that deposited silicates result in the local generation of oxidants in the lung. The surface of all silicates contains silanol (SiOH) groups. These dissociate,

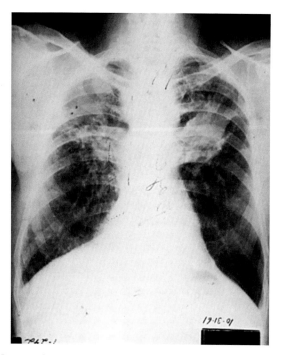

FIG. 13. Chest radiograph of a worker with complicated silicosis. There is a conglomerate shadow in left middle-upper lung zone.

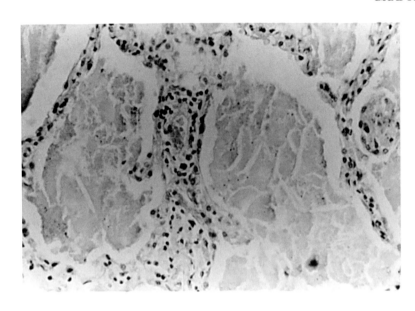

FIG. 15. Photomicrograph showing acute silicosis (silicolipoproteinosis) in the lungs in a sandblaster dying of acute respiratory insufficiency. Proteinaceous (pink) exudate fills all the alveoli. Interstitium is thickened by round-cell infiltration.

resulting in a net negative charge on the particle surface and allowing adsorption of organic and inorganic cations. In particular, ferric ions react and form complexes with silanol groups. Silanol groups found on silicates have the ability to attract ferric ions, forming silicate-iron complexes.

Reduction of iron in the complex results in the generation of hydroxyl radicals. These in turn oxidize cellular proteins and lipids, presumably resulting in the observed cytotoxicity. Thus, the surface of the ingested silicate particle brings together chelated iron, hydrogen peroxide, and a reductant such as superoxide to allow cytotoxicity to proceed. Experimentally, the toxicity of silica has been mitigated by coating the particles before exposing susceptible cells. In support of this theory, agents such as aluminum or polyvinyl pyridine N oxide, by changing the charge properties of the silica surface, block or markedly reduce the cellular toxicity. This theory also appears to account for the observation that different forms of silica exhibit differing toxicities.

Various inflammatory mediators have been implicated in the development of silicosis. The cytokine tumor necrosis factor (TNF-α) is produced by macrophages in response to exposure to silica in animal models, and antibodies to this particularly toxic cytokine block progression of disease. Some of the effects of silica may represent reparative responses to the ongoing cellular injury. For example, hyperplasia of type II pneumocytes helps to repopulate the alveolar surfaces. This process has been shown to be driven by transforming growth factor-α, a mitogenic cytokine released by macrophages.

The effects of inhaled silica are not limited to the lungs. They affect the immune system, with both cellular and humoral immune responses being markedly altered. Patients with silica exposure and silicosis frequently have elevated levels of circulating autoantibodies, such as antinuclear antibodies. Rheumatoid factor is usually not ele-

vated. This response is thought to represent a systemic response to continued tissue damage and release of nuclear components from dying lung cells. Further studies have shown that there is no reduction in the number or function of circulating T or B lymphocytes. Delayed hypersensitivity remains intact. A postulated decrement in suppressor T-cell function has been invoked to explain the prevalence of autoantibodies in silicosis. To understand genetic factors involved in the development of silicosis, human leukocyte antigen (HLA) phenotyping has been carried out in silica-exposed workers, mostly with inconclusive results. Experimental studies of the immunologic effects of silica delivered as an aerosol or a slurry instilled through the trachea of experimental animals have shown profound changes in immune function.

Diagnosis

The occupational history and radiographic findings almost always suffice to make the correct diagnosis of simple or complex silicosis. The occupational exposure to silica should be appropriately intense and prolonged, and the radiographic and/or CT features should be characteristic. Only in cases of mixed dust exposure might lung biopsy or other invasive studies be required. Isolated cases of acute silicosis may be an exception to this rule, as the disease progresses to respiratory failure so rapidly that lung biopsy may be required to rule out other or coexisting pulmonary disorders. If coexisting infection with *Mycobacterium tuberculosis* is suspected, bronchoscopy may be employed to collect cultures of organisms not found in sputum samples.

Treatment and Prevention

There is no effective treatment for silicosis. Palliative measures are nonspecific and similar to those offered to any patient with other severe restrictive pulmonary disorders and failure of the right side of the heart. Low-flow oxygen is recommended; however, there is no evidence that this prolongs life in patients with silicosis. Steroid therapy is probably of no benefit. Long-term steroid therapy may help patients with silicosis and a second pulmonary disorder that is steroid-responsive. Lung transplantation is offered to patients with end-stage pneumoconioses, including silicosis, and represents approximately 1% of lung transplants done in the United States.

Preventive measures are based on dust control through minimizing generation of respirable dust and providing adequate ventilation at the work site. Respirator masks may be used, but it is far preferable to provide adequate ventilation to remove airborne dust. Sandblasting remains particularly hazardous and has been outlawed in a number of advanced countries. Where allowed, sandblasting should be undertaken only when a positive pressure respirator with its own air supply is used.

Silicotuberculosis

Among the pneumoconioses, silicosis is unique in predisposing to tuberculosis and atypical mycobacterial disease. Miners and other workers with significant exposure to silica have long been known to have a high incidence of tuberculosis. Those parts of the world in which tuberculosis infection and disease rates have declined to low levels have seen a commensurate decline in silicotuberculosis. In contrast, in the emerging industrialized nations, silicotuberculosis remains a significant problem among miners and other exposed workers.

The presenting manifestations of silicotuberculosis are identical to those of tuberculosis and include anorexia and weight loss, fever, and cough. Radiographic features of the infection may be difficult to detect during its early stages, superimposed as they are on the features of silicosis. Later, the appearance is quite similar to that of classic tuberculosis. Silicotuberculosis may progress to cavitation quite rapidly (Fig. 16).

The inhalation of silica has long been recognized to impair the phagocytic functions of macrophages specifically. Because monocytes and macrophages are key effector cells in host defense against *M. tuberculosis* and other intracellular organisms, tuberculous infection tends to progress rapidly in the silicotic lung. Enhanced susceptibility to tuberculosis can be demonstrated in several ways in experimental animals: Initial infection can be established with relatively smaller numbers of organisms than are required to produce disease in control animals; counts of recovered organisms are higher, and there is a greater propensity for spread from subcutaneous inoculation sites to the lungs.

Under conditions of laboratory culture, there is no evidence that silica alters the growth properties or infectivity

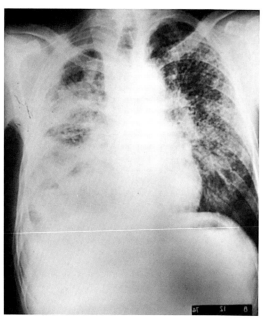

FIG. 16. Simple silicosis (ILO category 3/2) with tuberculous cavities in right middle and lower zones along with pleural effusion. This worker had been a borer and shot firer in a company that sank portals for deep coal mines.

of the tubercle bacillus itself. Nor does the inhalation and deposition of silica appear to interfere with other components of the immune response. Indeed, greater humoral and cell-mediated immune responses develop in animals exposed to silica than in control animals. Recently, it has been suggested that the increased incidence of tuberculosis in silica workers results from the accumulation of iron that forms complexes with silica dust particles in the lung. According to this hypothesis, silica particles may act as a local reserve of iron, which can be used by dormant mycobacteria as a virulence factor.

Mycobacteria other than *M. tuberculosis* have also been associated with silicosis. *M. avium-intracellulare* and *M. kansasii* have been isolated in subjects with silica exposure, even before overt disease is apparent on the chest x-ray film. When these atypical mycobacteria are detected in sputum samples, efforts must be made to determine whether they represent true pathogens or are simply opportunistic colonizing organisms.

The basic precepts of treatment of silicotuberculosis are the same as for treatment of tuberculosis in the absence of pneumoconiosis (Chapter 28). However, several important distinctions should be made. First, in severe cases of pneumoconiosis, the chest radiographic appearance may be dominated by the silicosis rather than by the tuberculosis. As a result, radiographic improvement during the course of chemotherapy may be minimal. Second, because macrophage phagocytic and killing functions are permanently impaired in silicosis, bacteriologic relapse is common despite the use of appropriate drugs and an adequate duration of therapy. Hence, more vigilance for relapse is in order after a full course of chemotherapy. Finally, disappearance of organisms from the sputum may be somewhat slower than in tuberculosis without accompanying silicosis.

All subjects with silicosis should be monitored with tuberculin skin tests. Those with a positive tuberculin skin test result but no mycobacteria in their sputum should receive routine isoniazid chemoprophylaxis (Chapter 28). Unfortunately, this is probably not as effective a preventive measure as in the general population. Some public health experts have therefore recommended that isoniazid be continued indefinitely in this disease; often, however, side effects preclude this approach.

A recent double-blinded, placebo-controlled trial of antituberculosis chemoprophylaxis was undertaken in 679 silicotic subjects in Hong Kong, where there is a high prevalence of both silicosis and tuberculosis. During the 5-year study, active tuberculosis developed in 27% of the placebo-treated workers and in 13% of those who received any of three chemoprophylaxis regimens. There were no significant differences between the several chemoprophylaxis regimens tested. There was no evidence that chemoprophylaxis led to the development of drug-resistant strains of bacilli. These data support the concept of decreased resistance of silicotic workers to tuberculosis and reaffirm the need for more effective antituberculosis chemoprophylaxis in this population.

Silica as a Potential Carcinogen

In recent years, the long-recognized possibility that silica might be a carcinogen has received renewed attention. Theoretical considerations consistent with this notion are derived from our understanding of the molecular biology of the silica-cell surface interaction. Reactions between silanol groups on the surface of silica particles, ferric iron, and cell surface components might be expected to activate intracellular signaling pathways involved in oncogene expression. However, there is little evidence that even advanced silicosis is associated with lung cancer. Indeed, during the early part of the twentieth century, when complex silicosis was much more prevalent, no association with carcinoma was apparent. Many studies have been unable to separate effects attributable to silica alone from those of other carcinogenic agents in the workplace, such as organic compounds, radon, and cigarette smoke. Animal studies are of limited value in answering these questions, given the relatively short term and high intensity of exposure necessary to elicit malignant responses in target species.

In summary, the evidence for an association between lung cancer and either silicosis or silica exposure remains quite controversial. If such an association exists, it is likely that silica has only a weak carcinogenic potential compared with such notorious carcinogens as cigarette smoke. The public policy consequences of any abatement projects would be prohibitively expensive. Moreover, the cost of diverting resources away from other more clearly hazardous dusts would be a societal tragedy.

Inflammatory and Immune Disorders Associated with Pneumoconioses

Progressive massive fibrosis seen in conjunction with rheumatoid arthritis is a syndrome described by A. Caplan in 1953 in Welsh coal miners with pneumoconiosis. Caplan's syndrome has occasionally been reported in association with silicosis and rarely with asbestosis. However, in the latter case the association may simply be the result of mixed exposure to silica or coal dust. The majority of reports of Caplan's syndrome come from the United Kingdom; the disorder appears rare in North America. Caplan's syndrome may occur in workers with elevated serum rheumatoid factor who do not have manifestations of arthritis.

Some investigators have suggested that rheumatoid arthritis and other connective tissue disorders are associated with silicosis. This is not surprising, given the regional and systemic alterations of the immune system associated with silicosis. Patients with silicosis often have elevated serum antinuclear activity. However, this activity may simply represent a marker of ongoing tissue damage rather than a sign of rheumatologic disease. It has been suggested that systemic sclerosis develops more frequently following silica exposure, although statistical support is lacking. Despite the possible associations between silica exposure and rheumatologic disorders, the majority of disabled workers have osteoarthritis, not rheumatoid arthritis, as a consequence of the heavy mechanical labor they perform during their careers.

DISEASES CAUSED BY NON-ASBESTOS SILICATES: THE SILICATOSES

In this section, the silicatoses other than asbestosis are discussed. Like silica, the various silicates are ubiquitous on the surface of the earth. As a result of mining and a wide variety of industrial processes, they become airborne and have the potential to be inhaled. The fibrous silicates are relatively long and narrow (i.e., their aspect, or length-to-width, ratio is >3). Both fibrous and nonfibrous silicates induce pneumoconioses but are generally far less fibrogenic than silica. Perhaps as a result of their lesser degrees of toxicity, descriptions of the clinical syndromes induced by the silicates are less clear-cut than those of asbestosis or silicosis. Furthermore, the silicates are often contaminated with more toxic minerals, such as tremolite, that produce effects that tend to dominate radiographic patterns and the course of disease.

Most silicates are nonfibrous (called *phyllosilicates,*

based on their leaflike structure). This group includes mica, kaolin, and vermiculite. Wollastonite, zeolite, and fibrous erionite are examples of the fibrous silicates. A number of silicates, such as talc, occur in both fibrous and nonfibrous forms. There is no substantial evidence that the nonfibrous silicates are in any way carcinogenic except when contaminated by asbestos.

Talc Pneumoconiosis (Talcosis)

Talc is a hydrated magnesium silicate having the chemical formula $Mg_6Si_8O_{22}(OH)_4$. It occurs in both fibrous and nonfibrous forms. Talc is mined in a number of parts of the United States, including Vermont, New York, Texas, and Montana. Talc deposits in the United States are contaminated with fibrous silicates such as tremolite, actinolite, and anthophyllite, but these are non-asbestiform variants of these minerals. As much as 40%–50% of some talc deposits may be contaminating minerals. In the United Kingdom, similarly impure talc ore was mined in the Shetland Islands. Talc has also been produced in Canada, Norway, Italy, France, and China.

Talc and mica have a platelike morphology that permits them to slide easily. This property makes them of value as lubricants and as a base for cosmetic powders. Talc is generally mined as soapstone, then milled and calcined. The latter process involves reduction of the milled material to a powder through heating at high temperatures (1200–1400°C). The finished product is used in the production of paints and ceramics, and as a lubricant in the roof-felting industry. It is also important in the production of pharmaceuticals and in the cosmetic industry, where it is used in face powder and talcum powder. High-grade talc from Italy, Vermont, and China is preferred for these uses.

Industrial exposure has been prominent in the rubber industry, where talc is frequently dusted into tire molds so that the finished tire can be more easily removed. Finely ground talc is used in the production of glossy paper. Low-grade talc is important in the fertilizer industry, where it is used for its anticaking properties and as a refractory filler.

Clinical Features of Talc Pneumoconiosis

Talcosis was described at the end of the nineteenth century. Like silicosis, simple talcosis causes few or no symptoms. Dyspnea and productive cough, when present, are usually a consequence of cigarette smoking, industrial bronchitis, or lung disorders other than the talcosis. However, when conglomerate shadows develop, the subject becomes increasingly dyspneic. Although it is clear that the talc itself (rather than its contaminants) is responsible for the pneumoconiosis seen in talc miners, it is far less fibrogenic than silica. Complicated talcosis with conglom-

erate shadows and disability is now a rare entity in North America, but it is still seen in Europe.

The chest radiographic appearance of chronic talc pneumoconiosis depends on the nature of the talc deposits to which the worker was exposed. When pure talc is involved, there is usually a mixture of rounded *q* and *r* shadows and irregular (*t* and *u*) shadows located in the middle zones, usually in a perihilar distribution. As the disease progresses with time, the shadows extend peripherally from the hila to involve the upper and lower zones. Small irregular shadows in the lower lobes are seen, particularly in cigarette smokers.

When talc deposits contain high concentrations of silica, the radiograph takes on a nodular pattern of shadows involving the middle and upper zones, more reminiscent of silicosis. The shadows are usually of the rounded *q* or *r* types and are located in the upper lobes.

Like asbestos, talc has the capacity to induce pleural plaques, and this can occur in the absence of contamination by asbestos. Pleural thickening is also seen in workers exposed to other silicates, such as sepiolite, wollastonite, kaolin, and zeolite. Such plaques often undergo calcification and are otherwise indistinguishable from those induced by asbestos.

Workers with talc pneumoconiosis who have not smoked have little or no impairment of pulmonary function. With advanced categories of simple talcosis, mild restrictive ventilatory impairment may be found. Only with the appearance of large conglomerate shadows is dyspnea likely to develop in the affected worker. The well-delineated plaques that occur in chronic cases are not associated with significant respiratory impairment. Diffuse pleural fibrosis is occasionally reported, but this is usually a consequence of a prior pleural effusion and so no calcified plaques are noted.

Pathology of Talcosis

Chronic inhalation of talc initially produces a mild alveolar inflammatory process. However, this process seldom progresses to alveolar fibrosis; talc particles are constantly being removed by alveolar macrophages and cleared from the parenchyma by the pulmonary defense mechanisms. With time, dust macules form. These are aggregations of dust-laden macrophages, foreign body giant cells, and epithelioid cells within the walls of the respiratory bronchioles. They resemble foreign body granulomas rather than the typical whorled nodule of silicosis. When these enlarge, small nodules may appear in the interstitial tissue in the same anatomic pattern of distribution as noted with silicotic nodules. Polarizing microscopy easily identifies an abundance of birefringent particles in the nodules. An unusual form of talc granulomatous lung disease occurring in intravenous drug users is associated with a typical vasculitis. Diffuse interstitial fibrosis and massive fibrosis have also been reported in talc pneumoconiosis but are exceedingly uncommon. The potential of talc as a carcinogen is minimal or nonexistent.

Silicatoses Other Than Talcosis

Kaolinosis

Kaolin pneumoconiosis was first reported in 1936 in the United Kingdom. Kaolinite, a complex hydrated aluminum silicate, is used for the manufacture of ceramics (china clay), glossy paper, soap, toothpaste, and medicine. As with silicosis, both simple and complicated pneumoconioses exist. The simple form is characterized by the development of rounded shadows in the lung (Fig. 17). Complicated kaolinosis evolves slowly and mimics silicosis on the chest radiograph (Fig. 18). Although kaolin is usually contaminated with silica, it is clear that the kaolin is responsible for the pneumoconiosis. Deposits of china clay are often heavily contaminated with silica. In the United States, kaolin is mined in the southeastern regions of the country. Intense exposure to kaolin is most likely to occur during the processing stages (drying and bagging). The simple and complicated pneumoconioses noted in shale miners may in part be a consequence of the kaolin content of shale.

The pathologic picture in the lungs varies somewhat from that of silicosis and includes both interstitial and nodular fibrosis as well as mild fibrosis of the alveolar wall. In simple kaolin pneumoconiosis, the lungs show

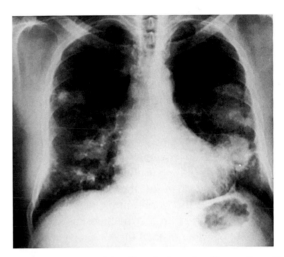

FIG. 18. Complicated kaolinosis in a kaolin worker. Conglomerate shadow appears adjacent to the heart.

grayish nodular lesions that are less prominent than those seen in silicosis. Simple kaolinosis is usually not associated with symptoms or alterations in pulmonary function parameters. However, as simple kaolinosis progresses to the complicated form, the patient notes the development of dyspnea. In complicated kaolinosis, a restrictive ventilatory pattern is present. Even more so than in silicosis, the profusion of shadowing on chest radiographs is more prominent than the degree of functional impairment.

Fuller's Earth Pneumoconiosis

Fuller's earth is a fine-grained absorbent clay originally used to remove grease and oil from wool (fulling). The highly adsorbent property of Fuller's earth makes it an ideal product to remove unwanted oil and grease. It has found use in oil refining and as a binder in foundry molding sands. It is also occasionally used as a filter and in cosmetic preparations. The various Fuller's earths are fine-grained calcium montmorillonite clays, attapulgite (palygorskite), and bentonite. Contaminating silica may be responsible for the development of disease, as Fuller's earth itself is innocuous. Fuller's earth is obtained by open-cast and underground mining. It is then dried, crushed, and milled. It is produced in the United Kingdom, Germany, and in the United States in the Midwest and Georgia (attapulgite).

Fuller's earth pneumoconiosis is a rare and little-studied clinical entity. It appears to occur in both simple and complicated forms. As with talcosis, only complicated cases appear to lead to impairment and disability. In the few autopsy-based studies available, the lungs contain large, peribronchial, black nodules, usually in the upper zones. Microscopically, there is a relative paucity of cellular reaction around the birefringent particles. The very few reports of Fuller's earth pneumoconioses that have

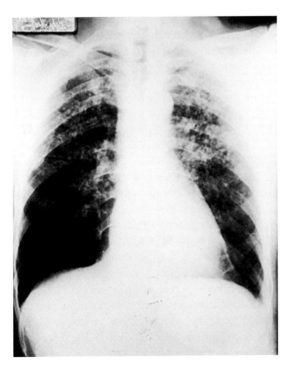

FIG. 17. Chest radiograph of simple kaolinosis. Pneumoconiosis is apparent in upper and middle zones.

been published suggest a benign course with little risk for symptomatic disease. Secondary users of materials containing Fuller's earths are not at risk for disease.

Bentonite Pneumoconiosis

Bentonite is a fine clay consisting mostly of calcium montmorillonite. It can swell inordinately when hydrated, giving it a high capacity for water absorption. It is this property that makes it so useful as a muddy slurry in oil well drilling and also in the refining of petroleum products. Much of the world mining of bentonite is done in Wyoming, with open-cast methods used, and in the nations of the northern rim of the Mediterranean. Bentonite is variably contaminated with quartz, shale, and sandstone.

Crushing and drying bentonite in ovens is dusty work and presents a hazard to workers. Bentonite pneumoconiosis can develop rapidly, be disabling, and result in fatal respiratory failure. Although bentonite is nonfibrogenic, it induces an abnormal pathologic change: the formation of foamy macrophages containing a periodic-acid-positive material. This pneumoconiosis is in large part a response to the cristobalite content of the product.

Anhydrous Aluminum Silicates

The anhydrous aluminum silicates include sillimanite, kyanite, and andalusite. They find important uses in the manufacture of refractory materials and in porcelain-containing materials such as spark plugs. Dust released during the preparation of these natural minerals can contain contaminating amounts of cristobalite. In general, radiographic changes have been minimal, but interstitial fibrosis appears to have developed in a few subjects. It is generally agreed that contaminating quartz is the underlying cause of the very few cases of mild pneumoconioses reported in sillimanite workers.

Miscellaneous Silicates

Mullite is a rare aluminum silicate that can cause pneumoconiosis. It occurs naturally but is also artificially produced for refractory construction. It also finds use in mortars, kilns, and furnaces. Prolonged exposure to mullite may cause mild pulmonary fibrosis, but probably only when dust exposure has been mixed.

Zeolites

The zeolites, which include fibrous erionite, are a group of hydrated aluminum silicates quarried from deposits of volcanic lava (tuffs). As a result of their marked adsorptive properties, they are used as molecular sieves, in gas chromatography, in the separation of radioactive gases, and as fillers in paper products.

Zeolites do not cause pneumoconiosis. However, during recent decades they have been implicated in the high rates of pleural fibrosis, pleural plaques, calcification, and premature malignant mesotheliomas seen in two villages in Turkey. Approximately half the deaths in this region have been caused by mesothelioma and lung cancer. In addition, pleural plaques, calcification, and fibrosis have been noted but have not resulted in deaths. Although these cases were initially thought to be the result of exposure to asbestos, more recent investigations have shown that ambient levels of fibrous zeolite are responsible for the epidemic. Erionite (a zeolite substance) is composed of long, thin mineral fibers and is extensively used in local building materials and stucco. Fibers of erionite have been found in the lungs of patients from the two villages concerned. Erionite has proved to be a particularly potent inducer of pleural disease in animal exposure studies. Of interest is the observation that many houses in the western United States and southern Mexico contain measurable amounts of locally mined erionite.

OTHER NATURAL FIBROUS MINERALS

Attapulgite

Naturally occurring clays such as attapulgite are composed of small, elongated, fiberlike particles and have not been shown to be harmful. Attapulgite is used as cat litter, in paints, and in fertilizers, and it is also pumped into oil wells to remove moisture during the drilling process. Palygorskite is a chemically related mineral consisting of longer, thinner fibers. It is quarried mainly in eastern Europe. Animal experiments have shown that palygorskite is capable of inducing mesothelioma in animals, as well as producing other effects induced by the amphiboles or asbestos.

Wollastonite

Wollastonite is a fibrous calcium silicate ($CaSiO_3$) sometimes contaminated with quartz. It is used in ceramics and paints. In recent decades, it has found an expanding market as a substitute for asbestos in insulation, wallboard, and brake linings. It is mined in the United States, Mexico, and Finland. An extensive survey of the wollastonite mines of the Adirondack Mountain region of New York State, one of the major production areas of the world, found no concentration relationship between respiratory symptoms and exposure. There was no evidence of fibrotic pulmonary disease or pleural disease. A follow-up study showed no change of chest radiographic patterns with time.

Vermiculite

Vermiculite is the name of a group of hydrated laminar magnesium aluminum silicates containing iron. More than twenty varieties occur in deposits that are quarried from open-cast mines.

Deposits of vermiculites are often contaminated by silica, talc, tremolite, or actinolite. These, rather than vermiculite itself, account for the pleural effusions and plaques found in vermiculite workers. Several studies have assessed the deleterious respiratory effects of exposure in vermiculite mining. Both positive and negative study results have been reported. Studies suggesting increased morbidity and mortality may reflect the contamination of vermiculite deposits by asbestiform minerals.

Artificial Fibers

During the past several decades, an effort has been made to replace asbestos with fiberglass and other artificial mineral fibers. Fiberglass is a continuous filament and therefore not respirable unless modified. Insulation wool is made from metal slag, igneous rocks, and glass, which are mixed and then melted down and spun into a fibrous mat. Many of the fibers produced in this process are in the respirable range. These ceramic fibers are produced from molten kaolin or from a combination of alumina and silica. Most of these artificial mineral fibers exhibit little or no toxicity.

Although these fibers may induce mesothelioma when implanted directly in the pleural or peritoneal cavity of experimental animals, they do not induce pulmonary fibrosis or tumors when given by inhalation. Moreover, fiberglass has been shown to undergo leaching and fragmentation and can therefore be removed from the lungs. Although a preponderance of evidence speaks against any increased risk from the use of artificial fibers, caution is wise. The mineralogic structure of these agents is fairly similar to that of other fibers known to be pathogenic or carcinogenic. Several factors limit the potential of these fibers to induce pneumoconioses. First, the factories producing these artificial fibers generate relatively few respirable fibers in the workplace environment; second, inhaled and deposited fibers are susceptible to fragmentation and leaching by pulmonary cells.

BIBLIOGRAPHY

Absher M, Sjöstrand M, Baldor LC, Hemenway DR, Kelley J. Patterns of secretion of transforming growth factor-α (TGF-α) in experimental silicosis: acute and subacute effects of cristobalite exposure in the rat. *Reg Immunol* 1993;5:225–231. *Transforming growth factor-α (TGF-α) from macrophages, a cytokine having potent mitogenic activity for epithelial and mesenchymal cells, may cause type II pneumocytes to proliferate and repopulate denuded epithelial surfaces during lung remodeling of silicosis.*

American Thoracic Society. The diagnosis of nonmalignant disease related to asbestos. *Am Rev Respir Dis* 1986;134:363–368. *An official statement offering clear and thoughtful criteria for the diagnosis of asbestosis and asbestos-related diseases.*

American Thoracic Society. Environmental controls in lung disease. *Am Rev Respir Dis* 1990;142:915–939. *An official statement presenting policies and regulations for the control of industrial dusts and other inhaled toxins, with a discussion of options for control.*

Becklake MR. Chronic air flow limitation: its relationship to work in dusty occupations. *Chest* 1985;88:608–617. *Exposure to irritant and toxic components in industrial dusts may be an important cause of chronic bronchitis.*

Becklake MR, Toyota B, Stewart M, Hanson R, Hanley J. Lung structure as a risk factor in adverse pulmonary responses to asbestos exposure. *Am Rev Respir Dis* 1983;128:385–389. *Anatomic features of the lung are one of the factors that make some workers more susceptible to pneumoconioses.*

Bégin R, Filion R, Ostiguy G. Emphysema in silica- and asbestos-exposed workers seeking compensation. A CT scan study. *Chest* 1995;108:647–655. *In this CT-based study from Quebec, there is a significant excess of emphysema associated with lung dysfunction among silica-exposed workers. In the nonsmokers, emphysematous changes appeared only in association with established pneumoconiosis; in smokers, emphysema developed even in the absence of pneumoconiosis.*

Browne K. A threshold for asbestos-related lung cancer. *Br J Ind Med* 1986;43:556–558. *See next citation.*

Browne K. Is asbestos or asbestosis the cause of the increased risk of lung cancer in asbestos workers. *Br J Ind Med* 1986;43:145–149. *The threshold for development of carcinoma is likely close to the threshold for development of asbestosis.*

Caplan A. Certain unusual radiological appearances in the chest of coal miners suffering from rheumatoid arthritis. *Thorax* 1953;8:29–37. *The original description of Caplan's syndrome, first recognizing the association between complicated pneumoconiosis and rheumatoid arthritis in Welsh coal miners.*

Churg AM, Warnock ML. Asbestos and other ferruginous bodies: their formation and clinical significance. *Am J Pathol* 1981;102:447–456. *A summary of the morphology and significance of ferruginous bodies.*

Craighead JE, Abraham JL, Churg A, Green FHY, Seemayer TE, Vallyathan V, Weill H. The pathology of asbestos-associated diseases of the lungs and pleural cavities: diagnostic criteria and proposed grading schema. *Arch Pathol Lab Med* 1982;106:544–596. *An attempt to set criteria for grading the number of asbestos particles in the lungs of exposed workers.*

Doll R. Mortality from lung cancer in asbestos workers. *Br J Ind Med* 1955;12:81–86. *Although a connection had been suspected for years, this was the first definitive report of the association between asbestos exposure and lung cancer.*

Gaensler EA. Asbestos exposure in buildings. *Clin Chest Med* 1992;13:231–242. *A thoughtful review of the risks from asbestos in public and private buildings, also touching on aspects of legislation and the costs of removal.*

Gaensler EA, Jederlinic PJ, Churg A. Idiopathic pulmonary fibrosis in asbestos-exposed workers. *Am Rev Respir Dis* 1991;144:689–696. *Careful correlation between the asbestos content of lung tissue and the presence of asbestos bodies assures the diagnostic value of the latter.*

Ghio AJ, Kennedy TP, Schapira, RM, Crumbliss AL, Hoidal JR. Hypothesis: is lung disease after silicate inhalation caused by oxidant generation? *Lancet* 1990;336:967–969. *The clearest explanation of the hypotheses regarding the toxicity of the silica surface for lung cells; the relevant biochemical pathways are traced.*

Graham WG, Weaver S, Ashikaga T, O'Grady RV. Longitudinal pulmonary function losses in Vermont granite workers. A re-evaluation. *Chest* 1994;106:125–130. *Contrary to findings in other studies, dust levels in the Vermont granite industry, which have been in compliance with Occupational Safety and Health Administration permissible exposure limits, do not accelerate pulmonary function loss.*

Hammond EC, Selikoff IJ, Seidman H. Asbestos exposure, cigarette smoking, and death rates. *Ann NY Acad Sci* 1979;330:473–491. *A ringing condemnation of cigarette smoking in the setting of asbestos exposure.*

Heintz NH, Janssen YM, Mossman BT. Persistent induction of c-*fos* and c-*jun* expression by asbestos. *Proc Natl Acad Sci USA* 1993;90:

3299–3303. *Exposure of lung cells to asbestos causes increases in levels of the proto-oncogenes c-fos and c-jun.*

Hong Kong Chest Service/Tuberculosis Research Centre, Madras/British Medical Research Council. A double-blind placebo-controlled clinical trial of three antituberculosis chemoprophylaxis regimens in patients with silicosis in Hong Kong. *Am Rev Respir Dis* 1992;145: 36–41. *An excellent recent study of chemoprophylaxis regimens in silicotic workers.*

Hughes JR, Weill H. Asbestosis as a precursor of asbestos-related lung cancer. *Br J Ind Med* 1991;48:229–233. *See next citation.*

Huuskonen MS. Asbestos and cancer. *Eur J Respir Dis* 1982:63(Suppl 123):145–152. *This and the previous citation—one from New Orleans, one from Finland—provide evidence for a threshold exposure to asbestos below which subjects are not at risk.*

Janssen YM, Barchowsky A, Treadwell M, Driscoll KE, Mossman BT. Asbestos induces nuclear factor κB (NF-κB) DNA-binding activity and NF-κB-dependent gene expression in tracheal epithelial cells. *Proc Natl Acad Sci USA* 1995;92:8458–8462. *This study suggests that NF-κB induction by asbestos is a key event in regulation of multiple genes involved in the pathogenesis of asbestos-related lung cancers.*

Lapenas D, Gale P, Kennedy T, Rawlings W Jr, Dietrich P. Kaolin pneumoconiosis. Radiologic, pathologic, and mineralogic findings. *Am Rev Respir Dis* 1984;130:282–288. *This small pathology study of five kaolin workers with complicated pneumoconiosis presents data derived by analytical scanning electron microscopy and x-ray diffractometry.*

McDonald JC. Asbestos and lung cancer. Has the case been proven? *Chest* 1980;78:374–376. *A review of the evidence that asbestos induces lung cancer.*

McDonald JC, Liddell FDK, Gibbs GW, Eyssen GE, McDonald AD. Dust exposure and mortality in chrysotile mining, 1910–1975. *Br J Ind Med* 1980;37:11–24. *A long-term study of mortality associated with chrysotile asbestos mining.*

Muir DC, Shannon HS, Julian JA, Verma DK, Sebestyen A, Bernholz CD. Silica exposure and silicosis among Ontario hard rock miners: I. Methodology. *Am J Ind Med* 1989;16:5–11. *See next citation.*

Muir DC, Julian JA, Shannon HS, Verma DK, Sebestyen A, Bernholz CD. Silica exposure and silicosis among Ontario hard rock miners: III. Analysis and risk estimates. *Am J Ind Med* 1989;16:29–43. *An epidemiologic investigation to determine the relationship between silicosis in hard rock miners in Ontario and cumulative exposure to silica (free crystalline silica—alpha quartz) dust. This report describes the analytic method and presents the risk estimates.*

Murray R. Asbestos: a chronology of its origins and health effects [see comments]. *Br J Ind Med* 1990;47:361–365. *A historical review of how asbestos, the "magic mineral" known in ancient times in Europe and Asia, became in the late nineteenth century an important industrial resource of particular interest to the navies of the world, and how its malignant effects gradually became apparent during the present century.*

Nicholson WJ, Perkel G, Selikoff IJ. Occupational exposure to asbestos: population at risk and projected mortality. *Am J Ind Med* 1982;3: 259–311. *Between 1940 and 1979, 27 million people were exposed to asbestos in the United States.*

Oghiso Y, Kagan E, Brody AR. Intrapulmonary distribution of inhaled chrysotile and crocidolite asbestos: ultrastructural features. *Br J Exp Pathol* 1984;65:467–484. *Fundamental differences in the histologic and ultrastructural effects produced by chronic inhalation of the amphibole crocidolite and the serpentine chrysotile can be demonstrated in experimental animal studies.*

Parkes WR. *Occupational Lung Disorders.* 3rd ed. Oxford: Butterworth-Heinemann; 1994. *Comprehensive descriptions of specific occupations associated with pneumoconioses, and a history of the study of dust-related diseases.*

Piguet PF, et al. Requirement of tumor necrosis factor for development of silica-induced pulmonary fibrosis. *Nature* 1990;344:245–247. *The cytokine tumor necrosis factor (TNF-α) is produced by macrophages in response to silica exposure in animal models; antibodies to this particularly toxic cytokine block progression of disease in mice.*

Reger RB, Morgan WKC. Silica: is it a carcinogen? *J Occup Health Safety Aust N Z* 1990;6:481–490. *A thoughtful review of the possible carcinogenicity of silica.*

Roggli VL, Pratt PC. Numbers of asbestos bodies on iron-stained tissue sections in relation to asbestos body counts in lung tissue digests. *Hum Pathol* 1983;14:355–361. *A detailed description of the methodology underlying a standard approach to the quantitation of asbestos bodies and free asbestos particles in tissue samples.*

Rom WN. Relationship of inflammatory cell cytokines to disease severity in individuals with occupational inorganic dust exposure. *Am J Ind Med* 1991;19:15–27. *Pneumoconioses caused by chronic occupational exposure to asbestos, coal, or silica are characterized by an alveolar macrophage-dominated alveolitis with exaggerated spontaneous release of mediators: oxidants, chemotaxins for neutrophils, and fibroblast growth factors.*

Silicosis and Silicate Disease Committee. Diseases associated with exposure to silica and nonfibrous silicate minerals. *Arch Pathol Lab Med* 1988;112:673–720. *A comprehensive review of the mineralogy and tissue diagnosis of silicosis and lung disease caused by silicates, with an overview of contemporary regulatory considerations.*

Sluis-Cremer GK, Bezuidenhout BN. Relation between asbestosis and bronchial cancer in amphibole asbestos miners. *Br J Ind Med* 1989; 46:537–540. *In a necropsy series of 339 amphibole asbestos miners, heavy smoking, age, and the presence of asbestosis were significantly associated with bronchial cancer.*

Staples CA, Gamsu G, Ray CS, Webb WR. High-resolution computed tomography and lung function in asbestos-exposed workers with normal chest radiographs. *Am Rev Respir Dis* 1989;139:1502–1508. *In asbestos-exposed subjects who have normal chest x-ray findings, high-resolution CT can identify a group with significantly reduced lung function, indicative of restrictive lung disease, in comparison with a group having normal or near-normal CT scans.*

Thurlbeck WM, Churg AM. *Pathology of the Lung.* New York: Thieme; 1996. *Detailed descriptions of pulmonary pathologic findings in asbestos- and silica-induced pneumoconioses.*

Wagner JC, Sleggs CA, Marchand P. Diffuse pleural mesothelioma and asbestos exposure in the North Western Cape Province. *Br J Ind Med* 1960;17:260–269. *Original description of the association between malignant mesothelioma and exposure to blue asbestos in South Africa.*

Wylie AG, Bailey KF, Kelse JW, Lee RJ. The importance of width in asbestos fiber carcinogenicity and its implications for public policy. *Am Ind Hyg Assoc J* 1993;54:239–252. *Human epidemiology, experimental animal implantation and inoculation studies, and lung burden studies show that fibers with widths of >1 μm are not implicated in the occurrence of lung cancer or mesothelioma.*

Textbook of Pulmonary Diseases, 6th ed.
edited by G.L. Baum, J.D. Crapo, B.R. Celli, and J.B. Karlinsky,
Lippincott–Raven Publishers, Philadelphia, © 1998.

CHAPTER

33

Occupational Lung Diseases: Coal Workers', Beryllium, and Other Pneumoconioses

W. Keith C. Morgan

COAL WORKERS' PNEUMOCONIOSIS AND RELATED CONDITIONS

Coal has been used as a source of fuel for hundreds of years. Initially, it was dug from outcroppings or augered from seams that came to the surface on the slopes of hills. It was the invention of pumps by Savery (1698) and Newcomen (1708) that made it possible to mine coal underground. Until the advent of the pump, there had been no means of controlling underground flooding or of providing adequate ventilation. Coal mining remains a major industry in the United States, Germany, France, Australia, the former U.S.S.R., China, India, and South Africa. Demand, however, has decreased, particularly in the United States and Britain, where the number of miners has been drastically reduced.

Work Force

Coal is mined extensively from both open-cast or surface mines and underground mines. In the United States, open-cast mines are mostly located in the Far West. With this method of mining, dust exposure is relatively limited. A few borers or shot firers who drill their way through rock before placing the explosive charges are exposed to high concentrations of silica, and the rapid development of silicosis has been noted in these workers.

The underground work force is usually subdivided into

W. K. C. Morgan: Chest Disease Unit, London Health Sciences Centre University Campus, London, Ontario N6A 5A5 Canada.

face workers, persons employed in transportation, workers concerned with the maintenance of machinery, and finally surface workers. Face workers include those who operate continuous miners and the cutting machines (Fig. 1), as well as roof bolters. Face workers have the dustiest jobs. Workers employed in transportation are responsible for moving coal from the face to the portal. They spend a considerable portion of time near the face, and their job is fairly dusty. Silicosis may develop in transportation workers, as they apply sand to the rails to provide traction for the diesel trains frequently used to carry the coal from the face to the portal. Behind and well back from the transportation workers are the miners whose responsibility it is to maintain equipment and carry out other miscellaneous jobs. This group includes electricians, welders, and mechanics. Finally, a few workers are employed in the lamp house and on the coal tipple. The latter is the site where the coal is washed before being transported for use. Surface coal miners, with the exception of drillers, have only very minor exposures to dust, and coal workers' pneumoconiosis is a rare finding in this group of people unless they have previously been employed underground. Drillers bore through rock strata and are subject to development of silicosis unless proper precautions are taken.

Respiratory Disease in Coal Miners

The hazards of mining were known to Agricola and Paracelsus in the sixteenth century. These early observers noted that Carpathian miners died of what was then known as *miners' phthisis*. It is also now abundantly clear that this term had a generic connotation and included a large number of diseases, ranging from silicosis on the

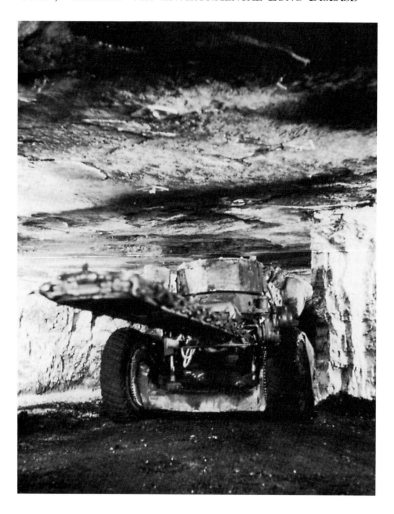

FIG. 1. Coal cutter in a U.S. coal mine.

one hand to tuberculosis, bronchitis, bronchiectasis, and probably lung cancer on the other.

Long-term exposure to coal dust leads to three chest diseases: (1) coal workers' pneumoconiosis (CWP), (2) silicosis, and (3) industrial bronchitis. Silicosis is seen uncommonly except in roof bolters, who bore through adjacent rock strata containing silica to place the roof bolts, and in transportation workers, who apply sand to the rails to provide traction.

Earlier in this century, it was noted that radiographic opacities, similar to those seen in silicosis, developed in the lung fields of Welsh coal miners. It was initially presumed that these radiographic features represented silicosis, as it was known that coal mine dust often contains a fair amount of free silica. However, it was observed that radiographic changes identical to those seen in the coal miner also developed in the coal trimmer, a type of stevedore who was responsible for the even distribution of the coal once it had been loaded into the holds of ships. The trimmers handled only coal that had been washed and, as such, contained virtually no free silica. Subsequent analysis of the lungs of some of these coal trimmers showed that they had no more silica in their lungs than did the inhabitants of Cardiff and Swansea. Confirmation

that inhalation of pure carbon could induce similar changes was subsequently noted. There is now compelling evidence to indicate that CWP is distinct from silicosis not only epidemiologically but also pathologically and in regard to prognosis.

CWP is best defined as the deposition of coal mine dust in the lung parenchyma and the reaction of tissue to its presence. It is customarily divided into simple and complicated pneumoconiosis, according to the radiographic features.

Simple Coal Workers' Pneumoconiosis

Simple CWP is recognized from its radiographic features plus a suitable history of exposure—that is, >10 years underground. The lung fields show the presence of multiple, small, rounded (regular) opacities. These usually appear first in the upper lobes and gradually spread all over the lung fields. Simple CWP is graded according to the profusion of small opacities on the chest x-ray film. Categories 1, 2, and 3 are recognized. The classification most commonly used was devised by a group of experts from the International Labor Office (ILO) and has received general acceptance. For epidemiologic purposes, a 12-point elaboration of the standard ILO classification was devised. Use of this 12-point elaboration is essential in the assessment of radiographic progression. Small opacities can be subdivided into *p*, *q*, and *r* types according to size, with *p* (punctate) being <1.5 mm in diameter, *q* (micronodular) being between 1.5 and 3 mm, and *r* being between 3 mm and 1 cm. Although there are occasions when all three types of opacity are present in a single radiograph, in general, a specific type predominates. In the vast majority of radiographs, the appearances tend to be fairly uniform, and one can detect only one type of opacity (Figs. 2 and 3). Larger nodules (*r*) are more commonly seen in silicosis than in CWP.

Symptoms

Simple CWP is not associated with symptoms, although many of those showing the characteristic radiologic features of the condition will admit to bronchitic symptoms—namely, cough and production of sputum. These symptoms are a consequence of either cigarette smoking or industrial bronchitis, should they happen to be present in nonsmokers.

Pathology

Simple CWP is a reaction to dust alone and does not progress in the absence of further exposure. By the same token, it probably never regresses, despite sporadic case reports purporting to demonstrate radiographic improvement. Most such reports are best explained by erroneous

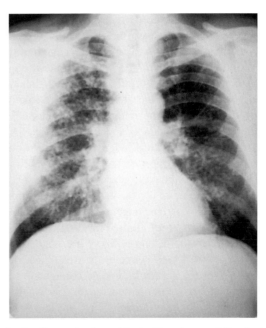

FIG. 3. Radiograph of a subject with category 3/2, *q/r* simple CWP.

diagnoses, such as sarcoidosis or welder's siderosis, which are known to regress, or by changes in technique in taking serial films. The value of the chest radiograph is that it provides an indication of the coal dust present in the lungs. Many investigations have shown that each successively higher category of simple CWP is associated with a comparable increment in the coal dust content of the lung. The mineral content of the lungs also influences the radiographic appearance, and it is of paramount importance to note that radiographic category is a direct reflection of the dust deposited and retained in the lung and an indirect reflection of cumulative dust exposure (Fig. 4). When coal dust particles are deposited in the

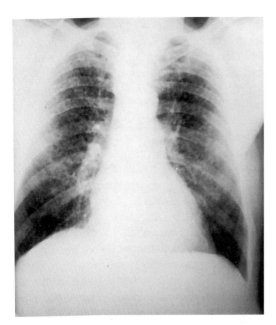

FIG. 2. Radiograph of a subject with category 2/2, *q/q* simple CWP.

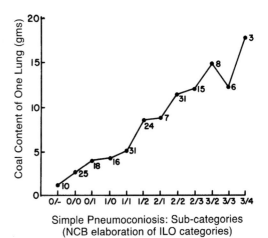

FIG. 4. Relationship between the coal content of one lung and the radiologic category of CWP. The numbers over the points on the graph denote the number of lungs examined within each category of simple CWP.

alveoli, they are taken up by the macrophages, which in turn convey the dust toward the respiratory bronchioles. The exact means whereby the macrophages migrate from the alveoli to the terminal bronchioles and to the interstitial tissue and the source of energy for their translocation are unknown. Provided dust exposure is not intense and prolonged, the clearing mechanisms usually remain effective, but in the face of high and prolonged exposure to coal dust particles, the dust-laden macrophages begin to accumulate at the portion of the respiratory bronchiole that lies adjacent to the pulmonary arteriole. Many subsequently die and liberate dust around the second-order respiratory bronchioles. This engenders a reticulin response and the development of limited fibrosis. Occasionally, with time, a few collagenous fibers are also formed. If the dust contains a high concentration of silica, then the fibrotic response is greater and more collagen is formed. The aggregates of coal pigment appear as small, black spots in large sections of the lungs and are known as *coal macules.*

Initially, the coal macule is small, but with prolonged exposure it slowly increases in size. This increase in size is accompanied by a concomitant increase in the amount of fibrous tissue present. Once this occurs, the smooth muscle in the bronchiolar wall atrophies and, as a result, the bronchiole dilates. It is uncertain what causes the dilatation, but it is probably a consequence of the application of extraluminal forces to the bronchiolar wall. The dilatation eventually becomes large enough to be seen by the naked eye and is then known as *focal emphysema* (Fig. 5). The location of the focal emphysema—namely, in the center of the secondary lobule—is similar to that seen in cigarette smoke-induced centrilobular emphysema. Whereas Gough and Heppleston distinguished focal from centrilobular emphysema and maintained that centrilobular emphysema induced by cigarette smoking is invariably accompanied by bronchiolitis, which is absent in focal emphysema, others maintain that the two pathologic conditions cannot be distinguished.

Recent investigations have suggested that the histologic appearance of the macules is affected by the composition and contents of the coal mine dust to which the miner has been exposed.

Lung Function

Although the ventilatory capacity of miners as a whole is decreased in comparison with that of persons of comparable socioeconomic status who are not miners, a higher category of simple CWP is not associated with a larger decrement in ventilatory capacity. If one studies non-smoking miners with simple CWP, it becomes evident that a variety of pulmonary impairments are present. These impairments include a disturbance in the distribution of inspired gas, which is manifested by a slight in-

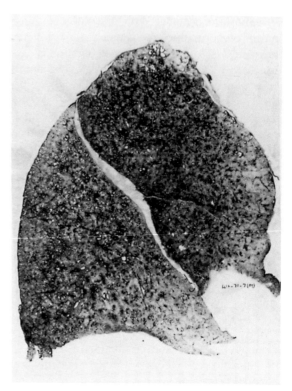

FIG. 5. Large lung section of a subject with CWP showing macules and focal emphysema.

crease in the alveolar-arterial pressure gradient, $P(A\text{-}a)O_2$; a minor reduction in the diffusing capacity, especially in subjects with type p opacity; and minimal hypoxemia caused by physiologic shunting in categories 2 and 3. With exercise, the $P(A\text{-}a)O_2$ may increase slightly, but in many instances it improves. The focal emphysema that accompanies categories 2 and 3 simple CWP is often associated with a minor loss of elastic recoil and a slight increase in the compliance of the lungs. In addition, an increase in the residual volume often occurs, which is probably related to the same factors mentioned earlier—namely, a change in the elastic properties of the lung (Figs. 6–8). The increase in residual volume occurs in subjects with and without airways obstruction and cannot be attributed to increased airways resistance.

In subjects with categories 2 and 3 simple CWP, as mentioned earlier, the diffusing capacity may be mildly reduced (Fig. 9). This is a consequence of ventilation-perfusion mismatching and is mainly present in type p opacities. Frans and associates have carried out more detailed studies in which the components of the diffusing capacity have been measured in subjects with simple CWP. They partitioned the diffusing capacity into the capillary blood volume (Vc) and the membrane component (Dm) and found that both were slightly reduced. Although pneumoconiosis had a slight effect on both these components, cigarette smoking had a far greater effect. An extensive study of the effect of CWP on the diffusing capacity was carried out by Kibelstis. He mea-

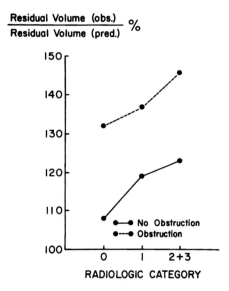

FIG. 6. The relationship of residual volume to radiographic category in coal miners with and without airways obstruction. (Reproduced from Morgan WKC, et al. *Thorax* 1971; 26:585.)

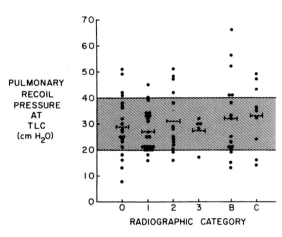

FIG. 8. Pulmonary recoil pressure of coal miners according to radiographic category. *Bars* represent mean values with standard deviation.

sured the steady-state diffusing capacity ($DLCO_{ss}$) at rest and during exercise. The vast majority of nonsmoking miners had a normal $DLCO_{ss}$. The effects of cigarette smoking far outweighed those of years spent working underground and the presence of pneumoconiosis.

Evidence of abnormal small-airways function is frequently observed in coal miners and appears to be unrelated to the presence of simple CWP. Abnormalities of closing volume and frequency dependence of dynamic compliance have been noted. It is likely that there is no one simple explanation for these abnormalities, and that small-airways obstruction, regional changes in compliance, and the mechanical properties of the lung all play a role. The presence of these small-airways abnormalities, however, cannot be regarded as disabling or of any clinical significance.

Complicated Pneumoconiosis or Progressive Massive Fibrosis

Unlike simple CWP, complicated pneumoconiosis is associated with symptoms, significant impairment, and decreased longevity. The condition is recognized by a large opacity or opacities 1 cm in diameter occurring on a background of simple CWP (Fig. 10). Although a number of investigators claim that progressive massive fibrosis (PMF) can occur on a background of category 0, the basis for this statement is somewhat suspect, in that other causes of large opacities cannot be excluded. Stage A (i.e., an opacity between 1 and 5 cm in diameter) is seldom

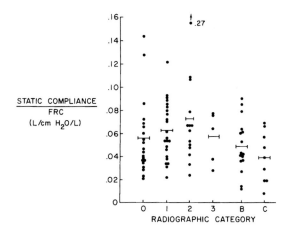

FIG. 7. Static compliance of lungs of coal miners according to radiographic category. *Bars* represent mean values with standard deviation. *FRC,* functional residual capacity.

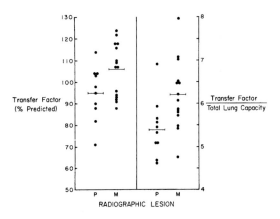

FIG. 9. The diffusing capacity (transfer factor) of a group of nonsmoking coal miners with simple CWP. *P,* punctate or *p*-type opacity. *M,* micronodular or *q*-type opacity. (Reproduced from Seaton A, Lapp NL, Morgan WKC. The relationship of pulmonary impairment in simple coal workers' pneumoconiosis to type of radiographic opacity. *Br J Ind Med* 1972;29:50.)

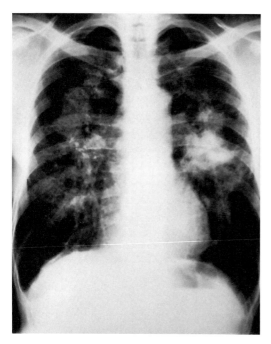

FIG. 10. Radiograph of a subject with stage C complicated CWP.

Lung Function

For the most part, no detectable abnormalities are present in stage A complicated pneumoconiosis. In stages B and C, the ventilatory capacity is reduced, and the reduction is usually proportional to the size of the conglomerate masses. Although both the FVC (forced vital capacity) and the FEV₁ (forced expiratory volume in one second) are decreased, the latter is sometimes reduced disproportionately. The ratio of FEV_1 to FVC ratio is generally reduced, especially in advanced stage C disease. The diffusing capacity is likewise affected, and the decrement observed is proportional to the size of the masses. The precise pathophysiologic explanation for the obstruction remains unclear, but it appears to resemble that occurring in far-advanced tuberculosis or widespread end-stage sarcoidosis. Large masses destroy both the vascular bed and many of the airways, and their effects on the former are responsible for non-hypoxemic pulmonary hypertension. Eventually, hypoxemia develops, but it is observed earlier and more frequently in those subjects who happen also to be cigarette smokers.

Pathology

As already mentioned, conglomerate shadows usually develop in the posterior segment of the upper lobes or the superior segment of the lower lobes. Macroscopically, they consist of large, black, amorphous masses that on section tend to liberate a jet-black grumous fluid. They are rubbery in consistency, and occasionally an irregular,

if ever associated with either symptoms or a significant decrease in lung function. Stages B and C, however, may be associated with both symptoms and a decrement in lung function. Stage B is defined as an opacity or opacities 5 cm in diameter but not extending over a third of the lung field. Stage C is defined as a large opacity or opacities occupying more than a third of one lung field (Fig. 11).

Symptoms

The usual symptoms of PMF are increasing shortness of breath, cough, and production of sputum, but again, the latter is probably a consequence of coincident bronchitis. Shortness of breath is seldom seen until stage B is fairly well advanced, but it becomes more evident as the disease progresses. In far-advanced disease, in which alveolar-capillary surface is lost, non-hypoxemic cor pulmonale often develops. This is associated with a right ventricular heave, the presence of large "a" waves, hepatomegaly, and peripheral edema. It must be stressed that cor pulmonale arising as a result of complicated CWP is an unusual finding in the United States at the present time and usually takes many years to develop.

Radiographically, the disease tends to appear in the axillary region of the posterior segment of either upper lobe. It then often slowly migrates toward the hilum at the same time as the hilum is retracted upward. It also is seen in the superior segment of the lower lobe, and the distribution of the massive fibrosis in this regard closely resembles that of tuberculosis.

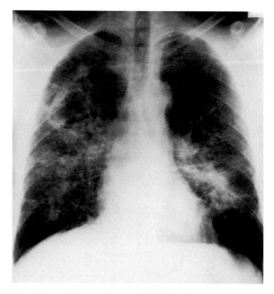

FIG. 11. Stage C complicated CWP with ischemic necrosis in the cavity in the left upper lobe. This subject had worked as a "slave laborer" for 4 years in the Belgian coal mines during the war.

thick-walled cavity may be present. The latter represents either ischemic necrosis or tuberculous infection.

Microscopically, the periphery of the masses seems to be composed of dense aggregates of fibrous tissue. Although formerly it was believed to be almost pure collagen, this is now known to be incorrect; the collagen bundles tend to be peripherally situated in the wall of the cavity. Even there, they are often separated by deposits of coal dust. The lung masses gradually encroach on and destroy adjacent airways and blood vessels. Remnants of former internal elastic laminae can be observed on microscopy. The pulmonary arteries, veins, and capillaries are all obliterated.

A rigid separation of simple from complicated pneumoconiosis is probably fallacious, and it is clear that the opacities of <1 cm in size gradually increase in diameter and form a large opacity. It has been shown that the hydroxyproline content of the large masses is only about 3%–4%, implying that the collagen content is about 25%–30%. In an analysis of fresh tissue from the center of conglomerate lesions, there was demonstrated a significant increase in calcium phosphate content and the presence of glycosaminoglycans such as hyaluronic acid and chondroitin sulfate in the mass lesion. These findings are supported by the normal urinary hydroxyproline content in both simple and complicated CWP. It also has been shown that fibronectin is an important component of the masses that characterize PMF.

Necessary for the development of PMF is a suitable dust burden and some factor or factors as yet unknown. Unlike simple CWP, PMF may develop after exposure has ceased, provided category 2 or 3 disease is present at the time the subject stops working. In addition, the disease may progress in the absence of further exposure.

Immunologic Aspects of Coal Workers' Pneumoconiosis

In 1953, Caplan described a syndrome in coal miners characterized by the presence of multiple rounded opacities in the lungs and associated with rheumatoid arthritis. Since then, the condition has been known as *Caplan's syndrome* or *rheumatoid pneumoconiosis*. The opacities differ from those in the usual form of PMF in that they tend to be peripherally situated and often appear in crops during a relatively short period. Moreover, they frequently occur on a background of category 0 or 1 pneumoconiosis. Although most of the patients who were originally observed had rheumatoid arthritis, subsequent studies showed that the condition may appear to antedate the development of rheumatoid arthritis. Typical nodules of Caplan's syndrome and the large opacities of PMF may be present in the same subject. The nodules are often accompanied by the typical rheumatoid nodules found on the Achilles tendon and elbows. Histologically, although

the nodules bear some resemblance to the rheumatoid nodules found on the elbows, there are distinct differences. It has been noted that there are concentric layers of dust and granulation tissue with a necrotic area in the center. Beside the necrotic area, there is often a cellular zone infiltrated with mononuclear cells and, in particular, lymphocytes and plasma cells (Fig. 12). Endarteritis is often present. This zone of active inflammation was named the *rheumatoid zone* by Gough and co-workers.

Through the years, a number of studies have compared the prevalence of rheumatoid factor in coal miners with that of a comparable referent population. Rheumatoid factor was present in about 70% with typical Caplan's syndrome. This far exceeded the prevalence in subjects with simple CWP. Furthermore, a significant proportion of those subjects with a radiographic appearance of Caplan's syndrome in whom rheumatoid factor was lacking when they were first seen subsequently tested positive for rheumatoid factor. Because of the fact that some subjects with Caplan's syndrome continued to test negative for rheumatoid factor, it was suggested that PMF existed in two forms: one form, much less common, associated with vasculitis, cellular infiltration, and rheumatoid factor in the serum, and a second form, nonspecific and associated with mild inflammation and obliteration of the vascular bed. The evidence in favor of this hypothesis is tenuous. Antinuclear antibody (ANA) is also frequently present in miners who have PMF.

Studies of immunoglobulin levels in miners with and without CWP have shown that the sera of anthracite min-

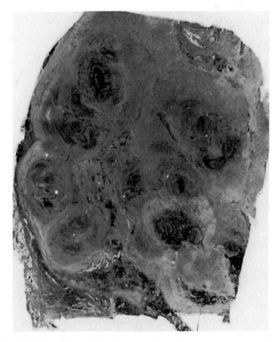

FIG. 12. Cluster of Caplan nodules from a large section of the lung of a deceased coal miner. Note the concentric layers of dust deposition in the nodules. The subject had severe rheumatoid arthritis, but only category 1/0 simple CWP.

ers with PMF contain relatively higher levels of complement (C3), α_1-antitrypsin, and immunoglobulins A and G (IgA and IgA) than do comparable sera from bituminous coal miners with PMF. Immunoglobulin levels, however, are normal in miners with simple CWP. Lung reactive antibodies have also been demonstrated in miners with CWP, but their role in the etiology of the condition is not apparent.

Emphysema and Coal Workers' Pneumoconiosis

Although there is no doubt that a form of emphysema usually referred to as *focal emphysema* occurs in coal miners with pneumoconiosis, the effects of this type of emphysema are presently a source of argument. Focal emphysema occurs in the center of the secondary lobule and, in this regard, resembles centrilobular emphysema. Gough and Heppleston maintained that focal emphysema is distinct from centrilobular emphysema as seen in cigarette smokers and does not lead to pulmonary hypertension. They also maintained that centrilobular emphysema of cigarette smokers is always accompanied by a bronchiolitis and in this respect differs from focal dust emphysema.

During the past few years, in a series of articles from South Wales, investigators have proposed that it is the emphysema in the lungs of coal miners that causes airways obstruction. The coal miners chosen for these studies were all disability claimants who had been reviewed by pneumoconiosis panels. As such, they can hardly be regarded as representative of coal miners as a whole. The investigators attempted to show a relationship between lung function in life and the extent of emphysema diagnosed at postmortem examination. They were, however, unable to demonstrate that obstruction increases with higher categories of simple CWP.

There are a number of compelling arguments to refute this hypothesis. It is well accepted that an increasing amount of dust deposited in the lungs is associated with a higher radiographic category. Similarly, it has been shown that the extent of focal emphysema increases in higher categories of simple CWP. If the focal emphysema is responsible for the obstruction, then a decrease in the ventilatory capacity should be noted with a higher category of simple CWP, but it is not. Second, extensive studies in which the hearts and lungs of deceased miners were examined have considered the relationship of antemortem smoking habits and simple and complicated pneumoconiosis. Right ventricular hypertrophy and cor pulmonale do not occur in coal miners if they have not been cigarette smokers or have not had PMF. Similarly, if the emphysema noted in the lungs of miners with simple CWP is truly disabling and leads to a reduction of the alveolar-capillary surface, then a significant reduction in the diffusing capacity should occur, but it does not. The

argument has been further developed in the Surgeon General's Report of 1985.

More recently, other investigators have endorsed the concept that the excess emphysema in the lungs of coal miners is responsible for the observed increase in airways obstruction. The proponents of this theory rely on a report of the findings in an autopsy study of the lungs of 1400 coal miners. The prevalence of emphysema was examined in 503 men, and a differentiation was made between panacinar and centriacinar (centrilobular) emphysema. Ninety-five nonsmokers were included, of whom 42 had some emphysema. The presence and type of emphysema were related to dust exposure, age, cigarette smoking, and bronchitis. Thirty-five percent (33 subjects) of the nonsmokers had centriacinar emphysema and 23% had panacinar emphysema. No relationship was found between the presence of panacinar emphysema and coal dust. Only 2 of the 21 nonsmokers who had no coal-induced fibrosis (i.e., no CWP) had centriacinar emphysema. Moreover, emphysema was regarded as being present when as little as 1/30 of the lung was involved. From this it might be inferred that many of those with emphysema had negligible involvement and were asymptomatic. Elsewhere, it has been shown that at least 20%−25% of the lung must be involved before the subject has symptoms of breathlessness.

The study defined three pathologic groups according to the presence of particular dust lesions. Group M included lungs showing circumscribed dust accumulations with minimal evidence of fibrosis. Most of these did not show radiographic evidence of CWP. Group F showed one or more fibrotic lesions between 1 and 9 mm in diameter. The third group comprised lungs from subjects with PMF having fibrotic lesions ≥ 1 cm in diameter. In a group of 257 miners who had undergone spirometry during life, only two nonsmokers had emphysema in the absence of PMF. Moreover, an exposure-response relationship was lacking between dust and extent of emphysema. Finally, the nonsmokers in the M and F groups, of whom there were almost none, showed no difference in lung function between those with and without emphysema. Thus, the report seems to provide little support for the hypothesis that centriacinar emphysema of nonsmoking coal miners produces airways obstruction, and in smoking coal miners it is clear that cigarettes are the main cause of obstruction.

Bronchitis and Coal Mining

There is no doubt that coal mine dust induces an increase in the size of the mucous glands and an increase in the number of goblet cells. These changes are associated with cough and production of sputum and a small reduction in ventilatory capacity. For the most part, only the large airways are affected. The reduction in ventilatory capacity is unrelated to radiographic category and is present in miners with no radiographic abnormality.

Relative Contributions of Dust Versus Cigarette Smoking and Airways Obstruction in Coal Miners

A number of cross-sectional and longitudinal studies have been carried out in coal miners comparing the effects of dust versus cigarette smoking. Most studies have shown that dust does have an effect, even in the absence of cigarette smoking. Two long-term studies, one carried out in Britain and the other in the United States, have reported that cigarette smoking has about three times the effect of coal dust on the development of airways obstruction. This conclusion is based on a comparison of the mean decrements induced by dust, cigarette smoking, age, and other factors. Unfortunately, such comparisons are misleading. It is well established that significant airways obstruction develops in only about 13%–15% of cigarette smokers. The vast majority of smokers are unaffected. In contrast, most miners who have spent 25 years in the coal mine (and this applies also to nonsmokers) have cough and sputum. Many of them have a small decrement in ventilatory capacity. Thus, when the effects of smoking are compared with those of dust, a significant and occasionally disabling decrement in a small percentage of subjects (13%–15%) is being compared with a much smaller decrement in a far greater proportion of subjects (40%–60%). There seems to be little doubt that coal dust in itself does not lead to disabling obstruction unless PMF is present. Moreover, as mentioned earlier, right ventricular hypertrophy and respiratory failure do not appear to occur in coal miners in the absence of cigarette smoking or PMF.

Lung cancer occurs less frequently in coal miners than it does in the general population. This is probably related to the fact that coal miners are not allowed to smoke in the mines, so that 8 hours of the day are spent in a smoke-free atmosphere. This observation has been made in numerous studies. Similarly, other studies have shown that heart disease occurs less frequently in coal miners than it does in the general population.

Effects of Coal Workers' Pneumoconiosis on Life Expectancy

A number of studies have been carried out showing that simple CWP has no effect on life expectancy, but that PMF is associated with decreased longevity. This has been observed in both Britain and the United States. It also has been noted that coal miners as a group have a normal life expectancy at the present time. Although the death rate from accidents and complicated pneumoconiosis is increased, this is counterbalanced by the decreased death rate from heart disease and lung cancer.

Radiographic Progression

Repeated observations have shown that increasing exposure, as measured by years underground or by cumula-

tive dust exposure, leads to radiographic progression. Originally, this was measured using the standard ILO 3-point scale (categories 1, 2, and 3), but it became apparent that the scale was not sensitive enough. As a result, Liddell and May elaborated their 12-point scale. The adoption of the more accurate gravimetric method of estimating coal mine dust, plus the use of the elaboration of Liddell and May, have made it possible to relate long-term dust exposure to the attack rate of pneumoconiosis and the likelihood that a person with pneumoconiosis will progress from a particular subcategory to another. Using such an approach, a dose-response relationship has been derived, both in Britain, by the National Coal Board, and in Germany. The results obtained in both countries were very similar despite completely different methods of measuring coal dust. Jacobsen has derived a series of curves suggesting that, provided the time-weighted average is kept below 2 mg/m³, category 2 disease or higher will develop in about 2% of miners who work 8 hours a day, 5 days a week, for a period of 35 years (Fig. 13). Hence, if one can prevent simple CWP, then there is every likelihood that PMF will not develop. The fact that the U.S. coal mines have a standard of 2 mg/m³ should mean the virtual elimination of CWP by 2005.

Bronchoalveolar Lavage Studies

A number of bronchoalveolar lavage studies of coal miners have recently been performed. Most have been poorly conducted, and the information yielded so far has not been particularly helpful in diagnosing or unraveling

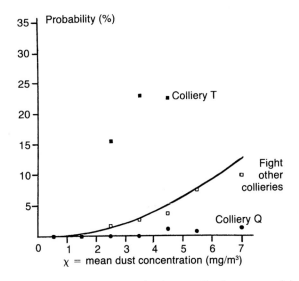

FIG. 13. The percentage of miners with disease evolving to category 2 or higher. This is based on 35 years of exposure for 8 hours a day, 5 days a week. (Reproduced from Jacobsen M. New data on the relationship between simple pneumoconiosis and exposure to coal mine dust. *Chest* 1980;78(Suppl):408.)

the mechanisms involved in the pathogenesis of CWP. There have also been a number of studies of tumor necrosis factor (TNF) in CWP, and it has been shown that in subjects with CWP the level of TNF is increased. Once again, the significance of increased levels of TNF is not understood. Although investigators have related the progression of CWP to increased levels of TNF, the authors of these studies have never been sure what constitutes progression—worsening of the radiograph or a decline in lung function.

OTHER PNEUMOCONIOSES

Several other pneumoconioses have been recognized. Most are relatively uncommon and the existence of some is questionable, but many of those that are well recognized result from the inhalation of metals.

Respiratory Conditions Associated with Exposure to Aluminum

Aluminum is mined as bauxite. Bauxite contains about 40%–50% alumina and other oxides, in particular iron. Deposits of bauxite are found in Jamaica, Australia, Guyana, and France. Metallic aluminum does not occur in a natural state but is found in combination with oxygen, silicon, and fluorine. It is frequently found as combined complex salts of silicic acid. Many minerals, including all types of asbestos, contain aluminum. Cryolite is aluminum fluoride and is found mainly in Greenland.

The production of aluminum involves two steps, the first of which is to convert the bauxite to aluminum oxide. This involves the digestion of bauxite with caustic soda at a high temperature and pressure. The resulting hydrate is then dried and calcined to the oxide. Subsequently, the alumina (Al_2O_3) is reduced by the Hall-Heroult electrolytic process. This takes place in the pot room, where the alumina is mixed with cryolite flux and the mixture placed in large steel pots into which carbon electrodes dip. With the passage of an electric current, the metal accumulates at the bottom of the pot while a crust of alumina and other impurities forms on top. The metal is subsequently removed from the pot.

A number of respiratory conditions have been attributed to exposure to alumina or metallic aluminum.

Shaver's Disease

This condition was first described in the Niagara Peninsula by Shaver. It was recognized in workers manufacturing the abrasive corundum. The process involves the mixing of bauxite with iron and coke and fusion in large iron pots at a temperature of 2000°C. During the process, dense white fumes are given off containing Al_2O_3 and amor-

phous silica. Subsequently, it was realized that during fusion some of the free silica had been converted to cristobalite and tridymite.

In a survey of four plants that were manufacturing alumina abrasives, Shaver and Riddell found 23 subjects with radiographic abnormalities. Those affected had shortness of breath and recurrent chest pain. Many also had a cough that was productive of some mucoid sputum. Subsequently, it became evident that the recurrent chest pain was often related to the development of spontaneous pneumothorax. On examination, the subjects were noted to have tachypnea, and cyanosis was present in those with advanced disease. Crackles were present in most, and occasionally signs of consolidation were noted.

The radiologic findings varied considerably. In most cases, both lungs were affected by a diffuse reticulonodular process. The upper lobes were most often involved, and with the passage of time, blebs began to appear and regional honeycombing became evident. In those in whom the condition developed rapidly, the first changes noted were those of an acinous filling pattern. This later resolved, but often only partially, and in doing so left a diffuse interstitial pattern.

Pathology

Macroscopically, the lungs appeared solid and were of a gray-black color, with much pleural thickening and frequent emphysematous bullae at the apex and elsewhere on the pleural surface. In the acute stage, alveolar edema and thickened septa were often present. Interstitial fibrosis developed later, but the classic whorled nodules of silicosis were absent.

Subsequent analysis of the fumes emitted showed that they contained about 70% aluminum and 4%–7% free silica. Initially, it was thought that the free silica occurred as amorphous silica and was probably harmless. However, it became evident later that at the high temperatures, some of the silica had been converted to cristobalite. The latter is one of the more fibrogenic forms of crystalline silica.

Shortly after Shaver described this outbreak, ventilation was improved, and since that time no further outbreaks have occurred. Moreover, numerous surveys of persons exposed to alumina, including those who work in aluminum plants that convert bauxite to alumina, have not revealed any additional cases of Shaver's disease or indeed pulmonary fibrosis. Furthermore, although the intratracheal injection of alumina has successfully induced fibrotic conditions in the lungs of animals, inhalation techniques using high concentrations of aluminum oxide have failed to induce fibrosis.

Aluminum Lung

Molecules of aluminum metal cannot exist in the air for any length of time because they are almost instantaneously oxidized to aluminum oxide. By the same token, larger particles of aluminum metal are invariably coated with aluminum oxide. It is this thin, self-generating coating that gives aluminum its corrosion-resistant properties. Every particle of aluminum is surrounded by a hard coating of alumina that is around 20 Å thick. When the coating is scratched off the surface of the particle so as to expose the metallic aluminum, it almost instantaneously regenerates.

For commercial use, aluminum particles are prepared in two forms. When fine metallic particles are necessary, aluminum is atomized. This process involves spraying a fine stream of molten metal into a high-velocity air jet, leading to the formation of granular particles with a smooth surface and a shape that is either ovoid or spherical. Granular aluminum particles have a number of uses, especially in the manufacture of pigments. A particular form of aluminum known as *flake* is used in the manufacture of paints and fireworks. This is also known as *stamped aluminum,* and it is processed into fine flakes by ball milling. Whereas granular aluminum particles have a limited surface area, the leaflike flake powder has a much larger surface area. A special type of flake powder known as *pyro* finds a particular use in the manufacture of fireworks and explosives. This is produced by ball milling flake aluminum into exceedingly fine particles that have a large surface area. During the ball milling of pyro, a lubricant is added to prevent impact welding, maintaining separation of the particles during stamping. The lubricant also increases and maintains the large surface area, a prerequisite for the manufacture of aluminum paints, and lessens oxidation. The lubricant that has been used predominantly for this purpose is stearin, a vegetable oil. Its addition during the stamping process causes the pyro flakes to be coated with aluminum stearate. The latter acts as a barrier between the flake surface and the atmospheric oxygen, thereby preventing further oxidation.

In wartime Germany and later in Britain, Sweden, and elsewhere, mineral oil (spindle oil) was substituted for stearin in the manufacture of pyro. The much-quoted reason for the substitution was a shortage of animal fats in Germany during wartime, but it seems that the real reason for the change was that mineral oil allowed more pyro powder to be packed into a cartridge so that the explosive effects were far greater. The latter property was desirable in the manufacture of fireworks.

Just before and during the war, Goralewski noted that pulmonary fibrosis developed in a number of German workers involved in the manufacture of pyro aluminum powder. As a result of Goralewski's experience in Germany, epidemiologic studies were subsequently carried out in Britain. No comparable condition was detected, and no explanation for the difference between the British and German findings was evident. Subsequently, however, a pulmonary fibrosis similar to that described by

Goralewski developed in several British subjects who were working with metallic aluminum powder. The various effects of aluminum on the lung and the history of aluminum-induced fibrosis of the lung have been well described.

Clinical Features

These are essentially the same as seen in Shaver's disease, namely, the onset of cough, production of sputum, and anorexia. Basal crackles are noted. As in Shaver's disease, the upper lobes tend to be predominantly involved. In the case of one subject who had pulmonary fibrosis, a diffuse toxic encephalopathy also was present. Radiographs show nodular and flocculent shadows in the upper lobes with an occasional pneumothorax.

Pathology

Macroscopically and microscopically, the changes are similar to those seen in Shaver's disease and most other forms of interstitial fibrosis. There does tend to be somewhat more involvement of the upper lobes than in most other types of interstitial fibrosis. Analysis of the lungs usually reveals a grossly increased aluminum content.

Pathogenesis

Corrin, in a series of in vitro and animal experiments, demonstrated that stamped aluminum powder reacts vigorously with water, whereas granular aluminum is almost entirely inert. The latter form of aluminum, as already mentioned, is coated with aluminum oxide, and this explains its relative inertness. Stamped aluminum, whether in the metallic form or treated with mineral oil, reacts vigorously with water, but the addition of stearin reduces this propensity. As mentioned earlier, during wartime in Germany mineral oil was substituted for stearin, and shortly thereafter Goralewski noticed pulmonary fibrosis developing in pyro workers. He correctly attributed the development of the pulmonary fibrosis to the substitution of mineral oil for stearin. Corrin also noted that it was only after stearin had been replaced by mineral oil that aluminosis began to occur in Britain.

This observation prompted Corrin to conduct a series of experiments in animals, in which he administered intratracheal injections of both granular aluminum and several forms of stamped aluminum, including stamped aluminum with stearin, stamped aluminum coated with mineral oil, and stamped aluminum with both lubricants removed. All three forms of stamped aluminum induced marked pulmonary fibrosis; however, granular aluminum was much less fibrogenic. He therefore concluded that all forms of aluminum powder were fibrogenic, although to differing extents. He still was of the opinion that stamped aluminum, when lubricated with mineral oil, was much more hazardous, but he could not completely exonerate stearin-treated pyro. He likewise realized that intratracheal injection did not necessarily reflect worker exposures, and in this regard he was remarkably prescient. Subsequently, in an attempt to prevent silicosis, metallic aluminum powder was administered by inhalation to many thousands of metal miners in Ontario and elsewhere, with no ill effects.

The patient described by McLaughlin and associates was believed to provide further confirmatory evidence that both stamped and granular aluminum powder could induce aluminosis. At the time this subject was given a diagnosis, he was working with pyro that had been treated with stearin, but it subsequently came to light that he had worked previously in the same factory at the time spindle oil was being used. Thus, it seems that aluminosis has been described only in subjects who have been heavily exposed to pyro treated with mineral oil. Similarly, granular aluminum is fibrogenic only when given by intratracheal injection, and this method of administration is not physiologic and should not be regarded as a suitable model for human disease.

Other Effects of Aluminum

Development of a granulomatous condition of the lung, attributed to the inhalation of alumina, has been described in two subjects. Once again, there was a lack of evidence to indicate that the disease was related to aluminum, although an increased aluminum content was noted in the lungs of both. As the aluminum content of the lungs is increased in virtually every subject who works with alumina or is involved in the reduction of alumina to metallic aluminum, this finding is of little significance.

A more recent study describes nine workers exposed to Al_2O_3 during the production of abrasives from alundum ore. Most had long-term exposure and all had abnormal chest radiographs (category 1/0 or higher). In three, the respiratory symptoms, prevalence of pulmonary impairment, and radiographic appearances were more significant than in the others, and as a result open lung biopsy was performed. In all three, interstitial fibrosis with honeycombing was seen. The lungs were found to contain a variety of metals, and in one case a significant amount of silica and an increased number of asbestos fibers. All three subjects who underwent biopsy had an increased aluminum burden in the lungs; however, the burden as measured by the number of aluminum particulates varied greatly. Five of the remaining six subjects had radiographs that showed changes of either category 1/0 or 1/1. All five were smokers. The finding of a high concentration of aluminum in the lungs is to be expected with long exposure and cannot be construed as indicating that the aluminum caused the fibrosis. Moreover, in most cross-sectional studies there has been no evidence whatsoever of restrictive impairment, decreased lung compliance, or other changes that indicate pneumoconiosis. All three subjects who underwent biopsy may well have had other forms of interstitial fibrosis, such as fibrosing alveolitis. It should also be borne in mind that radiographic changes have previously been demonstrated in workers exposed to aluminum oxide. The changes noted by these investigators were scanty, irregular opacities ranging from category 0/1 to 1/1 at the most, and predominantly, but not entirely, related to cigarette smoking. The circumstances in which aluminum may cause pulmonary fibrosis have been previously described by Morgan and Dinman and by Abrahamson and associates. The evidence that aluminum oxide produces pulmonary fibrosis is tenuous and unconvincing.

A subject with pulmonary alveolar proteinosis attributed to the inhalation of aluminum dust has also been described. The affected subject was a 44-year-old man seen with shortness of breath, radiographic infiltrates, and restrictive disease. A biopsy showed pulmonary alveolar proteinosis. The affected worker had been employed as an aluminum rail grinder for the prior 6 years. It was suggested that grinding rails generated a large quantity of aluminum particles, many of which were deposited in the lungs. The illustrations left little doubt that the subject had pulmonary alveolar proteinosis; however, the electron micrograph of the aluminum particles showed them to be completely spherical. It seems inconceivable that the particles generated by grinding would be spherical, and indeed the only way in which the aluminum particles could have been spherical is if they were generated as droplets of vapor at a very high temperature. It is well established that pulmonary alveolar proteinosis may develop after high exposure to a number of dusts, but there is no compelling reason to incriminate aluminum in this case report.

Potroom Asthma

An ill-defined and nonspecific form of airways obstruction has been reported in certain groups of potroom workers. This occurs relatively rarely and is completely absent in some aluminum plants. Whether it is a true form of asthma or industrial bronchitis is not definitely known. It has been suggested that the asthmatic symptoms may be a consequence of exposure to fluorides. Nevertheless, there is little doubt of increased evidence of chronic air flow limitation in potroom workers, which tends to worsen with continued exposure, so that by the end of the week a small decrement in lung function is often noted.

Antimony Pneumoconiosis

Antimony is a metal closely related to arsenic that has been used in the manufacture and plating of vases since the time of the Pharaohs. Antimony ore, before it can be used, has to be pulverized into a fine dust. A pneumoconiosis may develop in those workers, particularly at the furnace, who are exposed to the pulverized oxide. Although radiographic changes are present in the lung, pulmonary function does not seem to be affected, and similarly the lungs do not show any fibrosis.

Baritosis

The inhalation of barytes may induce a condition known as *baritosis*. Baritosis also has been described in the manufacture of lithopone, in which barytes is used. Some deposits of barytes are contaminated by significant concentrations of silica, and silicosis may be observed in such workers.

Baritosis is not associated with respiratory symptoms, but the radiographic appearances are quite striking. The deposits of barium appear as multiple, extremely dense, small, rounded opacities. Some radiographic clearing occurs with the passage of time.

Berylliosis

Beryllium is a rare metal. It is found in a number of naturally occurring minerals, of which beryl or beryllium aluminum silicate is the most important. Deposits of beryl are found in Argentina, Brazil, Zimbabwe, and South Africa. Beryllium is in demand as a metal that is often added to other metals to increase their tensile strength. It is nonmagnetic and transmits x-rays. It is frequently used in the manufacture of x-ray tubes as well as in the space program.

Two processes are used to extract beryllium from beryl. These are known as *sulfate* and *fluoride extractions*. The sulfate process involves melting beryl in an arc furnace at about 1700°C and pouring it through a high-velocity water jet to form frit. This is then treated with concentrated sulfuric acid and subsequently ammonia. Later, sodium hydroxide is added to form sodium beryllate, which is hydrolyzed so that beryllium hydroxide is precipitated. Beryllium hydroxide can be easily converted to metallic beryllium.

The fluoride process involves sintering in a rotating furnace a mixture of beryl sodium, silicofluoride, and soda ash. The sintered residue is pulverized, melted, and separated by leaching. Once again, sodium hydroxide is added and beryllium hydroxide is precipitated.

Exposure to beryllium can cause three conditions: dermatitis, acute pneumonitis, and chronic berylliosis.

Acute Berylliosis

The acute syndrome leads to the development of rhinitis, tracheitis, and pulmonary edema. The mucous membranes of the nose are swollen, ulceration may be present in the nasal mucosa, and septal perforation occasionally occurs. Tracheitis and bronchitis associated with a dry, irritative cough are common. When the exposure is severe, a chemical pneumonia develops and the subject becomes acutely short of breath; death is a frequent occurrence. Although many such cases were reported in the 1930s and 1940s, acute berylliosis has not been seen in North America for many years.

The subject with acute berylliosis is noted to be acutely short of breath, often with cyanosis and tachypnea, and in great distress. Crackles may be present all over the lungs. The chest x-ray film shows a bilateral acinous filling process with the appearance of noncardiogenic pulmonary edema. If the subject is capable of carrying out spirometry and other lung function tests, it will be observed that the lungs are stiff and that the patient has severe restrictive disease and a low diffusing capacity.

Treatment consists of giving supplementary oxygen and antibiotics to prevent secondary infection. In many instances, mechanical ventilation becomes necessary. Although steroids are given, usually in high doses, there is no conclusive evidence that they are of any use.

Subacute or Reversible Berylliosis

This entity has been described by Sprince and colleagues, who suggested that interstitial disease may develop in subjects exposed to high concentrations of beryllium that improves after the introduction of better ventilation and adequate industrial hygiene measures. Subacute berylliosis is a nebulous entity, and it remains somewhat unconvincing as a specific form of berylliosis.

Chronic Pulmonary Berylliosis

This condition was first described by Hardy and Tabershaw in 1946. It is a systemic disease associated with the development of granulomas throughout most of the body, but with a particular predilection for the lungs. Those initially affected were mainly involved in the manufacture of fluorescent bulbs for strip lighting; however, beryllium refineries now present the major hazard. Chronic berylliosis mainly develops in those working directly with beryllium, but there have been a few sporadic reports of berylliosis developing in wives of workers, presumably from beryllium dust brought home on their husbands' clothes. There also have been a number of so-called neighborhood cases, but most of these are not convincing. A latent period from first exposure to the development of the condition ranges from 2 or 3 to 15 to 20 years. Berylliosis is now a rare condition, but sporadic cases still occur, mainly resulting from exposure many years ago.

Clinical Features

Although most persons in whom the condition develops are currently working with beryllium, in a few cases it appears many years after exposure has ceased. This emphasizes the need for a detailed occupational history. The presenting symptoms are usually shortness of breath and a dry cough. Both are progressive and unremitting. Occasionally, skin lesions are also present. Physical examination usually reveals tachypnea and a small tidal volume. In the initial stages, few if any crackles are heard. With the passage of time, usually several years, and the development of fibrosis, crackles become evident. Initially, weight loss and fatigue are frequently present.

Berylliosis closely resembles sarcoidosis, and most of the features seen in the latter condition are common to both. Thus, lymphadenopathy occurs in both conditions, although generalized lymphadenopathy is much less frequent in berylliosis. Berylliosis, however, seldom presents without both parenchymal changes and hilar adenopathy. Hilar adenopathy by itself is rare. Granulomatous skin lesions are seen in both berylliosis and sarcoidosis, but the deforming facial rash leading to scarring that occasionally appears in sarcoidosis does not occur in berylliosis. Hepatosplenomegaly is present in both diseases, but parotid enlargement and cystlike bone changes are not seen in berylliosis. Renal involvement, including both nephrocalcinosis and hypocalcemia, occurs in both conditions. In contrast, the development of meningeal symptoms, peripheral neuropathy, and myocarditis indicates that the condition is likely to be sarcoidosis, and this is also true for uveitis and uveoparotid fever. Berylliosis does not seem to affect tuberculin reactivity. Similarly, spontaneous remission, although common in sarcoidosis, is extremely rare in berylliosis. Abnormalities of the plasma proteins occur in both sarcoidosis and berylliosis and do not help to distinguish them. Gamma globulin production is predominantly affected, and the IgG fraction is often elevated. It is also elevated in beryllium workers who have no evidence of berylliosis. As the disease progresses, the patient becomes more and more short of breath, the lungs become increasingly stiff, and the classic signs of cor pulmonale are noted. Pneumothorax may occur from bleb formation, and right ventricular hypertrophy is evident. The disease tends to progress slowly, and survival times of 15 to 20 years are frequent.

Radiographic Features

The most common radiographic presentation is one of miliary mottling, similar to that seen in miliary tuberculosis. Hilar adenopathy is distinctly uncommon. Large, blotchy, coalescent infiltrates resembling those seen in sarcoidosis also occur, and uncommonly, nodular infiltrates similar to those seen in nodular sarcoidosis may be observed. Gradually, the lungs become small, and the typical features of reticulonodulation and interstitial fibrosis develop along with honeycombing.

Pulmonary Function

Abnormalities typical of diffuse fibrosis are found—that is, stiff lungs and restrictive impairment. These abnormalities are entirely nonspecific. Obstruction does not occur except terminally, when minor degrees may be present. It has also been suggested that long-term exposure to beryllium is associated with the gradual reduction in pulmonary function. Such reductions are said to occur in workers who have no radiographic abnormalities. Moreover, it has been suggested that the alveolar-arterial oxygen difference gradually increases with cumulative exposure after controlling for age and smoking. The evidence for this, however, is tenuous and unconvincing.

Other Diagnostic Tests

In 1951, Curtis described a beryllium patch test. Results are usually positive in chronic berylliosis, but there is good evidence that its use may lead to a flare-up of the chronic pulmonary berylliosis. Metallic beryllium cannot be used for skin testing, and the patch test is best carried out by applying to the skin a piece of filter paper soaked in beryllium fluoride, sulfate, or nitrate. The Kveim test result is negative in berylliosis.

Tissue biopsy and spectrographic analysis of specimens for beryllium are not helpful. Increased levels are found in the tissues of most healthy workers in a beryllium refinery. This is true for the lungs only if exposure has been relatively recent, as beryllium is rapidly removed from the lungs and deposited in the bones and liver. It may be present in increased amounts in the urine, but usually only if the subject is currently exposed. Thus, analysis of tissue specimens cannot confirm the presence of disease. On the other hand, a lung biopsy specimen may have a normal beryllium content despite the presence of chronic berylliosis.

Pathology

Chronic berylliosis is characterized by the presence of noncaseating granulomas indistinguishable from those found in sarcoidosis. Eventually, as time goes by, the granulomas become organized and fibrotic. Blebs may develop late in the course of the disease, and these are frequently associated with some pleural thickening.

A number of cellular responses have been described following experimental exposure to beryllium. The alveolar macrophages take up beryllium particles by phagocytosis and in doing so are damaged and release lysosomal enzymes. Any beryllium deposited in the alveoli is cleared relatively slowly. Initially, macrophage activity is decreased, but subsequently activity rebounds and increases. There is also evidence that macrophages sequester beryllium in the lung and in doing so become more active, with resultant damage to the lung.

Treatment

In general, steroids are administered when the condition is diagnosed, but there is no convincing evidence that they have ever produced a cure. Usually, the subject is started on a high dose of prednisone (e.g., 75 mg/d), and this is gradually tapered to a maintenance dose of about 10 to 20 mg. The patient is best followed by serial tests of pulmonary function.

Pathogenesis

All the evidence presently available suggests that berylliosis is a hypersensitivity disease characterized by a cell-mediated immune response to beryllium. Differentiation between sarcoidosis and berylliosis is difficult. Marx and Burrell have suggested that lymphocytotoxins can be demonstrated in the cells of sensitized but not of unsensitized subjects. Production of migration inhibitory factor (MIF) has likewise been noted. The cellular and immune mechanisms of berylliosis were later studied by Deodhar and co-workers. They investigated blast transformation of lymphocytes in subjects with berylliosis. About 60% of their subjects showed this phenomenon, to which severity of disease appeared to be related. They found that the serum IgA level was elevated in about half their subjects, but in this their findings differed from those of Resnick and associates, who noted that the IgG fraction was increased.

A beryllium lymphocyte transformation test has been developed and has been used with some success in the diagnosis of berylliosis. Bronchoalveolar lavage also has been carried out in subjects with berylliosis, and the proportion of bronchoalveolar T cells has been noted to be increased.

The evidence currently available suggests a cell-mediated response to the inhalation of beryllium takes place that includes the following:

1. Microscopic features in the lungs and lymph nodes similar to those seen in other cell-mediated reactions
2. Skin sensitivity reactions
3. Blast transformation and MIF production from lymphocytes

4. Selective stimulation of T lymphocytes
5. Transfer in animal models of cutaneous sensitivity by lymphocytes but not by serum

Prevention

Dust control is of the utmost importance in preventing berylliosis. The present standard recommends that exposure should not exceed 2 g/m^3 of air during an 8-hour period. Whether this is entirely effective in the prevention of chronic berylliosis is unknown, as most of the evidence suggests that the condition is related to hypersensitivity. Although pre-employment and periodic medical examinations, including serial radiography and lung function tests, are recommended, there is no evidence to suggest that they are of any benefit in this disease, as the condition tends to come on rapidly and progress despite separation from exposure. Educating workers about the symptoms of chronic berylliosis and how to avoid exposure would seem to be much more effective methods of prevention.

Graphite and Carbon Pneumoconiosis

Graphite is a form of carbon and is also known as *plumbago* or *black lead*. It is mined or extracted in Austria, the former U.S.S.R., Sri Lanka, Norway, and Korea. Usually, it is found in veins that traverse igneous rocks. It occurs naturally in three forms: lump, amorphous, and flake. The latter is usually extracted by strip mining. Many deposits of graphite are contaminated by free silica, usually in low concentrations.

Graphite is used in the manufacture of steel and in lubricants, lead pencils, nuclear reactors, and electrodes. Because it also conducts electricity, it is often used in generator brushes. It was at one time used in the printing industry for duplicating plates.

It is now clear that inhalation of pure carbon may induce radiographic and pathologic changes indistinguishable from those associated with inhalation of coal. In some instances, the lung bases have been described as showing a fine reticulation, but more generally this disease appears as the typical nodulation seen in simple CWP. PMF likewise can occur. The pulmonary function abnormalities are similar to those seen in CWP.

Hematite Pneumoconiosis (Silicosiderosis) and Other Mixed-Dust Fibroses

Although iron oxide has been known for many years to produce a condition known as *siderosis*, it is also evident that a lung condition associated with radiographic changes may develop in iron miners. However, iron miners are not exposed to pure iron oxide, but to a mixture of dusts, often with a fair amount of free silica present.

The condition that occurs in iron miners is usually known as *silicosiderosis* and has been described in Cumbria in Britain, Germany, Bergamo in Italy, and Alsace-Lorraine. It seldom develops without at least 10 years of exposure.

The best pathologic description of the condition was given by Stewart and Faulds, who noted a diffuse rather than nodular fibrosis, although if the proportion of silica was high, then the latter type of fibrosis often occurred. The whole lung was noted to be brick red in color, with associated areas of focal emphysema. Radiographically, diffuse fibrosis appeared to predominate. Massive fibrotic lesions also were seen and were usually situated in the same regions of the lung in which conglomerate silicosis and PMF occur. As in the other two conditions, these fibrotic masses encroach on the blood and bronchial supply of the affected area. They also may undergo cavitation, either from ischemic necrosis or secondary tuberculous infection. Microscopically, aggregated particles of hematite and silica are seen lying in the alveolar walls. The lesions are situated in the same areas of the acinus that are primarily affected by silicosis, and peribronchiolar and periarteriolar fibrosis are common. Whorled nodules may be seen, especially along the lymphatic vessels. A fair amount of dense collagenous fibrosis is present, usually in association with the typical nodules of silicosis.

There is good evidence that cancer of the lung occurs more frequently in Cumbrian iron miners. Most of the evidence, however, suggests that the increase is related to radon daughters rather than to any inherent carcinogenic property of iron oxide. The symptoms of the condition are very similar to those of silicosis. The presence of iron in the inhaled dust leads to a situation in which, for a given cumulative dust exposure, radiographic abnormalities appear somewhat more rapidly than they would in workers exposed to other dusts containing free silica. A relatively similar condition can also develop in ochre miners.

A mixed-dust fibrosis is commonly seen in foundry welders and burners as well as in boiler scalers. These workers likewise are exposed to a mixture of iron, silica, and other dusts. Iron, with its high atomic number, tends to produce radiographic changes, and such changes are frequent in foundry workers. There is, however, an absence of significant fibrosis. Boiler scalers, on the other hand, are often exposed to dust containing a high content of free silica, and there is a tendency for a condition more closely resembling silicosis to develop.

Labrador Lung

An unusual form of mixed-dust pneumoconiosis known as *Labrador lung* has been described in the iron miners of West Labrador. These miners are exposed to iron, silica, and some anthophyllite. Lung biopsies have demonstrated increased amounts of iron and silica in the lungs and, in addition, a number of ferruginous bodies. The histologic appearances are frequently modified by the presence of anthophyllite.

Polyvinyl Chloride Pneumoconiosis

The manufacture of polyvinyl chloride (PVC) leads to the production of a varying number of respirable dust particles. When administered to animals, PVC may lead to bronchiolitis, some alveolitis, and the formation of granulomas. During the past 10 to 15 years, radiographic changes have developed in a number of subjects working with PVC. Many of these individual case reports have been far from convincing, but a number of epidemiologic surveys have demonstrated that PVC pneumoconiosis indeed exists.

PVC pneumoconiosis was first described in 1970 by Szende and associates. A number of studies have been carried out since Szende's description suggesting that radiographic changes take place. Other studies have indicated that respiratory symptoms and pulmonary impairment may occur. A well-designed study of a large group of workers exposed to PVC was published in 1980, showing a minimal increase in respiratory symptoms in those most heavily exposed and a similar minimal effect on the FVC and FEV$_1$. The radiographic changes, however, were subtle and consisted of small, scanty, rounded opacities. Pathologic changes in this condition indicated that there may be infiltration of the lung parenchyma with histiocytes and a few multinucleated giant cells, and, rarely, a little collagenous fibrosis may be seen. Macrophages migrate into the tissue and many contain PVC particles.

Shale Pneumoconiosis

Shale deposits are found in many parts of the world, in particular in the Midwest of the United States, Alberta in Canada, and to a lesser extent Scotland. Such deposits are a known source of oil. Shale consists largely of silicates, including a fair proportion of kaolin and mica. Either simple or complicated pneumoconiosis may develop in shale miners. The pathology resembles either CWP or kaolin pneumoconiosis. The simple form of the disease has little effect on lung function, but the complicated pneumoconiosis of shale workers leads to both restrictive and obstructive impairment, as is seen in CWP.

Siderosis (Arc Welders' Lung)

Siderosis was first described by Zenker in the late nineteenth century. Both his subjects had tuberculosis, and the fibrosis he noted was probably related to the infection rather than to the inhaled iron. Siderosis is caused by the deposition of iron in the lungs, usually in the form of iron oxide. It occurs in arc welders, oxyacetylene cutters, silver finishers, and magnetite pulverizers. During oxyacetylene cutting and arc welding, the iron that is being cut or welded melts and then boils from the heat of the arc or torch. This leads to the emission of fine particles of ferrous oxide, which on contact with the air are immediately oxidized to ferric oxide. They appear as bluish-gray fumes. Most of the particles present in these fumes are respirable, with many being submicronic in size. Prolonged inhalation and deposition of welding fumes leads to the development of siderosis, a condition characterized by radiographic changes somewhat similar to those seen in silicosis.

Silver finishers use a preparation (''jeweler's rouge'') to polish their products. Jeweler's rouge consists of iron oxide and is applied to the finished product with a buffer; this creates an aerosol of small iron and silver particles. Prolonged inhalation of such particles leads to a condition known as *argyrosiderosis*.

Welders' Siderosis

Welders' siderosis was first described in 1936 by Doig and McLaughlin. The weight of the evidence suggests that provided only iron oxide is inhaled, the condition is not associated with symptoms and does not lead to fibrosis. Morbidity and mortality statistics from the United States and Britain do not indicate any increased morbidity or mortality among welders other than from lung cancer. However, they do indicate that welders may be more prone to pneumonia and, in addition, frequently have metal fume fever. Nevertheless, sporadic case reports through the years have suggested that welding induces fibrosis and other problems. In certain instances, the welding has been reported to be associated with the development of restrictive impairment and pulmonary fibrosis, whereas in others it has been claimed that it leads to airways obstruction and emphysema. In none of these subjects was there any smoking history or were there any data regarding other exposures. The case reports of Charr described symptomatic welders at the Philadelphia shipyards, and the somewhat inadequate description of the pathology and the few photomicrographs available suggest that these men almost certainly had asbestosis. In fact, in one photomicrograph there appears to be an asbestos body. It must be recalled, however, that at that time it was not known that persons other than miners and millers were at risk for asbestosis. The subject described by Meyer and colleagues, although a nonsmoker, had been a sandblaster, and despite the presence of vast quantities of silica in his lungs, along with massive fibrosis, his disease was attributed to welding. This is not to say that all constituents of welding rods are harmless in all circumstances. The rods and other materials with which welders work contain carbon, manganese, aluminum, sili-

cates, and free silica. Arc welders also may be exposed to ozone, especially if they weld aluminum. Oxyacetylene cutters similarly may cut through cadmium-containing metal and thus be exposed to cadmium fumes.

In regard to the general health of welders, as already mentioned, they seem more prone to pneumonia and metal fume fever. The latter is a well-recognized cause of temporary morbidity. There also seems to be an excess risk for lung cancer that cannot entirely be accounted for by social class and smoking habits. However, many welders, including those studied by Beaumont and Weiss, have worked exclusively or for a long time in shipyards and thereby have had significant exposure to asbestos. Asbestosis is a well-recognized complication of shipyard welding.

Pathology

The pathologic effects of iron on the lung were first described by Harding and colleagues from autopsy findings of four arc welders and an oxyacetylene cutter. One of their subjects had coincident exposure to silica, and there was evidence of a mixed-dust fibrosis. The oxyacetylene cutter, however, showed no fibrosis. When fibrosis was found in the other subjects, it was not related to the deposition of iron oxide but to the other constituents of welding fumes or to other occupational exposures. Similar studies of silver polishers have shown an absence of fibrosis. Experiments in which animals have been exposed to the inhalation of iron have likewise failed to reveal any fibrosis.

The results of lung biopsies in seven welders described by Morgan and Kerr showed that although some of the iron lay free in the alveoli and respiratory bronchioles, most had been taken up by the macrophages and some could be seen in the lymphatic vessels. Fibrosis was entirely absent, except in the one subject who had had a mixed-dust exposure. An analysis of a portion of one subject's lung revealed an iron content 15 times greater than the normal level. Despite this, absolutely no fibrosis was present in the sections (Figs. 14 and 15).

A number of retrospective studies have been published purporting to show that welding fumes cause fibrosis. Of the 3600 cases referred to Liebow, nearly all of which were subjects with pulmonary fibrosis, it was possible to select 29 who were welders and who had fibrosis. No fewer than 14 were reported by Liebow as showing fibrosing alveolitis. Unfortunately, some have assumed that these cases are representative of welders as a whole, and this is clearly not the case. Others have assumed that low concentrations of the oxides of nitrogen induce pulmonary fibrosis, again with no scientific basis.

Radiographic Features

Radiographically, the lungs are characterized by small, rounded opacities widely distributed throughout both lung

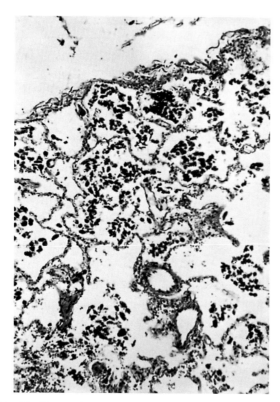

FIG. 14. Photomicrograph of a lung biopsy section taken from a welder. Note the absence of septal thickening and the pigment in the alveoli. Most of the latter is present in alveolar macrophages.

fields. The preponderance in the upper zones that occurs in silicosis is not usually evident. Moreover, the shadows tend to be somewhat smaller and of the *q* type rather than of the *r* type commonly observed in silicosis. Conglomeration can occur, but when it does, it is usually because of coincident exposure to silica (Fig. 16). Postmortem studies of the contaminants of the lung add little useful information other than giving an idea of the agents to which the welder was exposed during life. Serial observations of welders who have ceased exposure have shown that in certain instances the radiographic appearances tend to improve.

Pulmonary Function

Siderosis when not associated with the inhalation of other harmful agents is not related to significant pulmonary impairment. This is evident from the studies of Morgan and Kerr, who measured all aspects of pulmonary function except the diffusing capacity. Values obtained during subsequent measurements of the diffusing capacity were within normal limits. Stanescu and co-workers studied the pulmonary mechanics of a group of 16 welders who had abnormal radiographic findings. They were compared with a group of 13 unexposed healthy men. When certain of the more sophisticated parameters of lung me-

chanics were measured, including static and dynamic compliance of the lungs, values were slightly reduced. The minor abnormalities noted, however, do not cause symptoms.

A number of well-controlled epidemiologic studies of the respiratory status of welders have been carried out. These, for the most part, have shown that welding may be associated with a slight increase in airways obstruction, but this is present only in those welders who are smokers. There is also evidence that welders tend to smoke more often than does the general population.

General Health Effects of Welding

The biologic effects of exposure to welding fumes have generated considerable discussion during the past three to four decades. A fair number of articles have been published purporting to show that welding is a dangerous occupation associated with a number of conditions, ranging from lung cancer to dementia and motor neuron disease. The real and imaginary hazards of welding have been reviewed in detail.

The recognized and accepted hazards of welding can

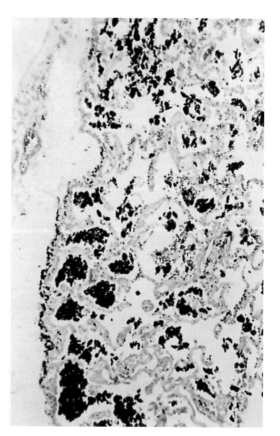

FIG. 15. Photomicrograph of a different section of the same lung as in Fig. 14, but on this occasion stained with Prussian blue. Note again the absence of fibrosis and the heavily stained deposits of iron, which appear intensely blue when viewed under the microscope.

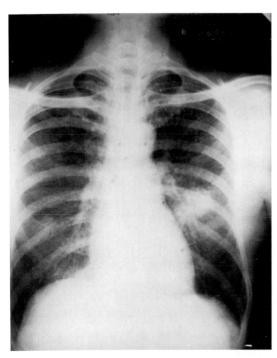

FIG. 16. Chest radiograph of a welder showing welders' siderosis. A large shadow is present in the left middle zone. The subject had a prior exposure to a number of mixed dusts, including some silica.

be grouped under (1) acute effects, (2) chronic toxic effects, (3) chronic respiratory effects, and (4) carcinogenic effects.

Acute Effects

A number of agents to which welders are exposed may produce acute effects. These include ozone, the oxides of nitrogen, cadmium fumes, phosgene, and metal fumes. There is little doubt that in exceptional circumstances all can be a respiratory hazard, and the effects of each are described elsewhere. Suffice it to say that exposure to the oxides of nitrogen does occur occasionally in welders working in confined spaces and has been noted in coal mines and elsewhere. Acute exposure to cadmium leading to the development of pulmonary edema and subsequently to emphysema also has been described. Metal fume fever is a recognized complication of welding and oxyacetylene cutting. It is entirely benign.

Chronic Toxic Effects

These occur as a result of exceptional circumstances. Manganese poisoning associated with central nervous system involvement has been described in the former East Germany and eastern Europe, but never in the West. Exposure to fluorides, lead, and various trace elements likewise may occur, but no reports of toxic effects from expo-

sures to these agents have appeared in the last 10 to 15 years.

Chronic Respiratory Effects

A number of chronic respiratory effects may occur as a result of welding. First and of most importance is welders' siderosis. This has already been described in detail.

There is a suggestion that cough and production of sputum are greater in welders than in a comparable general population. Although part of this may be explained by the fact that welders smoke more, little doubt exists that exposure to welding fumes leads to mild chronic bronchitis that is not associated with any significant pulmonary impairment.

Carcinogenic Effects

Evidence is fairly good that welders as a whole have a slightly greater risk for lung cancer than does the general population. Part of this can be explained by the fact that welders smoke more than does the general population; however, a significant proportion of welders have worked or still work in shipyards and have done so for many years. As such, these workers have been exposed to asbestos, and overt asbestosis has developed in many of them. The combination of excess smoking and exposure to asbestos almost certainly accounts for the increased incidence of malignant respiratory disease.

Silver Polishers' Lung

Silver polishers' lung differs from siderosis in that although silver polishers use iron oxide while buffing silver, the buffing tends to aerosolize both silver and iron oxide particles. As a result, inhaled iron and silver are both deposited in the lungs, and the lungs appear black at autopsy because of staining with silver. No physiologic abnormalities occur in this condition.

Magnetite and Limonite Pneumoconiosis

Radiologic changes similar to those seen in siderosis have been described in workers exposed to magnetite and limonite. The appearances radiographically resemble siderosis, and respiratory impairment has not been observed.

Stannosis

Tin is an important metal that is used frequently to form alloys. Both the Phoenicians and the Carthaginians traded with the inhabitants of Cornwall for the tin that was mined there. In the Middle Ages, most of the tin that was mined came from Cornwall, Saxony, and Bohemia, but at the present time, Malaysia, Bolivia, Zaïre, and Australia are the main sources. Although some tin is extracted by underground mining, in Malaysia the deposits are on the surface. Most Cornish tin mines are now closed down. Cornish miners, however, were not afflicted with stannosis, but rather with silicosis. The seams were usually located about 1000 ft below the surface, and the adjacent rock that had to be removed before reaching the seam frequently contained large amounts of free silica. Hookworm infection also was a problem. In Malaysia, tin is usually removed by open-cast mining.

The inhalation of tin oxide leads to a benign pneumoconiosis not associated with symptoms or respiratory impairment. Most of the subjects in whom the condition develops are involved in the bagging of concentrated oxide or in the smelting operation. During smelting, hot fumes are emitted that contain submicronic particles of tin. These are inhaled and lead to the development of stannosis.

The radiographic appearances of stannosis are so distinctive that it is difficult to confuse it with other conditions. The high atomic number of tin makes the opacities very dense, even denser than those noted in welders' siderosis and almost as dense as those noted in baritosis (Figs. 17 and 18).

Pathologically, blackish or grayish macules are widely distributed throughout the lungs. Gross pigmentation of the interlobular septa is frequent. The foci of dust are composed of dust-laden macrophages containing tin oxide

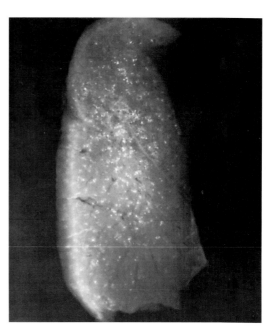

FIG. 18. Radiograph of a large lung section from a subject with stannosis. Death was caused by carcinoma of the prostate, not by stannosis.

and other agents. Focal emphysema occurs but is not as prominent as in CWP. Fibrosis does not occur.

Thesaurosis

Bergmann and colleagues in 1958 described several subjects with a chronic pulmonary disease that they termed *thesaurosis* or *storage disease*. They were generally young women exposed to hair spray, and Bergmann and associates attributed the condition to the inhalation of polyvinylpyrrolidone (PVP), a major constituent of hair sprays. Following their description, a series of subjects with so-called thesaurosis was described. Unfortunately, those who described thesaurosis seemed unfamiliar with Koch's postulates and certainly did not apply them when they weighed the evidence regarding the existence of this entity. In reality, the subjects described appeared to have sarcoidosis. Subsequent epidemiologic studies have provided absolutely no evidence that cosmetologists are at increased risk for the development of any lung condition other than chronic bronchitis and emphysema. The latter is related to the fact that the prevalence of smoking is exceedingly high in this trade.

Tungsten Carbide Pneumoconiosis (Hard Metal Disease) and Related Syndromes

Although the term *hard metal disease* is in common use, the available evidence at the present time suggests that it is not the tungsten carbide that leads to the respira-

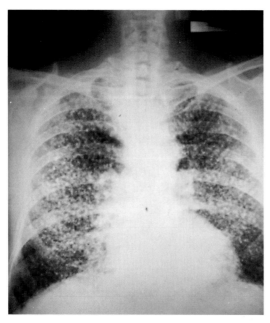

FIG. 17. Chest radiograph of a subject with stannosis. Tin oxide, having a high atomic number, shows up as intensely radiopaque deposits.

tory problems seen in hard metal workers, but rather the cobalt that is almost invariably present. Cobalt is frequently added to various alloys to increase their tensile strength. Hard metal is produced by metallurgic compounding of tungsten and carbon, with cobalt being added as a binder. Tungsten carbide, or hard metal, is extremely hard, second only to diamonds, and is used for cutting metals. It is particularly useful in the manufacture of dental drills.

Tungsten carbide is prepared by compounding extremely fine particles of tungsten and carbon. These particles are at the smaller range of the respirable fraction and are about 1 to 2 μm in size. The tungsten carbide mixture is then milled with the addition of between 3% and 25% cobalt. The tiny, hard metal crystals are deposited in the cobalt. Paraffin is added to provide body before the metal is pressed into ingots. The ingots are then sintered into hard metal, and the resultant tool is subsequently shaped as desired. Three respiratory diseases are produced by the inhalation of cobalt. These are (1) allergic alveolitis; (2) pulmonary fibrosis, or what is commonly called *hard metal disease;* and (3) a form of asthma.

In 1940, Jobs and Ballhausen noted that in a group of 27 German workers, abnormal chest radiographs developed in eight. A fine reticulonodulation was present. Subsequently, in an examination of 696 hard metal workers, Moschinski and colleagues found a high prevalence of bronchitis. Radiographic evidence of pneumoconiosis was found in a smaller percentage. Fairhall and associates surveyed 2000 tungsten carbide workers shortly after World War II and found that conjunctivitis, rhinitis, tracheitis, and bronchitis were frequent. In addition, pruritus and cobalt sensitivity occurred.

Cobalt-Allergic Alveolitis or Interstitial Pneumonitis

A description by Sjögren and colleagues of a syndrome similar to extrinsic allergic alveolitis in four subjects made it clear that an acute and reversible disease is induced by exposure to cobalt. All of Sjögren's subjects were grinders of hard metal, and symptoms and signs compatible with transient hypersensitivity pneumonitis developed in all. After an absence from work, the symptoms improved, the radiographic changes resolved, and the respiratory impairment decreased or in some instances resolved entirely.

The premonitory symptoms were cough, low-grade fever, muscle aches and pains, and generalized constitutional symptoms. These symptoms would often lead the subject to take several days off from work, during which time the symptoms would improve, only to recur on return to work. Medical examination during the acute phase would reveal basal crackles, low-grade fever, and in some subjects contact dermatitis. Of the four subjects described by Sjögren and colleagues, all had positive patch test

results. Of particular interest, it was shown that during the grinding, small particles of cobalt were disseminated in the air and dissolved in the coolants used to cool the metal being ground. Subsequently, when the coolant was applied during the grinding process, it became aerosolized, and the worker would inhale the aerosolized coolant containing large quantities of cobalt. It appears that the cobalt was very soluble in the particular coolants used. The pathology of this condition shows an alveolitis with marked response of type II pneumocytes. Frequently, there is a granulomatous reaction with giant cells present. With repeated exposures, the granulomatous pneumonitis slowly evolves into interstitial fibrosis.

Interstitial Fibrosis (Hard Metal Disease)

An excellent description of the clinical features of hard metal disease is that of Coates and Watson. These workers described 12 subjects with diffuse interstitial lung disease, of whom no fewer than eight died. The symptoms included cough, which was usually dry but occasionally productive of some scanty mucoid symptoms. Later, breathlessness developed that became progressively worse. On examination, the subjects had tachypnea and frequently clubbing of the digits. Basal crackles developed late in the condition. Lung function tests showed restrictive impairment, arterial desaturation, and a low diffusing capacity. With the passage of time, pulmonary hypertension developed, usually on the basis of hypoxemia, and eventually overt cor pulmonale appeared.

The disease was seldom seen without at least 10 years of exposure, but in retrospect, some subjects were found to have had repeated flare-ups of minor constitutional symptoms, suggesting recurrent attacks of interstitial pneumonitis.

Radiographically, the disease presents initially as a fine reticulonodular pattern in the middle and lower zones, with the nodules sometimes being quite large. As the disease progresses, the characteristic features of interstitial fibrosis are noted, and honeycombing may eventually result.

Although the radiograph usually suggests diffuse involvement, on biopsy or at autopsy the fibrosis may be seen to be distributed in a patchy fashion. The interstitial tissue is often infiltrated with histiocytes and plasma cells. The alveolar septa may be thickened. In a few instances, fibrosis may be associated with a granulomatous reaction and the presence of giant cells. The latter are found particularly frequently in this condition, and some believe they are almost pathognomonic. The alveoli contain what are assumed to be desquamated type II alveolar pneumocytes. Electron microscopy reveals the deposition of collagen and elastic tissue in the septa and the presence of multifaceted crystals thought to be tungsten carbide. In one series of subjects with interstitial pneumonitis and hard metal disease, a nongranulomatous process was described characterized by intra-alveolar exudate and some interstitial reaction. Bronchoalveolar lavage showed bizarre giant forms of the alveolar macrophage (Fig. 19).

Airways Obstruction or Asthma

Some subjects with interstitial pneumonitis may also have wheezing, cough, and shortness of breath. Such symptoms also occur in the absence of interstitial pneumonia. The symptoms tend to occur while at work. In most instances, they disappear on the weekends. When subjects return to work on Monday, they remain relatively free of symptoms until late in the afternoon, when symptoms recur. Once the symptoms have appeared, they usually slowly become more severe through the week, only to improve at the weekends. Most subjects with this type of response leave their jobs voluntarily. Those affected also may have itching and skin manifestations resulting from exposure to cobalt. Results of challenge studies with cobalt, but not tungsten, usually are positive, but not invariably so.

Treatment

There is no treatment for established hard metal disease characterized by extensive fibrosis. In contrast, the interstitial pneumonitis usually responds well to steroids and to separation from further exposure to cobalt. It will, however, recur should the subject return to work. Protective devices such as masks are seldom effective.

Etiology

Although a few persons still believe that tungsten carbide rather than cobalt may be responsible, the vast weight of evidence incriminates cobalt. Harding showed that powdered cobalt is toxic in animals, and it did not matter whether it was administered intratracheally or by inhalation. He also demonstrated that the metal was much more soluble in plasma than in saline solution. In contrast, tungsten carbide, when given to animals, is inert. Likewise, Harding was able to induce both an alveolitis and subsequently pulmonary fibrosis. Delahant was able to induce chronic bronchiolitis and metaplastic changes in alveoli with pulverized cobalt, but he failed to do so when he used tungsten carbide, titanium, and tantalum. Single exposures to cobalt during a short period induced granulomatous pneumonitis and bronchiolitis, but if exposures were continued for longer, interstitial fibrosis developed. The fact that cobalt is soluble explains why it may be completely absent in many biopsy specimens obtained from humans. There is little doubt that it is deposited in the lungs, but it is rapidly removed, and lung biopsy 1 month to 6 weeks later may show a normal cobalt content.

Miscellaneous Pneumoconioses

A number of miscellaneous pneumoconioses have been described. Most are of little clinical import. Nonetheless, when faced with a subject who has radiographic abnormalities, it is imperative to take a complete occupational history. Rare earths may induce pneumoconiosis, and cerium oxide is a recognized cause of radiographic abnormalities. Titanium likewise produces radiographic abnor-

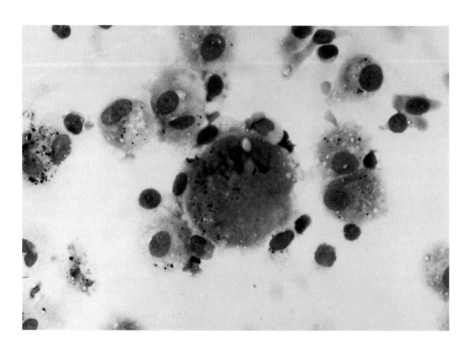

FIG. 19. Photomicrograph of bronchoalveolar lavage fluid showing a characteristic multinucleated giant cell with cytoplasmic vacuoles. Particulate matter is also present along with alveolar macrophages. Patient had hard metal disease.

malities, but no associated pulmonary impairment. The same is true of zirconium. Finally, it is important to remember that the esoteric habits of the "lunatic fringe" occasionally lead to the development of radiographic abnormalities and pulmonary impairment. Thus, the development of pulmonary fibrosis in a drug-snorting fire eater who played in a punk rock band serves to emphasize the importance of studying both avocation and vocation.

BIBLIOGRAPHY

Abrahamson MJ, et al. Does aluminum smelting cause lung disease? *Am Rev Respir Dis* 1989;139:242. *A relatively recent review of the literature relating to aluminum smelting and its possible hazards.*

Caplan A. Certain unusual radiological appearances in the chests of coal miners suffering from rheumatoid arthritis. *Thorax* 1953;8: 29. *The original description of Caplan's syndrome or rheumatoid pneumoconiosis.*

Carpenter RG, Cochrane AL, Clark WG, Jonathan G, Moore F. Death rates of miners and ex-miners with and without coal workers' pneumoconiosis in South Wales. *Brit J Ind Med* 1956;13:102. *A classic study of the effects of coal dust CWP on morbidity and mortality.*

Coates EO Jr, Watson JHL. Diffuse interstitial lung disease in tungsten carbide workers. *Ann Intern Med* 1971;75:709. *An early review of the clinical presentation of hard metal disease, emphasizing the airways effects.*

Cugell DA, et al. The respiratory effects of cobalt. *Arch Intern Med* 1990;150:177. *A more recent clinical description along with recent pathologic and radiologic correlations.*

Demedst M. Respiratory diseases from hard metal or cobalt exposure. *Chest* 1989;95:29. *The proof that cobalt rather than tungsten carbide is the pathologic agent.*

Doig AT, McLaughlin AIG. X-ray appearances of the lungs of arc-welders. *Lancet* 1936;1:771. *The original description of arc welders' lung or welders' siderosis.*

Goralewski G. Die Aluminiumlunge-eine neue Gewerbeerkrankung. *Z Gesamte Inn Med* 1947;2:665. *The original clinical description of aluminum-induced pulmonary fibrosis.*

Hardy HL, Tabershaw IR. Delayed chemical pneumonitis occurring in workers exposed to beryllium compounds. *J Ind Hyg Toxicol* 1946;28:197. *The first description of berylliosis.*

Jobs H, Ballhausen C. Powder metallurgy as a source of dust from the medical and technical standpoint. *Vertrauensartz Krankenkasse* 1940;8:142. *The original description of hard metal disease.*

Kriebel D, et al. The pulmonary toxicity of beryllium. *Am Rev Respir Dis* 1988;137:464. *The most complete recent review of the pathogenesis and effects of berylliosis.*

Lapp NL, Morgan WKC, Zaldivar G. Airways obstruction, coal mining, and disability. *Occup Environ Med* 1994;51:234. *A review of a large number of U.S. coal miners claiming pulmonary disability. The relationship of airways obstruction to radiographic category of CWP, cigarette smoking, and other factors is described. The data illustrate the rarity of significant chronic air flow limitation in the absence of complicated CWP and smoking.*

Liddell FDK, May JD. *Assessing the Radiological Progression of Simple Coal Workers' Pneumoconiosis.* London: National Coal Board Medical Services; 1966. *The original monograph describing the extended International Labor Office classification of the pneumoconioses. The 12-point classification made it possible to determine accurately the attack rate and rate of progression of CWP and thereby enable appropriate dust standards to be formulated.*

McMillan GHG. The health of welders in naval dockyards: welding, tobacco smoking and absence attributed to respiratory disease. *J Soc Occup Med* 1981;31:112. *An excellent review of respiratory morbidity in welders.*

Meiklejohn A. History of lung disease in coal miners in Great Britain. Part 1. 1800–1875. *Brit J Ind Med* 1951;8:127. Part II. 1875– 1920. *Brit J Ind Med* 1952;9:93. Part III. 1920–1952. *Brit J Ind Med* 1952;9:208. *A complete history of lung disease in coal miners throughout the ages. Relevant not only to British coal miners but to coal miners throughout the world.*

Morgan WKC. Industrial bronchitis and other nonspecific conditions affecting the airways. In: Morgan WKC, Seaton A, eds. *Occupational Lung Diseases.* 3rd ed. Philadelphia: WB Saunders; 1995: 503–523. *A recent review of the role of dusts, fumes, and gases in the induction of occupationally related bronchitis.*

Morgan WKC. On welding, wheezing and whimsy. *Am Ind Hyg Assoc J* 1989;50:59. *General health effects of welding.*

Morgan WKC. Other pneumoconioses. In: Morgan WKC, Seaton A, eds. *Occupational Lung Diseases.* 3rd ed. Philadelphia: WB Saunders; 1995. *Description of two rare pneumoconioses with reproductions of radiographs.*

Morgan WKC. Other pneumoconioses. In: Morgan WKC, Seaton A. *Occupational Lung Diseases.* 3rd ed. Philadelphia: WB Saunders; 1995. *Description of uncommon and often unrecognized pneumoconioses.*

Morgan WKC. Other pneumoconioses. In: Morgan WKC, Seaton A, eds. *Occupational Lung Diseases.* 3rd ed. Philadelphia: WB Saunders; 1995. *Composite review of the clinical, radiographic, and pathologic findings of hematite pneumoconiosis.*

Morgan WKC. Other pneumoconioses. In: Morgan WKC, Seaton A, eds. *Occupational Lung Diseases.* 3rd ed. Philadelphia: WB Saunders; 1995. *A history of stannosis with illustrations of the pathologic and radiologic features.*

Morgan WKC, Dinman BD. Pulmonary effects of aluminum. In: Gitelman NJ, ed. *Aluminum and Health: a Critical Review.* New York: Marcel Dekker; 1989:203–234. *A complete review of the effects of aluminum on the lung. The mechanism and etiology of pulmonary fibrosis and its relationship to aluminum dust, of Shaver's disease, and of pot room asthma are all described with the appropriate references.*

Morgan WKC. Other pneumoconioses. In: Morgan WKC, Seaton A, eds. *Occupational Lung Diseases.* 3rd ed. Philadelphia: WB Saunders; 1995. *A nondisease rendered inconsequential.*

Morgan WKC. Other pneumoconioses. In: Morgan WKC, Seaton A. *Occupational Lung Diseases.* 3rd ed. Philadelphia: WB Saunders; 1995. *A clinical, radiographic, and pathologic description of some of the less common pneumoconioses, including alleged pneumoconioses.*

Morgan WKC, Lapp NL. Respiratory disease in coal miners. State of the art. *Am Rev Respir Dis* 1976;113:531. *A state-of-the-art article describing the main features of CWP. The section on the effects of coal dust on the lung is the most complete review of the lung function abnormalities.*

Ortmeyer CE, Costello J, Morgan WKC, et al. The mortality of Appalachian coal miners, 1963–1971. *Arch Environ Health* 1974;29: 67. *A study of working and retired coal miners. The effects of dust exposure, CWP, both simple and complicated, and cigarette smoking are quantified.*

Robertson AJ. The romance of tin. *Lancet* 1964;1:1229. *The first description of stannosis.*

Ruckley VA, Fernie JM, Campell SJ, Cowie HA. *Causes of Disability in Coal Miners: a Clinico-pathological Study of Emphysema, Airways Obstruction, and Massive Fibrosis.* Edinburgh: Institute of Occupational Medicine; 1989:Report No. TM/89/05. *A detailed description of the relationship of dust exposure to and its effects on lung function, radiographic category, and the induction of emphysema in coal miners.*

Shaver CG, Riddell AR. Lung changes associated with the manufacturing of alumina abrasives. *J Ind Hyg Toxicol* 1947;29:145. *The first description of Shaver's disease, a pulmonary fibrosis related to the manufacture of abrasives and having little, if anything, to do with aluminum. There have been no further reports of the disease since adequate industrial hygiene measurements were put into effect.*

Sjögren I, et al. Hard metal lung disease: the importance of cobalt in coolants. *Thorax* 1980;35:653. *Recognition of hypersensitivity pneumonitis as a result of exposure to cobalt.*

Stewart MJ, Faulds JS. The pulmonary fibrosis of haematite miners.

J Pathol Bacteriol 1934;39:233. *The best description of the pathology of silicosiderosis.*

Surgeon General's Report. *The Health Consequences of Smoking: Cancer and Chronic Obstructive Lung Disease in the Work Place. A Report of the Surgeon General.* Rockville, MD: Office on Smoking and Health; 1985:287–313. *Encyclopedia on effects of smoking on health.*

Teculescu DB, Stanescu, DC. Carbon monoxide transfer factor for the lungs in silicosis. *Scand J Respir Dis* 1979;51:150. *A detailed review of the potential acute and chronic toxicity of welding along with an exegesis of the chronic respiratory and carcinogenic effects.*

Teculescu DB, Albu A. Pulmonary function in workers inhaling carbon monoxide. *Int Arch Arbeitsmed* 1973;31:163. *One of the few studies of the diffusing capacity in welders' siderosis.*

Van Ordstrand HS, et al. Beryllium poisoning. *JAMA* 1945;129:1084. *An early review of the clinical features of berylliosis.*

Wagner JC. Exiological factor in complicated coal workers' pneumoconiosis. *Am NY Acad Sci* 1972;200:401–404. *Description of the pathology of progressive massive fibrosis.*

Williams WJ. A histological study of the lungs in 52 cases of chronic beryllium disease. Br J Ind Med 1958;15:84. An early description of the pathology of berylliosis.

Williams WR, Williams WJ. Development of beryllium lymphocyte transformation tests in chronic beryllium disease. *Int Arch Allergy Appl Immunol* 1982;67:175. *A review of the immunologic mechanism and diagnosis of berylliosis.*

Textbook of Pulmonary Diseases, 6th ed.
edited by G.L. Baum, J.D. Crapo, B.R. Celli, and J.B. Karlinsky,
Lippincott–Raven Publishers, Philadelphia, © 1998.

CHAPTER

34

Occupational Asthma and Industrial Bronchitis

R. John Looney · Mark J. Utell

OCCUPATIONAL ASTHMA

Occupational asthma may be defined as reversible airways obstruction caused by specific agents in the workplace. It should be distinguished from pre-existing asthma that may be worsened by workplace exposures. The focus of this chapter is primarily on new-onset asthma induced by workplace exposures.

Occupational asthma may be immunologic or nonimmunologic in origin and may be caused by a wide spectrum of low- and high-molecular-weight substances delivered as fumes, gases, or particles. Different classifications are useful when various aspects of occupational asthma are considered (Table 1). One classification divides immunologically mediated occupational asthma into subsets based on type of antigen (high- versus low-molecular-weight agents; Table 2). A second classification divides occupational asthma into subsets based on pathophysiologic mechanisms. Typically, immunologically mediated asthma is associated with a latency period; in contrast, irritant-induced asthma (e.g., reactive airways dysfunction syndrome) occurs without any latency.

Epidemiology and Prevalence

Occupational asthma is now the most common form of occupational lung disease in many industrialized coun-

tries. In the United Kingdom and France, the number of claims for occupational asthma exceeds that of pneumoconioses. In the United States, asthma prevalence is increasing, involving approximately 5% of the population; recent studies indicate that 5%–10% of adult asthma is attributable to workplace exposures. However, disease prevalence varies greatly, as does the risk inherent to specific occupational exposures. For example, the prevalence of asthma can be as high as 50% for workers exposed to platinum salts and only 5% among workers exposed to either isocyanates or wood dust from western red cedar. Among 2500 asthmatic subjects ages 20 to 44 years studied in a large young adult Spanish population, the highest risk for occupational asthma was observed among laboratory technicians, spray painters, bakers, plastics and rubber workers, and welders; the risk for asthma attributed to occupational exposures after adjusting for age, sex, residence, and smoking status ranged from 5%–7%, depending on the definition of asthma.

It is difficult to estimate the true incidence or prevalence of occupational asthma. Many surveys have used questionnaire responses only, which may not accurately reflect airways hyperreactivity or its etiology. Cross-sectional studies of workers may underestimate asthma prevalence because of pre-employment screening to exclude sensitive workers and because of dropout of workers who become sensitized at work. Individuals who remain may reflect a healthy worker effect. Other workers may refuse to participate in epidemiologic studies for fear of losing their jobs.

Several risk factors that influence the development of disease have been identified. Genetic factors such as atopy predispose to the development of occupational asthma

R. J. Looney and M. J. Utell: Divisions of Immunology, Pulmonary/Critical Care, and Occupational/Environmental Medicine, Departments of Medicine and Environmental Medicine, University of Rochester Medical Center, Rochester, New York 14642.

TABLE 1. *Classification of occupational asthma*

Antigens
High-molecular-weight antigens
  Protein derived from domestic animals, insets, fungi, or
    vegetable matter
  Dextrans
Low-molecular-weight antigens
  Haptens such as platinum and other metal salts
  Penicillin and other drugs
  Toluene diisocyanate and other reactive chemicals

Pathophysiology
Immunologic—characterized by a latency
  IgE-mediated (seen with both high- and low-molecular-
    weight antigens)
  Non-IgE-mediated (seen only with low-molecular-weight
    antigens)
Nonimmunologic—no latency
  Pharmacologic—mast cells, sensory neurons, or
    smooth muscle as targets
  Irritants and toxins (reactive airways dysfunction
    syndrome)

in industries using high-molecular-weight antigens; the significance of atopy with low-molecular-weight compounds is less clear. In some studies, cigarette smoking has been linked to an increased risk for occupational asthma. The relationship between pre-existing airways hyperreactivity and development of occupational asthma is unclear but is under investigation.

Mechanisms

Asthma is a common disease affecting as many as 20 million individuals in the United States. Workplace exposures may exacerbate symptoms in persons with pre-existing asthma (work-aggravated asthma) or trigger new disease. The mechanisms by which occupational agents induce asthma are similar to those that are operative in non-occupational asthma. Important mechanisms include reflex bronchoconstriction, acute inflammation, and immunologic sensitization. For some agents, responses may be triggered through several pathways, whereas for others the mechanism by which the material causes asthma is undefined.

Work-Aggravated Asthma: Nonimmunologic Mechanisms

Work-aggravated asthma is defined as concurrent asthma worsened by gaseous or particulate irritants or physical stimuli in the workplace. Exposure to numerous industrial agents can cause reflex bronchoconstriction in asthmatic workers with hyperreactive airways. Sulfur dioxide, acidic aerosols, environmental tobacco smoke, chemicals, and automobile exhaust can precipitate cough or wheezing by stimulating irritant receptors. A striking

example of an acute exposure occurs with the gas sulfur dioxide (SO_2), which induces bronchoconstriction in asthmatic individuals at concentrations ≤ 1.0 ppm after exposures lasting only 5 min. In contrast, inhalation of SO_2 at concentrations 5 ppm causes only small decrements in airways function in normal subjects. Lung function responses to SO_2 in asthmatic persons are greater when SO_2 exposure is accompanied by increased ventilation, usually stimulated by physical labor or exercise. SO_2-induced bronchoconstriction can be further intensified by breathing cold air and/or dry air. Thus, the irritant response can be enhanced by conditions in the workplace.

At times, it may be difficult to draw a clear distinction between work-aggravated and *de novo* occupational asthma. This is particularly true in the case of atopic individuals who may become sensitized to allergens at work. The pathogenic mechanisms and perhaps even the genetic predisposition are similar for the work-related and non-work-related allergen exposure. For example, the physician may encounter an atopic, asthmatic individual with baker's asthma who is sensitized to aeroallergens outside the workplace, such as house dust mites, and also to aeroallergens encountered at work, such as protein antigens in flour. The severity of disease is determined by a combination of immunologic sensitivity and level of exposure to both work-related and non-work-related aeroallergens. The management of such cases needs to address both exposures or risk the possibility of inappropriate attribution; that is, residual symptoms of house dust mite exposure or other non-occupational allergens may be blamed on responses induced by exposure to flour antigens at work. On the other hand, a specific material may act as both an irritant and immunologically specific antigen. For example, isocyanates can cause cough or irritation to the eyes at high concentrations, but immunologic sensitization can also result, causing asthma at extremely low levels.

A second type of nonimmunologic or irritant-induced asthma is the reactive airways dysfunction syndrome (RADS). In 1981, Brooks and Lockey first used the term in an abstract that described 13 workers in whom symptomatic and physiologic evidence of bronchoconstriction developed within hours after a single toxic inhalation exposure. The symptoms were persistent, lasting at least 3 months and averaging 3 years after the time of initial exposure. A case of RADS was defined in the American College of Chest Physicians Consensus Statement, *Assessment of Asthma in the Workplace*, as meeting the following criteria: (1) a documented absence of preceding respiratory complaints; (2) onset of symptoms after a single exposure incident or accident; (3) exposure to gas, smoke, fume, or vapor with irritant properties present in very high concentrations; (4) onset of symptoms within 24 hours after the exposure with persistence of symptoms of at least 3 months; (5) symptoms consistent with asthma, such as cough, wheeze, and dyspnea; (6) presence of air

TABLE 2. *Causes of occupational asthma*

High-molecular-weight material		Low-molecular-weight compounds	
Plants		**Isocyanates**	
grain dust	grain workers, millers, dock workers	toluene diisocyanate	polyurethane, plastics
flour	bakers, millers	methylene diphenyldiisocyanate	foundries
soybean	farmers, dock workers	hexamethylene diisocyanate	spray paint, plastics
castor bean	dock workers, fertilizer workers	**Acid anhydrides**	
coffee bean	dock workers, food processors	phthalic anhydride	plastics, epoxy resins
tea	food processors	trimellitic anhydride	plastics, epoxy resins
hops	brewers	tetrachlorophthalic anhydride	epoxy resins
tobacco leaf	farmers and manufacturers	himic anhydride	fire retardants
latex	health care and laboratory workers	hexahydrophthalic anhydride	plastics, epoxy resins
cottonseed	bakers, fertilizer workers, manufacturers	**Metals**	
flaxseed	manufacturers	platinum	refining
linseed	manufactuers	nickel	metal plating
Animals		chromium	tanning, cement
laboratory animals	laboratory workers	cobalt	hard metal workers
birds	pigeon breeders and poultry workers	**Wood dust**	
eggs	food processors	western red cedar	carpenters, sawmill workers
milk	farmers and daily workers	California redwood	carpenters, sawmill workers
crabs	food processors	cedar of Lebanon	carpenters, sawmill workers
prawns	food processors	African maple	carpenters, sawmill workers
Insects		oak	carpenters, sawmill workers
house dust mites	office workers	mahogany	carpenters, sawmill workers
grain mites	farmers, grain workers, dock workers, bakers	African zebra wood	carpenters, sawmill workers
fowl mites	poultry workers	Central American walnut	carpenters, sawmill workers
silkworms	sericulture	**Soldering fluxes**	
mealworms	bait workers	colophony	electronics
cockroaches	laboratory workers	aminoethylethanolamine	aluminum solderers
honeybees	beekeepers	**Drugs**	
Enzymes		penicillin	pharmaceuticals
papain		cephalosporins	pharmaceuticals
subtilisin		spiramycin	pharmaceuticals
bromelin		tetracycline	pharmaceuticals
pancreatin		piperazine HCl	pharmaceuticals
pepsin		phenylglycine acid chloride	pharmaceuticals
trypsin		psyllium	pharmaceuticals
fungal amylase		**Miscellaneous**	
Vegetable gums		formalin	hospital staff, fur tanning, insulation
acacia	printers	ethylenediamine	beauty, plastic, rubber
tragacanth	printers	ammonium thioglycolate	beauty parlor
karaya	hairdressers		
guar	carpet manufacturers		

flow obstruction on pulmonary function tests; (7) presence of nonspecific bronchial hyperresponsiveness; and (8) other pulmonary diseases ruled out.

Histopathologic studies in RADS are limited but have shed light on the pathogenic mechanisms. In general, bronchial biopsy specimens have demonstrated only a mild inflammatory response, with sparse lymphocytes and polymorphonuclear cells and no eosinophils. However, biopsy results are variable depending presumably on type and severity of exposure, type of treatment, and time from injury to biopsy.

Although the acute symptoms following toxic inhalation are related to the resulting airways inflammation, the basis for the persistent bronchial hyperresponsiveness is not well explained. Hypotheses under investigation include altered receptor thresholds in the airways, increased airways permeability, smooth-muscle dysfunction as a result of massive mediator release, and persistent airways inflammation. The treatment of the patient with established RADS is no different from that of any other asthmatic patient.

Immunologically Mediated Occupational Asthma

Two observations suggest that immunologic mechanisms are involved in most cases of occupational asthma. First, there is clinical evidence of sensitization—that is, individuals do not experience respiratory symptoms when first exposed to an antigen, but repeated exposures begin to precipitate symptoms. Moreover, with repeated exposures, symptoms occur at extremely low concentrations. Second, there is immunologic evidence of sensitization. This is most easily seen with agents that induce an IgE response in which specific antibodies can be detected by immediate skin tests or radioallergosorbent test (RAST) and correlated with the development of allergic symptoms such as conjunctivitis and rhinitis in addition to asthma.

Antigens involved in occupational asthma fall into two categories. The first category consists of macromolecular antigens derived from animals, plants, microbes, and even recombinant DNA technology. These antigens resemble those responsible for atopic asthma and are mainly proteins. They are complete antigens containing both T- and B-cell epitopes, and they induce and elicit an immune response by themselves. Asthma secondary to these macromolecular agents is closely related to atopic/extrinsic asthma, as it is IgE-mediated. Indeed, atopy is a risk factor for the development of occupational asthma with at least some of these agents. Allergen-specific IgE is invariably found with occupational asthma caused by exposure to high-molecular-weight allergens. The second category consists of molecules of low molecular weight. These low-molecular-weight antigens are incomplete antigens—that is, they first haptenate macromolecules before they induce an immune response and therefore must themselves be chemically reactive molecules or metabolized to reactive intermediates. Asthma induced by some low-molecular-weight molecules is IgE-mediated. However, atopy is generally not a risk factor. Other risk factors have been sought and include, for example, cigarettes, which increase the risk for both immunologic sensitization to and occupational asthma with platinum salts. It is interesting that some low-molecular-weight molecules induce immunologically mediated asthma in which IgE antibodies appear to play no role. The mechanisms of non-IgE-mediated asthma are poorly understood.

Patterns of Cytokine Production

The importance of bronchial inflammation in asthma has become clear. Eosinophilic and lymphocytic infiltration is present in bronchial biopsy specimens of even mildly asthmatic subjects. A variety of proinflammatory substances are released into the airways tissues of asthmatic subjects, including lipids, proteases, bioamines, neurotransmitters, and cytokines. Of these mediators, cytokines are unique because they are primary effector mechanisms for T cells. The pattern of cytokine secretion appears to differ in the major categories of non-occupational asthma. Studies of cytokine production at the mRNA and protein levels indicate that in extrinsic asthma (allergic asthma) interleukin-4 (IL-4) is produced by mast cells and CD4 lymphocytes; IL-5 is produced by these cells and eosinophils. Intrinsic asthma (non-allergic asthma) has not been as extensively studied. Nonetheless, IL-5 and interferon-γ are found, but not IL-4. These patterns of cytokines fit with the immunopathology. IL-5 is essential for eosinophil production in the marrow and additionally is able to attract, activate, and enhance the survival of mature eosinophils. In both intrinsic and extrinsic asthma, IL-5 is produced in the airways mucosa, and both conditions are associated with prominent bronchial tissue eosinophilia. In extrinsic asthma, IL-4 is produced in the airways; in intrinsic asthma, interferon-γ is produced instead of IL-4. IL-4 is essential for IgE synthesis, whereas interferon-γ inhibits IgE production. Thus, extrinsic or atopic asthma is associated with a pattern of cytokines promoting IgE production, whereas the pattern of cytokines in intrinsic, non-allergic asthma inhibits the production of IgE.

The results of studies of IgE-mediated and non-IgE-mediated occupational asthma are remarkably congruous with those of studies of extrinsic and intrinsic non-occupational asthma (Table 3). In both IgE-mediated and non-IgE-mediated occupational asthma, airways inflammation is a predominant feature, and as in non-occupational asthma, eosinophils and lymphocytes infiltrate the tissue. Analysis of cytokine production in occupational asthma has been limited. In one interesting study, lymphocytes were harvested from bronchoalveolar lavage (BAL) fluid and grown in vitro after exposure to toluene diisocyanate (TDI), an agent that induces non-IgE-mediated occupational asthma. These TDI-elicited T cells were 80% CD8-positive and produced large quantities of IL-5 and interferon-γ but no IL-4. Challenge studies with non-occupational agents that induce IgE-mediated asthma elicit predominantly CD4 cells producing IL-5 and IL-4

TABLE 3. *IgE versus non-IgE immune-mediated occupational asthma*

	IgE-mediated	non-IgE-mediated
Eosinophilic bronchitis	++	++
T-cell infiltration of airways	++	++
Predominant T-cell subset	CD4	CD8
MHC presentation	Class II	Class I
Interleukin-5	++	++
Interleukin-6	++	−
Interferon-γ	−	++

MHC, major histocompatibility complex.

but no interferon-γ. BAL studies have not been done for IgE-mediated occupational asthma but presumably would be similar to those for IgE-mediated nonoccupational asthma. Thus, the two major differences between IgE-mediated and non-IgE-mediated asthma are the T-cell subset involved and the pattern of cytokine induced.

The preponderance of CD8 cells in BAL fluid after challenge with TDI was surprising, because previous studies of BAL fluid in asthmatic patients reported a predominance of CD4 cells. However, these previous studies used protein antigens, such as house dust mite or pollens. Exogenous protein antigens do not enter the cytoplasm of antigen-presenting cells and are therefore not presented via class I molecules to CD8 T cells. Instead, exogenous protein antigens are taken up into cytoplasmic vesicles, where they become bound to class II molecules and are then returned to the cell surface for presentation to CD4 T cells. Because TDI is not a protein but a reactive chemical, it can form covalent bonds with a variety of macromolecules. These macromolecules include self-proteins in the cytoplasm of the cell and even the class I molecules themselves. TDI-modified self-peptides from cytoplasmic proteins or TDI-modified class I molecules would be presented to CD8 T cells. It is interesting to note that although many low-molecular-weight antigens, such as TDI, western cedar, or colophony, induce asthma by non-IgE-mediated mechanisms, another group of low-molecular-weight antigens, such as platinum salts and acid anhydrides, induce antigen-specific IgE. It is tempting to hypothesize that a crucial difference between the chemicals that induce non-IgE-mediated versus IgE-mediated asthma may be presentation of antigen via class I or class II antigens, respectively.

Pathophysiology of Airway Responses

Classically, inhaled protein allergens such as those from cats (Fel d I) or mites (Der p I) induce an immediate hypersensitivity response with an early- and/or late-phase pulmonary response in patients who have asthma caused by these agents (Fig. 1). Both the early and late phase depend on allergen-specific IgE on the surface of mast cells. The early phase begins within minutes of exposure and typically wanes in an hour. Bronchospasm in the early phase is mediated by soluble factors produced by mast cells. The late-phase response occurs after several hours and then wanes by 12 to 24 hours. It is accompanied by a cellular infiltrate: granulocytes, especially eosinophils, initially and mononuclear cells later. Bronchospasm in the late phase is mediated by soluble factors produced by the infiltrating cells. The vast majority of patients with atopic asthma have an early-phase response, and asthmatic patients with a severe early-phase reaction are more likely to have a late phase. An isolated late-phase response occurs in 10% of atopic persons with asthma. Protein

allergens that induce occupational asthma are associated with the same airways changes as protein allergens that cause atopic asthma in the general population; typical IgE-mediated early- and late-phase responses are seen in challenge studies. The pattern of airways response is much more complicated in non-IgE-mediated occupational asthma. Although early- and late-phase responses occur, atypical patterns are also common. These can include isolated late responses, responses that peak early and then persist, responses that begin early and become progressively more severe, and responses that persist for several days (Fig. 1).

The pathophysiology of acute bronchospasm induced by TDI and similar agents in the absence of antigen-specific IgE is not well understood. TDI has direct biochemical effects, including the induction of substance P secretion. Moreover, TDI can induce the release of histamine-releasing factor by peripheral blood mononuclear cells from sensitized patients. However, neither of these effects provides an adequate explanation for TDI-sensitized patients with immediate bronchospastic responses. The direct effects on substance P or other mediators should not differentiate TDI asthma from asthma of other causes. In addition, histamine-releasing factor is produced slowly and is associated with the late- rather than the early-phase response. Clearly, additional work is needed to clarify the pathophysiology of non-IgE-mediated occupational asthma.

Diagnosis of Occupational Asthma

The two general requirements for a diagnosis of occupational asthma are (1) a diagnosis of asthma, and (2) documentation that the asthma is work-related. Although fulfillment of these criteria is conceptually simple, in practice it is often not straightforward. Several important diagnostic considerations may confound the evaluation of occupational asthma. First, other diagnoses, some of which may also be occupationally related, need to be considered. Second, pulmonary function test results vary considerably depending on whether the patient is currently exposed. Third, many factors in the workplace may act as nonspecific triggers in patients who have hyperreactive airways. Such individuals have work-aggravated asthma, and their management and prognosis differ from those of individuals with true occupational asthma. Finally, the diagnosis has important consequences for both worker and employer. Indeed, patients may either underreport or overreport symptoms for other than medical reasons. Our approach to the workup of occupational asthma is detailed below and illustrated in Fig. 2.

Defining the Problem

A complete medical history and physical examination are essential in the workup of occupational asthma. The

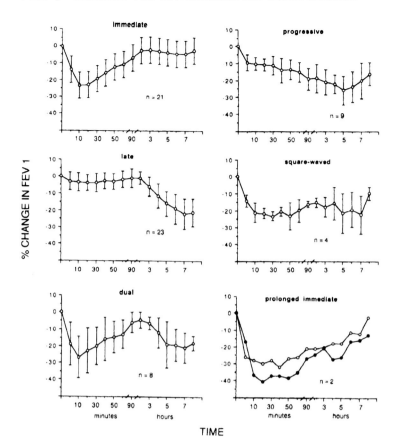

FIG. 1. Patterns of airway response to antigen challenge. (Adapted with permission from Perrin B, et al. Reassessment of the temporal patterns of bronchial obstruction after exposure to occupational sensitizing agents. *J Allergy Clin Immunol* 1991;87:630–639.)

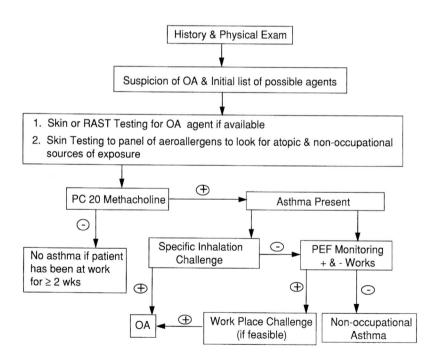

FIG. 2. Algorithm for the workup of occupational asthma. (OA = occupational asthma; PEF = peak expiratory flow)

four primary goals are to (1) establish that occupational asthma is sufficiently likely to require further workup, (2) identify alternative diagnoses, (3) assess the severity of illness and the need to eliminate further workplace exposure, and (4) identify likely etiologic agents. In other clinical situations, interventions might be started with just the data provided by the history and physical examination, but in the setting of occupational asthma, additional objective documentation is usually required.

History of the Present Illness

The interview should be open-ended, allowing the patient to raise concerns, and then focus on identified problems. A chronologic history of symptoms should be elicited, including both work-related and unrelated episodes. Particular attention is given to whether symptoms existed before the current job was started. Preceding asthma is rarely work-related except in the case of a common agent in the environment outside work or a previous work environment. Where and when in the workplace symptoms occur are important in tracking down an etiologic agent; for example, does the patient have problems only in certain areas, or are symptoms associated with a specific process or incidents, such as spills or other accidents? The temporal relationship between work and the occurrence or exacerbation of symptoms should be understood. Do symptoms begin immediately when the patient arrives at work, or do they appear only toward the end of the shift? Do they resolve after the patient has left work? Do they persist during the whole workweek but disappear during weekends or holidays? Are there eye or nasal symptoms, and how do these symptoms change in relationship to work? Are there known precipitants outside the work environment, such as a cat or other animal, damp basements, seasonal exacerbations? The severity and progression of symptoms determine the scope of the workup and whether continued exposure can be tolerated. Evidence of airways hyperreactivity, such as sensitivity to cold air or exercise, and the presence of symptoms that do not support a diagnosis of asthma, such as fever, weight loss, or peripheral edema and orthopnea, are important.

Past Medical History

The past history includes both the personal and occupational medical history. Previous medical records can be especially helpful in ascertaining whether symptoms developed before current workplace exposure. A history of smoking and atopy should be specifically elicited. Childhood respiratory problems such as bronchitis, asthma, frequent colds, hay fever, sinus problems, and allergies point to an atopic predisposition but do not rule out a diagnosis of occupational asthma. A listing of hospitalizations, medical emergencies, and medications should be ob-

tained. Time lost from work and the course of recovery from prior illness may provide insight into how the patient copes with illness. A family history for atopy and other inherited respiratory diseases should be obtained.

Occupational History

Identification of potential etiologic agents for occupational asthma begins with characterization of present and past work-related exposures. This includes a general characterization of the types of potential allergens (chemicals, drugs, metals, animal- or plant-derived proteins, recombinant proteins, or organic dust) and respiratory irritants as well as a general description of the job and the type of job site exposure. Some jobs, such as spray painting or handling animals, necessarily involve exposure to potential allergens. Precautions taken at the workplace, including use of protective gear and ventilation, may mitigate such exposure but can be offset by noncompliance and accidents. The intensity and duration of exposure should be noted. The clinician should also determine if other workers at the same work site have had work-related respiratory illnesses. Problems with ventilation and humidification systems, including contamination with microbes, are common sources of respiratory complaints in the workplace and should be carefully queried. Dampness, particularly when cloth such as carpeting or decaying organic material is involved, may lead to overgrowth of molds or even allergenic mites. Infesting rodents or cockroaches are also potential sources of allergen.

Nonoccupational Environmental History

Environmental factors outside the workplace need to be investigated. The nature and type of housing, type of heating and floor covering, and the presence of any new construction or excessive dampness should be determined. In addition, household pets and rodents or roaches are potential sources of sensitization. Hobbies may involve exposure to chemicals that are sensitizers.

Physical Examination

Normal findings on physical examination are compatible with a diagnosis of occupational asthma. Wheezing and irritation of the conjunctiva or nasal mucosa are the more common positive findings. Nevertheless, determination of vital signs, including the rate and pattern of respiration, examination of the skin, head and neck, heart, extremities, and abdomen, and a screening neurologic examination should be performed in all cases. The primary purpose of this examination is not to make the diagnosis of asthma but instead to exclude other diagnoses.

Confirmation of Asthma

Pulmonary function tests are essential for documenting airways obstruction and reactivity (Table 4). In some cases, the patient will have substantial abnormalities in baseline spirometry, and the diagnosis of asthma can be confirmed by demonstrating a 15% improvement in FEV_1 (forced expiratory volume in 1 second) with inhaled bronchodilators. More commonly, the results of baseline flow studies are normal. In these cases, assessment of bronchial airways hyperreactivity to methacholine, carbachol, or histamine should be undertaken. These tests have not been completely standardized, so the results from different laboratories are difficult to compare. It is therefore important that the individual laboratory have its own database ensuring that normal and asthmatic persons can be discriminated and that results in the same individual are reproducible. In a commonly used protocol in North America, methacholine in doubled concentrations (0.03, 0.06, 0.125, 0.25, 0.5, 1, 2, 4, 8, 16, and 32 mg/mL) is administered as an aerosol via nebulizer for 2 minutes at each dose. A practical problem with this protocol is that the large number of doses requires substantial time in the asthmatic patient with mild or moderate reactivity; often, shorter protocols are used. A major variable in these studies is the nebulizer itself. Use of the same nebulizer in an individual for repeated measurements helps reduce variability.

The end point for testing is generally a 20% decrease in FEV_1, and the results are expressed as the PD_{20}. Use of bronchodilators and ingestion of compounds containing bronchodilator agents (e.g., beverages containing caffeine) are stopped before testing. Most inhaled bronchodilators can simply be withheld beginning the evening (12 hours) before, but salmeterol and oral theophyllines should be stopped 24 hours in advance. If the patient is still working (i.e., has been going to work regularly for at least 2 weeks) and is still having work-related symptoms, then an absence of airways hyperreactivity essentially excludes the diagnosis of occupational asthma, and other diagnoses should be entertained. If the worker has been away from the work site for some time or if symptoms have been intermittent (perhaps because of the intermittent presence of the etiologic agent in the workplace), then the absence of bronchial hyperresponsiveness does not exclude asthma, and additional studies are required. One caveat is that the presence of bronchial hyperresponsiveness does not unequivocally mean asthma, because there are asymptomatic individuals with hyperactive airways. In addition, normal individuals may have bronchial hyperreactivity lasting for several months after a respiratory viral infection, such as influenza.

Identification of Potential Agents

Exposure assessment and immunologic testing are the primary tools in identifying potential agents. Exposure assessment begins with a careful history (see above). Additional sources of information include data from an industrial hygiene program, health and safety personnel, material safety data sheets (MSDS), other workers, and in some cases a visit to the work site. When contamination with microbes or mites is suspected, air and/or dust may be sampled for culture, microscopic identification, assays for endotoxin, mycotoxins, and chemicals, or immunoassays for aeroallergens.

Identification of the causative agent occasionally involves an immunologic assessment, because immunologic tests are available for only a few common allergens (Table 4). Asthma with a latency period is immunologically mediated. In immunologically mediated asthma, the immune response induces inflammation in the airways, and this inflammation results in nonspecific airway hyperresponsiveness. In some instances, it has been impossible to demonstrate immune sensitization by skin testing or in vitro assays. This has been particularly difficult with low-molecular-weight antigens, especially those that induce asthma via nonIgE-mediated mechanisms. With both high-molecular-weight antigens and low-molecular-weight antigens that sensitize via IgE, skin testing is still the most sensitive assay for demonstration of immediate

TABLE 4. *Confirmation of occupational asthma*

	Ease	Availability	Sensitivity	Specificity	Comments
Skin prick tests and RAST	++	++	+++	+	Poor correlation with bronchial reactivity. Usefulness and availability depend on antigen.
Spirometry	++++	++++	+	++	Often normal unless illness is severe.
PEFR, serially	++	+++	+++	+++	Very useful with cooperative patient, but compliance is a problem.
Bronchial reactivity (nonspecific)	++	++	++++	+	Very sensitive, standardized. Not specific for etiology.
Bronchial challenge (specific)	+	+	+++	++++	Potentially hazardous. Dose poorly controlled, but reproduces actual exposures.

PEFR, peak expiratory flow rate; RAST, radioallergosorbent test.

hypersensitivity. The problem in many cases is that the skin testing materials for these antigens are not standardized and frequently unavailable commercially. The investigators may then be faced with the task of manufacturing skin test reagents and/or verifying that they are active.

With some low-molecular-weight sensitizers, manufacture of material for skin testing may involve conjugating haptens to human serum albumin (HSA) and measuring the extent of derivation. Allergen-specific IgE can be measured in vitro using RAST with some allergens. The ability of RAST to quantify results and determine the degree of sensitization may be helpful. False-negatives are more common with RAST, and false-positives may occur in patients with very high total IgE levels. As with airways challenge testing, a database for the individual testing facility can be instrumental in validating skin test or RAST results. Although these tests document immunologic sensitization, sensitization neither proves a diagnosis of occupational asthma nor confirms the test antigen as the cause of symptoms. Generally, more individuals have positive skin test results and no symptoms than have positive skin test results with symptoms. Nevertheless, demonstration of positive immediate skin test results and increased nonspecific bronchial hyperresponsiveness in a patient with both appropriate symptoms and exposure is highly predictive of a positive result on airways challenge with a specific antigen. Moreover, negative skin test results with a valid skin test reagent is strong evidence against involvement of that agent in asthma. For many low-molecular-weight antigens, no skin test reagent has been developed, either because the asthma is not IgE-mediated or because the appropriate carrier or metabolite has not been identified. Skin testing to a limited panel of common non-occupational aeroallergens (in the Northeast a routine panel includes cat, dog, *D. farinae*, *D. pyterinisinus*, cockroach, mouse, mixed grasses, mixed trees, ragweed, *Alternaria, Helminthosporium, Aspergillus, Penicillium,* and any other pet) can be quite useful in the evaluation of patients suspected to have occupational asthma. Results of this panel are used to define atopic status and determine if non-occupational aeroallergens may play a role. In vitro testing for IgG antibodies may also be done in selected cases, but the presence of IgG antibodies is more helpful in the diagnosis of hypersensitivity pneumonitis than of asthma.

Establishing a Relationship to Work

Monitoring pulmonary function over time and challenges in the laboratory or at the work site are important in relating the workplace exposure to symptoms and physiologic changes and may help to identify the specific agent. Although pulmonary function monitoring to document changes related to work site exposure seems straightforward, there are many potential pitfalls. Perhaps the most significant problem is patient cooperation and compliance. With a highly motivated and reliable individual, useful data can be obtained by measuring peak flows periodically (every 2 hours in most studies, four times a day in some) for 2 weeks. Two studies have evaluated monitoring of peak flows using airways challenge as the gold standard. Peak flow monitoring in these studies was 86% and 87% sensitive and 89% and 84% specific. These results are excellent, but other studies provide evidence that patients are often unreliable and results fabricated up to 25% of the time. The use of computerized meters that record time and results automatically may improve the reliability of peak flow monitoring. Other problems with peak flow monitoring include instances in which exposure may be highly erratic and unpredictable, such as with accidents or equipment failure. In addition, when exposure results in prolonged or delayed respiratory problems, it may be necessary for the worker to be away from the job or on the job for several weeks before a change in function can be seen. Criteria for defining a positive response have often been subjectively based on visual assessment of the record. Objective criteria that have been proposed include (1) diurnal variation in peak flow of 20% or more, (2) occurrence of changes more frequently on days at work than on days not at work, and (3) designation of indeterminate recording when a 20% diurnal change occurs only once or when changes occur over several days rather than daily. By these criteria, 26% of recordings were indeterminate and the specificity and sensitivity of the remaining recordings were 90% and 93%, respectively. However, ''subjective'' assessment of the record was essentially equivalent to the more ''objective'' reading.

Airways challenges with specific antigens remain the gold standard for the diagnosis of occupational asthma. Under most circumstances, challenges can be avoided because of good correlation between positive skin test results plus nonspecific airways responsiveness or peak flow monitoring and airways challenges. Nevertheless, challenges are still a necessary tool for some patients. For example, in the patient with a history highly suggestive of sensitivity to a specific agent but in whom monitoring has been indeterminate or unreliable, airways challenge may clarify the issue. Similarly, if the suspected agent has not previously been reported to cause asthma or if the worker has been away from work for a long time, then airways challenge will document sensitization in a physiologically meaningful sense.

The overwhelming consideration in these specific challenges is safety. Laboratory challenges should be performed in specialized centers with trained personnel, often in an investigative setting. An intravenous line should be in place to provide access for medications. Oxygen, inhaled bronchodilators, steroids, and equipment for intubation and resuscitation should be at hand. Laboratory challenge involves several days of observation (Table 5).

TABLE 5. *Laboratory challenge*

Day 1: No exposure
    Baseline PFTs
    FEV₁ fluctuation <10%
Day 2: Exposure to control material
Day 3: Exposure to specific antigen
    For high-molecular-weight material:
        Increase doses of antigen every 20 minutes.
        Check FEV₁ every 10 minutes.
    For low-molecular-weight material:
        Increase doses of antigen on successive days.
        Check FEV₁ every 10 minutes for 1 hour, then
            every 30 minutes for another 2 hours, then
            every 1 hour for the rest of the 8-hour session.

PFT, pulmonary function test; FEV_1, forced expiratory volume in 1 second.

On the first day, bronchodilator medications are stopped and clinical status, baseline pulmonary function, and fluctuation of FEV_1 during several hours are determined. If the variation in FEV_1 is >10%, then the patient should return when more stable. On the second day, the subject is exposed to aerosolized diluent. Finally, on the third day, exposure to test material is begun. With high-molecular-weight materials, the patient can be exposed to progressively greater amounts of material throughout the course of the day (every 15 to 30 minutes), as isolated late-phase responses are unusual with this type of allergen. During these repeated exposures, FEV_1 should be measured every 10 minutes. With low-molecular-weight materials, isolated late-phase responses and atypical patterns of response are common. Therefore, the patient should be exposed to progressively greater amounts of test material only on successive days. On each of these test days, FEV_1 should be measured every 10 minutes for the first hour after exposure, then every 30 minutes for 2 hours, and finally every hour for the rest of the 8-hour session. The starting dose of test material has to be individualized based on the material to be tested, the severity of the reaction by history, and the patient's nonspecific airways hyperresponsiveness. A 20% fall in FEV_1 is considered a positive response.

If laboratory challenges are not feasible and peak flow monitoring is unreliable, it may be possible to have the patient return to the work site for progressively longer periods of time, with spirometry, and potential determination of airway responsiveness, performed before and after the exposures. If travel distance permits, these measurements may be made in the pulmonary laboratory, but more often a technician will have to visit the job site.

Although specific challenge tests may be considered the gold standard, false-negative and false-positive interpretations may result. Sources of false-negative results include testing with the wrong material or using an inadequate dose. In addition, nonspecific airways responsiveness decreases with time away from exposure, and a point may be reached at which several exposures are necessary before airway pathology is reinduced and a drop in FEV_1 occurs. Therefore, if there is no change in FEV_1 with exposure, nonspecific airways responsiveness can be measured at the end of the day and the next day to identify subtle changes. Such changes may be an indication for additional exposures. False-positive test results also occur; these may be caused by nonspecific irritation by the test substance or active asthma with a drop in FEV_1 that is independent of exposure. Suggestion may also play a role in airways responses. Indeed, there is some evidence that mast cell degranulation can be conditioned both in animals and humans. Thus, in some circumstances, blinding of both technicians and patient to the test substance may be an important consideration.

Management and Follow-up

The goals of medical treatment of occupational asthma are rapid control of symptoms, reversal of airways hyperresponsiveness, and prevention of irreversible changes to the airways leading to long-term persistence of symptoms.

In the management of occupational asthma, avoidance is the most important intervention. Once a person becomes immunologically sensitized, even infrequent low-level exposure may cause symptoms to persist. Therefore, patient and employer have to be advised that removal from the work site is essential. Interventions short of complete removal should be contemplated only if there is to be close follow-up and documentation of resolution of airways hyperresponsiveness. Such stringent environmental management may not be required in cases of work-aggravated asthma—that is, persons who do not have immunologic sensitization to workplace allergens. For these people, moderate improvements in workplace air quality may be sufficient to control work-related symptoms, especially if their non-occupational asthma is well managed.

Inhaled glucocorticoids are the cornerstone of the pharmacologic treatment of airways inflammation associated with chronic asthma. In a placebo-controlled trial, inhaled steroids have been shown to reverse the airways hyperresponsiveness that otherwise persists for many months after removal from exposure to TDI. It is too early to know whether the benefits of such treatment continue once the drug is stopped. However, if inflammation is the essential process in the development of irreversible changes in the airways, the sooner inflammation is eliminated, the lower the likelihood that permanent damage will result. At this point, it would seem prudent to treat occupational asthma aggressively with inhaled steroid for 6 months and then reassess; it may be reasonable to stop medication at that time and follow symptoms and airways reactivity.

Finally, it needs to be re-emphasized that a large number of diseases may mimic occupational asthma, and these need to be considered whenever the question of occupational asthma is raised. Such illnesses include asthma unrelated to occupational exposures, occupational or nonoccupational rhinitis, occupational or nonoccupational bronchitis, RADS, bronchiolitis obliterans, hypersensitivity pneumonitis, sinus disease, adductor spasm of the glottis, and other causes of extrathoracic obstruction. These alternative diagnoses need to be carefully excluded.

Specific Agents of Occupational Asthma

Low-Molecular-Weight Materials

With asthma induced by low-molecular-weight compounds (Table 2), atopy is not a risk factor. In these cases, IgE-mediated sensitization is unpredictable and may or may not be found. Because the antigens are incomplete antigens and need to haptenate a protein carrier, reagents for immunologic testing are often difficult to find. Several examples of asthma resulting from exposure to low-molecular-weight materials are considered below.

Isocyanates

Diisocyanates (TDI, toluene diisocyanate; MDI, diphenylmethane diisocyanate; HDI, hexamethylene diisocyanate; NDI, naphthalene diisocyanate) are used in spray painting, plastic molding, foundry work, and in the manufacture of polyurethane foams. Asthma occurs in 5%–10% of exposed workers. Diisocyanate-induced asthma does not appear to be mediated by IgE. Although RAST or skin testing will detect specific IgE in some workers, these tests do not predict clinical sensitization. Airways hyperresponsiveness to histamine or methacholine and eosinophilic inflammation of the airways are consistently found in sensitized workers. Once airways hyperresponsiveness has been established, it may persist for many years. Early detection of sensitization and removal from exposure are essential to prevent this long-term sequela. In addition to removal from exposure, treatment of sensitized workers with inhaled glucocorticoids accelerates resolution of airways hyperresponsiveness and inflammation. Airways challenge with diisocyanates frequently results in an isolated late-phase response. Atypical delayed and persistent responses are also common. Thus, in contrast to challenges with allergens that induce IgE-mediated sensitization, airway challenges with diisocyanates cannot be immediately repeated with an increased dose when an early-phase response is not observed. Hypersensitivity pneumonitis with pulmonary infiltrates has also been reported with diisocyanates (TDI, HDI, and MDI). In these individuals, specific IgG precipitins can be demonstrated.

Acid Anhydrides

Acid anhydrides (PA, phthalic anhydride; TMA, trimellitic anhydride; HHPA, hexahydrophthalic anhydride; HA, himic anhydride; TCPA, tetrachlorophthalic anhydride) function as hardening agents in the manufacture of epoxy resins used in adhesives, encapsulating agents, surface coatings, and plastics. Workers are exposed to these reactive compounds as fumes from heated resins, dust generated during the grinding of resins, and powdered chemicals added to reaction chambers.

Acid anhydrides are potent irritants that may cause eye, respiratory tract, and skin symptoms; permissible exposure limits for PA have been developed on this basis (6 mg/m^3). IgE-mediated allergic sensitization also occurs, and the permissible exposure level does not account for this. Conjugates of acid anhydride and HSA are sensitive reagents for skin testing, and RAST can also be performed. Results of airways challenge with acid anhydrides are typical of IgE-mediated sensitization; both an early-phase and a late-phase reaction are frequently seen. Specific IgE can persist for years after exposure. Acid anhydrides (TMA) are also associated with a late-onset respiratory systemic syndrome (LRSS) or with a syndrome of pulmonary hemorrhage and hemolytic anemia. These non-asthmatic pulmonary syndromes are associated with elevated levels of specific IgG.

Metals

Platinum salts can induce the production of specific IgE in a high proportion of heavily exposed workers, and this sensitization may lead to the development of skin rashes, eye and nasal symptoms, or asthma. Skin testing with platinum salts can be used to document sensitization, but high concentrations of platinum salts can cause nonspecific mast cell degranulation in unexposed controls. A RAST using malic dehydrogenase as a protein carrier has been developed. Asthma caused by exposure to a number of other metals has also been reported, including nickel, chromium, vanadium, cobalt, and fumes from steel welding and smelting of aluminum. There is evidence for an IgE mechanism with cobalt, chromium, and nickel in some cases, but the mechanisms involving vanadium or fumes from steel or aluminum are unknown.

Wood Dust

A wide variety of woods have been associated with occupational asthma, but the best studied example is red cedar. In red cedar asthma, sensitization is to plicatic acid, a reactive compound found in red and white cedar. Although specific IgE can be found in many workers, asthma appears to be non-IgE-mediated, and bronchial challenge is the only reliable test for immunologic sensitization. Delay in removal from exposure following the development of symptoms, particularly in older workers, has been linked with persistent airways hyperresponsiveness and dyspnea.

Solder

Colophony is used as flux in soldering, and electrical workers can become sensitized to colophony, with development of asthma. Colophony is a derivative of pine tree resin in which several reactive chemicals are found, namely abietic, pimaric, and dihydroabietic acids. As with wood dust, sensitization is not IgE-mediated, and airways challenge is the only reliable test for sensitization. Prolonged symptoms after removal from exposure have also been reported for colophony. Another component of solder flux, aminoethanolamine, can cause isolated late or dual responses.

Drugs

Occupational asthma can develop in workers exposed in the manufacture or use of a number of drugs (e.g., penicillin). Typically, these reactions are IgE-mediated and can be demonstrated with skin testing or RAST.

High-Molecular-Weight Materials

Atopy *is* a risk factor for sensitization to high-molecular-weight materials (Table 2). Typically, the sensitization is IgE-mediated. Because these materials are complete antigens, reagents for skin testing or RAST are usually available.

Foods

Asthma is a frequent occupational disease among bakers. Grain allergens are the usual cause, but sensitization to contaminants such as mold spores or grain mites has also been reported. Other foods causing occupational asthma include coffee beans, tea, soybeans, eggs, snow crabs, and cocoa. Castor beans containing the toxin ricin appear to be a special problem, and epidemics of asthma in nearby residents as well as workers have occurred.

Latex

Latex allergy among health care workers is an emerging problem. Although contact sensitivity is frequently caused by chemicals used in manufacturing, occupational asthma and other IgE-mediated reactions result from sensitization to protein antigens in native latex. Occupational sensitization to latex may have severe consequences for the health care worker who becomes a patient. Sensitized individuals should wear a medical alert bracelet.

Animals

Asthma caused by animal proteins in dander, saliva, or urine frequently develops in laboratory workers, farmers, and other people who handle animals. Such sensitization can occur to any warm-blooded animal.

Insects

Sensitization to the insects used in their work can develop in bee workers and bait workers. Less obvious exposures include sensitization of farmers, grain handlers, or bakers to storage mites, and sensitization of poultry workers to fowl mites.

Vegetable Gums

Vegetable gums represent another, less obvious source of allergens that may cause occupational asthma in workers in a variety of occupations, including printing, carpet manufacturing, and hairdressing.

Enzymes

Proteolytic enzymes used in detergents, meat tenderizer, and various manufacturing processes are potent sensitizers.

Course of Occupational Asthma

Occupational asthma allows investigators to view the entire natural history of asthma in response to a single, clearly defined etiologic agent. This perspective provides insight into the pace and variability of asthma development and also an opportunity to look at the resolution of asthma as workers are removed from exposures. Thus, occupational asthma provides a unique opportunity to study the pathophysiology of asthma. There have been several surprising findings in terms of the natural history of occupational asthma.

The variability in latency—that is, the time from initial exposure to development of symptoms—is well demonstrated in studies of occupational asthma (Fig. 3). The onset of symptoms follows an exponential curve. For example, the latency period for 50% of cases of sensitization to high-molecular-weight antigens is 3 years, but it takes 9 years to get to 75% of cases. There are even cases of occupational asthma developing in some workers after 30 years of exposure.

Another unexpected finding in occupational asthma is

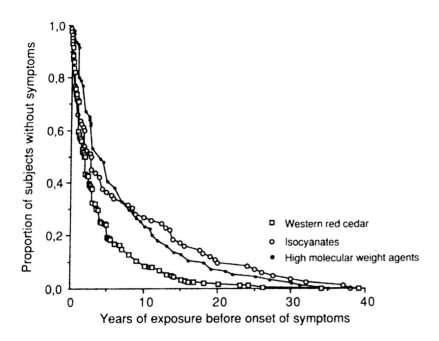

FIG. 3. Proportion of patients without symptoms as a function of exposure interval. (Modified with permission from Malo JL, et al. Natural history of occupation asthma: relevance of type of agent and other factors in the rate of development of symptoms in affected subjects. *J Allergy Clin Immunol* 1992;90:937–944.)

that symptoms are often not reversible when the worker is removed from exposure (Table 6). Even years after removal, airways hyperresponsiveness and inflammation persist in the majority of patients with occupational asthma studied in large series. The prognosis is worse for workers who stay on the job after onset of asthma and better for those workers who leave as soon as symptoms develop. These findings suggest a window of opportunity to remove the worker before irreversible changes take place. Although these results have been criticized because pre-exposure airways responses were often not available, in several workers with normal baseline function before exposure, airways hyperresponsiveness persisted long after removal from exposure. The relationship of inflammation to the irreversible stage of asthma is still controversial. However, an essential component of these irreversible changes may be the development of inflammation in the absence of exogenous antigen. Treatment with inhaled steroids induces resolution of inflammation and the hyperresponsiveness that persists after removal from exposure to TDI. At this point, there is no compelling reason to believe that occupational and non-occupational asthma differ in regard to pathogenesis of chronic effects. The

only real difference may be that it is easier to define the long-term effects in occupational asthma because symptoms persist despite removal from ongoing exposure.

INDUSTRIAL BRONCHITIS

Chronic bronchitis is defined as a productive cough lasting for >3 months per year for two consecutive years. Chronic bronchitis has been linked to cigarette smoke, which complicates the assessment of industrial bronchitis. Many workplace materials have been implicated as a cause of chronic bronchitis, including a variety of dusts (e.g., cotton dust), fumes, and vapors. The pathology of bronchitis is characterized by mucous gland hypertrophy and goblet cell hyperplasia in the large airways. There is an increase in mucus-secreting glands relative to serous acini, so that secretions tend to be more viscous and have less antibacterial activity. These changes in mucus may predispose to bacterial overgrowth. The role of inflammation in chronic bronchitis is not clear, although it may be important in the induction of mucous membrane metaplasia. In addition, one study indicates that sputum production correlates better with bronchial inflammation than with the structural changes in the mucous glands.

Many of the agents associated with industrial bronchitis have also been linked to an accelerated decline in FEV_1. The pathophysiology of this annual decline in FEV_1 is probably not bronchitis itself, which is a disease of the large airways. Instead, inflammation, mucous membrane metaplasia, and fibrosis in the small airways appear to be the pathologic features that lead to clinical airways obstruction. Thus, bronchitis and the development of small-airways disease with decreased FEV_1 are distin-

TABLE 6. *Irreversible asthma after occupational exposure*

Agent	No. of patients	Percentage with residual asthma	Follow-up
TDI	50	82%	>4 y
Red cedar	136	60%	4.3 y
Colophony	20	90%	29 mo
Snow crab	31	61%	1 y

TDI, toluene diisocyanate.

guished by their anatomic localization. They frequently occur together in the same person and often are both caused by exposure to the same agent. An agent inducing chronic bronchitis should alert the investigator to look for a decline in pulmonary function.

BIBLIOGRAPHY

Alberts WM, doPico GA. Reactive airways dysfunction syndrome. *Chest* 1996;109:1618–1626. *A comprehensive review of the clinical, pathologic, and epidemiologic presentation of RADS.*

Bardana E Jr. Occupational asthma and related respiratory disorders. *Dis Mon* 1995;3:144–199. *Excellent clinical review of occupational respiratory problems.*

Burge PS. Occupational asthma in electronics workers caused by colophony fumes: follow-up of affected workers. *Thorax* 1982;37:348–353. *Follow-up of 20 cases of colophony-induced asthma.*

Chan-Yeung M. American College of Physicians consensus statement: assessment of asthma in the workplace. *Chest* 1995;108:1084–1117. *Practical guidelines for the workup of occupational asthma.*

Chan-Yeung M, Lam S. Occupational asthma. *Am Rev Respir Dis* 1986;133:686–703. *State-of-the-art review of occupational asthma.*

Chan-Yeung M, MacLean L, Paggiaro PL. Follow-up study of 232 patients with occupational asthma caused by western red cedar (*Thuja plicata*). *J Allergy Clin Immunol* 1987;79:792–796. *Large series demonstrating the importance of early diagnosis and removal from exposure.*

Chan-Yeung M, Malo JL. Occupational asthma. *N Engl J Med* 1995;333:107–112. *Short but excellent recent review of occupational asthma.*

Frew AJ, Chan H, Lam S, Chan-Yeung M. Bronchial inflammation in occupational asthma due to western red cedar. *Am J Respir Crit Care Med* 1995;151:340–344. *Bronchial mucosal biopsy specimens from 9 patients with western cedar-induced asthma, 6 patients with atopic asthma, and 6 non-atopic, non-asthmatic controls were compared.*

Herd AL, Bernstein DI. Antigen-specific stimulation of histamine-releasing factors in diisocyante-induced occupational asthma. *Am J Respir Crit Care Med* 1994;150:988–994. *Peripheral blood mononuclear cells incubated for 48 hours with diisocyantes conjugated to HSA produced histamine-releasing factor.*

Hudson P, Cartier A, Pineua L, Lafrance M, St-Aubin JJ, Dubois JY, Malo JL. Follow-up of occupational asthma caused by crab and various agents. *J Allergy Clin Immunol* 1985;76:682–688. *Follow-up of 31 patients with occupational asthma related to crabs.*

Kogevinas M, Anto JM, Soriano JB, Tobias A, Burney P. The risk of asthma attributable to occupational exposures: a population-based study in Spain. *Am J Respir Crit Care Med* 1996;154:137–143. *Occupational exposures constitute a substantial cause of asthma in the young adult Spanish population.*

Lozewicz S, Assoufi BK, Hawkins R, Newman Taylor AJ. Outcome of asthma induced by isocyanates. *Br J Dis Chest* 1987;81:14–22. *Follow-up of 50 cases of diisocyante asthma.*

Maestrelli P, Del Prete GF, De Carli M, D'Elios MM, Saetta M, DeStefano A, Mapp CE, Romagnani S, Baffri LM. CD8 T-cell clones producing interleukin-5 and interferon-τ in bronchial mucosa of patients with asthma induced by toluene diisocyanate. *Scand J Work Environ Health* 1994;20:387–381. *An interesting article showing that CD8 T cells with a peculiar pattern of cytokine production predominate after challenge with TDI.*

Maestrelli P, DeMarzo N, Saetta M, Boscaro M, Fabbri LM, Mapp CE. Effects of inhaled beclomethasone on airway responsiveness in occupational asthma. *Am Rev Respir Dis* 1993;148:407–412. *An im-portant study showing that inhaled steroids can speed the resolution of nonspecific bronchial hyperresponsiveness in TDI asthma.*

Malo JL, Ghezzo H, D'Aquino C, L'Archevêque J, Cartier A, Chan-Yeung M. Natural history of occupational asthma: relevance of type of agent and other factors in the rate of development of symptoms in affected subjects. *J Allergy Clin Immunol* 1992;90:937–944. *Interesting epidemiologic analysis of 771 patients with occupational asthma.*

Mapp CE, Corona PC, DeMarzo N, Fabbri L. Persistent asthma due to isocyanates: a follow-up study of subjects with occupational asthma due to toluene diisocyanate (TDI). *Am Rev Respir Dis* 1988;137:1326–1329. *Follow-up of 30 patients with TDI asthma documenting persistent symptoms and airway hyperresponsiveness.*

Mapp CE, Saetta M, Maestrelli P, Di Stefano A, Chitano P, Boschetto P, Ciaccia A, Fabbri LM. Mechanisms and pathology of occupational asthma. *Eur Respir J* 1994;7:544–554. *Excellent short review of the pathogenesis of IgE and non-IgE occupational asthma.*

Paggiaro PL, Vagaggini B, Dente FL, Bacci E, Bancalari L, Carrara M, De Franco A, Giannini D, Giutini C. Bronchial hyperresponsiveness and toluene diisocyanate. *Chest* 1993;103:1123–1128. *Follow-up of 16 patients with TDI asthma showing persistent nonspecific airway hyperresponsiveness.*

Panhuysen CIM, Meyers DA, Postma DS, Levitt RC, Bleecker ER. The genetics of asthma and atopy. *Allergy* 1995;0:1–7. *Recent review of linkage studies for bronchial hyperresponsiveness and total IgE.*

Perrin B, Cartier A, Ghezzo H, Grammer L, Harris K, Chan H, Chan-Yeung M, Malo JL. Reassessment of the temporal patterns of bronchial obstruction after exposure to occupational sensitizing agents. *J Allergy Clin Immunol* 1991;87:630–639. *Analysis of the pattern of airway response after challenge of 69 patients with occupational asthma.*

Quirce S, Contreras G, Dybuncio A, Chan-Yeung M. Peak expiratory flow monitoring is not a reliable method for establishing the diagnosis of occupational asthma. *Am J Respir Crit Care Med* 1995;152:1100–1102. *Use of computerized peak flow meters demonstrates the shortcomings of peak flow monitoring.*

Saetta M, DiStefano A, Maestrelli P, DeMarzo N, Milani GF, Pivirotto F, Mapp CE, Fabbri LM. Airway mucosal inflammation in occupational asthma induced by toluene diisocyanate. *Am Rev Respir Dis* 1992;145:160–168. *Bronchial biopsy specimens from nine patients with TDI asthma and four unexposed controls without asthma were compared.*

Saetta M, Maestrelli P, DiStefano A, DeMarzo N, Milani GF, Pivirotto F, Mapp CE, Fabbri LM. Effect of cessation of exposure to toluene diisocyanate (TDI) on bronchial mucosa of subjects with TDI-induced asthma. *Am Rev Respir Dis* 1992;145:169–174. *Six months after exposure ceased, bronchial hyperresponsiveness and inflammation persisted but basement membrane thickening was reduced.*

Sheppard D, Saisho A, Nadel JA, Boushey HA. Exercise increases sulphur dioxide-induced bronchoconstriction in asthmatic subjects. *Am Rev Respir Dis* 1981;123:486–491. *Early demonstration of the interaction of air pollutant exposure and exercise in provoking changes in airway function.*

Virchow JC Jr, Kroegel C, Walker C, Matthys H. Cellular and immunological markers of allergic and intrinsic bronchial asthma. *Lung* 1994;172:313–334. *Short review of the pathophysiology, including cytokine profile, of extrinsic versus intrinsic asthma.*

Walker C, Bauer W, Braun RK, Menz G, Braun P, Schwarz F, Hansel TT, Villiger B. Activated T cells and cytokines in bronchoalveolar lavages from patients with various lung diseases associated with eosinophilia. *Am J Respir Crit Care Med* 1994;150:1038–1048. *Comparison of extrinsic and intrinsic asthma, eosinophilic pneumonia, bronchopulmonary aspergillosis, hypersensitivity pneumonitis, pulmonary fibrosis, and sarcoidosis.*

Walker C, Bode E, Boer L, Hansel TT, Blaser K, Virchow JC Jr. Allergic and non-allergic asthmatics have distinct patterns of T-cell activation and cytokine production in peripheral blood and bronchoalveolar lavage. *Am Rev Respir Dis* 1991;146:109–115. *Comparison of 10 allergic versus 10 non-allergic asthmatic patients.*

Textbook of Pulmonary Diseases, 6th ed.
edited by G.L. Baum, J.D. Crapo, B.R. Celli, and J.B. Karlinsky,
Lippincott–Raven Publishers, Philadelphia, © 1998.

CHAPTER 35

Byssinosis and Respiratory Disease Caused by Vegetable Dusts

William S. Beckett · Mark J. Utell

INTRODUCTION

The term *byssinosis* is applied to acute and chronic diseases of the airways occurring in persons exposed to three vegetable textile fibers: cotton, flax (which is woven into linen), and soft hemp (which is used for making rope and net). It is applied both to the acute syndrome of chest tightness, dyspnea, and reversible air flow obstruction that occurs at work within a few hours of exposure to cotton dust, and more broadly to the other respiratory effects of cotton, flax, and hemp dust. Because many more people worldwide are exposed to cotton than to jute and hemp dust, much of the following discussion focuses on cotton dust disease but also applies to the effects of the other vegetable fiber dusts.

With sufficient exposure, dusts from these materials may produce eye and nasal irritation, bronchitis, occupational asthma (with a characteristic pattern of worsening symptoms and air flow obstruction on the first day of exposure after a break from work), fever, chronic air flow obstruction, or combinations of these. The delayed febrile response to these dusts is now known as the *organic dust toxic syndrome (ODTS)*, which may occur after inhalation of a variety organic materials that have been kept in conditions permitting the profuse growth of contaminating micro-organisms (see below).

Long-term occupational exposure to a variety of vegetable dusts (including some grain and wood dusts) causes

airways symptoms of cough, expectoration of mucus, and wheeze, and with sufficient exposure leads to chronic air flow obstruction.

COTTON DUST DISEASE

Cotton is a plant-derived cellulose fiber. The long, thin, flexible cotton fiber consists of glucose units connected by glycosidic linkages containing reactive hydrogen groups. However, it is in large part the dust of the bract (dry, friable materials at the base of the cotton flower), leaf, and stem of the cotton plant, and the micro-organisms that grow on them, that cause disease (Fig. 1). Cotton dust may contain ground-up plant matter, fibers, bacteria, fungi, soil, pesticides, plant matter other than cotton, and other contaminants in varying proportions according to the conditions of plant growth and stage in the processing of cotton.

Although the relative importance of the different components of cotton dust in producing disease is controversial, the acute response of byssinosis correlates better with the measured exposure to endotoxin (from the cell walls of contaminating gram-negative bacteria), whereas chronic air flow obstruction correlates better with total cotton dust exposure.

Epidemiology

Cotton growing and production of cotton products are major industries worldwide. Hence, respiratory disease related to cotton dust will continue to be commonplace until dust control in these industries becomes more wide-

W. S. Beckett and M. J. Utell: Divisions of Occupational/ Environmental Medicine and Pulmonary/Critical Care, Departments Of Medicine and Environmental Medicine, University of Rochester Medical Center, Rochester, New York 14642.

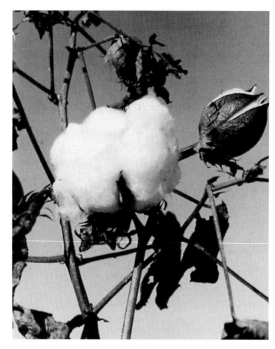

FIG. 1. The cotton plant, with cotton fibers supported by bract, leaf, and stem. A boll in the process of opening is seen in the *upper right.* In the *center,* the white cotton fibers are surrounded at the base by the brittle cotton bract. Cotton dust is composed mainly of bract, leaf, and stem.

spread. Among persons exposed to cotton dust are workers in cotton ginning, cottonseed oil mills, cotton thread and yarn manufacturing, cotton fabric manufacturing, and those working with textile waste used in padding, upholstery, and mattresses. Disease is not usually associated with the harvesting of cotton, flax, or hemp or with exposure only to cleaned cotton fibers once processed into their finished products (Fig. 2). In cotton textile production, where dust exposures are excessive, byssinosis may affect a large proportion of the exposed workers, reflecting a pharmacologic (rather than sensitizing) effect of inhaled materials in the airways. This pattern contrasts with that of typical sensitizing or latency occupational asthma, where fewer than 10% of exposed workers are usually affected.

Cigarette smoking is believed to be associated with an increased susceptibility to the adverse effects of cotton dust.

Clinical Presentation

Airways symptoms of cough, mucous production, or the development of chronic bronchitis are a common response to cotton dust exposure and occur in workers exposed to cotton dust who do not have the chest tightness and reversible air flow limitation of the acute syndrome; they are found in both smokers and nonsmokers. These syndromes have been observed repeatedly in carefully controlled studies of cotton textile workers in the absence of other symptoms of byssinosis.

The cardinal symptoms of the acute byssinosis syndrome are chest tightness and shortness of breath that occur on re-exposure to cotton dust after a weekend or several days away from work. This very common temporal pattern, ''Monday chest tightness,'' may also occur in previously unexposed persons on first contact with the dust. The temporal relationship of the onset of chest tightness to first exposure at work differs from the latency typical of occupational asthma; it often occurs 2 to 3 hrs after exposure to dust has begun, whereas in occupational asthma the early asthmatic response usually begins within the first hour, and the less common late asthmatic response occurs usually after 6 or more hrs. The chest tightness may be associated with a productive cough. In more severe cases or in older workers, dyspnea on exertion also may occur. Tolerance to cotton dust with a reduction in symptoms on subsequent mornings of the workweek is often seen, with loss of tolerance after 1 day or more away from work. With progression to more severe disease, symptoms of chest tightness and dyspnea may be

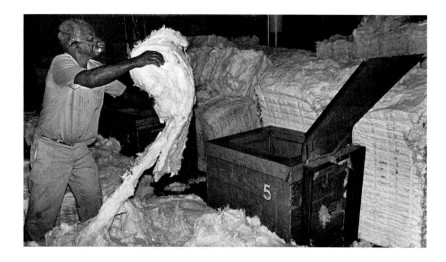

FIG. 2. Cotton mill worker opening a bale of cotton that has been ginned and shipped to the mill for further processing. Opening bales is one of the dustiest jobs in the cotton mill. (Photo copyright Earl Dotter, reproduced with permission.)

present each day at work, and eventually at all times. The severity of symptoms is enhanced if symptoms caused by chronic cigarette smoking are present, and both dust exposure and smoking contribute additively to chronic airways disease in cotton textile workers. Those with chronic air flow obstruction have the characteristic symptom of dyspnea on exertion, with reduction in exercise tolerance in proportion to the degree of air flow obstruction.

Thus, persons exposed to cotton dust may seek medical attention with a history of chest tightness occurring at work, intermittent or chronic bronchitis, acute fever occurring several hours after exposure to dust, or chronic dyspnea and exercise intolerance after years of exposure.

Pathogenesis

Byssinosis is a non-allergic airways disease. Bronchoconstriction and inflammation can be induced in previously unexposed persons with a first challenge to cotton dust extract. There are several theories regarding mechanisms, for which some experimental evidence exists. Local release of histamine from airways in contact with dust may result in the acute symptoms and air flow obstruction. A distinct inflammatory airways response to contaminating bacterial endotoxin, other bacteria-derived substances, or other components of cotton dust appears to be important in the chronic bronchitis associated with long-term exposure to cotton dust.

Physical Findings

Findings on chest examination are usually absent or minimal in patients with symptomatic dust disease, although wheezing may be heard. With chronic disease, the findings are chronic air flow limitation, weight loss, use of accessory muscles of respiration, prolonged expiration, and either a quiet chest or wheezing on expiration.

Laboratory Findings

No useful serologic markers have been found for byssinosis. Findings on chest radiographs in patients with byssinosis are usually unremarkable.

Pulmonary Function

In patients with the acute airways form of byssinosis, reversible air flow limitation may be demonstrated by comparing measurements made after a Monday work shift

with those made before (Fig. 3). Lung function may be normal between episodes of byssinosis. If spirometry is performed before and after the work shift throughout a week, the FEV_1 (forced expiratory volume in 1 second) and the ratio of FEV_1 to FVC (forced vital capacity) are reduced during the day of exposure in symptomatic workers with byssinosis. The absolute value of the fall in FEV_1 may be greatest on the first day of exposure, and less through the workweek as a result of adaptation. However, the baseline level of FEV_1 at the beginning of the day may be reduced with serial daily exposure through the workweek, only to return to the previously normal baseline on the next Monday morning. The magnitude of the reversible decline in FEV_1 in symptomatic patients may be relatively small (10%–20% during the acute episode) in relation to the degree of chest tightness experienced.

Patients with byssinosis have greater airways responsiveness to nonspecific challenge than do subjects without byssinosis from the same mill, and airways responsiveness has been demonstrated experimentally to increase across a Monday work shift in mill workers with byssinosis. The role or utility of nonspecific airways challenge in diagnosing byssinosis has not been defined.

Chronic air flow limitation with permanent impairment is seen as a result of long-term exposure to cotton dust through many years. The pattern cannot be distinguished on physiologic grounds from the chronic air flow limitation seen in cigarette smokers, and so the occupational history of exposure to cotton dust is important in establishing a diagnosis. Ascertaining the duration and levels of exposure to cotton dust, a history of acute respiratory symptoms, or a decline in FEV_1 across work shifts, as well as obtaining a complete smoking history, may be useful in determining the degree of chronic air flow limitation attributable to cotton dust versus that attributable to cigarette smoke in a cotton worker who has also smoked.

Treatment

Reduction in total exposure to cotton dust to prevent recurrence is the primary treatment of byssinosis. This can be achieved by control of airborne dust levels—for example, enhancing ventilation in areas with high dust levels. Prewashing of cotton has also been effective in reducing exposure to pathogenic dust.

When acute air flow obstruction is present, treatment with inhaled β-adrenergic agonist bronchodilators has been shown to reverse obstruction, and this treatment is advisable for the symptomatic patient in distress. The diagnosis of byssinosis is a sentinel health event indicating an excessive occupational exposure. Byssinosis is a reportable condition in many states and provinces, and the diagnosis is an indication for intervention in the workplace to reduce dust exposure for the symptomatic patient.

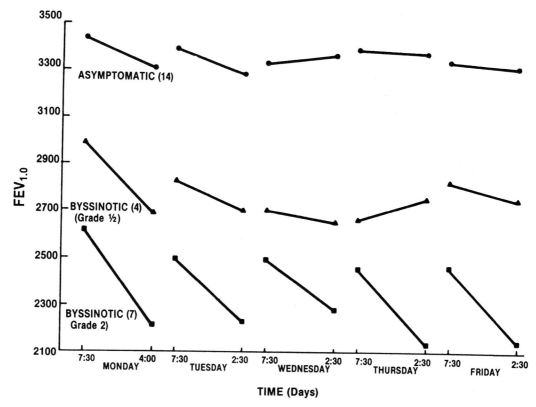

FIG. 3. Correlation of the grade (severity) of byssinosis with FEV_1 on spirometry during a work week in heavily exposed cotton mill carders. Grade 1/2 refers to those with occasional tightness or mild respiratory irritation on the first day of the work week. Grade 2 refers to those with usual chest tightness on the first day and other days of the week. Note that asymptomatic individuals also have work-related decrements in FEV_1. Carders with the higher grade of byssinosis have lower baseline lung function. *Numbers in parentheses* refer to the number of subjects in each group. (Reproduced with permission from Merchant JA, et al. Evaluation before and after exposure—the pattern of physiologic response to cotton dust. *Ann N Y Acad Sci* 1974;221:38–43.)

Because of the high attack rate in areas of overexposure, the diagnosis of one case indicates that many others are likely to be similarly overexposed and symptomatic. Occupational standards for dust in cotton-processing workplaces that do not produce acute symptomatic disease have been established and are enforced in many countries.

ORGANIC DUST TOXIC SYNDROME

The syndrome is characterized by prominent, delayed fever and systemic symptoms after an episode of inhalation of organic dust often described as moldy. The illness is self-limiting and without significant radiographic findings. It has been reported in a broad variety of circumstances, including in farmers unloading hay from silos and workers shoveling moldy wood chips. It is categorized among the inhalation fevers, which also include metal fume fever and (Teflon) polymer fume fever. ODTS is not an IgE-mediated allergic response, as it does not require previous sensitization and is characterized by tolerance to similar exposures on subsequent challenge. An

acute febrile response to inhaled cotton dust after a period of 2 days or more away from work (''mill fever'') is well described in cotton textile workers with heavier exposure to dust, and cotton dust is now recognized as one cause of ODTS.

GRAIN DUST DISEASES

Epidemiologic studies of agricultural workers exposed to a variety of grain dusts, both in harvesting and in storing, unloading, and transporting grain, have discovered an important association of allergic manifestations, acute and chronic bronchitis, and chronic air flow obstruction related to the levels and duration of dust exposure. A similar pattern has also been observed with at least one kind of wood dust. The clinical picture is often one of an inflammatory bronchitis with mucous gland hyperplasia, chronic hypersecretion of mucus associated with cough and phlegm, and, in cases of prolonged and heavy exposure, accelerated decline in lung function during a period of years. Because of the absence of specific physical, laboratory, or radiographic findings, the occupational history of recurrent exposure to dust (usually at levels that are easily visible in the workplace) may be the most important clue to the underlying cause of the patient's respiratory symptoms. A short course of anti-inflammatory medication, such as an inhaled corticosteroid, may be tried to treat the acute response, and interventions to reduce dust exposure through control technology or the use of respiratory protective masks (still markedly underutilized in agriculture) are necessary to prevent recurrent or progressive disease.

BIBLIOGRAPHY

Bouhuys A. Asthma and byssinosis. *Rev Allergy* 1966;22:473–476. *A concise clinical description of the differential diagnosis of byssinosis and other forms of occupational airways disease.*

Christiani DC, Ye TT, Wegman DH, Eisen EA, Dai HI, Lu PL. Cotton dust exposure, across-shift drop in FEV$_1$, and five-year change in lung function. *Am J Respir Crit Care Med* 1994;10:1250–1255. *Study of Chinese cotton workers demonstrating the relationship between dust exposure and the development of an irreversible accelerated decline in lung function.*

Enarson D, Vedal S, Chan-Yeung M. Rapid decline in FEV$_1$ in grain handlers. *Am Rev Respir Dis* 1985;132:814–817. *One of several studies indicating that those working in grain elevators and other areas of grain storage and transport may have an irreversible loss of lung function in addition to acute and chronic bronchitis and wheezing.*

Glindmeyer HW, LenFante JJ, Jones RN, Rando J, Abdel-Keder HM, Weill H. Exposure-related declines in lung function in cotton textile workers. *Am Rev Respir Dis* 1991;144:675–685. *This study found an accelerated decline in lung function in U.S. cotton textile workers, and also a synergistic interaction between cigarette smoking and cotton dust on the rate of decline in lung function.*

Merchant JA, Halprin GM, Hudson AR, Kilburn KH, McKenzie WN, Bermanzohn P, Hurst JH, Hamilton JD, Germino VH. Evaluation before and after exposure—the pattern of physiologic response to cotton dust. *Ann N Y Acad Sci* 1974;221:38–43. *The severity of cotton dust-related symptoms is correlated with a daily fall in FEV$_1$ when spirometry is performed in cotton mill workers before and after a workshift.*

Noertjojo HK, Dimich-Ward H, Peelen S, Dittrick M, Kennedy S, Chan-Yeung M. Western red cedar dust exposure and lung function: a dose-response relationship. *Am J Respir Crit Care Med* 1996;154:968–973. *In addition to causing occupational asthma in some exposed workers, the dust from this commercially important wood may produce a persistent decline in lung function in workers who do not have asthma.*

U.S. Department of Labor, Occupational Safety and Health Administration. Cotton dust. Title 29, Code of Federal Regulations, Part 1910.1043. *This government document outlines in detail an approach to the prevention of cotton dust disease based on measurement of air levels and regular testing of exposed persons.*

Textbook of Pulmonary Diseases, 6th ed.
edited by G.L. Baum, J.D. Crapo, B.R. Celli, and J.B. Karlinsky,
Lippincott–Raven Publishers, Philadelphia, © 1998.

CHAPTER

Occupational Pulmonary Neoplasms

36

David R. Graham · W. Keith C. Morgan

INTRODUCTION

Although the incidence of lung cancer is increased in certain occupations, the most important cause of this disease remains cigarette smoking. Even if one considers those cancers associated with a particular trade, the occupational risk is small compared with that of smoking. However, in the belief that something can be done to reduce the occupational risk, whereas many smokers seem powerless or too ignorant to help themselves, occupational lung cancer requires further consideration.

HISTORY OF OCCUPATIONAL CANCER

The first neoplasm noted to be related to a particular occupation was cancer of the scrotum. In 1775, Percival Pott observed that the disease characteristically occurred in chimney sweeps and concluded that it seemed to derive from a lodgement of soot in the rugae of the scrotum. Tumors of the skin were later described in cotton workers, shale oil workers, and aniline dye workers.

Harting and Hesse were the first to recognize cancer of the lung as a frequent cause of death in miners of copper, iron, and silver in Schneeberg. It was only later that the cause was found to be radioactive air in the mines. This same problem was identified in uranium mines, where the presence of radon daughters was shown to be associated with bronchogenic carcinoma. In more recent years, the risks associated with several other materials used in industry have been recognized. Lung cancer has

been shown to be associated with asbestos, arsenic, chromates, iron ores, coal gas, chloromethyl ethers, beryllium, nickel, and vinyl chloride. Several other substances are suspected, but as yet not proved, to be carcinogens.

EXTENT OF RISK: OCCUPATION VERSUS SMOKING

If the substances involved in producing human cancer can be identified and proved to be causally related, then those substances might be avoided. The portion of blame that can be attached to the various environmental factors thought to be carcinogens has been the topic of considerable debate during the last decade. Most of the work on this subject has been epidemiologic, relying on the incidence of cancers in various populations and countries. It has been suggested by some that environmental factors can account for up to 80% of human cancers. However, this figure is itself an exaggeration and includes not only the toxic materials of industry, but also factors such as diet, numbers of pregnancies, race, and so forth. Nevertheless, the figure of 80% has been used to suggest that exposure to chemicals and toxins such as asbestos is the major cause of cancer in Western society. This view is supported by Epstein, who goes further in stating that a cancer epidemic is in progress as a consequence of occupational and environmental exposures. Not surprisingly, these views have important political implications and have been supported by various governmental agencies. Bridbord and associates, under the auspices of the National Cancer Institute and the National Institute for Occupational Safety and Health (NIOSH), calculated the risk of exposure to six known carcinogens and concluded that occupational cancers comprise 23%–38% of the total number of cancers, with asbestos alone causing up to

D. R. Graham: Whiston Hospital, Prescot, Merseyside L35, DR, United Kingdom.

W. K. C. Morgan: Chest Disease Unit, University Hospital, London, Ontario N6A 5A5 Canada.

18%. To this figure must be added the effects of ionizing radiation and other known carcinogens not included in their calculation.

When these facts, together with the preceding data, were re-examined, basic flaws in the epidemiologic method used by Bridbord and associates were noted. One of the main faults was a disregard for dose and duration of exposure to particular carcinogens, resulting in gross overestimation of the risk. It may well be that the Occupational Safety and Health Administration (OSHA) article was written for political rather than scientific purposes, and that the figure of 38% for cancer deaths caused by occupation should be dismissed. It appears that there is no current cancer epidemic apart from the epidemic of lung cancer, which is largely a consequence of cigarette smoking.

A more realistic view of the situation suggests that 15% of lung cancers in men and 5% in women are attributable to some extent to contact with occupational agents. Of this 15% in men, a third are caused by asbestos, a third by fossil fuels, and the remaining third by other recognized agents, such as chromium, nickel, chloromethyl ethers, and ionizing radiation. Similar estimates of a 10% and 14% excess risk for lung cancer have been suggested. In fact, the figure of 38% of cancers being attributable to industry, noted in the 1978 federal report, has since been acknowledged to be an overestimate.

It is important to note that the results of the above studies are based on exposure to carcinogens in excess of those encountered in industry today. Overall, industrial hygiene has improved, exposure to asbestos is now under strict control, and the introduction of natural gas has, at least in the United Kingdom, decreased the numbers of workers involved with coke ovens. Future studies should show that the excess risk for lung cancer attributable to industry will continue to fall.

A systematic approach was used to examine the proportion of lung and bladder cancers resulting from occupation. An analysis of several large studies of various occupational groups between 1977 and 1988 showed that the proportion of lung cancers attributable to occupation varied by as much as 1%–40%. The main reasons for this large variation are the differences in levels of exposures to carcinogens in the various studies and countries. The criteria used to assess exposure have been improved but are not always precisely defined and may be the origin of any miscalculations.

INTERACTION OF SMOKING AND OCCUPATIONAL CARCINOGENS

A further consideration is the effect of the combination of smoking and exposure to a known carcinogen. The result of such a combination is best documented in the case of asbestos. The risk from exposure to asbestos alone can be demonstrated by examination of asbestos-exposed persons who have never smoked. However, because lung cancer in nonsmokers (including those exposed to asbestos) is rare, large populations are required to produce reliable results. Authors of several studies conclude that the risk for development of carcinoma in a nonsmoker as a result of asbestos exposure is very small, but this risk is approximately five times greater than that in an unexposed nonsmoker. The risk in a smoker exposed to asbestos is greatly increased, and not just additively; the level of risk can be calculated by multiplying the two separate risk factors. One view of this situation demonstrates that an unexposed nonsmoker has a mortality ratio of 1, a nonsmoking asbestos worker has a ratio of 5.17, and a smoking asbestos worker has a ratio of 53.3. The exposures also were quantified, and in smokers of more than one pack a day the mortality ratio rose to 87.4.

An interaction is also found between radon daughters and cigarette smoking, although it is not as clear as in the case of asbestos. It appears that there are two effects: first, an additive effect of the number of cancers induced by the two agents, and second, a hastening effect, so that the induction-latent period is shorter among smokers than among nonsmokers. Thus, cancers appear earlier in smokers.

Various explanations have been proposed for these interactions between cigarette smoke and carcinogens. Cigarette smoke is toxic to the ciliated epithelium, and the resultant loss of ciliary function with failure to clear sputum means that carcinogens can be in prolonged contact with the mucosa. Cigarette smoke can cause squamous metaplasia, and it also has been suggested that particles in cigarette smoke can absorb carcinogens and carry them farther down the bronchial tree. Conversely, the asbestos fibers may damage cells to allow entry of carcinogens present in cigarette smoke.

The overall conclusion is that no other known single measure would have as great an impact on the number of deaths attributable to cancer as a reduction in the use of tobacco. This view is supported by the Surgeon General of the United States, who stated that cigarette smoking is a greater cause of death and disability than the workplace environment. In occupations in which the worker is exposed to hazardous agents, control of both smoking and the agent itself provides the most effective means of reducing the risk.

INVESTIGATION OF OCCUPATIONAL LUNG CANCER

The investigation of a potential occupational carcinogen can be carried out in two ways: laboratory testing and epidemiologic survey. Under different circumstances, there is a place for both methods, although some agencies tend to give more weight to laboratory testing of animals than to epidemiology. This is a little surprising, as the majority of discoveries relating to occupational lung cancer have been made by astute observation backed up by epidemiologic confirmation. This approach not only led to the description of the first occupational neoplasm, but was also used by others to identify the associations between asbestos and lung cancer, asbestos and mesothelioma, nickel and lung and nasal cancer, and furniture work and nasal cancer.

Laboratory studies also have an important place, particularly when a carcinogen is suspected not because of an increased incidence in a certain trade but because a particular chemical has a structure similar to that of a known carcinogen. The experimental approach was used to identify the carcinogenicity of the chloromethyl ethers.

Laboratory Testing

If suspicion arises concerning a particular substance that physically or chemically resembles a known carcinogen, the approach should be in vitro testing, and if the suspicion is warranted, progression to animal exposure studies is appropriate. In vitro tests are the quickest and cheapest method of examining potential carcinogens. However, their use is limited, because their only function is to show whether or not a particular substance has any effect on DNA. They can be used as a screening test of new materials, or they can be used to show that one carcinogen is more dangerous than another. In *in vitro* testing, the ability of a substance to transform mammalian fibroblasts into particular colonies with malignant characteristics may be detected, or, as in the Ames test, a change in the rate of mutation of a nutritionally deficient strain of *Salmonella typhimurium* may be demonstrated. When such tests are used, known carcinogens will produce positive results nine times in 10. However, false-positive and false-negative results do occur, and no test is yet available that shows whether there is a threshold below which a suspected carcinogen is innocuous in humans.

Animal studies provide data that are more readily applied to humans. However, besides ethical considerations, there are important limitations; the production of tumors in animals remains uncertain and unpredictable and depends not only on variations between species but also on factors such as sex, diet, and age of the animals. Most animal experiments consist of a relatively short exposure of small rodents to substances at inordinately higher concentrations than those encountered in the workplace. Although valuable information can be obtained from animal experiments, as was the case with chloromethyl ethers, the results of carcinogenesis in animals cannot be blindly applied to humans.

The problem with laboratory studies as a determinant of carcinogenic properties lies in the process of carcinogenesis itself. There is evidence that certain compounds

act as initiators and induce mutation in the DNA of target cells (irradiation, halo ethers, mustard gas). Others are responsible for the second phase of carcinogenesis and act as promoters, inducing increased cell multiplication (asbestos). Most compounds act directly on DNA. However, nickel interferes with replication, and benzpyrene requires activation by the host before carcinogenic properties develop. It is clear that the basic mechanisms of carcinogenesis are incompletely understood, and for this reason, laboratory testing is, at best, a rough estimate of the risks that might be involved. Laboratory tests should not be used to declare a compound safe or unsafe, but rather should be used as an indicator of whether protection, surveillance, and further research are required.

Epidemiology of Occupational Lung Cancer

The value of epidemiologic study has been emphasized already. Of the known occupational exposures (Table 1) related to cancer of the respiratory tract, 11 were first detected by observation in particular working groups. Only in the case of the halo ethers was carcinogenicity first demonstrated in animal experiments and subsequently confirmed in epidemiologic studies.

As shown in the discussion of the relative parts played by occupation and smoking, the epidemiologic method most often used is that of mortality studies of cohorts. A cohort with a particular contact or exposure is identified and examined. Mortality rates and the causes of death of this cohort are then compared with those of the community in general, groups of smokers, and persons of a particular social class, race, and so on. The cohort can be further subdivided with reference to levels of exposure, age, and tobacco consumption, and thus groups within groups can be compared. The main problems encountered with this type of study are that numbers must be large and data, particularly concerning smoking and exposure contact, must be accurate. An alternative epidemiologic method is the case-control approach. In this method, persons with a certain disease are identified and compared in terms of occupational exposure with matched control subjects who do not have the disease in question. Again, numbers must be very large; for example, a study to estimate the proportion of lung cancer caused by occupation would require 10,000 cases and 10,000 controls.

In the study of occupational lung cancer, despite the disadvantages of requiring large numbers and resources and using retrospective information, epidemiologic studies have provided the bulk of information presently available, alerting industry to hazards so that preventative measures can be undertaken to avoid risks.

PREVENTION OF OCCUPATIONAL LUNG CANCER

Prevention is the most effective method of treating lung cancer, and the prevention of occupational pulmonary

TABLE 1. *Occupational hazards causing respiratory tract cancer*

Agent	Occupation	Tumor
Asbestos	Mining, weaving, utilization	Lung cancer, mesothelioma
Radioactivity	Uranium metal mining	Lung cancer
Nickel	Refining	Lung, nasal cancer
Chromates	Electroplating, tanning pigments, chemical industry	Lung cancer
Chloromethyl ethers	Fungicides, chemical industry	Lung cancer
Arsenic	Metal refining, sheep dip	Lung, skin cancer
Fossil fuels	Coal, coke, gas furnaces	Lung cancer
Mustard gas	Manufacture	Lung cancer
? Vinyl chloride	Manufacture, utilization	Lung cancer
? Beryllium	Utilization	Lung cancer
? Isopropanol	Manufacture	Nasal, ? lung cancer
? Printing ink	Utilization	Lung cancer
? Cadmium	Refining	Lung cancer
? Magnesium	Refining	Lung cancer
? Formaldehyde	Chemical industry	Lung cancer
? Diesel exhaust	Railroad, garage	Lung cancer
? Meat	Processing	Lung cancer

neoplasia cannot be realistically separated from the prevention of lung cancer as a whole. The majority of cases of pulmonary cancer are avoidable. The way to reduce the incidence of carcinoma of the lung is to avoid exposure to the relevant carcinogens. The link between smoking and carcinoma is well established. The American Cancer Society records a prevalence of lung cancer of 149,000 cases per year, and although approximately 10%–15% are associated with industry, the majority are caused by smoking. Within this 10%–15% attributable to industry, many cases will represent a combination of occupational exposure and smoking. In any discussion of prevention, these facts must be considered.

The responsibility for reducing the incidence of carcinoma rests with the medical profession, industry, the government, and the work force. The medical profession must make the facts available and educate industry, the government, and workers. It must continue both epidemiologic surveillance and research to identify new hazards. All this must be accomplished within the confines of available financial resources. Industry must accept advice from informed sources and do its utmost to protect the worker. The government must act responsibly, its first priority being the health of the work force.

The most important group, the workers, must be informed of the risks and must use all protective methods necessary. The most important fact, however, is that workers need to be aware of the risk of smoking, especially in the setting of an occupation with a known hazard.

SURVEILLANCE

Although prevention is the best approach to occupational cancer, another, albeit less effective, alternative exists—detection of early cases of disease in the hope that prognosis can be improved. There has been much debate concerning the value of screening for occupational cancer, and although the concept of medical monitoring has been received enthusiastically, it must be remembered that the value of screening programs is based on the assumption that early diagnosis is beneficial. Although this is true for most infections, it is not necessarily the case for occupational lung cancer. For example, is there any point in detecting mesothelioma earlier when no treatment or cure is available?

In 1968, the World Health Organization (WHO) produced guidelines for screening programs that still apply today. Although most of the criteria are relevant to occupational neoplasia, three require special mention. First, there should be an acceptable form of treatment for patients with recognizable disease. Second, the cost of case finding needs to be balanced economically in relation to possible expenditure for medical care as a whole. Finally, the benefits accruing to persons with true-positive findings should outweigh the harm done as a result of false-positive diagnoses. Added to the required standards of the screening program, the tests chosen must be accurate, sensitive, specific, and of predictive value.

The two tests available to screen for occupational lung cancer are the chest radiograph and sputum cytology. Although both these techniques are useful in detecting cancer, in practice many problems arise. Studies using serial radiography have not improved survival or at best have had only a minor effect. A particular problem is the case of patients with positive sputum cytology but no detectable tumor at fiberoptic bronchoscopy. Segmental bronchial lavage can be performed in an attempt to localize the tumor to a particular segment, but malignant cells can be obtained from several sites or even from both lungs, presumably as a result of spillover.

The results of an extensive three-center study on screening for lung cancer were published in 1984. There was little doubt that cancers could be detected earlier. The radiograph was the most sensitive method, with 40% of cancers identified as stage I (American Joint Committee on Cancer), whereas sputum cytology was effective at detecting early squamous cell carcinomas only. However, despite early detection, it was not clear that there was any subsequent decrease in mortality. A long-term study on chest x-ray screening in chromate workers demonstrated a modest improvement in 5-year survival of regular attenders; however, no significant improvement was seen in the 5-year survival when the total worker population was considered.

Finally, the cost of screening needs to be considered. In one reported experience, the cost per person per year was $135, and as the prevalence of detectable lung cancer is very low (1 in 2000 to 3000), the cost-to-benefit ratio becomes prohibitive. In an earlier series using the chest radiograph, the cost of detection of each cancer was $25,000, with no increase in life expectancy.

In view of all these facts, it may be that the money involved in such screening programs would be better used in preventing rather than detecting largely untreatable cancer.

MANAGEMENT

The treatment of occupational lung cancer is no different from that in the non-occupational setting. In general, the disease is incurable, but surgical resection is the treatment of choice and, if successful, affords a 20%–30% chance of surviving 5 years. The prognosis in occupational lung cancer is slightly worse for two reasons. First, there is a preponderance of small-cell and adenocarcinomas, both of which have a worse prognosis than the squamous cell type. Second, many workers have concurrent lung disease, such as fibrosis, which may make surgery less feasible. A relatively new concept is chemoprevention, and although no proven chemopreventative method exists, several substances, including vitamin A and selenium, have been under investigation. In any case, the improvements in prognosis with such methods are likely to be modest compared with the deleterious effect of smoking.

A problem peculiar to occupational cancer is that of medicolegal ramifications in the form of compensation to the worker or, as is sadly more often the case, to the family of the worker. However, such a discussion is beyond the scope of this chapter.

SPECIFIC CAUSES OF OCCUPATIONAL LUNG CANCER

Asbestos

It is quite clear that lung cancer and mesothelioma are associated with exposure to asbestos and that this association is dose-related.

Specific Occupational Risks

There is little doubt that weavers and certain users of the finished product, such as pipe fitters and laggers, are particularly at risk. In contrast, the risks associated with asbestos mining are significantly less, particularly for chrysotile miners in Quebec. This truism applies not only to mesothelioma, but also to asbestosis and lung cancer. One exception is the relatively higher risk in miners of crocidolite who were employed in the Wittenoom mine in West Australia. Shipyard welders and other workers, who may spend a good portion of their time in close proximity to pipe fitters and laggers, have either no increased risk or, at the worst, a slightly increased risk for asbestosis and lung cancer. Much the same can be said for railroad repair shed workers and, to a lesser extent, those who line furnaces. Garage mechanics working with brake linings do not appear to be at increased risk, and neither in general do persons who come in contact with asbestos merely through working in buildings that contain asbestos.

Asbestos as a Carcinogen

Asbestos is a cocarcinogen, and the presence of asbestosis, especially in smokers, is associated with a significantly increased incidence of lung cancer. The evidence suggests that asbestos is a promoter rather than an initiator of cancer. In regard to the excess of lung cancer that occurs in subjects with asbestosis, it is generally accepted that cigarette smoking is the usual initiator.

It has been estimated in the United States that about 430,000 construction workers and 648,000 workers involved in manufacturing have been significantly exposed to asbestos. Based on these estimates, it is calculated that asbestos plays a role in approximately 3% of all lung cancers that occur in the United States (i.e., 2501 deaths per year), but even then, asbestos acts synergistically with smoking, and the latter makes a greater contribution to the induction of the disease.

That lung cancer is a significant risk in asbestos workers is clear from Fig. 1. The relative risk in asbestos workers is said to be increased up to five to six times, irrespective of the smoking habit. It is now clear, however, that the risk of smoking in the induction of lung cancer was previously seriously underestimated. This is apparent from relating the calculated number of patients in whom cancer deaths were attributed to smoking to the number of cigarettes smoked per day. During the past decade, a number of studies have shown that provided the level of asbestos is kept below one fiber per cubic centimeter, the risk for development of asbestosis is negligible and the risk for development of lung cancer is not increased during a 35- to 40-year working life. In most of these studies, however, the population was exposed to

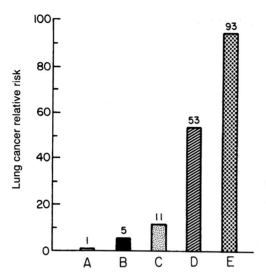

FIG. 1. The relative risk for lung cancer in persons exposed and not exposed to asbestos according to smoking habit. **A:** Unexposed nonsmokers. **B:** Nonsmoking asbestos workers. **C:** Unexposed workers. **D:** Exposed smokers, all. **E:** Exposed heavy smokers (20/d). (Based on data from Hammond EC, Selikoff IJ, Seidman H. Asbestos exposure, cigarette smoking, and death rates. *Ann NY Acad Sci* 1979;330:473.)

chrysotile only. Smoking has now been shown to play the pre-eminent role. In this regard, it must be remembered that lung cancer has been diagnosed in only about 30 or so lifelong nonsmoking workers with asbestosis. If the smoking histories in these subjects were inaccurate, as is often the case when compensation is being claimed, the excess incidence in nonsmokers would completely disappear. Moreover, great differences exist between the calculated relative risks of lung cancer obtained by different investigators. Such differences are to be expected in the absence of uniform and consistent protocols. Thus, the selection of subjects for studies has differed greatly, with some studies including only asbestos workers with prolonged exposure (i.e., 20 years) and others including all exposures of 6 months. In addition, the smoking habits of the various populations studied have varied greatly. Clearly, these variables will greatly influence the incidence of lung cancer. In certain studies, additional clinical, surgical, and autopsy information was collected from the asbestos-exposed group in whom lung and gastrointestinal cancer developed, but not from the control group. Without applying this refinement to both the groups, the introduction of bias is inevitable. Nonetheless, it is clear that the risk for development of lung cancer is related to the cumulative dose of asbestos; the greater the dose, the greater the risk. It is also evident that increased risk for lung cancer does not appear until the subject has had an exposure of at least 15 years plus asbestosis—that is, there has been a suitable incubation or latent period. The development of lung cancer in a subject who began to work with asbestos only 5 years before symptoms of the

tumor appeared indicates that the cancer is unrelated to the asbestos exposure.

In regard to the development of lung cancer in asbestos-exposed workers, the assumption of a linear relationship has received wide but somewhat uncritical acceptance. Such a hypothesis is convenient and simple, but it is not necessarily valid. Deductions based on observations of the risk for lung cancer in subjects with high cumulative exposures cannot, of necessity, be used to predict the response at lower doses. Back extrapolation of the regression line to the intercept at zero is often forced and contrived, as there are usually either no excess deaths or very few deaths occurring at the lower exposures. In many instances, there is just as much mathematical justification for drawing the regression line so that it has either a negative or a positive intercept. Moreover, it is impossible in practice to devise a study that will provide the necessary data to confirm the straight-line, no-threshold hypothesis. Much the same problem exists when the death rate from lung cancer in nonsmoking asbestos workers is considered. In general, the excess death rate in most studies is limited to one or two subjects.

An excellent review of this subject appeared in a supplement to *Thorax* (1996), which examines the article by Williamson et al. (1995) suggesting that excess cancer morbidity occurs without lung fibrosis, and then reviews the subject as a whole. The current evidence indicates that asbestosis (radiographic or histologic) is a prerequisite for excess lung cancer morbidity.

It is true that mining tends to be far less hazardous than weaving. In contrast, users of the finished product are at greater risk. Nevertheless, the apparent safety of mining probably results from the fact that most reliable studies have been carried out on chrysotile miners from Quebec and that chrysotile is less hazardous. There is now fairly compelling evidence to indicate that crocidolite is more carcinogenic than chrysotile, with amosite carcinogenicity in between. This applies not only to mesothelioma, but also to lung cancer. Indeed, it appears that the amphiboles are not only significantly more carcinogenic than chrysotile for a given exposure, but are also more fibrogenic and thus more likely to induce asbestosis. Australian crocidolite miners had a standardized mortality rate (SMR) of 247 for lung cancer after 15 years of exposure, whereas Quebec chrysotile miners with 20 years of exposure had an SMR of only 127. The various dose-response relationships that have been calculated from American studies are shown in Fig. 2.

All types of lung cancer are reported to occur in asbestos-exposed populations. The original descriptions suggested that asbestos-associated lung cancer was more likely to be peripherally situated and to be an adenocarcinoma. However, all histologic types are found, and it is impossible to sort out which cancers result from smoking alone, smoking plus asbestos exposure, and asbestos exposure alone (if the latter by itself ever causes lung can-

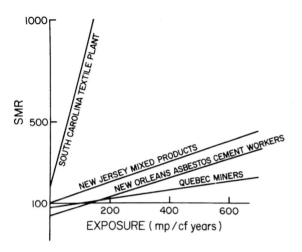

FIG. 2. The SMR for lung cancer in various exposed populations, showing a lesser risk in asbestos miners.

cer). Thus, the evidence from pathologic and epidemiologic studies would suggest that fibrosis and epithelial hyperplasia are essential for the induction of cancer. The inability of short fibers to induce fibrosis would explain why such fibers are not associated with the development of lung cancer, and the same is true for fiberglass. From this it can be inferred that the prevention of asbestosis likewise prevents asbestos-induced lung cancer.

Mesothelioma

Mesothelioma occurs either as a benign pedunculated pleural tumor, usually associated with hypertrophic pulmonary osteoarthropathy, or as a diffuse malignant tumor of the pleura or peritoneum. Rarely, the pericardium and tunica vaginalis are affected. Only the diffuse malignant mesothelioma is related to asbestos exposure. Epidemiologic studies would suggest at the present time that about 75%–80% of malignant mesotheliomas are associated with prior asbestos exposure. The tumor also has been associated with exposure to fibrous erionite, a zeolite that is a non-asbestiform mineral. The relationship between asbestos exposure and the development of mesothelioma was established by Wagner and co-workers in 1960.

Malignant mesothelioma usually develops many years after a subject is first exposed to asbestos. The incubation period varies from about 15 to 40 years, with the vast majority of mesotheliomas developing between 25 and 40 years after exposure commenced. In many instances, there has been no exposure to the mineral for 20 to 30 years. There is good evidence that once the lung has been primed by a sufficient dose of asbestos, the development of the tumor is inevitable. However, contrary to previous teaching, mesothelioma does not develop as a sequel to minute or minimal exposures. Although it is true that it may develop after short exposures, in the range of 3 to 24 months, such exposures have usually been intense.

Mesothelioma also has been reported in infants and in subjects with no history whatsoever of exposure to asbestos. Although mesothelioma is a rare tumor, it is estimated that it develops in about 1500 to 2000 subjects in the United States every year. In Canada, the figure is probably proportionally somewhat less, mainly because fewer Canadians were exposed to crocidolite in shipyards during World War II.

Mesothelioma and Fiber Type

Early experiments demonstrated that injection of asbestos fibers into the pleural space of animals induced development of mesothelioma. Abestiform fibers such as tremolite caused mesothelioma in the pleural space of rats, but equal doses of non-asbestiform fibers did not. Later, several non-asbestiform fibers, including fiberglass, were found to be capable of inducing mesothelioma provided the diameter of the fibers was 0.5 μm, but non-asbestiform actinolite, biotite, and talc failed to produce tumors. The relationship between fiber size and the development of mesothelioma was demonstrated, and it was concluded that fiber structure was a pre-eminent influence in the induction of malignant tumors of the pleura. Later experiments using various forms of asbestiform and non-asbestiform fibers, including fibrous glass and sundry fibrous clays, made it evident that carcinogenicity is related to the dimensional distribution of the fibers, which are longer than 8 μm and have a diameter of 0.25 μm.

For many years, it has been apparent that the likelihood of mesothelioma developing in chrysotile miners is less than in users of the finished product. It also became apparent that materials made from asbestos contained mixtures of different types, with varying proportions of amosite and crocidolite being added to Canadian chrysotile before weaving. Epidemiologic studies of the frequency of mesothelioma have shown that the tumor occurs much more frequently in persons exposed to the amphiboles and that crocidolite is particularly dangerous in this regard.

Radioactivity

The excessive mortality of Schneeberg miners was shown by Harting and Hesse in 1879 to be caused by lung cancer, but it had been appreciated three centuries earlier that men working in these mines died prematurely. Lung cancer may have accounted for 40% of deaths in these miners at a time before the introduction of cigarettes to Europe. A similar problem was identified in the uranium miners of Joachimsthal in 1930. The cause of the increased risk for lung cancer in these miners was unknown. However, Kennaway and Lindsey subsequently showed that the air in these mines contained high concentrations of radon and other radioactive elements.

Since that time, radioactive contamination of air or

water has been identified not only in uranium mines, such as those in Colorado, but also in several mines concerned with the production of nonradioactive substances, such as fluorspar mines in Canada, hematite and tin mines in the United Kingdom, hard rock mines in the United States, thorotrast mines in Denmark, and iron mines in Sweden.

Uranium

Uranium is mined in Colorado, Canada, Australia, Czechoslovakia, and Central Africa. It is mined on the surface and underground in the form of oxide or pitchblende, or as a compound oxide with vanadium and potassium known as *carnotite*. The ore, of which uranium constitutes 0.5%, also contains 5%–50% silica and hence is associated with a concurrent risk for silicosis.

After ore crushing, the uranium is extracted in the form of uranate known as *yellow cake*. This material is then packed for transport. Uranium is used mainly for the production of atomic energy (peaceful or otherwise), but it also has a minor use in the ceramic and chemical industries. The risk from uranium therefore applies to miners, uranium process workers, and users of the finished product, such as nuclear power plant workers and those who handle uranium in industry.

Mechanisms

Uranium itself is not, from a biologic point of view, dangerous, in that it emits mainly gamma rays, which are of such high energy that they pass through the human body. The problem occurs as uranium decays (Fig. 3). The first step in the decay series is from uranium 238 to radium 226, which in turn decays to radon 222. This element, which is one of the noble gases, decays into its daughters polonium 218 and 214, lead 214, and bismuth 214. Because these radon daughters are ionized metal atoms, they become attached to dust and water vapor. Thus, radon and its daughters can be inhaled into the respiratory tract, where they emit alpha radiation. Particularly important are the radon daughters that have a short half-life and so cannot be cleared from the respiratory tract before their energy is emitted. The alpha particles emitted have a range of 40 to 70 μm, sufficient at the site of impaction to damage the mucosal cells and initiate carcinogenesis. This action has been confirmed experimentally when lung cancer has been induced in rats with cesium 14.

Epidemiology

Apart from the observations described earlier, several detailed studies have examined the effects of uranium on the lung. Mortality rates of Colorado miners were examined during a 17-year period, and a mortality more than six times greater than expected was demonstrated. Even those miners with low exposure for several years had a fourfold increased risk for lung cancer. A further finding was that the increased total radiation exposure was associated with increasing frequency of undifferentiated small-cell carcinomas.

The interaction between cigarette smoking and radiation is important. Because the incidence of smoking was so high in the initial studies, it was initially believed that smoking was a prerequisite for cancer in uranium miners. However, further studies have shown that although uranium miners who smoke have a higher risk, nonsmoking miners still have an increased risk for lung cancer. From various studies, it is clear that the amount of radiation is

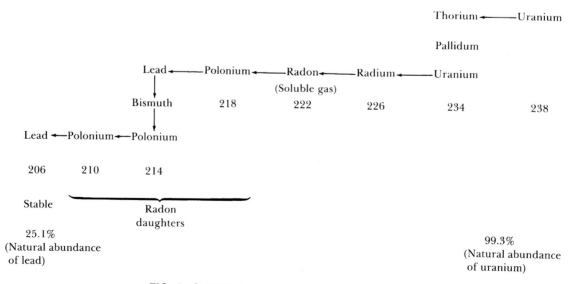

FIG. 3. Simplified natural decay series of uranium.

important, and for this reason an empiric unit, the *working-level month* (WLM), was derived. This unit is an exposure for 1 working month (170 hours) to a known concentration of radon daughters and thus reflects both intensity and duration of radiation. Risk factors were used to examine the problem in Swedish miners, and if normal nonsmokers had a risk for development of lung cancer of 1, then nonsmoking miners had a risk of 2.4. Smokers with no underground mining exposure had a risk of 6.8, and smoking miners had a risk of 18.2. Another study found that the excess cancer rate in nonsmoking miners was increased (18 observed deaths compared with 1.8 expected), but not as high as in smoking miners (32 actual, 11 expected). These figures suggest that the effects of smoking and exposure to radon daughters are additive. A further effect is the shortening of the induction-latent period, which results in an earlier appearance of cancer. This has been shown to be related to increasing age, increased exposure, and intensity of cigarette smoking, findings that have been confirmed in Sweden.

In summary, there is good epidemiologic evidence that the increased incidence of lung cancer in uranium miners is related to degree of exposure. However, increased incidence is also related to age and cigarette consumption.

Prevention

The atmospheric levels of radon daughters and exposure of workers to them must be kept to a minimum by providing ventilation, sealing off high-risk areas, and controlling water seepage. The work force should be monitored on an individual basis, and exposure should be controlled according to defined standards. In the United States, this is 4 WLM per year, with actual exposure levels being 1 to 2 WLM per year. Because the evidence suggests that the risks of smoking and uranium are at least additive, uranium workers must be strongly advised not to smoke. Some would even suggest that smokers not be employed in such high-risk situations. The question of surveillance is discussed elsewhere.

The preventative measures are not just for miners, but should also be applied to process workers, laboratory workers, and those employed in nuclear power plants.

Fluorspar

Fluorspar, or calcium fluoride, is used in the manufacture of steel and aluminum, in ceramics, and as a source of fluorine. The chief mining area of fluorspar is in Newfoundland, and it was here that the excess of carcinoma of the lung was first demonstrated. The cause of the increased mortality, which was 29 times that expected, was found to be related to radioactivity. Despite the fact that a nonradioactive material was being mined, radioactivity levels were comparable with those in uranium mines. The source was found to be radon daughters dissolved in water that had leaked into the mines.

Metal Mining

Lung cancer has been observed to be more common in certain metal miners. Mortality in hematite miners was found to be in excess compared with mortality in a control population of coal miners, and although initially it was thought that the carcinogens were iron and silica, these hematite mines were later found to be radioactive, much in the same way as the fluorspar mines in Newfoundland. This same problem has been identified in hard rock miners in the United States, metal miners in Sweden, thorotrast miners in Denmark, and tin miners in Britain.

Nuclear Power Plants

Through the years, the use of nuclear power as a source of energy has been an emotional issue. This is particularly so in respect to possible increased risks for cancers in workers, their families, and surrounding populations. Earlier studies have shown no evidence of an increased risk for carcinoma in nuclear power workers; it should be noted, however, that the data are being amassed for impending court cases concerning the possibility of the development of lymphoma in children of men exposed to radiation at a nuclear power plant in Cumbria, United Kingdom.

Nickel lung cancer was first identified as being related to nickel exposure at the Mond Nickel Works in South Wales in 1958. The findings were later confirmed. These workers also were observed to have an increased incidence of nasal cancer. Their risk was calculated to be increased five times for cancer of the lung and 150 times greater than expected for cancer of the nose. When the study was repeated, the mortality figures had fallen. Studies of other nickel workers also have shown increased risks, especially in smokers.

The agent responsible was thought to be nickel dust, but because the incidence fell as arsenic was eliminated from the process, this also has been implicated. In one autopsy study, however, there was no evidence of arsenic in the lungs of workers who died of cancer. Overall, the evidence suggests that the risk is increased with exposure to several nickel salts, in particular, nickel subsulfide.

Chromates

Chromium is used in the production of alloys, electroplating, pigment production, tanning, and the chemical industry. It is mined chiefly in the former U.S.S.R., Turkey, and South Africa, but it is processed on a much wider scale. A link between chromates and lung cancer was reported early in this century, but epidemiologic study confirmed the association only in the 1940s. A death rate 16 times greater than expected was reported in the United States. The findings were confirmed in the United Kingdom, and the risk was later shown to fall when exposure was reduced.

The risk for carcinoma of the lung and the nose seems to be related to exposure to the salts of chromium, particularly hexavalent compounds such as dichromates and chromium pigments rather than trivalent salts.

Prevention depends on enclosure, extraction, and the use of respirators.

Earlier studies have been updated and have again shown an increased risk for carcinoma of the lung and nose in chromate workers, and the subject has been approached from a different perspective in a later study. When the nickel and chromate content of lung tissues in patients with lung cancer was examined using atomic absorption analysis, significantly higher levels of both metals were shown in the lungs of patients with cancer than in control subjects.

Chloroethers

Chloroethers are compounds encountered in the manufacture of bactericides and fungicides, and two compounds in particular, bischloromethyl and chloromethyl ether, have been shown to be important carcinogens. The other causes of occupational lung cancer were identified by observation and confirmed epidemiologically, but the chloroethers are unique in that their carcinogenic potential was first shown in animal experiments. The effect on humans has since been confirmed, and it has been shown that bischloromethyl ether in particular is associated with oat-cell carcinoma, with risk ratios of 10 to 12 being reported with heavy exposure.

Arsenic

Arsenic has been known as a carcinogen for many years. It was thought to cause scrotal cancer among copper workers as early as 1820, and it was thought that therapeutic arsenic was responsible for skin cancer. Lung and skin cancer were described in 1934 in workers manufacturing arsenical sheep dip. These men were later investigated in detail, and it was found that most workers also showed the clinical manifestations of arsenical poisoning, with hyperpigmentation, warts, and hyperkeratosis.

Nowadays arsenic exposure has been reduced, but a risk still exists in the use and preparation of some pesticides, in metal refining, and in the chemical industry.

Fossil Fuels

The products of fossil fuels, including coal, coke, coal gas, and coal tar, have been shown to be related to an increased incidence of carcinoma. In 1959, lung cancer was shown to be approximately 15 times greater than expected in two studies of Canadian and London gas workers, findings that were supported in a prospective study. Oven top workers in the U.S. steel industry had a 10-fold increase in mortality from carcinoma of the lung, and similar studies have shown this same problem in coke oven workers in the United Kingdom. However, the situation is likely to be improved following the introduction of natural gas. Coke plant workers in the Netherlands were shown to have increased death rates from lung cancer and nonmalignant respiratory disease, but the study failed to examine smoking habits fully. Another study of a cohort of 10,000 foundry workers covering a period of 40 years showed an increased incidence of both lung cancer (SMR 147) and stomach cancer (SMR 137) in comparison with the general population.

Mustard Gas

Mustard gas ($\beta\beta'$-dichlorodiethyl sulfide) has been used as a weapon in warfare. A mortality 10 times greater than expected was shown in Japan, where the gas was manufactured during World War II.

Vinyl Chloride

Vinyl chloride is well-known to produce angiosarcoma of the liver, but it also has been implicated in lung cancer. However, the association is weak, and other studies have attributed the problem to smoking.

Beryllium

Beryllium has not been proved to be a human carcinogen, although the OSHA has recommended that it should be regarded as posing a carcinogenic threat.

Materials Considered Suspect

At the end of any discussion of occupational carcinogens, some compounds should be mentioned that are suspected but not proved to be carcinogens.

Diesel Exhaust

Diesel exhaust fumes have not been proved to cause an excess of lung cancer; however, some studies suggest that exposure to diesel exhaust can increase the risk. A small study showed an increased risk in Swedish garage workers, and a large study of U.S. railroad workers showed increased numbers of deaths from lung cancer in men exposed for 20 years. Further studies have shown a possible association between diesel exhaust fumes and lung cancer, whereas others have failed to demonstrate any increased risk.

Animal studies have also addressed the problem; squamous metaplasia developed in rats exposed to diesel exhaust for 2 years and lung tumors occurred in 16%, compared with no tumors in the control groups. The same study also examined the effect of coal oven flue gas and found a similar increase in the incidence of lung tumors. The possibility that diesel exhaust is associated with lung cancer requires further investigation.

Formaldehyde

Debate is ongoing as to whether formaldehyde causes lung cancer, and the data from a large group of industrial workers exposed to formaldehyde have been reanalyzed. According to the original interpretation of the data, excess mortality from lung cancer was not related to exposure to formaldehyde, but a repeated analysis suggested an association with formaldehyde. The final conclusion is that formaldehyde should be considered as a possible human carcinogen.

Other Materials

Several studies have examined the effects of silica and possible associations with lung cancer. Although it has been reported that the incidence of lung cancer is lower in miners with silicosis, other studies report increased numbers of deaths from lung cancer in men exposed to silica. Without more and better evidence, however, it is premature to conclude that exposure to crystalline silica has caused lung cancer in humans.

The links of several other compounds and processes with lung cancer remain doubtful. It has been suggested that cadmium is a carcinogen. Also, an increase in cancer has been noted in a group of workers exposed to magnesium.

Increases in lung cancer have been noted in the meat-processing industry and in Swedish bakers and pastry cooks, particularly those who work in small bakeries. Orchardists have been noted to have higher rates of lung cancer, although this is thought to be largely a consequence of cigarette smoking. A cohort of dry cleaners has been found to have a slightly increased incidence of cancer; however, the mortality was less than expected, and no significant increase in the numbers of lung cancers was found.

Isopropanol manufacture is associated with an increase in nasal cancer and possibly lung cancer. The agent suspected from animal studies is isopropyl oil. Suspicion also has been raised in Denmark and the United Kingdom about printing ink, as both printers and newspaper workers have been thought to have an increased incidence of carcinoma of the lung.

An increased risk for lung cancer was found in Swedish and Finish motor mechanics who had high blood levels of lead.

Several materials, such as glass fiber and fertilizers, have been studied and shown not to carry an increased risk for cancer. Cotton workers have been shown to have a decreased risk for lung cancer.

The subject of pulmonary occupational neoplasia is evolving. Further large, long-term studies must be carried out, and the constant review of the situation is necessary.

BIBLIOGRAPHY

Alderson M. *Occupational Cancer*. London: Butterworth; 1986. *Comprehensive factual monograph by the chief medical statistician of the Office of Population, Censuses, and Surveys that considers the entire subject of occupationally induced cancers. An examination of the epidemiology of specific agents and occupations is followed by a discussion of the etiology of specific cancers.*

Axelsson G, Rylander R, Schmidt A. Mortality and incidence of tumors among ferochromium workers. *Brit J Ind Med* 1980;37:121–127. *Investigation into the cause of death and incidence of tumors among almost 2000 workers in a ferochromium plant in Sweden. Workers were exposed mainly to metallic and trivalent chromium (Cr^{3+}), and there was no significant increase in respiratory tumors in the study population. Five cases of respiratory cancer were found, against an expected 7.2.*

Berlin NI, Buncher CR, Fontanna RS, et al. The National Cancer Institute Cooperative Early Lung Cancer Detection Program. Results of the initial screen (prevalence). Early lung cancer detection: introduction. *Am Rev Respir Dis* 1984;130:545–549. *Review of the incidence and detection of lung cancer, followed by a description of the design of a large, multicenter, cooperative lung cancer screening program involving three centers: Johns Hopkins, Memorial Sloan-Kettering, and the Mayo Clinic.*

Berry G, Newhouse ML, Antonis P. Combined effect of asbestos and smoking on mortality from lung cancer and mesothelioma in factory workers. *Br J Ind Med* 1985;42:12–18. *Study of mortality in 1600 asbestos factory workers between 1971 and 1980. The smoking habits were examined in relation to mortality from lung cancer and mesothelioma.*

Bidstrop PL, Case RAM. Carcinoma of the lung in workmen in the bichromates-producing industry in Great Britain. *Br J Ind Med* 1956; 260–264. *Report of a 6-year study on the mortality experience of workers in the chromates-producing industry in three factories in Great Britain, showing a statistically significant increase in mortality from carcinoma of the lung.*

Boffetta P, Harris RE, Wynder EL. Case-controlled study of occupational exposure to diesel exhaust and lung cancer risk. *Am J Ind Med* 1990;17:577–591. *Study comparing 2500 cases exposed to diesel exhaust with 5000 hospital worker controls. An association between exposure to diesel exhaust and an elevated lung cancer risk was not found.*

Boucot KR, Cooper DA, Weiss W. The role of surgery and the cure of lung cancer. *Arch Intern Med* 1967;120:168. *This review of the role of surgery in curing lung cancer in the 1950s and early 1960s tends to be realistic and pessimistic in view of the 5-year survival rate of approximately 5%.*

Buncher CR. Did formaldehyde cause lung cancer? *J Occup Med* 1989; 31:885. *Editorial discussing a large study by Blair et al. of 26,000 industrial workers exposed to formaldehyde. Their interpretation was that the excess mortality from lung cancer was not related to formaldehyde. In a repeated analysis of the data, Stirling et al. felt that the cumulative exposure to formaldehyde was related to high rates of lung cancer and death.*

Chovil AC. Occupational lung cancer and smoking: a review in the light of current theories of carcinogenesis. *Can Med J* 1979;121:548. *A review article considering modern theories of carcinogenesis as they apply to the induction of lung cancer in tobacco smoking and occupational exposure to carcinogens.*

Chovil AC. The epidemiology of primary lung cancer in uranium miners in Ontario. *J Occup Med* 1981;23:417. *Review of the epidemiology of lung cancer in uranium miners in northern Ontario whose cumulative exposure was relatively low and who were exposed for only a short period of time.*

deVilliers AJ, Windish JP. Lung cancer in a fluorspar mining community, radiation dust, and mortality experience. *Br J Ind Med* 1964;21: 94. *Description of the increased numbers of deaths from lung cancer in a small fluorspar mining community in St. Laurence, Newfoundland, apparently related to the high concentrations of radon and daughter products in air in the mines.*

Doll R, Hill AB. A study of the etiology of carcinoma of the lung. *Br Med J* 1952;2:171. *One of the earliest large epidemiologic studies of the etiology of carcinoma of the lung.*

Doll R, Peto R. Causes of cancer. Quantitative estimates of the avoidable risks of cancer in the United States today. *J Natl Cancer Inst* 1981;66: 1197. *Extensive monograph on the causes of cancer, with a particular emphasis on avoidable causes.*

Doll R, Peto J. *Asbestosis: Effects on Health of Exposure to Asbestos.* London: Her Majesty's Stationery Office; 1985 (Health and Safety Commission). *In-depth report reviewing the adverse effects of asbestos on health.*

Enterline PE, Marsh GM, Esmen NA. Respiratory disease among workers exposed to man-made and mineral fibers. *Am Rev Respir Dis* 1983;128:1–7. *Report of a study of workers exposed to fibrous glass and mineral wool. The respiratory cancer death rates were not excessive for fiberglass workers but were elevated for mineral wool workers.*

Epstein S, Swartz JB. Fallacies of lifestyle cancer theories. *Nature* 1981; 289:127–130. *An interesting alternative view suggesting that smoking is the major lifestyle factor causing cancer but that there have been substantial increases in lung cancer rates that cannot be accounted for by smoking.*

Hammond EC, Garfinkel L. General air pollution and cancer in the United States. *Prev Med* 1980;9:206–211. *Report from a conference on the primary prevention of cancer examining the effects of air pollution. The authors concluded, after standardization for age and smoking, that men with occupational exposures have increased rates of cancer (14%); however, general air pollution was thought to have very little, if any, effect on the lung cancer death rate.*

Hammond EC, Selikoff IJ, Seidman H. Asbestos exposure, cigarette smoking and death rates. *Ann NY Acad Sci* 1979;330:473. *Review article with extensive data on asbestos exposure, cigarette smoking, incidence of lung cancer, and death. The strong synergistic effect of exposure to asbestos dust and cigarette smoking on risk for lung cancer is clearly demonstrated.*

Harting FH, Hesse EW, Lungenkrebs DIE. Bergkrankheit Schneeberger Gruben. *Vjschr Gerichtl Med* 1879;31:102. *Historical reference. The first description of lung cancer as a frequent cause of death in metal miners.*

Higginson J. Present trends in cancer epidemiology. In: Morgan JF, ed. *Proceedings of the Eighth Canadian Cancer Conference.* Oxford: Pergamon; 1969:40–75. *Extensive review of cancer epidemiology, giving consideration to the proportion of human lung cancers that are preventable.*

Hill AB, Fanning EL. Studies of the incidence of cancer in a factory handling inorganic compounds or arsenic. *Br J Ind Med* 1948;5:1. *By 1948, the association between arsenic and carcinogenesis had long been suspected. This article describes the increased mortality attributable to cancer in comparison with that of other occupational groups.*

Jones RN, Hughes MJ, Weill H. Asbestos exposure, asbestosis and asbestos-attributable lung cancer. *Thorax* 1996;51(Suppl 2):S9–S15. *Excellent review that considers the excess deaths from lung cancer in persons exposed to asbestos.*

Kreyberg L. Lung cancer workers in a nickel refinery. *Br J Ind Med* 1978;35:109. *Study of lung cancer in nickel workers, emphasizing histologic types, development time, and tobacco smoking in addition to specific exposure to nickel dust and fumes.*

Liddel FDK, McDonald J. Radiological findings as predictors of mortality in Quebec asbestos workers. *Br J Ind Med* 1980;37:257–267. *Two cohorts of chrysotile miners and millers were studied in Quebec to determine the extent to which chest radiography during employment could be used to predict mortality.*

Machle W, Gregorius F. Cancer of the respiratory system in the United States chromate-producing industry. *Public Health Rep* 1948;63: 1114. *The first epidemiologic survey demonstrating a high death rate from cancer of the respiratory system in workers in the chromate-producing industry.*

Mattson ME, Pollock ES, Cullen JW. What are the odds that smoking will kill you? *Am J Public Heath* 1987;77:425. *Epidemiologic study calculating the long-term risks for smoking-related death in persons of various ages and smoking status.*

Morgan JG. Some observations on the incidence of respiratory cancer in nickel workers. *Br J Ind Med* 1958;15:224. *A study undertaken by the Mond Nickel Company Ltd. in Swansea, Wales, the largest nickel refinery in the country. The incidence of cancer of the lung and nose was found to be greater than that of the general population.*

Morgan WKC. Industrial carcinogens: the extent of the risk. *Thorax* 1979;34:431. *A review of the increased risks associated with industrial carcinogens. The details of the major publications on the subject are summarized, critically analyzed, and compared. Further consideration is given to the testing of carcinogens and the place of screening for disease.*

Morgan WKC. Early diagnosis of occupational lung cancer. *Eur J Respir Dis* 1982;123:139–144. *Review of early diagnosis and screening for occupational lung cancer that explains the principles of screening for disease (Wilson and Junger, WHO, 1968) and applies them to occupational lung cancer. The review also examines the costs and outcomes of screening programs.*

Nelson N. Carcinogenicity of halo ethers. *Newing J Med* 1973;288: 1123–1124. *Leading article discussing the occurrence of lung cancer in workers exposed to halo ethers.*

Pott P. *Chirurgical Works.* London: 1808:177 (vol 3). *Historical reference. The first description of a cancer attributable to an occupation—carcinoma of the scrotum in chimney sweeps.*

Radford EP, Renard KG. Lung cancer in Swedish iron miners exposed to low doses of radon daughters. *N Engl J Med* 1984;310:1485. *Retrospective study investigating lung cancer mortality from 1951 to 1976 in 1400 Swedish iron miners. The effects of smoking and exposure to radiation were almost additive.*

Saccomanno G, Archer VE, Auerbach O, et al. Histologic types of lung cancer among uranium miners. *Cancer* 1971;27:515. *Report of 121 cases of proven lung cancer from American uranium miners showing a higher incidence of undifferentiated carcinomas with increased radiation exposure. These confirm and extend the findings of early reports suggesting a relatively high frequency of small-cell undifferentiated carcinomas in miners exposed to radiation.*

Schilling CJ, Schilling JM. Chest x-ray screening for lung cancer at three British chromate plants from 1955 to 1989. *J Int Med* 1991; 48:476–479. *Large screening program lasting 34 years, with 229 employees given a diagnosis of carcinoma of the lung. Survival data from 124 cases (the study population) showed a modest improvement in 5-year survival in those who attended regularly for radiography.*

Seaton A. Occupational pulmonary neoplasms. In: Morgan WK, Seaton A, eds. *Occupational Lung Disease.* 2nd ed. Philadelphia: WB Saunders; 1984:657–675. *Chapter about occupational pulmonary neoplasms in a textbook of occupational lung disease. Consideration is given to the subject as a whole and to specific carcinogens.*

Selikoff IJ, Churg J, Hammond EC. The occurrence of asbestosis among insulation workers in the United States. *Ann NY Acad Sci* 1965;132: 139. *Report of a large study of 1500 asbestos insulation workers in the New York area. Evidence of asbestosis was noted in 339. Lung cancer was found to be seven times more common than expected.*

Selikoff IJ, Hammond EC, Churg J. Asbestos exposure, smoking and neoplasia. *JAMA* 1968;204:104. *Important report of a study of asbestos insulation workers. The authors state that it is quite clear that the risk for dying of lung cancer is extraordinary in asbestos workers who smoke.*

Sorahan T, Cooke MA. Cancer mortality in a cohort of United Kingdom steel foundry workers: 1946–1985. *Br J Ind Med* 1989;46:78–81. *Investigation of the mortality experience in a cohort of 10,000 United Kingdom steel foundry workers. The analysis showed an increased risk for lung cancer deaths in workers in the foundry area or fettling shop.*

Steenland NK, Silverman DT, Hornung RW. Case-controlled study of lung cancer and truck driving in the teamsters' union. *Am J Public Health* 1990;20:670–674. *Report of a large case-control study of lung cancer deaths in members of the teamsters' union, comparing the risks associated with different occupations within the teamsters. The study population comprised 996 cases and 1000 controls.*

Tomatis L. How many cancers are attributable to occupational exposures? *Arch Environ Health* 1991;46:5. *Editorial provides an overview of occupational carcinogens and raises interesting questions regarding the effect of low-dose exposure to carcinogens and the possible interaction between multiple low-dose exposures.*

Vineis P, Simonato L. Proportion of lung and bladder cancers in males due to occupation: a systematic approach. *Arch Environ Health* 1991; 46:6. *Review of studies conducted in several countries investigating the relationship of occupation and cancer in men. A standardized evaluation correcting for smoking was employed.*

Wada S, Miyanishi M, Nyshimoto Y, Kmbe S. Mustard gas as a cause of respiratory neoplasia in man. *Lancet* 1968;1:1161. *Report of an increased rate of deaths caused by neoplasia of the respiratory tract in factory workers engaged in the manufacture of mustard gas. Thirty-three deaths occurred, against 0.9 expected. The carcinomas were of the tongue, pharynx, sinuses, larynx, bronchus, and lung.*

Wagner JC, et al. Cancer mortality patterns among U.S. uranium miners and millers, 1950 through 1962. *J Natl Cancer Inst* 1964;32:787. *Study examining cancer mortality patterns in a group of uranium miners and millers in Colorado.*

Wagner JC. The discovery of the association between blue asbestos and mesotheliomas and the aftermath. *Br J Ind Med* 1991;48:399–403. *Historical review 30 years after the publication of* Diffuse Pleural Mesotheliomas and Asbestos Exposure in the North Western Cape Province *by the same author. Description of early cases and subsequent studies examining the relationship between asbestos and mesothelioma and carcinoma of the lung.*

Weiss W, Cooper DA, Boucot KR. Operative mortality in 5-year survival rates in men with bronchogenic carcinoma. *Ann Intern Med* 1969;71:59. *A study of 421 men who underwent surgery for bronchial carcinoma. In 265 who had resections, the operative mortality rate was 11% and the 5-year survival rate was 13%.*

Whitwell F, Scott J, Grimshaw M. Relationship between occupations and asbestos fibre content of the lungs in patients with pleural mesothelioma, lung cancer and other diseases. *Thorax* 1977;32:377–386. *Study examining asbestos fiber counts in lung specimens from patients with mesothelioma, asbestosis, benign pleural plaques, and lung cancer and from controls.*

Williams RL, Muhlbaier JL. Asbestos brake emissions. *Environ Res* 1982;29:70–82. *A brake-testing dynamometer was used to determine the importance of asbestos emissions from automobile brakes. The authors conclude that brake emissions are responsible for a minor fraction of ambient asbestos levels; however, there may be a noticeable increase in asbestos levels near high braking areas, such as toll booths.*

Textbook of Pulmonary Diseases, 6th ed.
edited by G.L. Baum, J.D. Crapo, B.R. Celli, and J.B. Karlinsky,
Lippincott–Raven Publishers, Philadelphia, © 1998.

CHAPTER

37 Noxious Gases and Fumes

David R. Graham

"Gas! Gas! Quick, boys! An ecstasy of fumbling,
Fitting the clumsy helmets just in time;
But someone was still yelling out and stumbling
And flound'ring like a man in fire or lime. . .
Dim, through the misty panes and thick green light,
And under a green sea, I saw him drowning."
—Wilfred Owen

INTRODUCTION

The deleterious effects of certain gases and fumes have been appreciated for many years. Indeed, several gases have been used specifically for their lethal effects as weapons of warfare. In the industrial setting, 20 or so gases and fumes may be encountered that are capable, after inhalation, of producing serious harm (Tables 1 and 2).

The SWORD (Surveillance of Work-related and Occupational Respiratory Disease) project, a register of cases of occupational lung disease in the United Kingdom, has shown that accidents involving inhalation account for approximately 10% of all industrial lung diseases.

MECHANISMS

The effects of a particular gas or fume can be anticipated by examining its physical and chemical properties. Inert gases cause harm by displacing oxygen, whereas toxic gases produce local irritation. The site of action of

D. R. Graham: Department of Respiratory Medicine, Whiston Hospital, Prescot, Merseyside L35 5 DR.

a toxic gas depends on its solubility. Soluble gases are absorbed in the upper airways, whereas those that are less soluble cause damage throughout the respiratory tract. Although brownian movement is a major factor in the dispersion of gases, the deposition of particulate matter is influenced more by gravity. Large particles (15 to 20 μm) deposit in the nose and upper airways, smaller particles (7 to 15 μm) deposit in the trachea and bronchi, and particles between 1 and 7 μm may reach the alveoli. Particles <0.5 μm are so small that they are influenced by brownian movement, and although deposition is limited, they are still able to cause harm.

The mechanisms by which toxic gases and fumes produce their harmful effects can be divided into four main groups.

1. Displacement asphyxia. The term *asphyxia* is derived from a Greek word that means "stopping the pulse." The condition is produced by a deficiency of oxygen in respired air, blood, or tissues. Asphyxia resulting from toxic gases or fumes can occur in two ways. In the first mechanism, oxygen is displaced from inspired air by high concentrations of other gases, such as nitrogen, carbon dioxide, and methane.

2. Oxygen-transport asphyxia. The second mechanism involves chemical interference with the process of oxygen transport, preventing either delivery to the vital organs or cellular respiration itself. Carbon monoxide combines with hemoglobin, reducing its oxygen-carrying capability, whereas cyanides block the cytochrome oxidase system, preventing respiration and thereby causing asphyxia at a cellular level.

3. Local irritation. Most toxic gases and fumes cause harm by local irritation. The more soluble substances,

TABLE 1. *Examples of inhaled chemicals known to cause pulmonary injury*

Chemical	Sources of exposure	Important properties	Injury produced
Acetaldehyde	Plastics, synthetic rubber industry	High vapor pressure; high water solubility	Primarily upper airway; rarely causes delayed pulmonary edema; also a CNS depressant
Acrolein	Plastics, textiles, and pharmaceuticals manufacturing	High vapor pressure; intermediate water solubility; extremely irritating	Diffuse airway and parenchymal injury
Ammonia	Fertilizers, chemicals, and pharmaceuticals manufacturing; refrigeration and oil refining	Alkaline gas; very high water solubility	Primarily upper airway burn; occasionally causes bronchiectasis
Anhydrides	Chemicals, paints, and plastics industries; components of epoxy resins	Water-soluble; highly reactive	Rhinitis, airway injury, asthma; pulmonary hemorrhage after high-dose exposure
Antimony trichloride; antimony pentachloride	Steel industry, organic catalysts	Highly corrosive	Pulmonary edema
Boranes	Aircraft fuel, welding, fungicide manufacturing	Water-soluble gas; diborane most corrosive of these compounds	Airway injury; pulmonary edema after high-concentration exposure
Bromine (hydrogen bromide)	Petroleum refining, chemical industry (as a catalyst)	Bromine is a liquid, hydrogen bromide a colorless gas at room temperature	Upper airway injury; rare pulmonary edema
Cadmium	Electroplating, paints, and pesticides manufacturing; cutting plated metals	Encountered as dry powder or mist	Diffuse airway and lung injury; renal injury; lung carcinogen
Chlorine	Chemical industry, transportation accidents, gas evolved from mixing chlorine bleach with acid cleaners, swimming pools	Potent oxidizing agent; forms HCl in presence of water	Diffuse airway and lung injury
Chromium	Alloy production, chrome plating, welding chromium-containing metals	—	Asthma; diffuse airway injury; lung carcinogen
Cobalt	Metal alloy manufacture, especially tungsten carbide; catalyst	Inhaled as a fine dust	Acute inhalation can cause pulmonary edema; chronic exposure may cause interstitial fibrosis
Copper sulfate	Vineyard sprayers	Inhaled as an aerosol during vineyard spraying	Patchy pneumonitis
Hydrochloric acid	Fires, welding, rubber manufacturing, metal refining	Inhaled as a gas or aerosol (volatile liquid at room temperature); extremely irritating; early warning of exposure	Upper airway injury
Hydrogen fluoride	Etching, welding, metal refining	Water-soluble gas at room temperature	Primarily upper airway; rarely causes pulmonary edema
Isocyanates	Polyurethane production; paints, varnishes, roofing; bathtub refinishing	Highly reactive; only moderately water-soluble	Asthma; diffuse airway injury; hypersensitivity pneumonitis
Lithium hydride	Rocket fuel, chemical industry, nuclear power plants	Highly corrosive gas	Pulmonary edema
Manganese dioxide	Chemical, battery manufacturing	Inhaled as dry dust	Parenchymal injury
Methyl bromide	Refrigeration, produce fumigation	Gas at room temperature; little early warning of exposure	Diffuse airway and lung injury; also causes CNS depression and seizures
Nickel carbonyl	Metal alloys, electroplating, welding	Volatile liquid at room temperature	Pulmonary edema; also causes headache, nausea, and vomiting
Nitrogen dioxide	Grain silos, mining fires, missile fuels	Brown gas at room temperature; insoluble in water	Airway injury; bronchiolitis obliterans; pulmonary edema
Osmium	Metal, chemicals industries	Evolves osmium tetroxide, a highly irritating, water-soluble gas	Upper airway injury
Ozone	Welding, high-altitude aircraft cabins, paper bleaching	Sweet-smelling gas; moderate water solubility	Airway injury, pulmonary edema at high concentrations
Polyvinyl chloride	Plastics, meat wrapping	Inhaled as dry particles or vapors	Asthma; pulmonary fibrosis

TABLE 1. *Continued*

Chemical	Sources of exposure	Important properties	Injury produced
Phosgene	Welding, chemicals industry, paint removal	Extremely water-insoluble gas	Pulmonary edema
Phosphine	Welding, chemicals industry	Foul-smelling gas; highly water-insoluble	Pulmonary edema
Selenium hydrochloride	Metal industry; paints, glass production	Gas at room temperature; water-soluble	Airway injury
Sulfur dioxide	Smelters, pulp mills, wineries, oil refineries, power plants	Highly water-soluble gas	Bronchoconstriction, mucous secretion; airway injury at high concentration
Titanium tetrachloride	Dyes, pigments, sky writing	Forms HCl in aqueous solutions	Upper airway injury
Trichloroethane	Waterproofing sprays	Insoluble in water; when combined with surfactants, forms a more soluble aerosol	Probable airway injury
Zinc chloride	Taxidermy, oil refining, galvanizing iron	—	Pulmonary edema

such as ammonia, dissolve in the mucus of the nose and upper airways, whereas the oxides of nitrogen, which are less soluble, exert their effects throughout the respiratory tract.

4. Toxic absorption. Some inhaled substances, in addition to producing immediate effects in the respiratory tract, are absorbed and may damage distant organs. Mercury and manganese damage the nervous system, whereas fluorides can harm the bones. Certain substances can produce long-term effects in the lungs; beryllium causes fibrosis, and cadmium has been associated with emphysema.

Displacement Asphyxia

Carbon Dioxide

Carbon dioxide is an odorless gas that is heavier than air and can be a hazard in any enclosed or ill-ventilated space. It is a particular hazard in coal mines when oxidation of the contaminants of coal occurs at unworked faces, particularly if a face is reopened.

Carbon dioxide was responsible for the deaths of 1700 people in Cameroon when a massive cloud of gas was released from Lake Nyos, a volcanic crater lake.

Inhalation of carbon dioxide causes hyperventilation, sweating, headache, and a bounding pulse with warm peripheries, followed by loss of consciousness. The treatment is to remove the patient from the source of the gas and administer oxygen. Mouth-to-mouth respiration is required if breathing has ceased. Carbon dioxide will extinguish a naked flame, and because of this property, safety lamps can be used to detect carbon dioxide in mines.

Nitrogen

Nitrogen constitutes approximately 80% of air; the remaining 20% is mainly oxygen. If the level of oxygen falls, as in oxidative processes that occur in mines, then the rest of the air is made up of nitrogen and carbon dioxide. If the oxygen level falls to 15%, dyspnea occurs on exertion. As the oxygen falls further to 10%, breathlessness occurs at rest, and at levels below this, collapse and even death may occur on minimal exertion. The way to detect a falling oxygen level again depends on the ability of the atmosphere to support combustion. The treatment is removal, administration of oxygen, and artificial respiration if required.

Methane

Methane, which is without taste or odor, is the product of decaying vegetable matter. It is known to miners as "firedamp" or "marsh gas." Methane was feared by miners not only because of its asphyxiant properties, but also because of its explosive potential when mixed with air. In the past, methane explosions were the cause of many mining disasters. However, in 1816, Humphrey Davy introduced a lamp that was able to detect methane, which burned with a blue flame.

Methane produces asphyxia by displacement of oxygen, much in the same way as carbon dioxide. The treatment is the same.

Oxygen-Transport Asphyxia

Carbon Monoxide

Carbon monoxide (CO) is the most commonly encountered noxious gas, because it is formed during the incomplete combustion of any carbon-containing material. As well as being an occupational hazard in mines, kitchens, and gas works, around furnaces, and in any situation where high concentrations of motor vehicle exhaust may be present, it is an important cause of death in burning

TABLE 2. *Summary of noxious gases and clinical correlations*

Agent	Principal occupations exposed	Main mechanism of injury	Level immediately dangerous to life or health, ppm
Acrylonitrile (cyanide)	Synthetic fiber, acrylic resin, rubber making	Toxic asphyxia	4
Ammonia	Fertilizer, refrigerator, explosive production	Direct action on mucosa of the eyes and respiratory tract, tracheitis and pulmonary edema	500
Cadmium fumes	Ore smelting, alloying, welding	Acute tracheobronchitis, pulmonary edema, emphysema, renal effects	
Carbon dioxide	Foundry work, mining	Displacement asphyxia	50,000
Carbon monoxide	Foundry work, petroleum refining, mining	Toxic asphyxia	2500
Chlorine	Bleaching, disinfectant and plastic making	Direct action on mucosa of the eyes and respiratory tract, tracheitis and pulmonary edema, possible chronic effect and airways obstruction	25
Copper fumes	Welding	Metal fume fever	
Formaldehyde	Disinfectant, embalming fluid use; paper and photography industry	Direct action on mucosa of the eyes and respiratory tract, dermatitis and asthma(?)	100
Hydrogen chloride	Refining, dye making, organic chemical synthesis	Direct action on mucosa of the eyes and respiratory tract, tracheobronchitis	100
Hydrogen cyanide	Electroplating, fumigant work, steel industry	Toxic asphyxia	50 mg/m^3
Hydrogen fluoride	Etching, petroleum industry, silk working	Direct action on mucosa of the eyes and respiratory tract, tracheitis	20
Hydrogen sulfide	Natural gas, paper pulp industries; sewage treatment; tannery work; oil well prospecting	Systemic and local effects, pulmonary edema, and toxic asphyxia	300
Manganese fumes	Foundry work, battery making, permanganate manufacture	Metal fume fever, predisposition to pneumonia, toxic to CNS	
Mercury fumes	Electrolysis	Direct action on mucosa of eyes, GI tract, and lung; interstitial pneumonitis; systemic effects; fever; rigor; CNS effects	28 mg/m^3
Nitrogen	Underwater work, mining	Displacement asphyxia	
Nitrogen dioxide	Arc welding, dye and fertilizer making, farming	Irritant, respiratory tracheitis, pulmonary edema, bronchiolitis obliterans	50
Osmium tetroxide fumes	Alloy making, platinum hardening	Direct irritation of respiratory tract	1 mg/m^3
Ozone	Arc welding; air, sewage, and water treatment	Direct irritation of respiratory tract	10
Phosgene	Chemical industry, dye and insecticide making	Direct irritation of respiratory tract, pulmonary edema	2
Sulfur dioxide	Bleaching, ore smelting, paper manufacturing, refrigeration industry	Direct action on respiratory tract, bronchitis, exceptionally pulmonary edema	100
Vanadium pentoxide fumes	Glass, ceramic, alloy making; chemical industry (catalysis)	Direct action on respiratory tract, bronchitis, asthma	70
Zinc chloride	Dry-cell making, soldering, textile finishing	Direct action on respiratory tract, irritant	200
Zinc oxide fumes	Welding	Metal fume fever	

buildings. In the United States, the number of people who die of carbon monoxide poisoning each year is estimated to be above 3,800. In Britain, 1,000 people are estimated to die annually because of the effects of carbon monoxide, which is the most frequent cause of poisoning in children.

The gas is odorless and lighter than air. It causes hypoxia by reducing the oxygen-carrying capacity of the blood and by directly poisoning the cytochrome oxidase systems. The affinity of carbon monoxide for hemoglobin is a 200 times greater than that of oxygen. Carbon monoxide not only forms carboxyhemoglobin and prevents oxygen transport, it also shifts the oxygen dissociation curve to the left, making less oxygen available to the tissue. The tissues most affected by carbon monoxide are those with the highest metabolic rates. Warning symptoms include dizziness and headache, but rapid loss of consciousness without premonitory symptoms often occurs; in fact, it has been estimated that up to 70% of fire-associated deaths in the United States are not caused by smoke or heat of the fire but rather by carbon monoxide poisoning, explaining why individuals with the opportunity to escape fires often fail to do so.

Breathlessness is not necessarily a feature, and physical examination is not particularly helpful. Cyanosis does not occur despite the hypoxia, but a cherry-red coloration of the mucous membranes, caused by carboxyhemoglobin, may be present. The pulse rate is usually elevated.

The chest radiographic findings may be abnormal in acute carbon monoxide poisoning in up to 30% of cases, the usual pattern being diffuse shadowing with a peripheral predominance. If levels of carbon monoxide are insufficient to produce acute carbon monoxide poisoning, then chronic carbon monoxide poisoning can occur. Chronic exposure to carbon monoxide causes headache, muscular weakness, and nausea. If the central nervous system is affected, extrapyramidal or psychiatric symptoms can occur. These features may also be seen in patients who recover from acute poisoning.

The deleterious effects of carbon monoxide are related to its concentration in the inspired air, the duration of inhalation, and the oxygen requirement of the exposed person (and therefore the degree of exertion at the time of exposure). An estimate of the saturation of hemoglobin by carbon monoxide can be obtained for use in, for example, contaminated mines when the concentration is not too high with the formula $b = 4ate/100$, where b is the saturation, a the concentration in parts per million (ppm), t the exposure time in hours, and e the exercise factor (1 for rest, 2 for walking, 3 for working). Even low concentrations of carbon monoxide (0.5%) breathed for 2 hours can cause death. Symptoms begin when the carboxyhemoglobin saturation reaches 20%. Unconsciousness occurs at 60% and death at 80%. High concentrations of carbon monoxide can be produced quickly from vehicle exhaust fumes; a lethal concentration can be reached in a single car garage within 10 minutes. Normal individuals have carboxyhemoglobin saturation levels of 0.5%, whereas smokers have levels of 5%–10%. Nonsmoking London taxi drivers had levels of 0.4%–3%, presumably because of exposure to exhaust fumes.

The traditional means of detecting the presence of carbon monoxide in mines relied on the observation of canaries falling off their perches. Although this method has been largely superseded by detector tubes or infrared analyzers, most mines still keep canaries.

The management of carbon monoxide poisoning is important and consists of prompt administration of the highest concentrations of oxygen available. Normally, this will be 100% oxygen delivered by face mask, but if available, hyperbaric oxygen expedites the dissociation of carboxyhemoglobin. The hyperbaric chamber is undoubtedly the most effective treatment, and such chambers should be available where the risk for carbon monoxide poisoning is high.

The diagnosis of carbon monoxide poisoning is often overlooked (30% in one series). Hence, it is important to measure blood carboxyhemoglobin or breath carbon monoxide in both the industrial setting and in persons who have escaped from fires; this should be followed by prompt treatment with oxygen.

Cyanides

Cyanide poisoning caused by sodium or potassium cyanate can affect persons who are involved in gold extraction and electroplating or who work in chemical and photographic laboratories. The greatest risk, however, occurs with the use of acrylonitrile (vinyl cyanide) in the manufacture of synthetic rubber. The fumes may be inhaled or absorbed through the skin, and workers engaged in loading and unloading or in the industrial process itself are at risk. Cyanides derived from burning seats and furnishings in combination with carbon monoxide were thought to be the cause of death in victims of a recent airplane fire disaster, and elevated levels of cyanide have been identified in persons involved in residential fires.

Cyanide blocks the cytochrome oxidase system. Thus, oxygen can no longer be transferred to the tricarboxylic acid cycle. Asphyxia, therefore, occurs at the cellular level. The symptoms are usually dramatic, with dizziness, nausea, and rapid breathing. This is followed by vomiting, chest and abdominal pain, confusion, and finally coma. Because of the rapid onset of symptoms, the subject is fortunately warned of danger, allowing escape before a fatal dose is absorbed. The saturation of oxygen is not disturbed, and cyanosis is not a feature until respiration is depressed. The diagnosis can be made by the characteristic odor of "bitter almonds" on the breath.

Cyanide poisoning is a medical emergency. Two antidotes are available: nitrites and cobalt. Amyl nitrite, which is inhaled, or sodium nitrite, which is given intravenously, combines with hemoglobin to produce methemoglobin. This combines with cyanide, which in turn combines with thiosulfate to produce the harmless thiocyanate. Thiosulfate is given intravenously with nitrites to augment this conversion. A better alternative therapy is cobalt, which forms stable, inert complexes with cyanide (cobalt cyanides). Hydroxycobalamin can be given intramuscularly, but very high doses are required, so the chelated cobalt dicobalt edetate is the drug of choice. It should be used only when the diagnosis is certain because of potential serious side effects.

A person poisoned with cyanide should be removed from the area, washed if the skin is contaminated, and given hydroxycobalamin intramuscularly and amyl nitrite to inhale as an immediate first aid measure. If the patient's condition remains severe (i.e., presence of neurotoxicity or depression of respiration), 300 to 600 mg of dicobalt edetate (Kelocyanor) should be given intramuscularly, with a further 300 mg if there is no recovery in 1 minute. Oxygen should be given in high concentration, as this has been shown to have a synergistic antidotal action, particularly when the nitrites are used. If the response is insufficient, then amyl nitrite should be inhaled every 2 minutes, with intravenous administration of sodium nitrite (10 mL of 3% solution) and sodium thiosulfate (25 mL of 50% solution). The patient may require inotropic support, artificial respiration, or even cardiac massage until the antidotes work.

Hydrogen Sulfide

Hydrogen sulfide has a characteristically unpleasant odor that has been used by generations of delighted schoolchildren to make stink bombs. In industry, it is a potential hazard in petroleum refining, the natural gas industry, tanning, the chemical industry, and in the preparation of fish meal.

Exposure to hydrogen sulfide causes conjunctivitis, blurred vision, keratitis, and blepharospasm, together with headache, dizziness, ataxia, nausea, and diarrhea. If the exposure is heavy or if the gas is inhaled, then cyanosis, confusion, pulmonary edema, convulsions, and coma occur. Severe acute exposure causes a greenish coloration of the face and chest. Coma and death result from toxicity of the central nervous system, because the gas binds iron and poisons the cytochrome oxidase system, preventing cellular respiration. Treatment consists of removal from the source with artificial respiration if required. Because the action of hydrogen sulfide is similar to that of cyanide, it would seem logical to give 10 mL of 3% sodium nitrite intravenously, as in cases of cyanide poisoning.

Irritant Gases

Ammonia

Ammonia is a widely used, highly irritant, highly soluble gas. It is utilized in refrigeration, fertilizer production, oil refining, and the manufacture of explosives and plastics. Exposure most commonly occurs as a result of industrial accidents in which tanks or pipes fracture.

The gas is very toxic, and because it is so soluble, its effects are manifested in the skin, conjunctivae, mucous membranes, and upper respiratory tract. Immediately following exposure, intense pain occurs in the eyes, nose, mouth, and throat, accompanied by a sense of suffocation. Stridor and aphonia are followed by cyanosis and ulceration of mouth, nose, and pharynx. Exposure to high concentrations for a minute or less will cause death.

Pathologic examination shows a severe acute inflammatory reaction characterized by edema, ulceration, and desquamation of mucous membranes. Death results from obstruction of the airway caused by edema of the larynx and blockage of the airways with desquamated epithelium. If the gas reaches the lungs, then the alveoli fill with blood and edematous fluid. Survivors have severe airways obstruction that can last for months, although in many cases the epithelial surface completely regenerates. Long-term impairment can occur and has been shown to be caused by bronchitis and bronchiectasis.

The treatment is rapid removal of the patient from the area by rescuers using breathing apparatuses. Weakly acidic mouth washes and eyewashes may help symptoms, but the main objective is to maintain oxygenation. All patients should be given oxygen therapy, and if the case is severe, tracheotomy and artificial respiration may be required. Severe ammonia burns require fluid to treat shock and antibiotics to prevent sepsis. The value of steroids and bronchodilators is unknown, but both tend to be used acutely.

Chlorine

Chlorine is another irritant gas that is widely used in industry in the manufacture of alkalis, bleaches, and disinfectants. It is less soluble than ammonia and is therefore more likely to affect the whole of the respiratory tract rather than just the upper airway. The gas is often stored or transported under pressure, and exposure occurs after accidents such as fracture of tanks or pipes.

Although the gas is less soluble, chlorine exposure still produces conjunctivitis and nasal irritation. However, the most serious effects occur in the lower respiratory tract. Acute exposure causes chest pain and breathlessness. Crackles and wheezes can be heard in the chest, and pulmonary edema with the production of a white or pink sputum can occur immediately or be delayed for several hours.

The degree of parenchymal damage is more severe than that produced by ammonia. Hence, the course of the acute illness is longer, with impairment of gas exchange for several days. Treatment is removal from the source and administration of oxygen, with intermittent positive-pressure ventilation if required. Steroids have been used, although benefit is not proved. Antibiotics are usually given to prevent infection, which may complicate the damaged respiratory mucosa.

Although chronic disability occurred in many victims of World War I gas attacks, this may have been a consequence of the sequelae of infection, as follow-up studies of persons poisoned by chlorine have not revealed permanent impairment of lung function. Nevertheless, there have been several recent isolated reports of persistent bronchial hyperreactivity and asthmatic symptoms (reactive airways dysfunction syndrome, or RADS) following a single large exposure to chlorine gas.

Similar situations have also been reported following a variety of particular smoke inhalations, such as from burning polyvinyl chloride (PVC). Thus, the development of prolonged obstructive airways disease after smoke inhalation is of concern to both fire victims and fire fighters.

Oxides of Nitrogen

Although nitrogen is capable of forming four oxides, the two forms of nitrogen dioxide, NO_2 and N_2O_4, are particularly hazardous. Nitrogen dioxide is a heavy, irritant, brown gas that is relatively insoluble. The gas occurs in several distinct situations in industry: silage production, arc welding, combustion of nitrogenous materials, and manufacture and transport of nitric acid.

Silage is used to feed livestock through the winter. It is produced from fresh green crops, such as grass, alfalfa, and corn, that are stored in a tower or pit at a controlled temperature of $\sim 38°C$. Nitrates derived from the soil or fertilizer are oxidized as a side reaction to the fermentation of vegetable matter, resulting in the production of nitrogen dioxide. The process begins within a few hours of filling the silo, peaks at 2 days, and subsides after a week or two. Farmers and their families are at risk for nitrogen dioxide poisoning at any time in the first week if the silo is entered or even simply approached. Poisoning has occurred up to 6 weeks after filling.

Arc welding, because of the very high temperatures involved, can cause atmospheric oxygen and nitrogen to combine to form nitrogen dioxide and causes a risk when carried out in confined spaces, such as inside tanks or ships' hulls.

Nitrogen dioxide also can be produced when nitrogen-containing materials are burned, as occurs during shot firing in coal and metal mines or the explosion of dynamite. In a particularly notorious episode of nitrogen dioxide poisoning at the Cleveland Clinic, the accidental burning of nitrocellulose radiographic film resulted in >100 deaths. The greatest risk from nitrogen dioxide fumes occurs in the chemicals industry, particularly in the manufacture, transport, and use of nitric acid. The hazard occurs after spills, as nitric acid gives off nitrogen dioxide on contact with organic material. There is also a risk when nitric acid is used to clean metals, in the handling of jet fuels, and in the nitrification of organic compounds.

In agricultural settings, nitrogen dioxide poisoning is known as *silo filler's disease*. However, the clinical features are similar whatever the source of the gas. The gas is not as irritating as ammonia, and low concentrations may produce only mild upper respiratory tract symptoms. The worker may be alerted to the danger by cough or by observing the characteristic brown gas. If the concentration of gas is high, choking and cough will cause the

worker to leave the site. Choking and cough are followed by the production of frothy sputum, increasing dyspnea, and within an hour frank pulmonary edema; death may occur at this stage. Alternatively, the onset may be less acute, with cough and dyspnea developing during a few hours, followed by gradual improvement within 2 to 3 weeks. Despite an apparent improvement, there may be a sudden relapse, heralded by fever and chills and followed by cyanosis, dyspnea, and generalized crackles. Death resulting from respiratory failure also may occur in this second stage, but if the patient survives, then recovery is usual, although obstructive defects with impairment of gas transfer have been reported.

Radiographic findings in nitrogen dioxide poisoning are variable. In the acute stage, the radiographic features can be normal or display the appearance of pulmonary edema, which initially may have a nodular component. As the patient recovers, the radiograph clears, but if a second stage occurs, then miliary mottling develops, which at times becomes confluent. In the acute phase, pathologic examination reveals mucosal edema, inflammatory cell exudation, dilated capillaries, and blood in the alveoli. The delayed lesion shows bronchiolitis obliterans.

Management is mainly preventative. Farm workers should be warned of the dangers of recently filled silos, welders should not work in poorly ventilated enclosed spaces, and in addition to the obvious precautions that must be taken in chemical works, even small exposures should be reported and workers observed for late sequelae.

Medical management includes the use of oxygen and ventilation if required. Steroids have been beneficial in case reports, although no controlled trial has proved their benefit. Antibiotics are given to prevent superinfection, but their effectiveness is unproved. Bronchodilators may be of some use in the acute attack.

Ozone

Ozone (O_3) is a constituent of photochemical smog and can be found in the cockpits of aircraft flying above 30,000 feet. It is also produced by high-tension electrical discharges in arc welding.

Serious poisoning by ozone has not been reported, but abundant work in animals has demonstrated that ozone produces structural and functional changes. In humans, low concentrations of the gas (0.3 to 0.9 ppm) produce cough, chest discomfort, and impaired pulmonary function of an obstructive type. Tolerance, however, appears to develop in persons exposed to repeated low levels of ozone, possibly as a result of increased superoxide dismutase.

The evidence that ozone is detrimental to health is increasing. Recent studies have confirmed that ozone causes adverse effects on the pulmonary function of healthy individuals and is particularly harmful to asthmatic patients, potentiating the allergic response even at low concentrations. The subject requires further study.

Phosgene

Phosgene, along with chlorine, was responsible for many of the deaths caused by gassing in World War I. It is a heavy, colorless gas that has a faint odor of newly mown hay. Because it is not particularly irritant, it may be inhaled for long periods without great discomfort. Phosgene is a hazard in the chemical industry, being formed as an intermediate in the synthesis of isocyanates and other organic chemicals. It also occurs when chlorinated hydrocarbons are heated, and cases of phosgene poisoning have been reported following an accident with a carbon tetrachloride fire extinguisher.

Phosgene is toxic to the pulmonary capillaries and causes pulmonary edema (Fig. 1). An exposed worker begins to cough and within an hour becomes breathless. Crackles develop throughout the lungs, and shock follows. Phosgene also appears to cause constriction of the pulmonary vasculature, increasing transudation through the already leaky capillaries and compounding the hypovolemic shock.

If the patient survives the acute episode, the pulmonary edema gradually subsides during a week. There is no definite evidence of long-term pulmonary damage.

Sulfur Dioxide

Sulfur dioxide occurs in the polluted urban atmosphere, being derived from the combustion of coal and gasoline.

In industry, it is encountered in paper production, oil refining, and the manufacture of food preservatives and bleach.

Sulfur dioxide is a heavy, irritating gas with a solubility similar to that of ammonia. The effects are therefore severe irritation of the mouth, eyes, nose, and upper respiratory tract. This is quickly followed by violent paroxysms of coughing. Heavy exposure to sulfur dioxide can cause death from pulmonary edema.

The treatment is much the same as for the other irritant gases, although sodium bicarbonate may provide local symptomatic relief. There is some evidence that sulfur dioxide can exacerbate chronic bronchitis, and long-term complications have included the development of obliterative bronchitis and bronchiectasis. However, a 10-year study of a group of paper workers showed no increase in mortality from either respiratory or other diseases.

Toxic Fumes

Metal Fume Fever

Metal fume fever is an acute febrile illness caused by the inhalation of metal oxides. It is variously known as *brass founders' ague, copper fever, brass fever,* and *Monday morning fever.* The disease is most commonly associated with zinc, copper, and manganese, but it is also seen in persons who work with cadmium, iron, nickel, selenium, tin, and antimony. The industrial situations include ship building, welding, electrical metal furnaces, zinc smelting, and galvanizing.

Metal fume fever is thought to be caused by the inhalation of finely dispersed particles (<1 μm in diameter)

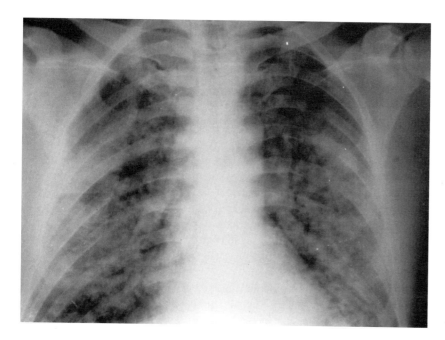

FIG. 1. Posteroanterior radiograph of a 55-year-old man with acute phosgene poisoning. Extensive alveolar shadowing is present, with a normal-sized heart and no evidence of diversion of blood to veins of the upper lobes.

that are produced by heating the previously mentioned metals. The disease invariably has an acute onset, and repeated bouts are common. Metal fume fever is usually worse on the first day at work, as transient resistance develops after a few days exposure, although this effect quickly wanes—hence the term *Monday morning fever.* Attacks can occur on first exposure to fumes without prior sensitization, indicating that a direct toxic action, possibly involving chemotaxis of neutrophils, rather than an immunologic mechanism is the most likely basis for the condition.

The symptoms begin within 4 hrs of exposure and include sudden onset of thirst with a metallic taste in the mouth. This is followed by rigors, fever, and muscular aches and pains associated with generalized weakness. All the symptoms settle spontaneously within 24 to 36 hours. The diagnosis of metal fume fever is based on clinical findings, as no test is specific, although a leukocytosis is often present. The disease is so common that the diagnosis is often made by the workers, who are well aware of the condition. No medical treatment is available, but drinking milk, for no known reason, provides symptomatic relief.

Polymer Fume Fever

Polymer fume fever is a condition similar to metal fume fever and is known as "the shakes." It occurs after exposure to the fumes produced during the manufacture of polytetrafluoroethylene (trademarks Teflon and Fluon). The condition, first described in 1951, begins several hours after exposure and is characterized by a sharp attack of chest tightness, choking, and a dry cough. Repeated attacks are common, as with metal fume fevers, and do not lead to permanent problems.

It is thought that inhalation of aliphatic and cyclic fluorocarbons, formed when polytetrafluoroethylene is heated to >250°C, causes leukocytes in the lung to degranulate and release endogenous pyrogens.

The vast majority of cases of polymer fume fever occur in smokers, and the incidence can be reduced if workers wash their hands before smoking. Better still, handlers of polytetrafluoroethylene should be strongly advised not to smoke.

Osmium

Osmium is a very dense metal that is closely related to platinum. It is found in Russia, Canada, Colombia, Australia, and the United States as the ore osmiridium. Osmium is used as a catalyst, as an alloy with iridium in nibs and compass needles, in photography, and for the staining of histologic sections.

The metal is innocuous, but osmic acid (osmium tetroxide) produces effects similar to those of the halogen gases, including severe conjunctivitis, tracheitis, and bronchitis. Blindness can occur from corneal damage, and prolonged exposure causes nausea and vomiting.

Trimellitic Anhydride

Trimellitic anhydride (TMA) is used in a variety of industrial processes, such as the manufacture of plasticizers, as a constituent of alkyl resins, and as a curing agent for epoxy resins. Asthma and bronchitis were the first problems reported with trimellitic anhydride. However, hemorrhagic pneumonitis also has been described. Workers with pneumonitis were exposed to fumes of trimellitic anhydride when a mixture with epoxy resin was heated; they presented with cough and repeated hemoptysis. Chest radiographs often showed patchy infiltrates consistent with blood in the lung. All patients had hemolytic anemia as well as respiratory problems. Pulmonary function testing showed hypoxemia, and although the diffusing capacity (DLCO) was occasionally raised initially because of blood in the lung, it was reduced as the anemia became more severe. Histologic examination in these cases showed a hemorrhagic pneumonitis with intravascular hemorrhage and alveolar cell hyperplasia.

Removal from the exposure usually results in resolution of symptoms. Treatment is supportive.

Mercury

The industrial hazard from mercury was appreciated as early as 1703 by Ramazzini, who reported that persons making mirrors became palsied and asthmatic from handling mercury. The inhalation of mercury vapor may cause inflammation throughout the respiratory tract, with tracheitis, bronchitis, bronchiolitis, and a pneumonitis. Exposure to this hazard occurs in extraction of the metal, in the manufacture of thermometers and tungsten-molybdenum wire, in the cleaning of tanks and boilers, and more recently, in the repair of sphygmomanometers.

Symptoms generally begin 1 to 4 hrs after acute exposure, with breathlessness and tightness of the chest. This is followed by development of paroxysmal cough, loss of appetite, fever, restlessness, rigors, and tremor. If the exposure is heavy, dyspnea can be severe and death may occur. If the exposure is small but repeated, the symptoms are of abdominal pain, diarrhea, erosion of the nails, gingivitis, and nonspecific neurologic symptoms such as tremor, irritability, or forgetfulness. Basal crackles may be heard in the lungs. The radiograph may show diffuse, patchy shadowing, and lung function tests show a mixed restrictive and obstructive defect. Mercury levels in the blood may be low, as it is fixed in the tissues. However, chronic exposure can be detected by finding raised levels in the urine. In severe cases, pathologic examination has shown tracheobronchitis and pneumonitis with alveolar edema and hyaline membrane formation. In infants, bronchiolitis and pneumothorax have been known to cause death. Occasionally, patients progress to pulmonary fibrosis. Management of the poisoning is supportive and includes oxygen and corticosteroids.

Manganese

Manganese is used as an alloy to harden steel. It is mined from a black ore containing manganese dioxide (pyrolusite) in Russia, India, Morocco, South Africa, and South America. Exposure to manganese occurs in smelting and the manufacture of dry-cell batteries and glass. The damage to the central nervous system caused by manganese is well-known; its effect on the lungs is not as clear. A high incidence of pneumonia and bronchitis has been observed in workers exposed to manganese, and animal experiments have confirmed its ability to cause pulmonary damage.

Cadmium

Cadmium is a soft, gray metal similar to zinc. It is produced chiefly in the United States, the metal being obtained from its own natural ore, greenockite, or from zinc, lead, and copper ores. Cadmium is also recovered from electrolytic zinc refining and from the fumes of lead and zinc smelting. Because it resists corrosion, cadmium is widely used for electroplating. It is also mixed with nickel and silver to form alloys used in nuclear reactors and batteries, and in the manufacture of jewelry.

Cadmium is toxic to humans. If the salts are ingested, nausea, vomiting, and diarrhea occur within 2 hrs. The most serious effects of cadmium, however, develop after inhalation of the fumes, which can occur at the time of smelting or if cadmium-plated metals are fired or welded. The effects can be either acute or chronic.

Acute exposure to high concentrations of cadmium fumes causes rhinitis, sore throat, cough, a metallic taste in the mouth, and retrosternal discomfort. Later, symptoms similar to those of metal fume fever develop, including malaise, rigors, and muscle pains, and, if the exposure is severe, dyspnea and hemoptysis. Physical signs include fever, tachypnea, cyanosis, and coarse or medium crackles in the chest. The chest radiograph shows vague infiltrates in the middle and lower zones or a pattern similar to that of pulmonary edema.

In fatal cases, pathologic examination shows damage to lung and kidney. The trachea and bronchi are inflamed, and the lungs are edematous. Histologic examination shows congestion with intra-alveolar exudate and hemorrhage. The kidneys are swollen with evidence of cortical necrosis. Glomerular vessels are often occluded by thrombi, and the tubules show widespread damage with proteinaceous and granular casts.

The effects of long-term exposure to cadmium are not as easily delineated. Nonrespiratory problems include anosmia, nasal ulceration, and discoloration of the teeth. Proteinuria occurs in 80% of workers with long-term exposure to cadmium and can be associated with severe tubular degeneration. Liver damage, anemia, and bone marrow depression have all been reported. The effect of long-term exposure to cadmium on the lungs is controversial. Some believe it causes emphysema, and although this may be the case, others argue that cadmium emphysema is in fact caused by cigarette smoking or is the aftereffect of an acute exposure. The situation is further complicated by the fact that cigarettes themselves contain cadmium. The symptoms of cadmium emphysema are much as expected, although there tends to be little in the way of accompanying bronchitis. Pulmonary function tests usually show obstruction, although one study by Smith and associates of heavily exposed workers showed a restrictive defect with evidence of pulmonary fibrosis in a minority of patients. These findings have not been observed by other investigators.

Pathologic examination of the lungs has shown marked emphysema without bronchitis, although there has not been unanimity concerning which type of emphysema is present, both panacinar and centrilobular patterns being reported.

No specific treatment is known for either acute or chronic cadmium poisoning, and both British antilewisite (BAL) and ethylenediamine tetra-acetic acid (EDTA) are thought to be contraindicated.

Vanadium

Vanadium is used to harden certain steels. It has been shown to cause industrial asthma, and after acute exposure, it can produce severe irritation of the eyes, nasal irritation, sore throat, cough, retrosternal discomfort, and bronchitis or a patchy bronchopneumonia.

Metal Fumes and Industrial Asthma

The list of substances that cause industrial asthma continues to increase and includes several metals, such as nickel, chromium, cobalt, and platinum salts. Industrial asthma is reviewed in Chapter 34.

MISCELLANEOUS AGENTS

Various agents are encountered in the workplace that do not necessarily fit into the classification of noxious gases and fumes discussed previously. Nevertheless, they deserve mention.

Diesel Emissions

Diesel emissions have been the subject of a number of investigations because they contain a complex mixture of harmful materials, including carbon monoxide, carbon dioxide, sulfur dioxide, formaldehyde, and nitrogen dioxide. However, despite the potential risks, several studies have failed to demonstrate serious effects. Coal miners showed no decrease in FEV_1 (forced expiratory volume in 1 second) or $FEF_{50\%}$ (forced expiratory flow, midexpiratory phase), railway workers exposed to short-term diesel exhausts showed no adverse effects, and iron ore workers in Sweden had no decrease in lung function after exposure to diesel fumes; an increased incidence of bronchitis was found in underground workers, although this was small compared with the effect of smoking.

Overall, diesel fumes, despite their hazardous potential, have not been proved to have any harmful effects, although surveillance should be maintained and any further complaints investigated. Diesel fumes are also considered in the chapter on occupational pulmonary neoplasms (Chapter 36).

Hexavalent Chromium Compounds

These compounds, used in pigments and tanning, cause nasal ulceration and perforation. In high concentrations they can induce severe tracheobronchitis and pneumonia. Recovery is usually rapid, but secondary infection can occur.

Hydrofluoric Acid

This acid is used in etching, in metal refining, and as a catalyst. It causes severe tracheobronchitis if inhaled.

Zinc Chloride

This compound can be a hazard in the manufacture of dry cells or in galvanizing. Its effects are similar to those of hydrofluoric acid.

Formaldehyde

This is a colorless, inflammable gas that has many industrial uses, including the manufacture of textiles, paper, rubber, adhesives, cosmetics, and insulation materials. It is used as a fixative and preservative in anatomy, in pathology laboratories, and by morticians. Formaldehyde is also present in cigarette smoke and automobile fumes. The irritant effects of formalin are well-known, with exposure causing lacrimation, nasal irritation, sneezing, sore throat, headache, and chest tightness. Evidence is increasing that formalin causes asthma. Formaldehyde has also been linked with cancer; this is discussed in Chapter 36.

Paraquat

This highly efficient herbicide is used worldwide, and although it becomes inactive on contact with soil, it is a serious occupational hazard. The devastating effects of ingestion of paraquat are well-known, producing an often-fatal pulmonary fibrosis. Occupational poisoning has occurred in agricultural workers spraying paraquat, and it is likely that absorption in these cases occurred through the skin. There is a single case report of a patient who survived poisoning by inhalation of aerosol.

Prevention is based on education of workers together with use of protective clothing and respirators. Treatment is supportive, including administration of steroids.

Methyl Isocyanate

Poisoning with methyl isocyanate (MIC) was not recorded until 1984, when a notorious accident occurred at a Union Carbide plant in Bhopal, India. This episode resulted in approximately 1,900 deaths, according to the official estimate of the Indian government; however, the true figure may have been as high as 2,500 to 5,000 deaths. Methyl isocyanate, which is used in the manufacture of pesticides, was thought to have escaped when water entered a tank of the gas. The exothermic reaction that resulted caused a massive escape in a densely populated area (100,000 people within a 1-km radius). The main effects were on the eyes and respiratory tract.

Pulmonary edema was followed by destructive lesions with cavitation, pneumomediastinum, and emphysema in affected individuals. Development of pulmonary hypertension has been reported in survivors, and the possibility of fetal damage and teratogenic effects has been raised. Because of the confusion following the disaster, records and data are incomplete, and many questions about the episode remain unanswered.

BIBLIOGRAPHY

Ahmad D, et al. Pulmonary hemorrhage and hemolytic anemia due to trimellitic anhydride. *Lancet* 1979;2:238. *Report of two cases of exposure to tremellitic anhydride complicated by pulmonary hemorrhage and hemolytic anemia. Review of the known cases, including immunologic studies.*

Ames RG. Acute respiratory effects of exposure to diesel emissions in coal miners. *Am Rev Resp Dis* 1982;125:39. *Examination of the pulmonary function tests of coal miners. Differences were seen between smokers and nonsmokers but not between persons exposed or not exposed to diesel fumes.*

Bardana EJ, et al. Formaldehyde: analysis of its respiratory, cutaneous, and immunological effects. *Ann Allergy* 1991;66:441. *Extensive review of the health risks of exposure to formaldehyde. Examination of biochemistry, exposures, and clinical problems, with an emphasis* on respiratory problems, cutaneous effects, systemic reactions, and immunology.

Barret L, et al. Carbon monoxide poisoning. *Lancet* 1981;2:996. *Letter highlighting the failure to recognize carbon monoxide poisoning. The authors suggest that better education of physicians would result in fewer cases of misdiagnosis of carbon monoxide poisoning.*

Battigelli MC. Effects of diesel exhaust. *Arch Environ Health* 1965;10:165. *Experimental exposure to diesel fumes at concentrations similar to those in locomotive workshops produced no significant effects in terms of symptoms and pulmonary function test findings. Smoking was more important than exposure to diesel fumes.*

Baxter PJ, Kapila M, Mfonfu D. Lake Nyos disaster, Cameroon, 1986: the medical effects of a large-scale emission of carbon dioxide. *Br J Med* 1989;298:1437–1441. *Description of a disaster caused by a massive release of carbon dioxide that killed approximately 1700 people. Discussion of the problems and mechanisms.*

Beach FXM, Jones ES, Respiratory effects of chlorine gas. *Br J Ind Med* 1969;26:231. *Detailed description of five cases of chlorine poisoning, with a review of the subject.*

Bonnell JA, et al. A follow-up study of men exposed to cadmium oxide fumes. *Br J Ind Med* 1959;16:135. *Discussion and results of a study of 100 men exposed to cadmium. Follow-up of an earlier study. Description of respiratory and renal problems.*

Carbon monoxide: an old enemy forgot. *Lancet* 1981;2:75. *A review of carbon monoxide deaths during a 10-year period, highlighting in particular problems with defective heating apparatus.*

Dalgaard JB, et al. Fatal poisoning and other health hazards connected with industrial fishing. *Ann Occup Hyg* 1964;7:223. *Report of fatalities and several cases of unconsciousness in the fishing industry, with interesting review of the subject. Suggests that the problem may be multifactorial, caused by combinations of asphyxia and carbon dioxide and hydrogen sulfide poisoning, possibly exacerbated on occasion by alcohol.*

Davies L. Manganese pneumonitis. *Br J Ind Med* 1946;3:111. *Extensive discussion of subject. Includes literature review and a description of manufacturing process, clinical features, environmental studies, laboratory work, and new cases.*

Doig AT. Respiratory hazards in welding. *Ann Occup Hyg* 1964;7:223. *Extensive review of the hazards likely to occur from exposure to gases and fumes generated during various welding processes.*

George M, Hedworth-Whitty RB. Nonfatal lung disease due to inhalation of nebulized paraquat. *Br Med J* 1980;280:902. *Case report of severe interstitial lung disease developing in a woman after inhalation of paraquat. She made a good recovery.*

Harris DK. Polymer fume fever. *Lancet* 1951;2:1008. *Description of the problems associated with exposure to polytetrafluoroethylene fumes (Teflon, Fluon), which produces a syndrome similar to metal fume fever.*

Health hazards in formaldehyde (annotation). *Lancet* 1981;1:926. *Review of the hazards of formaldehyde with recommendations for safe working practices. The clinical effects of skin contact and inhalation, including acute and long-term problems, are also discussed.*

Hendrick DJ, et al. Formaldehyde asthma. *J Occup Med* 1982;24:893. *Study of nurses on dialysis unit found to have formaldehyde asthma on provocation challenge testing. Removal from exposure led to cessation of symptoms, but continued exposure, even at low levels, was associated with persistence of symptoms and asthmatic responsiveness.*

Ide CW. Mercury hazards arising from the repair of sphygmomanometers. *Br Med J* 1986;293:1309. *Collection of case reports of patients exposed to mercury while repairing sphygmomanometers. Demonstration of significant absorption and exposure. Review of problems.*

Ilano AL, Raffin TA. Management of carbon monoxide poisoning. *Chest* 1990;97:165. *Extensive review indicating that carbon monoxide is a major cause of illness and death in the United States. The diagnosis of carbon monoxide poisoning is underestimated.*

Jaros F. Acute percutaneous paraquat poisoning. *Lancet* 1978;1:275. *Case report of a 44-year-old man who died with respiratory failure, acidosis, and renal failure after absorption of paraquat through the skin.*

Jones GR. Pulmonary effects of acute exposure to nitrous fumes. *Thorax* 1973;28:61. *Four case reports of acute exposure to nitrous fumes, with a review of the subject.*

Jones RD, Commins BT, Cernik AA. Blood lead and carboxyhemoglobin levels in London taxi drivers. *Lancet* 1972;11:302. *Study of blood levels of lead and carboxyhemoglobin in smoking and nonsmoking London taxi drivers. No differences were found in lead levels, but carboxyhemoglobin levels were significantly higher in smokers and day drivers than in night drivers.*

Jorgonsen H. Studies on pulmonary function in respiratory tract syndromes of workers in an iron ore mine where diesel trucks are used underground. *J Occup Med* 1962;4:152. *Study of workers exposed to diesel fumes in an iron ore mine. Underground workers had more bronchitic symptoms, particularly those who smoked. There were no changes in spirometry findings.*

Kerr HD, et al. Effects of ozone on pulmonary function in normal subjects. *Am Rev Respir Dis* 1975;111:763. *Report of a study of 20 adults exposed to 0.5 ppm of ozone in an environmental chamber. Symptoms (cough and chest discomfort) were found to be more common in nonsmokers. Changes in pulmonary function tests are described in detail.*

Koplan PK, Falk H, Green G, et al. Public health lessons from the Bhopal chemical disaster. *JAMA* 1990;264:2795. *Review of the 1984 chemical disaster in Bhopal, concentrating on public health aspects and what might be learned from the event.*

Kreit JW, et al. Ozone-induced changes in pulmonary function and bronchial responsiveness in asthmatics. *J Appl Physiol* 1989;66:217. *Study to examine the effects of ozone on normal and asthmatic subjects, showing significantly greater effects in asthmatics.*

Langford RM, Armstrong RI. Algorithm for managing injury from smoke inhalation. *Br Med J* 1989;299:902–905. *Management of thermal injury has improved, so that the management of inhalation of hot or toxic gases has become more important. The subject is related to experience of Kings Cross Fire in 1989.*

Leib GMP. Chronic pulmonary insufficiency secondary to silo filters disease. *Am J Med* 1958;24:471. *Description of a case of silage fume exposure, emphasizing the long-term effects.*

Levin PJ, et al. Pulmonary effects of contact exposure to paraquat: a clinical and experimental study. *Thorax* 1979;34:150. *Description of clinical and pathologic features of a fatal case of percutaneous paraquat poisoning. Investigation of less heavily exposed co-workers followed by animal experiment. Cutaneous absorption results in pulmonary arterial lesions.*

Lowry T. Silo filters disease: a syndrome caused by nitrogen dioxide. *JAMA* 1956;162:153. *Detailed description of a newly recognized syndrome, reporting four cases (two of them fatal) of silo filters disease. First description of bronchiolitis obliterans as part of the syndrome. Good review of subject.*

Mayes RW. The toxicological examination of the victims of the British Air Tours Boeing 737 accident at Manchester in 1985. *J Forensic Sci* 1991;36:179. *Review of the toxicologic analysis of body fluids of victims of an airplane accident. Concentrations of carbon monoxide were raised in all victims except one, and blood concentrations of cyanide and volatile substances were raised in all victims.*

McLaughlin, et al. Toxic manifestations of osmium tetroxide. *Br J Ind Med* 1946;3:183. *Review of the subject based on seven case reports of workers exposed to osmium tetroxide when refining osmiridium.*

Mehta RS, et al. Bhopal tragedy's health effects. A review of methyl isocyanate toxicity. *JAMA* 1990;264:2781. *An in-depth review of methyl isocyanate, including a description of toxicity and clinical and pathologic effects resulting from the Bhopal incident.*

Meredith SK, McDonald JC. Work-related respiratory disease in the United Kingdom, 1989–1992: report on the Sword Project. *Occup Med* 1994;44:183–189. *Description of a project to develop a national surveillance system for work-related respiratory disease relying on a reporting system comprising approximately 800 chest physicians throughout the United Kingdom. The Sword Project is ongoing and provides up-to-date information regarding the incidence of occupational lung diseases.*

Meredith TJ, Vale JA. Carbon monoxide poisoning. *Br Med J* 1988;296:77. *Excellent review of the subject of carbon monoxide poisoning, including epidemiology, mechanisms, clinical features, and treatment.*

Moisan TC. Prolonged asthma after smoke inhalation: a report of three cases and a review of previous reports. *J Occup Med* 1991;23:458. *Report of three cases of asthma developing after exposure to fumes from fires. Interesting review of a variety of conditions that follow exposure, but emphasis is mainly on airway responsiveness and asthma.*

Molfino NA, et al. Effect of low concentration of ozone on inhaled allergen responses in asthmatic subjects. *Lancet* 1991;338:199. *Original article examining the relationship between inhalation of ambient concentrations of ozone and airway reactivity and inflammatory changes in asthmatic subjects. Consideration of the effects of ozone in air pollution.*

Nichols BH. The clinical effects of the inhalation of nitrogen dioxide. *AJR Am J Roentgenol* 1930;23:516. *Review of clinical and radiologic features of nitrogen dioxide poisoning, including cases from the Cleveland Clinic disaster in 1929.*

Ozone: too much in the wrong place. *Lancet* 1991;338:221. *Review article giving a good overview of the subject of ozone. Discusses the literature and relates findings to clinical observations and air pollution.*

Ploysongsang Y, Beach BC, Dilisio RE. Pulmonary function changes after acute inhalation of chlorine gas. *South Med J* 1982;75:23. *Report of four young healthy adults exposed to chlorine who had significant symptoms and evidence of airway obstruction that cleared within 1 month and left no lung damage.*

Radford EP, Pitt B, Halpin B. Study of fire deaths in Maryland, September 1971–January 1974. Presented at the International Symposium on Toxicology and Physiology of Combustion Products, University of Utah, Salt Lake City, Utah, March 22–26, 1976. *Report from an international symposium on fire deaths. Examination of 107 fatalities from 85 fires. Carbon monoxide was a major contributor to death, with burns alone an infrequent cause of death. It is inferred that if these people had not been overcome by carbon monoxide, they would have escaped death. Excellent study supported by good data.*

Seaton A, Morgan WKC. In: Morgan WKC, Seaton A, eds. *Occupational Lung Diseases.* Philadelphia: WB Saunders; 1984:609–642. *An excellent chapter in a textbook on occupational lung disease that reviews the whole subject of toxic gases and fumes.*

Skalpe IO. Long-term effects of sulphur dioxide exposure in pulp mills. *Br J Ind Med* 1964:21:69. *Study examining the effects of chronic exposure of 54 workers to sulfur dioxide. Comparison with 56 control workers.*

Smith TJ, et al. Pulmonary effects of chronic exposure to airborne cadmium. *Am Rev Respir Dis* 1976;114:161. *Review of workers exposed to either high or low levels of cadmium. Questionnaire and examination of radiographs and pulmonary function tests. Concludes that a mild fibrotic reaction is associated with exposure to cadmium.*

Stokinger HE. Ozone toxicity: a review of research and industrial experience, 1954–1964. *Arch Environ Health* 1965;10:719. *Excellent, in-depth review of ozone. Includes discussion of effects in humans and animals, factors effecting toxicity, and mechanisms.*

Vale JA, Meredith TJ. Poisoning from hydrocarbons, solvents, and other inhalational agents. In: Weatherall DJ, Ledingham JGG, Warrell DA, eds. *Oxford Textbook of Medicine.* Oxford: Oxford University Press; 1983:6.27–6.33. *A chapter in major textbook on general internal medicine covering poisoning by a wide range of hydrocarbons, solvents, and inhalational agents and including details of clinical features and treatment.*

Williams N, Smith I. Polymer fume fever: an elusive diagnosis. *JAMA* 1972;219:1587. *Report of the case of a woman who had 40 attacks of polymer fume fever in a 9-month period. Describes features and recommends inclusion in causes of fever of unknown origin.*

Zeiss CR, et al. Tremellitic anhydride-induced airways syndromes: clinical and immunological studies. *J Allergy Clin Immunol* 1977;60:96. *Description of the spectrum of respiratory symptoms in workers exposed to tremellitic anhydride, followed by a discussion of immunologic studies.*

Zenz C, Berg BA. Human responses to continued vanadium pentoxide exposure. *Arch Environ Health* 1967:14:709. *Study of volunteers exposed to vanadium pentoxide in an environmental chamber. Demonstration of severe respiratory irritation, particularly on re-exposure.*

Textbook of Pulmonary Diseases, 6th ed.
edited by G.L. Baum, J.D. Crapo, B.R. Celli, and J.B. Karlinsky,
Lippincott–Raven Publishers, Philadelphia, © 1998.

CHAPTER

38

Pulmonary Effects of Radiation

Robert A. Nonn · Nicholas J. Gross

HISTORY

The discovery of x-rays in 1895 by Roentgen and a practical means of generating them led almost immediately to their use for diagnostic and therapeutic purposes. It also inaugurated the science of radiobiology. The first evidence of effects on the lungs came as early as 1898 in a study of guinea pigs by Bergonie and Teissier. The energy of therapeutic x-rays in the first decade of this century was so low that most was probably absorbed by the chest wall (even of guinea pigs), and the view at that time was that the lungs were relatively resistant to x-rays. During the second decade, however, higher-energy x-rays with more penetration were generated, and radiotherapists began to observe unusual lung reactions in their patients. It was the practice then to irradiate the chest wall of mastectomy patients with opposed anterior and posterior ports. The first suggestion of pulmonary reactions to this treatment was presented by Groover and colleagues in 1921 and described by them in the next 2 years. The same year as their first publication, 1922, Hines reported two cases with autopsy findings, and Tyler and Blackman reported seven cases, including some in which pleural changes were present; these were followed by Evans and Leucutia in 1925. There is some ambiguity in these reports, with early and late effects and pulmonary and pleural reactions being discussed simultaneously under the designation of "pulmonary fibrosis." However, these were neatly sorted out by Desjardins at the Mayo Clinic in 1926 in the first review article on the subject. His descriptions of the clinical and roentgenographic features and their differential diagnosis leave little room for additions in these areas more than 60 years later. The discoveries of the previous century had clearly resulted in the first lung disorder that was entirely of man's own making.

Subsequent developments can be summarized. The first detailed descriptions of pathologic changes following irradiation were presented by Engelstad and by Warren and Spencer; these were followed by experimental and clinical reports of Jennings and Arden and Smith. Shortly thereafter, in 1966, Phillips suggested that the major change of pathogenetic consequence was the effect on pulmonary capillary endothelial cells, a view that is no longer current.

The physiological effects of pulmonary x-irradiation were investigated by McIntosh and Spitz in 1939 and Freid and Goldberg the next year. But it was not until the era of relative sophistication in pulmonary function testing that a coherent picture of the functional changes emerged.

In the clinical sphere, corticosteroids were first used for treatment of radiation effects on the lungs by Cosgriff and Kligerman and for prophylaxis by Friedenberg and Rubenfeld. Although these and clinical studies by Bluestein and Roemer, Rubin and colleagues, and Whitfield and Bond suggested that corticosteroids might be of benefit, the report by Moss and co-workers appears to have confirmed this experimentally.

RADIOBIOLOGY

The following discussion of the physical and biological effects of ionizing radiation is intended only to provide a superficial background for the understanding of clinical events. For a more detailed and accurate account of the

R.A. Nonn and N.J. Gross: Departments of Medicine and Molecular Biochemistry, Stritch School of Medicine, Loyola University of Chicago, Maywood, Illinois 60153; and Medical Service, Hines Veterans Affairs Hospital, Hines, Ilinois 60141.

effects of radiation on biological tissues, the reader is referred to any text on radiobiology or radiotherapy.

The two most commonly used forms of ionizing radiation are x- or gamma rays and accelerated particles, of which the only variety of significance for pulmonary effects at present is fast neutrons. (Fast electrons are also in clinical use but, because of their limited penetration, cannot produce effects in the lungs from an external source.) X-rays and neutrons ionize the target by indirect processes. When an x-ray collides with an electron in the target, some of its energy is transferred to the electron, which is accelerated out of its orbit. Neutrons are more likely to accelerate hydrogen nuclei. In either case, fast-charged particles so generated ionize the atoms or molecules they collide with, resulting in ion pairs. These in turn react with adjacent molecules to produce free radicals. In biological tissue, where most of the molecules are water molecules, most of the free radicals will be hydroxy radicals, •OH, but free radicals also will be generated from more complex molecules. Free radicals, particularly •OH, have a great deal of excess energy because of their unpaired valence electrons. They can break covalent bonds to cause some of the biological effects of irradiation. It is in fact the free radical, which is much longer-lived and more energetic than the ion, that does the damage. However, the term *free-radical-forming radiation* is unlikely to displace the conventional term *ionizing radiation*. Although much damage can be rapidly repaired *in vivo*, the presence of oxygen in the target allows some of the free radicals to become oxidized. The result in the case of organic free radicals is an organic peroxide, which is less easily repaired than bond breakage without peroxide formation. Because the molecular injury is "fixed" by oxygen, most forms of radiation are much more damaging if the target is well oxygenated.

What is the target in biological systems? Although all molecules can be affected by the chain of events resulting from the absorption of ionizing radiations, the function of most of them is not important enough or not sufficiently altered to have serious consequences. Thus, a change in the viscosity of a mucopolysaccharide solution or an increase in permeability of a membrane could be corrected by replacement or repair of the damaged molecules. Doses in the range of thousands of rads are required to produce enough damage to nongenetic structures to seriously jeopardize the survival of most cells.

The damage to genetic material, DNA itself, is more important. Although the molecular events in genetic damage are not entirely clear, one can envision a number of points at which mutagenic or subsequently lethal effects could occur: single-strand breaks in DNA could be inadequately repaired, or base substitutions could be made in the repair process. Double-strand breaks could result in fragmentation or misalignment of the ends or cross-links between strands, all of which will occur in a small proportion of the population of irradiated cells. It is unlikely that such damage will be expressed in the cells until their next mitotic attempt. At that time, gross chromosomal damage may make it impossible for the chromatids to separate, resulting in anaphase arrest, or chromosomes may be divided unequally between the daughters, or major chromosomal aberrations such as ring forms, dicentrics, bridges, and fragments may appear. Equally fatal results may occur from deletions and point mutations. Genetic damage from radiation is therefore expressed as a loss of reproductive or clonogenic potential. This can occur at doses of a few hundred rads, in contrast to the thousands of rads needed to cause effects on nongenetic material.

Because ionizing radiations do not distinguish between normal cells and cancer cells, the history of experimental radiotherapy is the story of a search for methods to destroy the tumor cells without destroying the cells that make up the normal tissue around them and that will inevitably be irradiated in the process. This search has been considerably advanced by basic studies of the effects of radiation on cell survival (reproductive capacity). Loss of reproductive capacity is most satisfactorily studied in cultures of continuously dividing cells (i.e., HeLa cells, Chinese hamster cells, and mouse L cells), but similar experiments can be performed on the cells of certain organs *in vivo*.

Repair of Sublethal Damage

Following irradiation of cells *in vitro* or *in vivo* with different single doses of x-rays, a characteristic dose–response curve is generated (Fig. 1). There is an initial shoulder reflecting low doses, followed by a portion in which the fraction of cells that survive (divide) is inversely related to the dose. The initial shoulder indicates that a certain amount of radiation damage must be accumulated by cells for a lethal effect. This phenomenon is known as repair of sublethal damage. Above a certain threshold, reproductive death is a direct function of the dose absorbed. The amount of sublethal damage that can be repaired has been measured for many cell types, and there are techniques by which it can be measured *in vivo*. It has approximately the same value in many tissues and tumors *in vivo* and is equivalent to that produced by a notional dose (Dq) of 300 to 500 rads of x-rays (see Fig. 1); values for lung tissue also lie in this range. Furthermore, the survival curve following a second dose of x-rays given long enough after the first has the same shoulder as the first, indicating that sublethal damage must again be accumulated, and to the same extent, for a lethal effect. The phenomenon can be repeated indefinitely. The molecular mechanism of repair, like the mechanism of damage, is incompletely understood, but experiments in which the second dose follows the first by different times show that repair takes place rather quickly, within the first 4 to 6 hr and certainly within 24 hr. The fact that repair can be

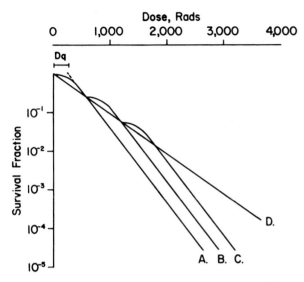

FIG. 1. Typical survival curves of cells in culture. Curve A represents survival (ability to reproduce) following various single doses of x-rays. The initial shoulder is due to sublethal damage, whose amount (Dq) can be calculated by extrapolation to the horizontal axis *(dashed line)*. Curve B shows the effect of a second exposure on a culture previously exposed to 600 rads, and curve C the effect of a third such exposure. The line D is the resultant effective survival after successive 600-rad fractions. In this example, a single exposure to 1800 rads would reduce the proportion of surviving cells to less than 10 whereas the same total dose in three equal fractions would reduce the proportion to only 10 - 2, illustrating the sparing effect of dose fractionation.

partially inhibited—for example, by low temperature—suggests it is a result of the activity of the cell's machinery. The implications of the repair phenomenon in the clinical situation are clear: the smaller the individual fractions, the larger is the total dose that can be administered in the course without destroying the organ, provided the fractions are separated by enough time for repair. Why a larger total dose in many fractions is good for the host cells and bad for the tumor cells may be related to the oxygen effect.

Oxygen Effect

That ionizing radiations are more damaging to a well-oxygenated target has already been mentioned. This is well demonstrated in survival curves (Fig. 2), which typically show less reduction of reproductive potential of cells *in vitro* that lack oxygen at the time of irradiation. Tumor cells are quite likely to be poorly oxygenated because cells toward the center of the tumor are separated from their blood supply. In fact, tumor cells more than 150 to 200 μm from stroma are likely to die of anoxia. Adjacent to the area of necrosis will be many tumor cells that are so poorly oxygenated that they will be relatively radioresistant; only at the periphery of the tumor will the cells

have the same radiosensitivity as the surrounding stroma. X-irradiation will destroy the well-oxygenated cells at the periphery of the tumor, thus bringing the hypoxic cells closer to the blood supply at the periphery and rendering them more susceptible in turn. Fractionation of the total dose of x-rays thus "reoxygenates" the more isolated hypoxic tumor cells while minimizing the lethal damage in normal stromal cells. This is particularly important in the lung, which is the best oxygenated of all tissues. It also explains why small tumors (which have a relatively large surface of well-oxygenated cells) are more likely to be amenable to x-ray control than large ones and why there is an interest in pharmacologic agents that sensitize hypoxic cells to x-rays.

Radiation Energy and Neutrons

The foregoing discussion assumes that all ionizing radiations have the same energy. X-rays have a wide spectrum of energies, however; most experiments in radiobiology were performed at energies of 250 kV or less, but current radiotherapy is almost universally performed at energies in the megavoltage range. Higher-energy radiation is more penetrating, and the oxygen enhancement effect is in general less. Because penetration and less protection from hypoxia are bad for tumor cells and less bad for normal stromal cells, it is understandable that radiotherapy should move in the direction of higher energies. Fast neutrons, depending on the way in which they are generated, have mean energies up to one order of magnitude greater than conventional x-rays and therefore offer advantages over x-rays in tumor therapy (Fig. 3). Heavier charged particles, such as accelerated nuclei, would be even more advantageous, but for economic reasons, they are most unlikely to make the transition from experimen-

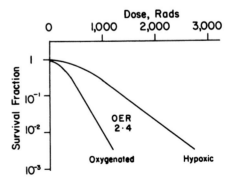

FIG. 2. Survival curves of cells in culture following exposure to various single doses of x-rays under hypoxic and oxygenated conditions. After each dose of x-rays, survival in the culture that was hypoxic at the time of exposure is 2.4 times greater than in the culture that was well oxygenated at the time of exposure. The oxygen enhancement ratio (OER) in this example is 2.4, a typical value for mammalian cells exposed to 250 kVp x-rays.

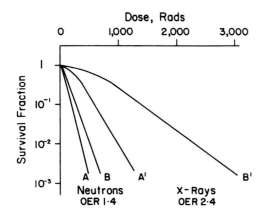

FIG. 3. Survival curves of cells in culture exposed to neutrons and 250 kVp, x-rays under oxygenated (A and A1) and under hypoxic (B and B1) conditions. Not only are neutrons more lethal than x-rays, dose for dose, but there is less sublethal damage (initial shoulder), and the oxygen enhancement ratio (OER) is less.

tal to therapeutic medicine in the time scale of this or the next edition of this text. For the present, fast neutrons are the only practical alternative to x-rays for deep therapy; experience with them is reviewed by Field. Although they appear to offer advantages in some tumor types, their use in lung tumors has been disappointing.

Units, Time, Dose, and Volume in Radiation Therapy

The unit of radiation exposure is the roentgen (R), but what matters to the patient is the amount of energy absorbed. This is a complex function of many factors, including density and thickness of the exposed tissue as well as energy of the radiation. In the case of x-rays, an exposure of 1 R to solid tissue results in an absorbed dose of approximately 1 rad, the unit of absorbed radiation. It is equal to 100 ergs absorbed energy per gram of tissue and has to be calculated on the basis of certain assumptions, tissue density, thickness, etc. It is important to note that the rad is the amount of energy absorbed per gram of tissue, so that a dose of 700 rads to both lungs is only a fraction of the energy absorbed when 700 rads is received by the whole body. The former would not produce any clinical effects; the latter would almost certainly be fatal. Another common misunderstanding is illustrated by the following: Suppose a patient received 5000 rads to a lung tumor and 5000 rads to the mediastinum. The total dose he or she has received is 5000 rads, not 10,000. The mass of tissue irradiated is thus quite as important as the dose of radiation because it is a determinant of the total energy absorbed. Because the only information that the clinician commonly receives, or takes notice of, is the total dose in rads, a unit, the megagram rad, was proposed. This is a mass integral of absorbed radiation energy and

has been used in correlating dose with effect, for example, in pulmonary function. This logical unit enjoyed a brief vogue in previous years but is not widely used now. Radiation scientists and therapists now use a new unit, the Gray (Gy), which is equal to 100 rads, and current reports and treatment plans use this unit instead of the rad.

Important as the total dose is, the way in which it is delivered is as important. As Fig. 1 shows, the phenomenon of repair of sublethal damage indicates that fractionation of the total dose will minimize the damage to normal tissues. The importance of fractionation is well illustrated by a case reported by Whitfield and colleagues of a patient with breast cancer. Following mastectomy, she received 1500 rads in a single dose to the axilla and, inevitably, to the underlying lung. If this dose had been delivered in five to ten fractions, it would have been unlikely to produce any symptoms, even if delivered to the entire volume of both lungs. As a single dose, however, it produced a severe radiation reaction in the underlying lung tissue.

Biological response is thus determined to some extent by the number of fractions a total dose is delivered in. To take account of the effect of fractionation, an isoeffect dose can be expressed as the total dose modified by fractionation factors. Because much of the original work was done by Frank Ellis, the formula that relates tolerance to dose and fractionation is known by his name (the original equation has been rearranged for the purpose of this discussion):

$$\text{NSD} = D \times N_{-9.24} \times T_{-0.11}$$

NSD stands for nominal standard dose; its unit is the ret (rad-equivalent therapy). Hypothetically, it is the number of rads equivalent to treatment as a single dose, but in reality, the formula cannot be extrapolated to fewer than about four fractions. It is the notional dose producing a certain biological effect, traditionally tolerance, resulting from a range of different dose-fractionation schedules. D is the total dose in rads, N the number of fractions, and T the overall treatment time. The Ellis formula (derived from experiments on skin) can be used to estimate the rets for tolerance in a large number of organs, including the lung. Phillips and colleagues reevaluated the exponents of N and T for the lung; in the equation form given here, they would be -0.377 and -0.058, respectively. (Actually, these will probably differ, if only to a minor extent, from one institution to another.) This formula indicates the importance of the number of fractions and, by comparison, the relatively small effect of the overall treatment time. It is used in treatment planning to calculate the total dose and fractionation to be used in irradiation of the entire lung, on the basis of the likelihood of pneumonitis. Thus, Wara and colleagues calculated that there is a 5% probability of clinical pneumonitis when 510 rets is delivered to the entire lung (Fig. 4). This dose is achieved by a wide range of alternative treatment schedules, for example, 1500 rads in 11 fractions over 20 days,

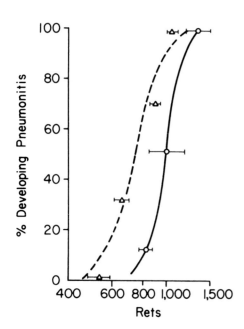

FIG. 4. The probability that pneumonitis will develop following whole lung irradiation at various nominal standard doses (rets) of x-irradiation, with (—△—) and without (-O-) concurrent actinomycin D therapy. (Redrawn from W. M. Wara et al. *Cancer* 1973;32:547. Reproduced from NJ Gross. Pulmonary effects of radiation therapy. *Ann Intern Med* 1977;86:81, with permission.)

2000 rads in 24 fractions over 24 days, or 2500 rads in 38 fractions over 40 days. Each of these will have the same biological effect on normal lung but probably different effects on the tumor (because of such factors as reoxygenation). In addition, there may be regional variation in the response to irradiation, with high-grade pneumonitis more frequently being seen after treatment for lower-lobe than upper-lobe tumors in both animal and human models of study. Concomitant therapy with cytotoxic agents (see Contributory Factors) alters radiation sensitivity, adding yet another dimension.

The Ellis formula applies, of course, to x-rays. The search for an equivalent formula for neutrons has been reviewed by Field; the exponent of N for neutrons is now -0.04. The greatly diminished weighting of the fractionation factor in fast-neutron exposure would be expected from the fact that repair of sublethal damage is much less following neutron exposure (see Fig. 3).

It should be apparent from the foregoing discussion that a great many factors determine the amount of biological damage inflicted on the tumor and the normal surrounding tissue by ionizing radiation and that all these factors have not been brought together into a single universal expression. There are also a number of assumptions and estimates about individual geometry and tissue density that will have to be made for each patient by each radiotherapist, with inconsistent degrees of success. Such judgments vary with the experience and knowledge of the therapist

and must entail a degree of error. Add to these such imponderable factors as errors in localization and field placement, and radiotherapy appears to resemble a thunderbolt with Zeus not completely in control.

PATHOGENESIS OF RADIATION PNEUMONITIS

Histopathologic Cellular Effects

The major clinical effects of lung irradiation are conventionally divided into two stages: radiation pneumonitis and radiation fibrosis. Although the relationship between these is discussed in more detail later (Clinical Syndromes Following Lung Irradiation), we can regard pneumonitis as the episode during which the specific effects of lung damage are expressed, and fibrosis as the subsequent wound-healing phase. Death from radiation of the lungs almost invariably occurs during the time of pneumonitis, 80 to 160 days after treatment. Beyond this time frame, death from radiation itself is uncommon. Moreover, inhibition of collagen synthesis (i.e., fibrosis) does not greatly reduce mortality in irradiated rats, indicating that fibrosis is not a factor in mortality from lung irradiation. Consideration of the pathogenesis of radiation reactions in the lung therefore concentrates on the mechanisms of the acute episode of radiation pneumonitis and the events leading up to it, a process that is probably similar in humans and experimental animals.

One can regard the cellular mechanism of lung damage as being principally a result of genetic damage to lung cells, especially because it is so distant in time from the clinical sequelae. Genetic damage is primarily expressed as a loss of reproductive potential leading to depletion of that cell type in the tissue. The damage sustained by an organ will therefore reflect the reproductive activity of its constituent cells and be expressed when a critical level of certain crucial cell type(s) is reached. In tissues where reproductive activity is minimal, typically highly differentiated tissues such as muscle, a large amount of genetic damage will remain latent; muscle cells have no mitotic future and thus proportionately little likelihood of expressing their genetic damage; such tissues appear to be radioresistant. Rapidly dividing tissues composed of stem cells such as bone marrow and intestinal crypt cells will express their genetic damage as soon as they reveal their incapacity to produce fully functional progeny at the rapid rate required by those organs. Such tissues appear radiosensitive. The principle that radiosensitivity varies directly with the rate of proliferation and the number of future divisions to maturity and inversely with the degree of morphologic and functional differentiation of a cell type was expounded in 1906 by Bergonie and Tribondeau. Much subsequent work has confirmed this general principle.

Discussion of the cellular basis of radiation pneumonitis can begin, therefore, with consideration of the turnover of cell types in the respiratory tract. The data that exist have been reviewed and are quite variable. The cells of the airways make up 10% to 15% of the total lung cell complement if neural, blood, and lymphatic cells are excluded. Turnover rates of individual airway epithelial cell types have not been measured, although these cells are all presumably derived from bronchial basal cells. For the airway epithelium as a whole, a turnover time (100% replacement of the population) has been estimated at 1 to 3 weeks. Bronchiolar epithelium turns over more slowly than bronchial epithelium.

The cells of the lung parenchyma make up 85% to 90% of the total lung complement, of which only a small fraction are alveolar epithelial cells, types I and II pneumocytes. Type I pneumonocytes provide over 90% of the alveolar epithelial layer; their complex three-dimensional structure (a single cell will often form the epithelium of two and possibly more adjacent alveoli) makes it practically certain that they cannot divide. They are fixed postmitotic end cells incapable of mitosis in growth or regeneration. Type II cells, in contrast, undergo mitosis at a slow rate; their turnover time in growing rodents is 4 to 5 weeks, but in response to injury such as exposure to high oxygen concentrations, oxides of nitrogen, or radiation, they can revert to a rapid reproductive cycle, repopulate the alveolar epithelium, and subsequently redifferentiate into type I cells. Thus, in addition to its important and well-known function in the synthesis and secretion of surfactant, the type II cell acts as a stem cell for the alveolar epithelium, capable of replacing alveolar epithelium when type I cells are destroyed.

Capillary endothelial cells comprise about a third of all lung cells. Like type I cells, they have an extended cytoplasm, but unlike type I cells, they are in a continuous process of self-renewal. Their turnover time has been estimated at 8 weeks; however, in regenerating lung they appeared to have the same mitotic activity as type II cells.

Pulmonary mesenchymal cells make up the bulk of total lung parenchymal cells but are themselves a heterogeneous group, at least some of which are fibroblasts and macrophage precursors. No figures are available for their turnover rate. Alveolar macrophages form another small but important sector of the population with interesting origins. The cell type is almost certainly derived from the bone marrow via the circulating monocyte. The monocyte leaves the circulation and enters the interstitial space. There it divides one or more times, possibly even residing as a stem cell, and differentiates into a tissue macrophage. In the lung, this process entails an increase in size as well as the development of an appropriate complement of lysosomal hydrolytic enzymes. The differentiated macrophage leaves the interstitial space and appears fully fledged in the alveolar space. There it performs its important defense functions, ultimately to bow out either via the mucociliary escalator or, less probably, via the pulmonary lymphatics. The turnover rate of macrophage precursors in the interstitium is not known. Their turnover time in the alveolar space is about 1 week, but this is due to traffic through the alveolar space rather than division therein.

Nearly all the preceding data have been derived from small mammals that grow continuously from birth to death. The cytokinetics in adult human lungs may therefore be different. From these data it appears that prime targets for radiation damage would be, in order of reproductive rate, the epithelial cells of the airway, the type II and capillary endothelial cells, and the interstitial macrophage precursors. The histologic and other evidence of radiation damage given below accord to some extent with the reproductive activity of cell types in the lung. However, the disproportionate degree of damage sustained by capillary endothelial and type I alveolar cells suggests that there is considerable nongenetic damage in these cells. This possibly results from their very extended cell processes, regions not richly endowed with organelles and in which repair or replacement of damaged nongenetic macromolecular structures such as cell membrane is limited.

Cytokinetic Studies

In the lung, the long latent interval between irradiation and the occurrence of radiation pneumonitis some months later strongly suggests that critical depletion of a crucial cell type is the mechanism of pneumonitis. Because type II cells and capillary endothelial cells are undergoing constant replication (albeit usually at a slow rate), they are thus both candidates for radiation damage. Endothelial cells have been shown to be sensitive to ionizing radiation; in fact, the radiosensitivity of capillary endothelial cells in an organ has been viewed as the limiting factor in radiation tolerance of that organ. Both capillary endothelial cells and alveolar type II cells perform crucial functions in the lung, the failure of which could conceivably produce the changes associated with radiation pneumonitis. However, a complete explanation of radiation pneumonitis in terms of the depletion of either of these cell types has proved elusive. Relatively little is known about the number of these two cell types following irradiation of the lungs because the systematic morphometric analysis of lung cell types following radiation has not yet been reported in detail. However, recent reports suggest there is a general depletion in all cell types 12 weeks after x-irradiation.

Relevant information also can be obtained by cytokinetic studies. The incorporation of precursors of DNA into the nucleus of a cell is evidence of imminent mitosis, and the proportion of cells in that population that are about to enter mitosis, the labeling index, indicates the replicative activity of that cell type. Cytokinetic studies on lung cells following small doses of radiation to the thorax show mitotic arrest in all cell types in the first week after irradiation. Following this, the labeling index of capillary endothelial cells rises severalfold above control levels for a few weeks and then gradually declines to control levels. The labeling index of type II cells also rises above normal levels after the first week and returns to baseline some 4 weeks later. However, from about 6 weeks on, it begins a steady climb to levels about four- to sixfold above normal throughout the period when pneumonitis is occurring. It is therefore difficult to imagine how significant depletion of either endothelial cells or type II cells could occur unless their loss through death also was accelerated. For the latter, there is no evidence. Thus, an explanation of radiation pneumonitis in terms of classic concepts of radiobiology has not been successful, at least with respect to either type II cells or capillary endothelial cells. Some other crucial cell type may become depleted and be responsible for radiation pneumonitis, but this has neither been suggested nor ruled out.

Nevertheless, there is some radiobiological evidence to implicate type II cells and exonerate endothelial cells as the target in radiation pneumonitis. Butylated hydroxytoluene (BHT) has been used to selectively expose various lung cell types to radiations. Administration of BHT in mice results in a brisk inflammatory response in the lungs, during which type II cells are the predominant proliferative cell at 2 days. At 6 days, the proliferative response resides mainly in the interstitial cells and capillary endothelial cells. Thus, irradiation at either 2 or 6 days should intensify the damage to type II cells or interstitial and capillary endothelial cells, respectively. Irradiation at 2 days only resulted in enhanced radiosensitivity, reducing the mean duration of survival from about 170 days to about 30 days and reducing the median lethal dose (LD$_{50}$) from 9.5 to 2.7 Gy. Irradiation at 6 days had no such effect and actually increased the LD$_{50}$ as compared to control mice not treated with BHT. This result argues in favor of the type II cell, and not the interstitial cell or capillary endothelial cell, as being the target for radiation pneumonitis, although it is possible that another unidentified cell type may have been stimulated to proliferate at 2 days and therefore was responsible for the enhancement of radiosensitivity following irradiation at that time.

Similarly, corticosteroids have been found to reduce the mortality of radiation pneumonitis (below). As they increase the replicative rate of type II cells in irradiated mice, it may be that their activity is functionally deficient in radiation pneumonitis (in the absence of corticosteroid stimulation). However, corticosteroids have many other effects on the lungs, for example, antiinflammatory effects (see below), and it may be that one of these other effects explains their protective role in radiation pneumonitis.

Biochemical Effects

Lipid studies are of interest because of the superficial resemblance between radiation pneumonitis and adult respiratory distress syndrome (ARDS) and because of histologic abnormalities in alveolar type II cells in the early stages of pneumonitis. Biphasic changes in lung total lipids of rats have been found in the first week after thoracic irradiation. Subsequent changes were not statistically significant, but the dose of x-rays, 800 rads, was well below that required to produce pneumonitis.

A transient increase in the content of lecithin has been noted in both lungs and alveolar fluid between 1 and 8 weeks after irradiation, and incorporation of precursors was probably constant throughout. These changes result from proliferation of type II cells, possibly as part of the regeneration of alveolar epithelium. At the stage of pneumonitis, 16 weeks after irradiation, the content of most phospholipids in the lung was increased up to 50%, and this increase was probably associated with increased phospholipid turnover. These changes were reflected in the alveolar lavage fluid; the degree of saturation of lecithin was normal throughout. These results do not suggest that radiation pneumonitis is associated with an abnormality of the surfactant system. Administration of corticosteroids from 2 to 3 weeks before the expected onset of pneumonitis further increased the phospholipid content of alveolar lavage fluid, increased the rate of incorporation of precursors into phospholipids, and normalized the surface tension properties of alveolar surface lining layer, both *in vitro* and *in situ*.

To identify patients at higher risk for radiation pneumonitis, a model was utilized that evaluated the production of free radicals in lipids after radiation exposure by measuring serum desferrioxamine-chelatable iron (free radical scavenger) and the percentage molar ratio of 9,11-linoleic acid and 9,12-linoleic acid (as an index of oxidation). After one week of radiotherapy, the group of subjects later developing pneumonitis exhibited significantly higher levels of desferrioxamine iron and a greater change in percentage molar ratio. This suggests that these assays might be useful indicators to identify patients more likely to develop radiation pneumonitis at a later time.

Coincident with pneumonitis, there is a five- to tenfold increase in microvascular leakage of plasma proteins into the interstitium and alveolar space, resulting in a chronic form of pulmonary edema. The amount of protein leakage is related to the dose of radiation, and its duration corresponds to that of pneumonitis. This probably explains the fall in lung compliance during pneumonitis. Corticosteroids had almost no effect on the amount of microvascular leakage, but mortality was substantially reduced. One speculates, therefore, that the steroid-mediated increase in surfactant phospholipids described earlier has a protective effect by promoting surfactant synthesis and delivery to the surface lining layer in sufficient amounts to counteract the inactivation or desorption of surfactant by plasma proteins. On the other hand, the beneficial effects of corticosteroids may be unrelated to surfactant production and may instead be secondary to some other action such as their antiinflammatory effect.

A cardinal feature of radiation pneumonitis is a fall in lung compliance that can be attributed to stiffness of the air–fluid interface of the alveolar lining. This may in turn be attributable to the leakage of plasma proteins into the alveoli with deleterious effects on the surfactant system as described above, a feature that radiation pneumonitis shares with any other forms of ARDS. It has now been shown that normal alveolar surfactant exists in several structural subtypes with different surface-active properties. The higher-density surface-active forms evolve into a lower-density form that is not surface active. The distribution of surfactant among these subtypes is greatly altered in radiation pneumonitis. Moreover, the metabolic evolution of surfactant subtypes, which is dependent on a unique serine protease that is secreted by the alveolar epithelium, is delayed in radiation pneumonitis. This may be the result of an 18-fold excess of α_1-antitrypsin (a serine-protease inhibitor) in the alveolar compartment that accompanies the microvascular leakage that characterizes this and other forms of ARDS.

Inflammatory Mechanisms

Following radiation to the lung there is an increase in the synthesis of prostaglandins and thromboxane, whereas in radiation pneumonitis there is an increase in the number of lymphocytes, possibly activated, in the bronchoalveolar lavage fluid. Experimental whole-body radiation results in early effects on cyclooxygenase products.

Phillips and co-workers were the first to show that corticosteroids reduced the mortality of experimental radiation pneumonitis, even when given many weeks after irradiation. Corticosteroids administered continuously to mice from 10 weeks after lethal thoracic irradiation substantially reduced mortality. However, if the corticosteroids were withdrawn during the period when pneumonitis was normally occurring, mortality increased and caught up with the mortality rate in the absence of corticosteroid administration. The protective effect of corticosteroids ceased after the time when pneumonitis normally occurs. Their effect, therefore, coincided with the phase of active radiation pneumonitis.

The inflammatory effects of irradiation can possibly be modulated by γ-interferon. Lung lavage fluid cellularity and protein content were monitored in treatment and control groups of animals. After 35 days, animals that were irradiated but did not receive γ-interferon had elevated protein and macrophage counts, whereas treated and irradiated animals did not vary significantly from unirradiated controls.

Studies carried out over 6 months after irradiation of rats are relevant to the mechanisms of late radiation damage. Among the findings were that prostacyclin (PGI_2) production by the irradiated lung increased progressively from a normal level at 2 months to a level two to three times higher than normal at 6 months. Coincident with this, there was a reciprocal decrease in perfusion of the irradiated lung. Because PGI_2 is a potent vasodilator and antithrombotic agent, the increase in its production is interpreted as consistent with a homeostatic response to impaired perfusion in the irradiated lung.

An alternative approach has been to study the effect of various antiinflammatory agents on mortality from experimental radiation pneumonitis when given well after irradiation but just before the time when pneumonitis normally occurs. The effect of corticosteroid administration is described above. The effects of a variety of agents that have more specific effects on arachidonate metabolism have been reported. In general, lipoxygenase inhibitors and leukotriene-receptor antagonists were markedly protective, more so indeed than corticosteroids. Cyclooxygenase inhibitors had variable effects; aspirin reduced mortality in a dose-dependent fashion, indomethacin markedly increased mortality, and other cyclooxygenase inhibitors had intermediate effects. These data were interpreted as suggesting that the protective effect of corticosteroids could be attributed to their antiinflammatory effects. They suggest that the mortality of radiation pneumonitis results from activity of the 5-lipoxygenase pathway and raise the possibility that clinical radiation pneumonitis can be mitigated by inhibitors or receptor antagonists of this pathway. This possibility has yet to be clinically tested.

PATHOGENESIS OF RADIATION FIBROSIS

The supposition in the past has been that radiation fibrosis was the natural consequence of lung damage expressed as pneumonitis. This is less clear now because of an apparent dissociation between some of the features of each. The connective tissue of the lung has been studied following x-irradiation both as a model of lung fibrosis and to determine the role of fibrosis in radiation reactions. Although the collagen content of the lungs is probably increased at the time of radiation pneumonitis, the increase at much later times is considerably greater, evidence that fibrosis is unlikely to play a major role in the pathogenetic mechanisms of pneumonitis.

One mechanism for the development of fibrosis is a progressive decrease in plasminogen activator activity that begins 1 to 2 months after lung irradiation. According to this hypothesis, the fibrinogen that leaks into the interstitial space as a result of radiation damage to the capillary endothelium, and is deposited as fibrin, is not adequately lysed by tissue fibrinolytic activity. The fibrin deposits act as foci for fibroblast stimulation and collagen secretion. Intricate cytokine and genetic pathways influencing fibroblast and fibrocyte maturation are well described. The ability of irradiation to induce a rapid and early maturation of fibroblasts as a result of genetic damage along with the enhanced production of cytokines by macrophages and type II pneumocytes has been substantiated. These stimuli together lead to an altered fibroblast-to-fibrocyte ratio, with an excess of fibrocytes favoring an increase in the production of collagen, leading in turn to fibrosis. Reduced fibrinolytic activity has also been demonstrated in irradiated lung and is caused by reduced plasminogen activator activity. Plasminogen activator is a product of both endothelial cells and alveolar macrophages. Either or both of these cells may be implicated in radiation fibrosis because endothelial cells irradiated *in vitro* exhibit impaired release of plasminogen activator and alveolar macrophages lavaged from irradiated rat lungs exhibit a time- and dose-related decrease in plasminogen activator activity.

The development of fibrosis in the lungs has been altered by a number of agents that affect collagen metabolism: triiodothyronine, colchicine, and β-aminopropionitrile. However, the best-studied agent is D-penicillamine, a reversible inhibitor of collagen cross-linking and maturation. Administration of D-penicillamine after irradiation of the rat hemithorax moderated late fibrosis in terms of histopathology, hypoperfusion, collagen accumulation, and lethality after 180 days, the latter being the conventional end of pneumonitis mortality. It also moderates the decrease in both angiotensin-converting enzyme and plasminogen activator activity described earlier. D-Penicillamine has been used in a number of other disorders in humans, but it has not been given prospective trials in patients undergoing radiation therapy to the lungs.

HISTOLOGIC CHANGES

Animals

The nature of radiation reactions in the lungs has been most often studied by microscopy. This is presented in summary form in Table 1. Changes are present at some time in virtually every structure within the thorax; therefore, only the main features are discussed.

It seems clear that damage to capillary endothelial cells is a consistent and significant feature. There is some disagreement as to when this first appears, either within hours in the form of vacuolation and blebs in the extended cytoplasmic processes or several weeks later. An early increase in capillary permeability suggests a functional lesion, even if it cannot be seen. Within a few weeks at most, the endothelial cells look definitely sick, raised from the basement membrane in some places and attenuated in others. Some cells are sloughed, leaving a denuded basement membrane and choking the lumen with debris and platelet and fibrin thrombi and, subsequently, colla-

TABLE 1. *Pulmonary effects of radiation: Histologic changes in animals*

Site	Immediate or early (0–2 months)	Intermediate (2–9 months)	Late (9+ months)
Capillaries	24 hr: Vacuolation of endothelial cells 2–7 days: Marked endothelial cell changes, separation from basement membrane, sloughing, obstruction of lumen with debris and thrombi, or normal 1+ month: Many capillaries swollen and obstructed	Marked abnormalities with widespread obstruction by platelets, fibrin, and collagen Capillary regeneration	Loss of many capillaries and regeneration of new ones
Type 1 pneumonocytes	Early degenerative vacuolation, death, and sloughing, or normal	Decreased number	Further decrease in number
Type II pneumonocytes	Early morphologic changes or normal redifferentiating into type I cells	Large increase in size and number, abnormal appearance	Return to normal size and number
Basement membrane	Early swelling, indistinct and later very irregular	Folded and thickened	Folded and thickened
Interstitial space	Edema and debris infiltrated with inflammatory cells and mast cells, slight increase in connective tissue	Infiltrated with mast cells, mononuclear cells, inflammatory cells, and collagen	Few inflammatory cells, large increase in collagen
Alveolar space	Fibrin, hemorrhages, and debris, increased number of alveolar macrophages, morphologically abnormal	Becoming smaller	Small, obliterated in places, distortion in architecture
Airway epithelium	Early transient inflammatory reaction, ciliary paralysis, increase in goblet cells, or normal	Epithelial proliferation	—

gen. Obstruction of the microvasculature is widespread. Arteriolar and arterial lesions resembling an immune vasculitis may be present. Around the damaged vasculature there is edema, cellular infiltrate, and possibly the beginnings of collagen deposition. Within about 6 to 10 weeks, there is evidence of repair. Some capillaries are recanalized, and new capillaries enter adjacent tissues, although perfusion probably remains reduced and permeability is increased (see Physiological Changes). Endothelial lesions are, in fact, a common feature following x-irradiation in many organs; indeed, many consider the endothelial damage to be the single or most important factor that determines the radiation tolerance of an organ. Evidence of damage to the basement membrane that subtends the vasculature may also be important in view of its role in providing a scaffold on which regeneration occurs and without which architectural reconstruction is abnormal.

Coincident with the endothelial changes are alveolar epithelial changes that may or may not be as functionally significant. Early vacuolation and blebs are seen by some in the type I pneumonocytes, which, like endothelial cells, are probably shed from the basement membrane, cluttering the alveolar space with debris. Infection in experimental rodents may have something to do with these early changes. Unlike endothelium, alveolar epithelium appears to have regenerative potential. Experiments in which damage to type I cells has been inflicted with such diverse agents as NO_2, oxygen, and bleomycin, as well as x-rays, indicate that the alveolar epithelium can be repopulated by type II cells that subsequently redifferentiate into type I cells. The large increase in the size and number of type II cells may reflect their role in regeneration of the alveolar epithelium. These cells appear to be relatively radioresistant by comparison with endothelial and type I cells. Nevertheless, the fact that they are stem cells and have important secretory functions warrants suspicion that they may play a role in the pathogenesis of radiation pneumonitis, as already discussed.

Some other features of the histologic changes are mentioned briefly. Cellular activity in the alveolar septum (interstitial space) is present early after irradiation: increased numbers of mast cells and mononuclear cells. There appears to be a paucity of acute inflammatory cells, although occasionally a brisk inflammatory response has been seen. Fibroblast activity can be seen within the first 2 months, when all the changes previously noted are at their height, but little collagen is laid down until about 6 months. At a later stage, dense fibrosis of alveolar septa dominates the histologic picture.

Little attention has been paid to the airway epithelium. The relatively rapid turnover of its cells, noted previously, would suggest early and extensive damage. This has only rarely been observed, however.

In summary, there are no characteristic histologic features; lesions in all cell types have been reported, but

damage to capillary endothelial cells and alveolar epithelial type I cells is fairly consistent. These changes can be found in damage from a wide variety of physical and chemical agents.

Humans

The picture in humans is complicated. Early and serial samples are not, of course, available, but at a late stage the dense fibrosis is entirely nonspecific. Again, material obtained at autopsy is likely to show superimposed changes from terminal heart failure or infection and postmortem artifacts. Changes in virtually all pulmonary structures have been reported in material obtained 4 to 12 weeks after completion of radiotherapy. As in the experimental studies, vascular damage is present. Arteriolar lesions are, however, more commonly mentioned. Changes in the alveolar epithelium are also present. Atypia, hyperplasia, sometimes bizarre, and desquamation into the alveolar space are noted, as well as other debris in the alveolar space and fibrin-rich exudate or hyaline membranes. Some observers considered them to be one of the most common and persistent of the abnormalities seen. Although animal studies frequently indicate abnormalities in the alveolar space, hyaline membranes as such are not reported. Possibly they are a terminal feature or secondary to other pathologic developments in humans.

The interstitial space is frequently thickened by edema and hypercellular because of a mononuclear infiltrate. A variable excess of collagen may be present, but inflammatory cells are usually absent. At 4 to 12 weeks after completion of a course of radiotherapy, abnormalities may be present in the airway walls. These include focal necrosis and squamous metaplasia.

Again, it can be seen that there is little that is characteristic about the histologic appearance in radiation pneumonitis. This is unfortunate because one of the more common clinical problems in diagnosis is the differentiation of a radiation reaction from tumor recurrence and infection. Now that the treatment of each of these alternatives is more aggressive, and lung biopsy by one or another route is so readily available, criteria for their differentiation would be most useful. Some criteria that have been suggested for diagnosis of radiation pneumonitis are (1) the presence within the sample of regions of greatly varying pathologic changes and (2) a combination of atypical alveolar epithelial cells, vascular changes, and widespread hyaline membrane formation. Possibly the absence of much evidence of inflammation and the presence of mast cells adjacent to regions of capillary damage can be added to the preceding features. It is highly unlikely that reactions will be found outside the irradiated regions, although there may be exceptions (see Associated Complications). A precise knowledge of the field placement and biopsy site is thus important.

Six months or more after the completion of a course of irradiation, the major abnormality is the huge amount of fibrosis interspersed with obliteration of alveolar spaces and vasculature, a picture that resembles end-stage lung damage of any etiology.

OCCURRENCE

It is difficult to assess how commonly radiation reactions occur in the lungs. No prospective studies have been performed to our knowledge, although in some studies this complication of treatment had obviously been anticipated in the investigative protocol and is reported in the subsequent publication. Published reports necessarily represent a population of patients highly selected by factors such as interest, awareness, and technique. The evolution of radiation therapy itself accounts for another factor of uncertainty. The trend toward more energetic and penetrating radiation deposits more energy in the lung and less in superficial tissues, but at the same time, dosimetry and field placement have become much more sophisticated. These and other technical factors are constantly evolving. Another difficulty in determining the occurrence of radiation reactions is semantic: some authors, particularly in the radiology literature, use the term radiation pneumonitis to denote a roentgenographic appearance; by others, particularly clinicians, it is used to denote the clinical syndrome, which is probably less common. Occasionally, the term is used without attempt at definition or distinction between pneumonitis and fibrosis. In fact, occurrence rates from 0% to 100% have been reported, raising the question of whether any incidence data are meaningful without definition of technical, clinical, and roentgenographic factors.

The principal conditions for which radiotherapy may expose the lungs to radiation are breast cancer, lung cancer, Hodgkin's disease, and lymphoma. The lungs may be exposed in treatment of other tumors such as cancer of the esophagus, but data are scant. The figures given below are based on selections from the literature that seem to provide some guide to occurrence in the era of megavoltage therapy.

Breast Cancer

The technique of tangential therapy of breast cancer minimizes damage to underlying lung, although wound healing, rib fractures, and chest wall necrosis are correspondingly more troublesome. The occurrence of roentgenographic changes in the lungs adjusted for numbers in each series is about 45%. The proportion of the total who had symptoms that may have represented radiation pneumonitis was 10%. Fatal reactions were not reported.

Lung Cancer

Although in lung cancer patients the occurrence of each of the radiation reactions is similar to that seen in patients with other malignancies, the incidence of lung cancer is extremely high (about 150,000 new cases per year in the United States). Because the majority receive lung irradiation at some stage, this group forms the largest portion of the population with potential or actual radiation damage.

Hodgkin's Disease and Lymphoma

Close cooperation between clinicians and radiation therapists in a number of large study groups has contributed to technical improvements in the treatment of Hodgkin's disease and lymphoma. A search for factors identifying patients at higher risk for radiation pneumonitis was undertaken by retrospectively evaluating 24 series of patients with over 1900 total subjects. The overall incidence of radiation pneumonitis was found to be 7.8%. Multivariate analysis suggested that fraction sizes greater than 2.67 Gy, once-daily dosing, and the total dose of radiation were associated with an increased risk of radiation pneumonitis. Field shaping (to fit the tumor) and field reduction during the course of treatment minimize the amount of normal lung exposed as it is brought into the field by the rapid reduction in size of the tumor mass.

The three malignancies just discussed contribute nearly all the cases of radiation reactions in the lungs. The figures in Table 2 indicate that roentgenographic changes are common in the early stage. Only a proportion of patients, maybe up to 15%, have clinical radiation pneumonitis, still a very large number. A small percentage of the total will die of radiation pneumonitis. In view of the number of patients who receive lung irradiation, radiation pneumonitis is a clinical problem of considerable size.

Brachytherapy and Interstitial Implantation of Isotopes

There is considerable interest in direct implantation of γ-emitting isotopes into the lesion. This innovation offers improved control of the dose and field. The usual isotope is iodine-125, which has a half-life of 60 days and a small volume of irradiation. Multiple sources are inserted directly into the lesion and not removed. Radiation pneumonitis was found in 9% of 46 patients receiving brachytherapy but was attributed to the external beam radiation delivered concomitantly. Experience with this form of radiotherapy is limited, and unfavorable reactions to it are as yet uncertain.

Accidental Irradiation with Isotopes

Intrapleural administration of isotopes with β-emission, such as radioactive gold, produces a local pleural reaction

TABLE 2. *Pulmonary effects of radiation: Occurrence of radiation reactions in the lungs (from selected reports)*

Primary diagnosis	Roentgenographic changes[a]	Clinical features[a]	Fatality due to radiation pneumonitis[a]	Roentgenographic changes of fibrosis[a]
Breast cancer	24.5	8		57
	20	13		60
	56	14		
	70	5		
	87			
Lung cancer	13 at 3 months	4.6	5	66 at 12 months
	33 at 6 months	15	2	100 at 30 months
	6	3	0.7	100
	100	5		
Hodgkin's lymphoma	65	6.4–33[b]	0.25–5.8[b]	65
		5		

[a] Figures are percentages of total number of patients in the series.
[b] Higher figures refer to cases with contributory factors, e.g., previous irradiation.

only. Inhalation of dust or particles containing γ-emitting isotopes can produce radiation damage. In the event of a nuclear disaster, this could be a long-term consequence. There is also a report of probable radiation pneumonitis, ending fatally, in a worker employed for 3 years in the production of radioactive luminous paint. The treatment with iodine-131 of thyroid malignancy, metastatic to the lungs, also has been associated with fatal radiation pneumonitis.

In patients being treated for inoperable hepatic tumors with intraarterial yttrium-90 microsphere infusions, five of 80 patients developed a syndrome resembling radiation pneumonitis 2 to 4 months after therapy. Technetium-labeled macroaggregated albumin studies were performed before the treatments, and the degree of intrahepatic shunt was quantified. Those who did not develop radiation pneumonitis had shunts of less than 1% to 15% with a median of 6%, whereas five of nine patients with shunts greater than 13% developed radiation pneumonitis. No patients developing radiation pneumonitis demonstrated shunts less than 13%.

CLINICAL SYNDROMES FOLLOWING LUNG IRRADIATION

Radiation Bronchitis

Courses of radiotherapy that typically call for 40 to 60 Gy take several weeks to administer and often include the central airways in the field. Dry irritant cough is very common toward the end of the course or during the next few weeks. From the cytokinetics of bronchial mucosa and the few histologic reports (see Histologic Changes), it seems conceivable that these symptoms are caused by radiation bronchitis. If symptoms are severe, the course of treatment may need to be suspended for a week or two, much as for radiation esophagitis. We are not aware of any detailed investigations into this possibility.

No serious complications ensue, and treatment is symptomatic.

Radiation Pneumonitis

Radiation pneumonitis develops insidiously. Although the symptoms can sometimes be traced back to a month or so after the completion of radiation therapy, it is uncommon for the patient to present less than 6 to 8 weeks after completion unless a contributory factor is present (see Contributory Factors). Roentgenographic changes may, however, be detected in advance of this if routine x-ray films are taken (Fig. 5). A useful rule of thumb is that roentgenographic changes can be expected 8 weeks after 40 Gy to a significant volume of lung and 1 week earlier for each 10-Gy increment above 40 Gy. Roentgenographic changes generally precede clinical features but do not, of course, make them inevitable. The early appearance of roentgenographic changes or symptoms, however, generally signifies a particularly severe episode.

The cardinal symptom of radiation pneumonitis is dyspnea. Mild and occurring only on exertion at first, it may progress in the course of a week or two to severe dyspnea on minimal effort or even at rest. Occasionally, the progression from mild dyspnea to severe respiratory distress may occur in only a few days, particularly if the lesion involves a large volume of lung. In our experience, these patients do badly. Other symptoms coincide with dyspnea but are overshadowed by it. Cough is common and initially dry and harsh. Small amounts of clear or pink sputum may be produced later, but purulent sputum or frank hemoptysis should be attributed to another cause. The sensation of a limitation of inspiratory capacity (doorstop sign) and fever, usually low grade but occasionally high and spiking, may be present. Vague chest pain is common but rarely troublesome unless caused by rib fracture (see Associated Complications).

The dominant physical signs are respiratory distress

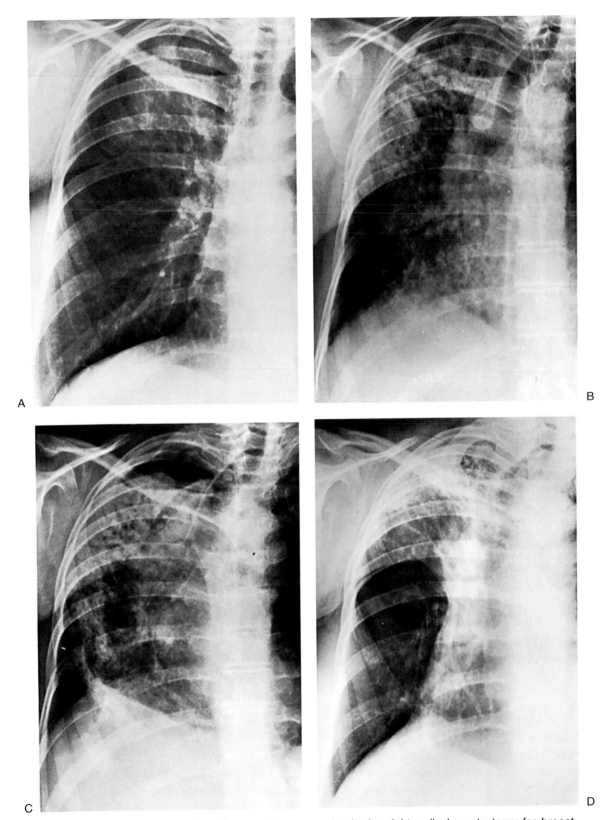

FIG. 5. Roentgenograms of a 54-year-old woman who had a right radical mastectomy for breast cancer and subsequent radiation therapy. **(A)** 3-19-73. Three weeks after completion of radiation therapy **(B)** 4-10-73. More extensive changes in parenchyma with retraction indicated by tracheal deviation, diaphragmatic elevation, and air bronchograms. Patient was symptomatic at this stage. **(C)** 4-30-73. More extensive changes of radiation pneumonitis with pneumothorax at right apex and a fluid level. Pneumothorax resolved spontaneously. **(D)** 12-11-74. Late roentgenographic appearance showing resolution of changes in mid and lower zones, radiation fibrosis at apex, marked tracheal deviation, and mediastinal shift. (Reproduced from NJ Gross. *Ann Intern Med* 1977;86:81.)

and tachypnea, particularly on mild effort, with or without central cyanosis. Finger clubbing may have been present because of underlying malignancy but does not develop at this stage. Examination of the chest often fails to elicit any signs. It is worth looking for the tattoo marks on the chest that radiotherapists sometimes use to outline the field and to compare these with the roentgenogram because the close correspondence between these and the roentgenographic changes is highly suggestive of a radiation reaction (see Roentgenographic Changes). However, there is no correlation between the severity of skin reactions such as pigmentation and desquamation and the presence of an underlying lung reaction. Occasionally, a pleural friction rub or rales are present over regions of pneumonitis. In a severe advanced case, features of respiratory distress syndrome with or without right-sided heart failure are present. Acute cor pulmonale is particularly ominous and usually indicates a fatal outcome. The typical course of radiation pneumonitis is protracted over several weeks or months, even if symptoms are mild. Commonly, symptoms persist for a month or more and subside even more gradually than they appeared.

The leukocyte count and red cell sedimentation rate are frequently raised, but not by very much. Blood gas studies are discussed in more detail under Physiological Changes; they commonly show arterial hypoxia and hypocapnia. Other data, such as results of enzyme studies, rheumatoid factor, and complement levels, are lacking. Pulmonary function abnormalities and roentgenographic abnormalities are discussed later; these are very likely to be present at the stage of radiation pneumonitis.

Radiation Fibrosis

Although fibrosis can be diagnosed with certainty only on histologic grounds, the term *radiation fibrosis* has come to be used in situations in which reasonable clinical grounds for it exist. Fibrosis is very likely, if not inevitable, in any region of the lung that has received therapeutic doses of radiation, whether or not radiation pneumonitis has occurred. Histologic (see Table 38-1), biochemical, and physiological evidence (see Physiological Changes) indicates that fibrosis begins as early as 2 months after irradiation and may take several months or years to become fully established. Whether or not pneumonitis was previously present, the roentgenographic features of fibrosis will gradually appear from 6 to 24 months after irradiation and will persist almost without change for the rest of the patient's life.

Clinical features are usually minimal. In a few patients—those with preexisting pulmonary function abnormalities and those who have experienced an episode of severe radiation pneumonitis—the additional burden of pulmonary fibrosis will result in chronic respiratory failure with dyspnea on effort and abnormal gas exchange.

Some patients so affected may even develop chronic cor pulmonale, but this is uncommon. More likely than this is a moderate exacerbation of preexisting symptoms such as a decrease in exercise tolerance. The majority will have no symptoms at all. Physical signs, if present, are explained on the basis of contraction of lung tissue in the region of fibrosis, for example, diaphragmatic elevation, mediastinal shift in the case of unilateral fibrosis, and loss of inspiratory excursion. Finger clubbing may develop.

ASSOCIATED COMPLICATIONS

Pleural Effusion

The possibility of pleural reactions following x-irradiation is most frequently suspected when the radiation given for breast cancer, possibly because of the tangential technique. The complication has been noted in 5.5% to 14% of patients so treated.

It is important to distinguish between a malignant effusion and a reaction to radiation. Radiation-induced effusions are invariably associated with and usually appear at the same time as pneumonitis. They may persist for long periods of time. Once they appear, they usually remain stable and rarely increase in size, unlike malignant effusions. The fluid is exudative in character but not blood-stained. Pleural biopsy specimens appear normal apart from a few nonspecific changes.

The mechanism of pleural effusions following radiation is unknown, but they occur with striking regularity in experimental radiation pneumonitis.

Pneumothorax

When pneumothorax occurs, it tends to be a feature of radiation pneumonitis and is found in the same side as pneumonitis. A typical case is illustrated in Figure 5. One would anticipate problems with expansion of the lung, but most reported pneumothoraces have reexpanded spontaneously.

Infection

In addition to its well-known suppressive effects on immunity, radiation impairs clearance mechanisms. In mice there is a transient drastic reduction in the number of alveolar macrophages between 1 and 8 weeks after a single dose of x-rays to the thorax. In addition, impaired phagocytosis and killing of microorganisms have been demonstrated. Although the morphology of macrophages is altered (they become transiently much larger), their individual functional abilities (phagocytosis, etc.) are retained. Thus, increased susceptibility to infection, which is present at this stage, is probably related to the transient reduction in their number.

Data in humans are hard to find. Furthermore, there often are other factors that more potently predispose to opportunistic infection, such as lymphoreticular malignancy or combination chemotherapy. No particular organisms have been associated with infections following irradiation.

Rib Fractures

Rib fractures may occur shortly after completion of the course of irradiation. They are found within the field of irradiation and appear to be more common when radiation is given for breast cancer. Possibly this is because the technique of tangential irradiation of the chest wall delivers more radiation to the rib cage than do opposed anterior and posterior fields. For the same reason, the fractures occur independently of radiation pneumonitis. They may be single or multiple and are usually painful. They heal spontaneously, although slowly if extensive necrosis of the chest wall is present.

Pneumonitis Outside the Field of Irradiation

One of the characteristic features of radiation pneumonitis is that it is confined to the region of lung that was irradiated. Nevertheless, there are a few reports of radiation reactions well outside the field and sometimes in the contralateral lung. This unusual and unexpected occurrence has raised speculations that include obstruction of the lymphatic drainage of the lungs and the induction of autoimmunity to lung tissue. Neither theory explains why the damage should be so widespread in a small number of patients and confined in the vast majority of cases. Hypersensitivity to radiation has been suggested, particularly when a severe reaction follows an apparently small exposure.

Of 17 patients evaluated by bronchoalveolar lavage (BAL) following lung irradiation, 13 (75%) exhibited bilateral lymphocytosis, with two demonstrating a more marked response leading to clinical radiation pneumonitis. In the remaining 25%, no lymphocytosis or immune response was detected. Changes in BAL lymphocyte populations as well as increases in radiolabeled gallium uptake were demonstrated bilaterally. It is proposed that these bilateral findings result from cytokines released from CD4$^-$ helper T lymphocytes recently activated in the irradiated lung exerting their effects in a widened area, which is more consistent with a hypersensitivity pneumonitis pattern. When large numbers of patients are treated according to strictly supervised protocols and closely observed, the number of cases of hypersensitivity diminishes to a fraction of a percent. One rare instance in which abnormal radiosensitivity has been established

(ataxia-telangiectasia) is discussed later (see Contributory Factors).

Radiation Carcinogenesis

It is reasonably well established in experimental animals that irradiation of the lungs enhances the formation of pulmonary metastases. The enhancement occurs briefly and transiently after each exposure and is thought to be related to changes in vascular perfusion or permeability. The phenomenon may be of considerable clinical importance in relation to prophylactic lung irradiation and postoperative irradiation for breast cancer.

An equally important but apparently unrelated phenomenon is the late appearance of a new primary tumor in a previously irradiated lung field. Figure 6 illustrates this phenomenon. If such cases are not coincidental, one can only speculate whether the mechanism involves radiation carcinogenesis, or is related to scar cancer.

Miscellaneous Complications

Acute obstruction of a large airway may occur when a tumor that occupies a large portion of its lumen is irradi-

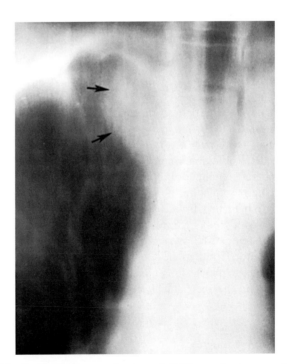

FIG. 6. Radiation carcinogenesis? The patient presented in 1968 with Hodgkin's disease of the right supraclavicular region, for which he received mantle irradiation with x-rays. Details of the treatments are not available, but the field probably resembled that shown in Fig. 8. He returned 8 years later with a lesion in the paramediastinal region of the right upper lobe, shown in this tomogram (*arrows*). The lesion was resected and found to be a primary lung carcinoma within the fibrotic region of previous irradiation. A few months later the patient was also found to have a malignant thymoma, again within the field of previous irradiation.

ated. This is because of edema of the tumor and can be prevented by administration of corticosteroids during the first few days of irradiation. Such cases may be mistakenly diagnosed as hyperacute radiation pneumonitis or pneumonia.

Hyperlucency of a lung after unilateral x-irradiation has been reported. Arteriograms show this to be related to hypoplasia of the pulmonary artery without obvious obstruction of its lumen.

Secondary pulmonary effects of cardiac damage from x-rays are, of course, not uncommon, but such a discussion falls outside the scope of this chapter.

Thoracic irradiation given before lung surgical procedures appears to cause few technical problems. In some series, however, there was a much higher incidence of complications related to delayed healing in previously irradiated tissues, i.e., bronchopleural fistula and empyema. At later stages after irradiation, a surgical procedure may be technically difficult because of fibrosis in the chest wall, pleura, and lung.

Phrenic and recurrent laryngeal nerve paralysis and Horner's syndrome do not occur following conventional radiation treatment of the lungs. Spinal cord damage, however, is a complication. Necrosis and cavitation of the lung do not occur except as a result of tumors, although radiation can cause fistulas between hollow viscera. Reactivation of granulomatous disease is rare.

PHYSIOLOGICAL CHANGES

In view of the delicate balance between the structure of the lung and its function, any pathologic condition that involves more than a very small portion will likely produce detectable abnormalities in overall function. Of the considerable number of reports in the literature, those that give the best picture of physiological events in humans concern patients with breast cancer. These patients, unlike those with lung cancer and Hodgkin's disease or lymphoma, can be presumed to have essentially normal lungs before irradiation.

Two principal lesions can be identified, the vascular lesion and the mechanical lesion, with resultant effects on gas transfer.

Vascular Changes

Changes in perfusion of the lungs have been studied by means of isotopes, either ^{131}I-labeled macroaggregates of albumin or xenon-133. A decrease in perfusion has been detected in the first few hours after irradiation, particularly following large single doses. This change appears to be transient and is of questionable clinical relevance (in view of the size of the dose needed to produce it). In the period from a few days to 14 days after irradiation. Some authors reported an increase, whereas others

reported a decrease, in pulmonary perfusion. A transient increase in diffusion capacity at this time supports increased perfusion. Permeability changes at this time are quite complex.

All authors have agreed that pulmonary perfusion is decreased from about 14 days on. Hypoperfusion is confined to the irradiated region and persists for a very long period, probably indefinitely. It is more marked following 15-MeV neutrons than γ-irradiation. The decrease in perfusion corresponds well with the capillary damage seen histologically and bears on the blood gas changes discussed below. In animals at the stage of pneumonitis there is a marked decrease in perfusion and a marked increase in permeability of the pulmonary vasculature that results in pulmonary edema. The mechanism of this is unclear, but a modest reduction in the perfusion defect can be brought about by long-term administration of the collagen antagonist D-penicillamine.

Mechanical Changes

Studies of pulmonary mechanics in both humans and experimental animals have uniformly shown a dose- and time-related fall in static compliance following irradiation (Fig. 7). This change is first evident at about 40 days, becomes more marked at the time of pneumonitis, and persists for many years. Static compliance of the thorax is the result of the compliance of three parallel elements: the thoracic wall, lung tissue, and lung surface. Studies of excised or exposed lungs of animals showed that the fall in total compliance was related entirely to a fall in the compliance of the lung itself rather than of the thoracic

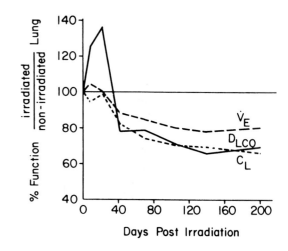

FIG. 7. Physiological effects of irradiation on one lung of dogs. Changes in diffusion capacity (D_LCO, *solid line*) compared with the preirradiation level of that lung. Changes in ventilation (VE, *long-dash line*) and compliance (CL, *short-dash title*) compared with those in the nonirradiated lung. (Redrawn from CD Teates. *J Appl Physiol* 1965;20:628. Reproduced from NJ Gross. *Ann Intern Med* 1977;86:81.)

wall. And this in turn was shown to result, at the stage of radiation pneumonitis, in increases in the surface tension of the alveolar surface. In fact, the alveolar fluid obtained by pulmonary lavage of irradiated mice behaves abnormally *in vitro,* and the stability of expressed lung bubbles is impaired. The abnormal behavior of alveolar fluid can be explained by the presence in the alveolar fluid of a large amount of protein of circulatory origin. It is known that extraneous protein, particularly fibrinogen, impairs surface activity. There is an alteration in the distribution of surfactant subtypes in radiation pneumonitis.

At later stages, low lung incompliance appears to result from development of fibrosis and a fall in static compliance of the lung tissue. This change can be regarded as permanent because it is present many years later.

Associated with the fall in lung compliance is a dose-related increase in the respiratory rate and a decrease in lung volumes, again long-lasting. Regional lung studies in patients have shown that volume loss was confined to the region of irradiation, where decreased perfusion also was present. The extent of overall changes in lung function in humans is therefore a function of the amount of lung affected by radiation. Airway resistance is normal or only minimally raised. Consistent with the fall in lung compliance, where present, the elastic work of breathing in humans is raised, and consequently, tidal volume tends to fall, and frequency tends to increase, resulting in a moderate overall increase in minute ventilation. However, decreases in lung volumes may not occur at all despite a successful response to radiation therapy.

Gas Transfer

Overall, gas transfer and blood gas changes again reflect the amount of lung affected. Within the irradiated region, perfusion changes are more severe than ventilatory changes, resulting locally in a high ventilation–perfusion ratio, little change in local gas transfer, and redistribution of pulmonary blood flow to other, unaffected regions. Where the volume of irradiated lung is small and the function of unirradiated lung is normal, overall gas transfer is not impaired, and blood gases are normal. If the volume of affected lung is large and/or the function of unirradiated lung is marginal, some abnormalities of gas transfer are found. In this situation, arterial blood gases typically show mild to moderate arterial hypoxemia with normal or reduced P_aCO_2, a reduced diffusion capacity for carbon monoxide, and an increased alveolar–arterial oxygen gradient. This is the most likely blood gas abnormality in patients with symptomatic radiation pneumonitis. Use of SPECT and CT scanning allows changes in local ventilation and perfusion to be determined relative to the three-dimensional dose distribution of the irradiated lungs. Standard pulmonary function testing noted a 20% decrease in vital capacity and 1-sec

forced expiratory volume (FEV_1). The average reduction of local ventilation and perfusion after radiation for all patients was approximately 10% below baseline values and was greater in those with clinically evident radiation pneumonitis. Correlations were demonstrated between decrease in perfusion, decrease in FEV_1, and the presence of radiation pneumonitis. In more severe degrees of radiation pneumonitis, greatly increased stiffness (decreased compliance) of the lungs may superimpose hypoventilation on mismatching, resulting in carbon dioxide retention and severe hypoxia, but this can be regarded as a terminal effect.

Symptoms of radiation pneumonitis are therefore a function of the volume of affected lung and are attributable to changes in the mechanical properties of the lung and associated blood gas abnormalities. Where only the apex of the lung is irradiated, as in postoperative irradiation for breast cancer, the symptomatic and physiological effects will be less because ventilation and perfusion are both lower at the lung apex. It may be possible, using modern refinements of radiation techniques, to ablate the gas exchange effects entirely.

It seems probable that routine clinical tests of pulmonary function such as lung volumes, diffusion capacity, and arterial blood gas tensions could provide early warning of symptomatic radiation pneumonitis, if they were regularly performed in patients at risk.

ROENTGENOGRAPHIC CHANGES

For detailed information on radiation effects in the lungs, the reviews of Rubin and Casarett and Libshitz and colleagues are recommended. As shown in Table 2, roentgenographic changes are very commonly seen following lung irradiation, more commonly than symptoms. They are also present before the clinical episode that may or may not subsequently occur.

The commonly recognized roentgenographic changes are first seen 4 to 8 weeks after completion of radiotherapy, possibly as much as 2 to 3 weeks before symptoms, if the latter should occur (Fig. 8). Initially, the lesion has a ground-glass or soft appearance, and the lung markings are hazy and indistinct. As the lesion evolves, the opacification may become micronodular and harder, with linear branching streaks a centimeter or more in length. These are usually radially oriented and may resemble Kerley B lines if the lesion is peripheral. Symptomatic pneumonitis is very likely to be present if and when these features are present. In the most severe lesions, the affected region may become densely opacified as the nodules and streaks become confluent. Air bronchograms may appear within this region, and pleural and interlobar effusions may occur. The outline of the mediastinum and cardiac shadow becomes indistinct when the lesion is adjacent to these structures. A most striking feature is a marked volume

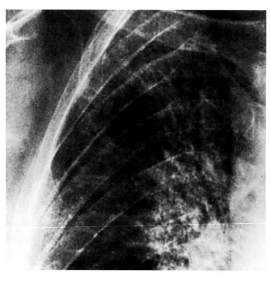
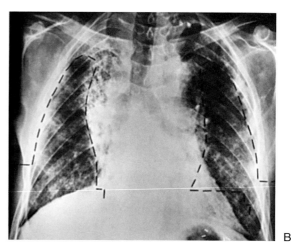
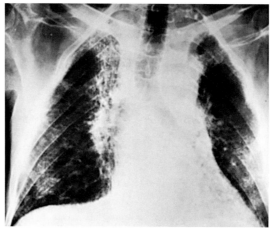

FIG. 8. Roentgenograms of a 64-year-old man with stage IIA Hodgkin's disease. **(A)** 5-15-72. Detail of right apex showing early appearance of radiation pneumonitis 5 weeks after completion of mantle irradiation. **(B)** 5-28-71. The outline of the lung shields from a treatment film (taken supine) has been traced onto a diagnostic roentgenogram (taken erect) to show the close topographic correspondence between roentgenographic changes and the field of irradiation around the lung shields. The patient had dyspnea, cough, and pyrexia at this stage. **(C)** 1-18-73. Roentgenographic changes of radiation fibrosis in the paramediastinal, apical, peripheral, and left basal regions, again corresponding to the irradiated regions of the lung. (Reproduced from NJ Gross. *Ann Intern Med* 1977;86:81.)

loss in the irradiated region. This is particularly obvious when irradiation was unilateral, as the trachea and mediastinum shift toward the lesion; elevation and tenting of the diaphragm and narrowing of the intercostal spaces are further evidence of contraction of the lesion. Cavitation is not seen in lung tissue, although it may occur in an irradiated tumor.

A cardinal feature of radiation pneumonitis is that the roentgenographic abnormality is limited sharply by the radiotherapy port (see Fig. 8). Roentgenographic changes outside the port are minor and adjacent to the port; if not caused by uncertainty of the port margins, they may be the result of scattered or oblique irradiation. Because the field of irradiation corresponds to the neoplastic lesion, the roentgenographic abnormality does not usually corre-

spond to anatomic boundaries in the lung. It is therefore of utmost diagnostic value for the clinician to have the treatment films or at least an accurate graphic description of the ports and to observe the skin marks corresponding to the port margins. With this technical information—chronology of treatment and symptoms and evidence of the evolution of lung changes—the diagnosis of radiation pneumonitis can usually be made with confidence. As with the clinical features described, the early appearance and rapid progression of the roentgenographic lesion generally signify a more severe clinical episode.

Like the clinical episode, the roentgenographic features of pneumonitis persist for long periods, possibly months. Depending on the extent and severity of the lesion, the roentgenographic changes gradually resolve and evolve into those of radiation fibrosis. The chest roentgenogram may not stabilize in less than 1 to 2 years. The irradiated region assumes a dense roentgenographic appearance, still limited to the margins of the treatment port but often contracted and further condensed (Figs. 5, 8, and 9). There may be linear streaks extending outside the port, but these are centered on the irradiated region, with compensatory hyperinflation in the adjacent or contralateral lung. Irradiated regions may adopt a bronchiectatic, cystic, or even honeycomb appearance and may be mistaken for active

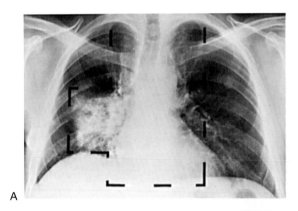

A

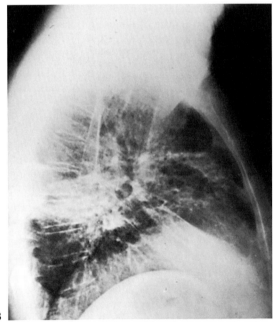

B

FIG. 9. Posteroanterior **(A)** and lateral **(B)** roentgenograms of a patient who initially presented with inoperable primary carcinoma of the right-lower-lobe bronchus, for which he received radiation therapy. These roentgenograms were taken on routine follow-up 7 months after therapy—the patient was asymptomatic. The outline of roentgenographic changes exactly follows the margin of the port, allowing for contraction due to fibrosis and the fact that treatment films are taken supine. The lateral picture **(B)** shows the opacity running the full depth of the lung, again corresponding to the x-ray beam. The patient received no further treatment and remained asymptomatic without roentgenographic progression of the lesion. Diagnosis: radiation fibrosis.

pulmonary tuberculosis. Calcification of lymph nodes has been reported, but hilar node enlargement does not occur. Conventional perfusion scans of the lung, whether with ^{131}I aggregates or ^{133}Xe, show decreased perfusion of the irradiated region in the stage of radiation pneumonitis. Hypoperfusion is likely to persist indefinitely.

In summary, roentgenographic changes of some sort are more likely than not to be present following irradiation of the thorax. These are usually strictly limited to the radiotherapeutic port and may or may not be associated with symptoms of pneumonitis. In the great majority, if not all patients, the roentgenographic changes of fibrosis will become evident over the subsequent year.

CONTRIBUTORY FACTORS

The enhancement of the effect of radiation by oxygen has already been mentioned. A number of other factors with similar effect but different actions are also known. Awareness of these is clinically important in modifying treatment planning as well as in recognition of unexpected complications.

Concomitant Chemotherapy

It has been recognized at least since 1959 that administration of actinomycin D enhances the undesirable effects of radiation on the lung. At equivalent radiation doses, pneumonitis is about 30% more likely to occur in patients who receive concomitant actinomycin D therapy (see Fig. 4). In view of the more aggressive current approach to tumor management and, in particular, the combination of multiple drugs with radiation therapy in treatment protocols, the phenomenon of unfavorable interactions has become one of increasing importance.

Lamoureaux reported a small number of lung cancer patients randomized into two groups. One group received mechlorethamine, procarbazine, and vincristine concurrently with radiation therapy; the other received radiation only in the same dose and schedule. All five of the chemotherapy patients had symptomatic radiation pneumonitis as compared to only one of the six patients in the nonchemotherapy group. Which of the three drugs was responsible for enhancing the effects of radiation is uncertain. In the nervous system, vincristine has been implicated, and the experiments of Phillips' group, discussed below, are consistent with such an effect in the lungs. Einhorn and colleagues reported severe radiation pneumonitis in five of 13 patients who received concomitant chemotherapy; three of these cases were fatal. Chemotherapy consisted of bleomycin, doxorubicin (Adriamycin), cyclophosphamide, and vincristine. Patients given chemotherapy alone suffered no pulmonary effects, nor did a further 20 patients who received radiation and the same chemotherapeutic treatment without bleomycin. Einhorn and associates therefore implicated bleomycin as the agent responsible for the extremely common occurrence of pneumonitis, a conclusion not supported by others. Soble and Perry reported a case in which fulminant fatal pneumonitis and bone marrow hypoplasia occurred 4 weeks after a course of 4000 rads to the mantle for Hodgkin's disease. The interesting feature was that the patient had received busulfan (480 mg total) over the previous 6 years. Although both pneumonitis and aplastic anemia can occur following busulfan in this dosage (15% to 20% probability), the sudden appearance of both complications shortly after radiation suggested to the authors that they were induced by interaction with radiation. It is possible that doxorubicin, which has marked effects on the myocardium, also may enhance radiation effects in the lungs. In the foregoing reports, pneumonitis started earlier than usual, was severe, sometimes preceded radiologic changes, and was evident outside the ports of irradiation.

Phillips and co-workers reported that significant enhancement of pulmonary lethality occurred with actinomycin (0.075 mg/kg of body weight), cyclophosphamide (75 mg/kg), and vincristine (0.5 mg/kg) given 2 hr before irradiation, but not with bleomycin, hydroxyurea, or BCNU. With actinomycin D there was significant enhancement of lethality, even when a small dose (0.015 mg/kg) was given 30 days before irradiation but not 30 days after it. Interestingly, the effect of these agents is not consistent between different organs. Nor is the list of drugs that potentiate the effects of radiation the same as the list that can cause pneumonitis in the absence of irradiation.

There is no obvious relationship between the mode of action of these agents and their potentiating effects on lung irradiation. Information on the time of administration of drug in relation to radiation, dose, and fractionation is fragmentary, although of clear clinical importance.

Corticosteroid Withdrawal

There is some controversy about the role of steroids in the treatment of radiation pneumonitis (see Management), and in clinical practice prophylactic steroid therapy is not used. Nevertheless, if steroids are being administered, their inopportune withdrawal appears to be capable of precipitating radiation pneumonitis. Cycles of chemotherapy that included prednisone are likely to be followed by episodes of pneumonitis. Thus, corticosteroids should be administered either continuously or not at all in the period following radiation. In lethally irradiated mice, deaths were markedly reduced by prophylactic prednisolone but occurred rapidly after its withdrawal at 160 days. The phenomenon can be interpreted either as unmasking of steroid-suppressed pneumonitis or, less likely, as precipitation, by the withdrawal itself, of a reaction that would not have been present at all if steroids had not been given.

Previous Radiation Therapy

It has been recognized from the earliest reports that retreatment is likely to precipitate radiation pneumonitis. For example, reirradiation of the mediastinum for inadequately treated Hodgkin's disease resulted in pneumonitis far more frequently than did a first course and that the episode occurred earlier and was more severe. It is not clear whether the phenomenon is a function of the total dose received or whether the lung is more susceptible after the first course.

Ataxia Telangiectasia

The rare disorder, ataxia telangiectasia, appears to be associated with abnormal sensitivity to ionizing radiation. This hereditary syndrome is characterized by cerebellar ataxia, oculocutaneous telangiectasia, immunologic deficiencies, and an increased occurrence of reticuloendothelial malignancy. Increased radiosensitivity can be demonstrated at the molecular, cellular, and clinical levels. Conventional doses of radiotherapy for the malignant complications are likely to be followed by severe radiation reactions. It has been postulated that the radiosensitivity results from defective DNA repair, which also accounts for another feature of the condition: chromosomal instability. This raises the possibility, as yet undemonstrated, of enhanced radiosensitivity in two other disorders characterized by chromosomal instability and predisposition to malignancy, Bloom's syndrome, and Fanconi's syndrome.

Other Contributory Factors

Age has been considered a factor that might modulate a patient's response to radiation. It is mentioned in many reviews but supported by only scant data. Gas transfer appears affected more in older patients. There appears to be an age-related increase in frequency and severity of roentgenographic changes in irradiated breast cancer patients. The grading was made on roentgenograms taken from 7 weeks to 30 months after the end of treatment. Whether atherosclerosis plays a role also has been considered, but data on this are absent. It does seem possible, however, that the lungs of children recover better than those of older adults from the effects of x-rays.

Underlying infection such as that which may be associated with chronic bronchitis also has been considered to be a predisposing factor to radiation intolerance. However, when patients with and without chronic bronchitis were compared, no change in the incidence of minor and major reactions was found, nor were subsequent functional changes different in the two groups. The commonly held view that patients with chronic obstructive lung disease tolerate radiotherapy poorly should be qualified: such patients are not more likely to experience radiation pneumonitis. Radiotherapy will add a certain amount of functional impairment to their already abnormal physiological state, but no more than in normal subjects. It is of interest that radiotherapy has been employed in emphysematous patients without malignancy as a means of reducing their excessive lung compliance—with only marginal success, but equally without much harm.

DIFFERENTIAL DIAGNOSIS

In a typical clinical setting, the patient who has received radiation therapy for a malignancy and subsequently develops pulmonary problems presents a diagnostic challenge. The differential diagnosis invariably includes radiation reactions, recurrent malignancy, infection, and possibly other entities such as drug-induced lung disease and thromboembolism. In view of the divergent therapeutic requirements of these conditions, their differentiation is of utmost clinical importance. It can often be made on the basis of clinical features and radiologic appearances.

The differentiation of radiation-induced pleural effusion from other effusions has been discussed (see Associated Complications). Differentiation of radiation pneumonitis from tumor recurrence is facilitated by the following criteria: recurrent malignancy is suggested by an interval of more than 4 months between radiation therapy and symptoms; steady progression of the roentgenographic changes, metastases elsewhere, anemia, and hemoptysis. Lymphangitic spread of tumor is usually associated with very severe symptoms, particularly dyspnea, and is more marked at the lung bases, where septal lines and long linear streaks from the hilus to the pleura are seen. Unlike radiation reactions, tumor recurrence is often roentgenographically manifest outside the field of irradiation.

Infections may present a more difficult problem. Criteria for differentiation of radiation reactions from tuberculosis have been suggested but have not been found to be particularly helpful. Usual features of other infections, pyrexia, leukocytosis, and purulent sputum, may or may not be prominent in infected patients who have been compromised by chemotherapy, corticosteroids, and tumors as well as by previous radiation therapy. The diagnosis rests on a combination of immunologic studies, stains, and cultures of bronchopulmonary secretions, and possibly histologic and microbiological studies of lung tissue.

The diagnosis of radiation reactions is greatly simplified by excellent roentgenograms and knowledge of the precise chronology, dose, field margins, and dose schedules in relation to the onset of subsequent problems. Microbiological backup is most helpful, but histologic samples obtained by bronchoscopy or open lung biopsy are particularly important in difficult cases. Even when these are available, differentiation between the various possibilities is not always straightforward.

MANAGEMENT

Because radiation pneumonitis rather than fibrosis is the major life-threatening event, management is principally directed toward this problem. Early recognition is important, as early treatment may affect the course of pneumonitis.

Untoward reactions following radiation could probably be anticipated in a large proportion of patients by roentgenographic monitoring and the more discriminating tests of lung function at the appropriate time. This has been considered impractical for routine purposes because of the extended time over which reactions can occur. Furthermore, the appearance of abnormalities does not necessarily inevitably lead to pneumonitis. Possibly patients who are at increased risk because of an unavoidable contributory factor should be so monitored.

Symptomatic

Patients whose symptoms are not severe or rapidly progressive and develop late (i.e., 10 to 12 weeks after completion of radiotherapy) will probably have a mild clinical course. For these patients, symptomatic therapy is all that is required: restriction of activity, cough suppressants, and observation during the 2- to 4-week period.

If an early reaction occurs and symptoms progress rapidly, additional therapy may be required, as follows.

Corticosteroids

The place of corticosteroids in the management of radiation pneumonitis remains controversial; no controlled clinical trials have been carried out to our knowledge. However, corticosteroids are widely used in clinical practice, and animal studies support their use.

Early clinical studies suggested that relatively small doses might be protective if given prophylactically, before the onset of pneumonitis, or early in its course. They were less beneficial if delayed much beyond the onset of symptoms. Pneumonitis may appear shortly after withdrawal of steroids, but there is a dramatic response of all patients shortly after restitution of prednisone, 20 to 80 mg/day.

Although early animal studies gave divergent views on the use of corticosteroids, it is now fairly clear that when corticosteroids are given before the onset of pneumonitis, mortality is significantly reduced. In a detailed analysis of this phenomenon in lethally irradiated mice, it was found that prednisone (4.0 mg/kg per day starting 10 weeks after irradiation but before deaths from pneumonitis normally occur) significantly reduced the mortality of radiation pneumonitis and was as effective as a larger dose in this respect. However, if steroids were withdrawn during the period when pneumonitis normally occurs, death rapidly occurred and caught up with that of mice that did not receive corticosteroids. But corticosteroids could be withdrawn at 30 weeks (after the usual period of pneumonitis) without resultant mortality. Prednisone had a lesser protective effect when given after the onset of pneumonitis. Steroids, therefore, reduce the mortality of lethally irradiated mice during the period of pneumonitis, even if commenced well after irradiation, a finding that suggests that their beneficial action is related to the suppression of the radiation response. There is evidence that their effect might be a result of suppression of the microvascular leakage that is characteristic of radiation pneumonitis.

The foregoing clinical and experimental data can be synthesized into a hypothesis concerning the place of steroids in radiation pneumonitis: There is a stage, probably following irradiation but preceding established pneumonitis, during which steroid administration prevents the progression of unfavorable cellular or biochemical antecedent(s) or trigger(s) to an abnormal physiological state. The antecedent event remains suppressed or deferred as long as steroids are administered. But once the event occurs, either primarily or because of steroid withdrawal, the physiological and clinical sequelae of radiation pneumonitis follow, and these are not amenable to steroid therapy. However, the antecedent event may occur over a long time span, several weeks, and the physiological sequelae may reverse spontaneously, if slowly. Use of steroids early in the period of emergent physiological derangement prevents further changes from occurring and allows normal repair processes to proceed. This hypothesis would explain the (1) protective effect of steroids, (2) unmasking of latent injury on steroid withdrawal, (3) abrogation of pneumonitis by early use of corticosteroids, and (4) relative inefficacy of steroids in reversing established pneumonitis. Current practice agrees with this hypothesis.

Prophylactic corticosteroids are rarely used in clinical practice. In general, large doses for long periods would be required to abolish all pneumonitis. If and when symptomatic pneumonitis occurs, and especially if early onset and rapid progression suggest a severe reaction, large doses of corticosteroids, for example, prednisone (100 mg/day in an adult), should be instituted as early as possible and maintained for several weeks. When symptoms have been absent or not clinically troublesome for a week or more, the dose can be cautiously reduced, but it must be raised promptly if relapse occurs. Subsequent tapering should be prolonged over several weeks. If respiratory failure ensues, the patient should be maintained by mechanical ventilation and supplemental oxygen in the expectation that the condition will ultimately remit spontaneously, provided the patient can be kept alive. It is, however, unlikely that corticosteroids will be of benefit to the patient who first comes under treatment at the stage of established respiratory failure. There are thus many instances in the literature and in common experience in which even large doses of corticosteroids failed to alter the course of radiation pneumonitis. The ideal would be to recognize pneumonitis early in its course, anticipate its severity, and treat appropriate cases as early as possible with large doses of corticosteroids. Agreement is universal that corticosteroids have no place at the stage of radiation fibrosis.

Other Forms of Therapy

A large number of other agents and procedures have been suggested or exposed to trial in the management of radiation pneumonitis. These are reviewed briefly.

It might have been anticipated that anticoagulants could prevent radiation pneumonitis in view of the prominence of the vascular damage that precedes pneumonitis. Daily injections of heparin given to rats from the time of irradiation did not provide protection against the physiological sequelae. We know of no controlled clinical trial, but oral anticoagulants were given without benefit to one series of patients.

Although there is experimental evidence of transient impairment of lung defense mechanisms, prophylactic antibiotic administration has also proved unable to offer protection against physiological changes or to alter mortality in experimental radiation pneumonitis. Administration of antibiotics to patients also would raise the possibility of superinfection with insensitive opportunistic organisms. When infection occurs as a complication of pneumonitis, it should be treated with the appropriate antibiotic.

Oxyphenbutazone, an antiinflammatory agent, also has been used prophylactically in one prospective double-blind trial on 116 patients receiving cobalt radiation therapy. Patients who received oxyphenbutazone experienced significantly less frequent or severe pneumonitis and fibrosis by roentgenographic criteria. As mentioned above, animal experiments strongly suggest that other antiinflammatory agents, particularly those that inhibit or antagonize the leukotriene pathway, may have a markedly beneficial effect on the survival from radiation pneumonitis.

L-Triiodothyronine has been given prophylactically to dogs, with small and nonsignificant effects on postirradiation thoracic compliance. β-Aminopropionitrile (BAPN), an inhibitor of collagen maturation, also has been studied as a prophylactic agent in rats. Although an increase in the collagen content of the lungs was prevented as long as BAPN was administered, mortality was not significantly diminished. Another inhibitor of collagen metabolism, D-penicillamine, also moderates the late effects of radiation on the lungs.

Pneumonectomy has been performed for severe unilateral radiation pneumonitis, and single lung transplantation might be considered in the current era.

Acknowledgment

This work was supported in part by grants from Veterans Administration Research Service and National Heart, Lung, and Blood Institute grant HL 45782-01.

BIBLIOGRAPHY

Adamson IY, Bowden DH. Endothelial injury and repair in radiation-induced pulmonary fibrosis. *Am J Pathol* 1983;112:224–230. *A study in mice showing that severe or prolonged regeneration of the endothelial cells is associated with the proliferation and activation of fibroblasts.*

Adamson IY, Bowden DH, Wyatt JP. A pathway to pulmonary fibrosis: An ultrastructural study of mouse and rat following radiation to the whole body and hemithorax. *Am J Pathol* 1970;58:481–498. *Shows the time course and sequence of epithelial damage and regeneration from type II cells and subsequent fibrosis.*

Bennett DE, Million RR, Ackerman LV. Bilateral radiation pneumonitis: A complication of the radiotherapy of bronchogenic carcinoma. *Cancer* 1969;23:1001–1018. *Reports seven unusual clinical cases (from a much larger total) in which bilateral pneumonitis occurred following unilateral irradiation.*

Boersma LJ, Damen EM, de Boer RW, Muller SH, Valdes Olmos RA, van Zandwijk N, Lebesque JV. Estimation of overall pulmonary function after irradiation using dose–effect relations for local functional injury. *Radiother Oncol* 1995;36:15–23. *Imaging and spirometry used to quantify the effects of irradiation.*

Cameron SJ, Grant IW, Pearson JG, Marques C. Prednisone and mustine in prevention of tumour swelling during pulmonary irradiation. *Br Med J* 1972;1:535–537. *A clinical study showing that corticosteroids given just before, during, and after the start of radiation therapy can prevent the obstruction of major airways by swelling of irradiated tumor.*

Castellino RA, Glatstein E, Turbow MM, Rosenberg S, Kaplan HS. Latent injury of lungs or heart activated by steroid withdrawal. *Ann Intern Med* 1974;80:593–599. *A large clinical study in which patients received cycles of combination chemotherapy including corticosteroids. Soon after the completion of a cycle, some patients were prone to show signs of radiation pneumonitis, suggesting that latent injury had been suppressed by steroids and unmasked by its withdrawal.*

Coultas PG, Ahier RG, Field SB. Effects of neutron and x-irradiation on cell proliferation in mouse lung. *Radiat Res* 1981;85:516–528. *A study in rodents showing the overlapping phases of alveolar epithelial and interstitial cells following x and neutron radiation.*

Elkind MM, Sutton H. X-ray damage and recovery in mammalian cells in culture. *Nature* 1959;184:1293–1294. *A classic study showing the dose–response cells irradiated in culture, repair of sublethal damage, and the effect of dose fractionation.*

Ellis F. The relationship of biological effect of dose-time-fractionation factors in radiotherapy. *Curr Top Radiat Res Q* 1968;4:359–388. *An explication of the Ellis Formula that relates the rad-equivalent dose of radiation to the total dose, number of treatment fractions, and overall treatment time.*

Emirgil C, Heinemann HO. Effects of irradiation of chest on pulmonary function in man. *J Appl Physiol* 1961;16:331–337. *A classic clinical study showing the development of stiff lungs and a restrictive ventilatory defect following radiation to the thorax.*

Evans ML, Graham MM, Mahler PA, Rasey JS. Use of steroids to suppress cellular response to radiation. *Int J Radiat Oncol Biol Phys* 1987;13:563–567. *A study in rats showing that the increased permeability of the endothelium of lung (and some other tissues) could be suppressed by administration of corticosteroids prior to pneumonitis but after irradiation.*

Field SB. An historical survey of radiobiology and radiotherapy with fast neutrons. *Curr Top Radiat Res Q* 1976;11:1–86. *A review of the experimental use of fast neutron therapy on many organs, showing that the oxygen effect and repair of sublethal damage are less with fast neutrons, which may be more effective at sterilizing tumors that are relatively radioresistant due to hypoxia.*

Freedman GS, Lofgren SB, Kligerman MM. Radiation-induced changes in pulmonary perfusion. *Radiology* 1974;112:435–437. *Shows the initial increase in perfusion followed rapidly by a progressive, prolonged decline consistent with pulmonary vascular damage.*

Graham MV, Purdy JA, Emami B, Matthews JW, Harms WB. Preliminary results of a prospective trial using three dimensional radiotherapy for lung cancer. *Int J Radiat Oncol Biol Phys* 1995;33:993–1000. *The risk of pneumonitis varies by lung region, being greater at the lung bases.*

Gross NJ. Experimental radiation pneumonitis: III. Phospholipid studies on the lungs. *J Lab Clin Med* 1979;93:267–237. *Total surfactant phospholipids are increased during the stage of pneumonitis, while their composition remains relatively normal.*

Gross NJ. Experimental radiation pneumonitis: IV. Leakage of circulatory proteins onto the alveolar surface. *J Lab Clin Med* 1980;95:19–31. *The physiological abnormality in radiation pneumonitis is due to a great increase in pulmonary vascular permeability and leakage of vascular proteins into the alveoli.*

Gross NJ. The pathogenesis of radiation induced lung damage. *Lung* 1981;159:115–125. *A review that synthesizes experimental findings in radiation pneumonitis, pointing to this as a form of adult respiratory distress syndrome (ARDS).*

Gross NJ. Altered surfactant subtypes in an experimental form of adult respiratory distress syndrome, radiation pneumonitis. *Am J Physiol* 1991;260:L302–L310. *An analysis of surfactant subtype composition showing that the heavy, large aggregate, subtype is much more abundant than normal in radiation pneumonitis.*

Gross NJ, Holloway NO, Narine KR. Effects of some nonsteroidal anti-inflammatory agents on experimental radiation pneumonitis. *Radiat Res* 1991;127:371–324. *The mortality of radiation pneumonitis is mitigated by some eicosanoid inhibitors, particularly those that inhibit the leukotriene pathway, in addition to steroids.*

Gross N.J, Narine KR, Colletti-Squinto L. Replicative activity of lung type II cells following lung X-irradiation. *Radiat Res* 1987;111:143–150. *In mice, the replicative activity of lung type II cells increases shortly after irradiation and remains high throughout the period of pneumonitis.*

Gross NJ, Narine KR. Experimental radiation pneumonitis: Corticosteroids increase the replicative activity of alveolar type 2 cells. *Radiat Res* 1988;115:543–549. *Corticosteroids given after radiation but before the stage of pneumonitis not only diminish mortality but further increase the replication of lung type II cells.*

Gross NJ, Narine KR, Wade R. Prophylactic effect of corticosteroids in radiation pneumonitis. *Radiat Res* 1988;113:112–119. *A study in lethally irradiated mice given steroids after radiation but before pneumonitis, showing that even moderate doses substantially reduce mortality provided they are continued through the period when pneumonitis would otherwise occur.*

Gustafson G, Vicini F, Freedman L, Johnston E, Edmundson G, Sherman S, Pursel S, Komic M, Chen P, Borrego JC, Seidman J, Martinez A. High dose-rate endobronchial brachytherapy in the management of primary and recurrent malignancies. *Cancer* 1995;75:2345–2350. *Brachytherapy effects on the lung—its pros and cons.*

Jack CIA, Cottier B, Jackson MJ, Cassapi L, Fraser WD, Hind CRK. Indicators of free radical activity in patients developing radiation pneumonitis. *Int J Radiat Oncol Biol Phys* 1996;34:149–154. *Variations in levels of markers of free radical activity correlate with pneumonitis.*

Kaplan HS, Stewart JR. Complications of intensive megavoltage radiotherapy for Hodgkin's disease. *Natl Cancer Inst Monogr* 1973;36:439–444. *A very large clinical experience describing the nature and incidence of a variety of complications of thoracic irradiation for this common malignancy.*

Lamoureux KB. Increased clinically symptomatic pulmonary radiation reactions with adjuvant chemotherapy. *Cancer Chemother Rep* 1974;58:705–708. *An early report detailing the enhancing effect of various chemotherapeutic agents on the development of radiation pneumonitis.*

Leung TW, Lau WY, Ho SK, Ward SC, Chow JH, Chan MS, Metreweli C, Johnson PJ, Li AK. Radiation pneumonitis after selective internal radiation treatment with intraarterial ^{90}Yttrium microspheres for inoperable hepatic tumors. *Int J Radiat Oncol Biol Phys* 1995;33:919–924. *Incidental pneumonitis from microsphere injections and pre-procedure risk-stratification.*

Liao Z, Travis EL, Tucker SL. Damage and morbidity from pneumonitis after irradiation of partial volumes of mouse lung. *Int J Radiat Oncol Biol Phys* 1995;32:1359–1370. *Animal model describing variation in pneumonitis with location of lung irradiation.*

Libshitz HI, Brosof AB, Southard ME. Radiographic appearance of the chest following extended field radiation therapy for Hodgkin's disease. *Cancer* 1973;32:206–215. *A useful description of the appearance of the chest roentgenograph, including time and dose relations.*

Morgan GW, Breit SN. Radiation and the lung: a reevaluation of the mechanisms mediating pulmonary injury. *Int J Radiat Oncol Biol Phys* 1995;31:361–369. *Comprehensive summary of the current biochemistry of radiation pneumonitis.*

Phillips TL. An ultrastructural study of the development of radiation injury in the lung. *Radiology* 1966;87:49–54. *An early but excellent review of the EM changes in lungs at several stages in the development of lung damage emphasizing endothelial cell damage.*

Phillips TL. Chemical modifiers of cancer treatment. *Int J Radiat Oncol Biol Phys* 1984;10:1791–1794. *A discussion of several chemotherapeutic agents and their potential in modifying the effects of radiation on the lungs.*

Phillips TL, Margolis L. Radiation pathology and the clinical response of lung and esophagus. *Front Radiat Ther Oncol* 1972;6:254–260. *An itemization of chemotherapeutic agents that interact with radiation on the lung.*

Phillips TW, Wharam MD, Margolis LW. Modification of radiation injury to normal tissues by chemotherapeutic agents. *Cancer* 1975;35:1678–1684. *A systematic study of the interaction of some chemotherapies and radiation on the mouse lung and other tissues. Actinomycin D, cyclophosphamide, and vincristine enhanced radiation damage, while bleomycin and hydroxyurea did not, and prednisone protected from radiation damage.*

Prato FS, Kurdyak R, Saibil EA, Rider WD, Aspin N. Regional and total lung function in patients following pulmonary irradiation. *Invest Radiol* 1977;12:224–237. *A controlled longitudinal study of the effect of radiation on lung perfusion in mastectomy patients. Function was markedly reduced for an indefinite period after radiation.*

Roach M, Gandara DR, Yuo HS, Swift PS, Kroll S, Shrieve DC, Wara WM, Margolis L, Phillips TL. Radiation pneumonitis following combined modality therapy for lung cancer: analysis of prognostic factors. *J Clin Oncol* 1995;13:2606–2612. *Important large scale study that identifies and quantifies specific risk factors for radiation pneumonitis.*

Rodemann HP. Cellular basis of radiation induced fibrosis. *Radiother Oncol* 1995;35:83–90. *Detailed descriptions of fibroblast maturation.*

Rosiello RA, Merrill WW, Rockwell S, Carter D, Cooper JA Jr, Care S, Amento EP. Radiation pneumonitis. Bronchoalveolar lavage assessment and modulation by a recombinant cytokine. *Am Rev Respir Dis* 1993;148:1671–1676. *Lung lavage evaluation of cytokine activity in pneumonitis in the presence of a cytokine inhibitor.*

Shapiro SJ, Shapiro SD, Mill WB, Campbell EJ. Prospective study of long-term pulmonary manifestations of mantle irradiation. *Int J Radiat Oncol Biol Phys* 1990;19:707–714. *A description of the sequence of changes in pulmonary function in the modern era. Pleural thickening and decreased perfusion was common within the port, but symptoms were mild or absent.*

Steinfeld AD, Ross WM. Bronchogenic carcinoma following postmastectomy irradiation. *Radiology* 1976;119:215–216. *Second primary bronchogenic cancer following radiation therapy and within the port margin, raising the possibility of radiation carcinogenesis.*

Tanaka Y. Effect of lung irradiation on the incidence of pulmonary metastases and its mechanism. *Acta Radiol Oncol Radiat Phys Biol* 1976;15:142–148. *A study in mice showing that lung irradiation results in a short period during which intravenously injected cells were more capable of growing into lung colonies. Possibly the transient increase in vascular perfusion favored the implantation of metastatic cells.*

Teates CD. Effects of unilateral thoracic irradiation on lung function. *J Appl Physiol* 1965;20:628–636. *A classic study of the sequence of decline in lung volumes, compliance, and gas transfer following unilateral radiation in dogs.*

Ts'ao C, Ward WF. Acute radiation effects on the content and release of plasminogen activator activity in cultured aortic endothelial cells. *Radiat Res* 1985;101:394–401. *A study on vascular endothelial cells in culture showing that irradiated cells release less plasminogen activator, a possible mechanism of defective fibrinolysis and in situ thrombosis following radiation of tissues.*

Ullrich RL, Meyer KR. The influence of butylated hydroxytoluene-induced cell proliferation on mouse lung damage after x-rays or fission neutrons. *Radiat Res* 1982;89:428–432. *Butylated hydroxytoluene was used to produce a proliferative response first in type II cells and later in vascular endothelial cells. Enhanced radiation sensitivity occurred after the former but not the latter. This result suggests that type II cells are the target of the effects of radiation in the lung.*

von der Maase H, Overgaard J, Vaeth M. Effect of cancer chemotherapeutic drugs on radiation-induced lung damage in mice. *Radiother Oncol* 1986;5:245–257. *With breathing frequency and mortality used as endpoints in mice, a variety of cancer chemotherapy agents were given immediately before or after lung irradiation. Adriamycin, bleomycin, cyclophosphamide, and mitomycin-C given either before or after radiation enhanced its effect by a factor of 1.5 to 2.5. In contrast, 5-fluorouracil, methotrexate, and cisplatin had no effects.*

Vracko R. Significance of basal lamina for regeneration of injured lung. *Virchows Arch A Pathol Anat Histopathol* 1972;355:264–274. *A study showing that where the alveolar septal basal lamina is destroyed by radiation, regeneration of the epithelium in a functional form cannot occur, suggesting that the basal lamina is essential for lung regeneration.*

Wara WM, Phillips TL, Margolis LW, Smith V. Radiation pneumonitis: A new approach to the derivation of time–dose factors. *Cancer* 1973;32:547–552. *Dose–response curves of the lung to radiations, derived from the Ellis formula, with and without concurrent actinomycin D. Showing the feasibility of predicting radiation effects based on total dose, number of fractions, and overall time of therapy.*

Ward WF. Radiation-induced pulmonary arterial perfusion defects: Modification by D-penicillamine. *Radiology* 1981;139:201–204. *Serial lung scans on lung-irradiated rats showed that the progressive hypoperfusion and perfusion defects could be delayed and mitigated by daily penicillamine treatment after irradiation, and recovery from vascular damage was accelerated.*

Warren S, Spencer J. Radiation reaction in the lung. *Am J Radiol* 1940;43:682–696. *An early and classic description of the sequence of histologic changes following lung irradiation.*

Whitfield AGW, Bond WH, Arnott WM. Radiation reactions in the lung. *Q J Med* 1956;25:67–76. *A differential diagnosis of lung lesions that may be seen following lung irradiation.*

Wohl ME, Griscom NT, Traggis DG, Jaffe N. Effects of therapeutic irradiation delivered in early childhood upon subsequent lung function. *Pediatrics* 1975;55:507–516. *A clinical and physiological report of children who received bilateral lung irradiation plus actinomycin D for metastatic Wilms tumor. Seven to 14 years later, mild restrictive defects with appropriate reductions in lung compliance and gas transfer were present. Therapeutic irradiation during the period of lung growth is well tolerated.*

Textbook of Pulmonary Diseases, 6th ed.
edited by G.L. Baum, J.D. Crapo, B.R. Celli, and J.B. Karlinsky,
Lippincott–Raven Publishers, Philadelphia, © 1998.

CHAPTER

39

Clinical Evaluation of Individuals with Suspected Indoor Air Quality Problems

Clifford S. Mitchell · Jonathan M. Samet

INTRODUCTION

The recognition of indoor air pollution as relevant to the practice of pulmonary medicine reflects the increasing time spent indoors, significant contributions of indoor environments to exposures to pollutants, the sealed environments of modern buildings, and the emergence of new clinical syndromes linked to indoor air pollution. Total personal exposure to pollutants represents a weighted average of the exposures received in indoor and outdoor environments, locations having homogeneous characteristics during the time that exposure is received. For many pollutants, indoor microenvironments make dominant contributions, e.g., radon and volatile organic compounds (VOCs). Even for some pollutants regulated in outdoor air, e.g., particles and nitrogen dioxide, exposures in indoor microenvironments may outweigh exposure received outdoors.

The spectrum of adverse respiratory effects of indoor air pollution is broad, ranging from symptoms and exacerbation of preexisting respiratory disease to acute and even fatal conditions that can be readily linked to indoor air pollution. The illnesses directly associated with indoor air pollution can be grouped as specific building-related illnesses and sick-building syndrome. The former includes such well-defined entities as hypersensitivity pneumonitis and Legionnaires' disease. The latter is a nonspecific syndrome, often having both respiratory and nonrespiratory elements. Indoor air is also widely contaminated by respiratory carcinogens: radon, environmental tobacco smoke (the mixture of sidestream smoke and exhaled mainstream smoke), and asbestos. Pulmonary physicians may be consulted concerning the risks posed by these agents and asked for guidance concerning control strategies.

SOURCES OF INDOOR AIR POLLUTION

Indoor air pollution has myriad sources including the materials from which the space is constructed, its furnishings, processes operating within the environment, biological agents, and even the occupants. Outdoor air pollutants can also penetrate indoors, as can soil gas. The broad source headings are combustion, evaporation, abrasion, biological, and radon. The principal combustion sources are gas cooking stoves, burning cigarettes, fireplaces, wood stoves, and unvented space heaters. Evaporation of volatile organic compounds from materials and products leads to ubiquitous contamination by these agents. Abrasion of friable asbestos is a principal source for this indoor contaminant. The biological agents are heterogeneous, extending from infectious organisms to pets and the occupants themselves. Radon comes primarily from soil gas.

The concentration of an indoor contaminant depends on the strength of its source, the rate of removal, the volume of the space, and the rate of exchange of air between the space and outdoors. This "mass-balance" formulation indicates that the concentration of a contaminant might be reduced by limiting source strength, increasing removal rate, or increasing exchange between indoor and outdoor air.

In the typical modern building, the exchange of indoor

C.S. Mitchell: Department of Environmental Health Sciences, Johns Hopkins School of Public Health, Baltimore, Maryland 21205.

J.M. Samet: Department of Epidemiology, Johns Hopkins School of Public Health, Baltimore, Maryland 21205.

779

with outdoor air is accomplished by a central heating, ventilating, and air-conditioning (HVAC) system. These systems are diverse, although all have the same purpose: the delivery of air of acceptable quality to building occupants. The volume of air to be delivered follows the recommendation of standards set by the American Society of Heating, Refrigerating, and Air-Conditioning Engineers (ASHRAE). In the majority of newer buildings, occupants can no longer control the temperature of the work environment, and in most buildings, occupants cannot open windows to increase air exchange. Most residences still rely on natural ventilation.

EVALUATING THE PATIENT

A patient presents to a pulmonary physician with non-specific complaints, perhaps cough and sore throat. When should indoor air pollution be suspected as a cause? How can the link to indoor air pollution be established? The same questions face the clinician for specific disease entities also caused by indoor air pollution, such as hypersensitivity pneumonitis, Legionnaires' disease, and worsening of asthma. For each, the diagnosis should raise questions about the role of the indoor environment.

For the physician evaluating and treating an individual patient, indoor air pollution often presents unusual challenges. First, the physician needs to think beyond diagnosis and management of the individual, to diagnosis and management of the specific environment. Interaction with other health and safety professionals may be needed to deal with problems of indoor environments. Second, because cases involving indoor air pollution often revolve around a workplace, physicians will frequently find themselves dealing with employers, unions, and other organizational entities and with complex nonmedical issues such as return to work, workers' compensation, risk communication and risk management. In some cases these "nonmedical" issues play a substantial role, and physicians should be familiar with the kinds of questions that will be asked (Fig. 1).

There is no "typical" presentation for individuals suspected of having health problems related to the indoor environment (Table 1). Patients may report the onset of new symptoms or exacerbation of a preexisting condition. In some cases patients will ask the physician about the possible relationship between symptoms and indoor air. In other cases, the clinician must be alert for diseases or patterns of symptoms that the patient does not necessarily link to a specific exposure or environment. In managing the patient, the physician's role includes five elements: first, diagnosing the clinical syndrome; second, characterizing the nature and magnitude of any exposures; third, deciding whether the clinical picture is consistent with the likely exposure; fourth, treating the condition; and fifth, managing nonmedical issues such as return to work,

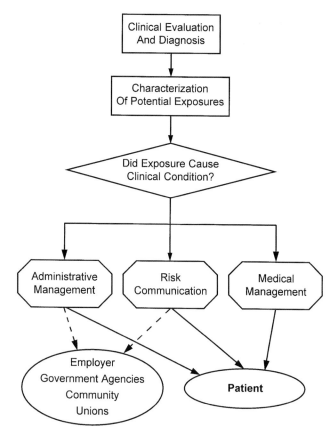

FIG. 1. Evaluation and management of indoor air quality problems.

compensation, and protection of other potentially affected individuals. Thus, the clinician will often need to consult with industrial hygienists, indoor air quality experts, public health officers, or others who can assist in characterizing indoor environments as well as employers, unions, and regulatory agencies in resolving issues such as return to work and workers' compensation. The physician's role may be complicated by tensions between involved parties such as employee unions and employers and the threat or presence of litigation.

Although patients may in some cases be convinced not only of the diagnosis but also of its relationship to a specific indoor exposure or environment, the physician should remain a "diagnostic skeptic." It is especially important to identify specific treatable and preventable conditions, not only for the patient but for others who may be potentially exposed to the same conditions.

A thorough history is the first and most important step in the clinical evaluation. In addition to the symptoms reported by the patient, the physician should elicit the temporal relationship between putative indoor exposure and the onset of symptoms. Do symptoms improve over weekends and vacations? Is there a pattern related to certain activities or locations? An attempt should be made to distinguish between upper and lower respiratory tract

TABLE 1. *Classification of the adverse effects of indoor air pollution[a]*

Clinically evident diseases: Diseases for which the usual methods of clinical evaluation can establish a causal link to an indoor air pollutant.
Exacerbation of disease: The clinical status of already established disease is exacerbated by indoor air pollution.
Increased risk for diseases: Diseases for which epidemiologic or other evidence establishes increased risk in exposed individuals. However, the usual clinical methods indicative of injury typically cannot establish the causal link in an individual patient.
Physiological impairment: Transient or persistent effects on a measure of physiological functioning that are of insufficient magnitude to cause clinical disease.
Symptom responses: Subjectively reported responses that can be linked to indoor pollutants or are attributed to indoor pollutants.
Perception of unacceptable indoor air quality: Sensing of indoor air quality as uncomfortable to an unacceptable degree.
Perception of exposure to indoor air pollutants: Awareness of exposure to one or more pollutants with an unacceptable level of concern about exposure.

[a] From Samet JM. Indoor air pollution. A public health perspective. *Indoor Air* 1993;3:219.

symptoms. For example, the presence of lower respiratory tract symptoms points away from sick-building syndrome and toward intrinsic lung disease such as asthma.

Physical examination should focus on the presence or absence of inflamed conjunctivae, sinus tenderness or congestion, signs of allergic rhinitis, nasal polyps, wheezing, and rales. In cases involving possible multiple chemical sensitivity or sick-building syndrome, symptoms may involve many organ systems, and a thorough physical examination is mandatory.

Laboratory testing should focus on the diagnosis of specific conditions, based on the presenting symptoms. Spirometry can be very useful in separating obstructive from restrictive physiology in relation to symptoms that involve only the upper respiratory tract. The presence of an elevated white count may suggest infection or hypersensitivity pneumonitis. Total serum IgE may be elevated in allergic disorders such as asthma and rhinitis. For allergic conditions in which an exposure is well documented or a particular agent is suspected, the use of specific antibody testing through RAST or epicutaneous tests is appropriate. However, the use of broad antigen panels, although they identify individuals with a range of allergies, may not help determine the specific agent to which the person is reacting in the indoor environment.

Because sick-building syndrome and multiple chemical sensitivity are diagnoses of exclusion, when these conditions are being considered there may be a tendency to "exclude everything" and to use tests that have not been adequately validated clinically. Use of appropriate diagnostic testing in sick-building syndrome and multiple chemical sensitivity is considered in more detail below.

Characterizing the responsible exposure will often require consultation with an industrial hygiene professional, an indoor air quality expert, and a heating, ventilation, and air-conditioning (HVAC) engineer. The evaluation of the indoor environment will in most cases involve interviews with the occupants, a walk-through evaluation, and sampling for common indoor pollutants including organics, bioaerosols, and, in some cases, particular substances such as pesticides or combustion products.

Measurements of temperature and humidity should be compared with ASHRAE standards. Ventilation rates, including air velocity and air changes per hour, should be measured. The HVAC system should be inspected carefully, including the air supply ducts, air-handling units, cooling towers, and air intakes (which can sometimes inadvertently be located near external sources of pollutants). The building should be examined for water leaks and other defects that often contribute to the development of bioaerosols and other indoor air pollutants. Other potential sources of indoor pollutants include photocopy machines (ozone, toner, VOCs), building construction material such as resin-containing particle boards (formaldehyde), and carpeting. Measurements of indoor air quality are rarely informative by themselves. If the setting is a workplace, and exposure to a particular chemical agent is at issue, the material safety data sheets should be reviewed. These are required under the U.S. Occupational Safety and Health Administration's hazard communication standard. Other factors may also be involved, including lighting of work areas, noise and/or vibration, ergonomics, and, importantly, work organization.

MANAGING INDOOR AIR QUALITY PROBLEMS

There are three aspects to successful management of indoor air quality problems: first, medical management of the affected individual or individuals; second, administrative management of both the individuals and the problem environment; and third, risk communication, a key aspect of medical and administrative management. Medical management depends on the diagnosis.

Whether the patient can return to work is of considerable significance. Patients with multiple chemical sensitivity or sick-building syndrome are often apprehensive that a return to the workplace will exacerbate their symptoms. However, although short-term removal from work may help to reduce symptoms and may also be useful diagnostically in linking symptoms to the workplace, there is a great deal of controversy over whether a return to the offending environment ultimately leads to increased morbidity. Some patients may benefit from supportive counseling or other psychological interventions to facilitate a return to an environment that produced symptoms.

Management of indoor air quality problems often involves more than individual medical therapy. When possible, the diagnosis of a building-related problem should prompt correction of the underlying problem. This generally requires the involvement of building engineers, HVAC professionals, and industrial hygienists. In cases in which a specific causal agent can be identified, the corrective action will usually be apparent. In most cases, however, an iterative approach is required, involving assessment of the design, operation, and maintenance of the HVAC system as well as appropriate decontamination or source control.

Communication is a critical component of successful management of indoor air quality problems. Communication with the patient should address (1) medical issues such as the diagnosis and recommended therapy and (2) administrative issues related to return to work. Although some physicians shy away from advising patients about workers' compensation, the physician should consider whether the employee is aware of workers' compensation and of what he or she should do to gain access to the system. This is particularly important because of the statute of limitations for some compensation claims.

Communication with the employer should include: (1) clear information on the ability of the employee to return to work, including any restrictions and need for follow-up; (2) if the condition is thought to be work-related, any recommendations related to identifying and fixing the source of the problem; and (3) whether there is a need to evaluate other employees who may potentially have been exposed.

The physician should consider not only the individual patient but whether other building occupants may have concerns about their risks. This includes individuals who may not be experiencing symptoms themselves. The communication program should include, at a minimum, disclosure of the findings from the evaluation of the building as well as a discussion of the clinical significance of the findings to the potentially exposed population.

RESPIRATORY HEALTH EFFECTS OF INDOOR AIR POLLUTION

As noted above, the spectrum of clinical responses to indoor air pollution is diverse. Table 2 describes some of the major categories of clinical responses, the responsible agents, and the setting in which they may be found. This section briefly describes these clinical responses, aspects of which are considered in greater depth elsewhere in this volume.

Asthma

Indoor air pollution both causes and exacerbates asthma. Exposure in the home to house dust mite antigen and to environmental tobacco smoke contributes to asthma. Similar exposures to these and a wide array of other biological agents, antigens from pets, rodents, cockroaches, molds, and fungi, may exacerbate asthma in the workplace. There may be exposure to molds and fungi that have contaminated moist surfaces of heating, ventilating, and air-conditioning systems. Volatile organic compounds, low-molecular-weight agents such as formaldehyde that are released from materials, furnishings, and office processes, may worsen asthma. Smoking adds particles and irritant gases to the air of public and commercial buildings.

Respiratory Infections

Indoor microenvironments are the principal locale for transmission of infectious respiratory diseases, including tuberculosis, influenza, and Legionnaires' disease. Risks reflect occupant density and the level of ventilation provided. Contamination of cooling towers and water systems, which aerosolize bacteria, has been linked to episodes of pneumonia and nonpneumonic disease caused by *Legionella* species. Diagnosis of Legionnaires' disease or Pontiac fever should prompt consideration of the source of the infection. Airborne transmission of tuberculosis has occurred in such diverse enclosed environments as ships, airplanes, and shelters for the homeless.

Lung Cancer

Three agents causally linked to lung cancer may contaminate indoor environments: radon, derived from decay of naturally occurring uranium and entering buildings in soil gas; asbestos fibers released from building materials; and environmental tobacco smoke from the smoking of occupants. Radon is estimated to cause approximately 14,000 lung cancer deaths a year, approximately 6000 to 7000 in never-smokers, and the estimate for mortality from environmental tobacco smoke is 2000 to 3000 lung cancer deaths annually in the United States. Exposures to asbestos in public and commercial buildings are generally low, and the associated cancer risks are likely far lower than for the other carcinogens. As yet, there are no specific markers for lung cancer caused by these agents.

Chronic Rhinitis

Chronic rhinitis related to indoor air pollutants can be a significant cause of morbidity and decreased quality of life for many patients. Causes of chronic rhinitis include annoyance reactions, allergic reactions, chemical irritation, and chemical corrosion. The estimated prevalence rate of allergic rhinitis is between 15% and 20%.

TABLE 2. *Pulmonary responses commonly associated with indoor air pollution*

Clinical responses	Causal agent	Specific incitants	Potential sources
Comfort	Environment	Temperature, humidity	HVAC system
Nonspecific irritation	Chemicals	Volatile organic compounds	Building materials (adhesives, caulking compounds, carpeting, particleboard, plywood, upholstery, paints, stains, varnishes, wallpaper, floor and wall coverings)
			Office supplies and equipment (carbonless copy paper, duplicating machines, laser printers, marker inks, rubber cement, typewriter correction fluid)
			Pesticides
	Combustion products	Environmental tobacco smoke	
		NO_X, SO_X, O_3, CO_X	Outdoor air pollution (all); indoor combustion sources (for NO_X, SO_X, CO_X)
Asthma and rhinitis	Bioaerosols	Dust mites	Ubiquitous
		Spiders	
		Insects	
		Animal dander	Pets, laboratory animals
		Pollens	Indoor, outdoor plants
		Protozoa	Humidifiers (humidifier fever)
		Fungi	Wet or water-damaged environments (basements, foam insulation, carpeting, ceiling tiles)
		Enzymes	Detergent and pharmaceutical manufacture
	Chemical sensitizers	Latex, sterilizing agents	Health care industry
		Other chemicals	Specific industries
Reactive airways dysfunction syndrome (RADS)	Chemicals	Various	
Hypersensitivity pneumonitis	Bioaerosols	Animal, bird proteins	Attics, warehouses, other unoccupied spaces
		Organic dusts	
	Chemicals	Acid anhydrides	
Humidifier fever	Biological agents	Various bioaerosols	
Infectious diseases		*Legionella pneumophila*	Contaminated water sources (humidifiers, cooling towers)
Pontiac fever		*Legionella* spp.	
Mycotoxicosis	Trichothecene-producing fungi	*Stachybotrys.* spp.	Wet or water-damaged environments (basements, foam insulation, carpeting, ceiling tiles)
Sick building syndrome	Unknown	Unknown	New or "tight" buildings, renovated buildings
Multiple chemical sensitivity	Unknown	Multiple chemicals	Pesticides, tobacco smoke, gasoline fumes, other organic chemicals
Cancer	Radiation	Radon	Infiltration from soil
	Combustion products	Environmental tobacco smoke	
	Fibers	Asbestos	Building materials, insulation

Hypersensitivity Pneumonitis

Hypersensitivity pneumonitis, caused by inhalation of organic dusts and immunologically active chemicals, has usually been associated with building air-handling systems, although room humidifiers have also been implicated in some cases. Humidifier fever has been considered a separate entity because of the absence of chest x-ray findings in the latter condition.

SICK-BUILDING SYNDROME

Sick-building syndrome is a widely used term to describe a constellation of symptoms associated with exposure to an indoor environment, typically a modern office building. The syndrome is characterized by mucous membrane irritation, respiratory complaints, and sometimes skin, central nervous system, or gastrointestinal effects. There is no generally agreed on case definition, and no unifying pathophysiological mechanism has been advanced to account for all of the symptoms (Table 3). Although occupants of buildings where sick-building syndrome (SBS) has occurred often have a very high symptom prevalence, there is no consensus regarding the percentage of occupants who must be symptomatic in order for the building to qualify as a ''sick'' building. Affected occupants may be only a minority of the total occupants, but they may be clustered geographically in one area of the building.

The prevalence and incidence of SBS have been studied in a number of different indoor environments. In several studies of office building workers, the prevalence of symptoms was quite high, over 80% for at least one SBS symptom. However, as noted above, there is no agreement that a certain percentage of occupants must be affected in order for the building to qualify as ''sick.'' Risk factors associated with the development of symptoms consistent with sick-building syndrome include female gender, a history of asthma or rhinitis, occupation (clerical workers are at increased risk compared with managers), high psychosocial stress, and jobs involving use of carbonless copy paper and visual display terminals.

Thus far, the etiology of sick-building syndrome remains uncertain, although volatile organic compounds, bioaerosols such as bacterial endotoxins or β-1,3-glucan, work organization and other psychosocial factors, and unpleasant odors have all been suggested as possible causal or contributing factors (Fig. 2). There is also disagreement whether and under what circumstances the amount of building ventilation affects the development of sick-building syndrome. However, poor maintenance of the HVAC system has been found in many buildings with occupants affected by SBS.

The clinical presentation of SBS is highly variable. Patients may complain only of irritation, or they may have a wide range of symptoms. Sick-building syndrome is characterized by the presence of symptoms in the building and resolution when exposure ceases. The persistence of symptoms outside the suspected building should increase suspicion that another underlying process is involved. In some individuals, symptoms will initially be present only in the building, but over time the symptoms become more generalized, triggered by a variety of chemical exposures. Eventually, some of these patients may become indistinguishable from patients with multiple chemical sensitivity. Individuals with sick-building syndrome usually do not have evidence of any abnormality of respiratory function. The upper respiratory tract has been the focus of considerable attention as a likely target organ. The presence of lower respiratory tract symptoms, particularly cough, wheeze, or dyspnea, should prompt examination for the presence of airways hyperresponsiveness.

Sick-building syndrome is a diagnosis of exclusion. A careful history and physical examination should be conducted. Keys in making the diagnosis are an appropriate relationship between symptoms and occupancy of the building and an appropriate epidemiologic context with similar problems in other persons working in the same building. The physician should be particularly alert for signs or symptoms of allergic disorders because these may be misdiagnosed as SBS and not adequately treated.

There is no specific medical treatment for SBS. Rather, the physician must consider management issues related to the individual patient, the building, and the work environment (including, frequently, psychosocial aspects of the environment). Management of the individual patient often involves some form of reassurance that the problem is being addressed seriously, that there is no long-term health threat, and that, where appropriate, additional therapeutic modalities such as supportive psychological counseling will be available. Symptoms should not be minimized or trivialized, either by the physician or by the building management. Some patients may insist that the cause of the problem be identified and removed, and these

TABLE 3. *Proposed case definitions for sick building syndrome*

Component	World Health Organization	American Thoracic Society
Symptoms	1. Sensory irritation in eyes, nose, and throat 2. Neurotoxic or general health problems 3. Skin irritation 4. Nonspecific hypersensitivity reactions 5. Odor and taste sensations	1. Eye irritation 2. Headaches 3. Fatigue 4. Throat irritation 5. Chest burning, cough, sputum production in the absence of exposure to tobacco smoke 6. Wheezing or chest tightness 7. Malaise 8. Rhinitis
Population affected	Majority of occupants	Substantial proportion of a building's occupants, or of the occupants of a particular space within a building

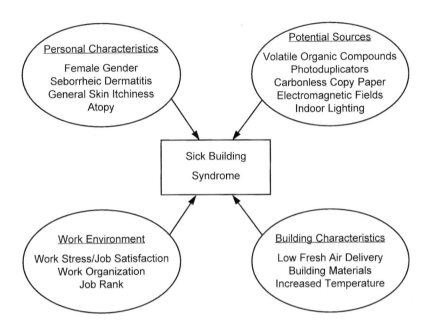

FIG. 2. Contributing factors in sick-building syndrome.

patients may require considerable reassurance and support if they are to successfully return to work.

One of the most important aspects of management is effective communication among patient, physician, and employer. Resolution of SBS may require that the physician contact the employer; this needs to be done with the patient's knowledge and approval. If several occupants appear to be affected, and industrial hygiene or building engineering is undertaken to correct a problem, the affected individuals should be kept informed of all findings and corrective actions, along with appropriate interpretations of the probable clinical significance of the findings.

Prevention of SBS requires both proper building design and maintenance, particularly of the HVAC system. Changing uses of the building should prompt careful analysis of the impact on occupants. Overloading of HVAC capacity by increasing occupant density or adding new equipment may lead to SBS, as may failure to address moisture problems, which facilitate microbial growth. Use of low-emission products and allowing emissions from new building materials to dissipate before occupying the building may also reduce the likelihood of SBS. This can be accomplished through a bake-out period before occupancy.

MULTIPLE CHEMICAL SENSITIVITY

The earliest references to multiple chemical sensitivity (MCS) as a distinct clinical entity date to 1987, although some clinicians have for years postulated that there are certain individuals who have a "sensitivity" or "allergy" to environmental chemicals. Other terms for this condition have included "environmental illness" or "chemical hypersensitivity or hypersusceptibility." The most com-

mon clinical and epidemiologic definition used for MCS was developed by Cullen:

> [An] acquired disorder characterized by recurrent symptoms, referable to multiple organ systems, occurring in response to demonstrable exposure to many chemically unrelated compounds at doses far below those established in the general population to cause harmful effects. No single widely accepted test of physiologic function can be shown to correlate with symptoms.

Patients with MCS may consult pulmonary physicians because of respiratory symptoms.

There is no scientific consensus regarding the etiology and pathogenesis of MCS. Physiological, psychological, psychophysiological, and sociologic models have been proposed to explain MCS. It has been described as a chemical sensitization of the central nervous or immune system, a conditioned response, a panic attack, or a post-traumatic stress response to odors, as a misdiagnosis of psychological or physical illness, and as an illness "belief system." Clinical studies of patients diagnosed with MCS have not found any consistent abnormalities in physiological, immunologic, neurologic, or psychological parameters.

The upper respiratory tract has been the focus of considerable attention as a likely site involved in the pathogenesis of MCS. Attention has focused on inflammatory changes detected in some patients by rhinolaryngoscopy and on the possible role of a hypothesized but as yet unconfirmed relationship between inflammation and distant neurophysiological effects.

Typically, a patient will present with symptoms in a number of organ systems that are triggered by exposure to perfumes, cigarette smoke, cleaners, automobile and truck exhaust, and other chemicals with strong odors. Common symptoms include headache, fatigue, confusion,

TABLE 4. *Diagnostic evaluation of patients with multiple chemical sensitivity*[a]

A. History
    Detailed exposure history (workplace and other environmental exposures)
    Industrial hygiene data (Material Safety Data Sheets, results of exposure monitoring, etc.)
    Current and past medical illnesses and results of previous diagnostic workups and treatments
    Review of prior medical records
B. Physical examination
    Rule out other illnesses in the differential diagnosis
C. Diagnostic testing
    There is no established diagnostic testing for MCS
    Rule out other illnesses in the differential diagnosis
    The following tests are currently not validated for clinical use to confirm the diagnosis of MCS:
        Environmental challenge testing (unblinded, uncontrolled)
        Quantitative electroencephalography
        Brain electrical activity mapping
        Evoked potentials (brainstem, visual, sensory)
        Positron emission tomography scanning
        Single photon emission computed tomography scanning
        Immunologic testing
        Measurement of trace concentrations of volatile organic compounds or pesticides in blood (parts per billion)
        Neuropsychological testing
D. Consultation
    Occupational and environmental medicine specialist
    Psychiatrist
    Other specialists as appropriate to rule out other medical conditions in the differential diagnosis
E. Other
    Symptom diary
    Short-term removal from exposure

[a] Adapted from Sparks PJ, et al. Multiple chemical sensitivity syndrome: a clinical perspective. II. *J Occup Med* 1994;36:733–734.

memory problems, shortness of breath, arthralgias/myalgias, and nausea. Symptoms may also be triggered by a particular location such as an office, and it may be difficult to distinguish MCS patients from patients with sick-building syndrome. Although many patients report that their condition was triggered by a specific inciting event, some state that the condition developed gradually.

The evaluation of patients with symptoms characteristic of MCS (Table 4) is often time-consuming, and consultation with a specialist in occupational medicine may be helpful. Because symptoms are by definition multisystem, patients with symptoms in only or primarily one organ system should be carefully evaluated for another diagnosis. The presence of concomitant or explanatory psychiatric diagnoses should be established. Some patients with symptoms characteristic of MCS may also meet many of the criteria for chronic fatigue syndrome, but there is as yet no consensus regarding any relationship between the two entities.

Treatment of patients with MCS is typically difficult and best accomplished by a multidisciplinary team that includes a psychologist or psychiatrist. Many patients are concerned about any possible chemical exposures, and it is not uncommon for patients to resort to increasing social isolation in an attempt to prevent exposure. Just as there is no agreed-on case definition, there is also no agreed-on therapeutic regimen. Most treatment has been aimed at relief of symptoms, which can of itself have a significant

salutary effect. The issues that have engendered the greatest controversy over management of patients with MCS are (1) whether to remove patients from exposure, and if so for how long; (2) the use of behavioral therapies; and (3) the role of desensitization or chemical detoxification. In the experience of the authors and of most of the scientific literature, short-term removal from exposure may be helpful both as a diagnostic test and therapeutically, but there is little evidence that long-term removal improves clinical outcome. The use of behavioral therapies has been hotly debated. There have been no controlled trials of behavioral therapy, although case reports suggest that some patients respond favorably to the use of biofeedback or other supportive modalities. No controlled trials have validated the use of chemical desensitization (sometimes termed "neutralization") therapies.

BIBLIOGRAPHY

Allred EN, Bleecker ER, Chaitman BR, Dahms TE, Gottlieb SO, Hackney JD, Pagano M, Selvester RH, Walden SM, Warren J. Short-term effects of carbon monoxide exposure on the exercise performance of subjects with coronary artery disease. *N Engl J Med* 1989;321:1426–1432. *Key investigation of the health effects of low-level exposure to carbon monoxide in a susceptible group, persons with coronary artery disease.*

American Thoracic Society, Committee of the Environmental and Occupational Health Assembly, Bascom R, Bromberg PA, Costa DA, Devlin R, Dockery DW, Frampton MW, Lambert W, Samet JM, Speizer FE, Utell M. Health effects of outdoor air pollution. Part 1. *Am J*

Respir Crit Care Med 1996;153:3–50. Part 2. *Am J Resp Crit Care Med* 1996;153:477–498. *This recently published state-of-art review covers the principal outdoor air pollutants; the literature on carbon monoxide and nitrogen dioxide is directly relevant to the indoor environment. There is extensive coverage of the toxicology of air pollutants in the respiratory tract.*

American Thoracic Society. Environmental controls and lung disease. *Am Rev Respir Dis* 1990;142:915–939. *Provides guidance for clinicians. A report from a second workshop on the topic is expected to be published in 1997.*

Ashford NA, Miller CS. *Chemical Exposures: Low Levels and High Stakes.* New York: Van Nostrand Reinhold, 1991. *Describes the history of multiple chemical sensitivity as well as some of the theories advanced to explain the condition.*

Burge H, Center for Indoor Air Research, ed. *Bioaerosols.* Boca Raton, FL: Lewis Publishers, 1995. *This edited volume covers the complex topic of bioaerosols. It touches on sources, measurement, and health effects.*

Coultas DB, Lambert WE. Carbon monoxide. In: Samet JM, Spengler JD, eds. *Indoor Air: A Health Perspective.* Baltimore: Johns Hopkins University Press, 1991. *Provides a general introduction to carbon monoxide including the pathophysiological mechanism underlying its adverse effects on health.*

Cullen MR. The worker with multiple chemical sensitivities: an overview. *Occup Med State Art Rev* 1987;2:655–661. *First article to describe and name multiple chemical sensitivity as a distinct condition.*

Darby SC, Samet JM. Radon. In: Samet JM, ed. *Epidemiology of Lung Cancer.* New York: Marcel Dekker, 1994. *A general overview of radon and lung cancer.*

Elsom DM. *Atmospheric Pollution, a Global Problem,* 2nd ed. Cambridge, MA: Blackwell Publishers, 1992. *A general textbook on air pollution that provides broad coverage of the history of air pollution regulation throughout the world.*

Godish T. *Indoor Air Pollution Control.* Chelsea, MI: Lewis Publishers, 1989. *Broad coverage of the topic.*

Godish T. *Sick Buildings: Definition, Diagnosis and Mitigation.* Boca Raton, FL: Lewis Publishers, CRC Press, 1995. *A recent book that provides comprehensive coverage of the sick-building syndrome. Covers medical aspects and causes and control of this new and difficult problem.*

Guerin MR, Jenkins RA, Tomkins BA, Center for Indoor Air Research, eds. *The Chemistry of Environmental Tobacco Smoke: Composition and Measurement.* Chelsea, MI: Lewis Publishers, 1992. *This book provides extensive coverage of environmental tobacco smoke, the mixture of sidestream smoke and exhaled mainstream smoke inhaled by nonsmokers. It includes voluminous information on various markers for environmental tobacco smoke and on levels of these markers in public and private buildings.*

Hasselblad V, Kotchmar DJ, Eddy DM. Synthesis of environmental evidence: Nitrogen dioxide epidemiology studies. *J Air Waste Manage Assoc* 1992;42:662–671. *A meta-analysis of the epidemiologic studies on adverse respiratory effects of nitrogen dioxide.*

Health Effects Institute, Asbestos Research Committee, and Literature Review Panel. *Asbestos in Public and Commercial Buildings: A Literature Review and a Synthesis of Current Knowledge.* Cambridge, MA: Health Effects Institute, 1991. *Key report on indoor asbestos. Covers toxicologic and epidemiologic evidence and exposure to asbestos in public and commercial environments.*

Hodgson M. The medical evaluation. *Occup Med State Art Rev* 1995;10:177–194. *General discussion of the clinical evaluation of patients who believe their illness to be building-related.*

Hodgson M. The sick-building syndrome. *Occup Med State Art Rev* 1995;10:167–175. *Review of sick-building syndrome literature.*

Hoge CW, Reichler MR, Dominguez EA, Bremer JC, Mastro TD, Hendricks KA, Musher DM, Elliott JA, Facklam RR, Breiman RF. An epidemic of pneumococcal disease in an overcrowded, inadequately ventilated jail. *N Engl J Med* 1994;331:643–648. *An interesting report showing that inadequate ventilation increases infection risk.*

Institute of Medicine, Committee on the Health Effects of Indoor Allergens, Division of Health Promotion and Disease Prevention, Pope AM, Patterson R, Burge H, eds. *Indoor Allergens: Assessing and Controlling Adverse Health Effects.* Washington, DC: National Acad-

emy Press; 1993. *An important committee report that covers the general topic of indoor allergens.*

Landrigan PJ, Kazemi H. *The Third Wave of Asbestos Disease: Exposure to Asbestos in Place. Public Health Control.* New York: The New York Academy of Sciences, 1991. *Report of a symposium on the possibility of a third-wave of asbestos-related disease caused by exposures in public and commercial buildings.*

Lippmann M. Asbestos and other mineral fibers. In: Lippmann M, ed. *Environmental Toxicants: Human Exposures and Their Health Effects.* New York: Van Nostrand Reinhold, 1992. *This chapter provides a general introduction to fibers and their toxicity.*

Lubin JH, Boice JD Jr, Edling C, Hornung RW, Howe G, Kunz E, Kusiak RA, Morrison HI, Radford EP, Samet JM, Tirmarche M, Woodward A, Xiang YS, Pierce DA. Lung cancer in radon-exposed miners and estimation of risk from indoor exposure. *J Natl Cancer Inst* 1995;87:817–827. *Presents the findings of a pooled analysis of the major cohort studies on radon and lung cancer in underground miners. Offers a new risk model and estimates the burden of lung cancer in the population caused by indoor radon.*

Mauderly JL, Samet JM. General environment. In: Crystal RG, West JB, eds. *The Lung: Scientific Foundations.* New York: Raven Press, 1991. *Provides an introduction to the epidemiologic and toxicologic approaches used to investigate the health effects of air pollution.*

Mendell MJ. Nonspecific symptoms in office workers: A review and summary of the epidemiologic literature. *Indoor Air* 1993;3:227–236. *Comprehensive synthesis of the literature on symptoms in building occupants. Addresses ventilation.*

Miller JD. Fungi as contaminants in indoor air. *Atmos Environ* 1992;26A:2163–2172. *Reviews clinical effects, biologic settings in which fungal contamination plays a role.*

Molhave L. Volatile organic compounds and the sick building syndrome. In: Lippmann M, ed. *Environmental Toxicants: Human Exposures and Their Health Effects.* New York: Van Nostrand Reinhold, 1992. *Provides an excellent overview of the topic with an emphasis on health effects.*

Mossman BT, Bignon J, Corn M, Seaton A, Gee JBL. Asbestos: Scientific developments and implications for public policy. *Science* 1990;247:294–301. *A controversial report that addresses the public health significance of indoor asbestos.*

National Research Council, Committee on Passive Smoking. *Environmental Tobacco Smoke: Measuring Exposures and Assessing Health Effects.* Washington, DC: National Academy Press, 1986. *Another one of the key reports on passive smoking.*

National Research Council, Committee on the Biological Effects of Ionizing Radiation. *Health Risks of Radon and Other Internally Deposited Alpha-Emitters: BEIR IV.* Washington, DC: National Academy Press, 1988. *Comprehensive report on radon and lung cancer risk associated with radon. Will be supplanted by BEIR VI in 1997.*

National Research Council, Committee on Advances in Assessing Human Exposure to Airborne Pollutants. *Human Exposure Assessment for Airborne Pollutants: Advances and Opportunities.* Washington, DC: National Academy Press, 1991. *This report lays out the conceptual basis for considering exposures for environmental pollutants, including air pollutants. Provides coverage of measurement methods.*

National Research Council, Committee on Risk Assessment of Hazardous Air Pollutants. *Science and Judgment in Risk Assessment.* Washington, DC: National Academy Press, 1994. *Although the focus of this volume is on outdoor air pollution, it provides an up-to-date review of this method for quantifying health risks, which is widely applied to indoor carcinogens.*

Nero AV Jr. Radon and its decay products in indoor air: An overview. In: Nazaroff WW, Nero AV Jr, eds. *Radon and Its Decay Products in Indoor Air.* New York: John Wiley & Sons, 1988. *Provides a broad perspective on the problem of indoor radon.*

Pershagen G. Passive smoking and lung cancer. In: Samet JM, ed. *Epidemiology of Lung Cancer.* New York: Marcel Dekker, 1994. *This chapter covers evidence on passive smoking and lung cancer through the early 1990s.*

Reinikaneinen LM, Jaakkola JJK, Seppänen O. The effect of air humidification on symptoms and perception of indoor air quality in office workers: a six-period cross-over trial. *Arch Environ Health* 1992;47:8–15. *Workers reported fewer symptoms of dry skin and mucosa, allergic reactions, and sensation of dryness when indoor humidity was increased from 20–30% to 30–40%.*

Rylander R, Persson K, Goto H, Yuasa K, Tanaka S. Airborne beta-1,3-glucan may be related to symptoms in sick buildings. *Indoor Environ* 1992;1:263–267. *Endotoxin and β-1,3-glucan levels in two schools, a post office, and a day-care center were correlated with sick-building syndrome symptoms.*

Samet JM, Utell MJ. The risk of nitrogen dioxide: What have we learned from epidemiological and clinical studies? *Toxicol Indust Health* 1990;6:247–262. *Nitrogen dioxide is a ubiquitous indoor air pollutant released by combustion sources. This paper synthesizes the evidence through 1990.*

Samet JM, Spengler JD. *Indoor Air Pollution. A Health Perspective.* Baltimore: Johns Hopkins University Press, 1991. *This book provides a comprehensive treatment of the principal indoor air pollutants, covering sources, patterns of exposure, and health effects. There is also coverage of issues in the control of indoor air pollution.*

Samet JM. Nitrogen dioxide. In: Samet JM, Spengler JD, eds. *Indoor Air Pollution. A Health Perspective.* Baltimore: Johns Hopkins University Press, 1991. *An overview of the health effects of exposure to nitrogen dioxide in indoor environments.*

Samet JM. Indoor air pollution: A public health perspective. *Indoor Air* 1993;3:219–226. *Provides broad consideration of the range of health effects associated with indoor air pollution. Offers a classification of the health effects of indoor air pollution.*

Samet JM, Speizer FE. Introduction and recommendations: Working Group on Indoor Air and Other Complex Mixtures. *Environ Health Perspect* 1994;101:143–147. *This paper provides the overall findings of a workshop that addressed indoor air pollution and other complex mixtures. The workshop proceedings provide useful coverage of a number of methodologic issues.*

Samimi BS. The environmental evaluation: commercial and home. *Occup Med State Art Rev* 1995;10:95–118. *Summarizes elements of indoor environmental evaluation, including current standards.*

Smith KR. *Biofuels, Air Pollution, and Health. A Global Review.* New York: Plenum Press, 1987. *Provides a broad perspective on indoor air pollution and its causes and consequences in the developing countries.*

Sparks PJ, Daniel W, Black DW, Kipen HM, Altman LC, Simon GE, Terr AI. Multiple chemical sensitivity syndrome: a clinical perspective. I. Case definition, theories of pathogenesis, and research needs. *J Occup Med* 1994;36:718–730. *Reviews theories regarding the etiology of multiple chemical sensitivity.*

Sparks PJ, Daniell W, Black DW, Kipen HM, Altman LC, Simon GE, Terr AI. Multiple chemical sensitivity syndrome: a clinical perspective. II. Evaluation, diagnostic testing, treatment, and social considerations. *J Occup Med* 1994;36:731–737. *Reviews the use and misuse of diagnostic testing in multiple chemical sensitivity as well as the advantages and disadvantages of various management options.*

Spengler JD, Samet JM. A perspective on indoor and outdoor air pollution. In: Samet JM, Spengler JD, eds. *Indoor Air Pollution. A Health Perspective.* Baltimore: Johns Hopkins University Press, 1991. *This chapter provides a broad perspective on the impact of outdoor and indoor air quality on human health. It introduces key concepts related to personal exposure to air pollutants.*

Taylor AE, Johnson DC, Kazemi H. Environmental tobacco smoke and cardiovascular disease: A position paper from the council on cardiopulmonary and critical care, American Heart Association. *Circulation* 1992;86:1–4. *Statement of the American Heart Association on passive smoking and heart disease.*

Tunnicliffe WS, Burge PS, Ayres JG. Effect of domestic concentrations of nitrogen dioxide on airway responses to inhaled allergen in asthmatic patients. *Lancet* 1994;344:1733–1736. *A report that documents synergistic interaction between nitrogen dioxide and inhaled allergen. The exposure scenario addresses the real-world problem of mixtures.*

Turner WA, Bearg DW, Brennan T. Ventilation. In: Seltzer JM, ed. *Effects of the Indoor Environment on Health.* Philadelphia: Hanley & Belfus, 1995. *Provides a brief introduction to the ventilation (delivery of outside air) of buildings. Inadequate ventilation and other problems with the heating, ventilating, and air-conditioning system contribute to the occurrence of the sick-building syndrome.*

US Department of Health and Human Services. *The Health Consequences of Involuntary Smoking: A Report of the Surgeon General.* Washington, DC: US Government Printing Office, 1986. *One of the key reports on involuntary smoking. Concluded that involuntary smoking causes lung cancer in nonsmokers. Also covers exposure and toxicology and nonmalignant diseases.*

US Environmental Protection Agency. *Indoor Air Pollution.* Washington, DC: US Government Printing Office, 1991. *A brief introduction to the topic.*

US Environmental Protection Agency. *Technical Support Document for the 1992 Citizen's Guide to Radon.* Washington, DC: US Government Printing Office, 1992. *Describes EPA's approach to assessing the risk of indoor radon.*

US Environmental Protection Agency, Office of Research and Development, and Office of Air and Radiation. *Respiratory Health Effects of Passive Smoking: Lung Cancer and Other Disorders.* Washington, DC: US Government Printing Office, Monograph 4, 1993. *Key report on the health effects of involuntary smoking. Covers the evidence on lung cancer and effects on children.*

Wallace LR. *The Total Exposure Assessment Methodology (TEAM) Study: Summary and Analysis.* Washington, DC: US Environmental Protection Agency, Office of Research and Development, 1987. *A key study advancing our understanding of the contributions of indoor and outdoor sources to personal exposures to pollutants.*

Wallace LA. Volatile organic compounds. In: Samet JM, Spengler JD, eds. *Indoor Air Pollution. A Health Perspective.* Baltimore: Johns Hopkins University Press, 1991. *This chapter provides an introduction to the volatile organic compounds, a ubiquitous group of indoor air pollutants.*

Wolkoff P. Volatile organic compounds—Sources, measurements, emissions, and the impact on indoor air quality. *Indoor Air* 1995;3:9–73. *A recent and extensive review of the volatile organic compounds. Includes extensive listings of the agents.*

Subject Index

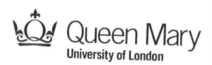